Eighteenth Annual

Symposium on Computer Applications in Medical Care

NOTICE

Transforming Information, Changing Health Care

Eighteenth Annual

Symposium on Computer Applications in Medical Care

A Conference of the American Medical Informatics Association

November 5–9, 1994
Sheraton Washington Hotel
Washington, DC

Edited by Judy G. Ozbolt, Ph.D., RN
Program Chairman

HANLEY & BELFUS, INC.
Medical Publishers
Philadelphia

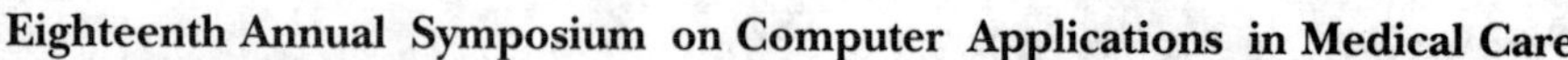

Eighteenth Annual Symposium on Computer Applications in Medical Care

Published by Hanley & Belfus, Inc.

Printed in United States of America

1 2 3 4 5 6 7 8 9 0 MALMAL 9 8 7 6 5 4 3

Library of Congress Number 79-641114

ISSN: 1067-5027

ISBN: 1-56053-123-1

This book was prepared camera-ready.

Port City Press was printer and binder.

American Medical Informatics Association Board of Directors

18th Annual SCAMC Program Committee

Program Chair
Judy G. Ozbolt, Ph.D., RN
University of Virginia
Charlottesville, Virginia

Evening Workshops
Reed M. Gardner, Ph.D.
LDS Hospital/University of Utah
Salt Lake City, Utah

Poster Session/Demonstrations
Roy L. Simpson, RN
HBO & Company
Atlanta, Georgia

Student Paper Competition
James J. Cimino, M.D.
Columbia-Presbyterian Medical Center
New York, New York

Tutorials and Panels
Mark S. Tuttle
Lexical Technology
Alameda, California

Tracks

Database Methods and Delivery
Christopher Chute, M.D., Dr.P.H.
Mayo Foundation
Rochester, Minnesota

Image and Signal Processing
Alan H. Rowberg, M.D.
University of Washington
Seattle, Washington

Instructional Technology
Susan Sparks, Ph.D., RN
National Library of Medicine
Bethesda, Maryland

Issues in Designing Health Care Information Systems
Reed M. Gardner, Ph.D.
LDS Hospital/University of Utah
Salt Lake City, Utah

Library Information Science
Mary Ellen Sievert, Ph.D.
University of Missouri
Columbia, Missouri

Networks and Standards
W. Ed Hammond, Ph.D.
Duke University Medical Center
Durham, North Carolina

Nomenclature and Coding
James J. Cimino, M.D.
Columbia-Presbyterian Medical Center
New York, New York

Simulation, Modeling, and Research Support
Joyce A. Mitchell, Ph.D.
University of Missouri
Columbia, Missouri

Support for Clinical Practice and Decision Making
Suzanne B. Henry, D.N.Sc., RN
University of California
San Francisco, California

Support for Health Care Administration
Samuel Schultz, Ph.D.
University Hospital Consortium
Oakbrook, Illinois

System Description, Selection, and Evaluation
Robert P. Spena, D.S.W.
American College of Physicians
Philadelphia, Pennsylvania

Preface

The theme of the Eighteenth Annual Symposium on Computer Applications in Medical Care is **"Transforming Information, Changing Health Care."** Advances in technology are producing dramatic growth in our ability to transform information from raw data to knowledge, decisions, and actions. In this environment, informatics has become a tool for changing health science and health care. It is not merely a means of doing more efficiently what would have been done in any case. Clinicians and biomedical researchers, armed with better information and greater access to knowledge than ever before, can confront difficult challenges in new ways.

Health science librarians and information service professionals use electronic tools to put knowledge and information at the fingertips of health care providers and researchers. Educators and students have new tools for searching and presenting knowledge. In basic science as in clinical studies, new approaches to acquiring, analyzing, interpreting, and presenting information enable researchers to discover knowledge for significant improvements in health and health care. Increasingly, health care practitioners have the ability to study their own behaviors and to compare their practice with that of others to identify more effective, less costly treatments. Standards and guidelines can be retrieved for consideration virtually wherever and whenever they are needed.

But if current trends in medical informatics are rich with potential, they are also fraught with dilemmas. Transforming the information of health science and health care raises issues related to ethical, economic, and professional conduct. We must respect and protect privacy, information use, and responsibility for research, clinical judgment, and personalized care. With the increasing technological power to transform information comes the vital imperative for the medical informatics community to develop the innovations, implement the systems, and contribute to the policies that will change health science and health care for the better.

SCAMC '94 chronicles these changes and the response of our community. The symposium begins with tutorials on Saturday, November 5 and Sunday, November 6, with material for both novices and experts in medical informatics. Evening workshops on Saturday and Sunday provide opportunities for participants to discuss shared concerns. Always exciting, the Student Paper Competition on Sunday afternoon scales the heights of excellence. The finalists in this competition present their papers again in regular sessions throughout SCAMC. Monday morning's Plenary Session includes awards and the keynote address by Kathryn Hannah, Ph.D., internationally recognized for her contributions to health informatics. Scientific sessions with papers, theater-style demonstrations, and panel discussions begin after Monday's Plenary Session and continue until noon Wednesday. (The papers in the *Proceedings* are grouped in the same way as in the sessions.) Tuesday morning includes a second Plenary Session, for which the distinguished speaker is C. Everett Koop, M.D., Sc.D., former Surgeon General of the United States. Late Tuesday afternoon is devoted to paper and electronic posters. From Monday through Wednesday, the Exhibit Hall displays the latest commercial applications. Interspersed throughout SCAMC are meetings of the membership and committees of the American Medical Informatics Association (AMIA), Working Group meetings and receptions, and special ""Meet AMIA" sessions for getting acquainted with and questioning AMIA officers, Board members, and committee representatives. Tuesday evening's SCAMC reception offers fun and relaxation. Wednesday's closing session, organized by the American College of Medical Informatics (ACMI), includes awards for outstanding work presented at SCAMC and a talk by the ACMI Distinguished Lecturer, Nina W. Matheson, M.L., Director of The Johns Hopkins University's Welch Library.

This symposium would not have been possible without the dedicated and expert work of the staff of the AMIA office: Gail E. Mutnik, M.P.A., Executive Director; Jeanne Nevin, M.B.A., Associate Executive Director; Denise J. Herich, Director, Member Services; Ellen Cooper, Consultant, Meetings; Renée Fleuette, Database Administrator; Donna J.B. Barber, Membership Assistant; Debbie Preusse, Accountant; Y. Michelle Daniels, Receptionist. All these people worked unstintingly to give the maximum flexibility to authors, reviewers, and the Program Committee, while still meeting the necessary deadlines. Their graciousness in working long hours cheerfully was an inspiration. The members of the Program Committee gave generously of their personal and professional time, gladly volunteering for work beyond their normal responsibilities; it has been an honor and a joy to work with them: Christopher Chute, M.D., Dr.P.H.; James J. Cimino, M.D.; Reed M. Gardner, Ph.D.; W. Ed Hammond, Ph.D.; Suzanne B. Henry, D.N.Sc., RN; Joyce A. Mitchell, Ph.D.; Alan H. Rowberg, M.D.; Samuel Schultz, Ph.D.; Mary Ellen Sievert, Ph.D.; Roy L. Simpson, B.S.N., RN: Susan Sparks, Ph.D., RN; Robert P. Spena, D.S.W.; and Mark S. Tuttle. Of course the *sine qua non* of SCAMC is the authors who submitted their work and the reviewers who provided thoughtful and constructive critique. They have my profound thanks, for it is they who give substance, quality, and integrity to the symposium. Finally, my thanks to my colleagues at the University of Virginia and to my family for bearing with my absences and my distraction as I prepared for SCAMC, and for providing the support, encouragement, and irrelevant delights that made the endeavor feasible. Enlightened and inspired by the wisdom and beauty of these people, I deeply hope that SCAMC '94 and these Proceedings may enlighten and inspire others to develop and use informatics to improve health care.

Judy G. Ozbolt, Ph.D., RN
Chair

1994 SCAMC Reviewers

Jos E.C.M. Aarts
Joseph L. Abrego
Michael J. Ackerman
Anthony R. Aguirre
Jack W. Alexander
Constantin Aliferis
Raymond D. Aller
Eric Alper
Rita Altamore
Russ B. Altman
Peter C. Amadio
Margret Amatayakul
Seyamek Amin
James G. Anderson
David B. Aronow
Jeffrey S. Augenstein
William R. Ayers
E. Andrew Balas
Marion J. Ball
Richard Banvard
Gary P. Barnas
Stephen P. Bartold
Jackie D. Bastille
F. Scott Beadenkopf
George W. Beeler
Douglas S. Bell
Mary Benhase
Gary Berg-Cross
Charles W. Bishop
Gordon C. Black
Mary B. Blackwelder
Pamela J. Blaesing
Leslie A. Blide
Barry Blumenfeld
John M. Boehme
Norman K. Bohrer
Omar Bouhaddou
Michael W. Breene
George M. Brenckle
Patricia F. Brennan
Naomi C. Broering
Austin Brown
Gregory Buffone
Pat Bush
E. Sonny Butler
Patricia S. Button
Dean E. Calcagni
Keith E. Campbell
Paul C. Carpenter
Jerome H. Carter
Val Catanzarite
Ifay F. Chang
Kathleen G. Charters
Arjun B. Chatterjee
Wei-Tih Cheng
Homer L. Chin
William M. Chop
Christopher G. Chute
Christopher Cimino
James J. Cimino
Susan Clark
William G. Cole
George S. Conklin
Greg Cooper
Larry D. Cousin
John J. Crawford
Charles R. Croft
Helen Cronenberger
Diana J. Cunningham
Roger W. Dahlen
Ruth E. Dayhoff
Beatriz de Faria Leao
Jocelyn DeWitt
Patrice Degoulet
Catherine L. Delmain
Gregory L. Denison
Cecil Denney
Randall Dickson
William R. Dito
Herbert J. Doller
Francis Dumler
Thomas D. East
Linda Edmunds
Eric L. Eisenstein
John P. Enterline
Jack Erhart
R. Scott Evans
Danielle Fafchamps
Stephen Fath
Andrew Friede
Charles P. Friedman
Mark E. Frisse
Reed M. Gardner
Merryellen Giger
Joe D. Gillespie
Michelle Godin
Julian M. Goldman
Paul N. Gorman
Andrew M. Grant
Hugh D. Greenbaum
Robert A. Greenes
Ruby Grewal
Perry W. Grigsby
Ira J. Haimowitz
Joseph W. Hales
Priscilla D. Hall
W. Ed Hammond
Kathryn Hannah
Terry J. Hannan
Anna M. Harbourt
Peter J. Haug
Robert R. Hausam
Lawrence L. Heidenberg
Barbara R. Heller
Michael Henderson
Steven J. Henkind
Suzanne B. Henry
William R. Hersh
Kristine Heyrend
Daniel B. Hier
Edward J. Hinman
Earl F. Hoerner
Lloyd E. "Gus" Hoffman
John Holmen
Margaret W. Hougland
George M. Hripcsak
Peter F.M. Hu
Donna L. Hudson
Edward Humphrey
Betsy L. Humphreys
Joan S. Huntley
Patrice M. Jackson
Patrick W. Jamieson
Chiang S. Jao
Holly B. Jimison
Merida L. Johns
Kevin B. Johnson
Neill Jones
Judith A. Joy
Charles E. Kahn
Joel A. Kahn
Michael G. Kahn
Joel B. Karlinsky
Michael Kattan
J.P. Keating
Karen Keniston
Barbara Kerlin
Debra Ketchell
Christopher Y. Kim
Lawrence C. Kingsland
John R. Kludt
Ken Kobayashi
Isaac S. Kohane

Gilad J. Kuperman
Steven E. Labkoff
Curtis P. Langlotz
James L. Latimer
David Lawson
Robert S. Ledley
Harold P. Lehmann
Jerome A. Levin
Zongrong Li
Michael J. Lincoln
Craig N. Locatis
Henry J. Lowe
Henry Lundsgaarde
Joseph P. Lyons
Katarzyna J. Macura
Robert T. Macura
Thomas A. Marciniak
Robert S. Marcus
David Margulies
Yolan N. Marinez
Tom Marlin
Brian Ray Marrs
G. Daniel Martich
Daniel R. Masys
Pam Matthews
Katherine G. Mazzuckelli
Mary McAlindon
Robert C. McClure
Elizabeth McColligan
Alexa T. McCray
Clement J. McDonald
Mary L. McHugh
Claudia McKenzie
Roberta M. McKnight
Janet McLaughlin
William L. McMullen
Doug McNair
Judith Messerle
Perry L. Miller
Randolph A. Miller
Rodger S. Miller
Mary Etta Mills
Joyce A. Mitchell
Jochen Moehr
Pat Molholt
Terry Montlick
Gretchen Murphy
Les Muse
Mark Musen
Frank Naeymi-Rad
Lynn M. Nagle
Ernest R. Navara
Donald A.F. Nelson
Stuart J. Nelson
Susan K. Newbold
Bruce R. Niebuhr
Lucila Ohno-Machado
Frank Olken
Sidney Ontai
Richard Orr
Helmuth F. Orthner
Judy G. Ozbolt
Miranda Lee Pao
Ralph Pascualy
Vimla L. Patel
Alan N. Peiris
Kim R. Pemble
Daniel F. Peters
Lawrence Peterson
Claude S. Poliakoff
John B. Posey
Ronald N. Price
Marlon L. Priest
Stephen L. Priest
Fred W. Prior
T. Allan Pryor
Gretchen P. Purcell
Ian Purves
Elaine S. Reber
Lori Reed-Fourquet
James A. Reggia
Glenn Rennels
Mary Anne Rizzolo
Edward N. Robinson
Mitra Alipour Rocca
Roberto A. Rocha
Nancy K. Roderer
R.P. Channing Rodgers
Carol A. Romano
Kevin Rosenberg
David J. Rothwell
Alan H. Rowberg
Donald Rucker
Thomas A Russ
Robert M. Ryder
Charles Safran
Naomi Sager
Daniel Z. Sands
Karyn V. Sanford
Jean-Raoul Scherrer
Richard D. Scheyer
Robert M. Schmidt
Samuel Schultz
Jerry Seidenfeld
Adam Seiver
M. Michael Shabot
Yuval Shahar
Anne Shanney
Bern Shen
Richard N. Shiffman
Theodore M. Shoemaker
Edward H. Shortliffe
Michael Shwe
Robert V. Sideli
Mary Ellen Sievert
Ida Sim
Lori Simon
Diane J. Skiba
Glenn E Snelbecker
Mark M. Snyder
James Sondheimer
Gail Sorrough
Susan M. Sparks
Robert P. Spena
A. Robert Spitzer
Michael E. Spoon
Padmini Srinivasan
Thomas Stair
Klaus J. Staisch
Timothy Stettheimer
Frank W. Stitt
Paul Eric Stoufflet
David P. Strum
Walter Sujansky
Walton Sumner
Paul C. Tang
Barry A. Tanner
Thomas G. Tape
Jonathan M. Teich
Linda Tetzlaff
Philip Tibbs
Patricia Tikkanen
Ann K. Tinker
Maria A. Tovar
Mark S. Tuttle
Paul A. Upham
Jan H. van Bemmel
Michael W. Vannier
Michael M. Wagner
Jonathan S. Wald
Kirt Walker
Fred D. Wallace
Richard F. Walters
Bruce G. Warr
Judith J. Warren
Charles W. Webster
Wladimir Wertelecki
Frederick Westbrook
Diana F. Willson
Linda Woolery
Julian Zelingher
Ivan Zendel
Rita D. Zielstorff
Judy A. Zimmet

Contents

Section II **Vocabularies and Nomenclature**

Issues in Modeling Clinical Vocabularies

Methodologies for Coding Clinical Information

Evaluation of Clinical Vocabularies

Experiments in Coding Clinical Information

**Student Paper Competition Finalist*

Clinical Data Applications

Time & Decision Support

Ethical Issues in Access to Data

**Student Paper Competition Finalist*

Tools for Managing the Clinical Enterprise

Tools & Approaches for Contemporary Problems in Health Administration

Section IV **Networks and Standards**

Regional Health Information Networks

Networking for Clinical Data Interchange

Computer-Based Patient Records: Capturing the Data

Making Standards Work for Sharing Patient Data

Computer-Based Patient Models & Concepts

**Student Paper Competition Finalist*

Section V **Support for Clinicians**

Support for Clinical & Social Services

Clinician-Directed Systems: Design, Implementation & Enhancement

**Student Paper Competition Finalist*

Computer-Based Approaches to Knowledge Acquisition

Application of Fuzzy Logic & Neural Networks to the Clinical Domain

Belief Networks

Formalizing & Implementing Practice Guidelines

Linking Knowledge-Based Tools with the Computer-Based Patient Record

Evaluating the Impact of Decision Support Systems in Clinical Care

Support for Research & Imaging Neural Networks

**Student Paper Competition Finalist*

**Student Paper Competition Finalist*

Visualization of Data

Section VII **Posters**

Section IX **Theater-Style Demonstrations**

Section I

Issues in Education

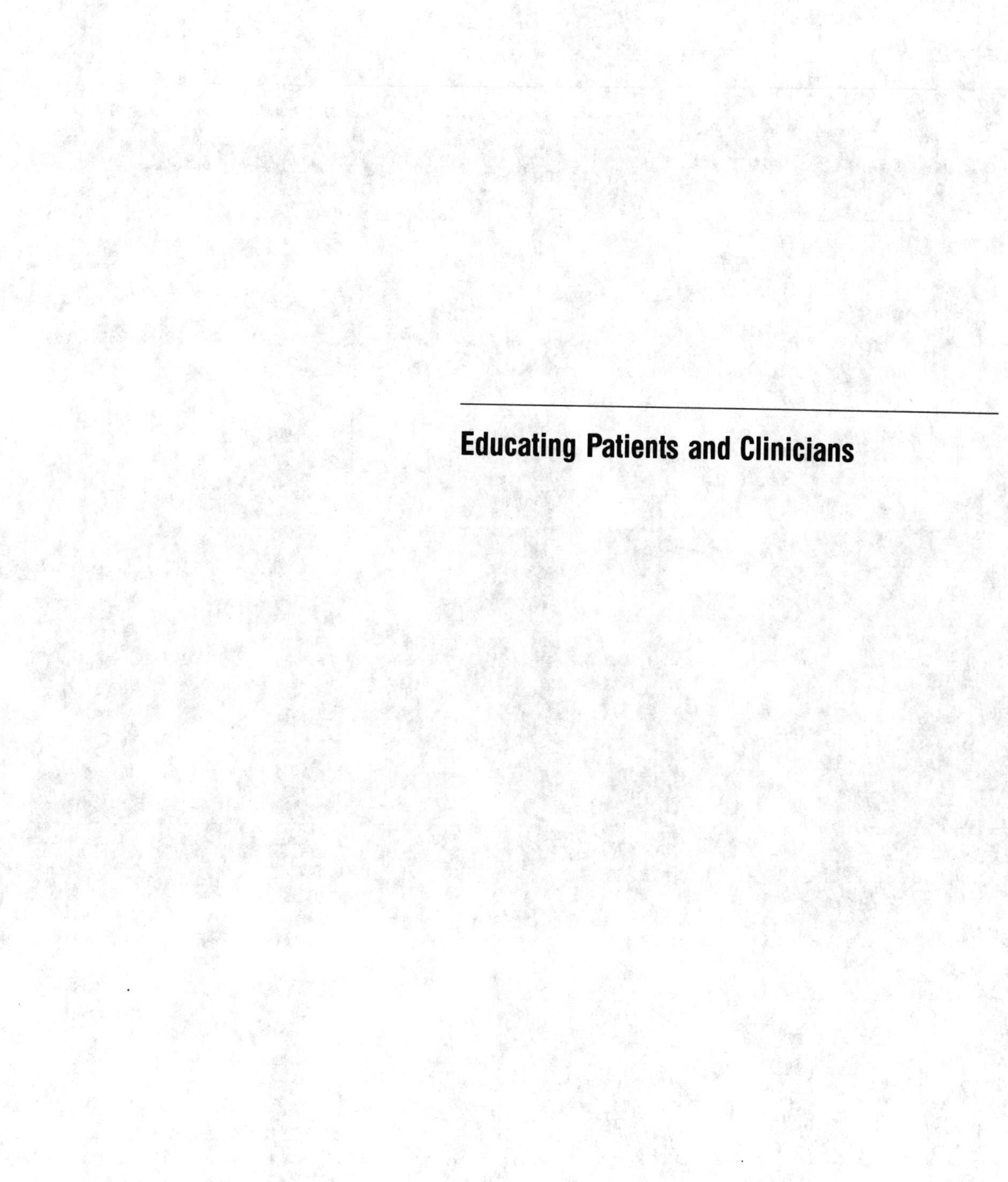

Educating Patients and Clinicians

Generating Patient-Specific Interactive Natural Language Explanations

Giuseppe Carenini Vibhu O. Mittal Johanna D. Moore
Intelligent Systems Laboratory, University of Pittsburgh, Pittsburgh, PA 15260

Patient compliance is a significant problem and is strongly correlated with the patients' understanding of their condition and prescribed treatment. Since doctors typically do not have large amounts of time to educate patients, and impersonal, voluminous patient handouts are largely ineffective, we propose the use of a sophisticated computer-based information system to generate tailored, interactive handouts to communicate with patients. Our system uses text planning and user modeling techniques to generate natural language descriptions of migraine, its symptoms, triggering factors and prescriptions. The system is capable of handling follow-up questions requesting further information, and generating responses in the context of previously supplied information – a capability unavailable in previous patient information systems. The system tailors its interaction to: (i) the class of migraine patients, (ii) the individual patient, and (iii) the previous dialogue. Preliminary evaluation of the system indicates that patients find it useful and informative. More extensive evaluation is in progress.

Introduction

Patient noncompliance is a significant problem with both economic and quality of life implications. A number of studies have shown that patient compliance is strongly correlated to the patients' understanding of their condition and prescribed treatment, e.g., [7, 11]. It is essential, therefore, that communication with patients be structured carefully to maximize the possibility of their comprehension. The importance of doing so is further underscored by research indicating that patients often do not understand important documents (such as 'informed-consent' forms) that they are asked to read and sign [6, 13]. Facilitating patient education is one way of overcoming these problems. However, doctors typically do not have large amounts of time to either explain their diagnostic procedures, or discuss their rationale for the prescribed therapy [10–12]. Unfortunately, handing out lengthy descriptions of different illnesses and possible treatments is unlikely to ameliorate the condition; a number of studies have shown that impersonal, decontextualized information has negligible impact on patients as compared to the selective presentation of relevant, patient-specific information, e.g., [2, 14]. It has also been observed that handouts are not very effective unless clinical personnel review them with patients to ensure comprehension and answer follow-up questions [12]. Therefore handouts can address only part of the problem. One possible solution is to use a computer-based system to select and present patient-specific information in an appropriate manner. This paper describes how a system can tailor the patient interaction – both the explanations generated, as well as the follow-up questions – to maximize patient education.

The authors are listed in alphabetical order.

System Requirements

A patient education system must be able to:

- take into account patient characteristics and select relevant information,
- present the information in a manner both comprehensible and acceptable to the patient, and
- engage in follow-up dialogues, and facilitate queries for clarifications, elaborations, etc. in the context of the on-going conversation.

While a number of previous efforts have investigated the possibility of using computer-based information delivery systems, e.g., [1, 7, 9–11] none of these systems attempted to incorporate advanced natural language generation capabilities to tailor the interaction – not just the content, but also the organization and the phrasing of the explanations – to individual patients. Furthermore, they did not allow patients to query the system to receive further elaboration or clarifications.

We have designed a sophisticated information delivery system that meets these requirements. The system is based on a text planning framework [15] that dynamically selects and structures the information to be presented in each case. Since we are unable to parse free-form text, the system has a large library of possible questions[1]. The patient can ask questions by clicking on mouse sensitive portions of the text and by selecting available questions from menus [15]. Both the menus containing questions that the user may ask, and the responses produced, are generated in a context sensitive manner, taking into account both the patient model and the previous dialogue [5].

Conceptually, the migraine system [3] consists of three main components: (a) an interactive **history-taking module** that collects information from patients prior

[1] The set of questions was determined from an ethnographic analysis of a large number of doctor-patient interactions; the field work and analysis was conducted by Forsythe, Brostoff and Bee [8].

0195–4210/94/$5.00

to each visit and builds a patient model[2] (b) an intelligent **explanation module** that produces an interactive information sheet containing explanations in everyday language tailored to individual patients, and that responds intelligently to follow-up questions, and (c) an **interaction manager** that presents the interactive information sheet on the screen and manages the subsequent interaction with the patient.

In addition to presenting individual patients with information specific to their case, it is also important for the system to communicate information important to all migraine patients. For instance, ethnographic field studies have found that migraine sufferers are concerned about the possibility of more serious causes for their headaches, such as brain tumors or stroke [8]. The system is designed to address these concerns as well. Thus, the system tailors the explanation not only to the individual patient, but also to the larger class of migraine patients.

Patient Modeling in Migraine

The **interactive information sheet** provides patients with information about migraine, their specific condition, the prescribed treatment and its implications. The system can respond intelligently to follow-up questions about topics covered in the information sheet. The content and organization of the information sheet are based on three sources: (i) results of ethnographic research [8], (ii) sample information sheets written by the physician on our research team, and (iii) sample information sheets being given out in local hospitals and clinics. For example, because of the ethnographic findings, the information sheet deals with global concerns before going on to instruct patients about how to follow their therapy regimen. However, the actual contents that are included when covering each topic will vary for each patient, because the system is sensitive to the data stored in the patient model. The information sheet produced by our system displays the following information:

- a statement about the diagnosis,
- an explanation of how the diagnosis accounts for the patient's symptoms,
- a discussion of situations and substances that act as migraine triggers for the patient, and information to help patients identify additional triggers,
- a set of instructions about the patient's individual treatment plan, and
- a discussion of the possible side effects of the prescribed therapy with instructions.

Each of these points is tailored to the individual patient. A snapshot of the system is shown in Figure 1.

Tailoring the Output to Individual Patients

In order to adapt explanations to a patient, the explanation facility must have access to a stored description of relevant features: the patient model. Information about the patient that would typically be gathered using a questionnaire on their first visit – such as the symptoms, past treatments, relevant habits, and other current medical treatments – is gathered by a computerized version of such a questionnaire (the history-taking module) and translated into a patient model that can be used by the explanation component. Information about the patient's diagnosis and prescribed therapy is provided by the physician or other clinical personnel immediately after the visit with the physician. The system uses this patient model to generate customized explanations at every possible step. For example, the patient's symptoms, as well as specific supporting evidence, such as family history of migraine, are used to corroborate the physician's diagnosis:

If the patient's migraine attacks are characterized by a severe, throbbing headache, the system generates: *"One of the most common symptoms of migraine is a severe, throbbing headache ... "*. If there were no *throbbing* sensation for another patient, the system would modify it to: *"One of the most common symptoms of migraine is a moderate to severe headache."* In cases of migraine characterized by the visual aura alone, the system can generate: *"A strong indicator of (classic) migraine is a disturbance in the visual field, known as an aura."*

The system uses information about the patient's physical examination to further reassure the patient that the condition is not a life-threatening one. The fourth paragraph in Figure 1 shows part of the description generated for a pre-menopausal, female patient. If the patient had been post-menopausal, the system would generate an explanation along the lines of, *"Migraine often gets better with age, since hormones play a role in making the attacks more severe"* without mentioning the role of menopause.

The description of migraine triggers is also tailored: it takes into account information about the gender and age of the patient, as well as any specific triggers reported by the patient:

"Migraine triggers ... *you were not aware of any trigger factors, except possibly stress and sleeping late on weekends. Stress is difficult to avoid, but try maintaining a regular sleep pattern ...*"

[2]The information collected here is also used to summarize the patients' status for their physicians.

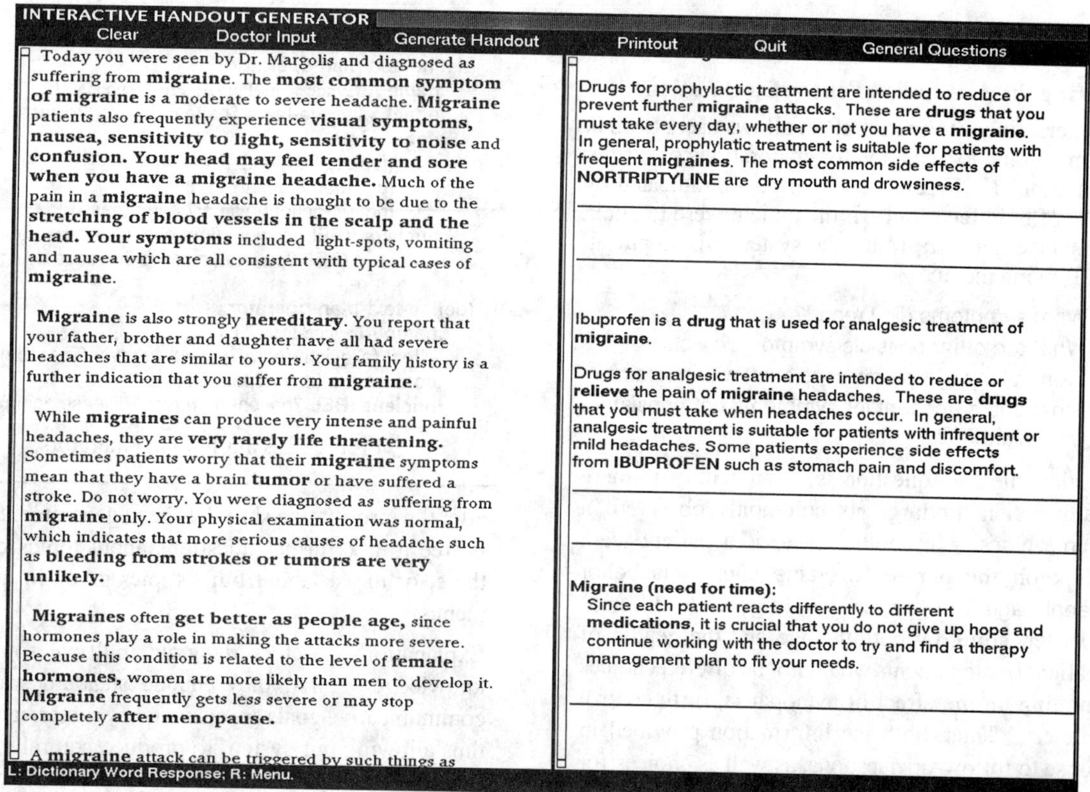

Figure 1: A snapshot of the system.

Similarly, the section addressing the prescribed treatment takes into account the drugs that are already being taken by the patient (for conditions other than migraine), as well as information about their possible effects on the patient's life style. For instance, among the side-effects of the drug Inderal are a reduced maximum heart rate and lowered arterial blood pressure. This side-effect does not noticeably affect patients with a sedentary lifestyle, but can result in individuals with an active life style no longer being able to indulge in strenuous activities to the same extent as before. The system elaborates on this side-effect of the drug differently depending on aspects of the patient's lifestyle, as determined during the history-taking session.

This scenario illustrates how patient information is used not only to determine *how* to phrase pertinent information, but also to determine *what* aspects are to be elaborated upon; if the patient specific information had not been taken into account, the handouts generated would have been quite different, with identical descriptions of the triggers, drugs and their side-effects, information on hormonal effects, and so forth, irrespective of the patients' age, gender, lifestyle, and other factors.

Tailoring the Output to the Patient Class

In addition to tailoring the description to individual patients, the generated handout also contains information that pertains to the general population of migraine patients as a whole. Ethnographic studies in the project have shown that migraineurs have both fears and concerns about their condition. For instance, migraineurs are usually worried about the possibilities of more serious problems such as cerebral haemorrhages, brain tumors or strokes as a result of the symptoms they experience [8]. It is important to address these fears explicitly in the information sheet. Migraine patients also worry about the dangers of taking hormonal medicines for other conditions (for instance, birth control pills), possible job discrimination, avoiding food/drink triggers in social situations, etc. These fears and concerns may be specific to migraine, and may not be applicable to other types of headaches (sinus, tension, cluster, etc). Initial results from the field suggest that different types of headaches cause patients to worry about different issues. Since our intention is to generalize the system to be able to deal with other headache types as well as migraine, issues such as these (pertaining to the general migraine population) must also be represented explicitly so that the system's coverage may be expanded without undue difficulty.

The result of this modeling of the patient class can be seen in the first three sentences of the third paragraph of the handout shown in Figure 1. Such information would typically be included for all migraine cases, but would change for patients with a different diagnosis.

Tailoring the Answers to Follow-Up Questions

The interactive information sheet allows users to click on terms in the explanation for elaborations or further information. (In Figure 1 such terms are indicated by the use of bold face font). If the patient were to click, for instance, on **symptoms**, the system would put up the following menu:

- What symptoms did I report?
- What are other possible symptoms?
- Were all my symptoms consistent with migraine?
- What could account for symptoms not consistent with migraine?

Note that the last question is offered only if there are any patient findings not commonly observed in migraine cases. In another case, if a patient were to click on the phrase "migraine often gets better as people age," the system would generate different menus depending on both the age and the gender of the patient (male patients would not be offered choices elaborating on the effect of menopause, birth control pills, etc.). Thus, both the information provided in response to follow-up questions, as well as choices for further information are tailored based on the patient model.

The System: Issues in Tailoring

A detailed description of the system is beyond the scope of this paper. A description of the overall system may be found in [3]; the text planning framework used in generation is described in [15]; our knowledge representation framework is described in [4]. In this section, we briefly highlight techniques necessary for tailoring explanations to the individual patient and discourse context.

The system uses a text planning framework to guide the presentation of information – we adopted this framework because it facilitates the fine-grained tailoring required in our system. The explanation planning process begins when a communicative goal (e.g., "make the hearer believe that the diagnosis is migraine," "make the hearer know about the side effects of Inderal") is posted to the text planner. Posting a goal leads to the retrieval of knowledge units (facts, operators) which are useful in attaining that goal; the attempt to apply those knowledge units may result in the posting of further goals. Planning continues until all communicative goals have been refined to speech acts (e.g., `INFORM` and `RECOMMEND`) that can be "executed" to produce the actual English text. In our system, there are two ways that a communicative goal may be posed to the text planner. First, when the interaction begins, the goal to generate the information sheet for the current patient-user is posted. Second, after the information sheet has been generated, the user is free to ask further questions about topics covered there, or to ask about other topics given in question menus.

```
(define-text-plan-operator
    :name Alleviate-fears-Female-Pre-Menopausal
    :effect (alleviate-fears ?patient (forever ?disease))
    :constraints
        ((female ?patient)
         (pre-menopausal? ?patient)
         (not (in-patient-history? estrogens)))
    :nucleus ((BEL ?patient (improve ?disease (after menopause)))
              (BEL ?patient (improve ?disease aging))))

(define-text-plan-operator
    :name Alleviate-fears-Male
    :effect (alleviate-fears ?patient (forever ?disease))
    :constraints (male ?patient)
    :nucleus (BEL ?patient (improve ?disease aging)))
```

Figure 2: Sample Plan Operators.

Explanation operators integrate multiple sources of knowledge. First, they encode standard ways that communicative goals are achieved by rhetorical means, thus allowing our system to produce natural explanations. Second, operators contain applicability constraints that specify the knowledge that must be available if the operator is to be used. These criteria can refer to the system's medical knowledge base, the patient model, or the dialogue history. Figure 2 shows two (simplified) plan operators used in the system. The first operator applies only if the patient is female, premenopausal and does not have a history of estrogen drugs. The second operator satisfies the same goal as the first, but is only applicable to male patients. The explanations generated for the two cases differ substantially, with the first patient being provided information about the effect of menopause on migraines in addition to the information on aging. The system currently contains approximately 280 operators dealing with different situations. The majority of these operators refer to the patient model in their applicability constraints.

System Evaluation

The usability and utility of the migraine system has been evaluated in three preliminary studies. Two of these studies are relevant to the evaluation of the interactive information sheet. In the first study, 3 patients used the system in the context of an actual visit with a neurologist. In the second study, 13 persons with headache and one or more symptoms of migraine interacted with the history taking and the interactive information sheet without seeing the neurologist. In both of these studies, the patients were observed using the system, and were also interviewed afterwards regarding their session with the system. While we recognize that this is an evaluation of patients perceptions, and not a study of outcomes, we nevertheless believe that the results are helpful and encouraging. Table 1 shows an excerpt of patients' assessment of the interactive information sheet.

Questions	*Answer Category*	
	Yes	No
Did you like using the program?	16 (1.00)	0 (0.00)
Did all of the information presented make sense?	13 (0.81)	3 (0.19)
Did you feel comfortable about using a computer to get this kind of information?	16 (1.00)	0 (0.00)
Was the computer itself easy to use?	14 (0.88)	2 (0.12)
Did the program tell you anything you did not already know?	15 (0.94)	1 (0.06)
Do you think this information will help you manage your headaches better?	9 (0.56)	7 (0.44)
Did you learn anything that you would not have asked your doctor?	12 (0.75)	4 (0.25)

Table 1: Responses on the Interactive information sheet Follow-up Interview.[3]

Conclusions and Future Work

Studies have shown that patient compliance with the prescribed therapy significantly increases with understanding. We have demonstrated how a text planning framework can be used to automatically synthesize tailored, interactive information sheets for migraine patients. In generating these information sheets, the system takes into account characteristics of both the individual patient as well as the general class of migraine patients. In addition, the system takes the patient model into account in dynamically generating menus of follow-up questions, as well as answers to them.

The usability and utility of the MIGRAINE system has been evaluated in three preliminary studies. These studies were aimed at assessing patient and physician perceptions about the system. While the results from these studies have been encouraging, we are aware that a more thorough and objective evaluation is necessary.

Finally, we also plan to extend the coverage of the system to handle other types of chronic headaches in addition to migraine. Since the knowledge base and text plan operators used in the system were designed in a modular fashion, we expect that a reasonable percentage of these knowledge sources can be re-used in a larger patient education system.

Acknowledgments

This work is supported by grant number R01 LM05299 from the National Library of Medicine, NIH. Its contents are solely the responsibility of the authors and do not represent the official views of the NLM. We gratefully acknowledge the contributions of the other members of the Migraine project: G. Banks, N. Bee, M. Brostoff, B. Buchanan, D. Forsythe, S. Ohlsson and E. Rees. The ethnographic results that the paper draws upon are due to field-work and analyses by Forsythe and Brostoff.

[3]The numbers in parentheses represent the percentage of respondents who gave a particular answer.

Reference

[1] ARMSTRONG, M. L. Orchestrating the process of patient education. Methods and approaches. *Nursing Clinics Of North America 24*, 3 (Sept. 1989), 597–604.

[2] AUERBACH, S. M., MARTELLI, M. F., AND MERCURI, L. G. Anxiety, information, interpersonal impacts, and adjustment to a stressful health care situation. *Journal Of Personality And Social Psychology 44*, 6 (June 1983), 1284–96.

[3] BUCHANAN, B. G., MOORE, J., FORSYTHE, D., CARENINI, G., BANKS, G., AND OHLSSON, S. Using Medical Informatics for Explanation in the Clinical Setting. Tech. Rep. Number CS-93-16, Computer Science Dept., Univ. of Pittsburgh, 1994.

[4] CARENINI, G., AND MOORE, J. D. Using the UMLS semantic network as a basis for constructing a terminological knowledge base. In *Proceedings of SCAMC-93* (Washington, D. C., 1993).

[5] CARENINI, G., AND MOORE, J. D. Generating Explanations in Context. In *Proceedings of the International Workshop on Intelligent User Interfaces* (Orlando, Florida, Jan. 1993), pp. 175–182.

[6] CASSILETH, B. R., ZUPKIS, R. V., SUTTON-SMITH, K., AND MARCH, V. Informed Consent: Why are its goals imperfectly realized? *New England Journal of Medicine 302* (1980), 896–900.

[7] FISHER, R. C. Patient education and compliance: a pharmacist's perspective. *Patient Education and Counseling 19*, 3 (June 1992), 261–71.

[8] FORSYTHE, D. E. Using Ethnography in the Design of an Explanation System. *Expert Systems with Applications (in press)* (1994).

[9] GILLISPIE, M. A., AND ELLIS, L. B. Computer-based patient education revisited. *Journal Of Medical Systems 17*, 3 (Aug. 1993), 119–125.

[10] JONES, R. B., MCGHEE, S. M., AND MCGHEE, D. Patient on-line access to medical records in general practice. *Health Bulletin 50*, 2 (Mar. 1992), 143–50.

[11] KAHN, G. Computer-Based Patient Education: A Progress Report. *M.D. Computing 10*, 2 (1993), 93–99.

[12] KAHN, G. Computer-Generated Patient Handouts. *M.D. Computing 10*, 3 (1993), 157–164.

[13] LEEB, D., BOWERS, JR., D. G., AND LYNCH, J. B. Observations on the Myth of Informed Consent. *Plastic Reconstructive Surgery 58* (1976)

[14] MARSHALL, W. R., ROTHENBERGER, L. A., AND BUNNELL, S. L. The efficacy of personalized audiovisual patient-education materials. *Journal Of Family Practice 19*, 5 (Nov. 1984), 659–63.

[15] MOORE, J. D. *Participating in Explanatory Dialogues: Interpreting and Responding to Questions in Context.* Cambridge, MA: MIT Press., 1994.

A Comparative Study Between A Computer-Aided Education (ISIS) and Habitual Education Techniques For Hypertensive Patients

BEN SAID Mohamed, MD,
Service d'Informatique Médicale ◇ Hopital La Pitié-Salpétrière ◇ Paris - France
e-mail:bensaid@biomath.jussieu.fr

CONSOLI Silla, MD
Unité Médico-Psychologique ◇ Centre de Prevention Cardio-Vasculaire
Hopital Broussais ◇ Paris - France

JEAN Jocelyne, RN
Service d'Hypertension ◇ Hopital Broussais ◇ Paris - France

Abstract

ISIS is a patient education computer program about hypertension. It aims to be complementary to the habitual educational techniques by bringing into patient education the facility of multimedia features. Its efficiency in improving the knowledge about hypertension was tested among 158 hypertensive patients. Their prior knowledge was evaluated using a questionnaire. They were then randomly separated in a control group (CG) which had the regular education program and ISIS group or (IG) which, in addition, had an interactive session using ISIS. Two months after discharge, all the patients were asked the same questions over the telephone. A total of 138 observations (69 CG, 69 IG) were reported in the final analysis. The initial scores were significantly improved for both groups. The improvement is more evident in the IG, particularly among patients whose initial score was low and patients whose hypertension was discovered for more than 6 months. ISIS is actually used by hospitalized patients and by nurse students.

INTRODUCTION

Patient education is an important step toward the patient understanding of preventive measures. Building a patient educational program is a difficult task which involves decisions about knowledge representation and communication strategies. The use of computers as a medium for patient education is even a more difficult choice, as evaluation studies are uncommon in the litterature [1]. These difficulties were emphasized by physicians at the Departement of Hypertension (Professors Corvol P., Ménard J.) at Broussais Hospital in Paris-France, as they decided to develop a computer-aided education program for hypertensive patients about hypertension and cardiovascular risks. The computer-aided education as a neutral medium, will help address communication biases [2] such as patient passiveness and misinformation about the disease, which in turn will improve the complex patient-educator relationship. This latter is particularly influenced by the way the patient lives with the disease, the suddeness of its discovery and the willingness to comply with the constraining therapy and prevention. The fact of being sick and in need of health care, "infantilizes" the patient in the presence of a "healthy" and "knowledgeable" health care educactor. The "infantilization", is transformed into passiveness which masks the patient real knowledge about the disease, and retains unexploited potential information. By providing more autonomy, the computer-aided education will comfort the patient in the role of actively controlling the access to the knowledge. The easiness and the pleasure in using it and the recollection of the contents after, will determine the success of this method.

A computer program called ISIS[1] [2] was developped in the period of 1990-1992 and a comparative study in

[1] ISIS: Initiation Sanitaire Informatisée et Scénarisée

[2] ISIS is also a personage from the ancient Egypt

1993, showed its high performance particularly among categories of hypertensive patients. It is actually used patients with other methods in the Department of Hypertension, where emphasis is put on the patient education given the context of hypertension.

Background

Hypertension represents a major risk factor for coronary, cerebral and renal vascular diseases. It has a high prevalence among populations and plays a major role in the aggravation of the overall risk of premature cardio-vascular diseases [3, 4]. The severity of the disease imposes a rapid and long term drug treatment. Statistical findings [5, 3] show the benefits of associating a serie of a non-pharmacological therapies such as diet, quitting smoking, preventing overweight and sedentariness, controlling reaction to stress and improving the quality of life. In summary, the success of hypertension therapy requires important behavioral changes. *" Still the inherent agreement between the physician and the patient are at the basis of the success in the treatment"*[3]. Unfortunately, statistical findings, reveal a failure among patients, to comply with the long term therapy [6] and make the the health education of hypertensive patients even more necessary.

Specifications

The following specifications identified the scope and the context of using ISIS:

- the computer-aided education will be used without the educator full-time assistance,
- the patients will pilot their own progress in finding out about hypertension and associated risks,
- the educational contents will use accurate, up-to-date knowledge, as identified by a team of experts,
- the educational contents will be represented and communicated, in an easy-to-access way, considering age variation, diversity of cultural bakgrounds and unfamiliarity with computers,
- the educational contents will avoid direct instruction and will use "agreable" and appropriate ways in informing about the disease and prevention,
- the computer-aided education will provide ways of evaluating itself, and evaluating the patient educational progess.

MATERIAL AND METHODS

Development Phase

Hardware, Software

ISIS is developped on a color MacIntosh, and uses the following software to create graphics (MacPaint, PixelPaint), to create animations (MacroMind Director) and to digitize sound (MacRecorder). To the best of our knowledge, these were the most adapted tools to develop an aplication that meets the specifications. ISIS runs on MacIntosh II and higher and requires 8 megabytes of RAM, a coprocessor and a color monitor of 13 inches. It takes 32 megabytes of disk space and is organized into 30 MacroMind Director files or "movies". Macros and scripts use a high level language ("Lingo") to navigate between files and to keep track of the patient performance. Creating animations is trivial and sophisticated scenarios are not difficult to develop using the "Lingo" programming language.

Design consideration

ISIS combines graphical symbols and icons with texts into a real communication language. The icons design and arrangement on the screen had to address design issues. We will use the outline in [7] to describe them:

- *Lexical issues or how icons are produced ?* The icon size, shading, corner angle, line thichkness, color brightness, are about the same and few style variations, such as differences in shapes and colors, are used in different modules. Textual labels are associated with the icons.
- *Syntactic issues or how do the signs appear in space and time ?* The icons are used when asking questions, for immediate answer feed-back, for explanations, for help and for navigation. Each category appears in the same position in the screen and respectively in the same context.
- *Semantic issues: to what do the signs refer ?* Depending on the context, the icons point to concrete objects such as body organs, food, medical equipement, therapeutical objects; or to abstract objects, such as age, time, stress, therapeutical function, physiological function, social life, life style, daily events and familiar objects, etc.
- *Pragmatic issues: How the signs are used ? Icons legibility is favored under typical viewing distances and ambient lighting.* They have to be easy to identify *both individually and within groups.*

The advantage of using icons is that they can be understood immediately, faster than reading textual information. They do not depend on a language, and do not require a prior study. They have to be precise though, avoiding ambiguities and unnecessary details. They also have to be frank, carrying warm expressions and leaving the viewers with pleasant sensation. Familiarity and simplicity generally add weight to their meaning, humor and wittiness favor their acceptance among viewers [8]. The use of a grid, facilitates consistency in the screen design and the objects arrangement. There are minimal variations in the answer modes and the general mode of using ISIS is reduced to learn how to use the mouse click, which is explained by the nurse, Mrs Jean, at the beginning of the interaction.

ISIS tries to capture the user attention and to take her/him away from the anxiounsess and the stress of the context of the disease. It proposes a diverting educational moment.

The Computer Program Contents

The educational program alternates relaxing interludes with educational messages. The patients discover the educational program as they progress through an imaginary trip in the ancient egyptian world. At any time, they may look how far they went in the trip by consulting a map, or look how far they went in the educational part by consulting a list of visited modules. Leaving the program can be done at any time, and a patient identifier number allows to continue where left off.

The interludes help relax and refresh the attention between two educational interactions. A guide: "ISIS" will accompany the patient along the trip. At each step three referees present the rules to clear obstacles and if successful, the patient will be rewarded by a pleasant view along with a selected music.

The educational part consists of series of questions (three to five) presented to the patient and require a response. Animated messages of "Bravo" or "Inexact" follow and a performance score summary is presented after each serie of questions. The patient may then consult an explanation, usually a graphical animation that illustrates the experts messages in the specific context of the questions. The patient may review the questions, move to the following section or just leave the program. Six modules covering educational topics in hypertension and cardio-vascular diseases, constitute the educational part. They are:

Arterial pressure General notions about arterial pressure are presented in this module. Blood pressure physiology, systolic and diastolic pressures measures and variations with day time, age, environment, are described in a first part. In a second part, the arterial pressure measurement and the underlying physiology, are described to the patient.

Epidemiology In this module, notions such as: hypertension severity, prevalence, etiology, heredity, dietary prevention and the organic lesions hypertension causes, are explained to the patient.

Heart This module includes explanations about the heart physiology, gross anatomy, systemic and pulmonary circulations.

Athersoclerosis A first part covers the physiology of the arterial sclerosis and its evolution with age. A second part describes the atheroma pathophysiology and complications.

Risk factors This module describes the factors that could be modified, including nutritional and life style habits, to prevent from the risk of premature cardiovascular diseases. Realistic scanned images illustrate varieties of aliments and dishes, presented as function of their amounts in fat.

Treatment This module describes the drug mechanism of action using analogies with daily life scenes. The drug classes and their specific mode of action are described in a second part.

The patient will interact with a number of educational modules and if successful, will obtain enough bonus points to access to a secrete room in a symbolic edifice: the "Pharmacy" which is the final step of the imaginary trip. The patient will recieve from ISIS some symbolic objects as a reward to the quest of knowledge, and which will accompany her/him in another imaginary trip. During the development phase physicians experts, psychologists, nurses, dieticians, at the Department of Hypertension, and medical informatics professionals in Broussais Hospital provided valuable feed back. They helped reach a consensus about the contents, their representation and the communication methods developped in ISIS program.

Evaluation Phase

Methods

A pre-study phase helped refine ISIS program and prepare the final evaluation. It was organized into two phases: first, the ISIS program was shown to a large number of health professionals working in the Department of Hypertension. The general reaction was favorable and additional refinements were incorporated into the program. A second phase focused on the reaction of a small group of 30 patients who had an exploratory interaction with ISIS program. A preliminary questionnnaire was proposed and helped prepare the final evaluation questionnaire.

The objective of the final evaluation was to anlayze the effect of using ISIS program as a complement to the already existing patient education methods, on the patient knowledge about hypertension. A randomized study was undertaken during the period between March 1, 1993 and September 30, 1993 and included 158 hypertensive patients among hospitalized patients for initial check-up or therapeutic adjustment. They were randomly separated into two groups, a control group (CG), (79 patients) and an intervention group or ISIS group (IG), (79 patients). An initial evaluation of the patients knowledge about hypertension was made after admission to the Department. A questionnaire of 28 items prepared in collaboration with experts in hypertension and cardio-vascular diseases, was proposed to the 158 patients. The CG then followed the regular educational activities which consist of educational sessions, dialogs with physicians, nurses, dieticians and access to health information through brochures, posters and videotapes. The IG in addition to the regular educational activities had during 30 to 60 minutes, an interactive educational session using the ISIS program. Two months after discharge, the same investigator: Mrs Jean, asked the 158 patients over the telephone the same series of 28 questions. Some of the patients missed a follow-up questionnaire and were dropped from the final analysis. The results of only 138 patients are reported in the final analysis. They are distributed into, 69 in the IG and 69 in the CG and their socio-demographic and clinical characteristics are described in table 1.

RESULTS

From the beginning we explored the links between the initial health score and sex, age or general instruction.

Table 1: *Study Population:General Characteristics.*

population	138	
sex	65 men	73 women
age	50.4	± 12.4
duration of hypertension	less than 6months	51
	6 months - 2years	26
	more than 2 years	61
general instructional level	high school	51
	finished high-school	35
	college - university	51
initial test	14.3± 4.2	

Table 2: *Comparative evolution of health knowledge.*

study group	ISIS	Control	P
total poulation (138)	3.8 ±3.6	2.4 ± 3.2	0.02
Initial score=<16 (89)	4.8 ±3.6	2.9 ± 3.0	0.008
age =<65 years (118)	4.2 ± 3.4	2.6 ± 3.3	0.01
Women (73)	4.6 ± 3.7	2.4 ± 2.9	0.006
hypertension more than 6 months (87)	3.8 ± 3.5	1.8 ± 3.0	0.006

Prior health knowledge: The mean score of prior health knowledge tested with the first questionnaire was 14.3 ± 4.2 (extremes : 4 to 25), which corresponds to approximately 50% of correct answers. This score is positively correlated to the patient *age* (Pearson's r= 0.31; p=0.0002), to the level of *general instruction* (Spearman's rho = 0.36; p=0.0001) and linked to the *sex* (p=0.027). The mean score of prior health knowledge is higher among men (15.1 ± 4.6; p=0.027) than among women (13.5 ± 4.7; p=0.027); the level of general instruction being also higher in the men subpopulation. The evolution of the health knowledge was estimated by calculating the difference of the global scores between the first and the second questionnaire.

Evolution of health knowledge score in the global population: The mean score is significantly improved in both groups (17.4 ± 3.5); the mean difference between the two tests is (3.1 ± 3.5) (p=0.0001; Student's t test for paired groups). The improvement is negatively correlated with the duration of hypertension (rho = -0.19; p=0.04) and with the initial health knowledge score (r = -0.32; p<0.0001).

Comparative results between the intervention and the control group: Table 2 illustrates the differences between the two groups. The improvement in hypertension knowledge is higher the IG than in the CG (using test t of Student for impaired groups). The differences are more evident among the patients whose *initial score* was *less than* or *equal* to 16, among the patients who are *less* than *65 years* old and among the patients whose *hypertension* is discovered for *more* than 6 months.

DISCUSSION

Despite the peculiarity of its context (hypertensive patients, hospitalized for a short stay in a specialized health center), the evaluation of ISIS program brings many arguments together in favor of this method as a complement to the habitual educational techniques. The patients who started with *average* or *low initial score* have more chances to significantly ameliorate their performance in the second test. The same argument explains the fact that women progressed more than men, between the two tests. The more important receptivity observed among the patients whose *age is less than 65* years is not surprising. It is however interesting, to notice the difference between the habitual education techniques and the significant benefit brought by ISIS to the patients whose *hypertension is known for more than 6 months.* In other words, the hypertensive patients who discovered their disease for less than 6 months are more curious, more concerned and more receptive regardless of the educational method, than the long-term hypertensive patients, for whom the habitual education techniques efficiency "dries up" and the interactive education, with relaxing interludes, represents an interesting complementary method.
The role of the *nurse* in the organization of the evaluation protocol, and in encouraging the patients to use the computer, was certainly an essential factor in the relative success of ISIS program.

FUTURE PERSPECTIVES

The evaluation study, still preliminary, encourages experimentation in other specialized health centers, and among a more representative hypertensive population. It needs to be demonstrated however, that the health knowledge improvement, and the pleasure and the activeness the patients manifested in using ISIS program, will promote a better compliance with the therapy, and a better quality of life. A long term evaluation of this method will elucidate these hypotheses.

ISIS is actually used by hypertensive patients hospitalized in the Department of Hypertension, and by nurse students, as part of their academic curriculum. The text messages in ISIS are in french language and prototype versions in english and in arabic are available. Finally, the development and implementation of ISIS, is an encouraging collaborative experience between medical informatics professionals, a team of pshychiatrics and psychologists, physicians, nurses, dieticians, and communication professionals associated with the Departement of Hypertension at Broussais Hospital.

References

[1] A. Roca-Cusachs, D. Sort, J. Altimira, R. Bonet, E. Guilera, J. Monmany, and J. Nolla. The impact of a patient education programme in the control of hypertension. *Journal of Human Hypertension*, 5:437–441, 1991.

[2] P. Hanna, K.J.and Conley-Price, D. Fenty, E. McKiel, Soltes D., Hogan T., and D. Wiens. Computer applications for staff development patient education. *Methods of Information in Medicine*, 28(4):261–266, 1989.

[3] E. Braunwald. *Heart Disease - a Textbook of Cardiovascular Medicine.* W.B. Saunders Company, Hartcourt Brace Jovanovich, Inc. the Curtis Center Independence Square West, Philadelphia, PA 19106, 1992.

[4] F.P. Plouin, G. Chatelier, J.Y. Pagny, and T. Lang. Hypertension arterielle (epidemiologie, hemodynamique et physiopathologie, strategie de l'exploration et de la prise en charge. *Encycl. Med. Chir. (Paris, France), Coeur-Vaisseaux, 11302 A19, 9-1986, 12 P.*, pages 1–12, 1986.

[5] J. Marley, N. Davis, and M. Joy. Is the nonpharmacological treatment of hypertension neglected ? *Journal of the Royal Society of Medicine*, 84:540–541, September 1991.

[6] S.M. Consoli and M.E. Safar. Predictive value of the patient's psychological profile and type of patient-practitioner relationship in compliance with antihypertensive treatment. *Arch Mal Coeur*, 81 (Suppl HTA):145–150, 1988.

[7] A. Marcus. Graphic design for electronic documents and user interfaces. *ACM Press Eds*, pages 60–63, 1992.

[8] 0. Yukio. Pictogram design. *Kashiwashobo Eds*, pages 90–92, 1987.

A Survey of Patient Access to Electronic Mail: Attitudes, Barriers, and Opportunities

Douglas B. Fridsma MD[1], Paul Ford MD[2], Russ Altman MD PhD[1]
[1]Section on Medical Informatics, Stanford University School of Medicine
MSOB X-2105, Stanford, CA 94305-5479
[2]Department of Medicine, Stanford University School of Medicine
900 Blake Wilbur Rd., Stanford, CA 94305-5430
fridsma@camis.stanford.edu, ford@camis.stanford.edu, altman@camis.stanford.edu

ABSTRACT

The use of electronic mail (e-mail) is increasing among both physicians and patients, although there is limited information in the literature about how patients might use e-mail to communicate with their physician. In our university-based internal medicine clinic, we have studied attitudes toward and access to e-mail among patients. A survey of 444 patients in our clinic showed that 46% of patients in the clinic use e-mail, and 89% of those with e-mail use it at work. Fifty-one percent would use e-mail all or most of the time to communicate with the clinic if it were available, and many of the communications that currently take place by phone could be replaced by e-mail. Barriers to e-mail use include privacy concerns among patients who use e-mail in the workplace, choosing the appropriate tasks for e-mail, and methods for efficiently triaging electronic messages in the clinic.

INTRODUCTION

The use of electronic methods of communicating medical information is increasing. Physicians already use electronic mail (e-mail) to consult with their colleagues [1, 2], to review and disseminate medical journals [3], and to obtain hospital laboratory information [4]. In Europe, the 3I Project represents a large collaborative effort to link general practitioners with pharmacies, hospitals, and consultants using standard electronic data interchange formats [5]. In most circumstances, however, these systems are designed to connect physicians with their peers or with physician-specific information resources, not to connect physicians to their patients.

Among patients, there is a similar growth in health-related electronic communication: bulletin boards and electronic forums for AIDS patients [6], caregivers of Alzheimer patients [7], and disabled patients [8] have been previously described. Although these computer bulletin boards provide a variety of health-related information and database functions, the e-mail or communication features were the most popular and widely used by participants. These bulletin board systems were designed primarily for peer support among patients, and although some had the capability to ask questions of a medical expert, this expert was not the patient's personal physician.

Recently, a study by Neill [9] explored the use of patient–physician e-mail. In this survey study, Neill found that communication via e-mail was positively perceived by patients for many routine tasks, and 90% of patients who used e-mail to communicate with their physician used it to discuss a medical problem (N=10). It is likely that as the use of e-mail increases among patients, additional demands may be placed on physicians for this kind of access.

All physicians in our university-based internal medicine clinic have access to e-mail, and use it routinely to discussion patients and patient problems with other clinic physicians. Informally, we have noted an increase in the use of e-mail between a subset of computer-literate patients and their physicians. However, a large number of patients with e-mail access to their physician could become problematic if physicians are overwhelmed with messages and are ill-equipped to triage these messages effectively. Adoption of e-mail in this setting might be impaired.

An informal study conducted in 1993 (Ford, 1993 unpublished data) suggested that there may be a large number of patients willing to use this medium for communication: 54% of clinic patients surveyed indicated they would use e-mail to communicate with their physician if this option were made available. In anticipation of more widespread use of e-mail within our clinic, we completed an exploratory survey to examine potential strategies for the successful adoption of this new form of communication between physicians and patients.

METHODS

The university-based internal medicine clinic in which the study was performed has 70% of patients enrolled in managed-care plans, 25% with Medicare health insurance, and 5% of patients with Medicaid insurance. Although some medical house officers have their outpatient clinic in this setting, most patients are seen by full-time clinical faculty. A survey comprising 18 questions was distributed during a two-week period to all patients when they checked in for their scheduled appointments in the clinic. Questions were grouped into three main categories: (1) patient demographics and current health care use patterns, (2) current methods used by patients to communicate with the clinic, and (3) access and attitudes toward e-mail for communication with their physician. Patients completed the survey while waiting to see their physician, and all patients that had completed at least part of the survey were included in the study. Responses were coded into categorical observations for analysis. For ranking questions, the mean ranks were tabulated for each question. In all circumstances, calculations were based on the number of patients that completed a particular question.

RESULTS

Survey Response Rate

A total of 444 of 770 patients (58%) completed at least part of the questionnaire while they waited to see their physician. Since all patients did not answer or rank every question, the total number of responders varied for individual questions.

Demographics and Health Care Utilization

A total of 177 (41%) of the patients were men, 257 (59%) where women. The median age group was 40 to 50 years old for men and 30 to 40 for women. For more than half the patients (55%), this was the only university-based clinic in which they received care. Most patients (58%) visited the clinic every 6 months or less and talked with their physician or nurse with about the same frequency.

Current Mediums of Communication

Patient were asked to rank from 1 to 5 (1 signifying most common, and 5 least common) the principal mediums through which they communicated with the clinic. Not all patients ranked all categories; the number of patients that provided any rank for the question is listed in Table 1. Most patients used the telephone as their primary medium of communication, and of the 119 patients who ranked e-mail as a medium of communication, most ranked it last.

Table 1. How Patients Communicate with the Clinic

Medium of Communication	No. of Patients Ranking	Mean Rank
telephone	404	1.1
office visit	233	2.2
mail	150	3.9
fax	118	4.8
e-mail	119	5.0

Similarly, when the clinic staff wanted to communicate with patients, the telephone was the principal medium they used (Table 2). Only 17 patients indicated that they currently received information from the clinic staff via e-mail.

Table 2. How the Clinic Staff Communicates with Patients

Medium of Communication	No. of Patients Ranking	Mean Rank
telephone	310	1.2
office visit	162	1.7
mail	103	2.1
e-mail	17	4.1
fax	14	4.0

Each patient was asked what was the typical purpose of the communication when they contacted the clinic. These results are summarized in Table 3. Nearly all patients ranked scheduling a routine visit as the most common reason for contacting the clinic. Other reasons for contacting the clinic were specific to each patient, so no obvious ranking for all patients was obtained.

Table 3. Purpose of Patient Communication

Purpose of Communication	No. of Patients Ranking	Mean Rank
schedule routine visit	337	1.2
schedule urgent visit	246	2.8
medical advice	240	3.1
medication refill	215	4.2
obtain test results	194	4.4
HMO authorization	196	4.5
emergency visit	169	5.5

Electronic Mail Access and Attitudes

Of patients surveyed, 194 (46%) used e-mail. Of those, 43 patients (23%) used in-house e-mail systems that could only be used within their workplace. The remaining 151 (77%) had the ability to send messages to people outside their workplace or from home. Men and women had similar levels of e-mail access: Of patients with e-mail, 91 (46%) were men and 103 (54%) were women. Patients between 20 and 50 years of age constituted more than 83% of patients with e-mail, although patients as old as 80 used e-mail.

Table 4 shows patient e-mail use stratified by age with percentages within a stratification indicated by parentheses. None of the patients less than 20 years old used e-mail. Patients 20 to 30 years old used e-mail more frequently than any other group. Access to electronic mail decreased as age increased, although all age groups over 20 years of age had at least some patients that used e-mail.

Table 4. Patient E-mail Access by Age

Age	Responders	Use E-mail	Don't Use E-mail
<20	3	0	3
20-30	66	43 (65%)	23 (35%)
30-40	129	69 (53%)	60 (47%)
40-50	102	49 (48%)	53 (52%)
50-60	53	18 (34%)	35 (66%)
60-70	38	9 (24%)	29 (76%)
70-80	27	5 (19%)	22 (81%)
>80	5	1 (25%)	4 (75%)
Total	423	194 (46%)	229 (54%)

Most patients used e-mail primarily at work. Of all patients who used e-mail, 169 (89%) used it at work, 62 (33%) used it at home, and 46 (24%) used e-mail both at work and at home. A total of 95 (49%) patients that used e-mail indicated that even though e-mail was available to them, they would not use it for personal or family matters. In this subset of patients, only 11 used e-mail at home. The remaining 84 (88%) patients used e-mail primarily at work.

All patients, regardless of whether they currently used e-mail or not, were asked if they would use e-mail to communicate with the clinic if they had access to it (Table 5). Ninety-nine (51%) patients who currently use e-mail said they would use it all or most of the time; 48 (24%) patients without e-mail said they would use it to communicate with the clinic staff.

Table 5. Patient Estimated Frequency of E-mail Use

Estimated Frequency of Use	Responders	Currently Use E-mail	Currently Don't Use E-mail
all the time	60	41 (68%)	19 (32%)
most of the time	97	58 (60%)	39 (40%)
occasionally	110	58 (53%)	52 (47%)
rarely	50	18 (36%)	32 (63%)
never	62	13 (21%)	49 (79%)
Total	379	188 (50%)	191 (50%)

Finally, patients were asked what would prevent them from using e-mail to communicate with their physician. For those patients who used e-mail primarily at work, 48 patients (38%) would not use e-mail for reasons of privacy or convenience. Only 7 (10%) of the patients who used e-mail at home listed privacy as a barrier to the use of e-mail to communicate with their physician.

DISCUSSION

Despite our response rate of 58%, our study population is likely representative of our clinic population. Patients were given time to complete the questionnaire only between the time of check in and seeing their physician, and it is likely that those not completing the questionnaire were unable to do so because of time constraints, rather than selection bias. Despite the random error introduced by sampling, it is encouraging that this study confirms our findings in our previous study of 200 patients (Ford, 1993 unpublished data).

Our clinic population is composed primarily of patients in health maintenance organizations (HMOs) and is similar to other clinics in the San Francisco area, that have a significant HMO patient population. Our location in Silicon Valley is reflected in the high levels of e-mail sophistication among this population of patients, and this specialized population may serve as a test bed for research into computer-mediated patient–physician communication.

Work by Neill [9] indicates that patient–physician communication via e-mail is "positively perceived" by patients and that e-mail is suitable for simple and non urgent problems. In our study, there are two primary ways in which patients receive information from their physician: by telephone and through office visits. Other data collected in our clinic suggest that the purpose of more than 40% of telephone calls is the management of simple or non urgent problems that may be appropriately managed using e-mail.

Substituting e-mail for simple communication tasks is not without potential problems, however. In the computer-science literature, there is a noteworthy body of work on media richness and choosing the most appropriate medium for communication [10, 11]. This computer science literature suggests that fact retrieval tasks can be done with a medium such as e-mail, but tasks that require negotiation and uncertainty are best performed with telephone conversations or face-to-face meetings. In medicine, the distinction between these two types of tasks can be blurred. A test result that is either positive or negative may be classified as a simple fact retrieval task, but may require a great deal of explanation to an anxious patient. Scheduling of routine appointments and return of normal laboratory results may be appropriate uses for e-mail, further investigation of other medical tasks that are suitable for this medium is warranted.

E-mail has the potential to benefit both physicians and patients. Physician-initiated e-mail might be used to remind patients of routine health care screening that they might otherwise miss. In other circumstances, e-mail may allow patients to obtain needed information without an office visit. In a study at the Harvard Community Health Plan, patients with access to electronic medical information in their home tended to call the physician's office more frequently, but often these calls could be handled by nurses [12]. Electronic mail would be a natural extension of these information systems and could provide personalized answers to the questions that patients have.

There are some fundamental problems that we have identified as well. Most patients use e-mail at work and there are many issues surrounding ownership of the messages and privacy that are situation specific [13]. This controversy may limit patient enthusiasm for this medium for discussion of personal medical issues. In our study, those patients who used e-mail at home were less concerned with issues of privacy and convenience than those who used e-mail at work, but represented a small subset of all patients who used e-mail.

The expanded use of e-mail by patients may have a profound effect on clinic operation. If we analyze our data to determine an upper and lower bound of e-mail use by patients, we can determine a range of potential e-mail usage among patients. Assuming all non-responders do not use e-mail, we can calculate a lower bound for e-mail use among our population. A conservative upper bound can be calculated by extrapolation of our study results to the rest of our patient population. Using a lower bound analysis, at least 25% of clinic patients have access to e-mail and of these patients, 51% would use e-mail all or most of the time to communicate with the clinic. In our clinic population of 20,000 patients, this would mean that at least 2,500 patients (and as many as 9,000) would use e-mail as their primary method of communication. Extrapolating from current phone usage, we estimate that 50 to 100 e-mail messages a day could be generated by this population. If methods for intelligent sorting, authenticating, and triaging of incoming messages are not employed, physicians and nurses could quickly become overwhelmed by the number of e-mail messages they receive. Further work in these areas is needed to anticipate the expansion of e-mail use.

Although our population may not be representative of the country as a whole, it may serve as a model for the future. The Internet, the prototype of the information superhighway, is growing exponentially, with new system connections occurring every 20 minutes [14]. As patients become more sophisticated users of e-mail, they may demand electronic access to their physician. If electronic communication is to be successfully introduced, additional information about the barriers and potential problems must be obtained. Access that is both private and secure is important, and an environment that allows an honest and candid interchange should be fostered. This may mean that the current access to e-mail that patients have at work may not be adequate unless there are mechanisms to assure confidentiality. Additional mechanisms for intelligent triage of messages will also become necessary to prevent overwhelming current clinic operations. Only then can we use this new technology to improve patient care.

Acknowledgments
This work was supported by grant LM-07033 from the National Library of Medicine. Computing services provided by the CAMIS resource, grant LM-05305. Russ Altman is supported by NIH LM-05652 and the Culpeper Foundation. Nora Sweeny provided editorial assistance.

References

[1] Branger PJ, van der Wouden JC, Schudel BR, et al. Electronic communication between providers of primary and secondary care. *British Medical Journal* 1992, 305(6861):1068-1070.

[2] Sands DZ, Safran C, Slack WV, Bleich HL. Use of electronic mail in a teaching hospital. In Safran, C. (ed.),*Proceedings of the Seventeenth Annual Symposium on Computer Applications in Medical Care* Washington, D.C.:McGraw-Hill, 1993:306-310.

[3] Kassirer J. Journals in bits and bytes: electronic medical journals. *New England Journal of Medicine* 1992, 326:195-197.

[4] Antti-Poika M, Korpela M. Computer-supported cooperation of health care staff: the Peijas-Rekola case. In Degaulet P. et.al (ed.), *MEDINFO 92. Proceedings of the Seventh World Congress on Medical Informatics.* Amsterdam, Netherlands: North-Holland, 1992:106-111.

[5] Hasman A, Ament A, Arnou PC, Van Kesteren AC. Inter-institutional information exchange in healthcare. *International Journal of Biomedical Computing* 1992,31(1):5-16.

[6] Gustafson DH, Bosworth K, Hawkins RP, Boberg EW, Bricker E. CHESS: a computer-based system for providing information, referrals, decision support and social support to people facing medical and other health-related crises. In Frisse, ME. (ed.),*Proceedings of the Sixteenth Annual Symposium on Computer Applications in Medical Care* Baltimore, MD: McGraw-Hill, 1992:161-165.

[7] Brennan PF. Computer networks promote caregiving collaboration: the ComputerLink Project. In Frisse, ME (ed.), *Proceedings of the Sixteenth Annual Symposium on Computer Applications in Medical Care* Baltimore, MD: McGraw-Hill, 1992:156-160.

[8] Hassett M, Lowder C, Rutan D. Use of computer network bulletin board systems by disabled persons. In Frisse, ME (ed.), *Proceedings of the Sixteenth Annual Symposium on Computer Applications in Medical Care* Baltimore, MD: McGraw-Hill, 1992:151-155.

[9] Neill RA, Mainous III AG, Clark JR, Hagen MD. The Utility of Electronic Mail as a Medium for Patient-Physician Communication. *Archives of Family Medicine* 1994, 3:268-271.

[10] Kydd CT, Ferry DL. Electronic mail, social presence and information richness. In Milutinovic V , et. al. (ed.), *Proceedings of the Twenty-Fifth Hawaii International Conference on System Sciences* Los Alamitos, CA, USA: IEEE Comput. Soc. Press, 1991, 4: 380-391.

[11] Zack MH. Electronic messaging and shared context in an ongoing work group. In Mudge TN et.al. (ed.), *Proceeding of the Twenty-Sixth Hawaii International Conference on System Sciences* . Los Alamitos, CA, USA: IEEE, 1993, 4:528-537.

[12] Gareiss R. Electronic Triage. *American Medical News* 1994, 4/25/94:23-27.

[13] Castagnoli C. Someone's been reading my E-mail! Privacy protection for electronic mail users in the US and the EC. *Tolley's Computer Law and Practice* 1993, 9(6):215-220.

[14] Rutkowski AM. A Year in the Life of the Internet. *Internet Society News* 1994,2(4):9.

A Computer-Based Interview to Identify HIV Risk Behaviors and to Assess Patient Preferences for HIV-Related Health States

G.D. Sanders[2], D.K. Owens[1,2], M.D., M.Sc., N Padian[3] Ph.D., A.B. Cardinalli[1,2], A.N. Sullivan[1,2], R.F Nease[4], Ph.D.

[1]Section of General Internal Medicine, Department of Veterans Affairs Medical Center, Palo Alto, CA and [2]Section on Medical Informatics and Division of General Internal Medicine Stanford University School of Medicine, Stanford, California

[3]University of California San Francisco, Department of Obstetrics and Gynecology San Francisco, California

[4]Center for the Evaluative Clinical Sciences, Department of Community and Family Medicine, Dartmouth Medical School, Hanover, New Hampshire

ABSTRACT

We developed a computer-based utility assessment tool to assess the preferences of patients towards HIV -related health states and identify risk behaviors (both sexual and drug related) of the patient being interviewed. The reliability of the computer-based interview was assessed through comparison with person-to-person interviews.

Our pilot study included 22 patients. Twelve of these patients were also interviewed by the research assistants in person-to-person interviews. The agreement between the person-to-person and computer-based interviews was excellent (3 discrepancies of 180 compared answers), and the majority of the patients preferred to use the computer to disclose sensitive information regarding risk behaviors. Our study suggests that assessment of patient preferences and risk factors can be performed reliably through a computer-based interview.

INTRODUCTION

Screening for human immunodeficiency virus (HIV) infection is valuable for two reasons. It allows the HIV infected person to obtain early medical intervention, and it may also provide a public health benefit if screened HIV infected persons alter their risk behaviors. Widespread screening of all patients in all populations is not cost-effective however [1]. Guidelines that customize HIV screening for particular clinical settings may be more cost-effective than generic guidelines that do not take into account differences in patient populations [2].

To investigate the factors that influence the cost-effectiveness of screening for HIV infection, we developed a probabilistic decision model that estimates both the health benefits and costs of a screening program [3]. The screening strategy is represented by a 21-state Markov model; the no-screen strategy is modeled by a 9-state Markov model. The model accounts for changes in length and quality of life caused by HIV infection, transmission of HIV infection to sexual partners, the direct costs of screening, the incremental costs of medical therapy, and the cost savings that accrue when HIV infections are prevented.

The model represents the natural history of HIV disease as progression through three health states: HIV infection without symptoms, HIV infection with symptoms (but without symptoms or complications that meet the case definition of AIDS), and AIDS. We account for the detrimental effect of HIV infection on quality of life by applying quality adjustments to each of these health states. Our analyses with this model indicate that three factors have a critical impact on the cost-effectiveness of a screening program for HIV infection: the prevalence of HIV infection in the screened population, the prevalence of risk behaviors (high risk sexual practices and injection drug use), and the beliefs of the screened persons about the quality of life with HIV infection.

The prevalence of risk behaviors is an important determinant of the cost-effectiveness of screening because it affects the public health benefit that may accrue from testing and counseling. For example, if testing and counseling promotes a decrease in high risk sexual behavior, the potential benefit is greater in a person who has many sexual partners than in a person with one partner. In addition, a screening program that identifies a person with HIV infection may either positively or negatively affect quality of life. These effects of screening on quality-of-life should be considered when evaluating the cost-effectiveness of a screening program.

Although HIV seroprevalence has been studied widely, risk behaviors and patient preferences have not been studied in many populations that are candidates for screening. Since assessment of these population characteristics is essential to determine the cost effectiveness of HIV screening, we developed an instrument to perform such assessments. Our purpose in designing the tool was to collect data for determining the cost effectiveness of screening. The tool also could be used, however, in clinical settings in which clinicians wanted to elicit risk.

We used a utility assessment tool, U-titer, to assess patient preferences for HIV-related health states and to identify HIV risk behaviors. U-titer is an automated, modular utility assessment Hypercard software package [4]. The U-titer software allows the programmer to implement several different methods of assessing patient preferences such as the standard gamble and time trade-off. The programmer is also able to significantly tailor each of these methods. U-titer is a generalized utility assessment tool and has been used in several studies and settings, including assessment of utilities among patients with angina, psoriasis, and atrial fibrillation.

SYSTEM DESCRIPTION

Our version of U-titer adapted for HIV preference and risk assessment consists of a 45 to 60 minute computer-based interview. The interview has three sections. The first obtains demographics: gender, ethnicity, income, average distance traveled, and waiting time for physician visits, level of education, and employment. The second assesses the patient's preferences for the three HIV-related health states: asymptomatic HIV infection, HIV infection with symptoms, ands AIDS.

The interview uses time tradeoff and standard gambles to assess preferences; both are standard approaches for assessment of utilities. We used the utility assessments to calculate the quality adjustments for the HIV-related health states. The HIV-related questions are preceded by a pair of questions on the patient's preferences concerning being blind (monocular and binocular blindness); these questions allow the patient to become familiar with the method of questioning as well as ensure that they understand the utility assessment questions.

The final group of questions identifies patient risk behaviors: type, and frequency of sexual activity (vaginal, oral, and anal intercourse), use of sexual barriers (such as condoms), number of sexual partners, length of sexual relationships, use of drugs (specifically, use of needles), and frequency of needle sharing. The results of the questions are stored in a result file that records both the patient's answers and the time spent answering each question.

Questions are branched so that a patient is only asked those questions that are relevant based on their answers to previous questions. For example, if a patient answers "No" to the question "Other than insulin prescribed for you by a physician, have you ever injected or used needles to take drugs of any kind", the program skips over more specific drug questions to the next series of questions.

The interface was designed so that questions could be answered using a mouse or trackball; patients were not required to type.

METHODS

We recruited patients from the Internal Medicine Clinic and the inpatient services at Stanford University Medical Center. Once patients agreed to participate and gave informed consent, they completed the computer-based interview. The research assistant stayed with the patient for the first few questions to assure that the patient understood both how to operate the computer and, more specifically, that they understood the preference assessment questions. Once the assistant felt comfortable that the patient was capable of completing the interview successfully, the assistant left the patient alone. We believe that in a more private atmosphere patients are more likely to answer the risk behavior questions truthfully.

We used several methods to assess the reliability of the computer-based interview. Internal consistency was assessed by creating several questions that asked for similar information but were worded differently. An example of a pair of questions that were designed to detect possible contradictions is the following (asked of a heterosexual male):

> Question A: "When was the last time you had sex with your partner?"
>
> Question B: "Over the last year, on average, how often did you have vaginal sex with your partner?"

If the patient answered, "Within the last six months" to Question A, yet answered "Never" to Question B (as well as similar questions asking how often the patient and his partner had oral or anal intercourse) then we were able to flag this as an inconsistent patient response.

To assess reliability we interviewed 12 patients in person after they completed the computer-based interview and compared the answers from the computerized interview and the answers obtained in a person-to-person interview. After this personal interview, the patient was asked his or her preferred interview format.

RESULTS

Demographic characteristics of the subjects are shown in Table 1. Ninety-five percent had completed high school. Only 14% of the patients were working either part time or full time. The patients were of varying ethnicities: 41% were White; 36% were Black; 14% were Asian; and 9% were Hispanic.

Table 1 Patient Characteristics

Characteristics	Average or proportion	Range
Age	55.1 years	30 to 82
Education	13.8 years	8 to 20
Gender	0.77 female	-
Income	$24,431	$0 to $90,000

Table 2 Time Tradeoff

	Average	Range	*p* value
HIV+, Asx	0.63	0 to 0.995	0.0013*
HIV+, Sx	0.51	0 to 0.979	0.0636†
AIDS	0.21	0 to 0.896	0.0129‡

HIV+ = HIV infected, Asx = Asymptomatic, Sx = Symptomatic. *p* values calculated with one-sample sign test. Calculations with one-sample t-test were similar.
* HIV+ , Asx compared with AIDS
† HIV+ , Asx compared with HIV+, Sx
‡ HIV+ , Sx compared with AIDS

The quality adjustments (based on the time-tradeoff questions) for the HIV health states are as shown in Table 2. The quality adjustment can vary between 0 and 1.0, with 0 indicating that the health state is equivalent to death, and 1.0 indicating that the health state is equivalent to usual health. The quality adjustments decreased with progressively worse health states, which suggests that the majority of the patients understood the task and the descriptions (Figures 1-3). Differences in the quality adjustments between the health states were statistically significant with the exception of the difference between HIV infection without symptoms and HIV infection with symptoms. This borderline significance is not surprising given our small sample size.

All of the respondents reported having had sex. The average number of lifetime sexual partners was approximately 25 for men and 5.4 for women. During the last year, 11 of 22 (50%) reported having had vaginal intercourse, 6 of 22 (27%) having had oral intercourse, and 1 of 22 (4%) having had anal intercourse. Overall, 27% reported using condoms; the frequency of condom use varied from "occasionally" to "always." Most respondents were in long-term relationships, with 73% reporting relationships that lasted more than three years. Three of 22 patients had used needles to take drugs.

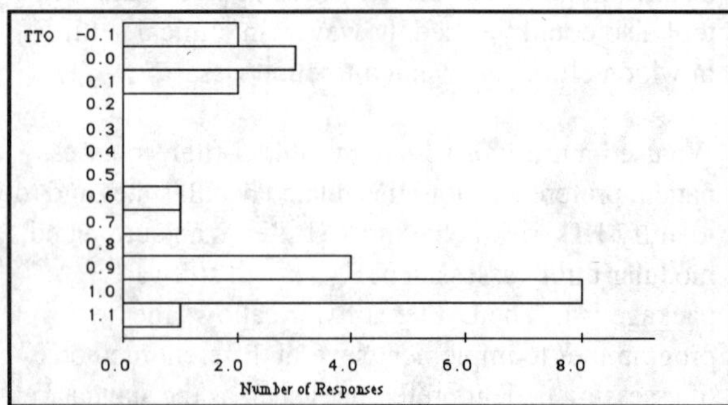

Figure 1 HIV+ Asymptomatic Time Tradeoff Histogram. Utility of -0.1 corresponds to patient who would rather die immediately than live for any length of time with asymptomatic HIV infection. Utility of 1.1 corresponds to a patient who viewed HIV infection without symptoms to be at least equivalent to their current health state.

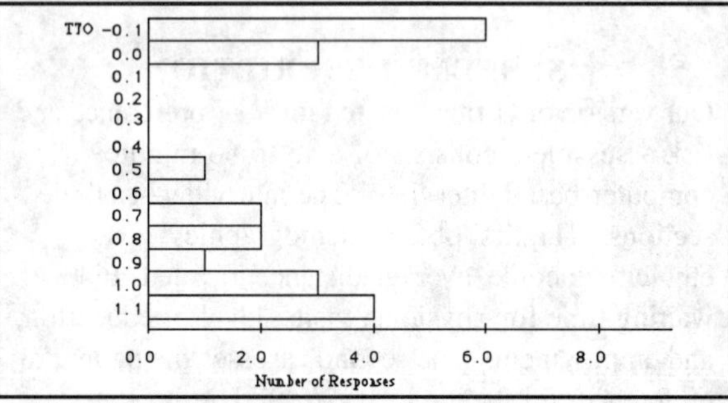

Figure 2 HIV+ Symptomatic Time Tradeoff Histogram. Utility of -0.1 corresponds to a patient who would rather die immediately than live with symptomatic HIV infection. Utility of 1.1 corresponds to a patient who viewed HIV infection with symptoms to be at least equivalent to their current health state.

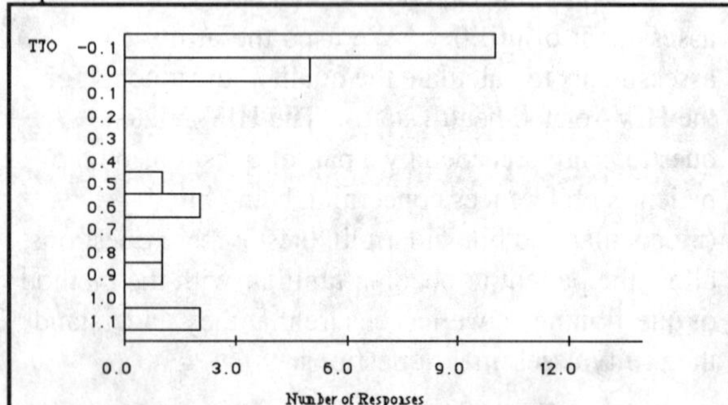

Figure 3 AIDS Time Tradeoff Histogram. Utility of -0.1 corresponds to a patient who would rather die immediately than live with AIDS. Utility of 1.1 corresponds to a patient who viewed AIDS to be at least equivalent to their current health state.

Approximately 24% of outpatients contacted by telephone agreed to participate in the interview. The most commonly cited reason for not participating was lack of time. Seventy-five percent of the inpatients approached agreed to perform the interview. Of the patients who began the interview, 100% completed it.

Table 3 Reported Sexual Behavior

	Average or proportion	Range
Lifetime No. of Partners:		
men	25	16 to >25
women	5.4	1 to >25
Length of partnership	19.44 years	1 night to 58 years
Practicing safe sex	0.27	-
Exclusive partnerships*	0.94	-

* Exclusive partnerships are those where the patient reported having a steady monogamous partner.

The reliability of the assessment tool, assessed by comparing questions asked in person and by computer was excellent. The 12 patients who were interviewed in person answered a total of 180 questions about risk behaviors. In only three of 180 questions (1.7%) did answers differ between the computer-based and the person-to-person interview. In these three questions, respondents declined to answer the question on total number of lifetime sexual partners during the computer-based interview. However, each of these respondents answered the person-to-person questions about current partners. Of the 12 patients who were interviewed in person after the computer-based interview, 9 preferred the computer interview, 2 were indifferent, and 1 preferred the person-to-person interview. Seven other patients who only took the computer-based interview were asked their preference. Of these patients, 4 said they would prefer the computer, and 3 said they would be indifferent.

To illustrate how the data from these interviews will be used, we evaluated the cost-effectiveness of screening in our decision model using data from the interviews as inputs. For example, if we use the low end of the range of quality adjustments for the health state "HIV infection without symptoms" (0, which indicates that the health state is equivalent to death), then screening for HIV infection actually reduces quality-adjusted life years when compared to not screening. That is, the screening strategy not only costs more, but the total health benefit, measured in quality adjusted life years, decreases. If we use the high end of the range for this quality adjustment, however, screening not only increases the number of quality-adjusted life years, but is also reasonably cost effective ($55,700 per quality-adjusted life year saved). The number of current sexual partners a person has also affects the attractiveness of screening. For example, the cost-effectiveness of screening varies from $56,300 to $38,500 per quality-adjusted life year saved as the number of current sexual partners if varied from one to three (the highest number observed in our sample).

DISCUSSION

In this pilot study, we developed and tested a computer-based instrument that assessed patient preferences for HIV-related health states and identified HIV risk behaviors. Our study suggests that a computer-based interview is a viable method for assessing patient preferences and identifying HIV risk behaviors. Although Nease and colleagues [5] showed previously that U-titer is a reliable instrument for utility assessment, our study is the first to use this tool to incorporate the assessment of sensitive risk behaviors into a preference assessment interview. In addition, our instrument is the first computer-based tool developed to assess quality of life with HIV infection.

Elicitation of HIV risk behaviors is important in several contexts. Our short-term objective in eliciting this information was to provide essential inputs for the Markov model used in our analyses of the cost-effectiveness of HIV screening. However, identification of risk behaviors is also important in clinical practice because the initiation of individual clinical or counseling interventions may depend on such knowledge. In addition, identification of risk behaviors is a mainstay of efforts to protect the blood supply — it is used to exclude potential blood donors who may be at increased risk of HIV infection.

The identification of HIV risk behaviors, although important, is also notably difficult. Patients often are unwilling to disclose behaviors which may be stigmatized, or personal, or both [6]. A study of a computer-based interview of blood donors, however, found that the computer-based interview was more effective than the person-to-person interview in identifying risk behaviors [7]. In that study, and in ours, the majority of participants indicated that they preferred a computer-based interview to a person-to-person interview. Thus, we have preliminary evidence that computer-based instruments are preferred to traditional approaches, and may be more effective in identifying risk behaviors.

Our findings indicate that this group of patients understood the description of the health states and the utility assessment task. The decreasing utilities for the health states (asymptomatic HIV infection, symptomatic HIV infection, AIDS) suggest that patients were able to effectively use the computer-based interview to express their preferences for the different HIV-related health states. The subjective impression of the interviewers, however, was that many patients had little familiarity with HIV-related disease. In addition, some patients rated life with HIV-related health states as better than their usual state of health. To facilitate the subjects' understanding of the assessment task, we have since developed more detailed descriptions of the health states. During the patient interviews, we also ask subjects factual questions about the health states to ensure that they have read carefully and understood the descriptions of each state. We have used these strategies previously, and each contributes to the reliability of the utility assessments. The program also assesses whether the subject has misordered the HIV health state utilities — for example if they have stated that they would prefer to live with HIV with symptoms rather than HIV without symptoms. If such a misordering is found then the program alerts the subject and allows them the opportunity to make the relevant time tradeoff decisions again. We also plan to assess test/retest correlation on a sample of 30 subjects.

The use of the utility assessment and risk behavior assessment in determining cost-effectiveness of screening is contingent on the reliability and validity of our computer-based interview. Ideally we would document people's true risk behaviors and compare this with their reported behavior; this task is difficult since we can not directly observe their behavior. Therefore we assessed reliability as compared to the current standard which is the person-to-person interview. The agreement between the computer interview and the person-to-person interviews was excellent as shown by concordance in 98% of the questions.

We plan to further refine the interview based on the results of this pilot study. We will then interview patients at three clinical centers (both inpatient and outpatient) to obtain the desired HIV health state preference assessment and risk behavior information. Data from the interviews will be used to determine the necessity of guidelines for voluntary screening for HIV infection that are customized for particular clinical settings. The cost-effectiveness of these customized screening guidelines will then be estimated and ultimately used to guide screening practices at the participating institutions.

ACKNOWLEDGMENT

Dr. Owens is supported by a Career Development Award from the Health Services Research and Development Service, Department of Veterans Affairs. Dr. Nease is a Picker/Commonwealth Scholar. Our thanks to Lynda Hynes for help with the pilot test, to Michael G. Walker and Nora Sweeny for comments on the manuscript, and to Ryan A. Harris for help with the analyses. Computing facilities were provided by the Center for Advanced Medical Informatics at Stanford, which is supported by grant number LM5305 from the National Library of Medicine.

Reference

[1]. Brandeau ML, Owens DK, Sox CH, Wachter RM. Screening women of childbearing age for human immunodeficiency virus infection: A model-based policy analysis. Management Science 39:72-92.1993.

[2]. Owens DK, Nease RF, Harris RA. Use of cost-effectiveness and value of information analyses to customize guidelines for specific clinical practice settings [abstract]. Medical Decision Making 13:395. 1993.

[3]. Owens DK, Nease RF, Harris RA. Screening for HIV infection in acute-care settings: Determinants of cost-effectiveness [abstract]. Medical Decision Making 13:395. 1993.

[4]. Sumner W, Nease R, Littenberg B. U-titer: A utility assessment tool. Proceedings of the Fifteenth Annual Symposium on Computer Applications in Medical Care 701-705. 1991.

[5] Nease R, Kneeland T, O'Connor G et al. Variation inpatient preferences for outcomes of stable angina: Implications for practice guidelines. Clin Res 41:181A. 1993..

[6]. O'Campo P, De Boer MA, Faden RR et al. Discrepancies between women's personal interview data and medical record documentation of illicit drug use, sexually transmitted diseases, and HIV infection. Med Care 30:965-71.1992.

[7]. Locke SE, Kowaloff HB, Hoff RG, Safran C, Popovsky MA, Cotton DJ, Finkelstein DM, Page PL, Slack WV. Computer-Based Interview for Screening Blood Donors for Risk of HIV Transmission. JAMA 268(10):1301-1305. 1992.

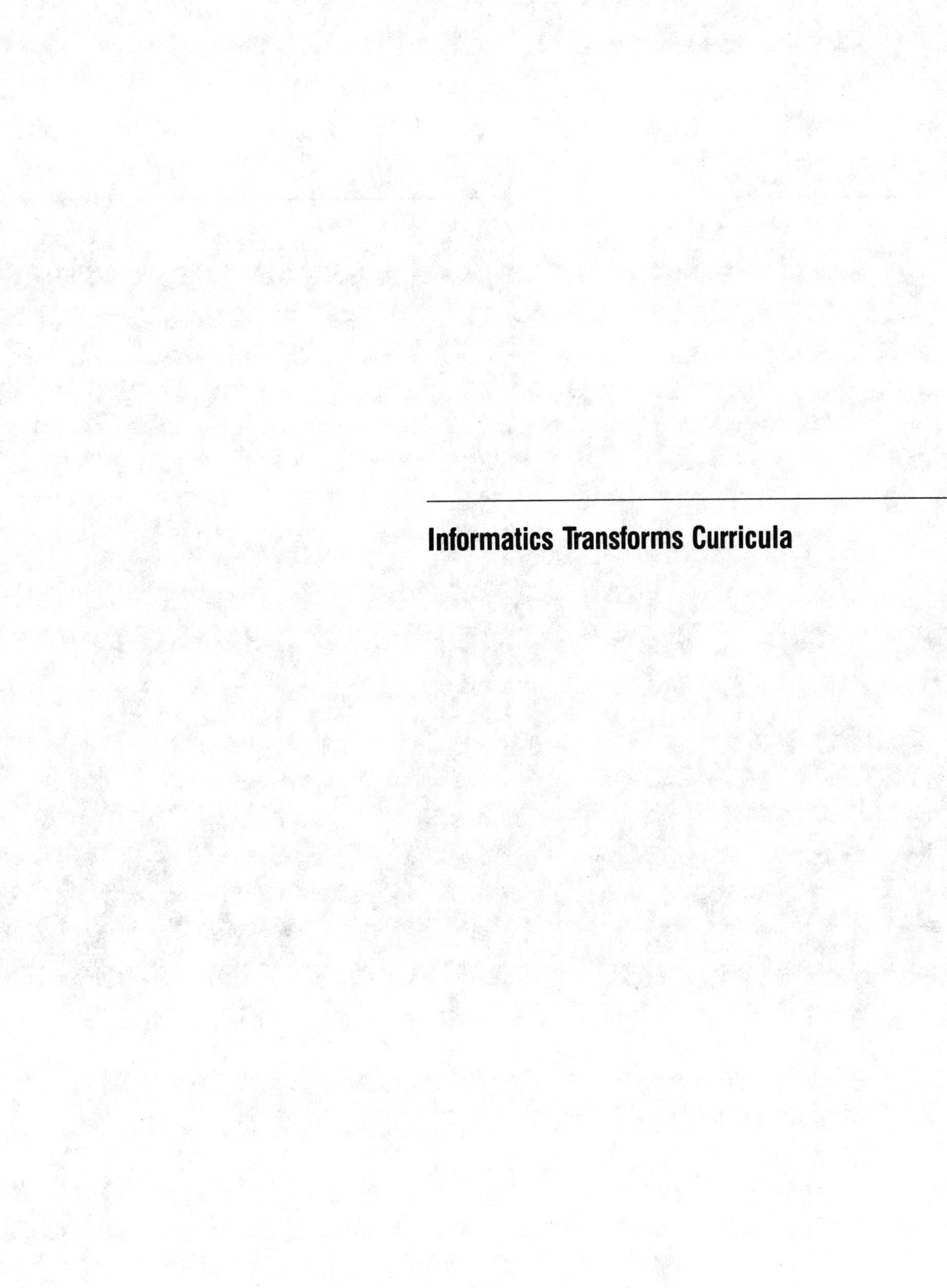

Informatics Transforms Curricula

Developing AJN Network: Transforming Information to Meet the Needs of the Future

Mary Anne Rizzolo, EdD, RN, Director, Interactive Technologies
American Journal of Nursing, Co.

Karen DuBois, MSN, RNC, Project Coordinator, Special Projects Grant
American Journal of Nursing Co.

In September of 1993 the American Journal of Nursing Company was awarded a three-year Special Projects Grant from the Division of Nursing, Department of Health and Human Services to develop a national information service to provide a variety of formal and informal continuing education services to nurses in medically underserved communities. ***AJN Network*** *went "live" in March 1994. Using a train the trainer approach, over 150 trainers were oriented in rural areas of our pilot states: North Carolina, Nevada and Wisconsin. This core group is now going out to rural hospitals to train other nurses on the system.*

During the first year of operation, ***AJN Network*** *has been be available through a dial in service. Beginning in September 1994 it will be offered over the Internet, an international network linking hundreds of smaller computer networks throughout the world. This project will make use of the High Performance Computing and Communications (HPCC) initiative which provides a backbone extending across the country, capable of transmitting data at tremendous speeds.*

Services that are currently available on ***AJN Network*** *are described along with plans for future development.*

INTRODUCTION

In September of 1993 the American Journal of Nursing (AJN) Company was awarded a three-year Special Projects Grant from the Division of Nursing, Department of Health and Human Services to develop a national information service to provide a variety of formal and informal continuing education services to nurses in medically underserved communities. The grant proposal was generated from an awareness of the pressing need for access to information in rural areas. A search of the literature and a needs assessment that included a survey of Area Health Education Centers (AHECs) across the country documented the suspected need.

AJN Company had been considering the feasibility of providing various services in an electronic format for several years. The Company has access to a large and ever increasing amount of clinical content and other valuable information for nurses. The proliferation of bulletin boards and Internet access by and for health care providers indicated that the time was right to institute a national information service.

NEED FOR THE PROJECT

Literature Search

Health in Rural America. A search of the literature revealed that the health of rural Americans has been steadily declining. Increasing poverty, loss or lack of insurance coverage, and difficult transportation needs all combine to significantly limit rural residents' access to the healthcare that is available to them. In this environment, it is not surprising that rural residents experience consistently higher rates of chronic illness, disability, and maternal and infant mortality compared to urban residents [1]. In addition, the increase of the geriatric population with related health problems and the increase in new illnesses, such as the 37% increase in AIDS cases in rural areas from 1988 to 1989 [2], have placed a serious burden on the already stretched rural health care system. All of this has only added to the demands made of the rural nurses.

Rural Nursing. The rural environment places special demands on the rural nurse. Isolated geographically, rural nurses are affected by the factors of excessive autonomy, lack of adequate staffing, lack of organizational resources, and limited technology [3]. Clinically, rural nurses need to be proficient in all areas. The rural nurse is often the lone practitioner and the generalist, having to meet any need presented by a patient. Yet, "recent employment data show that nurses in rural settings have less professional education than those employed in agencies within a metropolitan area" [4].

The nurse in a rural community has both opportunities and limitations for development and fulfillment. The nurse can be a community leader and decision maker in health policy and community projects. Nevertheless, low salaries, longer hours of service and being on-call, less time off, and less access to continuing education are realities to be borne [5]. The consequences of this are becoming even more dramatic as advances in healthcare knowledge and new technologies have quickened in the last decade.

Continuing Education Needs. The demands of handling a variety of healthcare situations and of keeping up with the latest information and technology have increased the needs of rural nurses for continuing education. New graduates, inactive nurses returning to work, nurses expanding into new areas, and experienced nurses all need educational programs offered at frequent intervals to meet the need for keeping up to date with healthcare advances. Currently, 22 State Boards of Nursing require that nurses and/or nurse practitioners acquire a defined number of continuing education hours in order to renew their licenses to practice. With or without a legal mandate, the rapid changes in healthcare now mean that nurses must stay current in order to practice safely.

Access to the necessary continuing education for rural nurses remains difficult, however. The factors of distance, travel and course cost, and the lack of personnel to provide coverage all contribute to reducing the ability of rural nurses to pursue continuing education [6]. In addition, in-house educational programs that can cost as much as $5,000 per nurse have been the first to be cut as rural hospitals struggle to remain financially viable. Furthermore, there is not enough time for rural nurses to devote to education purposes when hospitals cannot cover the costs of replacement staff and cannot even spare senior staff for on-the-job mentoring.

Needs Assessment

A questionnaire was developed and administered to key personnel in Area Health Education Centers (AHECs) across the country. Both the telephone and electronic networks (Health Alaska, Virtual Medical Center in Montana, ALF - the Rural Information Center electronic bulletin board, ET Net, and the Internet) were used to collect data. . We assembled information from 25 sites in 22 states representing all geographic regions of the United States. The survey revealed that the major concern of rural nurses was **access** to continuing education and information. We learned that nurses isolated in extremely rural areas have problems traveling to conferences when swampy roads are covered with water and mountain passes are filled with snow. We heard about small rural hospitals without any library facilities or access to recent books and journals. While access to computers and modems is limited in some rural areas at this time, when asked if nurses would use computers for CE, the answer was "yes." The recent efforts of several AHECs and other state nursing organizations in exploring new electronic network technology speaks to the need for further improving access to continuing education for nurses via technology.

ELECTRONIC NETWORK SOLUTIONS

Individuals and organizations have started to implement electronic networks and bulletin board systems to attempt to meet the information needs of nurses. We investigated the offerings of the several of these including ET Net, the American Nurses Association's WAIS (Workplace Advocacy Information System), Sigma Theta Tau's Electronic Library, the "Healthcare building" of Denver Free-Net, Nurses Corner (Florida), Nurses Station (Kentucky), FITNET (Fuld Institute for Technology in Nursing Education), PC Nurse (Delaware), Trilogy (Maryland), SON*NET (Texas), KARENET (Texas), and CAMEL (Nevada). We found these electronic networks valuable, but generally limited in scope and their ability to address continuing education needs of rural nurses.

The use of electronic media to disseminate information has been strongly recommended by several experts in rural nursing [7]. The proliferation of state and local electronic networks for nurses with different purposes indicates that there are growing numbers of nurses who are able and willing to use the new communications technologies. In addition, PC costs are plunging, making new hardware technology more readily available. Therefore, programs must be developed to meet the capabilities of the new technologies and the needs of those who will use them. The AJN *Network* is being designed to meet that need.

PROJECT OBJECTIVES

Based on the information gathered, the objectives of the project were developed as follows:

1. to develop a computer network system, reachable through personal computer modems, which will serve the needs of nurses on a national level;

2. to provide access for nurses to information that will assist them in providing effective nursing care, including direct patient care, management, and promotion of community health by

   a. establishing a nurse consultant help-line with expert nurses who will respond to specific inquiries from nurses;

   b. establishing a Bulletin Board system for nurses to ask their peers for answers to specific nursing care and management questions and to share information;

   c. making available AJN Co.'s library of patient information so that nurses can print this information directly for patients;

   d. establishing a special consultation service on HIV/AIDS which will provide prevention information and increase the knowledge and skill of nurses caring for persons who are HIV positive or who have AIDS;

   e. establishing a special consultation on sociocultural diversity for nurses to gain cultural competence which will assist them in providing care to members of diverse cultural groups;

3. to provide greater access for nurses to continuing education by

   a. offering computer assisted instruction (CAI) programs on topics relevant to (and selected by) the users;

   b. establishing a feature article of the month and a time during which nurses from anywhere can talk to the author through synchronous conferencing--the author can also respond to questions posted through the Bulletin Board;

   c. offering on the network continuing education articles and tests which are available on a monthly basis in the *American Journal of Nursing, MCN, The American Journal of Maternal Child Nursing*, and other publications;

   d. creating new continuing education course offerings from user input on the bulletin board;

4. to provide assistance to nurses in accessing the large, existing resources of healthcare information already available by

   a. converting information from a variety of sources that currently exist in print format to searchable digital databases;

   b. providing access to or information from existing digital databases available on the Internet and elsewhere;

   c. establishing a special feature section that provides national and international news affecting nurses and healthcare in medically underserved areas.

PROGRESS TO DATE

To initiate the development of our information service, we recruited the remaining personnel for the project, began the identification of content, and the selection of equipment and software.

Software/Hardware Selection

Following an extensive review of commercially available software and hardware for bulletin board systems project staff selected Res Nova software and a Macintosh platform. We also selected a program called Ripterm that provides communications software with a graphical user interface.

Network Content

In order develop content that would be responsive to the needs of rural nurses in our pilot states of North Carolina, Nevada and Wisconsin, we developed a learning needs assessment that was mailed to the pilot sites, returned, and summarized. We used the results of this assessment, along with suggestions from our Advisory Panel members to plan the offerings on the AJN *Network*. Much of the work in this first year of the grant has been devoted to setting up the process, policies and procedures for putting content on AJN *Network* and to make that process as automated as possible.

Forums. One of the most active areas to date has been the Forums. Forums are intended to be used for professional support and peer education purposes. At this time, we have Forums for typical clinical areas, such as Medical/Surgical, Maternal-Child, Emergency, Gerontology, and Psychiatric/Mental Health Nursing. In addition, Forums have been added for Rural Health, Administration/Management, HIV/AIDS, Medications and Cultural Issues. Nurses with experience in these areas have volunteered to act as moderators of these Forums and encourage discussion among Forum users. Forum messages will be monitored and evaluated carefully. Additional Forums will evolve based on user input.

Nursing Consult. The goal of the Nursing Consult area of AJN *Network* is to provide consultation on clinical care problems. In preparation, a database of nurse experts has been designed and implemented on AJN Company's local area network. The editors of AJN Company journals are in contact with authors on virtually every nursing subspecialty. The Convention Manager has an extensive list of speakers who have expertise in a wide range of nursing areas. These nurses entered their list of nurse experts into the database. It now contains over 2000 names. When a nurse in a pilot site posts a question in our "Nursing Consult" section, the database will be used to locate an appropriate person to respond to the query. Legal advice is under consideration regarding policies and procedures that would govern information that is posted in the "Nursing Consult" section.

Continuing Education. Continuing education (CE) offerings currently on AJN *Network* consist of computer-assisted instruction programs and CE print products that have been converted for downloading.

Computer-Assisted Instruction. Four CAI programs are now available for downloading only in the pilot states. We are entering into agreements with other companies to have portions of a program (one case study for example) available for distribution on a wider basis. We see this as a way for software developers to beta test programs and to make demonstration copies available. Eventually it can be a way to distribute programs.

CE Articles. The Project Coordinator meets regularly with the AJN Director of Continuing Education to identify CE offerings in print that are relevant to the project users. These are converted to a digital format that is usable on the network and set up so that they can be downloaded and printed at the user's site. Conversion procedures and instructions for users on downloading and printing have been developed. Plans are in motion to have CE tests returned electronically for automated processing and quicker response time.

Journal Club. We believe it is not sufficient to just convert print materials to an electronic format. Each medium has its own characteristics and strengths that should be matched to the content. In an effort to convert our beliefs into practice we are initiating a Journal Club.

An AJN article will be available for users to download and read, then the author will respond to questions posted on AJN *Network* about that article for the following 30 days. One or two hours during that month will be set aside for a synchronous conference -- the author will log onto AJN *Network* and answer questions as network users post them during that hour. AJN *Network* can currently support 103 simultaneous users.

AJN Company's journal editors have been working with Project Staff to identify authors who might participate in "Journal Club." Our intent is to offer a "Journal Club" for each of AJN Company's journals *American Journal of Nursing, MCN, The American Journal of Maternal Child Nursing*, and *Nursing Research.* We are pursuing relationships with other journals who may also want to establish a "Journal Club" with their own authors and articles.

We are also working with our CE Director to offer CE credit for participation in "Journal Club." Our software will allow us to track the amount of time each individual user spends in the synchronous conference with the author as well as time they spend posting and reading messages about the Journal Club article. If the amount of time equals 50 minutes or more, we may be able to offer CE credit. This matter will be pursued in more detail in Years 2 and 3, after we have more experience with the software and examine more carefully how users are responding to Journal Club.

Another plan to provide innovative, timely and responsive continuing education offerings involves using our Forum Moderators and Project Coordinator to monitor bulletin board messages and analyze the type and frequency of questions. From this information, the Project Coordinator will determine what topics are significant enough to warrant a course offering. The Project Coordinator will then work with the Program Director, the Director of Continuing Education, and editorial staff to create a new CE course offering. An example might be the pulling of questions and answers on HIV/AIDS from various parts of the network and the creation of an article on "Rural Nurses' Major Questions and Concerns About HIV/AIDS." This objective will be developed fully in Years 2 and 3, after our user base expands.

Databases. Two databases are now functional: a list of nursing organizations and a listing of nursing conferences with over 400 listed. A full search Apple search engine is used to search for entries. More databases are planned.

News. Segments from Nurse Executive Newscan, a monthly audiotape distributed by AJN Co. are currently available in the Administration/Management Forum. Plans are in progress to have AJN Company's news editor to identify news that will be of most interest to the user population, post it on AJN *Network,* and encourage forum discussions on topics. Once a regular system for handling this is established, the service will be ongoing in the second and third years of the project.

Patient Information. Patient information sheets on a variety of topics have been converted to digital data and set up so that the sheets can be downloaded and printed at the user's site. Plans for acquiring and posting other patient focused materials are under discussion.

FUTURE PLANS

We will devote considerable time to examining resources on the Internet in Year 2, evaluating information available through the Internet and informing our users about other valuable sources of electronic information. We will investigate incorporating digitized audio, still images, and motion images as well as text.

Our goal is also to make AJN *Network* as user friendly as possible. We have already instituted a help line that users can call for personal assistance in logging on or using the Network. A database is used to log problems that users encounter so that we can include these in our manual. We have begun preliminary discussion of a graphic motif or metaphor that will provide an easy graphical interface for users.

Guided by an eminently qualified Advisory Committee, and in response to continued surveys that are conducted on the network, AJN *Network* will continue to add new resources and endeavor to meet the information needs of nurses throughout the world. At the conclusion of the grant period AJN *Network* will be offered as a subscription service to generate revenue for continued development.

REFERENCES

[1] Bigbee, J.L. (1993). The Uniqueness of Rural Nursing. *Nursing Clinics of North America, 28,* 131-144.

[2] Carwein, V.L., Sabo, C.E., & Berry, D.E. (1993). HIV Infection in Traditional Rural Communities. *Nursing Clinics of North America, 28,* 231-239.

[3] Muus, K.J., Stratton, T.D., Dunkin, J.W., & Juhl, N. (1993). Retaining Registered Nurses in Rural Community Hospitals. *JONA, 23,* 38-43.

[4] Bushy, A. (1990). Rural Determinants in Family Health: Considerations for Community Nurses. *Family and Community Health, 12,* 29-38.

[5] Turner, T.A., & Gunn, I.P., (1991). Issues in Rural Health Nursing. In Bushy, A. (ed.) *Rural Nursing, Volume 2,* 105-127.

[6] Anderson, J., & Kimber, K. (1991). Meeting the Continuing Education Needs of Nurses in Rural Settings. *The Journal of Continuing Education in Nursing, 22,* 29-34.

[7] Parker, M., Quinn, et al. (1991). Case Management in Rural Areas: Definition, Clients, Financing, Staffing, and Service Delivery Issues. In Bushy, A. (ed.) *Rural Nursing, Volume 2,* 29-40.

Building Internet Accessible Medical Education Software Using the World Wide Web

John A. Kruper[1], Marc G. Lavenant[1], Manisha H. Maskay[2], and Thomas M. Jones[2]
[1]Biological Sciences Division Academic Computing, The University of Chicago
[2]Department of Medicine, The University of Chicago
Chicago, IL 60637

We describe work to enhance existing software protocols and develop a suite of new software utilities based upon a set of standards known as the World Wide Web (WWW). Specifically, we have developed an effective X-windows based WYSIWYG WWW browser/editor and a prototype for integrated wide-area authentication and authorization support for delivery and maintenance of WWW service. These software development activities, along with parallel work in content development, are empowering individuals to better use the Internet as a resource to easily author, publish, and access materials.

As an illustrative application, we describe one Web-based self-instructional unit designed to increase users' knowledge of hazardous substances in the environment. This on-line monograph was adapted from a series of paper-based case studies developed by the Agency for Toxic Substances and Disease Registry of the U.S. Department of Health & Human Services. The on-line version illustrates many of the innovative features provided by the Web, and demonstrates how such materials can significantly impact medical education at all levels.

INTRODUCTION

With over thirty years of active development, the announcements, reviews, and scholarly papers describing Computer Assisted Instruction (CAI) and other technology-based medical education efforts would fill volumes. However, in general, the impact of instructional technology on the medical school and generalist science curricula has been at best modest [1, 2].

This fact notwithstanding, there is today ample proof that, in the *proper* setting and in the hands of *properly* trained users, computer supported learning *can* work [3, 4]. Hypermedia systems are one particularly promising CAI tool. These have the potential to let students experience an active, personalized, and inquiry-based exposure to medical content and problem solving. When empowered with appropriate hypermedia tools, students can selectively discover, access, and retrieve relevant information from the content overload they currently face [5].

Such systems have the promise to dramatically impact medical education, yet they suffer from a devastating drawback. Due to the proliferation of computers in classrooms, laboratories, dormitory rooms and homes, and to the parallel growth in the number of proprietary hypermedia software tools and applications running on these systems, a modern day technological Tower of Babylon has been created. As a result, the computer functions as an information island, unable to tap into the wider web of an ever growing communal knowledge base.

Recently though, two significant developments in information technology have occurred that make the goal of seamlessly accessing and integrating the many distributed networked information resources and services realizable.

THE INTERNET & WORLD WIDE WEB

The first is the government sponsored effort to establish "information superhighways" using the established Internet networking infrastructure and protocols. This effort has already linked 100% of the American Research Level I Institutions; improvements in Wide Area Networking technologies are allowing additional sites -- from the home office to the local high school to the rural primary care clinic -- to join this networked world-wide community.

The second development is the creation of the World Wide Web (WWW). The World Wide Web project merges the techniques of information retrieval, hypermedia, and open standards to build an easy but powerful global information system. Originally developed at CERN for the High Energy Physics community, it has spread to many other areas and attracted much interest in user support and resource allocation. It is currently the most advanced information system deployed on the Internet, and it offers the greatest promise for future development of wide area information platforms and collaborative "groupware" applications. Significantly, its application and potential use in the academic medical community has not gone unnoticed [6].

The Biological Sciences Division office of Academic Computing (BSDAC) at the University of Chicago has begun enhancing existing software protocols and developing a suite of new software utilities based upon the World Wide Web architecture. This effort in total is named the Phoenix Project; its aim is to develop an integrated academic information system providing full Internet connectivity and wide-area distributed hypermedia authoring services to the students, teachers, researchers, clinicians, and administrators who comprise BSDAC's user base.

Our efforts toward these goals include two significant areas of enhancements to the WWW: an effective X-Windows based What You See Is What You Get (WYSIWYG) WWW browser/editor, and a prototype for integrated wide-area authentication and authorization support for WWW-based file service.

The Phoenix WWW Editor

Aside from a number of conversion utilities (rtf2html, LaTeXtoHTML, ps2html) and rudimentary HTML editors (tkWWW, NextStep editor, the WYSIWYG Hypercard Stack, EMACS HTML-mode), no easy to use WYSIWYG WWW editor exists. Because our goal is for content experts and novices alike to directly author their own materials for publication on the WWW, we first needed to develop a WYSIWYG WWW editor.

Figures 1 and 2 show "browsing" and "authoring" views, with supporting feature explanations, of our first generation Phoenix client. This software currently runs as an X-windows application, and is thus accessible from the three preferred operating systems on our campus: Macintosh, MS DOS/Windows, and UNIX.

Besides supporting an easy to use WYSIWYG interface, an important feature of Phoenix is its ability to share the contents of its clipboard with a remote client's clipboard. This both reinforces a common interface between the PC and Phoenix environments, and facilitates the integration of the Phoenix editor within the user's local (primarily Macintosh and MS DOS/Windows) application environment.

Another unique feature of Phoenix centers on its handling of the underlying WWW file system. Because conventional distributed file systems (Appleshare, NFS, etc.), typically represent systems that support standalone documents lacking a comparable degree of integration found in the WWW environment, we have departed from the standard file system interface and instead *transparently* provide file services to Phoenix users. By using aliases, all basic file operations can be performed via indirect references to the underlying WWW file locator identifiers (called URLs for Uniform Resource Locators), user and group names that use existing URL aliases (such as Hotlist, and History items), as well as novel aliases corresponding to users and groups.

We have also included support for a suite of "second generation" (HTML+) WWW information features, including in-line images (GIF format) and ISMAPs, in both browse and edit modes.

Enhanced Security Features

Currently, WWW users enjoy read-write access to existing information services provided by WWW servers according to the authoring/browsing permissions governing the underlying WWW documents (predominantly world-read, local-write). Integrated organization of these distributed information resources is thus achieved using existing features in the WWW framework (HTML, for Hypertext Markup Language, and HTTP, for Hypertext Transfer Protocol). However, in a wide-area multi-server authoring environment in which users belonging to multiple groups can selectively browse and edit information, the existing HTML/HTTP implementation requires extension in the areas of user authentication and authorization.

We have thus implemented a prototype for integrated wide-area security support for maintaining information placed on the WWW framework. This implementation addresses two key deficiencies of the current WWW, namely support for abstracting personalized views of information resources and (due to the lack of a robust WYSIWYG editor), the ability to selectively edit and add to information or other computing resources.

BIOMEDICAL CONTENT DEVELOPMENT

With the enabling Phoenix software utilities in hand, we have set about building a suite of information resources in the area of primary care medicine. The content providers for this work are the clinical faculty in the University Health Service (UHS), the general medicine clinic and student and employee health service at the University of Chicago Medical Center (UCMC). As we have described previously [7], the primary care practice at the UHS represents an unparalleled resource in which to design and test new patient and student centered curricular and care programs. It is in support of these efforts that we have developed a prototype content repository and organization for clinical and health education materials.

"Case Studies in Environmental Medicine" is a suite

of self-instructional units designed to increase a user's knowledge of hazardous substances in the environment. The on-line resources were adapted from a series of paper-based case studies developed by the Agency for Toxic Substances and Disease Registry of the U.S. Department of Health & Human Services.

In addition to providing the same information as the paper units, the on-line counterparts contain additional graphics and supporting information utilities such as a full featured glossary. They also contain links to relevant "in-house" resources, such as the UHS Health InfoLine, a WWW-based collection of health information materials available to the University of Chicago community. Demonstrating the leveraging rewards available when using the Internet-wide WWW framework, the case studies contain links to appropriate off-site information resources. Finally, using the forms features of the WWW, the on-line versions support drill and practice presentations including multiple choice questions with corrective feedback; this feature also enables users to electronically submit post-test responses for automatic assignment of credit.

In designing the delivery platform for these materials, we have employed a number of innovative and unique WWW enhancements, including:

•the use of relational database technology to support a fine grained data schema. This approach allows information content to be viewed from multiple perspectives, with those perspectives determined by the aims and needs of the individual user. A novice student accessing a Lead Toxicity unit in support of a Health Education class would necessarily both want and need a different view on the content than the practicing clinician using the unit to diagnose lead poisoning in a patient;

•dynamically built page 'mosaics' instead of static WWW documents. Because the case studies information content resides in a database repository, individual pages can be dynamically "assembled" on the fly. This enables the multi-perspective data views mentioned above, as well as allows for easy maintenance of the content. When information is updated in any of the underlying databases, the resulting documents will automatically reflect any changes. As new software features are added, a simple modification to the script that generates a page modifies all appropriate documents; and

•consistent design format. The top of every page displays a consistent organization and presentation of graphics that in addition to providing visual anchor clues to the user, also provides links to appropriate higher level information pages. These features help prevent the "lost in hyperspace" condition often experienced in rich hypermedia systems.

These efforts demonstrate how integrated hypermedia systems can be built using non-proprietary international standards. Indeed, it may be that this approach is the first to fully realize the goals of efforts such as the National Library of Medicine's IAIMS project to provide institution-wide access to appropriate bibliographic and knowledge databases and present them in an integrated fashion [8]. Together, these utilities suggest that a new dawn in the use of information technology is at hand.

References

[1] T. E. Pimme. "Computer Assisted Learning and Evaluation in Medicine." *JAMA* 1988; **260**:367.

[2] J.D. Rootenberg. "Information Technologies in U.S. Medical Schools: Clinical Practices Outpace Academic Application." *JAMA* 1992; **268**:3106.

[3] Report on the Effectiveness of Technology in Schools: 1990-1992. Software Publishers Association, Baltimore MD 1993.

[4] H. C. Lyon, J. Healy, J. R. Bell, J. F. O'Donnell, E. K. Shultz, M. Moore-West, R. S. Wigton, F. Hirai & J. R. Beck, "Plan Analyzer, an Interactive Computer-Assisted Program to Teach Clinical Problem Solving in Diagnosing Anemia and Coronary Artery Disease." *Academic Medicine* **67**(12) pp821-828, 1992.

[5] S. Muller. (Chairman) "Physicians for the Twenty-First Century: Report of the Project Panel on the General Professional Education of the Physician and College Preparation for Medicine." *J. Med. Educ.* **59**, Part 2, November, 1994.

[6] E. S. Metcalfe, M. E. Frisse, S. W. Hassan, & J. L. Schnase, "Academic Networks: Mosaic and World Wide Web." *Academic Medicine* **69**(4) pp270-273, April, 1994.

[7] J. A. Kruper & T. M. Jones, "The Centennial Patient Care Program: Binding Patient, Student, and Clinician-Teacher in a Learning Triad." In the *Proceedings of the 17th Annual Symposium on Computer Applications in Medical Care*, pp. 752-756, 1993.

[8] T. Detre (Chairman). "Integrated Information Management Systems in Health Care." Association of Academic Health Centers, Washington, D.C. 1991.

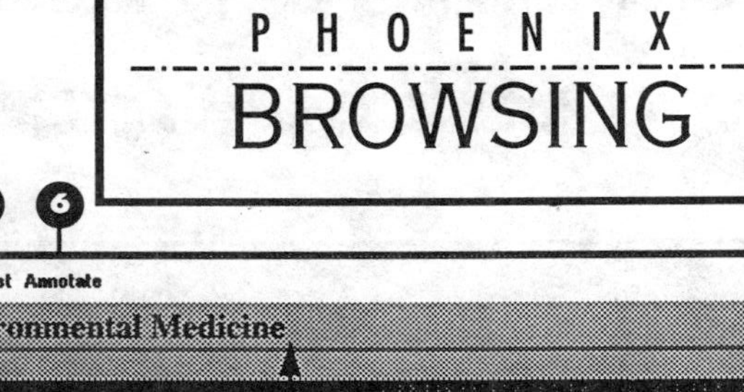

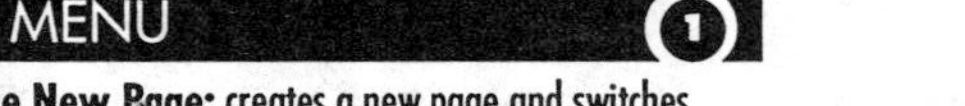

FILE MENU ①

Create New Page: creates a new page and switches Phoenix to author mode

Open: opens a document residing on the local machine (bio-3.bsd.uchicago.edu for Phoenix users at the U of C)

Goto URL: Opens a document via HTTP; you must specify the full address (Uniform Resource Locator, URL) of the document you wish to access. The URL for the BSDAC home page, for instance, is *http://bio-3.bsd.uchicago.edu/index.html.*

Get info: invokes an inormation dialog box describing the features of the current page.

Save As... : invokes a save file dialog for specifying the desired destination to which the current page is to be saved in HTML format.

Save Text...: as above, except that the document will be saved as TEXT-ONLY.

Print: Prints the current document to the printer specified in the popup dialog box.

Mail: mails the current document to the recipient specified in the popup dialog box.

Quit: Closes the given Phoenix window; it does not affect other Phoenix windows.

View HTML: Displays document Hypertext Markup

BROWSE MENU ②

Copy: copies the current selection to the Phoenix clipboard (it also copies selected text to the Macintosh clipboard, if Phoenix is run using MacX).

Find: invokes a dialog box in which to specify keywords for a Wide Area Information Services (WAIS)

Change Fonts: pops-up a font selector dialog box

HISTORY MENU ④

This menu lists the titles of the documnets through which you have browsed with the current Phoenix window (if the document does not have a title, the URL is listed instead). Selecting a given menu item from here will retrieve the corresponding document in the current Phoenix window.

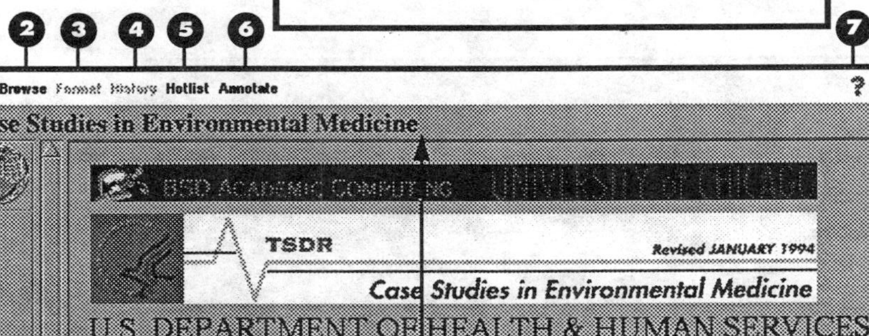

BUTTONS

A Mode : Switches Phoenix between browse and authoring modes.

B Previous: displays the previous document

C Find: invokes a dialog box in which to specify keywords for a Wide Area Information Services (WAIS) search. *This feature is only available for certain documents!*

D Mark: Adds current document to hotlist.

E Refresh: redraws the document window.

F Clone: launches a new browser window displaying the current document.

G Quit: closes the current document window.

H Nest: Return to Home Page

HOTLIST MENU ⑤

The hotlist is a list of bookmarks enabling the rapid retrieval of your favorite world-wide-web documents

Add Page to Hotlist:
adds the current document to the hotlist.

Delete from Hotlist:
deletes the current document to the hotlist.

ANNOTATE MENU ⑥

Annotation are private text-only notes you can attach to documents on the web.

Add Annotation:
adds annotation to the your view of the current window.

Edit Annotation:
edit current annotation (You must be viewing the annotation to edit it)

Go to Annotation:
displays the annotation selected from the pull-down menu

HELP MENU ⑦

Provides access to Help for Phoenix, Phoenix-browser, and Mail

APPLICATION MENU ⑧

The application menu is used to launch applications, to navigate between Phoenix windows, to set your Phoenix password, and to exit Phoenix.

Web-Browser:
provides a pull down menu of active Web-browser windows.

Mosaic:
launches the NCSA web-browser (usefull for viewing documents containing HTML forms)

XV: launches the XV image viewing/editing software

Medline:
launches a telnet session to the Ovid Medline server (You will need a Ph alias and password to use this resource).

Configure: use this to change your password

Exit Phoenix: terminates you current Phoenix session, logging you out of the Phoenix server.

Figure 1. Overview of Phoenix Browsing Features

FILE MENU ①

New: creates new document

Save As... : invokes a save-file dialog for specifying the desired destination to which the current page is to be saved in HTML format.

Save Text...: as above, except that the document will be saved as TEXT-ONLY.

Quit: Closes the given Phoenix window; it does not affect other Phoenix windows.

View HTML: Displays document Hypertext Markup

EDIT MENU ②

Cut: removes the current selection from the document, and places it in the clipboard (it also copies selected text to the Macintosh clipboard, if Phoenix is run on a Macintosh using MacX).

Copy: copies the current selection to the Phoenix clipboard (it also copies selected text to the Macintosh clipboard, if Phoenix is run on a Macintosh using MacX).

Paste: pastes the contents of the Phoenix clipboard into the location of the cursor.

Clear: removes current selection from the document, without placing it in the clipboard

Select All: selects all of the text between consecutive Images in the neighborhood of the cursor.

Select none: deselects the current selection.

Edit Anchor: invokes the Edit-Anchor dialog for setting the target (destination) of a link. The anchor of the link (text selection at the time the Edit-Anchor item is clicked) appears at the top of the dialog box. The destination of the anchor can be set manually by typing the Uniform Resource Locator of the target in the address-field of the dialog box, or can be set automatically by selecting the appropriate target entry from the History or Hotlist menus. Click OK in dialog box to complete.

Insert Image: invokes a dialog box with which to select an image title to be inserted

Change Fonts: invokes a font selector dialog box

PHOENIX AUTHORING

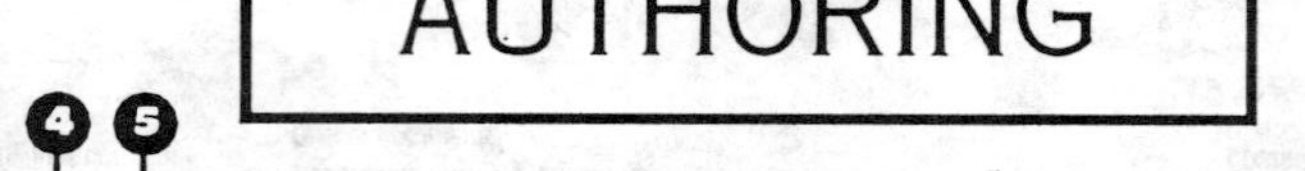

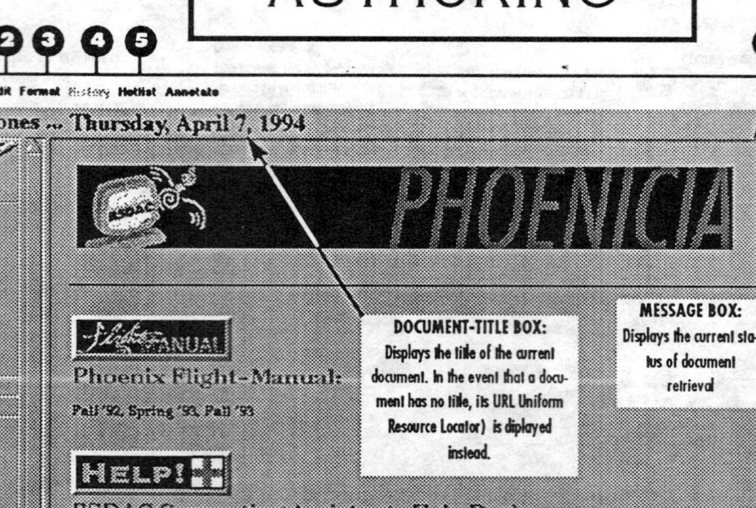

BUTTONS

Ⓐ Mode : Switches Phoenix between browse and authoring modes.

Ⓑ Refresh: redraws the document window.

Ⓒ Clone: launches a new browser window displaying the current document.

Ⓓ Quit: closes the current document window.

Figure 2. Overview of Phoenix Authoring Features

FORMAT MENU ③

Format commands are used to format text selections in edit mode.

HISTORY MENU ④

This menu lists the titles of the documents through which you have browsed with the current Phoenix window (if the document does not have a title, the URL is listed instead). Selecting a given menu item from here while creating or editing a link in *Authoring Mode* will define the corresponding document as the target (destination) of the link.

HOTLIST MENU ⑤

The hotlist enables easy linking of the selected text in the current document to your favorite documents around the world-wide-web (see the *Edit Anchor* menu item in the *Edit Menu* section).

HELP MENU ⑥

Provides access to Help for Phoenix, Phoenix-browser, and Mail

APPLICATION MENU ⑦

The application menu is used to launch applications, to navigate between Phoenix windows, to set your Phoenix password, and to exit Phoenix.

Web-Browser: provides a pull down menu of active Web-browser windows.

Mosaic: launches the NCSA web-browser (usefull for viewing documents containing HTML forms)

XV: launches XV image viewing/editing software

Medline: launches a telnet session to the Ovid Medline server (You will need a Ph alias and password to use this resource).

Configure: use this to change your password

Exit Phoenix: terminates you current Phoenix session, logging, you out of the Phoenix server.

Undergraduate Health Care Informatics Education: A needs analysis and proposed curriculum

Deborah Foy, Kip Canfield, John Schwartz
Department of Information Systems
University of Maryland, UMBC

ABSTRACT

This paper describes a needs analysis and resulting curriculum in Health Care Informatics. It is implemented as a track for the BS degree within the Department of Information Systems at the University of Maryland, Baltimore County. The track in Health Care Informatics is an interdisciplinary specialty within the broader field of Information Systems which is itself an interdisciplinary field. The needs analysis shows current thinking by practitioners and educators in the new field of Health Care Informatics. It also presents a survey of undergraduate students to monitor interest in and knowledge of this field. A curriculum design is presented that addresses these needs.

INTRODUCTION

The curricula for interdisciplinary studies are difficult to design for a number of reasons, two of which are listed below:

- Student prerequisites
- Academic respect

Students face a difficult adjustment to a field that has broad and shifting boundaries. It is very difficult to get the prerequisites in all component disciplines of an interdisciplinary field and at the same time, without these, one risks dismissal by practitioners and students of each component discipline. Academic respect is a function of the previous observation. Students and faculty risk being viewed as "non-rigorous" in their approach to their field. It should be mentioned that political problems result from the financial and "turf" implications of creating a new interdisciplinary field in academia but these are beyond the scope of this paper. These realities for interdisciplinary studies are discussed below with special reference to Health Care Informatics as an undergraduate academic discipline.

Undergraduate education has the further requirement of training students broadly in a field. It is widely regarded as a mistake to specialize undergraduate studies too narrowly. This paper describes a needs analysis and resulting curriculum in Health Care Informatics. It is implemented as an optional track for the BS degree within the Department of Information Systems at the University of Maryland, Baltimore County. The track in Health Care Informatics is an interdisciplinary specialty within the broader field of Information Systems which is itself an interdisciplinary field. We are also considering a modified version of this track as a minor for majors in other disciplines.

Information Systems as an academic discipline is growing out of Computer Science and various domain areas that use information systems technology. As computer science (itself a relatively new discipline) has tried to more strictly define itself as a basic science, applications-oriented computing research suffered under tenure evaluation in many Computer Science departments. Information Systems as an academic discipline is a response to these developments. It was first made popular as a subdiscipline in the Business School as Management Information Systems. It has since become more interdisciplinary such as the department at Baltimore. The unifying theme of these information systems studies is that they are grounded in specific domains and applications of information technology. As such, it is more philosophically aligned with academic engineering schools than basic science ones.

Health care is a broad (and interdisciplinary) field that requires significant use of information technology. Furthermore, health care has special characteristics that information systems professionals need to be aware of to effectively design, develop, and implement information technology. We have developed a curriculum in Health Care Informatics that addresses these needs. The remainder of this paper describes the needs analysis for the Health Care Track in Information Systems and the details of the resulting curriculum.

NEEDS ANALYSIS

The needs analysis had two phases:

- Content analysis
- Survey of student interest and knowledge

The content analysis for the proposed track in Health Care Informatics had two components: informal interviews with educators and professionals in the field and a more formal evaluation of the proposed track by Denis Protti.

The informal interviews consisted of discussions with both information systems and health care professionals about the educational needs for undergraduates who will enter the field. These discussions targeted this undergraduate population and not dual training in information systems and a health care specialty such as nursing or medicine. The broad results of these interviews are categorized below:

- Balance technical and organizational issues
- Practical training in CO-OPs
- Keep the curriculum broad

Successful implementation of information systems in organizations is a complex set of tasks that requires many skills. Information systems are equally about communication in organizations and technical implementation. It is possible to create an information system that meets the technical requirements but fails to succeed. A mix of management, technical, and organizational behavior education is needed for Health Care Informatics. At the same time, this program is geared towards undergraduates seeking entry-level jobs. This requires a heavy emphasis on practical technical competence in the areas that are used to build health care information systems. It is a common failing in interdisciplinary fields to slight the technical issues. This is seen in many business-oriented programs in Management Information Systems where graduates learn more "why" than "how." The basic technologies that must be emphasized in Health Care Informatics are analysis and design methods, database development, and networking the organization.

Because the undergraduate education in Information Systems is not typically in a health care school, there is consensus that students must gain domain experience in health care environments. They can do this with independent studies directed by faculty in a health care school or through CO-OPs at health care institutions. CO-OPs are cooperative education programs common at universities that allow students to earn credits for work in industries relevant to their studies.

The specialty in Health Care Informatics must also be tempered with the need for undergraduate students to remain fairly flexible in their major training. They must be mainstream information systems professionals that could go into any area, but have special training and experience in health care.

Denis Protti [1] is a Professor of Health Information Science at the School of Health Information Science at the University of Victoria in Canada. He heads a program that offers the undergraduate degree in Health Informatics. This degree is the first of its kind and their experience with the degree was considered valuable for our program. Dr. Protti came to the University of Maryland to evaluate our proposed curriculum. He supported the informal results given above and refined these ideas. Dr. Protti emphasized that the information links and flow patterns in health care are more complex than those found in business and that the graduates in Health Care Informatics need to be prepared to deal with this complexity. "What distinguishes health care paths of information from others is the high intensity and responsiveness required of information in the horizontal dimension, particularly in matters concerning patient information." [2] He also corroborated the need for practical student experience in CO-OPs. He observed that the specialty training in Health Care Informatics increases the probability that our graduates would be successful change agents in health care in the United States.

The second phase of the needs analysis consisted of a survey to measure the interest and general knowledge about health care informatics of undergraduates at the University of Maryland, Baltimore County (UMBC). We developed two surveys: one for current majors of Information Systems and one or majors in other areas. The survey for Information Systems majors was to measure interest in the proposed track and the non-major survey was to measure interest in a (non-implemented) minor in Healthcare Informatics. Information Systems is the largest major on this campus with approximately 700 undergraduate students.

Each survey consisted of 15 questions and was administered by the instructor of a course during class time. The surveys were designed to show the level of interest in Health Care Informatics in a general way to aid in designing the track. Responses are reported for a subset of the questions below. The surveys were given only to upper division undergraduate students.

350 survey questionnaires were distributed to UMBC students with the following distribution of majors:

Biology/(Bio-)Chemistry	87
CS/Engineering	10
Information Systems	46
Psychology	42
Unknown/Other	54
Total	239

Of the 239 respondents 88 were males and 131 were females (with 20 unreported genders). The reasons for non-response were not captured. Responses for the following subset of questions are reported for *Information Systems* (IFSM, n=46) majors:

1. Do you consider yourself to have a content area specialty in your major? (y/n)

2. Would you be interested in a track in IFSM that allowed you to specialize in a field such as scientific computing or health care? (y/n/maybe)

3. The study of information systems in health care is often called Health Care Informatics. Do you think this is important to your major in IFSM? (y/n/maybe)

4. Would you be interested in a track in Health Care Informatics that allowed you to specialize your IFSM major? (y/n/maybe)

5. Do you think that you may get a job related to health care? (y/n)

Q#	yes	no	maybe	no response
1	24	21		1
2	17	7	22	0
3	23	14	9	0
4	9	17	20	0
5	12	33		1

IFSM majors only report having a domain area specialty about 52% (24/46) of the time. The survey went on to determine that the majority of these students reported business as their specialty. 85% (39/46) of the students wanted a specialty or wanted more information on them. 67% (31/46) of the IFSM students were possibly interested in Health Care Informatics and 63% (29/46) were interested in a formal track (or more information on it) for the major. Finally, 26% (12/46) of the students thought that they would get a job related to health Care. These results indicate that there is interest in the student population of Information Systems majors for education in Health Care Informatics.

Responses for the following subset of questions are reported for *Other*(non-IFSM, n=193) majors:

1. How important do you think computers and information systems are to your field? (y/n/maybe)

2. Are you interested in studying information systems applications in your major field? (y/n/maybe)

3. Would you be interested in a minor in information systems that allowed you to specialize in your major field? (y/n/maybe)

4. The study of information systems in health care is often called Health Care Informatics. Do you think this is important to your major field? (y/n/maybe)

5. Do you think that you may get a job related to health care? (y/n)

Q#	yes	no	maybe	no response
1	168	3	21	1
2	154	34	0	5
3	65	54	73	1
4	114	26	51	2
5	139	47		7

In the case of non-IFSM majors, 87% (168/193) of the students reported that information systems were important to their major field. 80% (154/193) of the students wanted to combine their major field with the study of information systems. 34% (65/193) were interested in a minor in Information Systems. 59% (114/193) of them thought that Health Care Informatics was important to their major field and 72% (139/193) thought they might get a job related to health care. The large number of students in Biology and (Bio-)Chemistry is probably responsible for the interest.

These results are encouraging not only for a minor in Health Care Informatics but for the general idea that one could obtain a minor that allowed information systems study that was tailored to the student's major field of study. The sample was too small and the survey conditions too uncontrolled to be able to stratify the results by major area etc.

CURRICULUM

Based on the needs analysis, we designed a curriculum that allowed an undergraduate specialty in Health Care Informatics with broad training in Information Systems. The curriculum is shown in detail in Appendix 1. The content of each class is generally obvious from the title. The health care specific classes include a year long course in Health Care Informatics, an independent study or CO-OP, a course in Health Economics, and one in the Politics of Health (Policy). The first course in Healthcare Informatics follows a departmental or intra-organizational view with sections on particular areas in the health care enterprise (lab, nursing, CPR, etc.). The second course takes an inter-organizational view with an emphasis on network communications and policy (CHINs, payment, research repositories, etc.). The track is approved and begins in the Fall of 1994.

This curriculum balances organizational issues with technical ones, includes practical training in health care environments, and remains a broad program within Information Systems. It can serve as training for Information Systems professionals who typically go on for a masters degree or a pre-professional program for students wishing to enter health care post-graduate study [3]. Ball [4] has suggested a classification for Health Informatics curricula as:

- Health-based curricula
- Informatics-based curricula
- Dedicated and integrated curricula

Each of these types of curricula have an important place in graduate and undergraduate education. The health-based curricula are deployed primarily as components of professional education in health care such as the Nursing Informatics program at the University of Maryland. Dedicated and integrated curricula have equal emphasis on the health domain and the information systems theory and technology. These are also typically graduate programs such as the MS/PhD in Medical Informatics at the University of Utah. The informatics-based curricula (such as this one) are particularly relevant to undergraduate education since they allow broad education in information systems and exposure to the domain of health care. (The authors would like to acknowledge the work of Tony Norico and Marion Ball for help in developing this curriculum.)

CONCLUSIONS

The needs analysis reported here shows a coherent rationale for an undergraduate track in Healthcare Informatics within a major in Information Systems. The survey component of this analysis shows acceptable demand from the student population. In addition to majors in Information Systems, majors from other areas show interest in applying the study of Information Systems to their own major field of study. This squares nicely with the vision of Information Systems as a domain area-based field of study. The field tries to balance technical and organizational/management study to produce practitioners that will be more successful in designing, developing, and implementing information systems for enterprises.

The curriculum developed from this needs analysis for Health Care Informatics addresses the issues of breadth in information systems and practical experience in health care. This curriculum places Health Care Informatics in the mainstream of the field of Information Systems to reduce the problems associated with class pre-requisites and academic respect. There is definitely an important place for informatics education in the curricula of the health care professions, but due to time constraints, it is very difficult to become a true health information systems professional in the course of a graduate clinical education.

Reference

[1]. Protti, D., C. Anglin, The continuum of health informatics education: Where do existing curricula fit?, MEDINFO92, K. Lun et al. eds., Amsterdam:North-Holland, 1992, pp1066-1071.

[2]. Protti, D., Personal Communication, 1993.

[3]. Ranum, D., "Pre-Medical" Informatics, 17th SCAMC, C. Safran ed., 1993, pp743-746.

[4]. Ball, M., J. Zimmerman, Informatics Education and the Professions, *J. Am. Soc. Inf. Sci.* 40 1989, pp.368-377.

APPENDIX 1

Health Care Informatics Track

27 Hrs in Information Systems

IFSM 202—Systems Analysis Methods
IFSM 310—Software and Hardware Concepts
IFSM 410—Database System Development
IFSM 420—Advanced Database Concepts
IFSM 436—Structured Systems Analysis & Design
IFSM 460—Health Care Informatics I
IFSM 461—Health Care Informatics II
IFSM 468—Project in Health Care Informatics
and one of:
IFSM 450—Data Communications and Networks
IFSM 425—Decision Support Systems

8 Hrs in Computer Programming

CMSC 201—Computer Science I for Majors
CMSC 202—Computer Science II for Majors

18 Hrs in Economics and Management

ECAD 210—The Practice of Management
ECON 101—Principles of Economics I
ECON 102—Principles of Economics II
ECON 467—Health Economics
POLI 452 —The Politics of Health
ENGL 393—Technical Writing

13 Hrs of Mathematics and Statistics

MATH 151—Calculus and Analytic Geometry I
MATH 221—Introduction to Linear Algebra
IFSM 300—Introduction to Management Science
STAT 351—Applied Statistics

The Effects of an Undergraduate Nursing Informatics Curriculum on Students' Knowledge and Attitudes

Lucille L. Travis, PhD, RN, CNA, Frances Payne Bolton School of Nursing
Case Western Reserve University, Cleveland, OH
JoAnne Youngblut, PhD, RN, Frances Payne Bolton School of Nursing
Case Western Reserve University, Cleveland, OH
Patricia Flatley Brennan, PhD, RN, FAAN, Frances Payne Bolton School of Nursing
Case Western Reserve University, Cleveland, OH

This paper describes the fourth stage of a process to design, implement and evaluate the nursing informatics courses incorporated into a baccalaureate nursing program. The challenge is to structure the nursing informatics curriculum so as to provide the nursing professional with the basis with which to impact health care delivery. The basic components of the framework are information, technology, and clinical care process. Students in the fourth course worked closely with agency personnel to design, implement and evaluate clinical application projects.

Preparing health care professionals to utilize information technology is a challenge that needs to be addressed by educational programs. Therefore this paper will describe the design, implementation and evaluation an integrated informatics curriculum currently in place in a baccalaureate nursing program. First time implementation of the fourth course of a required four course sequence will be discussed as well as the ongoing evaluation of the first, second and third courses of the curriculum.

BACKGROUND AND REVIEW

In the Fall of 1990, the inaugural class of a new baccalaureate program in nursing was admitted. Previous to the admission of the first class of this new program, nursing educators recognized an opportunity to formally incorporate information science into a university curriculum through a required sequence of four courses. Preparation of nursing professionals to face the challenges of health care in the 21st century rests on educational programs well grounded in the sciences that support nursing. Increase in the use of computer technology and information science in nursing practice, education, and administration demands a new approach in the preparation of nurses for the use of information technology [3,11]. However, the ability to implement the necessary changes in curriculum to address the demands of complex clinical practice characterized by escalating information management challenges is difficult [2,3]. Additionally, the report of Priority Expert Panel E: Nursing Informatics [6] continually challenges faculty to produce a baccalaureate graduate who utilizes information technologies in their clinical judgement to improve the patient care process and join the cadre of nursing professionals needed to change health care.

Of particular interest to this audience is the innovative inclusion of nursing informatics throughout the four years of baccalaureate curriculum. Other key aspects of the program include a focus on acute and critical care nursing, a bedside nursing emphasis, strong clinical experience throughout all four years beginning in the first semester of the curriculum, a development of identity with professional nursing through personal link-ups with nurses in clinical settings, and well defined linkages to the three consortium hospitals that provide the clinical experiences for the students. Each student is placed in a single clinical site for the entire four-year educational program which allows the student to become integrated in the organizational culture and social climate of the hospital.

CHALLENGE

The implementation of the fourth course placed in the last semester of the fourth year of the program provided the following challenges:
1) To assist the students to view the integration of information technology as a tool in support of the patient care process in the broader venue of health care. 2) To develop and implement the fourth course and closely align it with other nursing courses.

DESIGN

In the development of the curriculum, we faced a challenge to produce a new type of university graduate destined for excellence in clinical practice in acute and critical care through effective use of information technologies. Argyris and Schon [1] suggest that the clinical field experience in a professional nursing program should not be designed merely to give students experience in the real clinical setting to learn accepted practices, but should also provide the student with the opportunity to try out new approaches and modalities of care. In addition, the recommendations set forth by Peterson & Gerdin-Jelger [8] and Ronald & Skiba [10] were reviewed for guidance in the design.

Consequently, the nursing informatics courses are designed to articulate with the clinical experience and comprehensive course progression followed by the baccalaureate students. The three basic components of the model identified to provide a framework are information, technology, and clinical care process. A model was developed to illustrate the three aspects of nursing informatics in the undergraduate curriculum (See Figure 1). Each of the four courses address the three components, however, the emphasis regarding each component is dependent on the specific course. In order to successfully focus the curriculum, faculty consciously worked to develop all nursing courses whereby nursing informatics and nursing science theories would be integrated throughout the curriculum. There is a total of 122 credits in the undergraduate nursing curriculum. Seven credits are in the required informatics sequences. Of the 122 credits required, 81 are nursing credits.

The first course in the sequence is Introduction to Nursing Informatics (2 credits). The emphasis is on information and technology with an overlap in the clinical care process (see Figure 1). This course focuses on helping students identify the content, flow and processing of patient information within the hospital [12]. In Nursing Informatics II (1 credit), the primary emphasis is on information and the clinical care process with secondary emphasis on technology (see Figure 1). This course prepares the student to handle the increased quantitative information encountered in the clinical area [13,14]. In the third course, Nursing Informatics III: Clinical Nursing Information Systems (2 credits), the focus is on the overlap of the three components: information, technology, and clinical care process (see figure 1). The emphasis is on the use of information technologies to support nursing management in clinical applications [14]. The culminating course in the nursing informatics sequence is Nursing Informatics IV: Applications (2 credits). This course is designed to provide hands-on experience for the student in selected areas of application in nursing informatics. The course is conducted as a project-based course, in

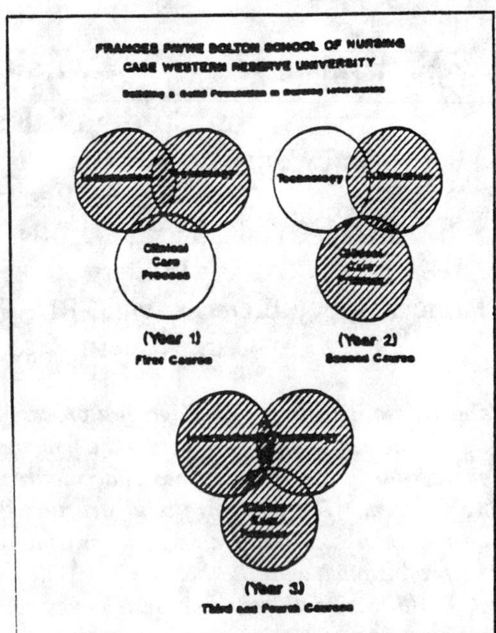

Figure 1

which students are grouped into teams of five-to-seven members to work on agency-specified projects. Our curriculum reflects the advances in technologies and demands of the marketplace as outlined in Neighbors & Eldred [7] and reported by those who have endorsed specific level requirements for informatics in baccalaureate and graduate educational programs [3,4,9].

It is important to acknowledge the ability to implement these courses is in part due to the fact that the Case Western Reserve University has a well developed fiberoptic network (CWRUNET) that supports a variety of teaching strategies. Students can access the university network from student, laboratories and from their dormitory rooms. If they have a computer each dormitory room is equipped with a faceplate giving them immediate access to the network. From previous surveys, we found that approximately 60% of incoming freshmen owned computers [12,13]. On the other hand, the consortium hospitals are all in the process of selecting a nursing information system. Therefore, students continue to have varied opportunities to observe applications in the nursing practice environment.

IMPLEMENTATION

The projects that formed the core activities of Nursing Informatics IV were projects that originated in the consortium hospitals and met needs emergent within the hospital environment. In addition, for the purposes of learning nursing informatics, the previously explained long-term relationship of the students with the clinical agency help students better understand the nature of information management within the agency, and meaningfully participate in informatics projects. To initiate project design, the course instructor met with key personnel in each of the participating agencies. These personnel included nurse administrators, clinical nurse specialists, and information systems coordinators. The concept of nursing informatics projects was explained to encompass any work required to enhance nurses' ability to obtain, manage, store, or manipulate the data and knowledge necessary for practice. Agency personnel were asked to identify 4-6 projects per hospital, and to provide the following information for each project: Project title, objectives, deliverables, special considerations, and deadlines. Projects requiring approximately six-weeks of work (about 200 person-hours) were sought.

Nineteen suitable projects were identified from the three consortium hospitals. Listed below is a sample of the project activities:
1) Develop a scantron-form for recording the critical path of patients with cardiac surgery. 2) Construct a database to help a nurse practitioner-lactation consultant manage her practice. 3) Propose a data access policy for a large university teaching hospital. 4) Create a database to enable staff on a psychiatric inpatient service to conduct follow-up on patients. 5) Generate charts and graphs from a mainframe-stored hours-worked data set. 6) Devise a database and screening system to predict patients at risk for discharge planning challenges. 7) Establish the information flow of an out-patient ultrasonography service. 8) Provide off-hours backup and training support for a hospital bringing up a new hospital information system. 9) Define the information requirements necessary to support a continuous quality improvement project.

The projects varied in terms of the extent of computing skill necessary to conduct the work, and the amount of face-to-face interaction required to complete the tasks. Some informatics projects had absolutely no need for computer systems; others, such as the database creation activities, required specific computer skills. All of the projects challenged students to work with an agency staff member to define project deliverables, to interact with peers in a task-focused manner, and to apply prior nursing informatics knowledge to solve real-world problems.

After reviewing the projects available within their respective agencies, students within each consortium hospital group self-selected into project teams. Students participated in four class sessions in which the content focused on team building, project planning, and organizational communication. Under the direction of the course instructor, students spent six weeks preparing a project work plan and obtaining the necessary skills and materials to carry out the work plan. Once a project team received written approval from the course instructor and the agency contact person, the team implemented the work plan.

Students' teams provided weekly electronic mail updates of project status to the course instructor. Addressed in each e-mail message were the progress towards objectives, accomplishments of the week, and any obstacles to progress with a plan for managing the obstacles. The course instructor provided weekly feedback. Each project team also maintained a three-ring binder of materials related to the project, including background reading and drafts of work. These binders were kept in a public place accessible to all students.

EVALUATION - NURSING INFORMATICS IV

Seventeen of the 19 projects were initiated and completed within the academic semester. Two of the projects were withdrawn by the agencies before work had begun. Students presented the results of their projects to classmates and selected faculty through a variety of methods i.e. posters with detailed explanation of output presented, demonstration of developed programs on computers, and presentation of deliverables agreed on by project group. Students' reactions to the projects were predictably mixed: many students voiced pleasure at their own skill in nursing informatics, some evaluated the projects as being 'not clinical', and therefore not relevant to their work. In addition, students reported that due to a variety of reasons, it appeared that the outcome from some of the projects might not be operationalized immediately which was somewhat disappointing to them. However, the agency personnel interacting with the student groups were very complimentary and appreciative of the efforts of the groups.

UPDATE ON INFORMATICS I, II, III

The students continue to value the self-paced computer simulation packages used in Nursing

Informatics and other nursing courses. These packages require students to use the technology. Specifics of the packages have been discussed in previous articles [13, 14]. Assignments continue to reflect application of information technology to patient situations.

PROGRAM EVALUATION

This is the fourth stage of a longitudinal study that has extended over a four year period. Evaluation of outcomes with respect to both students' attitudes and knowledge acquired has occurred after each stage. In addition to following the first cohort of students through the four year period, a comparison between the first group of students and succeeding student cohorts will occur. At the end of the present courses, the survey previously developed [13] to evaluate the students' knowledge and attitudes toward computers and nursing informatics has been readministered so that an ongoing evaluation of changes in knowledge and attitude has been captured.

The instrument to be used for this study is a 30 item questionnaire adapted from McConnell, O'Shea, and Kirchhoff [5], to measure knowledge and attitudes toward computers. Students rate each item on a five point Likert scale. Factor analysis on the first sample supported a three factor structure and deletion of six items. The three scales are scientific use of technology, common misconceptions associated with technological advances, and clinical care process. The scientific use scale is composed of four items regarding the advantages of computer technology in the health care setting. Higher scores indicate more positive knowledge and attitudes. Cronbach's alpha for the scale is .58. The common misconceptions scale has eight items which describe commonly held fears and concerns regarding advances in technology in the workplace. Lower scores indicate more negative knowledge and attitudes. Cronbach's alpha was .83. The 12-item clinical care scale addresses the application of technology to support the nurse in providing patient care. Higher scores indicate more positive knowledge and attitudes. Cronbach's alpha was .85.

Each cohort was assessed at the end of each academic year on knowledge and attitudes. Data analysis was conducted to answer two research questions: 1) Do students' responses change after completion of each of the four courses? and 2) Are students' responses following each course different for each cohort? Ratings for the first cohort after each of the four courses were compared with oneway Analysis of Variance (ANOVA) and Scheffe tests for post-hoc comparisons. Repeated measures analysis is not possible as we collected data in a way to maintain anonymity for students. Their scores on the Clinical Care Process scale were significantly lower after the fourth course than after each of the other three courses, $F\ (3, 272) = 8.43, p < .001$. Differences on the Scientific Use and Common Misconceptions scales were not significant, $F\ (3, 277) = 1.38$, $p =$ NS and $F\ (3, 278) = 1.80$, $p =$NS, respectively. The lower scores on Clinical Care Process after the fourth course likely represent the students' attempts at responding to the "gap between education and practice" [11]. Indeed, scores on this scale were significantly lower for each subsequent year, indicating a continuing process of reconciling the theoretical content presented in class with the reality of the clinical setting.

This finding is consistent with our previous analysis with this group of students [14]. Obtaining differences on this scale and not on the other two may indicate that the Scientific Use and the Common Misconceptions scales represent a broader base; that is, the knowledge and attitudes tapped by these two scales are less central to the daily clinical reality and, thus, are less influenced by the education-practice gap.

To address the second research question, a series of oneway ANOVAs with Scheffe tests were used to compare students' ratings after the first, second, and third informatics courses across cohorts. In the comparisons of scores after the first course, the fourth cohort (current freshmen) had significantly lower scores on the Clinical Care Process scale than each of the other cohorts, $F\ (3, 306) = 12.30$, $p < .001$. The other two scales were not significantly different across cohorts. In the comparisons of scores after the second and third courses, none of the cohorts were significantly different on any of the three scales. There are several possible reasons for the finding. First, some changes were made to the first course based on our experience with previous classes. Specifically, the source of readings was changed from primarily articles to primarily textbook. In addition, increased emphasis was placed on electronic communication, which may have diminished attention on clinical applications. Second, the timing of administration of the instrument was changed with the fourth group. In the three previous cohorts, we had students complete the instrument upon entering the first course so that we could evaluate the level and content of this first course. These three previous cohorts gave us sufficient data about our students' sophistication with information technology to identify the appropriateness of the course plan and the teaching strategies. However, it is possible that this pretest served to direct students' interest or attention to the application of information technology to the clinical setting, thus increasing their overall knowledge and attitude level. If so, this change in measurement protocol may have resulted in students' in the fourth cohort having lower scores than their predecessors. These findings are consistent with the third reason, that students integrate information obtained in the classroom with experience in the clinical area. Thus, students' knowledge and attitudes about nursing informatics becomes less idealistic and more practical with increasing exposure to the clinical arena.

SUMMARY

The challenges of equipping nursing professionals for delivery of health care in the 21st century are many. However by incorporating information technology in the didactic and clinical portions of courses, faculty have ensured a blend of information, technology, and the clinical care process. Consistent with the results obtained after the students completed the third course, student scores on the clinical care process scale continued to decrease. The students' ability to complete complex application projects suggest they do indeed have the skills and knowledge to use information technology in the clinical setting. This ability in conjunction with the scores supports our previous hypothesis that students are reconciling the education-practice gap through application of their critical thinking skills.

References

[1].Argyris, C. & Schon, D. (1974). A Theory in Practice: Increasing Professional Effectiveness. Joffey-Bass, San Francisco.

[2].Bryson, D. M. (1991). The computer-literate nurse. Computers in Nursing, 9(3), 100-107.

[3].Heller, B.R., Romano, C. A., Damrosch, S., & Parks, P. (1985). Computer applications in nursing: implications for the curriculum. Computers in Nursing. 3(1), 14-21.

[4].Heller, B.R., Damrosch, S., Romano, C. A., & McCarthy, M.R. (1989). Graduate specialization in nursing informatics. Computers in Nursing. 7(2), 68-77.

[5].McConnell, E.A., O'Shea, S.S., & Kirchhoff, K.T. (1989). RN attitudes toward computers. Nursing Management, 20(7), 36-40.

[6].National Center for Nursing Research (1993). Nursing Informatics: Enhancing Patient Care (NIH Publication No. 93-2419). Bethesda, Maryland: U.S. Department of Health and Human Services.

[7].Neighbors, M. & Eldred, E.E. (1993). Technology and nursing education. Nursing and Health Care, 14(2), 96-99.

[8].Peterson, H. & Gerdin-Jelger, V. (1988). (Eds.) Preparing Nurses for Information Systems: Recommended Informatics Competencies. (NLN Publication No. 14-2234). New York: National League for Nursing.

[9].Romano, C., Damrosch, S., Heller, B. Parks, P. (1989). Levels of computer education for professional nursing: Development of a prototype graduate course. Computers in Nursing, 1(7), 21-28.

[10].Ronald, J.S., & Skiba, D.J. (1987). Guidelines for Basic Computer Education in Nursing. (NLN Publication No. 41-2177). New York: National League for Nursing.

[11].Sparks, S. M. (1990). Computer-Based Education in Nursing [Monograph]. U.S. Department of Health and Human Services, National Institutes of Health, National Library of Medicine. 90-1.

[12].Travis, L., et al. (1991). An integrated informatics curriculum in baccalaureate nursing program. In Proceedings of Fifteenth Annual Symposium on Computer Applications in Medical Care. McGraw-Hill, New York.

[13].Travis, L., et al. (1992). Supporting collaboration through a nursing informatics curriculum stage II. In Proceedings of Sixteenth Annual Symposium on Computer Applications in Medical Care. McGraw-Hill, New York.

[14].Travis, L., & Youngblut, J. (1993). Supporting collaboration through a nursing informatics curriculum stage III. In Proceedings of Seventeenth Annual Symposium on Computer Applications in Medical Care. McGraw-Hill, New York.

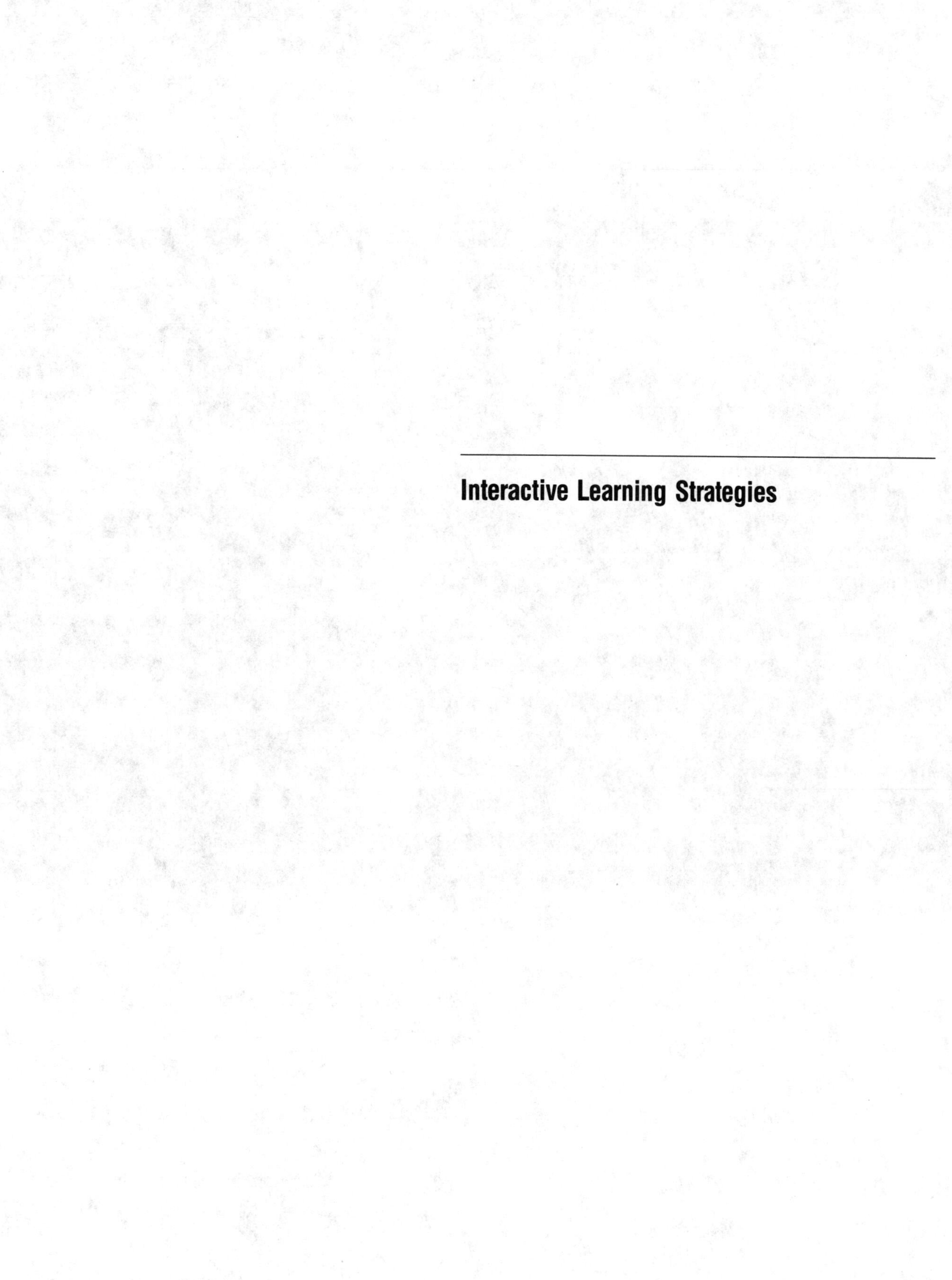

Interactive Learning Strategies

An Interactive Learning Environment for Health Care Professionals*

Elizabeth Cobbs, MD[1], Pierre Pincetl, MD[2,3], Barry Silverman, PhD[2,4], Ren-Lan Liao, MS[2], and Camille Motta, MS[4]

The Departments of Health Care Sciences[1], Computer Medicine[2], and Medicine[3].
Institute for Artificial Intelligence[4]
The George Washington University, Washington DC 20052

* Supported by a grant for Model Education Projects for Health Professions, HRSA # 1D31AH53006-01

ABSTRACT

This article summarizes experiences to date with building and deploying a clinical simulator that medical students use as part of a 3rd year primary care rotation. The simulated microworld helps students and health care professionals gain experience with and learn meta-cognitive skills for the care of complex patient populations that require treatment in the biopsychosocial-value dimensions. We explain lessons learned and next steps resulting from use of the program by over 300 users to date.

1) INTRODUCTION

The purpose of this effort was to create a learning environment that provides experience and knowledge about the management of complex patient populations. The target users of this environment include medical students and physicians as well as allied health care professionals. A number of quite good computerized training programs are available commercially, however, virtually all of them focus narrowly on the diagnosis and/or treatment of strictly the biomedical dimension of patients' problems (e.g., see RxDx series, QMR patient simulator, or the Slice of Life videodisc). In complex patient populations (e.g., elderly, chronically ill, cognitively-impaired, aids, or dying), clinical decision making is strongly influenced by non-biomedical factors such as patient preferences, psychological, and social resources. Depending on the settings of these factors, the clinician often must alter the treatment decisions.

For these reasons we created a new clinician training environment, one useful to health care professionals seeking to learn how to think about, problem solve for, and better manage complex patient populations. In doing this, we encountered and attempted solutions to a number of decision structuring, pedagogical, human-computer interaction, artificial intelligence, and usage evaluation issues. To begin our efforts, we developed a version of the learning environment for geriatric patient populations. This paper explains the lessons learned to date.

2) HEALTH CARE FRAMEWORK

Complex patients often defy the application of a straightforward (biomedical) decision approach. For example, among other difficulties, there may be impediments to communications, and there may be written directives about unexpected care desires. There often is no way to cure them. This presents an unsettling situation for MDs used to being in control and focusing on the (biomedical) solutions. Traditional decision structuring process breaks down and they become unsure of what to replace it with.

To work with complex patient populations requires the MD to adopt a reasoning framework broader than biomedicine alone. For geriatric patients the framework includes four dimensions that must be combined to isolate the best plan of care [7]:

(1) Biological (B) -- This is the traditional area where clinicians label the etiology and physiology of the patient's complaints. For non-complex patients, treatment is linked to this diagnosis in the "fix-it" approach to medical decision making [3].

(2) Psychological (P) -- This provides insight into the patient's mental outlook, coping styles, personality, stress level, and so on. How will the patient manage current and future medical problems?

(3) Social (S) -- This dimension encompasses support the patient will receive from the immediate and larger social network around them. It also concerns the cultural and social class mores concerning care. Are there family members or others to act as caregivers? Any cultural factors?

(4) Value/Cost (V) -- The patient's beliefs, fears, and preferences about pain, stress, disfigurement, death represent an important dimension of health care decision making. What are the patient's concerns about being a cost (financial and care) burden to the

family? What value and cost will the alternative medical intervention plans pose to the patient?

The goal of our training environment is not so much to teach the student the correct answer, but to fundamentally alter the decision processes the student uses. Thus, they must learn that in a clinical setting it is vital to collect and evaluate answers to questions along all four of these BPSV dimensions. This requires the clinician to elicit references from the patient, or a surrogate in the determination of the best possible outcome and intervention plan.

3) PEDAGOGICAL ISSUES

In the 1980s, prevailing wisdom (e.g., [1]) would cause us to design our environment to lecture the users on the biopsychosocial-values dimensions, and closely drilled them on practice cases. By the end of the 1980s, however, the medical schools in North America began to shift from instructionism to constructionism, or problem based learning. At the same time, intelligent tutoring systems fell out of favor in the field of computer science. The idea of constructivist environments caught on (e.g., see [6]).

Constructivist environments, like problem based learning (PBL), favor student-centered learning, self-discovery of clinical insights, and personally experiencing realistic patient cases albeit in a simulated microworld. The more the microworld mimics the real world, the easier the learner can transfer the lessons to actual practice. Also, in constructivist microworlds, if any tutors exist (and often they don't), they act more as facilitators, temporary cognitive apprenticeship, and meta-cognitive aids that focus on learning to learn skills.

4) INTERACTIVE LEARNING SYSTEM

The learning environment consists of (1) a case base of patients that can be visited, (2) a simulator of the patient, their support group, and clinical personnel, and (3) a graphical user interface that lets the student conduct exams, give orders, monitor progress/results, consult collaborators, update the patient record, and so on. This section presents each of these in turn. The system runs on IBM 386 compatibles with MS Windows. The system is programmed in Assymetrix Toolbook using DB III for the databases. Our architecture is generic to any of the domains mentioned in the introduction. By editing the case and databases, one can adapt the simulator to a new domain. The simulator engine and graphical user interface do not need to be altered.

The Case Base -- The case base currently consists of eight geriatric cases, each containing 100s of possible dialogue, diagnosis, and intervention options. Each case may be described in terms of a state space representation scheme where the patient's situation comprises the states, and students' actions determine state transitions. The student controls the simulator clock, so there is ample wall-clock time to explore a given state and alter one's decisions and/or interventions before simulator time advances. To manage the computing complexity, each patient case is indexed into about 6 to 10 overall states, including a starting state, a successful end-state(s), a failed-end state(s), and the remainder being intermediate states. Intermediate states, may be (1) steps in the right direction but from which the student could still branch to either a successful or failed end-state, (2) commonly committed, contra-indicated actions that are important to teach about (and that are recoverable from), or (3) default states that are reached by advancing the clock with either no interventions, or with none of the interventions that lead to the other intermediate states. If the student reaches the default state twice in a row, s/he follows the default path and terminates in a fail-state.

The Simulator -- It is one thing to learn an abstract decision structuring framework in class. It is another to know how to apply the framework in a clinic. The simulator causes the student to struggle with how to structure the biopsychosocial-values dimensions in the context of managing the patient situation.

The student begins the simulated "rounds" by selecting a patient and starting a new case. The simulator's 5 step algorithm then ensues. In step 1, the case is instantiated with 100s of pieces of information from three databases including the patient history DB, the possible orders (and exams, workups, labs, transports, etc.) db, and the canned text dialog strings of about 3 dozen possible case collaborators (e.g., attending nurse, clinical specialists, family members, attorney, etc.). In standard constructivist mode, the students browse as much of this material as they deem warranted. They can examine a teaching message from the system, but this is at the meta-cognitive level (e.g., something about decision structuring) and it says nothing about the specific way to solve the current case. In step 2 the student advances the clock, and the simulator collects the student's actions to date and helps them eliminate any violations (e.g., can't send to ER if already at ER). In step 3, the student receives a blank screen that inquires about their clinical impressions thus far. Next the case stack database (DB) is updated in step 4, and the state index is advanced. With the new state index, step 5 consults the DBs and reinstantiates the 100s of items the user previously browsed in step 1. If an end state has not yet been reached, the student returns to browse mode (step 1), and the algorithm repeats this time showing the student the progress to date. If an end state has been reached, the case stops, the student DB gets an update, and any final case messages are loaded, including detailed explanations and in-depth on-line references for further study. If the end state is a fail-state, the attending nurse takes proper action so the patient outcome is the desired one. The student can browse the final state at their leisure and proceed to another case when ready, or terminate rounds. An example of how all this works can perhaps best be illustrated in the context of the screens the student sees.

The Graphical User Interface -- Our student interface design follows widely used conventions that many students may already know. This includes use of pull down menus, list boxes with scroll bars, push buttons, and a simple 2 column window layout. As an assist, there is also a tutorial and practice session under the F1 help key for learning to use the mouse and the features just mentioned. The main pull-down bar of the interface leaves the control of the case in the student's hands, rather than forcing them through a fixed protocol. The pull downs let the student (1) change the file to a new case, (2) access the patient chart, (3) conduct a physical, (4) examine the history of the current illness, past illness and lab results, and current and past medications, (5) order new labs and workups, instruct the patient, and advance the clock, (6) transport the patient to the ER, Hospital, LTC, or residence, (7) consult a variety of individuals, (8) inspect the teaching messages, and (9) obtain help.

In general, after making a physical, orders, transport, or consult selection from the pull-down bar the student enters a 2-column screen. The left column is a menu of further detailed selections. The right column posts the responses. These also get posted to the patient chart and history. In a future version we hope to add audio-visual features that will give the student practice in interpreting the raw data directly (e.g., actual chest xray image). Results in the right column also are stored in the patient history file for later re-browsing by the student. When the student advances the clock, the 2-column format is replaced by windows that collect the student's clinical impression, convey lab results, and offer various dialog messages (e.g., from health care professionals, the patient/surrogate, and the tutor). At the end of the case, the student pages through teaching material starting with case answers and objectives and evolving to broad principles and reading citations.

Example geriatric case, Mrs. Brown -- The nursing home nurse complains that Mrs. Brown is agitated and needs sedation (start-state, Brown-100). The patient herself is noncommunicative (in this case). Selecting FAMILY will put the student in touch with Mrs. Brown's niece, Lucy her Durable Power of Attorney for Health Care, who would explain some of Mrs. Brown's wishes. The clinician must determine that the underlying condition causing the agitation is pneumonia, and send Mrs. Brown to the ER (successful End State, Brown-200). Ordering a chest xray, oxygen, or antibiotics are successful intermediate states labelled Brown-400 and -500 that suggest the student is on the right path (another intermediate state is being added of a blood oxygen detector), but these must be reached the first time the simulator clock is allowed to advance or else they will be too late to help the patient. If the student fails to send the patient to ER after Brown-100, -400, or -500, the simulator advances the case to Brown-300. Here the student has one last chance to assess the situation and send to ER, or the case terminates in a fail state, Brown-600. If the student ends up in the fail-state, the night nurse would take over the patient's care. Thus the student would hear how the patient was brought out of trouble, and is doing better at the ER. Alternatively, if the student sent the patient to the ER, Figure 3e is a report from the ER physician, and a thank you from niece Lucy.

5) STUDENT USAGE RESULTS

To create an environment that permits exploration and self-discovery, also holds the opportunities for students to get lost, in trouble, and frustrated. To minimize these obstacles, the Director, Div. of Aging Studies & Services (Dr. Cobbs) works with the student users as they come through a 6 week primary care rotation which includes geriatrics as one of the topics. The software with the 8 cases is currently required of all 150 3rd year medical students per year when they go through this rotation. On the first day of the rotation, they get an orientation to the software and instructions to complete the 8 cases before the 6 weeks are up. They also take a pre-test of their geriatric knowledge (see below). Sometime during the rotation, they spend about 2 hours with the preceptor in a 12 person group discussion of caring for the elderly and of solving cases both in the computer, and in practice. This discussion centers around the BPSV framework, though the framework is never formally presented. On the last day of the rotation they retake the test as a post-test. Neither time do they learn the correct answers to the test.

The students generally use the computer with a set of books and articles on the table next to them. The goal of the computer program is to help the students gain experience and confidence in applying the BPSV framework so they will better be able to utilize it in practice. The results to date are promising, but also show that there are a number of improvements needed. Let us examine a few of these results in this section and then return to the implications for improvement of the software in the last section.

To date, we have collected four types of evaluation measures from the 300 plus student users: (1) software usage patterns, (2) transfer of experiential learning across similar cases, (3) before and after usage performance scores, and (4) student reactions. We are still analyzing the bulk of this data, and can only give a few indications of what it conveys.

Software Usage Patterns -- Looking at the Mrs. Brown case, discussed earlier, in a recent sample of 18 students, 13 students (72%) reached the successful end state. Yet, 85% of these 13 visited a non-fruitful intermediate state (Brown-300) and probably got to the success-state by reading teaching messages and the nurse's suggestions, rather than by diagnostic effort. None of these (or the 5 failed students) viewed the broader framework that would have led to the correct end-state. If they had consulted the family, for example, they would have seen that the family did not want the patient to be treated by all medical means short of life-support or resuscitation. A trip to the ER would meet the needs of the family.

Only one of the students actually appeared to use the psychological framework. This student asked to look at the history of the patient, the history of Mrs. Brown's mental status as well as her psychiatric history. After referring to all of the historical information, the student examined the patient's heart and lungs and ordered her transported **immediately** to the ER. It is most interesting to note, as mentioned earlier in this paper, the software was designed to help teach a framework broader than biology alone and that the most successful student in the Brown case, attained success by doing exactly what the software is trying to teach - that is by seeing the patient in the broader reasoning framework.

Knowledge Transfer Across Cases -- One of the goals of the computer program is to have the students learn from (simulated) experience. Did they pick up any insights about the framework that they are now transfering to and using on subsequent cases? We should be able to detect if this is happening by comparing the same students' performance on a similar case. One of the 8 existing cases, that of Mrs. Johnson, bears some useful similarities to Mrs. Brown's case. Mrs. Johnson has advanced Alzheimer's disease. The students need to administer a swallow test to detect she is in the final stage, after which they must follow family directives and allow her to die in peace.

In contrast to the Brown case, the students both examined the history of the patient, including mental status and neurological, as well as consulted with family members. After doing so though, only 1 student ordered a swallow test. The rest of the students seemed to find it difficult to do nothing for Mrs Johnson, as the family preferred, and they proceeded to order a feeding tube or a hospital admission. Thus as the students progress from case to case, we do see an improvement in the process that they use for treatment of elderly patients. The software seems to lead to knowledge transfer of the framework. However, old habits die hard. The software fails to dampen the biomedicine-only tendencies instilled in the students over the years.

Performance Score Improvements -- Another goal of the software is ultimately to help the students perform better after their (geriatrics) rotation. The pre- and post-test is an instrument currently in use to determine if the students are benefiting from the rotation. The test includes (a) a self-rating of knowledge about sub-aspects of the BPSV framework, (b) a series of multiple choice and true/false questions on care of the elderly, and (c) a short geriatric case followed by a request for a list of the patient's current problems and how the doctor should help the patient for the very near future. Although it was never designed into an experiment for measuring the value of the software, we can glean some insights from the testing data.

Comparing the self-rating forms on part (a) shows the students rate themselves about 30% higher after using the software. This is a crude measure that the software seems to help the students, at least with their confidence in the knowledge. However, the computer has no impact that is measurable by multiple choice/true-false (MC/TF) tests (part b). This should not be surprising since the computer aims at experiential learning of a framework rather than memorization of facts. Finally, their answers to part (c) of the post-test reveal the students rarely structure their answers into or even show they're using the BPSV framework. This may be related to the fact the BPSV framework is never formally taught, either in the rotation or in the software (although it is discussed in the recommended readings including Dr. Cobbs' book). Not formally teaching the biopsychosocial-values framework is consistent with the constructivist pedagogy (students should discover it). Yet this pedagogy may not be ideal if it is important to transfer a stronger skill in BPSV decision structuring within the 6 week rotation, especially in light of the students' prior bias to use the biomedical-only portion of the framework. More on this shortly.

Reactions -- At the end of their rotation, the students complete a 1 page evaluation form on their experience. Comments on the software generally fall into two categories: human-computer interaction and pedagogy. The human computer interaction comments show the software is not yet working as well as it needs to. There are problems with synonym lookup, free text translation, user confusion, and saving and printing functions. In terms of pedagogy, the students frequently request more quick info, greater teaching/hinting guidance, and finer-grained evaluation.

6) DISCUSSION AND NEXT STEPS

The results presented above are leading us to a number of changes and improvements in the computing, pedagogy, and evaluation areas. The computing changes include, but aren't limited to: an alternative to the free text input of orders and requests (e.g., a pick and click form, a word wheel, or a robust style synonym checker); program and printer speedup and other efficiency improvements; more flexible entry/deletion options; and an improved on-line tutorial that helps the student understand what to get from the system. To improve doctoring skills, we are also exploring the addition of multimedia representations of (1) raw patient sign and symptom data, (2) lab results, and (3) conversational interaction with family and surrogates.

In terms of the pedagogy and instructional capabilities of the software, the students are enthusiastic about the clinical simulation and the ability to learn to react in a practical setting. The students seem to want more of an instructional approach, though, and less of a dependence on exploration and self-discovery. This is an area where a delicate balancing is required. On the one hand, we do not want to just cave in to the students' search for facts to memorize. The theory is well established that knowledge one discovers and experiences is personalized, whereas memorized facts are soon forgotten. The results of the student usage patterns and cross case knowledge transfer show that the constructivist pedagogy is having some success, plus the self-ratings on the post-test indicate their confidence is increased. On the other hand, the balance of the pre- and post-results show the students aren't learning enough meta-cognitive skills. At best, they discover and integrate only part of the BPSV framework for elderly patient care into their decision structuring processes.

To improve this situation without falling into the fact-memorization pit, we would like to add several meta-cognitive apprenticeship and temporary mental scaffolding features at key points in our environment. For example, we would like to add a meta-cognitive "influencer" lesson they can consult prior to (or during) any case. This influencer would interactively explain the BPSV framework, and point to the teaching objectives of this rotation, including references to the accompanying handout materials. In each case we would also like to add an active meta-cognitive teaching assistant that can explain the case learning objectives and how to achieve them. We would also like this agent to engage the students in two-sided argumentation, challenging them to explain and defend the framework they are using and why.

Once we accomplish these and some automated analysis changes to the software, we expect the results will begin to bear out our current beliefs that self-exploration of computerized microworlds can support medical student experiential knowledge and meta-cognitive decision structuring skills. If we reach this point we should have a teaching and learning tool that can be widely disseminated to support the ongoing clinical training of health care professionals, not just medical students, in the care of a variety of complex patient populations. By replacing the appropriate case and data bases, the Gericase simulator can teach and let students experience the biopsychosocial-values framework in any domain where its relevant (e.g., Aids, terminal cancers, and severe hypertensives), not just geriatrics. That is the larger value of our research.

REFERENCES

1. Clancey, W., Knowledge Based Tutoring: The Guidon Program, MIT Press, 1987.

2. Lajoie, S.P., Derry, S.J., Computers as Cognitive Tools, Hillsdale: Erlbaum, 1993.

3. Lynn, J., "Goals of Care," in Yoshikawa, T.T., Cobbs, E.L., Brummel-Smith, K., Ambulatory Geriatric Care, St. Louis: Mosby, 1993, pp. 2-8.

4. Pincetl, P., Cobbs, E., et al., "PC CLIN-SIM: A Toolbook Based Clinical Simulation Environment," Proc. SCAMC, 1992, pp. 793-4.

5. Silverman, B.G., Critiquing Human Error, London: Academic Press, 1992.

6. Soloway, E., (Editor), "Technology in Education: Special Issue," CACM, v. 36, n. 5, May 1993.

7. Yoshikawa, T.T., Cobbs, E.L., Brummel-Smith, K., (eds.), Ambulatory Geriatric Care, St. Louis: Mosby, 1993.

Interactive Electronic Whiteboards in the Medical Classroom

Nilesh L. Jain, MS[1,4], John F. Murphy, MD[2], Scott W. Hassan, BS[3],
Edward L. Cunnius, MS[3], Edward S. Metcalfe, BA[3], John L. Schnase, PhD[3,4],
Paul A. Schoening, MS[3], S. Andrew Spooner, MD[1], and Mark E. Frisse, MD[1,3,4]
[1]Division of Medical Informatics, Department of Internal Medicine; [2]Division of Cardiology,
Department of Internal Medicine; [3]Advanced Technology Group, School of Medicine Library;
[4]Department of Computer Science; Washington University, St. Louis MO 63110

Most research on computer-assisted instruction has concentrated on developing systems to be used outside the teaching environment to supplement or complement in-class teaching. We believe that interactive large-screen computers can be used effectively in the classroom *as electronic whiteboards to more effectively teach select medical school courses. We describe our experience with one such device, the Xerox LiveBoard™, to teach a course on computer-assisted clinical decision analysis to a group of first-year medical students.*

INTRODUCTION

Since the early 1960s, researchers have envisioned the promise of computer-assisted instruction (CAI) and have developed many systems for use by medical students and other health professionals [13]. Development and implementation of CAI systems is a major focus of medical school curriculum committees in both the United States and abroad [8, 15]. However, the instructional media used in the medical school classroom generally remain limited to blackboards, 35mm slides, and overhead transparencies, supplemented by the occasional use of video. This range is expanding with the advent of new computer hardware and broadband communications [14].

For example, researchers in the computer-supported cooperative work (CSCW) community are developing interactive large-screen computers for use in collaborative work environments. Although the primary intent of these devices is to support group meetings, presentations, and remote collaboration, we believe that such devices can also be used effectively as electronic whiteboards for teaching purposes [5,8].

Most CAI research has focused on developing systems to supplement or complement the role of teachers, either through out-of-class tutorials or, less often, through in-class computer laboratories which reduce the teachers' role to the management of instructional material [2]. We have sought instead to augment the practices of educators, aiding, in this case, classroom interaction with students and information. Apart from one very early endeavor [1], little research has been done on taking the computer into the medical classroom for use in teaching. In this paper, we describe our experience using the Xerox LiveBoard™ to teach a course on clinical decision analysis to a group of first-year medical students.

THE XEROX LIVEBOARD

The LiveBoard is a large-screen pen-based computer developed by researchers at Xerox Corporation's Palo Alto Research Center (Figure 1) [5]. In its standard configuration, the LiveBoard is powered by an Intel 486-based computer. The image is produced by projecting a liquid crystal display (LCD) onto a 4-ft by 3-ft rear-projection screen with a standard VGA display. Input to the LiveBoard is through wireless pens, and through the keyboard and mouse. Pens can be used

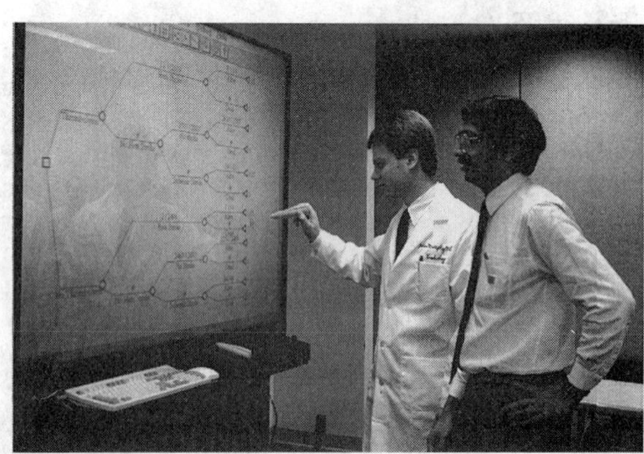

Figure 1: View of the LiveBoard being used by two instructors in a course on clinical decision analysis to create a decision tree.

both by touching their tips to the screen and from distances of several feet from the screen.

The standard LiveBoard software configuration includes Microsoft Windows® and Microsoft Pen Extensions for Windows™. The LiveBoard is capable of running all software compatible with Microsoft Windows. The Pen Extensions provide support for handwritten character recognition and gesture-based interaction with software. The LiveBoard also features multimedia support through an audio system as well as full-motion video.

A key advantage of the LiveBoard is the size of its display, which enables collaborative work at a common location by creating a large, shared workspace for group interaction. In addition, multiple LiveBoards in different locations can be connected using existing data communication technologies to permit simultaneous remote collaboration. Using the time-space taxonomy of groupware systems, the LiveBoard supports "same time/same place" as well as "same time/different place" interaction [4]. The Washington University School of Medicine, through the Advanced Technology Group (ATG) in the School of Medicine Library, is studying the use of LiveBoard technology in digital libraries, computer-supported collaborative work, and education [11].

CLINICAL DECISION ANALYSIS AND THE LIVEBOARD

The curriculum for first-year medical students at Washington University School of Medicine includes a six-session elective mini course on clinical decision analysis. Effective teaching of clinical decision analysis requires the use of software to interactively construct decision trees, elicit probabilities and utilities, calculate expected utilities in real-time, and perform one-way and two-way sensitivity analyses [16]. It also requires the presentation and annotation of such didactic material such as diagrams, images, and text.

The LiveBoard is a useful technology to combine these activities and media, and was a logical choice as the teaching medium for the clinical decision analysis mini course. Wireless pens can be used to "write" on the LiveBoard facilitating its use as a whiteboard. Slides made in Microsoft Powerpoint® can be displayed and annotated using the pens. Spreadsheets made in Microsoft Excel® can be displayed and used for real-time interactive calculations.

TIDAL—TEAM INTERACTIVE DECISION ANALYSIS IN THE LARGE-SCREEN ENVIRONMENT

We surveyed existing software packages such as DATA™ (TreeAge Software, Inc., Boston, MA), Decision Maker© (Division of Clinical Decision Making, New England Medical Center, Boston, MA), and DPL™ (Applied Decision Analysis, Inc., Menlo Park, CA). However, none of these are easily modifiable to support gesture-based input which is an essential form of pen interaction, and to create hypermedia links to electronic information sources. Hence, we developed TIDAL—Team Interactive Decision Analysis in the Large-screen environment.

TIDAL is a "groupware" application for team-based decision analysis. In its current version, TIDAL supports the interactive construction and manipulation of decision trees using pen-based gestures, menus, and keyboard commands. A tree is constructed by creating the structure of the tree, labelling the nodes and arcs, assigning probabilities to the arcs emanating from chance nodes, and assigning utilities to the outcome nodes (Figure 2). Analysis in TIDAL consists of real-time calculation of expected utilities, and rapid one-way and two-way sensitivity analyses.

TIDAL uses a generalized multimodal graphical editor to implement a direct manipulation user interface. The system was written in Microsoft Visual C++ and supports OLE 2.0 (Object Linking and Embedding). At its core, the TIDAL system supports generalized computations over graph-based formalisms. In addition to decision analysis, the system will eventually support compartment modelling.

MINI COURSE—COMPUTER-ASSISTED CLINICAL DECISION ANALYSIS

The goal of the mini course was to teach students an analytic methodology to solve difficult clinical problems and arrive at informed medical decisions. The analytic methodology—clinical decision analysis—combines pathophysiology, diagnostic test interpretation, treatment efficacy, patient preferences, and cost-effectiveness. Fourteen students signed up for the course. The following topics were covered in six sessions:

1. Diagnostic test interpretation [7]
2. Decision tree construction [10, 16 pp. 147–61]
3. Utility assessment for health outcomes [17]
4. Biases in utility assessment
5. Probabilities and sensitivity analysis [18]

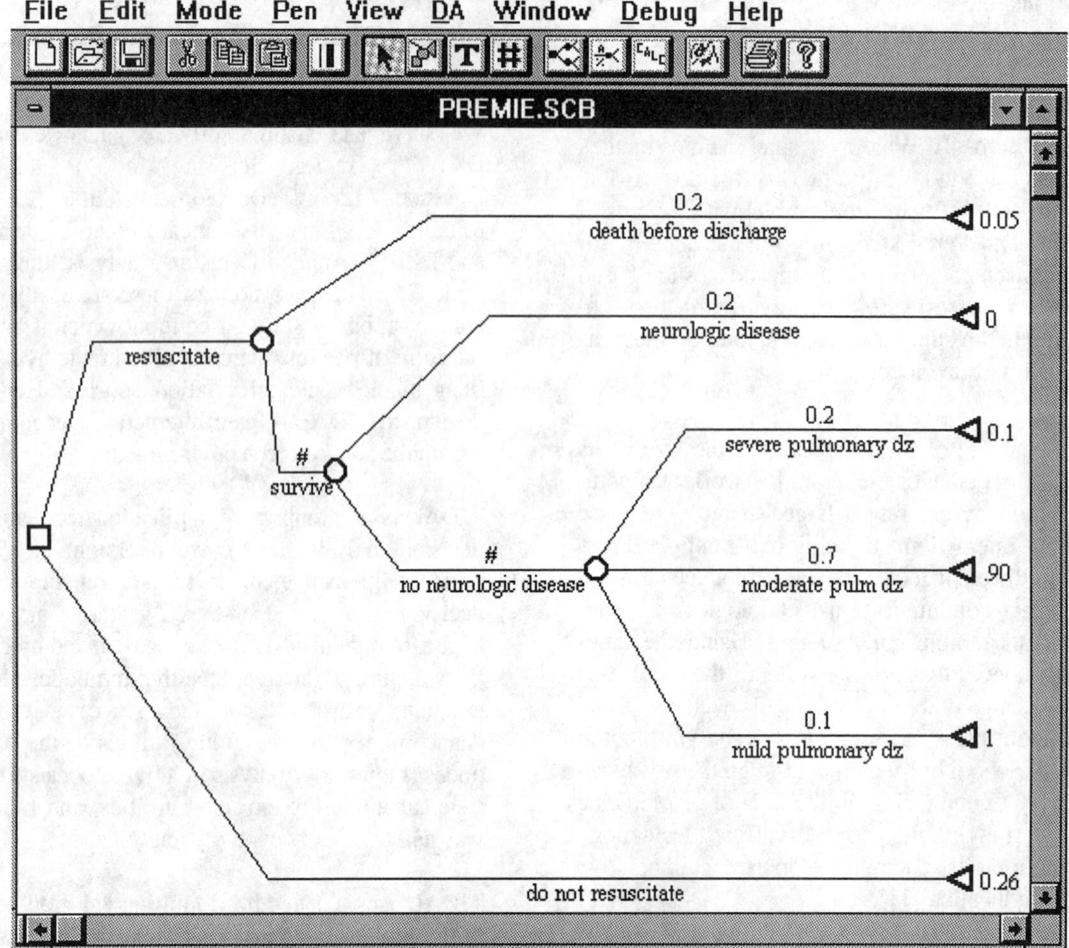

Figure 2: A screen view of TIDAL. This example is a decision tree used for analyzing the decision to resuscitate a premature baby.

6. Cost-effectiveness analysis [3].

The LiveBoard and Powerpoint slides were used in teaching all sessions. Additionally, we used Excel in the first session and TIDAL in the second through sixth sessions. For the third session on utility assessment, we used "Gambler" from the New England Medical Center in Boston [6]. Unlike traditional media, we could simultaneously execute and easily switch between all these applications. All sessions were videotaped for retrospective review.

Several clinical examples were used to illustrate the concepts being taught in class. For diagnostic test interpretation, the examples included: anti-nuclear antibody test to diagnose systematic lupus erythematosus; magnetic resonance imaging or auditory brain stem response to detect an acoustic neuroma in unilateral sensorineural hearing loss; and screening for prostate and breast cancers. Excel macros were written to compute positive and negative predictive values given the sensitivity and specificity of a diagnostic test and prior probability of the disease.

For the construction and evaluation of decision trees, elicitation of probabilities and utilities, and sensitivity analyses, the decision scenarios included: administering thrombolytic therapy to acute myocardial infarction patients with elevated blood pressure [12]; activity recommendations for athletes at risk for sudden cardiac death; resuscitation of an extremely premature infant (Figure 2); and performing surgery for a suspicious pancreatic biopsy. TIDAL was used to demonstrate the features of a decision tree such as decision nodes, chance nodes, and outcome nodes, and other aspects of decision analysis such as calculating expected utilities, and performing one- and two-way sensitivity analyses. The interactive nature of TIDAL allowed us to construct the decision trees in class with active participation from all the students. We were also able to demonstrate expected utility calculation and sensitivity analysis in real-time. This would not have been possible with the use of traditional 35mm slides, overhead transparencies, or a blackboard where it would have been necessary to create decision trees and perform analyses before class. Using TIDAL and the LiveBoard also taught students the necessity of collaboration and iteration in medical decision making and made the sessions more interesting.

For the assessment of utilities, we used the health outcomes in the following decision scenarios: administration or withholding of thrombolytic therapy for acute myocardial infarction patients; surgery or radiation therapy for prostate cancer; and toe or below knee amputation in diabetic patient. All four utility elicitation methods present in Gambler were taught, and students worked on the LiveBoard to perform the utility assessment for the last two examples.

STUDENT EVALUATION

We conducted two course evaluations to assess the views of the students on the use of the LiveBoard and TIDAL for teaching clinical decision analysis. An interim course evaluation was given at the end of the fourth session, and a final course evaluation at the end of the sixth session.

In the interim course evaluation, most students (83%) responded that the LiveBoard was better than the conventional teaching methods that they had experienced previously. Most students (92%) found TIDAL to significantly enhance their understanding of decision trees, and all students (100%) found Gambler to improve their understanding of utility assessment.

In the final evaluation, students were asked to rate features of the LiveBoard which we felt were important for its suitability as a teaching device. Table 1 shows the averaged responses of the students. Most students (91%) wanted to have TIDAL made available to them or installed on computers in the Library's media center.

In both evaluations, students were asked to write in comments on aspects of the LiveBoard or TIDAL that they liked or disliked. Features that most students liked were the real-time calculation of expected utilities enabling them to see immediately the results of a different set of probabilities or utilities in the same decision tree. They also liked the real-time calculation and display of sensitivity analyses which summarized the decision over a range of probabilities or utilities. Many students found the LiveBoard to be novel and different, and found the course to be more interesting due to the increased interactivity provided by this new technology. A few students added that the LiveBoard would be an excellent teaching device in courses where the number of students is small. When asked to identify other courses where they would like to use the LiveBoard, many students suggested medical genetics. Some students wanted to use its multimedia capability to visualize simulations of common physiologic processes or to interactively explore the quantitative relationships among the different components of the physiologic system.

Table 1: Average responses of the students on the various features of the LiveBoard. The following scale was used for the responses to the evaluation:
1: Very helpful; 3: Somewhat helpful; 5: Not helpful

LiveBoard / TIDAL features	Avg. rating
Drawing decision trees during lectures	2.0
Entering probabilities and utilities interactively during lectures	2.0
Calculating expected utilities instantaneously	1.4
Displaying sensitivity analyses graphs	1.7
Using Gambler for utility assessment	2.0
Handwritten character recognition	3.5
Switching instantaneously between slides and course software	2.4
Readability and quality of the display	2.2
Lack of simultaneous use of a blackboard/ chalkboard	1.9

Students were critical of handwritten character recognition and felt that it added unnecessary time to the process due to the number of mistakes it made. Students also criticized glare from the screen surface and the low resolution which occasionally made it difficult to read the contents on the screen.

FUTURE WORK

Given the success of the course and the positive feedback from the students on the LiveBoard and TIDAL, we plan to use it again next year for teaching this mini course. We want to design a system whereby students in the class can follow the instruction on their own portable computers, thus allowing them better interactivity with the course software and ready access to the course material outside class hours.

We are planning to extend TIDAL to incorporate hypermedia links to electronic sources of information such as MEDLINE to point directly to objective sources of probabilities in the literature. We will also extend TIDAL to support group decision making by collaborators located in different places.

ACKNOWLEDGMENTS

We would like to thank the students in the mini course for their constant enthusiasm and active participation, Steven Norkaitis and Pat Wells for videotaping the sessions of the mini course, and Dr. Mark H. Eckman of the New England Medical Center, Boston for providing us with "Gambler" (version 1.05) to demonstrate the utility elicitation techniques.

Dr. Murphy is a cardiology fellow supported by a training grant from the NHLBI. Dr. Spooner is an American Academy of Pediatrics Fellow of the Pediatric Scientist Development Program.

Reference

[1] Abdulla AM, Watkins LO, Henke JS, et al. Classroom use of personal computers in medical education: A practical approach. Med Educ 1983; 17: 229–32.

[2] Blickhan DS. The teacher's role in integrated learning systems. Educ Tech 1992; 32(9): 46–8.

[3] Eddy DM. Cost-effectiveness analysis. A conversation with my father. JAMA 1992; 267: 1669–75.

[4] Ellis CA, Gibbs SJ, Rein GL. Groupware: Some issues and experiences. Comm ACM 1991; 34: 9–28.

[5] Elrod S, Bruce R, Gold R, Goldberg D, et al. Liveboard: A large interactive display supporting group meetings, presentations and remote collaboration. In: Bauersfeld P, Bennett J, Lynch G, eds. Proceedings of the Conference on Computer Human Interaction (CHI '92). Reading MA: Addison-Wesley; 1992: 599–607.

[6] Gonzalez EF, Eckman MH, Pauker SG. "Gambler": A computer workstation for patient utility assessment. Med Decis Making 1992; 12: 350.

[7] Griner PF, Mayewski RJ, Mushlin AI, Greenland P. Selection and interpretation of diagnostic tests and procedures. Ann Intern Med 1981; 94: 553–600.

[8] Grudin J, ed. Special Section on Computer-Supported Cooperative Work. Comm ACM 1991; 34(12): 30–90.

[9] Hendricson WD, Payer AF, Rogers LP, Markus JF. The medical school curriculum committee revisited. Acad Med 1993; 68: 183–9.

[10] Kassirer JP. The principles of clinical decision making: An introduction to decision analysis. Yale J Biol Med 1976; 49: 149–64.

[11] Leggett JJ, Schnase JL. Viewing Dexter with open eyes. Comm ACM 1994; 37(2): 76–86.

[12] Murphy JF, Jain NL, Kahn MG, Parvin CA, Romero, Jr. CA. The impact of hypertension on the risk of hemorrhagic stroke in thrombolytic therapy: An appraisal and hypothesis. Submitted for publication; 1994.

[13] Piemme TE. Computer-assisted learning and evaluation in medicine. JAMA 1988; 260: 367–72.

[14] Soloway E, ed. Special Issue: Technology in Education. Comm ACM 1993; 36(5): 28–90.

[15] South M, Nolan T. Computer-assisted instruction in Australian medical schools. Med J Aust 1993; 159: 175–6.

[16] Sox, Jr. HC, Blatt MA, Higgins MC, Marton KI. Medical Decision Making. Boston MA: Butterworth-Heinemann; 1988.

[17] Torrance GW. Measurement of health state utilities for economic appraisal: A review. J Health Econ 1986; 5: 1–30.

[18] Tversky A, Kahneman D. Judgment under uncertainty: Heuristics and biases. Science 1974; 185: 1124–31.

Multimedia Clinical Simulation based on Patient Records: Authoring, User Interface, Pedagogy

Ramon M. Felciano[1] and Parvati Dev PhD[2]
[1]Section on Medical Informatics, Stanford University School of Medicine
MSOB X-215, Stanford, CA 94305-5479
[2]SUMMIT, Stanford University School of Medicine
MSOB X-329, Stanford, CA 94305-5470

Abstract: As an alternative to available computer-based clinical simulations that mimic patient encounters, we developed a clinical case simulation that more closely resembles the patient record. Our system, implemented in a Macintosh program called Short Rounds, features rapid and customized case authoring by editing a structured text file, a dynamic user interface that presents a case-specific screen layout, and a pedagogical model that is suitable for teaching third-year medical students. We believe this approach allows faculty members to create multimedia case simulations in shorter periods of time than in available clinical simulations.

INTRODUCTION

Computer-based clinical simulations have been used extensively to give medical students experience in medical problem solving, establishing diagnoses, and performing clinical procedures. A wide variety of approaches have been used to model and present patient case information; most require either extensive data entry or formal knowledge modeling. We developed a third system that focuses on presentation and on rapid authoring of clinical materials, and which greatly reduces data entry and eliminates formal knowledge modeling.

BACKGROUND

Computer-based clinical simulations have been difficult and tedious to program. Authoring approaches include manual authoring of each case [6]; manual authoring of the baseline values for a healthy individual with patient variables as a subset of the normal values [8]; and automatic authoring from a knowledge base [7]. Our work is based on the manual approach to authoring.

In all of the previously mentioned authoring approaches, the granularity of the data are the individual symptoms or findings and modifiers of the findings. The advantage of realism is counterbalanced by the tedium of authoring and checking a large number of findings, both normal and pathologic. For the system architect, creating a usable interface for each clinical domain usually means that different versions of the system must be maintained.

From the user's point of view, while some clinical simulations provide a wealth of findings for each case [2, 7], this data-rich format often leads to an awkward user interface. The user is required to scroll through long lists or move through several levels of menus to reach a particular finding. Evidence suggests that this "high fidelity" model, which provides responses to a large number of user queries, may not be best suited to use by third year medical students and that a "pedagogic" model that provides explicit cues on the nature of the case is more appropriate for students just being introduced to clinical medicine. [5]

A second problem in authoring is that the author must usually learn a new computer program that forces him transform his clinical knowledge into a form the computer can use. These authoring tools can be tedious to use because they often force authors to think about the case differently than they are accustomed to doing. Clinical faculty want to make their knowledge available to students but resist modeling it explicitly (as in knowledge-based or expert systems [1]) or presenting it in a fixed format (as in many multimedia presentation systems [3, 4, 8]).

OBJECTIVES

We set out to design a system that addressed some of the limitations of existing computer-based clinical case simulations and their authoring environments. Our target user group was third-year medical students who were just learning clinical medicine; our target author group was the clinical faculty members who taught them. Our goals were to develop a system that provided (1) a pedagogy and scope of clinical information suitable for third year medical students, (2) rapid case authoring in a manner that was natural to the author, and (3) a case-specific user-interface that let students go through cases quickly.

Pedagogy and Scope of Information

Our central information goal was to focus the student user on the pedagogical points of the case. Clinical simulation programs such as Real Problems and DxR provide a detailed data-driven model of a patient case [8]. The Chest Pain module in Real Problems, for example, has a data set of over 200 items that define a patient case (30 history items, 49 physical findings, etc.) DxR includes a similarly exhaustive set of findings [Irwin, personal communication]. Therefore, these programs have a rigid model of a patient case, where the findings available through the user interface do not vary on a case-by-case basis. Consequently, students face a diffuse body of information and are not guided to the essential insights in the case. In contrast with high fidelity simulations such as DxR, the data granularity in our simulation is a cluster of findings rather than a single finding.

Thus, our system should allow authors to transform the existing clinical information in the patient cases into the user interface of the program, displaying an author-definable selection of findings to the user, and presenting broad rather than deep selection of information. By allowing faculty to integrate existing case materials such as patient records and student handouts, and allowing them to control how this information gets displayed, we hope to encourage the development of a large library of shareable clinical cases.

Case Authoring

We focused on developing a rapid and simple authoring mechanism that would transform the author's clinical information into an interactive presentation for the student. Our goal was to develop a system that would enable the faculty member to spend less than 3 hours to author a single clinical case, including data entry and testing, and that supported the author's personal model of case presentation.

Because obtaining high-quality digital media is difficult (they are hard to locate, and usage rights are complicated [Dev & Felciano, unpublished work]), our system presented information textually, using a graphic interface and page layout techniques, with media as an option, not crucial, feature.

User Interface

The user interface of our system had to present clinical information in a way that communicated the case author's pedagogic goals, and allowed students to review the cases in under 20 minutes per case. Given these constraints, we needed a system that lets faculty control the presentation and flow of information without much formal programming or explicit direction. We did this with a special layout algorithm, described in the next section, that builds the user interface based on the structure of the clinical case.

In order to facilitate access to patient-case data, we decided that all user prompts should be immediately visible on the screen, and not hidden in popup menus or dialog boxes. Furthermore, wherever possible, user interaction is in the form of a single click. We expect the single-click focus of the interface to simplify the porting of the interface to other platforms, especially mobile platforms where interactions such as double-clicking or dragging with a pen may be more difficult to perform. [4]

We also decided that any piece of information would be available within two mouse clicks, regardless of what part of the patient case the user was viewing. This meant the presentation module would need a screen layout that presented only the clinical information relevant to the case, and allowed for single-click navigation between screens.

SYSTEM OVERVIEW

We have attempted to achieve these goals by building a program called Short Rounds. Short

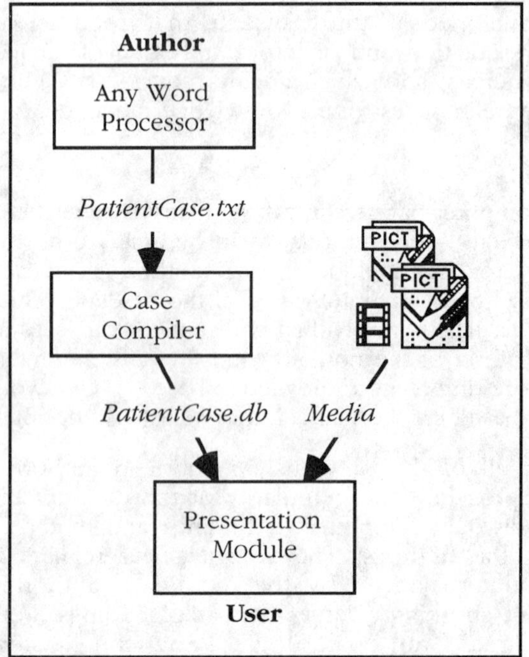

Figure 1. Short Rounds System Design

Rounds consists of a case compiler and a presentation module (Figure 1), both implemented as HyperCard stacks. The case compiler takes an author's text file and compiles it into a database format for the presentation module to use. Compiled cases typically occupy less than 50K of disk space (not counting media files).

The presentation module reads a single compiled case and displays it to the user in a graphic interface. Media files are stored in a separate directory that accompanies the file; they are combined with the textual elements of the case by the presentation module.

User Interface

Short Rounds displays patient information from one of three categories: History and Physical, Tests, and Diagnosis and Treatment. Each screen is separated into two areas: a fixed header bar along the top (A in Figure 2), and a content area underneath. The content area is further separated into an button area on the left (B. in Figure 2) and a findings area on the right (C. in Figure 2).

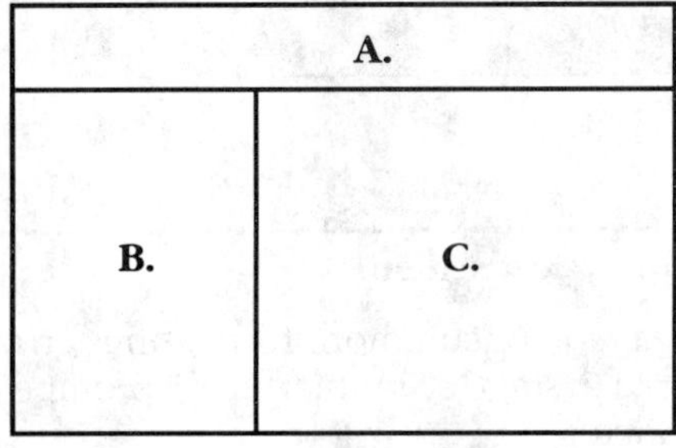

Figure 2. Screen Areas

Each screen displays a single category of information; the button area contains button panels that split this information into sub-categories. Figure 3 shows a History and Physical category with three subcategories: History, Physical Exam, and Systems Exam.

The header bar contains the case name and three navigation buttons to move between categories. The header bar also provides buttons to load a new case, access on-line help, and get a basic overview of the program goals. Users click on a category button to move to the screen of their choice.

One or more button panels on the left side of the content area prompt the user to what findings are available. When the user clicks on a button in the panels, text, graphic, and/or sounds relevant to the finding are displayed in the center of the content area.

Finding results that the user has displayed are marked with a bullet (•) in the button panel. In Figure 3, the user has asked about Present Illness, Family/Social History, has done a General, Skin, and HEENT exam, and is currently viewing the patient's Past History.

Once the user has taken a history, performed the physical examination, and ordered tests, he/she can establish a diagnosis and order treatment. Treatment cannot be ordered until a diagnosis has been indicated. The user is given immediate feedback as to whether a correct, incorrect, or possible correct diagnosis was chosen. A summary button that displays a case write-up is available once the user is finished.

Authoring

Authors create Short Rounds cases by editing a structured text file using any word processor on any platform. This allows authors to use text editing software they are familiar with, and obviates training them on a new tool.

The text file contains natural language prompts that are parsed by the Short Rounds program. Special delimiters indicate the start of each cluster of clinical findings. Each such cluster contains text that may be entered in the patient record as well as file names for media that amplify the text, such as the x-ray image, the patient's heart sound, or a digital movie. The media elements are optional; cases can be entirely textual.

The specific guidelines for developing a case are purposefully simple. Double-bullets (••) mark the names of Categories and Sub-categories. Single bullets (•) indicate clinical findings. Special prompts, such as "Picture:", are used to point to media file names. The resulting text file is both human and machine readable, and, most importantly, resembles a conventional case write-up.

Figure 4 shows an excerpt defining entries in the "History" sub-category of the "History & Physical" screen.

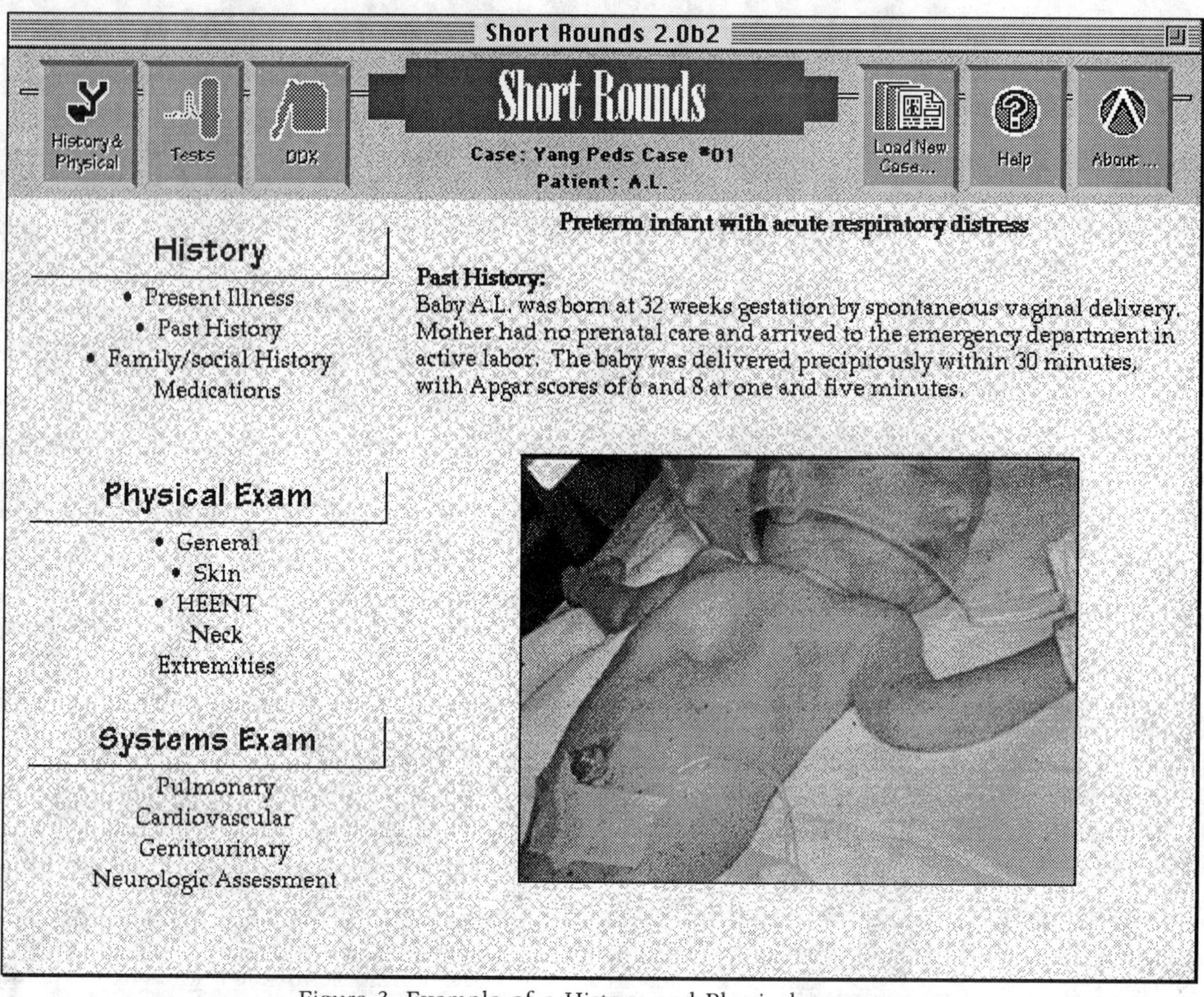

Figure 3. Example of a History and Physical screen

•• History & Physical : History
• Present Illness
Baby A.L. is a two-hour-old preterm male infant with sudden onset of respiratory distress while in the Neonatal ICU. He is breathing rapidly, cyanotic, and has mild nasal flaring and audible grunting on expiration. (Sound heard is grunting on expiration).
Picture:Baby A.L.
Sound: Grunting

• Past History
Baby A.L. was born at 32 weeks gestation by spontaneous vaginal delivery. Mother had no prenatal care and arrived to the emergency
etc ...

Figure 4. Sample Case File

Case Compiler

The case compiler verifies the basic structural integrity of the file, and converts it into a more compact database format. Because there is no data or format verification done by the word processor, the compiler attempts to strip out superfluous data such as trailing spaces, and ignores some common formatting errors (for example, using "*Graphic:" as a prompt instead of "•Picture:").

Authors usually save in a compiled format for the presentation module to load. During the authoring stage, however, the compiler can be integrated with the presentation module. This allows authors to load an un-compiled case into the presentation module and have it compiled just before it is displayed. Since this compilation can take as long as two minutes for large cases, cases are typically distributed in compiled form once they are complete.

Presentation Module

The presentation module dynamically constructs the screen layout of the content area from the structure of the patient case file. This process involves (1) linking the user interface elements to clinical content and (2) positioning the user interface elements on the screen. Loading a compiled case and preparing the screens typically takes less than 7 seconds.

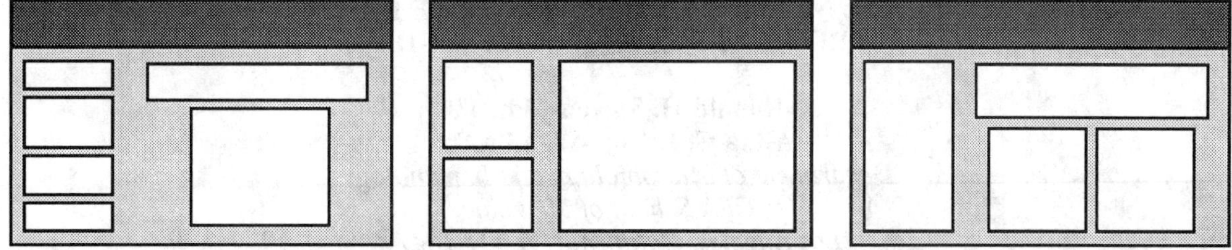

Figure 5. Alternate Layouts

The layout algorithm uses the number of finding subcategories, the number of media elements, and the types of media to build the layout. During a first pass, the program parses each cluster of findings in the patient case, creates a button on the fly for that cluster, and links text and pertinent media (images, video clips, or sounds) to the button. During a second pass, the program organizes all the buttons in an aesthetic layout in the window. Each panel of findings and result display is a rectangular panel that can be moved or resized on the screen. The layout algorithm preserves a consistent graphic design by maintaining proportional sizing and spacing on the screen. Representative layouts (Figure 5) show how panels could be arranged to display different combinations of subcategories and findings.

Since all findings are listed along the left side of the screen and the navigation buttons are preserved in the header bar, users can get to any finding by clicking no more than twice: once on the category and once on the finding.

USAGE

Short Rounds is currently in the development stages, and has been used to develop six neonatal intensive care cases. During this initial development process, we have found it easy to enter the clinical information such as history and physical findings. Informal discussions with faculty have indicated a need for Short Rounds cases to include an explicit teaching element in addition to the clinical information; this teaching element would allow faculty to explain why this is a good teaching case.

ACKNOWLEDGMENTS

The authors thank Michael Walker, Tom Rindfleisch, and Philip Constantinou for guidance and support. Lawrence Mathers, MD, provided the initial set of clinical cases. Nora Sweeny provided valuable editorial comments on earlier drafts of this paper. This work was sponsored by the Stanford University Medical Media and Information Technologies (SUMMIT) laboratory, and partially supported by a gift to SUMMIT from Dr. Peter Bing and Mrs. Helen Bing. Some computing services were provided by the CAMIS resource at Stanford, NIH grant No. LM-05305.

REFERENCES

[1] Chin, H.L. and Cooper, G.F., Case-based tutoring from a medical knowledge base. *Comput Methods Programs Biomed*, 1989. 30(2-3): p. 185-98.

[2] Cundick, R., *et al.* ILIAD as a patient case simulator to teach medical problem solving. in *13th Annual Symposium on Computer Applications in Medical Care*. 1989. Washington, DC: American Medical Informatics Association.

[3] Dichter, M.S., Greenes, R.A., and Bergeron, B.P. Authoring multimedia clinical problem-solving exercises with CaseBase. in *Proc Annu Symp Comput Appl Med Care*. 1991.

[4] Felciano, R.M., Daane, S.P., and Dev, P. Clinical Pearls and Short Rounds: Two Shells for Multimedia Case Presentations. in *AMIA Spring Congress*. 1994. San Francisco, CA: AMIA.

[5] Friedman, C.P., France, C.L., and Drossman, D.D., A randomized comparison of alternative formats for clinical simulations. *Med Decis Making*, 1991. 11(4): p. 265-72.

[6] Lyon, H.J., *et al.*, PlanAlyzer, an Interactive Computer-assisted Program to Teach Clinical Problem Solving in Diagnosing Anemia and Coronary Artery Disease. *Academic Medicine*, 1992. 67(12): p. 821-828.

[7] Miller, R.A., *et al.*, The INTERNIST-1/QUICK MEDICAL REFERENCE Project—Status Report. *The Western Journal of Medicine*, 1986. 145 (6): p. 816-22.

[8] Perper, E.J., Felciano, R.M., and Dev, P. Real Problems: A Layered Approach to Constructing a Patient Simulation. in *17th Annual Symposium on Computer Applications in Medical Care*. 1993. Baltimore, MD: American Medical Informatics Association.

ARTIFICIAL NEURAL NETWORK COMPARISON OF EXPERT AND NOVICE PROBLEM-SOLVING STRATEGIES

Ronald H. Stevens, Ph.D.,
Alina C. Lopo, M.D., Ph.D.
Department of Microbiology and Immunology
UCLA School of Medicine
Los Angeles, California 90024-1847

The successful strategies of second-year medical students were electronically captured from computer-based simulations in immunology and infectious disease and were used to train artificial neural networks for the rapid classification of subsequent students' and experts' strategies on these problems. Such networks could categorize problem solutions of other students as successful or non-successful >85% of the time. These neural networks, however, performed poorly (as low as 13%) when classifying experienced immunologists' or internists' successful performances, suggesting an ability to distinguish between novice and expert strategies. The neural networks also identified a group of students who framed the infectious disease problems correctly, but had difficulty discriminating between differential diagnoses.

INTRODUCTION

We have been exploring the ability of artificial neural networks to classify the performances of medical students who are engaged in problem solving in multiple disciplines and have shown that neural networks trained with the successful problem performances of students can accurately recognize the strategies of new students on these same problems > 85% of the time [1].

This success rate would not be unusual were separate neural networks trained for each problem in each discipline and if subsequent students performances were evaluated by these individual neural networks. In fact however, within each discipline, a single neural network has encapsulated successful student strategies across the 6-7 different problems composing the problem set. This suggest two distinct abilities of the trained neural networks, the ability to recognize successful strategies from problem performances, and the ability to discriminate each problem from the others in the set, even when they are quite close conceptually.

These broad capabilities suggested that neural networks trained with students' performances could provide revealing information not only about the nature of students approaches to the problems, but also about the nuances constituting various levels of expertise. To pursue these studies we have used two very different problem spaces, immunology and infectious disease.

The IMMEX::IMMUNOLOGY problem set is basic-science-oriented and students need an understanding of molecular immunology as well as knowledge of the principles of flow cytometry, RFLP, gel retardation etc. Studies of student performances on these problems reveal considerable search and the generation and discarding of alternative hypotheses. By contrast, the IMMEX::INFECTIOUS DISEASE problems are clinical and diagnostic in scope.

In this study we wanted first to determine how suitably trained neural networks would classify new students performances in these two different problem domains to determine sources of predictive error, and then to determine if such neural networks could perhaps distinguish expert from novice performances.

METHODS

The IMMEX Problem-Solving Format

The approach is based on the cognitive principles of having a starting condition (i.e. Case History), a goal condition (i.e., Diagnosis) and the access to the information needed to transit these conditions. Each problem starts with a patient history which contains sufficient information for the generation of hypotheses regarding the possible immune defect or in the case of the infectious disease problems, a process and infectious agent involved. Students performing these problems then access additional information and laboratory tests from 50-70 different menu items which can be used to verify/reject hypotheses. When they are confident of the patient's immune defect/disease process, a diagnosis can be made. The details of the software and its implementation have been described in detail [2].

During the problem solving, a transaction database records the student's selection of information, time, score, diagnosis, etc. This can be accessed by search-path mapping software which displays the students sequential requests for more information and can therefore reconstruct individual or group problem solving performances [3]. The IMMEX::ANALYSIS software also saves the test selections returned from queries made to the database and prepares them for insertion into the IMMEX::NEURAL software for generation of artificial neural networks and the classification of subsequent performances.

Construction and Training of Artificial Neural Networks with Student Performances

Multi-layer backpropagation neural networks were trained using over 400 performances of students who solved one or more of seven different problems in immunology or six problems in infectious disease. The training data for the back propagation neural networks [4] were from individual student problem solving performances which had been collected under conditions requiring students working on their own.

The input data for the neural network was derived as follows. As students progress through the problems the sequence of their test selections was recorded in the form of two-test classifying characteristics. For instance in Figure 1, the classifying characteristics would be "Start To FACS CD4/CD3", " FACS CD4/CD3 TO T-Cell Proliferation", "T Cell Proliferation TO MHC mRNA" etc. Each unique classifying characteristic of the training set constitutes an input node. In Immunology the neural network constructed consisted of 533 input neurons (one for each classifying characteristic), 40 hidden neurons, and output neurons, one for each problem in the problem set. These layers were fully interconnected by weighted links; the momentum was 0.9, the learning rate was 0.06 and the network was trained to a 0.005 sum of errors [1]. During testing, a student's test selection is presented to the neural network and the problem-specific output weights collected. The problem-specific output weights range from 0 to 1. This process is repeated for each test selection made by the student until the completion of the problem, resulting in a series of output weights for each problem which can be displayed as histograms. Successful performances are indicated by high output weights for the relevant problem and low for the other problems (Figure 1). Unsuccessful, and false negative performances are often indicated by low output weights across all problems.

For the infectious disease problems, the number of input classifying characteristics was 654, the number of hidden nodes was 20, and there were six problem specific output neurons. The learning rate and momentum were as for the immunology problems.

Collection of Expert Immunologists and Infectious Disease Internist's Performances

Two different approaches were used to collect expert problem performances. In Immunology, anonymous problem performances by experienced immunologists were collected over a 3-day period at the 1993 American Association of Immunologists meeting. Seventy-six percent of the participants held the title Assistant Professor or higher, providing an indication of the level of expertise. Of the problems completed by experts, there were 123 performances where the problem was solved and 55 instances where the diagnosis was missed. This frequency of solutions (69%) was slightly higher than that of UCLA second-year medical students under testing conditions (302/450 or 67%) this past year. While this expert performance value may seem low, consideration should be given to the fact that each student had over 10 hr. practice on similar problems and their performance during the exam would account for 50% of their total grade. Of these 178 immunologists' performances, 87 were on problems where student performances were used to train artificial neural networks. These performances constitute the testing data for this part of the study.

Expert performances on the infectious disease problems were collected from individuals holding the position of Chief Resident or higher in the Department of Medicine at UCLA or its affiliated hospitals. The frequency of solutions of the internists (81%) was slightly lower than that of UCLA second-year medical students (87%), again most likely for the reasons mentioned earlier.

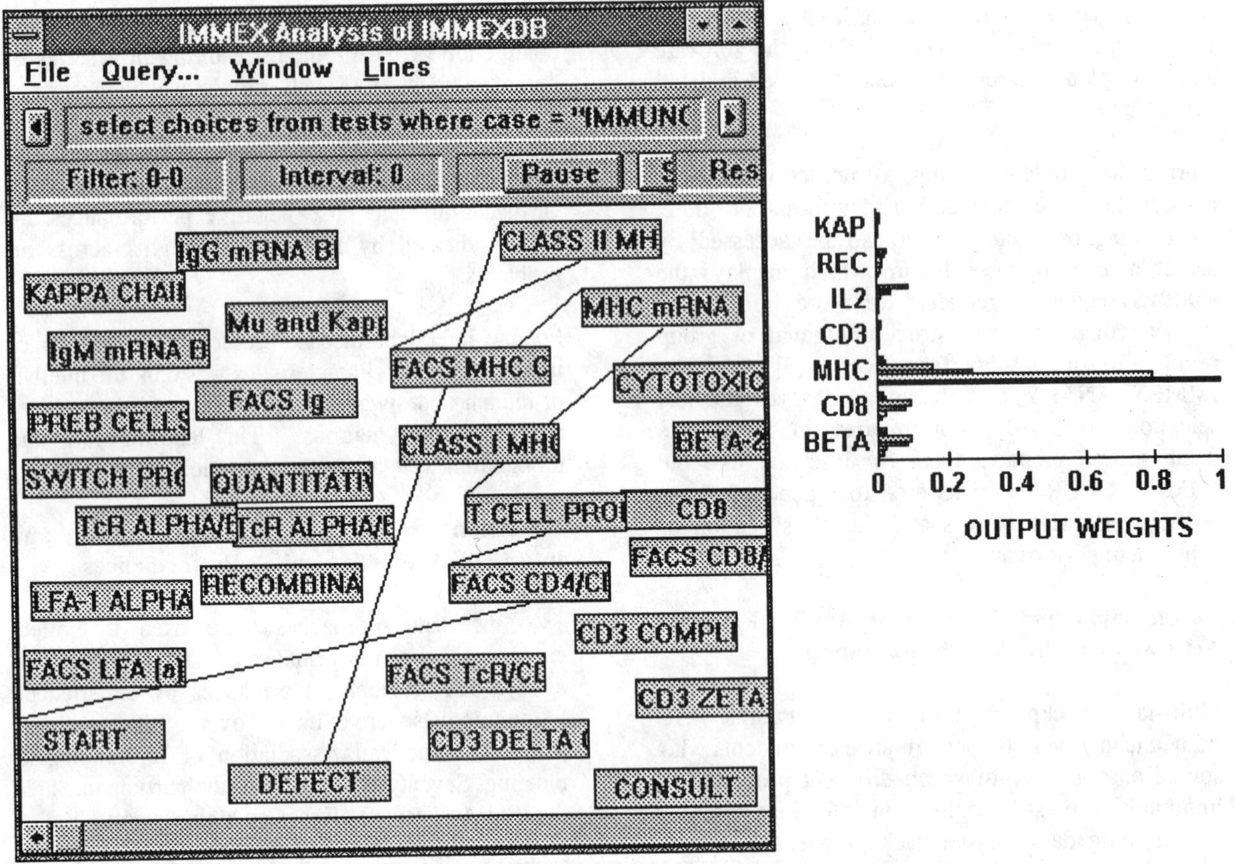

Figure 1 A Comparison of IMMEX::ANALYSIS search path mapping and IMMEX::NEURAL which provides an interpretation of the analysis output. These figures follow the progression of one student as tests were selected during solving an immunology problem. The lines connecting the boxes show the sequence of a student's tests. The histograms show the output weights returned from a trained neural network as each of these test selections were presented to the trained neural network.

RESULTS

A. Expert Immunologists' Performances

True negative performances (where the correct diagnosis was not obtained) of both the students (47/49) and immunologists (20/21) were accurately detected by the artificial neural networks trained with student performances (Table 1). The neural networks identified 33/44 (75%) true positive performances (where the diagnosis was made) of second-year UCLA medical students and 18/26 (69%) true positive performances of first-year George Washington University medical students, all of which were obtained under testing conditions. Thus subsequent student performances when presented to the trained neural networks, were correctly classified as having solved or not solved a particular problem >85% of the time. In contrast, only 23/66 (35%) of the immunologists' performances were identified by the student trained neural networks. The true positive immunologists' performances which were detected by the neural networks were not uniform across the problems but ranged from a high of 75% to a low of 13% (Table 1). The above results indicate that the sequence of actions employed by immunologists in solving the same problems are not well encapsulated by neural networks trained on students' successful problem performances.

TABLE 1

		STUDENTS' PERFORMANCE	
		TRUE +	TRUE -
NETWORK CLASSIFICATION	+	46	2
	-	17	47

		IMMUNOLOGISTS' PERFORMANCE	
		TRUE +	TRUE -
NETWORK CLASSIFICATION	+	23	1
	-	43	20

Table 1. Contingency Tables of Student and Immunologists Problem Performances as Classified by Student-Trained Artificial Neural Networks trained on IMMEX Immunology problems.
The sensitivity for the individual problems performed by the immunologists was: Bare Lymphocyte Syndrome (27%), CD3 Complex Deficiency (13%), Beta-2 Microglobulin Defect (25%), Recombinase Defect (27%), and IL-2 Promoter Defect (75%). Varying the neural network output weight decision threshold values between 0.45 and 0.65 did not produce significant differences in the above classifications. The student and immunologist distribution of true positive and false negative were significantly different (Pearson $\chi^2 = 18.46$ $P<0.0005$).

B. Infectious Disease Problems

As discussed earlier, the infectious disease simulations differ significantly from the immunology problems in that they more closely parallel the clinical diagnostic process. As such, we were as much interested in the sensitivity and specificity performance of the student trained artificial neural networks as we were in how well they would discriminate between expert and novice performances. Forty-three percent (62/144) of the student true negative performances were classified by the infectious disease trained neural network as positive. This was in direct contrast to the immunology performances and suggested an appropriate strategy was being used but an incorrect diagnosis was resulting. Visual analysis of these student performances by search path mapping using IMMEX::ANALYSIS confirmed the inability of these students to clearly distinguish between related differential diagnoses. The infectious disease internists did not have this difficulty (Table 2).

Similar to the immunology problems, the student-trained neural networks identified 176/253 (70%) of true positive performances for medical students. These same neural networks identified internists performances 61% of the time. As with the immunology basic science problems, the true positive internists' performances detected by the neural networks were not uniform across the problems but ranged from a high of 100% to a low of 17%.

CONCLUSIONS

Artificial neural networks have had a broad applicability in medical decision making [5]. Our studies extend these efforts to medical education and indicate that appropriately trained artificial neural networks may be useful tools which can be used not only for routine (and rapid) evaluation of student problem solving performances, but also which may be used to discriminate between novice and expert performances, particularly on the more difficult problems.

We are currently acquiring a sufficient number of immunologists' and infectious disease experts' problem performances to train "expert" artificial neural networks. With these networks, in an evaluation setting, student "passing" may consist not only of solving a series of problems, but by solving them with a strategy better represented in the expert neural network rather than the novice-trained neural network.

TABLE 2

		STUDENTS' PERFORMANCE	
		TRUE +	**TRUE -**
NETWORK CLASSIFICATION	+	176	62
	-	77	82

		ID INTERNISTS' PERFORMANCE	
		TRUE +	**TRUE -**
NETWORK CLASSIFICATION	+	33	3
	-	21	12

Table 1. Contingency Tables of Students' and Infectious Disease Experts' Problem Performances as Classified by Student-Trained Artificial Neural Networks.
The sensitivity for the individual problems performed by the ID experts was: Bacterial endocarditis (57%), Rheumatic Fever (100%), Listeria (57%), Disseminated M. tuberculosis (83%), M. avium intracellularae (17%) and Salmonella osteomyelitis (83%). Varying the neural network output weight decision threshold values between 0.45 and 0.65 did not produce significant differences in the above classifications.

REFERENCES

[1]. Stevens RH, Najafi K. Artificial neural networks as adjuncts for assessing medical students' problem solving performances on computer based simulations. *Computers & Biomedical Research* 1993; 26:172-187.

[2]. Stevens RH, McCoy JM, Kwak AR. Solving the problem of how medical students solve problems. *MD Computing.* 1991; 8:13-20.

[3]. Kwak AR, Stevens RH. Administering a microcomputer-based problem-solving examination. *Journal of Biological Computing* 1990;17(3):9-13.

[4]. Rumelhart D, Hinton GE, McClelland JL. *Parallel Distributed Processing*, 1, Ch. 2, The MIT Press, 1986.

[5]. Reggie, J. Neural Computation in Medicine. *Artificial Intelligence in Medicine* 1993; 5(2):143-158.

ACKNOWLEDGMENTS

Supported in part by funding from the United States Public Health Services, Bureau of Health Professions. Special thanks to Drs. Phyllis Kind, Barbara Dau and Ann Linton at GWU for providing student performances, to the immunologists who participated in the IMMEX Problem-Solving Software Workshop at the 1993 AAI meeting in Denver, and to the infectious disease experts at UCLA, the UCLA Affiliated Hospitals, and the Health Sciences Center, University of Texas at San Antoino

Benefits for Users

TOWARD A DEFINITION OF INFORMATION THERAPY

Donna J. Mitchell
Medical Informatics Fellow
University of North Texas, Denton, Texas

ABSTRACT

In these days of healthcare reform, there is an increasing need to control the costs of medical care. Preventive medical care can help by providing information to the patient, not only for illnesses, but for prevention and wellness. "Information Therapy" is a new term for supplying patients with health information, enabling them to make informed decisions about their health and care, participate in their own well-being, and thus decrease the utilization of healthcare resources. The formal definition for Information Therapy is presented and the basis for defining it lies in bibliotherapy, patient education, consumer health trends, patient's rights, and the Freedom of Information Act. The parameters and coverage of Information Therapy are discussed, the roles that Information Therapy can play in healthcare are explored, and the dual nature of its goals is presented. Barriers to its implementation are listed, however, the electronic age with its information superhighways is expected to provide a unique delivery system for Information Therapy.

INTRODUCTION

In a 1992 article in JAMA, Lindner introduced the phrase "information therapy," although she gave no formal definition for it[1]. The focus of her article concerned the use of the medical library by the public, and she stated that "every scrap of information leading patients in the direction of discovering more about their disease becomes 'information therapy' ". This paper presents as a formal definition that Information Therapy is "the therapeutic provision of information to people for the amelioration of physical and mental health and well-being." To support this definition, various aspects of information and its provision will be explored, along with the roles Information Therapy can play in healthcare, and the goals it should strive for.

THE ROOTS OF INFORMATION THERAPY

Bibliotherapy

The basis for beginning to define Information Therapy starts with a look at bibliotherapy. The term *biblio* means book, and therapy is derived from *therapeia*, which means to serve and to help medically. Sadie P. Delaney, one of the early practitioners of bibliotherapy, defined bibliotherapy in 1938 as "the treatment of a patient through selected reading"[2]. Bibliotherapy has been called "helping with books"[3], "the use of selected reading materials as therapeutic adjuvant in medicine and in psychiatry" and "the use of reading as an ameliorative adjunct to therapy"[4]. Bibliotherapy is generally regarded as directed reading with a therapeutic dialogue or interaction between the patient and a facilitator, often a librarian, who has received special training. The idea of bibliotherapy goes back to the early Greeks, who recognized the healing value of reading and placed inscriptions over their library entrances that meant "place of healing for the soul." In addition, as early as the 1800s, Dr. Benjamin Rush recommended the Bible as therapeutic reading. Just as reading can have a therapeutic benefit in bibliotherapy, the possession of information can have a therapeutic effect on mental and physical health and well-being in Information Therapy, and its definition should contain some reference to the therapeutic value of information.

Patient Education

Another aspect of Information Therapy can be derived from a look at patient education. A 1984 definition by Johnson states that patient education is "designed to assist patients to cope voluntarily with the immediate crisis response to their diagnosis, with long-term adjustments, and with symptoms; to gain needed information about sources of prevention, diagnosis, and care; and to develop needed skills, knowledge, and attitudes to maintain or regain health status."[5] Green defines health education more broadly than patient education, stating that it is "a combination of learning experiences designed to predispose, enable, and reinforce" behavior in the general public.[6] Therefore, the term 'patient education' is seen to be too restrictive, and should be replaced with the term 'Information Therapy'. Squyres makes a differentiation between health education and health information, in that, health education is designed to teach and change behavior, whereas health information is simply meant to be informing. In addition, his definition of health education encompasses both patient education for diseases and health promotion for wellness and prevention.[7] These definitions supply three central tenets that should be included in the definition of

0195–4210/94/$5.00

Information Therapy. The first idea is the provision of information, regardless of whether it is intended simply to inform or whether it is meant to change behavior. The second tenet is that Information Therapy can be centered either on the patient or directed toward the general public. Last, Information Therapy should not be limited to information directed toward a specific disease, but could also include information of a preventive nature. In this way, the aim of Information Therapy is to increase the knowledge of the general public and to create a sense of responsibility in patients for preserving and maintaining their own wellness. A key word seen in one of the definitions of patient education is enable, which also means to empower. By providing patients with information, we are enabling or empowering them to take an active role in their own healthcare. By utilizing information received through Information Therapy, people can provide some self-care and accept responsibility for their health and well-being.

Consumer Trends

The current consumer trends provide another basis for defining Information Therapy. The best seller *Megatrends*,[8] describes an increase in societal pressure for health information as people are shifting from institutional reliance to self-reliance. In order for health conscious consumers to be self-reliant, they must be provided with information. The new Information Age with its information "super highways", should provide consumers with endless access to massive amounts of health information. Also emerging is a new field, called Consumer Health Informatics, which studies the development and implementation of computer and communication systems designed to be used by consumers themselves. This growing trend of individuals who are actively seeking information about health is discussed by Ferguson [9]. The three categories of health consumers that he describes are: passive patients, concerned patients and health-active, health-responsible patients. Passive patients are individuals who feel that there is nothing they can do to manage their illness. An example of this type of consumer is the cancer patient who gives up without a fight. These patients rarely seek information about their condition, or how to manage it. Concerned patients are individuals who occasionally ask questions, but simply do whatever their doctor recommends. These patients will seek information from sources other than their doctor, but only if they feel that their physician approves. Health-active, health-responsible patients are individuals who are motivated to play active roles in their own care. They will actively seek information from a variety of sources. Ferguson states that "these are the most enthusiastic and tireless seekers of health information."(p.10) They refuse to relinquish control, and demand to play a role in the decisions that have to do with their care. He estimates that by the year 2000, one in four consumers will be active information seekers. These people will benefit most from Information Therapy.

Patient's Rights

Another basis for defining information therapy is the patient's right to be informed. Recognizing this need, the American Hospital Association developed *A Patient's Bill of Rights* in 1972. Of this list of rights, half relate to receiving information about diagnosis, prognosis, treatment, medical procedures, personnel, or the hospital itself.[10] "Informed consent" requires that patients be provided with the necessary information to make decisions about their health care and involves a written legal document verifying that the patient has received information and has had the opportunity to ask and receive answers to any questions. Hospitals are adamant about fulfilling these moral obligations, but the obligation to provide information to people should extend beyond healthcare providers, and constitutes a fundamental basis for Information Therapy.

Freedom of Information Act

The roots of Information Therapy must also lie in the Freedom of Information Act, which guarantees that people have access to information. To deny a patient health information would be a breach of this Act, and would be a limitation of their right to know. Hafner states that in democratic societies today, "it is well established that the individual, as a patient, family member, or concerned consumer, is entitled to free and unrestricted access to information."[11] Legal obligations to provide information are well established in other consumer arenas such as lending laws, and the labeling of food products, toys, and the provision of pharmaceutical information and interactions to patients. Therefore, a moral as well as legal obligation to provide health information to consumers through Information Therapy is not an unreasonable concept.

THE ROLES OF INFORMATION THERAPY

Many terms have been used for the delivery of information to a patient concerning their health: health education, health information, patient education, patient teaching, patient counselling, and now, a new term "Information Therapy". The use of these differing terms can be confusing and in some cases inappropriate. However, the term "information therapy" appears to be the most descriptive, the richest in possible meanings, and the broadest in scope. Although this term was originally and exclusively used by Lindner [1], a 1993 symposium concerning "Information Therapy" was held in New York, where the meanings and uses of information therapy were discussed, and publication of the proceedings from this symposium should help to clarify and advance this term.[12]

Brenda Dervin, a communications specialist, sees information as anything a person finds informing.[13] Individuals cope by trying to make sense of their world, and drawing upon resources available, such as what they have heard, read, seen or experienced. If these resources are inadequate, they seek additional information from other sources. The information may not be acted upon or utilized in any way, but it appears that just having the information provides people with a sense of control and power. The information provided may not need to apply to any specific disease or illness, as Lindner [1] has suggested, but may be of a general nature or may be information regarding wellness or prevention of a disease. Therefore, the scope of the term Information Therapy is expanded beyond disease-specific information, and beyond patient education. The parameters of Information Therapy should include: disease-specific information targeted toward an individual such as the causes, symptomatology, and treatments available for multiple sclerosis; health information on a general topic such as breast cancer or heart disease; or preventive health information targeted to the general public on topics such as smoking cessation, nutrition and vitamins, exercise and wellness issues. Thus, virtually any information dealing in any way with medicine, health, wellness or quality of life that can be informing, increase skills or improve the attitude of a person can be termed Information Therapy.

The coverage of Information Therapy, as should be for all information of any nature, is universal. Healthcare reform policy is concerned with universal access to healthcare, and in the same manner, Information Therapy should be accessible to every individual. Unfortunately, in the past this has not been the case, as Lindner [1] describes that she was unable to deliver information to patients because the "policy" of the medical library where she worked prevented her from giving specific information to patients without their physician's consent. The *President's Commission on Ethical Practices in Medicine* in 1982 has mandated that medical libraries be open to health consumers, and the Medical Library Association's Code of Ethics includes an ethical obligation to advocate access to information for all people.

Information Therapy is meant to increase the general public's knowledge concerning health issues, and should help to create a sense of responsibility in them for their own health. In this way, one of the roles of Information Therapy is to provide patients with informational services and support that will provide facts and decision-making assistance, which will empower them to manage their health, illness, acute or chronic disease, life-threatening situations, or a loss. The Planetree Health Resource Center, located on the San Francisco campus of California Pacific Medical Center, was founded on the belief that "access to information can empower people and help them to face health and medical challenges."[14] This Resource Center is a medical library which is open to the public and promotes individual responsibility for health through the provision of information. Armed with information, people are able to provide more self-care and to accept self-responsibility for their health and well-being. Pingree et.al. states that "for people diagnosed with life-threatening illnesses, obtaining necessary information, making effective plans and decisions, and locating sources of support can play a key role in coping with the crisis." [15]

Another important role Information Therapy can provide to people is assistance with self-care. Levin defines self-care as "an intentional behavior that a lay person takes on his or her own behalf, or on behalf of the family, friends, or community to promote health or to treat illness."[16] The practice of self-care includes a variety of activities such as: self-diagnosis based on previous experience, seeking advice from friends and family, self-medication with over-the-counter medicines and home remedies, consulting books and magazines, asking the advice of pharmacists, or consultation with a healthcare professional.[17] Ferguson [9] proposes a framework for understanding an individual's attempt at self-care and the impact information can have on self-care. This model is shown in Figure 1.

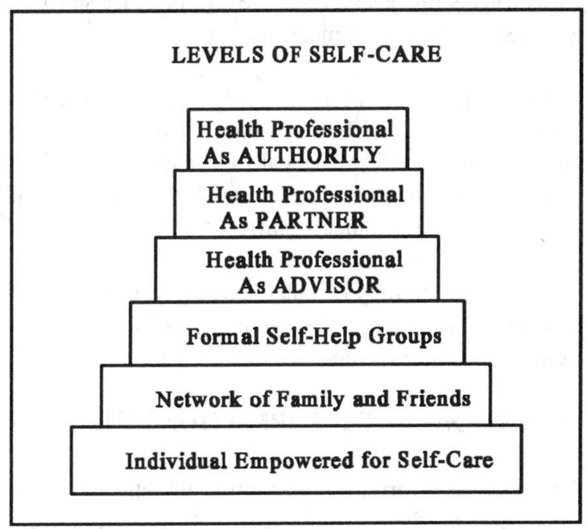

Figure 1 (adapted from Ferguson, <u>The Futurist</u>, Jan-Feb, 1992)

The first step is when individuals, before consulting a physician or other healthcare professional, conduct a search for information on how to manage on their own. They utilize self-care, therebysuccessfully dealing with health problems by providing self-therapy. The next step is when the individual utilizes information from family and friends, thereby successfully dealing with a health problem through therapy given by family members or friends. Next is the level of formal self-help groups, where groups of individuals with similar health problems administer therapy to each other. The fourth step is the initial contact the individual has with a health professional who serves only as an advisor and realizes that with the appropriate information therapy and support, patients can effectively manage their own care. The fifth step utilizes the health professional as a partner, and occurs when the patient and healthcare provider as equal partners decide on an appropriate therapy. The top level utilizes the health professional as an authority, and is when the healthcare provider is the authority who manages the therapy for the patient. According to Ferguson, this top level is appropriate in less than 0.1% of health problems. An Elliott-Binns study [18] of 1,000 patients in an English general practitioner's office concluded that 96% of patients had received advice or treatment before coming to the physician. Most health problems can be handled with therapy in the bottom two or three steps of this framework. Thus, the more Information Therapy people receive, the more active role they can play in their healthcare and can push self-care into one of the bottom levels of the model. This model is not meant to circumvent healthcare providers, but merely to empower people for self-care and free the provider for those whose care must be managed for them. By providing Information Therapy in this way, healthcare costs will decline because people will increase self-care and decrease usage of medical care.

A third role for Information Therapy is to decrease the usage of scarce healthcare resources. Kemper's meta-analysis of the effect medical self-care interventions demonstrated that self-care is in widespread use, and that its use can produce significant effects in terms of utilization of healthcare and reduction of costs.[17] Information Therapy can play a major role in assisting people with self-care, and should be a part of healthcare reform to reduce the costs of medical care.

THE GOALS OF INFORMATION THERAPY

The idea of information becoming therapy may be a new use of the term therapy. However, various departments in a healthcare setting provide therapy to patients: physical therapy, occupational therapy, speech therapy, etc. Whatever form it takes, the essential purpose of all these departments is to help the patient resume (or maintain) the normal activities of independent living. New uses of the term therapy are also seen in areas such as dance therapy, music therapy, art therapy, vitamin therapy and aroma therapy. While these uses of the term therapy may not fit our traditional definition, their intent is also to help the patient maintain normal activities, oftentimes in the absence of any disease. In this way, information is also seen to provide the patient with the means for self-care when there is an illness, self-help with decision making, and self-wellness in the area of prevention. Brown made this application of bibliotherapy, stating that "reading guidance can be regarded as bibliotherapy even though there is no physical or mental disorder requiring help."[3] Thus, information can be utilized as a therapeutic device, whether for illness or health.

The goals of Information Therapy can be separated into two categories: those that relate to the patient, and those involving medical care. The goals relating to the patient are: (1) to provide people with a sense of control; (2) to provide coping and disease management skills; (3) to improve the capacity to respond; (4) to enhance psychological as well as physiological well-being; and (5) to enable people to provide self-care. These goals, centered on the patient, are of a proactive rather than a reactive stance.

The goals of Information Therapy which apply to medical care are: (1) to enhance the doctor-patient relationship by patients being better informed; (2) to increase patient question-asking, allowing the doctor to provide information therapy; (3) to decrease usage of hospital and physician services by people utilizing self-care; and (4) to prevent costly acute and chronic complications of disease by patients' awareness and self-responsibility.

CONCLUSION

There are several barriers to the widespread use of Information Therapy that must be addressed. These include: the quality of the content of the information; liability and confidentiality issues; a person's ability to filter large amounts of information and determine its usefulness; a needs assessment as to the usability of Information Therapy, both from the patient's point of view and from the healthcare professional's view; and the cost of provision of Information Therapy, including the possibility of third-party reimbursement.

The information superhighways can provide a unique delivery system for Information Therapy. Online systems, bulletin boards, the Internet, and other systems can provide people with access to health information. In addition, the telephone can utilize information lines that are already in place, and can provide a platform for people to acquire information. More studies are needed to assess the impact of these systems in the delivery of Information Therapy.

The initial usage of the term "information therapy" by Lindner [1] has been expanded in this discussion of a definition for Information Therapy, the role Information Therapy can play in this era of healthcare reform, and the goals that Information Therapy should strive for. The formal definition presented here is that Information Therapy is "the therapeutic provision of information to people for the amelioration of physical and mental health and well-being." Thus, for physicians, medical librarians, healthcare professionals, and indeed anyone, the admonition in the title of Lindner's article[1] still resounds that we should "Encourage Information Therapy".

Reference

[1] Lindner, K. (1992) Encourage Information Therapy. Journal of the American Medical Association, 267(19), 2592.

[2] Brown, E. F. (1975) Bibliotherapy and Its Widening Applications. Metuchen, N. J.:The Scarecrow Press, Inc.p.9.

[3] Stephens, J. W. (1981) A Practical Guide in the Use and Implementation of Bibliotherapy. Great Neck, N. Y.: Todd & Honeywell, Inc.

[4] Brown, op.cit.,p. 10.

[5] Johnson, J. & Blumberg, B. (1984) A commentary on cancer patient education. Health Education Quarterly, 10, 7-18.

[6] Green, L. (1986) Prevention and Health Education. In: Last J. ed. Public Health and Preventive Medicine. 12th ed. East Norwalk, Conn: Appleton-Century-Crofts.

[7] Squyres, W. (1983) Challenges in Health Education Practice. Journal of Biocommunication, 10, 4.

[8] Naisbitt, J. (1982) Megatrends. New York: Warner.

[9] Ferguson, T. (1992,January-February) Patient, Heal Thyself. The Futurist, pp. 9-12.

[10] Fernsler, J. & Cannon, C. (1991) The Whys of Patient Education. Seminars in Oncology Nursing, 7(2), 79-86.

[11] Hafner, A. (1994) Introduction: Patient Access to Medical Information. Bulletin of the Medical Library Association, 82(1), 44-45.

[12] Mitchell, D. (1993, November) A Conceptual Model of Patient Centered "Information Therapy" in the Primary Care Setting. Proceedings of the Symposium on "Information Therapy" I. (in press) Columbia-Presbyterian Medical Center, New York City.

[13] Dervin, B., Harlock, S., Atwood, R. Garzona, C. The human side of information: an exploration in a health communication context. In: Nimmo, D., ed. Communication Yearbook 4. New Brunswick, N.J.: Transaction Books, 1980, 591-608.

[14] Cosgrove, T. (1994) Planetree health information services: public access to the health information people want. Bulletin of the Medical Library Association, 82(1), 57-63.

[15] Pingree, S., Hawkins, R., Gustafson, D., Boberg, E., Bricker, E., Wise, M., Tillotson, T. (1993) Will HIV-Positive People Use an Interactive Computer System for Information and Support? A Study of CHESS in Two Communities.Proceedings of the Seventeenth Annual Symposium on Computer Applications in Medical Care. October 30-November 3, 1993. Washington, DC.

[16] Levin, L., Katz, A., Holst, E. (1979) Self-Care in health: lay initiatives in health. New York: rodist.

[17] Kemper, D., Lorig, K. Mettler, M. (1993) The Effectiveness of Medical Self-Care Interventions: A Focus on Self-Initiated Responses to Symptoms. Patient Education and Counseling, 21, 29-39.

[18] Elliott-Binns, C. (1973) An Analysis of Lay Medicine. Journal of the Royal College of General Practitioners, 23, 255-264.

Performance Evaluation of a Distance Learning Program

D.J.Dailey*, K.R. Eno** and J.F. Brinkley**
Depts. Electrical Engineering* and Biological Structure**
University of Washington, Seattle, WA 98195

ABSTRACT

This paper presents a performance metric which uses a single number to characterize the response time for a non-deterministic client-server application operating over the Internet. When applied to a Macintosh-based distance learning application called the Digital Anatomist Browser, the metric allowed us to observe that "A typical student doing a typical mix of Browser commands on a typical data set will experience the same delay if they use a slow Macintosh on a local network or a fast Macintosh on the other side of the country accessing the data over the Internet." The methodology presented is applicable to other client-server applications that are rapidly appearing on the Internet.

INTRODUCTION

Interest in applications that access information over the Internet is growing, as demonstrated by the many browser-like implementations such as Wais, Internet Relay Chat, and Xmosaic, as well as medical applications in the areas of telemedicine, teleradiology, online access to databases, and distance learning [1]. One of the factors in the usefulness of these network based programs is the response time due to the network distance between the client and the server. This factor becomes especially important when images are transferred, because of the large file sizes.

In this paper we describe a methodology for quantifying network performance delay, and apply the methodology to a network-based application, called the Digital Anatomist Browser, that we have been developing for distance learning in anatomy [2].

During a one year experiment with the National Library of Medicine (NLM), a Browser client was placed at NLM in Bethesda, Maryland, and used to access images and other structural information stored on a server in Seattle. Measurements of the mean response time for various student actions were made and combined with the probability of the actions to produce a metric. This metric expresses the overall performance, at various network distances, as a single number. The performance evaluation methodology, developed for this experiment and presented here, is applicable not only to our own Digital Anatomist Browser, but to other wide-area applications whose operations can only be analyzed nondeterministically.

THE DIGITAL ANATOMIST BROWSER

The Digital Anatomist Browser is one module of our overall Digital Anatomist Framework, which is a client-server architecture, in which various problem-solving programs access an evolving knowledge and database of structural information.[2]

The Browser is currently used as an image-based reference atlas for neuroanatomy. Students pick from a list of subjects, each of which consists of a series of image frames, usually depicting a set of serial sections through an anatomical region of the brain. Associated with each image is a set of contours depicting active areas on the image. When the user clicks on an active area the computer displays the name of the object, as well as any textual descriptions about the object. The Browser can also quiz the student, asking him or her to point on the screen to named objects. All information utilized by the Browser is stored on the server, and is sent over the network to the client, which for this study was a Macintosh program written in Supercard.

The Browser has been used to teach neuroanatomy for several years at the University of Washington. In addition several demonstration versions have been installed at remote sites around the country. The performance results in this paper

0195-4210/94/$5.00 © 1994 AMIA, Inc.

were obtained using local clients at the University of Washington, and a remote client at the National Library of Medicine in Bethesda, Maryland.

QUANTIFICATION METHODOLOGY

The goal of the performance evaluation methodology is to develop a single number (or metric) that takes into account not only the mean delay time for various possible user actions, but also the probability that a user will choose each action. Since the particular sequence of actions taken by the user cannot be predicted in advance, and since network load will cause delay times that vary from one session to the next, the metric is presented as a probabilistic measurement over multiple sessions.

Our general approach is to estimate mean values for each of the time delay components (T_j) associated with each possible user action and from these estimate a mean total delay (T) which is our performance metric. The mean value is estimated using,

$$T = \sum_{j=1}^{M} p(a_j)T_j \tag{1}$$

where $p(a_j)$ is the probability of action j (of M possible actions), and (T_j) is the mean value for the jth delay.

The probabilities are used as weights to reflect the assumption that the overall delay should not be unduly influenced by actions that are performed only rarely, even if those actions have a long delay. The next sections describe the methodology for estimating the components of this metric.

Probabilities of Actions

The usage pattern of the Browser, in terms of the sequence and frequency of actions taken, will vary by student. Our quantification of the Browser performance is designed to represent some "typical usage." This typical usage is a probabilistic representation of the usage patterns and would not necessarily duplicate any one student's particular experience. Therefore observation of a group of students using the Browser over an extended period is an appropriate way to gather data on the usage patterns. The data set generated by such observations provides the information necessary to construct a statistical description of the actions taken by the students when using the Browser. The particular statistics needed for our performance metric are: (1) the probabilities for the actions taken by the student when using the Browser and (2) the probabilities associated with the likelihood of selecting particular images and anatomical information.

The possible actions are shown in Table 1. The probability of choosing each of these actions is based on the frequency of occurrence of each action. The frequency interpretation of the probability for the occurrence of action a_i of the N available actions each having been observed m_i times is,

$$p(a_i) = m_i / \sum_{i=1}^{N} m_i \tag{2}$$

In particular the mix of the three actions enumerated in Table 1 have probabilities for each action: (1) Choose subject $p(a_1)$, (2) Choose frame $p(a_2)$, and (3) Choose structure $p(a_3)$. These quantify the probability of students taking each of the three actions identified in Table 1 during the course of a typical session.

We approximate the probability of accessing the ith file (having size f_i) of the N files that make up the available Browser images using

$$p(f_i) \approx n_i / \sum_{i=1}^{N} n_i \tag{3}$$

where n_i is the number of times file i has been accessed in our test data set. The same approximation is used for $p(c_i)$, the probability of accessing c_i contours associated with the ith image file.

Mean Delays

Our overall performance metric combines the probabilities developed in the last section with measured quantities. To quantify the performance we need to define several observed rates and delays.

In the case of file transfer across the network, the observables are the size of the file (f_i) and the rate at which data is transferred across the network (r^f) in bytes per second. The mean file size is calculated,

$$\bar{f} = \sum_{i=1}^{N} p(f_i)f_i \tag{4}$$

and the mean rate is established by observing a number of data transfers and calculating the sample mean,

$$\bar{r}_f = \frac{1}{N}\sum_{i=1}^{N} r_i^f . \tag{5}$$

Table 1: Actions and Associated Delays

Action	Description	Associated Variables	Delay Type
a_1	**Choose subject** - This is the selection of the subject area to be considered. This is principally a dynamic type of action that has an observable network delay.	S_c	Dynamic
a_2	**Choose frame** - This is the selection of the specific image to be viewed. This action contains both static and dynamic delays delays associated with:		
	Retrieval of image information.		
	Retrieve image size and filename.	I_s	Dynamic
	Retrieve structure names associated with the contours.	t_n	Dynamic
	Retrieval of image:		
	File transfer	t_f	Dynamic
	Image retrieval overhead	I_o	Static
	Retrieval of contours:		
	Transfer shapes (xy coordinates)	t_s	Dynamic
	Contour retrieval overhead	C_o	Static
	Frame overhead	F_o	Static
a_3	**Choose structure** - This is the selection of individual structures on the anatomical slide presented. A delay is introduced by the retrieval of information about the selected structure.	G_d	Dynamic

These values $\bar{f}$ and $\bar{r}_f$ are combined to get a mean delay time,

$$t_f = \frac{\bar{f}}{\bar{r}^f}. \tag{6}$$

This presumes a linear relationship between the size of the file and the time it takes to transfer the file. Testing over a range of file sizes supports the validity of this hypothesis.

In the case of contours it is the number of contours (c_i) that is the observable to be used in constructing a metric for performance. The mean size for the contours is,

$$\bar{c} = \sum_{i=1}^{N} p(c_i)c_i. \tag{7}$$

The rates for "getting names" (r^n), and "getting shapes" (r^s), are used with the mean contour size to quantify the delays. The mean contour transfer rates are equal to the sample mean of a large number of observations,

$$\hat{r}^n = \frac{1}{N}\sum_{i=1}^{N} r_i^n \qquad \hat{r}^s = \frac{1}{N}\sum_{i=1}^{N} r_i^s. \tag{8}$$

These produce the contour related delays,

$$t_n = \frac{\bar{c}}{\bar{r}^n} \qquad t_s = \frac{\bar{c}}{\bar{r}^s}. \tag{9}$$

Static and Dynamic Delays

We divide the time delay penalty into two major categories: static delays (T^s) and dynamic delays (T^d)

$$T = T^s + T^d. \tag{10}$$

The activities that are heavily dependent on the network performance are assigned to the dynamic category, and those that depend primarily on local CPU performance are assigned to the static category. In reality each dynamic operation must have some static (local CPU) overhead in addition to the network activity but we are assuming that dynamic delays are dominated by the network performance.

Static delays

The static time delay is composed of:

1. Operating system overhead on contour retrieval (C_o) whose average value is obtained in performance tests.

2. Operating system overhead on frame acquisition (F_o) whose average value is obtained in performance tests.

3. Image overhead (I_o) whose average value is obtained in performance tests.

These delays are weighted by the probability of the "choose frame" action that initiates these functions so that,

$$T^s = (C_o + F_o + I_o)p(a_2) \tag{11}$$

is the static delay metric.

Dynamic delays

The dynamic delay is composed of:

1. The delay due to the retrieval of structure names (t_n).
2. The delay associated with the retrieval of contour outlines (t_s).
3. The delay due to image file transfers (t_f).
4. The delay in retrieving image size and filename (I_s).
5. The time to get descriptive information for the material in the current frame (G_d).
6. The time delay (S_c) introduced by the "choose subject" activity.

The dynamic delays above are weighted with the probability for the action that precipitates the delay and then summed to calculate the overall dynamic delay,

$$\begin{aligned} T^d &= (t_n + t_s + t_f + I_s)p(a_2) \\ &+ S_c p(a_1) + G_d p(a_3). \end{aligned} \tag{12}$$

The sum of the static delays (equation (11)) and dynamic delays (equation 12)) is a metric for performance. Separating the delay into static and dynamic components allows the relative effect of network delays to be quantified.

RESULTS

To demonstrate the performance metric just presented, we instrumented the Browser, and recorded the time for each of the values in table 1 for three different situations: (1) the Browser operating locally on a Macintosh Quadra, (2) the Browser operating at the NLM using a Macintosh Quadra, and (3) the Browser operating locally using an older Macintosh IIX. These three simple cases allow the trade off between CPU power and network distance to be discussed in a quantitative manner.

At the University of Washington the users were students in a neuroanatomy during one 10 week quarter. Users at NLM were NLM staff who were demonstrating the Browser at the NLM Teaching Learning Center. Because of the difference in user population the usage probabilities were obtained from the UW students and applied to the delays measured both locally and at NLM, in order more realistically simulate expected usage in a class situation at both sites.

The action probabilities are used with the file sizes and contour sizes to produce mean file and contour size values shown in equations (3) and (9). In the test data set there are 5058 accesses of images, each of which retrieved one of the 105 images available.

The numerical values for the static and dynamic delay components of the Browser as developed in the previous sections are shown in table 2. Table 2 presents the static and dynamic time delays for the individual actions unweighted by the probability of that action. The second column of table 2 indicates the action with which the delay is associated. The third column lists the values for the probability of the actions $p(a_i)$ that precipitate the delays. The static (T^S), dynamic (T^D), and overall (T) delay metric for the two sites and two CPU's are shown in bold in table 2.

For two Macintosh Quadra CPU's of essentially the same speed located at different sites on the internet the static delays (T^S) are nearly equal but the dynamic delays (T^D) are vastly different. The static delays on the slower Macintosh IIX computer are a factor of four larger than those on the faster CPU. However, the dynamic delays are also larger for the slower computer at the UW site. This is behavior is expected since it is difficult, in the case of the dynamic delays, to separate the CPU speed effect from the network performance.

DISCUSSION

The value for the overall metric provides a quantitative comparison of the performance of the Browser when operating on different platforms and at different locations. The values from Table 2 suggest that the overall performance on a slower local machine is similar to a faster CPU that uses the Internet to obtain the structural information from the other side of the country. This result demonstrated to us that the local machine configuration is very important in determining the performance delay. For that reason we recently completed a new version of the Browser, written in C rather than Supercard, that is much faster than the version evaluated in this study. We are

Table 2: Delay results

DelayType		a_i	$p(a_i)$	Location/Computer UW/Quadra	NLM/Quadra	UW/Mac IIX
Static Delays						
Contour Overhead	C_o	a_2	0.14	1.42	1.38	6.32
Frame Overhead	F_o	a_2	0.14	1.09	1.18	2.94
Image Overhead	I_o	a_2	0.14	0.46	0.80	5.45
Static Delay	T^S			**0.416**	**0.475**	**2.06**
Dynamic Delays						
Get Descriptions	G_d	a_3	0.83	0.74	1.50	1.69
Choose Subject	S_c	a_1	0.025	0.45	1.07	1.12
File Transfer	t_f	a_2	0.14	1.37	29.81	6.9
Get Names	t_n	a_2	0.14	0.34	0.48	0.48
Get Shapes	t_s	a_2	0.14	1.27	2.94	2.06
Image Setup	I_s	a_2	0.14	0.45	1.21	1.50
Dynamic Delay	T^D			**1.10**	**6.08**	**2.96**
Delay Metric	T			**1.52**	**6.55**	**4.96**

currently collecting performance data on the new version, and expect to see much smaller overall delay because of the reduced static component.

We plan to use the methodology embodied in the Browser metric to quantitatively compare Browser performance at different remote sites. A questionnaire we are developing will ask students to qualitatively rate the acceptability of the perceived delay. Correlations between these qualitative assessments and the measured metric will allow us to determine an acceptable threshold value for Browser performance. We also plan to incorporate a network model, described at last year's SCAMC [3], that will allow us to predict the Browser metric without actually installing the Browser client. Such a methodology should be very helpful in determining the potential acceptability of the Browser at remote sites, and in analyzing the tradeoff between network upgrades and faster local machines.

The same methodology is applicable to other non-deterministic client-server applications that are becoming increasingly prevalent on the Internet. The advantage of this kind of performance evaluation is that it allows the tradeoffs between network and machine upgrades to be analyzed in terms of working applications, rather than more abstract measurements such as network bandwidth.

Acknowledgments

This work was funded by National Library of Medicine Contract N01-LM-1-3506.

References

[1] E. Braun. *The Internet Directory.* Fawcett Columbine, New York, 1 edition, 1994.

[2] J.F. Brinkley, K. Eno, and J.W. Sundsten. Knowledge-based client-server approach to structural information retrieval: the digital anatomist browser. *Computer Methods and Programs in Biomedicine*, 40:131–145, 1993.

[3] D.J. Dailey, K.E. Eno, G.L. Zick, and J.F. Brinkley. A network model for wide area access to structural information. In *17th Symposium on Computer Applications in Medical Care*, pages 497–501. SCAMC, 1993.

Explaining Information Technology Use with the Usefulness Scale: A Comparison with User Age

Michael W. Kattan[1] and Dennis A. Adams[2]

[1]Departments of Urology and Information Technology, Baylor College of Medicine, Houston
[2]Department of Decision and Information Sciences, University of Houston

ABSTRACT

Understanding and predicting the use of information technology is an important problem in healthcare management. The relationships among user characteristics and information technology have generally been weak. This paper describes a recently developed scale that measures perceived usefulness of information technology. Following this description, the scale is compared with user age in ability to explain information technology use. The results suggest perceived usefulness explains a significant proportion of the variance in use ($r^2 = .13$, $p \leq 0.0001$), while age was not a significant predictor. Implications and suggestions for use of the usefulness scale are discussed.

INTRODUCTION

Many studies have examined use of medical and non-medical information technology. Generally, the purpose of these studies is to explain and/or predict voluntary use of information technology. A technology that is not used cannot be effective [1]. Explaining technology use can be excellent feedback for technology designers or can help diagnose problems with technology that are leading to poor acceptance. Predicting technology use could greatly assist information technology managers in selection among competing packages. Prediction of technology use might also benefit IS trainers by indicating the possible superiority of a particular training methodology.

Physicians have historically not used information technology in their daily routine [2-4]. While many reasons have been proposed, age of the user has received considerable attention [5,6]. However, age itself would seem to be a proxy for some underlying factor (e.g., reticence [5], lack of training). Theoretically, age is not the important factor, but a convenient measure for something that perhaps correlates with age. To attempt to measure this underlying theoretical factor, a perceived usefulness scale has been derived by Davis [7,8]. This usefulness scale is compared here with age in explaining use of information technology.

METHODS

A summary of the development of the usefulness scale is presented here, and details can be found in [7]. Based largely on the theory of reasoned action, perceived usefulness is defined as "the degree to which a person believes that using a particular technology would enhance his or her job performance." A useful technology should have a positive use-performance relationship. Initially, 14 job performance items were candidates for the usefulness scale, though rigorous psychometric analysis [7-9] suggested that 6 items were sufficient to capture the semantic content of the usefulness construct. The final usefulness scale appears in Table 1.

Table 1. Items of the Perceived Usefulness Scale

1. Using [Technology X] allows me <u>to accomplish tasks more quickly</u>.
2. Using [Technology X] enhances my <u>effectiveness</u> on the job.
3. Using [Technology X] improves my <u>job performance</u>.
4. Using [Technology X] makes <u>it easier to do my job</u>.
5. Overall, I find using [Technology X] to <u>be advantageous in my job</u>.
6. Using [Technology X] increases my <u>productivity</u>.

These items seem to capture many of the variables speculated by others [5] to affect information technology use. For example, a large amount of time required to use the technology [10] is reflected in items 1 and 6. A lack of value in using the technology [11] seems similar items 3 and 5, as well as perhaps items 2 and 4.

The usefulness scale is designed to be domain and technology independent. That is, the theory behind the scale suggests that a physician would not use medical information technology that he/she does not perceive as useful, nor would an auto mechanic use an automotive diagnostic technology that he/she does not perceive as useful. For this reason, we chose to measure perceived usefulness, age, and information technology use by individuals across a variety of industries, including healthcare. Approximately 80% of the respondents held professional to executive levels in their respective organizations. Nearly 80% were college educated. The average age of the respondents was 35.5 years; 41% of the respondents were female; and the average time with their current employer was 8.2 years. The technologies selected were voice mail (v-mail) and electronic mail (e-mail), and the particular systems used varied across and within organizations. Each respondent evaluated his or her specific v-mail and/or e-mail system (e.g., PC Eudora).

Confidential pencil-and-paper questionnaires were administered to 260 individuals across 10 organizations, and 118 questionnaires were returned, for a response rate of 45%. Given the theoretical technology independence of the usefulness scale (described above), we chose to report pooled results of the e-mail and v-mail systems, yielding 170 observations. (Of the 118 respondents, 52 used both e-mail and v-mail systems.) The usefulness items were each measured on 7-point Likert scales, ranging from "Strongly Disagree (1)" to "Strongly Agree (7)". The usefulness scale is the equally weighted sum of the six individual items. Age was self-reported in years. Use was self-reported as the sum of the number of messages sent and received on a typical day.

RESULTS

As a preliminary check of the multi-item usefulness scale, reliability was verified. Cronbach's alpha was high, at .93, indicating that respondents' scores across the usefulness items tended to covary. The individual items appear to address the same construct as scores on the individual items move together across respondents.

Separate regression analyses were performed to investigate the explanatory powers of age, perceived usefulness, and the individual items of the perceived usefulness scale. Respectively, the results appear in Figures 1, 2, and 3a-3f.

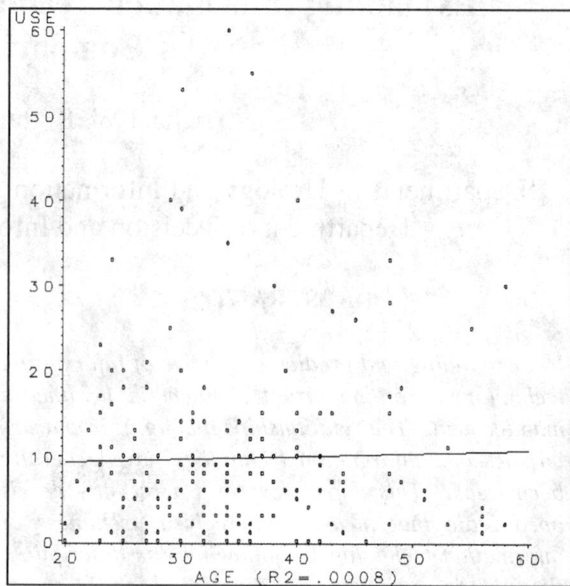

Figure 1. Use Regressed on Age

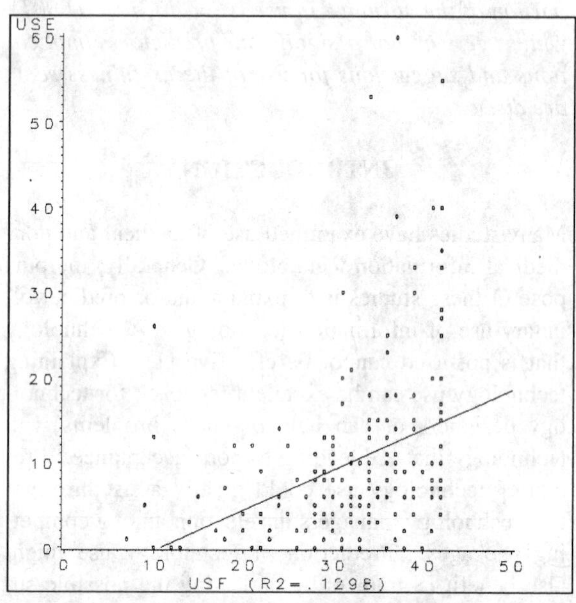

Figure 2. Use Regressed on Usefulness

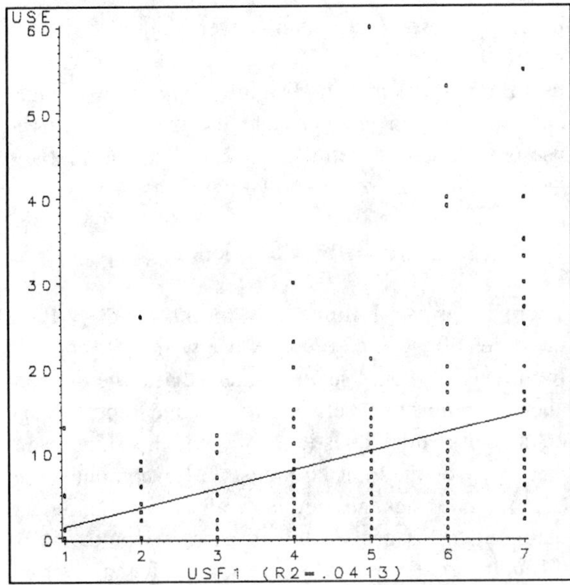

Figure 3a. Use Regressed on "Accomplish Tasks More Quickly"

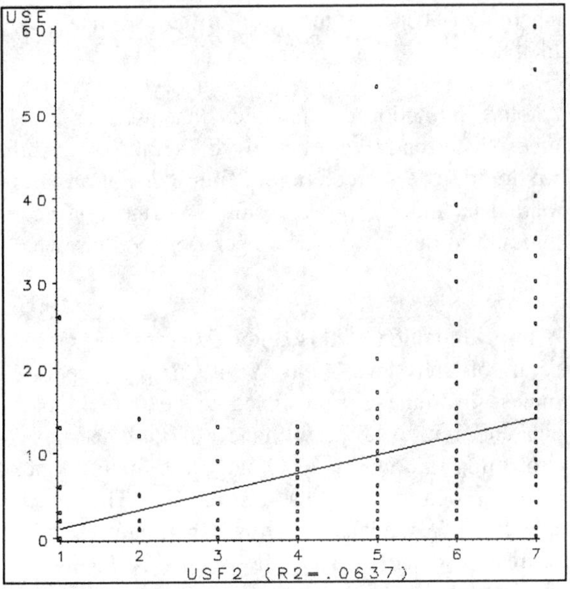

Figure 3b. Use Regressed on "Enhancing Effectiveness"

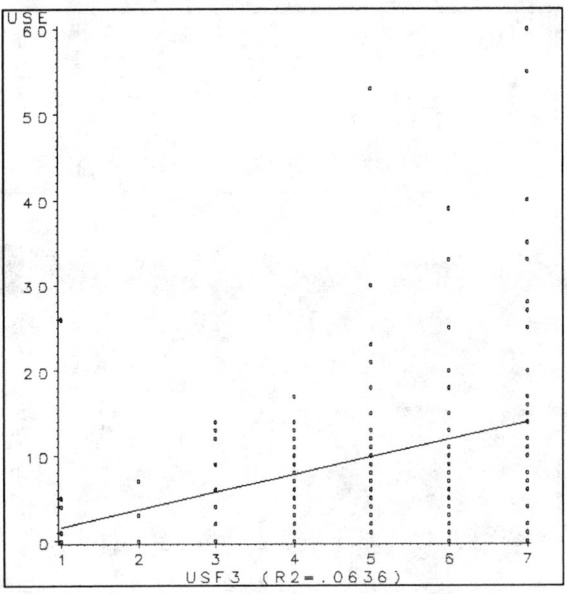

Figure 3c. Use Regressed on "Improving Job Performance

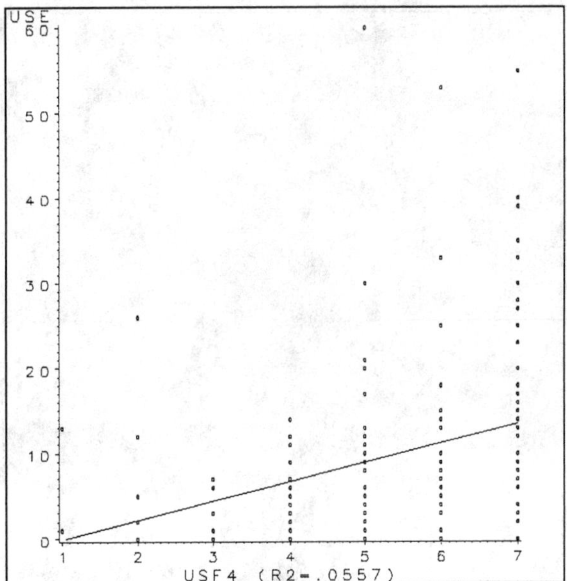

Figure 3d. Use Regressed on "Easier to do Job"

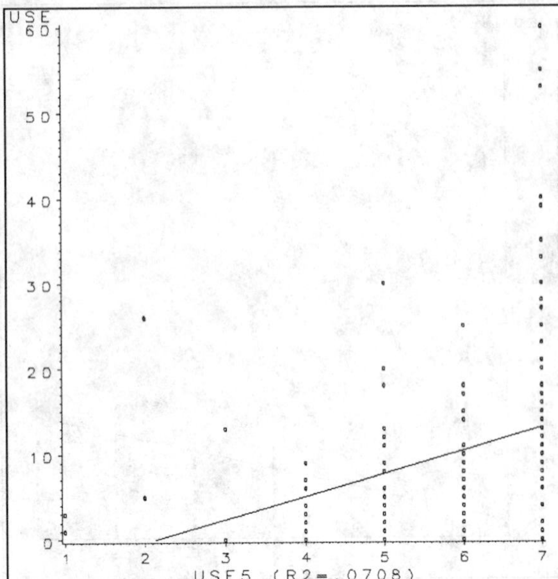

Figure 3e. Use Regressed on "Advantageous to my Job"

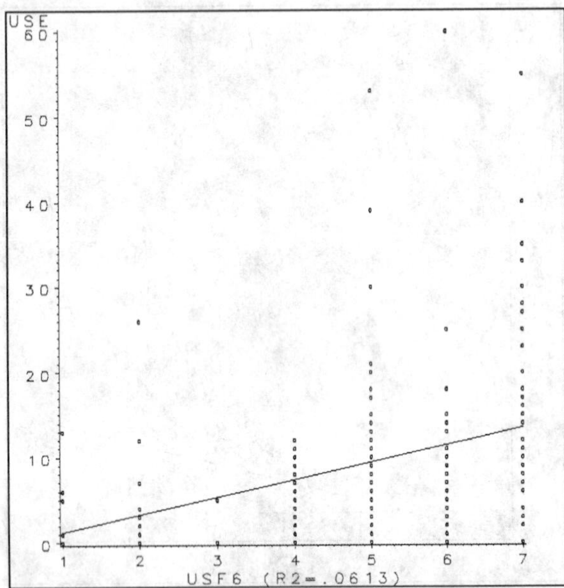

Figure 3f. Use Regressed on "Increases Productivity"

The model that regressed use on age (Figure 1) was a poor fit (p>.05). Only 0.08% of the variance in use was explained by age. In contrast, the model that regressed use on perceived usefulness (Figure 2) was significant (p≤.0001), and 13% of the variance in use was explained by usefulness. The effect of age after controlling for usefulness was examined by adding age to the regression model containing usefulness. The effect of age again was not significant (figure not shown). Regression models of use on each of the perceived usefulness items were significant (all p≤.01, Figures 3a-3f). Thus, each of the perceived usefulness items provided significantly more variance explanation than did age, and the overall perceived usefulness score seems to provide a substantially better fit than any of the individual items.

DISCUSSION

There are several limitations to this study. First, measures of age and computer use were self reported. Intuitively, it would seem unlikely that large discrepancies would arise between actual and reported age on a confidential questionnaire, but the same argument may or may not be plausible for computer use. Some e-mail packages automatically log outgoing and incoming messages, in which case it would not be difficult to determine a good estimate for an average number of messages sent and received per day. This is probably not a feature of most v-mail systems, and there is no assurance that respondents checked the e-mail logs for verification of message estimates. Therefore, at least some error in the use measure is likely.

Another limitation of this study that use was measured concurrently with perceived usefulness. While we do not assess prediction of future use of an information technology, good results with the usefulness measure in this regard have been obtained elsewhere [7].

A third limitation of this study concerns the specific nature of a physician's job. While the perceived usefulness instrument is designed to be domain independent, improved performance of the measure in explaining information technology use might be possible through tailoring the instrument. That is, the specifics of usefulness to physicians might be better addressed in the items of the scale. Such tailoring was not performed here because we were interested in assessment across industries, including healthcare.

These limitations aside, the usefulness measure did show a strong relationship with information technology use. Each of the individual items was significant, though not as strongly as was the overall usefulness measure, as would be expected with a multi-item scale [12]. The relationship for age was weak, as found previously [5]. These findings have implications for different areas of healthcare management.

The usefulness measure may be the best available predictor of subsequent computer use. This would be important information for information technology managers who must predict user load in advance of software procurement when optimal pricing might be available through volume discounts. This measure may also be useful to software trainers who desire immediate feedback on the quality of training. This measure could easily be administered following a training session, and the results would indicate training effectiveness, as users should understand the usefulness of a technology if they have been effectively trained to use the technology and understand the role of the technology within the organization. For example, trainees could be randomized into one of two training programs, and perceived usefulness could be measured following training.

The usefulness measure was shown to capture the effects of several other variables that have been speculated to be influential in explaining information technology use. Many other variables exist, and some would fall under the category of "ease of use" (e.g., prior experience [13], skills [14]). While it might be tempting to investigate the additional contribution of ease of use, previous research has suggested that ease of use explains little beyond that explained by usefulness [7, 9]. One reason offered for this is that individuals may feel that a technology is more useful once they find it easy to use. For example, as someone gets better at MEDLINE searching (ease of use increases), use of MEDLINE would help the individual work more quickly (a usefulness item). Thus, ease of use affects usefulness, which in turn affects use. Still, more research is needed to compare usefulness with other measures (e.g., Hudiburg's Computer Technology Hassles Scale [15]).

In conclusion, the usefulness scale predicts use well and may play an important role in the management of information technology. While a large degree of use of information technology remains unexplained, usefulness explains a significant portion. Refinement of the usefulness scale and a better understanding of its fundamental properties are needed Nonetheless, we believe this paper demonstrates the potential value of the perceived usefulness scale.

References

[1]. K. Mathieson. Predicting User Intentions: Comparing the Technology Acceptance Model with the Theory of Planned Behavior. Info. Sys. Res. 2:173-191.

[2]. R. Haynes, M. Ramsden, K McKibbon, C. Walker, N. Ryan. Review of Medical Education and Medical Informatics. Acad. Med. 64:207-212.

[3]. T. Massaro. Introducing Order Entry at a Major Academic Medical Center: I. Impact on Organizational Culture and Behavior. Acad. Med. 68:20-30.

[4]. J. Williamson, P. German, R. Weiss, E. Skinner, F. Bowes. Health Science Information Management and Continuing Education of Physicians. Ann. Intern. Med. 110:151-160.

[5]. P. Clayton, G. Pulver, C. Hill. Physician Use of Computers: Is Age or Value the Predominant Factor. Proceedings of the 17th SCAMC. 301-305.

[6]. E. Drayton, quoted in Inside Healthcare Computing 3(March 22, 1993):8.

[7]. F. Davis. Perceived Usefulness, Perceived Ease of Use, and User Acceptance of Information Technology. MIS Quarterly. 13:319-340.

[8]. F. Davis, R. Bagozzi, P. Warshaw. User Acceptance of Computer Technology: A Comparison of Two Theoretical Models. Mgmt. Sci. 35:982-1003.

[9]. D. Adams, R. Nelson, P. Todd. Perceived Usefulness, Ease of Use, and Usage of Information Technology: A Replication. MIS Quarterly. 16:227-247.

[10]. W. Tierney, M. Miller, J. Overhage, C. McDonald. Physician Inpatient Order Entry Writing on Microcomputer Workstations. JAMA. 269:379-383.

[11]. R. Friedman, D. Gustafson. Computers in Clinical Medicine, a Critical Review. Comput. Biomed. Res. 10:199-204.

[12]. J. Nunnally. Psychometric Theory. McGraw-Hill, New York, NY, 1978.

[13]. M. Pao, S. Grefsheim, M. Barclay, J. Woolliscroft, M. McQuillan, B. Shipman. Factors Affecting Students' Use of MEDLINE. Comput. Biomed. Res. 26:541-555.

[14]. R. Haynes, A. McKibbon, C. Walker, N. Ryan, D. Fitzgerald, M. Ramsden. Online Access to MEDLINE in Clinical Settings, A Study of Use and Usefulness. Ann. Intern. Med. 112:78-84.

[15]. R. Hudiburg. Psychology of Computer Use: VII. Measuring Technostress: Computer-Related Stress. Psych. Rep. 64:767-772.

Acknowledgment

This research was supported in part by a grant from the National Library of Medicine (1T15LM07093).

Interface for the Documentation and Compilation of a Library of Computer Models in Physiology

Richard L. Summers, MD and Jean-Pierre Montani, MD
Department of Physiology and Biophysics
University of Mississippi Medical Center
Jackson, MS 39216-4505

ABSTRACT

A software interface for the documentation and compilation of a library of computer models in physiology was developed. The interface is an interactive program built within a word processing template in order to provide ease and flexibility of documentation. A model editor within the interface directs the model builder as to standardized requirements for incorporating models into the library and provides the user with an index to the levels of documentation. The interface and accompanying library are intended to facilitate model development, preservation and distribution and will be available for public use.

INTRODUCTION

Computer models are used by both the research scientist and the educator for the study of physiological systems. Hence, there are a large number of models currently being developed in many academic institutions. These models represent the distillation of our knowledge of the dynamic functioning of biological systems and serve as a statement of hypothesis or theory [1,2]. Because of this increasing important role for computer models in the biological sciences their development and preservation now deserve special consideration. Some of these models make their way into the formal literature but many are kept within the creating institute for local use. We have found within our department an increasing need to better document and preserve the models we create in order to provide consistency to the knowledge base concerning the theoretical mechanisms of functioning of these systems. Better documentation delineates the assumptions and methods used in the development of the model or theory, whereas a systematic method of compiling these models into an organized library system allows for better distribution of available models. Since models are often built upon a common database of existing experimental evidence from the literature, this approach will hopefully prevent the continual "reinvention of the wheel" by the modeler and provide a starting point for the theorist. While a single model may look at one particular system or organ, a modeling library has the potential to allow us to compare and combine models and systems and take a more integrated view of the structure and workings of the overall organism. A similar approach has been used for the library database of the human gene map [3].

THE COMPUTER MODEL LIBRARY

The idea for a computer model library came from the necessity to better organize and document the modeling efforts within our own department. Computer modeling has been an integral part of our department beginning in the late 1950's and has been used in collaboration with experimental studies to develop hypotheses concerning the mechanisms of physiological systems [4]. Some of these models include the well known Guyton cardiovascular model [5] and HUMAN developed by Coleman [6]. Since those early beginnings, our department has developed hundreds of models of a variety of types. While some of these models are quite large, consisting of several hundred equations, many of these models are small models designed to facilitate a particular research project or to assist a student in learning. Many of these models are often lost over the years or are too poorly documented for others to

0195–4210/94/$5.00

use. The purpose of the computer model library is to provide a mechanism for preserving these models and to standardize a methodology for their documentation. This is in the hope that we might better collaborate our theoretical efforts and build upon existing ideas by using these models in computer simulation studies. This goal is in part the mission of Project 1 of our departmental Program Project Grant HL-11678 from NIH.

Standardization

In determining the best methods for standardizing documentation within the library, we considered three classes of library users. The library will first be used by established modelers as a reference point for developing more models. As noted before, models are a statement of hypothesis. Any such statement should have listed the basic assumptions used in the development of the hypothesis. Hence, the library should include a mechanism for detailing the intricate structure of the model through equations and block diagrams along with annotation as to the assumptions by which these relations were derived.

The second class of library user will include the student or novice modeler who might want to dissect and study the model and incorporate parts into new models. Therefore, it was felt that the contents of the library should be very portable and easily manipulated within the environment of today's mainstream software and word processors.

Finally, there are some users with no modeling experience who are only interested in the results of the models and their theoretical implications. The library then will be required to be dynamic and capable of easily using the models in computer simulation studies to test new ideas. We have utilized VisSIM, a commercially available simulation package and MODSIM, a simulation support software developed in our department [7,8]. However, a library by tradition has all types of books. Likewise, a computer model library should be flexible enough to hold all types of models and methods of simulation. This will help assure the greatest usefulness and prevent the alienation of a group of modelers and limit the scope of the library. These were the considerations used in the development of the software interface and led to the development of a standard set of rules for inclusion into the library.

Library rules

A set of rules for standardization were drafted and are presented in outline form.

1. Required Basic Ingredients for any accepted model.
   - a. Title Page
     - 1. Title
     - 2. Author
     - 3. Affiliation
   - b. Keywords
   - c. Abstract
   - d. Schematic of model system. VisSIM diagram or standard electrical engineering format.
   - e. Equations
     - 1. FORTRAN
     - 2. C language
     - 3. Alphanumeric
   - f. Parameter set - baseline values with units specified
   - g. References - AJP format
   - h. Compiled executable form
   - i. Optional - desired features
     - 1. References for individual equations.
     - 2. Graphical representations of model parts
     - 3. Annotation on model derivation

2. Other Library Components - accepted additions to the library

   - a. Executable forms of models where the author does not want to reveal the equations.

     Minimum requirements
     - a. Title page
     - b. Keywords
     - c. Abstract
     - d. References

   - b. Function curves of organ systems
     - a. Title page
     - b. Equation
     - c. Parameter set
     - d. References
     - e. Optional -Schematic/graphic

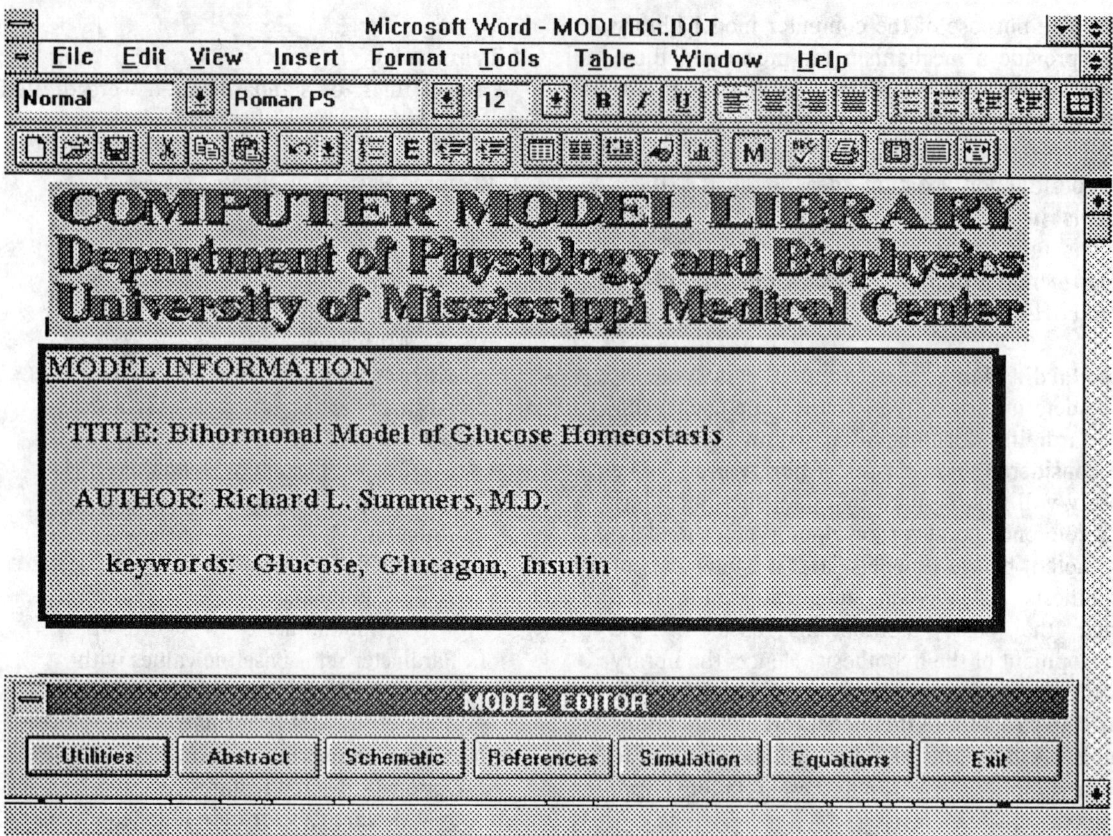

Figure 1. Model Library interface title page with Model Editor

LIBRARY INTERFACE

The software interface for the library was developed as an interactive template for Microsoft's Word for Windows. This flexible word processor allows the user to program macros within a template document using a language called WordBasic which is similar to the Visual Basic used by windows programmers [9]. The macros within the template enable the Word document to act as an interactive program with popup menus, buttons and bookmarks. These functions can be used to direct operations in the word-processing environment. Subroutines within the macros also allow the user to run Windows applications from within the document. Using these utilities, a full featured Model Editor was developed that has the flexibility of a word processor with the power of the Windows application functions. Upon execution of the Model Library icon, the interface template and model editor are installed in a window and are ready for use in model documentation (see Figure 1).

Model Editor

The functions of the Model Editor reflect the requirements stated in the library rules. Selecting a function key brings the user to the appropriate subsection of the model document and calls forth a nested set of additional function keys. Within the abstract section the user is directed to input a title, author and keywords for the model. These inputs are saved and installed in the global context of the word processor and serve as the database for indexing in our library. The equation, schematic and references subsections provide frameworks for documenting these model features with annotation windows for detailed clarification if needed. The word processing environment allows for full feature editing including transfers to and from the clipboard and importation of equations into simulation support software packages. The utilities and equation sections also provide access to graphics and calculator accessories available within Microsoft Word. Since an executable form of the model is the ultimate goal of the library, a simulation subsection is necessary. In our department the Model Editor has been programmed to shell out to either VisSim or MODSIM for simulation purposes. This feature can readily be adapted to accommodate almost any simulation support software that the user desires. It is our wish that the library be open to any type of modeling or simulation as long as the basic requirements for documentation are met.

Once the fully documented new model is saved it can exist alone as a separate template to be used at a later date.

FUTURE GOALS

At present a variety of previously developed models are being incorporated into the model library using VisSim and the present library interface. New models within the department are also being developed using the model format as outlined by the model editor. As the library expands it is our plan to develop a catalog system that uses the global variables of the keywords along with author and title information to index the library and make it more user friendly. The model library will be placed in our departmental and university network system and hopefully will be available on the Internet in the future.

CONCLUSION

As biomedical scientists increasingly use models to describe and communicate their ideas, the development of a library that can document and preserve these models will be very important. Since modeling and systems analysis in general is an integrative task, a standardized method for communicating these models is needed. This paper describes a dynamic software interface developed for a computer model library based upon a standard set of library rules. The interface is felt to be flexible and can accommodate many kinds of models. As the library is further developed it is the desire of the authors that the interface will serve as a medium for the dissemination and reception of a variety of models from within the scientific community at large. (Microsoft and VisSim are licensed trademarks) (Supported by HL-51971)

REFERENCES

1. Summers, R.L. and J-P. Montani, Computer Simulation Studies in Systemic Physiology and Pharmacology. Alternative Methods in Toxicology Book Series, Vol. 8, Editor: A.M. Goldberg, Mary Ann Liebert Inc., Publishers, New York, N.Y., pp. 479-484, 1991.

2. Summers, R.L. and J-P. Montani, Hypothesis Testing in Physiology: A Proposed Methodology Using Computer Simulation Studies. J. of Ms Acad. of Sciences, 35:49-54, 1991.

3. Miller, P.L., Ball, S., and K.K. Kidd, The Human Gene Mapping Library Database: Representational Challenges Posed by New Bioscience Technologies and by Evolving Biomedical Knowledge. Proceedings of the Thirteenth Annual SCAMC, IEEE Computer Society Press, Washington, D.C., pp. 81-84, 1989.

4. Montani, J-P., Adair, T.H., Summers, R.L., Coleman, T.G., and A.C. Guyton., Physiological Modeling and Simulation Methodology: From the Mainframe to the Microcomputer. J. of Ms. Acad. of Sci. 34:15-24, 1989.

5. Guyton, A.C., Coleman, T.G., and H.J. Granger, Circulation: Overall Regulation. Ann. Rev. Physiol. 34:13, 1972.

6. Coleman, T.G., and J.E. Randall, HUMAN - A Comprehensive Physiological Model., The Physiologist. 26:15-21, 1983.

7. VisSim User's Guide, Visual Solutions, Inc., Westford, MA, 1993.

8. Montani, J-P., Adair, T.H., Summers, R.L., Coleman, T.G., and A.C. Guyton., A Simulation Support System for Solving Large Physiological Models on Microcomputers. Int. J. of Biomedical Computing. 24:41-54, 1989.

9. Microsoft Word for Windows: User's Guide, Houghton Mifflin Company, pp. 763-787, 1990.

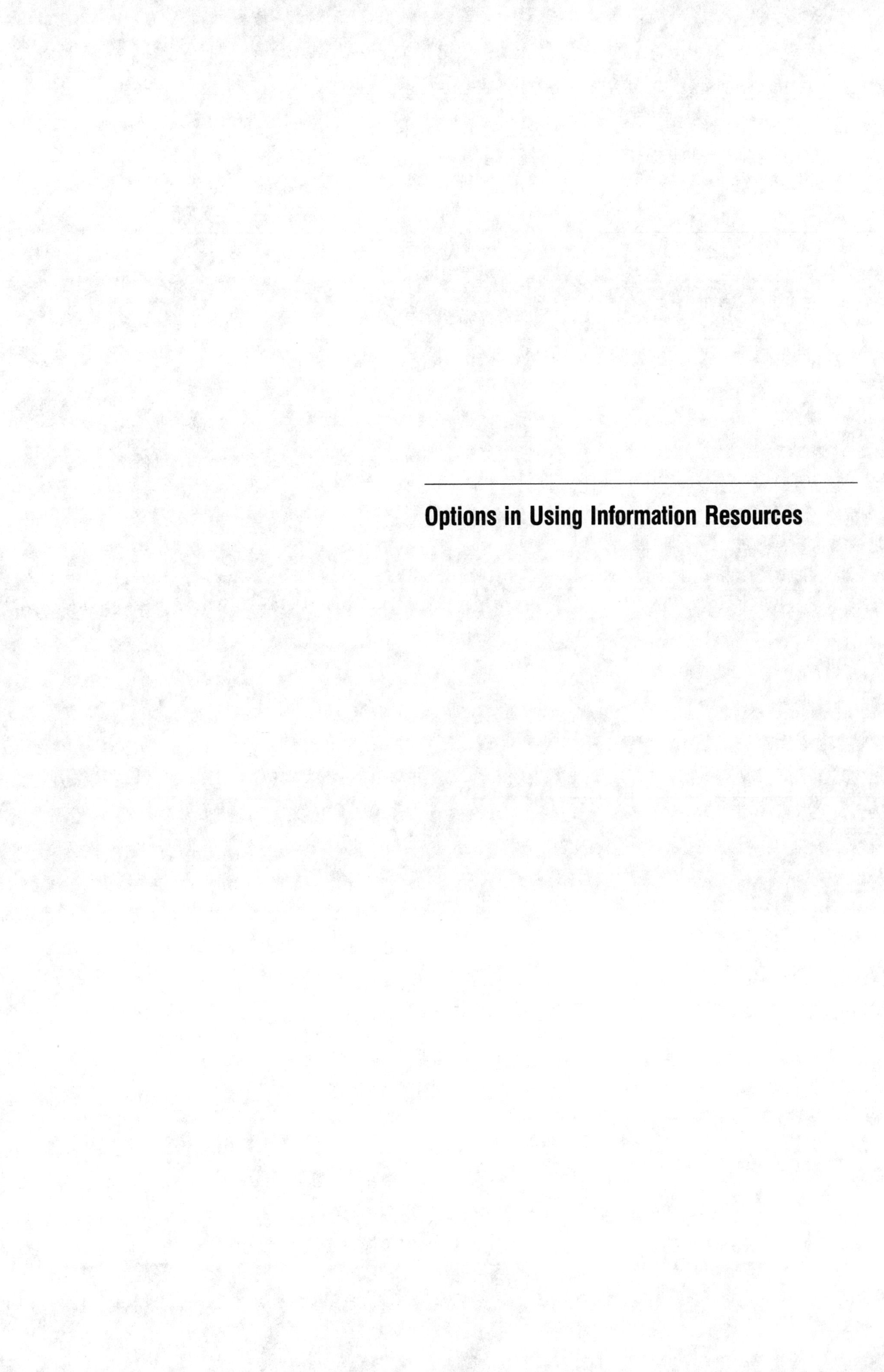

Options in Using Information Resources

Classifying and Identifying Servers for Biomedical Information Retrieval

Timothy B. Patrick, Ph.D.[1] and Gordon K. Springer, Ph.D.[2]
[1]Medical Informatics Group, University of Missouri-Columbia
[2]Department of Computer Science, University of Missouri-Columbia

Useful retrieval of biomedical information from network information sources requires methods for organized access to those information sources. This access must be organized in terms of the information content of information sources and in terms of the discovery of the network location of those information sources. We have developed an approach to providing organized access to information sources based on a scheme of hierarchical classifiers and identifiers of the servers providing access to those information sources. This approach uses MeSH tree numbers as both classifiers and identifiers of servers. MeSH tree numbers are used to indicate the information content of servers, and also as OSF/DCE server identifiers. This allows the identity and location of a server providing access to a given information source to be determined from the information classification of that information source.

A basic goal of the Medical Informatics community is the development of distributed information systems that will facilitate truly useful retrieval of biomedical information from large distributed information spaces [1],[2]. Such systems should be based on sufficiently general paradigms of information retrieval. They must, for example, treat retrieval of information from document information sources (e.g., Medline) equally with retrieval of information from computational information sources (e.g., molecular sequence analysis tools.) Such systems must also facilitate the use of combinations of information sources [3]. And above all, such systems must have a sound logical foundation that allows for systematic, organized access to information sources wherever, and whenever those information sources are available [4]. Systematic and organized access to information sources requires two types of organization. First, access to information sources must be organized in terms of the information content of information sources. Second, access to information sources must be organized in terms of the discovery of the network location of information sources.

Several very useful tools for browsing the Internet are currently available, most notably Gopher and Mosaic/World Wide Web [5]. These tools support information retrieval from large distributed information spaces. Using user menus and hyper-links, these tools support information retrieval that is organized in terms of the information content of information sources. In addition, these tools may be used to retrieve information equally from both document information sources and computational information sources. However, as currently utilized, these tools suffer from two defects. First, in order to access a specific information source, a user may be required to follow a circuitous and time-consuming path from menu to menu or hyper-link to hyper-link [6]. Second, rather than determining the network location of a server providing access to a desired information source at the time access is requested, these tools *hardcode* the network location of a server in the identifier of an information source [7]. A disadvantage of this approach is that if the network location of the server has changed, and the identifier of the information source has not been updated, an attempt to access the information source will fail.

We have developed an approach to information source access which uses standard MeSH tree numbers [8] as both hierarchical classifiers and hierarchical identifiers of the servers providing access to information sources. This approach supports organized access to information sources both in terms of their information content and in terms of the discovery of their network location. The identity of a server providing access to an information source is determined directly from the information classification of the information source. The network location of the server is determined at the time access to the information source is requested.

OVERVIEW

Our approach provides support for information retrieval from large distributed information spaces. The information space is assumed to consist of multiple possibly overlapping information domains. An information space is represented by one or more hierarchical information vocabulary trees. Information domains are represented by subtrees of the information space. We use the MeSH vocabulary trees to represent the biomedical information space and MeSH subtrees to represent particular biomedical information domains. MeSH codes are used to classify the information content of both information sources and servers providing access to information sources. The appropriate server class for a desired information source is determined from the MeSH codes used to classify the information source. The MeSH code used to classify the server is transformed to provide a server identifier. A *name service* is used to lookup the current network locations associated with the server identifier. The server instances at the reported network locations are queried for current support of the desired information source. When a positive response is received, a request to access the information source is sent to the corresponding server instance.

IMPLEMENTATION

We have implemented this approach in a client/server, distributed information system, *MUinfo* [9]. *MUinfo* is based on the Open Software Foundation/Distributed Computing Environment (OSF/DCE) [10],[11]. *MUinfo* is currently in testing with servers running on DEC Alpha and IBM RS/6000 workstations at the University of Missouri-Columbia and on an RS/6000 and the Cray Y-MP C90 at the Pittsburgh Supercomputing Center.

MUinfo

The main components of *MUinfo* are (1) an information sources database (ISDB) the entries of which describe application programs, (2) a set of utilities for processing the entries in the ISDB and for combining information sources, (3) a standard type of client and server which provide command string access to information sources, where an information source is an application program, (4) a set of intermediary servers which provide gateways to environments other than OSF/DCE, and (5) a Motif user interface. The ISDB is similar to the National Library of Medicine Information Sources Map [2], except that the ISDB entries describe application programs rather than databases. The ISDB entries include sufficient information to build command strings to access the application programs. The ISDB utilities provide a means for constructing command strings. The ISDB utilities also support the use of combinations of information sources by allowing data to be filtered from the results returned by one information source so that it may be used as input to another information source. The standard type client and server allow a constructed command string to be sent to an appropriate server in order to execute a desired application program. Such an application program may itself be a client which accesses a remote server. One example of this is a telnet script that we use to retrieve gene map information from Online Mendelian Inheritance in Man (OMIM.) The intermediary servers provide a means to access information sources that are not directly accessible by means of OSF/DCE. An example *OSF/DCE to FTP* intermediary server is described by [12].

OSF/DCE Server Identifiers

An OSF/DCE server is identified by a standard form Object Universal Unique Identifier (Object UUID) and a standard form Interface Universal Unique Identifier (Interface UUID). A UUID consists of 32 hexadecimal digits. An Object UUID and Interface UUID pair may be used to uniquely identify a server. The following is an example Object UUID and Interface UUID pair.

Object 03746500-0000-0000-dddd-08002b37598d
Interface 10000000-0000-0000-dddd-08002b37598d

Using an Object UUID and Interface UUID pair, OSF/DCE servers register themselves with the OSF/DCE *name service*. The OSF/DCE name service may be used to look up the network locations currently associated with a particular Object UUID and Interface UUID pair. A helpful discussion of the OSF/DCE name service may be found in [11].

Classification and Identification of Servers

In *MUinfo* we use the Object UUID to encode the *information domain* supported by a server and we use the Interface UUID to encode the *server type*.

Information domains are represented by MeSH subtrees. A server is classified by the MeSH tree number that is the root of the server's information domain. The Object UUID of a server is derived from the MeSH tree number used to classify the server. For example, Figure 1 depicts the derivation of the server Object UUID

Object 03746500-0000-0000-dddd-08002b37598d

A server with this Object UUID is associated with the information domain represented by the MeSH subtree

Mouth Diseases (C7.465)
Periodontal Diseases (C7.465.714)
Alveolar Bone Loss (C7.465.714.150)

A server providing access to information sources in this domain is classified with the root of the domain, i.e., *Mouth Diseases (C7.465)*. The Object UUID assigned to a server providing access to information sources in this domain is derived from the MeSH tree number *C7.465*. As shown in Figure 1, the initial portion of the Object UUID, "03746500-0000-0000", is derived from the MeSH tree number for the MeSH heading "Mouth Diseases"-- C7.465 -- with the "C" mapped to its alphabetic position, i.e., "03". The latter portion of the Object UUID, "dddd-08002b37598d", is a common UUID stub.

(1) The information domain *Mouth Diseases* is represented by the MeSH subtree

Mouth Diseases (C7.465)
Periodontal Diseases
Alveolar Bone Loss

(2) C7.465 is mapped to the UUID fragment

03746500-0000-0000

(3) The UUID fragment is concatenated with the UUID stub.

03746500-0000-0000 + dddd-08002b37598d

(4) The resulting Object UUID is

03746500-0000-0000-dddd-08002b37598d

Figure 1 Derivation of an Object UUID

Different types of servers may be associated with the same information domain. A server's Interface UUID encodes its *type* and implies the protocol that must be used to make requests of the server. For example, the protocol that must be used to make requests of a standard type *MUinfo* command string server is a particular set of OSF/DCE Remote Procedure Calls (OSF/DCE RPC.) We adopted the Interface UUID

Interface 10000000-0000-0000-dddd-08002b37598d

to represent that server type. Thus, the Object UUID and Interface UUID pair

Object 03746500-0000-0000-dddd-08002b37598d
Interface 10000000-0000-0000-dddd-08002b37598d

identifies a server that is of the *MUinfo* OSF/DCE RPC command string server type and that provides access to information sources in the information domain represented by the MeSH subtree

Mouth Diseases (C7.465)
Periodontal Diseases (C7.465.714)
Alveolar Bone Loss (C7.465.714.150)

Servers which support that same information domain but which require a different access protocol (e.g., a different set of remote procedure calls) have the same Object UUID but a different Interface UUID. In principle, even servers which require an access protocol other than OSF/DCE RPC (e.g., a Gopher server or a Mosaic/World Wide Web server) could register themselves with the OSF/DCE name service. The OSF/DCE name service could be used to lookup the network locations currently associated with such servers. The protocol implied by the server type could then be used to make requests of the server. In this way, an Object UUID and Interface UUID pair is analogous to an *unbound* URL (Uniform Resource Locator) [7]. An Object UUID and Interface UUID pair is an *unbound* URL in the sense that the network locations associated with it are determined at the time access to the corresponding server is required. Part of our current development effort is directed to building a Mosaic/World Wide Web server which is able to register itself with the OSF/DCE name service.

Organized Access to Information Sources

The *MUinfo* ISDB entries index information sources (i.e., application programs) with MeSH codes. Such indexing *locates* an information source in an information domain. The location of an information source in an information domain is used to determine the Object UUID of a server that will provide access to the information source. For example, consider an information source indexed with

Alveolar Bone Loss (C7.465.714.150)

The information source is located in the information domain represented by the MeSH subtree

Mouth Diseases (C7.465)
Periodontal Diseases (C7.465.714)
Alveolar Bone Loss (C7.465.714.150)

The root of that MeSH subtree is *Mouth Diseases (C7.465)*. A server classified with *Mouth Diseases (C7.465)* provides access to information sources located in that information domain. The Object UUID of such a server is

Object 03746500-0000-0000-dddd-08002b37598d

The initial portion of this Object UUID is constructed from the MeSH tree number "C7.465", with the "C" mapped to its alphabetic position. Given this Object UUID, and given the Interface UUID for the type of server desired, the OSF/DCE name service is used to determine the current network locations associated with that Object UUID and Interface UUID pair. The server instances at each of the reported network locations are queried for current support of the *Alveolar Bone Loss* information source. Given a positive response, a request to access the information source is sent to the corresponding server instance. In the case of the standard *MUinfo* servers, that request is a command string required to execute the *Alveolar Bone Loss* information source.

Server Hierarchies

The approach we have developed allows us to use MeSH trees to represent not only information domains, but also logical hierarchies of types of servers, where the type of server is represented by a particular Interface UUID. Each node in a MeSH tree may represent a server Object UUID. Different levels in the tree may represent different levels of server responsibility. For example, Figure 2 depicts a server hierarchy corresponding to the MeSH subtree

Mouth Diseases (C7.465)
Periodontal Diseases (C7.465.714)
Alveolar Bone Loss (C7.465.714.150)

Subject to the length constraint on UUID's, a server Object UUID is constructed from the MeSH tree number of each non-terminal node in the subtree (e.g., *Mouth Diseases* and *Periodontal Diseases*.) These UUIDs are constructed in the usual way (see Figure 1.)

Organized Searching for Information Sources

Our representation of logical hierarchies of types of servers provides a basis for organized searching for information sources. The search is organized by the information classifications of information sources. For example, suppose we are searching for an information source to provide information in the category *Alveolar Bone Loss*. Furthermore, suppose that we intend to access that information source using an *MUinfo* OSF/DCE RPC command string server, i.e., a server with Interface UUID

Interface 10000000-0000-0000-dddd-08002b37598d

Using the server hierarchy depicted in Figure 2, we could first use the DCE name service to search for a server providing access to information sources in the information domain *Periodontal Diseases*. We could search for a server with Object UUID and Interface UUID

Object 03746571-4000-0000-dddd-08002b37598d
Interface 10000000-0000-0000-dddd-08002b37598d

If a server instance were available, it could be queried for an *Alveolar Bone Loss* information source. If such a server were not available, or did not provide access to an *Alveolar Bone Loss* information source, then the next server class in the hierarchy could be processed. That is, the DCE name service could be searched for a server providing access to information sources in the information domain *Mouth Diseases*. We could search for a server with Object UUID and Interface UUID

Object 03746500-0000-0000-dddd-08002b37598d
Interface 10000000-0000-0000-dddd-08002b37598d

If such a server were available, it could be queried for an *Alveolar Bone Loss* information source.

Mouth Diseases (C7.465)
Object UUID
03746500-0000-0000-dddd-08002b37598d
Interface UUID
10000000-0000-0000-dddd-08002b37598d

Periodontal Diseases (C7.465.714)
Object UUID
03746571-4000-0000-dddd-08002b37598d
Interface UUID
10000000-0000-0000-dddd-08002b37598d

Alveolar Bone Loss (C7.465.714.150)

Figure 2 A Hierarchy of Standard *MUinfo* Servers

In the case of the standard *MUinfo* servers, such a query takes the form of a keyword search of an ISDB maintained at the server. For example, a query for an *Alveolar Bone Loss* information source takes the form of an ISDB search using the keyword *Alveolar Bone Loss*. If a matching entry is found in the server's ISDB, the ISDB entry is returned for processing by the client's ISDB utilities. A command string for the information source is constructed. The information source is accessed by sending the command string back to the server.

SUMMARY AND CONCLUSION

We have developed an approach to providing organized access to information sources both in terms of their information content and in terms of the discovery of their network locations. Our current implementation of this approach uses standard MeSH tree numbers as hierarchical classifiers and also as hierarchical identifiers of the servers providing access to information sources. This approach allows the identity and location of a server providing access to an information source to be determined from the information classification of that information source. We hypothesize that this approach may be extended to standard public vocabularies other than MeSH, and to information domains other than biomedical information domains.

Our approach allows the use of MeSH trees to represent logical hierarchies of servers. These hierarchies of servers may be systematically searched for a server providing access to an information source in a desired category.

Although the use of MeSH trees to represent logical hierarchies of servers appears promising, serious questions remain about the best way to understand those hierarchies and the relationship between the classification of servers and the classification of information sources. In particular, the extent of the responsibilities, or the scope of the content, of any given server must be determined. We must ask, for example, whether a server identified by a given node in a MeSH tree is responsible for providing access to all information sources classified by descendants of that node. In the logical extreme, this policy would require a server associated with the ultimate root of a MeSH tree to provide access to any information source classified with any node in that tree. While this policy seems to us unacceptable, the details of an acceptable, systematic alternative remain an open question.

ACKNOWLEDGEMENTS

This work was supported in part by grants LM07089 and LM05513 from the National Library of Medicine, and also by Pittsburgh Supercomputing Center grant number NCR930001P from the NIH National Center for Research Resources.

Reference

[1] Miller PL, Frawley SJ, Powsner SM, Roderer NK. Enfranchising the User for Network Exploration: The Yale Pilot UMLS Information Sources Map. In: Proceedings of the American Medical Informatics Association 1994 Spring Congress. Bethesda, MD: American Medical Informatics Association, p. 126.

[2] Masys DR, Humphreys BL. Structure and Function of the UMLS Information Sources Map. In: Lun KC, Degoulet P, Piemme TE, Reinhoff O, eds. MEDINFO 92. Amsterdam, The Netherlands: North Holland, 1992:1518-21.

[3] Lynch LA. The Client-Server Model in Information Retrieval. In: Dillon M, ed. Interfaces for Information Retrieval and Online Systems: A State of the Art. Westport, CT: Greenwood Press, 1991:301-318.

[4] Garrett JR. Digital Libraries, the Grand Challenges. EDUCOM Review, July-August 1993, pp.17-21.

[5] Obraczka K, et al. Internet Resource Discovery Services. IEEE Computer, Sept. 1993, pp. 8-22.

[6] Bowman CM, Danzig PB, Manber U, Schwartz MF. Scalable Internet Resource Discovery: Research Problems and Approaches. Comm. ACM, 37(8), pp. 98-114.

[7] Metcalfe ES, Frisse ME, Hassan SW, Schnase JL. Academic Networks: Mosaic and World Wide Web. Academic Medicine, 69(4), pp. 270-273.

[8] National Library of Medicine. Medical Subject Headings. Bethesda, MD: NLM, 1994.

[9] Patrick TB, Springer GK, Sista SM, Davison S. Methods for Shared Access to Medical Internet Information Sources. In: Proceedings of the American Medical Informatics Association 1994 Spring Congress. Bethesda, MD: American Medical Informatics Association, p. 123.

[10] Open Software Foundation (OSF). Introduction to OSF/DCE. Englewood Cliffs,NJ: Prentice-Hall, Inc., 1992.

[11] Open Software Foundation (OSF). OSF/DCE Application Development Guide. Englewood Cliffs,NJ: Prentice-Hall, Inc., 1993.

[12] Shirolkar S. Intermediary Servers. MS Thesis, Computer Science Department, University of Missouri-Columbia, 1994.

CPMCnet: An Integrated Information and Internet Resource

Robert M. Kahn, Ph.D., Pat Molholt, M.L.S., Jeff Zucker, M.A.
Office of Scholarly Resources, Health Sciences Division
Columbia University, New York, NY

The Network and Computer Systems department of the Health Sciences Library developed CPMCnet, an UNIX-based information and Internet server at Columbia-Presbyterian Medical Center. The project linked Gopher and World-Wide Web protocols as well as clients into an integrated application, providing the advantages of both. Development and use of CPMCnet has opened new channels of communication among information providers and end-users.

"...Strategic advantage is often provided by the ability to restructure through the power of electronic integration. This integration comes in several forms, integration of formerly distinct transaction processes, integration of multiple forms of data representation and knowledge, and integration of groups through communication. Such integration is enabled by two dominant properties, improved interconnection and improved, shared data access. Technology creates new integration possibilities through interconnection and shared data" [1].

Many universities and health sciences centers have embraced the concept of a campus-wide information system (CWIS) to provide "one-stop shopping" for information, and the information is often full-text as opposed to fielded data [2]. At CPMC, mission-critical full-text files were mounted in a DOS application called Folio Views. Folio Views allowed a great deal of control over hypertext links, indexing, full-text searching, and printing, but these features were only available to DOS clients [3]. While a Macintosh client was promised "down the road", the need for wider accessibility to the data prompted an assessment of other technologies.

Columbia University's Academic Information Systems unit had developed a UNIX-based CWIS called ColumbiaNet [4] that incorporated advanced features such as Kerberos-based access control and line-mode cut-and-paste. Mounting files on ColumbiaNet was considered, but having local control over the Medical Center's applications promised greater responsiveness to local needs.

Thus, the Network and Computer Systems department of the Health Sciences Library, part of the Office of Scholarly Resources at CPMC, developed a UNIX-based CWIS called CPMCnet, designed to complement ColumbiaNet and focusing on the needs of the Medical Center. CPMCnet is both a physical and a virtual repository, providing local storage for CPMC full-text data files as well as pointers to biomedical resources on the Internet. The development of CPMCnet has been an integrative effort in both the technical and the socio-political realms, incorporating multiple retrieval technologies, creating new links between departments, and merging many functions into an integrated whole.

TECHNICAL INTEGRATION

Clients and Servers

It has become clear in the last year that the client-server/distributed information model is well suited for providing both local (campus) and wide-area (Internet) information services [4]. Less clear was which server and which client to implement.

On the server side, Gopher [5] and the World-Wide Web [6] were both well established in global academic computing, both presented standard interfaces to information sources, both had powerful mechanisms for searching the Internet, and both could be combined with other important tools such as FTP, Telnet and WAIS. Gopher allowed quick and easy display of text files which could be mounted without major text processing. It also provided a very simple hierarchical menu structure that was well suited to the needs of beginning computer users. The World-Wide Web (WWW) required more effort in the realm of text processing and maintaining links between documents, but allowed greater flexibility of cross-referencing and was better suited for multimedia displays.

On the client side, line-mode clients allowed text access to users regardless of their computer brand or method of connecting to the Internet. Graphics

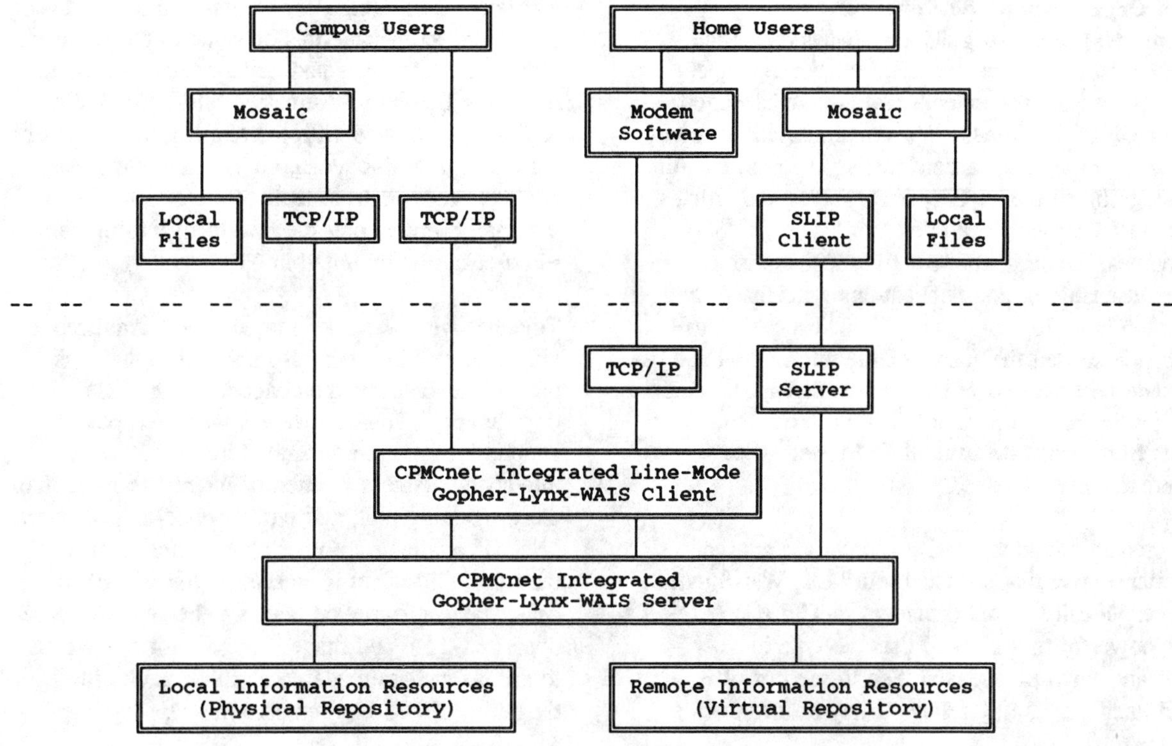

Figure 1: CPMCnet connections, clients, and servers

clients, on the other hand, required direct Internet connections, and depended on the capabilities of each individual computer: the local computer must be on the Internet, have graphics capabilities, and be among the computers for which stable clients have been released.

We decided that the richest computing environment would be obtained by combining the best of each of the available tools. Several products were introduced in 1993 that made an integrated approach viable. The University of Minnesota, developers of the original gopher protocol, introduced Gopher+ clients and servers which, among other improvements, had the ability to indirectly connect with Web clients. Gopher+ clients could recognize documents in HTML (Hypertext Markup Language) and hand these over to say, Lynx, a WWW client/server application developed at the University of Kansas. This meant that a single document directory structure could carry both Gopher-style and Web-style documents; in addition, switching between the two protocols could be carried out automatically by the software.

A second development was the introduction in 1993 of Mosaic clients for Macintosh and Windows computers. Mosaic, the World-Wide Web graphic client developed by the National Center for Supercomputer Applications (NCSA) at the University of Illinois at Urbana/Champaign, had previously only been available for X-Windows computers. Windows and Macintosh clients meant that we could extend UNIX-based multimedia capabilities to much of the campus based on the HTML protocol.

Thus, our goal for the CPMCnet client was to allow users the ability to seamlessly access hierarchical Gopher menus, a mode familiar to nearly everyone; to navigate WWW hypertext links; and to carry out robust full-text searching in both domains. To accomplish this, we customized the source code of the Gopher+ and Lynx clients. We made the keystrokes for navigation, searching, printing, and help identical in the two clients. Additionally, we incorporated WAIS full-text searching which is accessed from both the Gopher+ and Lynx portions of the integrated client. Finally, users with Mosaic or other graphics clients could use CPMCnet as a starting point to navigate multimedia applications. This will be increasingly important as we develop a graphics-rich electronic curriculum environment at CPMC [7]. (See Figure 1.)

Data Organization and Retrieval
Gopher text processing did not always create the kind of data structures we desired. For example, Gopher's menus presented a partially alphabetized list of UNIX filenames. We superimposed our own formats, propagating a standard organization for all online publications in CPMCnet. Texts and articles were listed by their full titles, not by UNIX filenames. Documents were fully alphabetized (case-insensitive), and publications were listed in reverse chronological order. We added tags onto each title so that the source of the information and the date became part of the title as displayed. This was particularly important when a search retrieved items from disparate parts of CPMCnet. (See Figure 2.)

We created a comprehensive search option at the top menu level that searched a full-text WAIS index of every locally-stored document on CPMCnet. This powerful tool allowed users to type in a Boolean search phrase, and then to see how it is distributed across a dazzling variety of information sources.

As an example, a WAIS search for the word 'renal' brought up i) the full-text of an article from P&S Medical Review on sickle cell disease; ii) abstracts of several SCAMC papers presented by Columbia University affiliates; iii) a Medical Logic Module on renal failure; and iv) sections of a CPMC Campus Profile text that reflected which departments on campus were involved in renal-related research. Because of the tags in each title mentioned earlier, a WAIS search that brought up the 'renal' articles showed which journal the articles were from as well as the date of publication.

Problems
Some problems have proved intractable for a small development group. For example, for resources that are restricted to Columbia and/or CPMC affiliates, Medical Center users still must telnet to ColumbiaNet, which has robust Kerberos-based authentication capabilities. A second problem is that widespread installation of Mosaic awaits an upgraded hardware base at the Medical Center.

SOCIO-POLITICAL INTEGRATION

Having a unified client and effective presentation format, all we needed was data! The Offices of Grants and Contracts and External Relations were early converts. Both departments had a long history of creating print materials of value to the campus. Grants and Contracts had collaborated with us in mounting Funding Information into Folio Views, and while delighted with the application, they were frustrated that Macintosh, UNIX, and VMS users couldn't access it from their office or lab. Their materials were among the first local information resources to be mounted in CPMCnet.

Together with these departments we formulated a philosophy of information stewardship that was useful in explaining the concept to other departments. The basic tenets were deceptively simple: Information generated in the course of university business is often of interest to more than the originating unit, and within guidelines, it should be made available to other appropriate units for their use; CPMCnet is an *information switching center*, and information that is to be shared can be deposited there and made available for other units to use, as well as made accessible for viewing by the entire CPMC community when appropriate.

Information Provider Agreements
Other departments came on board, and we were soon faced with telling them that their information was "in the queue". The large number of departments and information sources that provided data to CPMCnet meant that the task of processing text became complicated and time consuming; in order to handle this flow of information with limited staff, it was vital to streamline both the processing and the delivery of the text.

The first problem encountered was the diversity of software used by information providers. Materials for CPMCnet were received in a variety of different word processing packages, in desktop publishing format, in straight ASCII, in database and other software formats on Macintosh, UNIX and MS-DOS platforms. A second problem arose with the page layout and markup of each text. There was, to start, no consistency in the way chapters and sections were marked and virtually every document had a different font size and margin setup. A third problem arose with the physical delivery of information; documents were delivered via UNIX email, MS-DOS email, FTP, hand-delivered on disks, and, in a few cases, via hard-copy. To foster participation as we got started, we took information however we could get it.

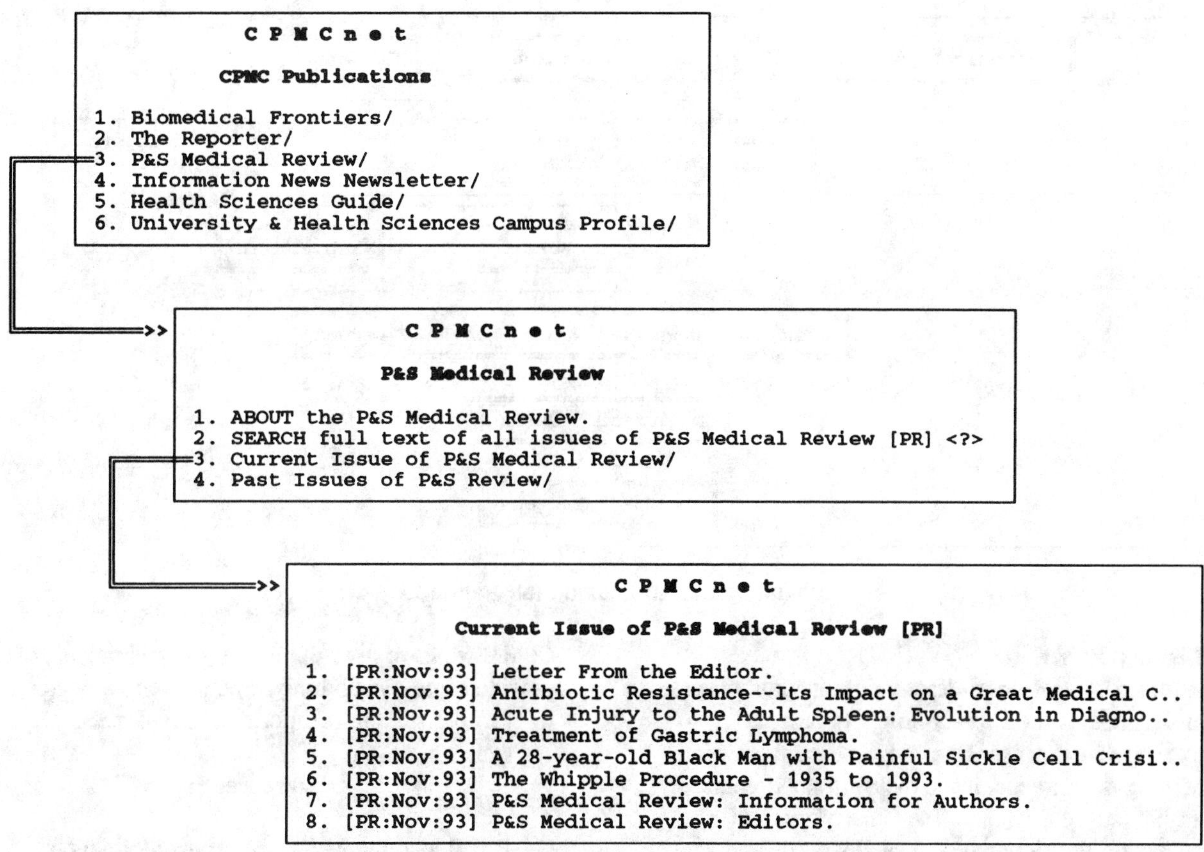

Figure 2: Integrated interface for publications on CPMCnet

In order to manage the flow of information, we developed a two-way "Information Provider Agreement" which specified the respective responsibilities of the departments that provide information and of the Office of Scholarly Resources, which manages the information. The agreement was adapted for each information source so that it was as specific as possible for each source. The finished agreement specified the software source of the information, the page layout and markup of the documents, and the timeline and method of delivery of updates. The agreements provided clear instructions for the providing department about how to prepare and deliver documents. Since each information source is slightly different, we have not created a single monolithic agreement which all must abide by, rather we customize the agreement for each source. This does mean that each source involves a development process unique to itself; however, once the initial development has taken place, future updates can remain consistent and require less development effort.

New Lines of Communication

Another kind of integration was provided by feedback options distributed throughout the CPMCnet menus. Users could quickly send comments and questions to the CPMCnet developers or suggest new information sources. More importantly, patrons could quickly send questions or comments to the diverse and geographically dispersed providers of the information, crossing barriers of buildings, elevators, streets, and departments. To facilitate this, all full-text sources have an 'About' file that describes who is responsible for maintaining the information. Several departments asked us to incorporate "feedback" options in their menus. (See Figure 3.)

When navigating resources beyond CPMC, the user was often unaware of where the information resided. We decided that references to the origin of a data file should be provided on the menus in order to clarify the notion of responsibility for information and/or for its presentation or format.

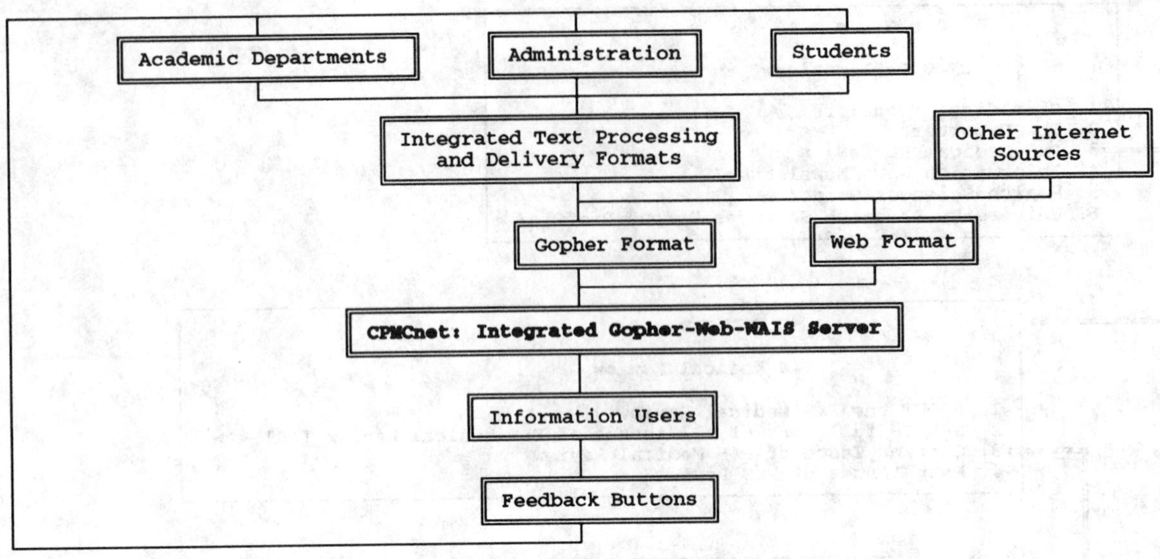

Figure 3: The information integration loop

Library Expertise
Another kind of cross-department integration can be anticipated as the Library brings to bear its expertise in end-user searching and cataloging, helping departments make their information more usable and retrievable. The Library's role in collection development and cataloging is seen as key to providing sensible and navigable pathways to the mass of information on the information superhighway. It is possible to organize the menus by subject area, by geographic location, and so on. Librarians, who routinely work with end users, already understand how information is sought and used by CPMC faculty and students. Translating this into the provision of electronic pathways simply uses the skills of librarians in new ways.

CONCLUSION

"The link between information and influence has often been noted; data are a political resource and building a database is often a political act" [8].

This rather telling quote makes clear that multiple agendas sometimes conflict. As we work to integrate information across administrative departments and academic units, to form new collaborative relationships between the library, its network and computer division, and the rest of the campus, and to move the academic enterprise forward in its rational and productive use of information, the road is not totally smooth. At CPMC we have used the notion of integration to provide some overarching principles and a degree of logic to the sharing of information resources.

References

[1]. R.I. Benjamin, M.S.S. Morton. Information technology. *INTERFACES*, 18:3, May-Jun 1988, 97.
[2]. J.J. Branin, G. D'Elia, T.W. Shaughnessy. Implementing an integrated information center in an academic setting: Research in progress. *Proceedings of the 56th Annual Meeting of the American Society for Information Science*, 30, Oct 1993, 217-220.
[3]. J. Zucker, R.M. Kahn, N. Narayanan. Clinical, scholarly, and campus information hypertext tools at Columbia-Presbyterian Medical Center. *Proceedings of the 17th Annual Symposium on Computer Applications in Medical Care*, Oct 1993, 539-543.
[4]. Campus computing environment: Columbia Univ. *CAUSE/EFFECT*, 16:2, Summer 1993, 34-37.
[5]. F. Anklesaria, et. al. The Internet Gopher protocol. *Internet RFC 1436*, March 1993.
[6]. T.J. Berners-Lee, R. Cailliau, J-F Groff, B. Pollermann. World-Wide Web: The information universe. *Electronic Networking: Research, Applications and Policy*, Spring 1992, 52-58.
[7]. P. Molholt. Integrating libraries into the curriculum: The CHIPS project. *Emerging Communities: Integrating Networked Information into Libry. Svcs.*, Ann P. Bishop (ed), 1994, 275-84.
[8]. P.G.W. Keen. Communications in the 21st century: Telecommunications and business policy. *Organizational Dynamics*, 10:2, Autumn 1981, 65`.

OncoLink: A Multimedia Oncology Information Resource on the Internet

E. Loren Buhle, Jr. Ph.D., Joel W. Goldwein, M.D., Ivor Benjamin, M.D.
University of Pennsylvania School of Medicine, Philadelphia, PA

ABSTRACT

This paper describes OncoLink, the first multimedia World-Wide-Web (WWW) and gopher server focusing on cancer information for both the health care professional and the patient. OncoLink provides an internetworked hypertext and multimedia resource linking people, computers and information together in an easy to use fashion. Our objective in developing OncoLink is to provide comprehensive and timely information about many aspects of oncology for both patients and healthcare providers.

Specifically, OncoLink's purposes are: (1) the rapid dissemination of information relevant to treatment of cancer and concomitant problems; (2) education of health care personnel (at all levels) in the field; (3) education of patients and families of patients who have cancer; (4) posting of clinical trials and eligibility criteria; (5) the rapid collection and dissemination of quality, peer-reviewed information pertinent to oncology in general and specific subspecialities; (6) provide a well-organized, frequently updated hypertext system to access other quality cancer information resources on the Internet. OncoLink attempts to provide one-stop shopping for the patient, healthcare provider, researcher or Internet browser searching for cancer-related information.

Since its inception on March 7, 1994, OncoLink has averaged more than 36,000 accesses per month from around the world. While also accessible by text-based gopher servers, preliminary observations infer increased use of multimedia and hypertext documents over traditional text-only resources. From the large following of users, it is clear that electronic dissemination of high quality, peer-reviewed cancer information is very popular.

We conclude OncoLink is both useful and has wide interest in the international community. We believe, in the future, such systems will become common media for the international dissemination of cancer and other medical information.

INTRODUCTION

The Internet is a global computer network that facilitates educational, corporate, government and private communications throughout the world. Currently, there are an estimated 20 million users, with many more with potential access. One of the components on the Internet is World-Wide-Web

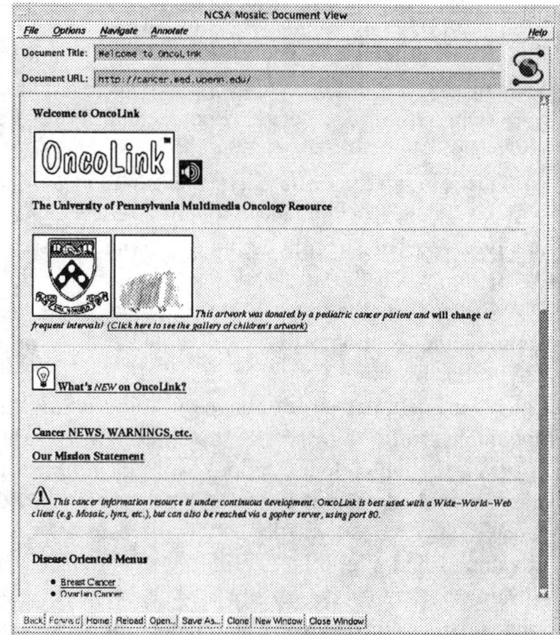

Figure 1 - Top of OncoLink's home page.

(WWW) servers[1,6], providing a mechanism for the distribution and navigation through multimedia information.

World-Wide-Web clients, such as the public domain browser Mosaic, allow users to easily navigate information available on the Internet. Mosaic is an ongoing software project of the National Center for Supercomputing Applications (NCSA) at the University of Illinois. One of their goals is to implement the emerging standards that unify the various Internet data browsing and retrieval services (Wide Area Information Server (WAIS), gopher, Archie, WWW, etc.) as they are developed by the Internet Engineering Task Force (IETF). The NCSA calls Mosaic a "networked information system for wide area distributed asynchronous collaboration and hypermedia-based information discovery and retrieval." After installing the WWW client, such as Mosaic, it is fairly trivial to browse audio, graphic images, and video, as well as make use of hypertext links between information resources. The hypertext elements are activated by a simple point-and-click on underlined "key" portions of the displayed text or images, causing Mosaic to retrieve the related document and display it.

WWW software is based on three primary

components: Hypertext Markup Language (HTML), Hypertext Transport Protocol (HTTP) and Uniform Resource Locator (URL). Both HTML and HTTP are drafts, not yet officially published as part of the Internet Request for Comments (RFC) process.

The Hypertext Markup Language (HTML) is a non-proprietary document tagging language based on the International Standard 8879:1986 Standard Generalized Markup Language (SGML). HTML allows an author to structure a document with several levels of headings, graphics and typographical emphasis, indicating where hypertext anchors or links will be placed. The author also specifies how the link is resolved -- where to find the image, sound, movie or document when the user chooses to follow the link. HTML supports the inclusion of graphical, video and audio elements into the document, either "inline" or as a hypertext resource. Currently, only GIF and X-bitmap images are supported for images residing within the document (*inline graphics)*, but through separate programs called Helpers, various types of multimedia files -- such as QuickTime, MPEG movies, JPEG images, and AU audio files can be accessed. NCSA developed and supports X Window, Macintosh, and Window client versions of Mosaic. Others have contributed World-Wide-Web clients for NextStep, VMS, and DESQview/X, and non graphical terminal screen windows (e.g.Lynx, www).

Hypertext Transport Protocol (HTTP) is a relatively simple data communications protocol designed for speedy transport of text files, graphics and the like over wide-area networks. The heart of the World-Wide-Web is the server, which commonly is the HTTPD, or Hypertext Transport Protocol Daemon. Other WWW servers include GN [3] and the Perl implementation, Plexus. Microsoft Windows NT WWW servers are under development in several locations [2]. HTTP runs on top of TCP and maps each request to a TCP connection (default TCP port of 80).

The third component of WWW is the concept of the Uniform Resource Locator (URL), sometimes called the Universal Resource Locator or Unified Resource Locator. The URL provides a standardized specification for objects or resources on a network. The URL allows both document retrieval and full-text search operations as an HTTP object. HTTP objects are identified by the HTTP protocol type, the corresponding server's name, and the path name to the file where the objects' contents reside. Parts or subsections of a document can also be specified. If a search operation is requested, the URL or HTTP object identifier carries the set of specified keywords instead of the path name.

An example of a URL for obtaining a document containing an inline image is the following: "http://www.mit.edu:8001/usa.html" will connect to the WWW at MIT via port 8001 and obtain the file usa.html, a weather map of the United States. The first part of this URL is the protocol specification, in this cast is "http". The second part of the URL is the name of the host where the resource resides. If there is a colon after the resource name, this is the particular port to be used to access the file following the final "/". The port number may be optional. Other URL protocols include telnet, File Transfer Protocol (FTP), WAIS, gopher[4], and Network News Transport Protocol (NNTP). Depending on the protocol other pieces of a URL may be optional.

MATERIALS AND METHODS

The WWW server GN software [3] was implemented on an existing DEC 3000-800 computer running Digital Equipment Corporation's implementation of the OSF/1 operating system. The GN server allows rapid dissemination of both hypertext and plain-text information to both WWW and gopher clients, respectively. The GN server software was selected on the basis of its simplicity of design, efficiency of serving documents to both the WWW and gopher clients, and the security it afforded the server.

OncoLink is accessed at no charge by WWW clients via the URL: http://cancer.med.upenn.edu/. Gopher clients can access OncoLink by pointing to cancer.med.upenn.edu. The security offered by the GN server software is due to tight control of server behavior by allowing only the behavior specified in a menu file. While this menu file is cached to provide speedy service, no externally suggested documents or actions are supported if they are not explicitly stated in this menu. This arrangement tightly controls the behavior of the WWW server and appears to preserve the integrity of the computer and its resources.

OncoLink's top level menus are divided into four general categories: (1) disease sites (e.g. Breast Cancer, Ovarian Cancer), (2) medical specialty (e.g. Pediatric Oncology, Gynecologic Oncology), (3) news items (e.g. What's New, Public Announcements, etc.), and (4) links to other cancer-related resources on the Internet. Extensive hypertext links between the documents contained within OncoLink and documents contained elsewhere on the Internet enhance the navigational value of WWW in seeking information. The user may start in a promising document and follow hypertext links to other documents by merely clicking on the hypertext keys, focusing their attention on seeking specific information and not concerning themselves with logistics of accessing documents.

In order to track usage patterns, a detailed log

of all accesses to OncoLink is recorded. The log contains the Internet name, resource requested, and the time of the request for each OncoLink access. This log is a very important and powerful aspect of information publishing via the Internet, providing a passive feedback to OncoLink's authors and maintainers. In addition to furnishing an insight to OncoLink's most popular resources, the time between hypertext key requests and the path between the selection of one key and the next hypertext key gives an insight to the information sought, what portions the documents were viewed and how long the requester spent on each section of a document. By examining the interchange between the WWW client and OncoLink, as well as the gopher client and OncoLink, this log also revealed how many requests were from (a) graphical WWW clients, (b) text-based hypertext capable WWW clients and (c) gopher clients. This detailed tracking information is invaluable in assessing OncoLink's use.

We define an access as a specific request for a document or resource within OncoLink. A gopher client requests a minimal number of OncoLink resources (ie. one access per document), while a multimedia WWW client such as Mosaic, may request five or six items to download a document containing four or five inline images (i.e. one for the document, and additional accesses for each inline image or icon). Since these accesses are logged only with the Internet name of the WWW or gopher client (and not the specific user), we cannot further quantitate the actual number of individuals using OncoLink. Like a scientific journal subscription, a single copy of journal to a library may be read by many people while a single copy of a journal to an individual is read by only a few people. In the case of commercial services like America OnLine, the usage is represented by 2-3 addresses accessing extensive portions of OncoLink with great frequency.

RESULTS

OncoLink was released on the Internet as a WWW and gopher server in the evening of March 7, 1994. Between March and July 31, 1994, a total of 233,784 accesses were recorded from more than 62 identifiable countries around the world. Approximately 80% of these access were from WWW clients. On a month by month analysis, March yielded 34,972 accesses, increasing steadily to 63,956 access in July of 1994. The average weekday access rate is generally three times heavier than weekend use. Within a given day, OncoLink is accessed heaviest between 8am to 11pm EST, though use between 1-6am EST typically is typically heaviest from Australia, New Zealand, and Japan, reflecting their working hours.

From the Internet names, we have determined the scope of OncoLink users to be international, with accesses from countries originate from essentially all settled continents., even if English is not the primary language of the country (e.g. Japan, Germany, Poland, Israel, Brazil, etc.). OncoLink has only been advertised in the electronic environment, with minimal conventional print-media announcements.

Gopher access could be discerned by the selection of the non-HTML files. In the early days of OncoLink, the cancer resources served by gopher and WWW were essentially identical, the gopher resources lacking only the multimedia and the hypertext. As OncoLink developed, the gopher menus were extended to allow access to contents formerly only available within the hypertext keys of HTML documents. Documents such as the "Pediatric Oncology Case of the Month" progressed in a more non-linear direction, requiring access to hypertext keys to access the treatment given, etc. While still represented in the classical linear or sequential fashion present in the printed literature (i.e. the entire document is laid out in a chronological sequence), the hypertext documents such as the "Case of the Month" remains the most popularly requested document.

When the HTML files are selected, inline images were sent to the multimedia capable WWW clients. WWW clients operating in a text-mode do not request the inline images, allowing our discrimination of multimedia and text-only WWW clients. Approximately one third of the WWW clients accessing OncoLink appear to be text-only clients. This is reflected by their predominate selection of non-image based hypertext keys.

The choice of image based hypertext keys, existing as small icons of what was to follow, appeared to be more popular than a text-based keys. In the March "Case of the Month", the diagnostic pathology and radiology used pictorial icons of the resource contained in the hypertext keys. These icons were selected much more frequently than when the hypertext key was the text: "a CT reveals...". This observation was made on only two case studies and does not take into account the newness of OncoLink, the novelty of icons in an image, the interest of the case to the reader, etc. Further study is necessary to evaluate the correlation of pictorial hypertext keys versus text-based hypertext keys and use.

Large documents were subdivided to allow the user to read the document in a non-linear or arbitrary order. This subdivision was performed for both gopher and WWW services. While this was originally done to allow certain subdivisions of a document, such as "Coping with Survival" to be the hypertext destination of other HTML documents, we observed most users read the documents in a non-linear fashion. For larger documents (e.g. >30 printed pages), the user frequently viewed approximately 10% of the document before selecting another OncoLink hypertext key (sending the user to a different part of the same document or another document). Tracing the hypertext pathway of a user's session revealed a focus on acquiring particular information. Users proceeded through the disease oriented documents, navigating through the chemotherapy agents used for the particular disease, searching the support lists for groups relevant to the particular disease, etc. Qualitatively, we believe that increasing the number of hypertext links to documents contained elsewhere on OncoLink increased their frequency of being viewed. Documents accessed only by descending through several menus appeared to be accessed less frequently than documents at a similar menu hierarchy containing many hypertext links. This observation is very preliminary and must be taken only in a qualitative sense. This observation appears to reflect the greater ease of navigation using hypertext links, versus the requirement of choosing relevant documents from a menu.

In late May, OncoLink won the international award for "Best of the Web'94" in the Professional Services division, clearly setting the pace for future World-Wide-Web development.

DISCUSSION

OncoLink was originally constructed around the medical specialties of pediatric oncology, radiation oncology, medical oncology, surgical oncology, medical physics, psycho social support and other resources. These subjects reflected the expertise of two co-Founders at the University of Pennsylvania Cancer Center (ELB and JWG). Gynecologic Oncology was added as the result of a strong contributing interest from another member of the Cancer Center (IB). Within the Pediatric Oncology menu, several submenus appeared, including a "Case of the Month", medical manuscripts, surveys (e.g. Pediatric Radiation Oncology Sedation Survey, Cancer Survivor Survey), and teaching files for instruction in pediatric oncology. Hypertext links to other documents, such as specific keys to documents discussing side-effects of chemotherapy, were liberally placed throughout these documents to enhance the navigational value of WWW in seeking information. This forum also provides the opportunity for education and wide distribution of "rare" entities, such as the short movie clip of opsoclonus, a fairly rare condition seen only in large medical centers. Nonetheless, physicians are still expected to recognize this condition.

While this model using medical specialties appeared to suit the academic community well, patients and other users of OncoLink informally requested (via email) a disease oriented approach. The contents of the disease oriented menus, such as breast cancer, were rapidly assembled from existing resources present in medical, surgical and radiation oncology sections.

The issue of presentation and navigation through the immense quantity of information regarding cancer make resources like OncoLink valuable. Despite large amounts of journals, pamphlets, etc. on cancer, patients and physicians alike comment on the difficulty in accessing and understanding this information. Printed information may be outdated and thus no longer reflect current practice. In addition to providing original material, OncoLink functions as a lens to focus the bewildering array of cancer-related Internet resources for the information browser. The benefits for patients and healthcare providers of being able to easily access timely and detailed cancer-related information via a multimedia point-and-click interface is formidable.

The selection and placement of information on OncoLink was largely a function of the interests and expertise of its founders. Currently, OncoLink material is solicited for original publication on OncoLink either from within the University of Pennsylvania or from outside authorities. Other sources of OncoLink material include information reprinted (with written permission) from other sources, reports from cancer and medical agencies (e.g. FDA, CDC, etc.), and unsolicited material of interest to the OncoLink audience. All material is peer reviewed prior to release on OncoLink.

While electronic dissemination of cancer information has advantages in both speed and the ability to navigate through immense quantities of information, OncoLink is only as good as the quality and timeliness of information it contains. Peer review has worked well in the areas for the limited number of specialties covered to date. Rapid peer review of the contents of OncoLink is critical. In cases where there is controversy, we believe the controversy should be noted and the cogent aspects of each side presented in a fair fashion. We are in the process of establishing an editorial board of experts in a wide-variety of cancer-related disciplines. This will broaden the appeal and usefulness of OncoLink to patients and healthcare providers.

To our knowledge, there are only a handful of resources devoted to cancer on the Internet: the National Cancer Institute's PDQ gopher (helix.nih.gov) and the gopher at the M.D. Anderson Cancer Center (utmdacc.utgh.tmc.edu) (see [8] for a review of online resouces). While there will certainly be more gopher servers providing detailed cancer information in the future, we believe gopher severs are hampered by their inability to present multimedia information and provide hypertext navigation through the potentially vast quantities of information available on cancer. WWW servers devoted to a particular topic currently seem to be developing along lines following the discipline of Diagnostic Radiology[7]. However, most WWW servers located at major medical centers devote most of their resources to information pertaining to the facility, academic programs of the facility and the research pursuits of their faculty. Very few WWW servers are devoted to particular topics of broad interest to the international population, a feature that makes OncoLink stand out among the rapidly increasing number of WWW participants.

Electronic manuscripts must be recognized modes of publication, akin to publication in conventional peer reviewed journals. While issues such as copyright clearly must be addressed [5], the ability to rapidly communicate cancer information to a wide population in a easily navigated fashion addresses many of the problems of cost, storage and timeliness in conventional medical libraries.

CONCLUSION

OncoLink is a electronic library of cancer information potentially available to millions of people throughout the world. OncoLink addresses physicians, health care personnel, patients and their supporters on both medical and non-medical issues related to cancer. Using a simple point-and-click interface, Oncolink allows the user to navigate the rich multimedia resources maintained locally within OncoLink as well other oncology related Internet resources. We believe OncoLink is the first WWW and gopher server devoted to detailed information regarding cancer.

Based on our results, we believe: (1) There is a significant interest in cancer-related resources in the Internet community; (2) we believe users tend to browse cancer related information in a non-linear fashion; (3) we believe the graphical hypertext links stimulate users to browse documents more frequently and extensively; (4) we feel the content of OncoLink should be carefully peer-reviewed by experts spanning the various cancer-related disciplines. Therefore, we intend to expand the editorial board of OncoLink.

We conclude that OncoLink as a medical information resource is both useful and has wide interest in the international community. We believe, in the future, such systems will become common media for the international dissemination of cancer and other medical information.

References

[1] T. Berners-Lee et al. "World-Wide-Web: The Information Universe", Electronic Networking: Research, Applications, and Policy, Vol 2, No. 1, Spring 1992, pp. 52-58.

[2] HTTPS is a multithreaded Windows NT "service" accessible by anonymous ftp from enwac.ed.ac.uk and is available for both Intel and DEC Alpha architectures. HTTPS was produced as part of the European Microsoft Windows NT Academic Centre (EMWAC) project. HTTPS supports HyperText Transport Protocol (WWW) and gopher services under Microsoft Windows NT.

[3] The GN software is available by anonymous FTP or by setting a WWW URL to ftp: // ftp.acns.nwu.edu/ pub/gn/ gn-2.12.tar.gz. A later version may be present on this server, so the "2.12" may be different. GN was written by: John Franks from: Dept of Math. Northwestern University.

[4] Gopher originated at the University of Minnesota as a campus-wide online information system. Gopher is based on using a hierarchy of menus to access information contained either locally or elsewhere on the Internet. The information retrieved by a gopher server is usually text based, though there have been some discussions of extending the support to other types of information.

[5] The Journal of Medical Imaging has written a whitepaper on electronic publications in the medical imaging community. This document is accessible on the WWW by: http://jmi.gdb.org/JMI/ejourn.html.

[6] T. Berners-Lee, R. Cailliau, A. Luotonen, H.F. Nielsen, A. Secret, "The World-Wide Web", Comm. ACM 37:76-82(1994).

[7] J.R. Galvin, M.P. D'Alessandro, W.E. Erkonen, T.A. Knutson, D.L. Lacy, "The Virtual Hospital: A New Paradigm for Lifelong Learning in Radiology" Radiographics 14:875-879(1994).

[8] K. Nagy, "Cancer Information Seekers Cruise the 'Highdays'" J. NCI 86:1115-1118(1994).

A Quantitative Method for Measuring Library User Journal Needs: A Pilot Study Using CD Plus MEDLINE Usage Statistics

Kathel Dunn, M.S.L.S., Cheryl Chisnell, M.A., Suzanne Szak, B.A., Dean F. Sittig, Ph.D.

The Informatics Center, Eskind Biomedical Library
Vanderbilt University, Nashville, Tennessee

Objective: To develop a quantitative method for measuring library user journal needs based on an analysis of bibliographic search results. Design: Retrospective bibliometric comparison of citation selections generated by users in the library. Measures: Number of times each journal was identified by library users during multiple bibliographic search sessions. Results: Library users identified 4907 journal titles. The top 200 journal titles accounted for 55% of the library user journal needs. Of the 1380 unique titles identified, 652 were selected once. Conclusion: Our pilot study demonstrated that analysis of bibliographic search results can be used to identify library user journal needs. Such a method could also be used to estimate user requirements for online, full-text scientific journals.

INTRODUCTION

One of the hottest topics in corporate America today is customer service. Many organizations have hired expensive management consultants to help them identify their customers, determine their needs, and identify the requirements of those needs. Libraries are no exception. For hundreds of years, librarians have struggled with the decision of which journals they should have in their collection to best serve their customers. Now that the National Library of Medicine indexes over 3600 different journals, the decision is even more difficult. Only the largest and best endowed libraries can even consider having all these journals in their collection.

We hypothesize that it may be possible to assess the library customer's needs by watching what they do and learning from their actions. Our scenario for a given user's actions is this: a searcher sits at a computer and accesses a bibliographic database of a particular field. The searcher looks up a topic and selects the citations that are the most relevant to his/her work.

This study was undertaken to develop a quantitative method for measuring these library user needs based on a retrospective bibliometric analysis of their bibliographic search patterns.

BACKGROUND

A review of the literature reveals a number of attempts to establish a relationship between the user and the library collection. In constructing the library collection, for example, librarians develop criteria for the selection and deselection of materials for a particular collection [1,2]. Although a criteria list may include as many as ten items, the library user is generally only referred to in an oblique manner: as the "demand" [1] or as the "communal" [3]. Where there is mention of meeting user needs, there is little description of exactly how these interests and needs are determined. Certainly, traditional criteria cannot be abandoned and collections built solely on user wants, but more objective data are required to help in the selection of the materials.

Other researchers have used bibliometric methods for assessing a collection and in turn, establishing a relationship between what a user wants and the library collection. Two of the methods used include citation analysis and journal use studies. Citation analysis can either examine the work of one author, or set of authors, to determine publication patterns or it can determine the publications that have the highest number of cited articles, i.e., the most heavily used journals [4,5]. Citation analysis is only available for work that has been published and does not address the needs of the unpublished researcher or practicing clinician utilizing the library's collection in support of patient care.

In a similar manner, researchers will select a subject, for example, pediatrics, and then determine which journals produce the highest concentration of articles on the given topic [6,7,8,9]. While work of this nature has provided valuable insight into

0195-4210/94/$5.00

publishing patterns and established the concept of core journals in a field, it presupposes that users needs were completely met by the cited works.

The next step in these lines of study is to establish a closer link between the user and the collection in a quantitative, objective manner. With the advent of computers, researchers have been able to take advantage of new technology to assess collection development practices. CD-ROM and database management play a major part in moving collection development toward more quantitative, objective methods [10].

DESIGN/METHOD

Data Selection The Eskind Biomedical Library at Vanderbilt provides access to MEDLINE using CD Plus' Ovid software. Access is available to any workstation connected to the Medical Center network. This includes 400+ shared workstations scattered throughout the hospital and clinics as well as twenty-eight public workstations in the library. For the purpose of this pilot study, bibliographic search data were obtained from all CD Plus' MEDLINE searches conducted in the library on one day (March 17, 1994), using the last five years of the MEDLINE database (MEDL).

Data Manipulation A usage report for one day's bibliographic searches in MEDL was created. See example below. A "C" program was written to extract data from this report.

File Access:
medl

Citations browsed:	159
Citations printed:	1
Citations downloaded:	1254
Sets created:	9

Last search sets:

1 - Diastolic Dysfunction.tw.	303
2 - compliance/ and ventric$.tw.	82
3 - relaxation.tw. and heart/	323
4 - (relaxation and left ventr$.tw.	740
5 - 1 or 2 or 3 or 4	1476
6 - limit 5 to english language	1186
7 - diastol.$.tw.	11533
8 - 6 and 7	754
9 - limit 8 to review articles	116

A large, single search (*Search1*) comprised of all 870 separate search statements recorded in that file was constructed. *Search1* was executed in CD Plus' MEDLINE (1990-1994) to re-create the results obtained by the original searchers. In this way the search revealed not only the number of citations retrieved, but also the citations themselves. Since the intent of this pilot study was to quantify library user needs, it was necessary to limit the results of *Search1* by making some assumptions about which of the retrieved citations were actually wanted by the user. These assumptions were written as rules that were used repeatedly over all search statements to eliminate the user's intermediate results yet retain his/her final results.

For example, a user searching for the effects of vitamins during pregnancy might construct the following search:

Example Search in MEDL

	Search Word	No. of articles found
1	Vitamins/	797
2	Pregnancy/	49033
3	1 and 2	75

We infer from the above search that the user wanted the citations from search statement number 3 and not the citations retrieved from either statement 1 or 2. That is, the user was only interested in the terms vitamins and pregnancy together. Thus, the results of the first line (797 hits) for vitamins and the second line (49033 hits) for pregnancy are only part of the process in obtaining the final result of 75 hits. A rule reflecting the search above would be written, "Do not use results of any search statements that are used in a subsequent search statement." This rule was modified and other rules added to it as more searches, including more complex searches, were examined. The rules used to assess *Search1* are listed below:

Rules

1. If the results of any search generate 100 hits or more, then do not use these results. The default printing limit at our library is 100 citations.
2. If a search statement is used in a subsequent search statement, then do not use the earlier intermediate results. Searches that are used in earlier lines most likely represent only a portion of a thought process.

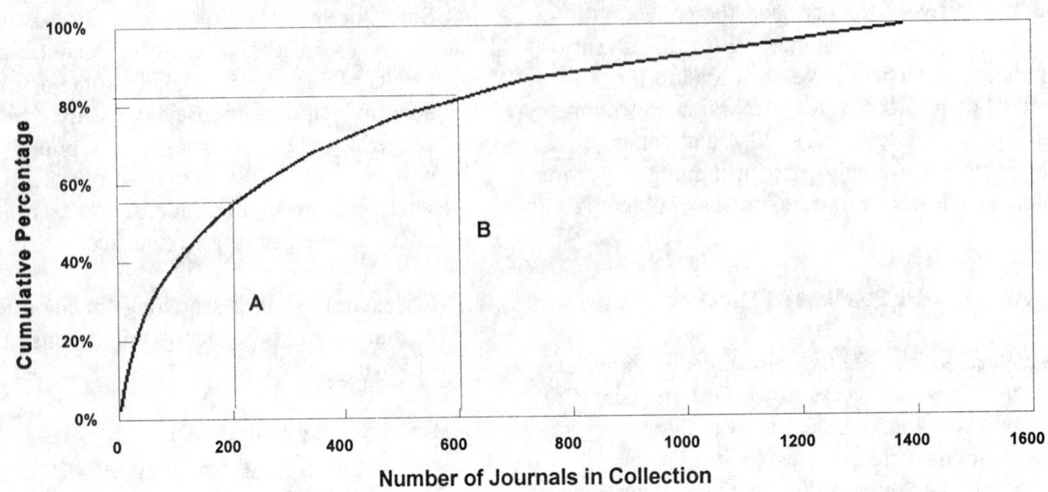

Figure 1

3. If a combined search statement results in 0 hits, then ignore Rule 2 and keep the results from the individual searches used in the combined search statement. The result of 0 hits probably required some rethinking on the part of the searcher, most probably requiring him/her to go back to the previously used statements.

Examples of the rules process:

	Search Word	No. of articles found
1	cocaine.tw.	3337
2	abruptio placentae/	103
3	1 and 2	10
4	from 3 keep 4,10	2

In the above search, lines 1 and 2 are eliminated because they have over 100 hits. Line 3 would normally have been kept as a result since it produced under 100 hits, but it is used again in line 4 -- "from 3 keep 4,10". Thus, line 3 is eliminated. The only results retained are those from line 4. Another example:

	Search Word	No. of articles found
1	(atropine and pa2).ti,ab,sh.	70
2	1 and muscarinic.ti,ab,sh.	48
3	from 2 keep 3,8,13,15,19-20,22-23, 25-26,28-29	12

In the above search all of the search statements produced hits of under 100, but line 1 was used in statement 2 and line 2 was used in statement 3, thereby eliminating the results of lines 1 and 2 from the final results set.

RESULTS

The Vanderbilt collection is split among several libraries, including the Stevenson Science Libray, the Heard Library and the Eskind Biomedical Library. Eskind Biomedical Library's journal collection numbers 2072. The MEDLINE database indexes 3600 journals and of that number, Vanderbilt holds 1884 titles. The total number of journal citations identified by library users was 4907. Of that number, 4140 are held in the Vanderbilt collection. A total of 1380 unique journal titles were identified by the users, of these 652 were selected once. Of the top 100 journals identified in this study, Vanderbilt holds 97% in its collection. The top 200 journal titles accounted for 55% of the library user journal needs.

Figure 1 shows the cumulative percentage of non-unique biomedical journals titles identified by library users from the current MEDLINE (1990-1994) file. Of particular interest is line A which shows the cumulative percentage of non-unique journal titles that came from the top 200 journals. Line B represents the top 600 journals.

Table 1. The top 32 journals identified.

Table 1

#	Journal Title	# of times ident
1	Journal of Biological Chemistry	133
2	Proc. Nat. Acad. of Sciences U.S.A	100
3	Development	42
4	Molecular & Cellular Biology.	41
5	Biochem.& Biophys. Res, Comm.	39
6	Journal of Bacteriology	39
7	Nature	34
8	Oncogene	34
9	Jour. of Pharm. & Exp.Ther.	33
10	Infection & Immunity	42
11	Nucleic Acids Research	33
12	EMBO Journal	32
13	Journal of Clinical Investigation	32
14	Science	38
15	FEBS Letters	32
16	Cancer Research	29
17	Biochemical Journal	28
18	Circulation	28
19	Radiology	27
20	American Journal of Physiology	27
21	European Journal of Pharmacology	26
22	Biochemistry	26
23	Endocrinology	25
24	Biochimica et Biophysica Acta	25
25	European Journal of Biochemistry	24
26	Journal of Virology	23
27	Magnetic Resonance in Medicine	23
28	Gastroenterology	23
29	Cell	23
30	New England Journal of Medicine	23
31	Ann. New York Acad. of Sciences	23
32	American Journal of Roentgenology	23

Figure 2 shows the number of times the library users selected unique journal titles.

DISCUSSION

The method developed in this pilot study represents a potential breakthrough in quantitatively defining the relationship between a library's users and its collection. By examining CD Plus' usage log of bibliographic search sessions, we can determine the final result sets identified by users as well as the contents of those sets. From a user's point of view, the final result set is exactly what s/he wants. We quantify what the user wanted and, more importantly, whether or not s/he obtained what s/he wanted. This quantitative method for measuring library user journal needs serves as an indicator for the development of a library's journal collection. Also, the method could serve as an indicator of whether or not a journal should be maintained in paper or received in an online, full text format.

Returning to the scenario described earlier, after the user has selected his/her chosen citations, s/he then attempts to retrieve them from whatever library collection is available. It is in stepping away from the computer that a user is frequently met with disappointment: the library collection does not have his/her selected items. The choice of selected items is usually modified and changed, based on the availability of items in a particular library's collection. At this point, knowledge of what a user wanted is forever lost.

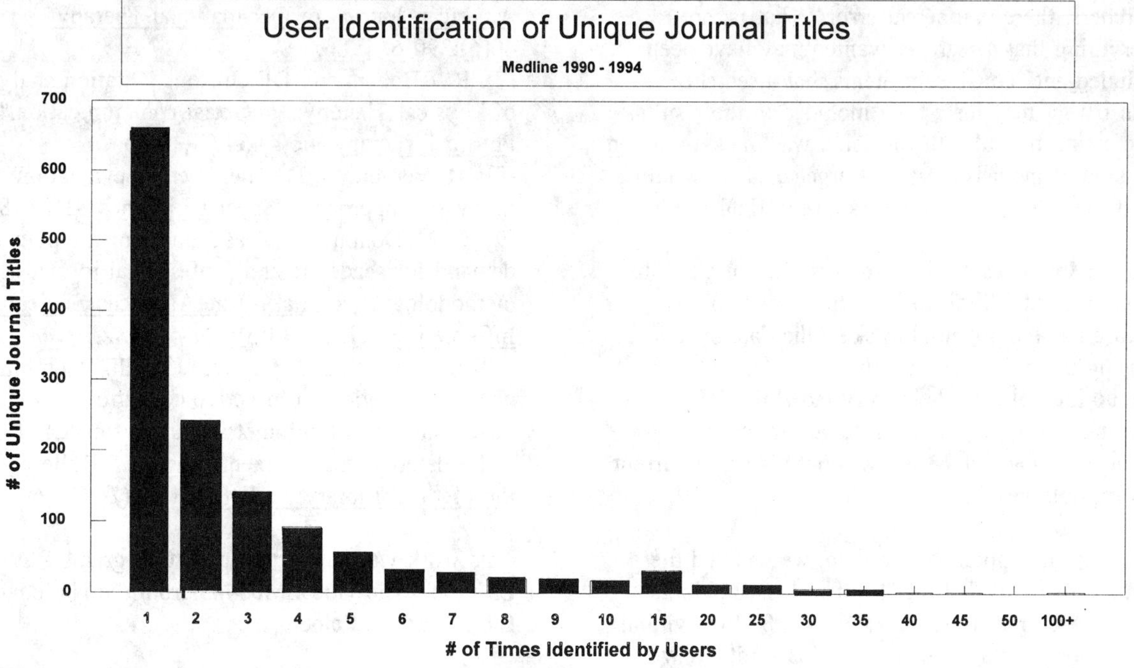

Figure 2

Limitations with this method

Data For the purposes of testing this method and assessing its feasibility, we used only one day's worth of MEDLINE (MEDL) searches conducted in the library. In order to draw more meaningful conclusions, a larger set of data is necessary. A longer time period with searches done by a wider variety of individuals will not only produce more data, but will further validate the use of this method as a collection development tool. Including other data in the study, such as journal usage studies and document delivery statistics, will further define and validate the relationship between the user and the collection.

Other research has concentrated on whether or not library users have chosen the most appropriate database and/or searched it well. Our method, designed to assist in the collection development process, concentrates on the customers' needs rather than on the process by which those needs are identified. Regardless of whether or not the searcher chose or searched well, under our rules, s/he still identified the particular journal titles that s/he wanted and hence that our library should have.

Rules The rules used in this method were crucial to the outcome. The rules determined what data were chosen and what were left out. Given that the rules were applied on search statements that represent the thought processes of any number of different searchers, there is inherent error. That is, not everything that a searcher wanted may have been included and, conversely, items that a searcher didn't want may have been included in the results. In creating the rules the decision was made to err on the side of inclusiveness. A larger data set would limit the effect of these errors on the final results.

System Features An important feature of CD Plus is its ability to "limit to local holdings." This feature has the potential to skew the data by 1) causing us to overestimate the percentage of non-unique journal titles held by Vanderbilt and 2) limiting our ability to measure accurately what library users actually want without regard to current library holdings.

To assess this potential problem, we counted the number of times that the "limit to local holdings" feature occurred in *Search1*. Of the 870 individual search statements, 30 contained this limit. If we assume that a complete search session contains, on average, 5 individual search statements, then only 17% of the search sets identified by users were affected.

Implications for further research
The next step in our research is to test this method with more data. We hope to also test this method against other collection development methods including citation analysis, journal use studies, inter-library loan and circulation statistics.

REFERENCES

[1]. J. Rutledge., L. Swindler. "The selection decision: defining criteria and establishing priorities." College and Research Libraries. 48(2):123-31, 1987.
[2]. RK Hunt. "Journal deselection in a biomedical research library: a mediated mathematical approach." Bulletin of the Medical Library Association. 78(1):45-8, 1990.
[3]. R. Atkinson. "The citation as intertext: toward a theory of the selection process." Library Resources and Technical Services. 28:109-19, April-June 1984.
[4]. ME Fang. "Journal rankings by citation analysis in health sciences librarianship." Bulletin of the Medical Library Association. 77(2):205-11, 1989.
[5]. L. Bronars., K. Branch. "Cost-cutting uses of new Scisearch feature." Database 13(6):53-8, 1990.
[6]. KS. Johnson., DJ Leising. "The literature of occupational therapy: a citation analysis study." American Journal of Occupational Therapy. 40(6):390-6, 1986.
[7]. RW Bohannon., DF Gibson. "Citation analysis of Physical Therapy: a special communication." Physical Therapy 66(4):540-1, 1986.
[8]. M. Berger., J. Devine. "Serials evaluation: an innovative approach." Special Libraries 81(3):183-8.
[9]. C. McDonough. "Measurement of the potential demand for academic and professional journals: a methodology." Journal of the American Society for Information Science 33(5):321-4, 1982.
[10]. J. Burnham., B. Shearer. J. Wall. "Combining new technologies for effective collection development: a bibliometric study using CD-ROM and a database management program." Bulletin of the Medical Library Association. 80(2):150-6.

This work was supported in part by grants R29 LM05284 and G08 LM05443 from the National Library of Medicine.

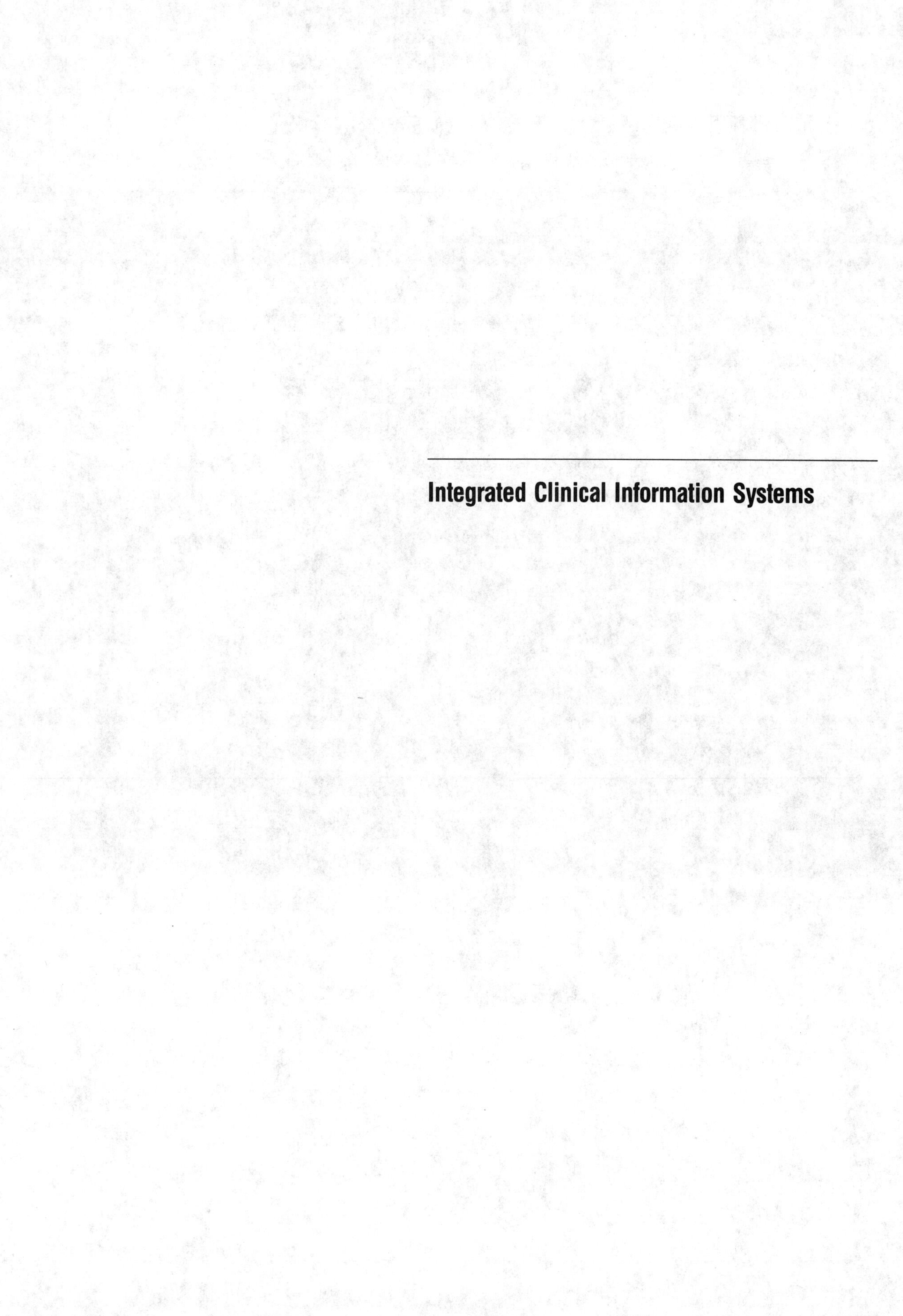

Integrated Clinical Information Systems

From HIS to IAIMS: Expanding the Scope of Information Processing Applications in a German University Hospital

H.U. Prokosch, Ph.D., B. Puhle, M. Müller, R. Wagner, Ph.D., G. Junghans, Ph.D., K. Marquardt, Ph.D., J. Dudeck, M.D.

Department of Medical Informatics
University of Gießen
Germany

Since the mid eighties the department of medical informatics at the University Hospital of Gießen (Germany) has been engaged in the development of a comprehensive hospital information system. The installation of a campus wide network has set the basis to provide not only clinical patient-oriented information, but also general information resources for research, medical education and administrative purposes, thus creating an environment which in the U.S. became known as an integrated academic information management system (IAIMS). The underlying concept of the whole approach is to provide one-stop information shopping capabilities at the clinicians and administrators desktop in order to meet the increasing information needs of health professionals with the emerging reality of the potential benefits of computer and communication technologies. This paper describes the various steps performed to realize this concept at Gießen University Hospital and the evaluation results derived from analysis of the acceptance of these new technologies among our hospital staff.

INTRODUCTION

Gießen University Hospital is a 1,350 bed hospital which has about 36,000 inpatient admits and 320,000 outpatient visits per year. There are 4,000 employees and staff. During the last two years the HIS at Gießen University Hospital (WING [1]) has emerged from the phase of prototype and pilot implementations towards the state of a routinely used system with comprehensive coverage of inpatient departments and outpatient clinics. In the same time, the scope of information processing applications which were accessible for clinical and academic users was continuously expanded. These efforts have led to a set of information resources, covering clinical and administrative patient data, various clinical and administrative information services and a number of medical education programs. Even though in Germany an official analogue to the U.S. IAIMS grant program does not exist, this integrated institutional approach for the implementation of an information management system for clinical practice, medical education and biomedical research has constituted an IAIMS-like system (according to the terminology of Lindberg et al.[2]).

THE WING/GISNET STATUS

The design, development and implementation of the HIS at Gießen University Hospital can be divided into four phases. These are (1) the phase of isolated departmental systems (1975-1985), (2) the HELP evaluation phase (1986, 1987), (3) the prototyping phase (1988-1991) and (4) the production phase (since 1992). Even though, we appreciated the general concept (e.g. a central medical data dictionary and integrated decision support functions) of the HELP system very much, organizational differences between German and American Hospitals (and accordingly the requirements for HIS functionalities) proved to be too large, so that we finally discarded the idea of adapting this American HIS to our hospital environment. The decision was made to start with own HIS developments, keeping in mind all our HELP experiences and the basic ideas and concepts of the HELP system (for more details compare [1]). This new HIS development approach was named WING (which is the abbreviation of the German terms for 'knowledge based information network in Gießen'). While, during the prototyping phase, the first WING functions could only be tested in three nursing units, the opening of a new premise for the surgery department (fully connected to the backbone network (GISNET)) and the extension of the network in the internal medicine department in 1992, initiated a widespread HIS usage throughout the whole hospital campus. Today (August 1994) about 500 clinical workstations in more than 100 different nursing units and various laboratories and outpatient clinics are connected to the network and are accessed by more than 1000 clinical users.

The network (GISNET) is geographically distributed across an area of about 2 square kilometers with 25 different medical and administrative buildings. It encompasses 2 Tandem mainframe computers, a Tandem Unix server, a HP 9000, two AEG Modcomp computers, about 20 SUN workstations and servers, 15 Novell file servers, a CD-ROM server, about 350 DOS PCs, the same number of printers and a growing

0195-4210/94/$5.00 © 1994 AMIA, Inc.

number of Macintosh computers. The network is based on ethernet with a backbone moving to ATM within the next years. It supports TCP/IP, IPX, Netbios and DEC-LAT-protocol.

ONE-STOP INFORMATION SHOPPING

While expanding the information processing capabilities throughout the Gießen University Hospital during the last two years, we were pursuing the goal, to implement the concept of "one-stop information shopping" (as described for example by Clayton et al. [3]). This means that EDP workstations (discless DOS PCs) with an attached printer are available at all nursing stations and physician offices as well as numerous laboratories, outpatient clinics and secretary offices. Thus, the hospital staff has access to various information resources from their desktop through the GISNET main menu and 4 sub-menus. The available information resources comprise (1) clinical patient data (e.g. laboratory data, diagnosis and physician discharge summaries as well as specialty specific medical documentation of oncology and cardiology data), (2) administrative patient data, (3) medical and administrative information services (e.g. the drug information system edited by the German pharmaceutical industry (Red List), the Micromedex information systems (DRUGDEX, POISINDEX, MARTINDALE, TOMES), a medical terminology dictionary, a diagnostic consultation system and the German train schedule), (4) library services (MEDLINE), (5) medical education programs (e.g. cardiac emergency case simulations, physiology question catalog) and (6) standard Novell/ DOS software (e.g. MS-Word, Harvard-Graphics, Microsoft Windows, Excel, electronic mail).

GISNET INFORMATION RESOURCES

The functionality of the clinical information system WING and some of the integrated clinical subsystems has been extensively described elsewhere (e.g. [1, 4, 5, 6]). In the following we will present our approach to make non-patient-related information accessible for clinical care, biomedical research and medical education.

Medical Information Services

Drug information is usually the most often required information to support the physician in defining his/her therapeutic strategy. Traditionally, the German pharmaceutical industry yearly publishes a book with drug information for all the brands currently available at the German market and provides this book to every German physician. Because of its red cover this book is called the "Rote Liste" (Red List). Lately the information provided within the book is additionally available within a PC-based drug information system. The information contents is updated every six month. The network version of the Red List has been installed on a GISNET Novell fileserver in spring 1992 and is available at every connected workstation. For a more comprehensive and scientific coverage of drug information the pharmacy of Gießen University Hospital has decided to provide access to the DRUGDEX database from Micromedex additionally to the Red List. DRUGDEX together with POISINDEX, MARTINDALE, REPRORISK and DRUG-INTERACTIONS are stored on one CD-ROM and supplied with a common user interface.

Library Services

Another goal of our developments was to provide a system for quick and easy access to bibliographic references of the medical literature. We therefore connected a CD-ROM server to the network with 14 CD-ROM players attached to it. Using the Silverplatter software package we thus provide access to medical literature references from 1966 up to now stored within the MEDLINE database. Retrieval results may be downloaded on the user's privat file server directory or printed on a freely selectable GISNET printer. A customized program supports the automatic generation of the official library ordering form for books or journal articles.

Hospital Internal Information Services

In 1994 the clinical users asked us to additionally provide some means for hospital internal information services. In regard to this, a first step was done by installing an online version of the hospital's weekly updated cafeteria menu plan. Until today the hospital kitchen regularly distributes a paper-based plan in hundreds of copies throughout the whole hospital. In all locations connected to GISNET this plan can now directly be reviewed (and printed) from the staff's desktop workstation, thus eliminating the need for a paper-based distribution.

After this successfull first implementation it was decided to develop a generic framework for the creation, maintenance and access to hospital internal "electronic books". This framework comprises an editor module (to define the book's structure and search index), a reader module (to access an electronic book from the GISNET workstations), a bulletin board module (which serves as a communication function between the readers and the editor of a book) and an analysis module (to derive various statistics on the usage of an electronic book).

The first book created with these tools and integrated into the GISNET environment is related to WING/GISNET itself. It shall provide an easy way to inform the hospital staff on activities associated with information processing developments, program updates and new installations, user instructions as well as seminars and other courses, thus serving as an IAIMS newsletter within the Gießen University Hospital. Furthermore, three more electronic books are under development by clinical departments, focusing on "infectious disease information", "adverse drug events" documented at our hospital and the pharmacy's "drug formulary".

Medical Education Programs

During 1993 a close cooperation between the department of medical informatics and the medical faculty was established in order to analyse and propose a new and innovative structure for the medical curriculum applying modern hard- and software technologies. In this cooperation different scenarios for the integration of medical education programs into the medical curriculum have been evaluated. A proposal for a long term strategy is currently under development. In the meantime several small steps have already been accomplished to investigate the attitude of students but also teachers on the usage of new electronic media and to provide campus wide access to a preliminary set of medical education programs throughout the GISNET interface. Thus, since July 1993 three case simulation programs for cardiac emergency situations have been implemented on a Novell file server and made accessible within a GISNET submenu. After first positive responses to the installation of these programs three more programs (case simulations on reanimation and abdominal pain as well as a physiology questions catalog) were added in February 1994.

To perform a formal evaluation of the usage of these programs and the users attitudes towards such medical education programs a short electronic questionnaire was developed. Thirteen questions were asked in order to determine the user´s background, general attitude towards computers and computer usage in medicine, the duration of the current session, a rating for the program he/she has just used and if he/she would recommend the program to colleagues and wishes to have more computer-based medical education programs accessible at the GISNET workstation. During February and March 1994 this questionnaire was automatically presented to every user of any of the six programs.

Administrative Information Services

As an information service mainly focused on secretaries and administrative staff the complete German train schedule and the German postal code reference system have been implemented in summer 1993. The latter was especially helpful in the second half of 1993 since in July 1993 the German postal code system has been completely revised and changed from a four-digit to a five-digit system.

RESULTS

Different approaches have been choosen to evaluate the various steps performed in broadening the scope of information services at Gießen University Hospital. First of all, an internal logging mechanism keeps track of every usage of any of the newly established services. Secondly, a paper-based questionnaire has been sent to all physicians of the two departments which have had the longest experience with the WING/GISNET functionalities, trying to investigate the attitude of the clinical users to electronic data processing in general, but also specificly to the services provided to them through the GISNET workstations. Finally, the attitude to the six medical education programs was investigated by the means of an electronic questionnaire which was appended to each of the implemented education programs during the months of February and March 1994.

The GISNET Logfile

The following presents the analysis results for the logfile entries during the first quarter of 1994. Among the newly established GISNET services MEDLINE is the most widely used (47 calls per day). Second in usage is the German drug information system (37 calls per day). The cafeteria menu is reviewed 26 times per day and train schedules are retrieved 18 times per day. The medical dictionary, the medical diagnostic consultation system, the postal code reference system and the American drug information system DRUGDEX are less often accessed (with 11, 9, 7 and 4 calls per day).

In total an average of 159 daily calls to any of the above mentioned information services have been logged during the first three months of 1994 and the medical education programs have been used in average 38 times per day. Among these programs one (the cardiac emergency case simulation program) seems to be more attractive (with about 10 daily calls), whereas the other five are about equally often used (five to six calls per day).

The WING/GISNET Questionnaire
One section of the questionnaire send to the physicians of two major departments at Gießen University Hospital was related to the physician's frequency of use and their rating of the available information sources. Analysis of the responses confirmed the results from the logfile analysis. On a scale between 0 and 5 (where 5 denotes "very helpful") MEDLINE and the German drug information system Red List received average ratings of 4.38 and 4.35 respectively (the second best ratings after the WING module for laboratory results review) and were the most often used GISNET resources. 43% of the physicians reported that they access the Red List at least once a day, whereas the majority of the physicians (38%) retrieve bibliographic information from MEDLINE several times a week (14% reported accessing it once or more times per day). The requests for additional information sources given as responses to this questionnaire have stimulated the implementation of some of the newer GISNET resources (e.g. the medical dictionary and the diagnostic consultation system).

The Medical Education Programs Questionnaire
Even though the GISNET workstations are generally not accessible for medical students (since they are usually installed in clinical environments and not in any location open to students) the medical information programs installed on a GISNET file server were positively received among the GISNET users. During the two months period of formal evaluation with the electronic questionnaire we received a total of 1315 responses. One surprising result was that nursing staff were the favorite users of these programs (39% of all calls), followed by medical students (25%), physicians (19%) and others (17%).

Further analysis showed that 11% of the users have used a program more than 5 times, 20% have used it between 2 and five times and 69% have used it for the first time. In 83% of all uses a single user was working with the corresponding program whereas in 17% of the calls the program was used by a group of users. In most cases (51% of all calls) the program was only used for a time period of less than 15 minutes (which may just be sufficient to work through one case simulation). Nevertheless, 37% reported a working time between 15 minutes and 1 hour and 12% of even more than an hour. In 62% of the calls the users reported that they had fully completed a session, whereas in 38% they had quit the program without finishing a simulation case (however, no reason for this was specified).

In order to get a rating for the six programs the questionnaire distinguished between the overall quality of a program, the users benefit from using the program and the ease of handling. On a scale between 1 and 6 (where 1 is the best rating) the programs received average ratings for the overall quality ranging between 2,1 and 3,6. The average ratings for the user's benefit ranged from 2,4 to 2,9 and finally the ratings for the ease of handling ranged from 2,6 to 3,4. Finally, 68% of the users reported that they would recommend the corresponding program to other GISNET users and 78% of them requested that further medical education programs should be implemented within GISNET.

DISCUSSION

The evaluation analysis has shown that there exists a broad spectrum of information needs amongst health professionals which is not only limited to patient related data. The information services provided within the GISNET environment have been widely accepted throughout the hospital staff. We even got the impression, that next to the laboratory results review module, these services helped some people to reduce eventually existing acceptance barriers and attracted them to integrate a computer workstation as a natural tool within their daily work environment.

Networking was the fundamental supposition for this movement towards an IAIMS-like environment. It offered the technical platform which was necessary to integrate a variety of different information sources. In future a vast number of both local and national computer-based information resources will be accessible and may be integrated in the environment of clinical or academic workstations with relatively small technical efforts and low costs. However, this does not mean, that all problems in information management are already solved. Our investigations have also revealed several challenges for further improving the IAIMS environment.

First of all, even though more than ten information resources can currently be directly accessed from the clinicians desktop, together replacing an enormous amount of traditional paper-based information sources (e.g. books) from which some were not even available anywhere in the hospital in former times, clinicians already claimed that finding the relevant piece of information sometimes takes minutes and may be cumbersome, since switching back and forth between different information resources is time consuming and requires formulating similar search commands multiple times in different environments.

Solutions to this problem may be given with different levels of comfort for the information retriever. A first short term approach is, to substitute the current DOS-based GISNET menu environment by a WINDOWS-based environment supporting the simultaneous opening of multiple information sources in different windows of the screen (thus eliminating the need to go back and forth through different menu screens and wait during the processes' startup time). However, this might not only bring improvements, since the WINDOWS-environment will also increase the complexity of the user interface and may confuse some of the novice users. The implementation of a drug therapy documentation module [4] has already discovered problems with windows hidden behind each other, adaption to using the mouse or even space problems for the mouse on a desktop already covered with numerous forms and patient charts. Nevertheless, the advantages and the problems related to such a new GISNET user interface will be investigated this summer during a pilot installation on two nursing stations of our hospital.

A second long term strategy is to integrate relevant information sources directly into the environment of clinical HIS applications and render context-sensitiv information access without the need (for the user) to know from which information resource such information may actually be derived from. However, this is a highly complex endeavour which first needs to tackle the questions of "which information is relevant in which clinical context?" (compare e.g. [7]) and "how can the local terminology be mapped to the vocabularies of external information resources?". Research results of the UMLS (Unified Medical Language System) project [8] hopefully may provide answers at least to the latter question in the near future.

References

[1] H.U. Prokosch, J. Dudeck, G. Junghans, K. Marquardt, P. Sebald, A. Michel. WING - Entering a New Phase of Electronic Data Processing at the Gießen University Hospital. Methods of Information in Medicine 1991, 30:289-298.

[2] D.A.B. Lindberg, R.T. West, M. Corn. IAIMS: An Overview from the National Library of Medicine. Bull Med Libr Assoc 1992, 80:244-246.

[3] P.D. Clayton, R.V. Sideli, S. Sengupta. Open Architecture and Integrated Information at Columbia Presbyterian Medical Center. MD Computing 1992, 5:297-303.

[4] D. Wieczorek, H.U. Prokosch, B. Neidhart, H. Kreckel, J. Dudeck. One Year of Experience with EDP Support for Drug Threrapy at Gießen University Hospital. Proceedings MIE 93, Freund Publishing House Ltd. 1993, 322-325.

[5] A. Michel, H.U. Prokosch, J. Dudeck. Some Experiene with the Implementation and Operation of a Hospital Wide Online Diagnosis Documentation and Coding System. Proceedings MEDINFO 92, Elsevier Science Publishers 1992, 1311-1315.

[6] B. Neidhart, D. Wieczorek, J. Dudeck. Neue Wege in der Entwicklung von Subsystemen im Universitäts-Klinikum Gießen. Proceedings GMDS 1993, MMV Medizin Verlag München, 1994, 50-53.

[7] J.J. Cimino, S.B. Johnson, A. Aguirre, N. Roderer, P.D. Clayton. The Medline Button. Proceedings SCAMC 1992, McGraw Hill 1993, 81-85.

[8] B.L. Humphreys, Lindberg, D.A.B. Lindberg. The Unified Medical Language System Project: A Distributed Experiment in Improving Access to Biomedical Information. Proceedings MEDINFO 92, Elsevier Science Publishers 1992, 1496-1500.

Effect of Physician Reminders on Preventive Care: Meta-Analysis of Randomized Clinical Trials

Suzanne M. Austin, M.H.A.*, E. Andrew Balas, M.D., Ph.D.*†, Joyce A. Mitchell, Ph.D.†, Bernard G. Ewigman, M.D., M.S.P.H.‡

Program in Health Services Management *, Medical Informatics Group †, and Family and Community Medicine ‡, University of Missouri-Columbia, Columbia, MO

The objective of this study was to assess the clinical value of the physician reminder, an information intervention, in increasing compliance for selected preventive health care measures. Meta-analysis was used to combine the quantitative evidence from randomized controlled clinical trials meeting the eligibility criteria.

The trials included in this meta-analysis were conducted in a family or internal medicine clinic. Physician reminders were used in the trials to influence utilization and compliance of preventive health care activities. The use of physician reminders for preventive health care activities resulted in a homogeneous effect for the subcategories of cervical cancer screening (test for heterogeneity $X^2_2 = 4.122$*, non-significant) and tetanus immunization (test for heterogeneity* $X^2_2 = 3.139$*, non-significant). Similarly, the odds ratio from the combination of evidence from the three cervical cancer screening trials was significant (1.180, 95 percent CI: 1.020 to 1.339). The resulting odds ratio from the combination of evidence from the three tetanus immunization trials was significant (2.819, 95 percent CI: 2.664 to 2.975).*

The results of the meta-analyses for cervical cancer screening and tetanus immunizations indicate that physician reminders are an effective information intervention and can improve compliance for these two preventive health care procedures. Based on the results of this meta-analysis, further trials testing the effect of physician reminders on tetanus immunization would be unnecessary and probably unethical.

INTRODUCTION

The continuously evolving standards of medical practice create a clinical need to decrease the use of some procedures and to increase the use of other clinical procedures. Changes in physician practice patterns can be promoted through the provision of information. Information is a relatively inexpensive intervention used to change the process and outcome of patient care. Utilization can be effected by providing information at crucial points during the process of care.

An information intervention is referred to as a reminder when it arrives at the time of the decision making. A reminder is often delivered as an alert, effectively prompting the physician to make a decision. A reminder can also be presented in the form of immediate feedback. This method provides the physician with information when the decision is made.

The objective of this study was to assess the clinical value of the physician reminder intervention in increasing compliance with preventive health care measures. This objective was met through the conduction of a meta-analysis and an exploration of the effect of physician reminder intervention on utilization and compliance.

METHODS

The trials selected for this study were abstracted from the Columbia Registry [1]. The Columbia Registry includes over 300 randomized controlled clinical trials from the areas of information and utilization management. Database searches, manual searches, and informal contacts have been used to create the registry. To meet eligibility criteria for inclusion, the published study must be: i) a randomized controlled clinical trial; ii) a comparison of information or utilization management intervention in the study group with no similar assistance in the control group; and iii) an evaluation of the change in the process and/or outcome of patient care. The Columbia Registry trials containing a physician reminder intervention were selected for this study. Of the physician reminder trials, the focus for the meta-analysis became the effect variables of cervical cancer screening and tetanus immunization.

The qualitative information and quantitative utilization data were abstracted from the eligible trial reports. The utilization data were abstracted in the form of the number of clinical actions performed and the number of clinical actions not performed for the control group and the physician reminder intervention group. If additional trials met the selection criteria, but did not contain the utilization data in a form to be abstracted and transformed into an odds ratio, the authors were contacted.

This meta-analysis used the odds ratio method to compare utilization. Utilization was calculated as the ratio of preventive cancer screening or immunizations performed compared to preventive cancer screening or immunizations not performed. The odds ratio for single study confidence levels and the pooled odds ratio for intervention success used the Peto modification of Mantel-Haenszel method described by Yusuf [2]. The method assumes identical effects in the pooled studies (homogeneity of treatment effect), and variances around each mean effect depend on the size of the study. The Breslow-Day chi square test for heterogeneity was used to determine if the binary end-point variables of the selected physician reminder trials constituted a homogeneous sample [3]. In estimating odds ratios, 95 percent confidence intervals were calculated for the individual studies and also for the combined effect. The tolerance was calculated using the method proposed by Rosenthal [4].

RESULTS

Ten eligible trials were identified from the Columbia Registry that measured either cervical cancer screening, tetanus immunization, or both of these preventive health care procedures. However, the appropriate data were not available from six of the trials. These eligible trials were eliminated from the analysis when only percentages or means were listed in the results, and a crucial number, such as total number of patients, was missing from the trial report. However, data in an appropriate form was available for three of the cervical cancer screening trials [5] [6] [7] and three of the tetanus immunization trials [6] [7] [8]. With the exception of one report on cervical screening, all eliminated trials indicated significant positive results.

Table 1 contains the qualitative description of the four articles included in the meta-analyses of cervical cancer screening and tetanus immunization. The sites of the four trials were family or internal medicine clinics in the countries of United States, Canada, and Israel. The providers were either family or internal medicine physicians. In addition to the physician reminder contained in all four trials, two trials also examined the effect of patient letter reminders and patient telephone reminders [5] [7]. The four trials also examined blood pressure recording compliance, smoking status assessment, thyroxine screening compliance, fecal occult blood screening compliance, and pneumococcal immunization status in addition to the preventive care procedures of interest to this meta-analysis.

Figure 1 graphically represents the odds ratios with 95 percent confidence intervals for cervical cancer screening compliance in each of the studies and the overall effect. The three trials were homogeneous (test for heterogeneity $X^2_2 = 4.122$, non-significant). The primary effect variable in two of the trials had a non-significant effect variable because 1.000 was included in the

Trial	Providers	Patients	Effects
McDowell 1989	family medicine physicians	family medicine 662 patients	cervical screening
Rosser 1991	family medicine provider teams	family medicine 2874 patients	cervical screening
			tetanus immunization
Tape 1993	internal medicine residents	internal medicine 1809 patients	cervical screening
			tetanus immunization
Weingarten 1989	family medicine physician, nurse	family medicine 222 patients	tetanus immunization

Table I Characteristics of the trials

95 percent confidence interval [5] [6]. One trial had a significant odds ratio and 1.000 was not included in the 95 percent confidence interval [7]. However, when the three trials were combined, the overall odds ratio became significant (1.180, 95 percent CI: 1.020 to 1.339).

Figure 2 graphically represents the odds ratios with 95 percent confidence intervals for tetanus immunization compliance in each of the studies and the overall effect. The three trials were homogeneous (test for heterogeneity X^2_2 = 3.139, non-significant). The primary effect in all three trials was significant because 1.000 was not included in the 95 percent confidence intervals for any of the three trials. When the three trials were combined, the overall odds ratio was significant (2.819, 95 percent CI: 2.664 to 2.975).

The tolerance of the three studies combined in the meta-analysis of cervical cancer screening was 0.794. This is below the level of 25 studies recommended by Rosenthal [4]. This number indicates that a few cervical cancer screening studies with negative effect could overturn the results of this meta-analysis. On the other hand, the tolerance of the three studies combined in the meta-analysis of tetanus immunization was 105.220. This number substantially exceeds the threshold level calculated by the Rosenthal method [4].

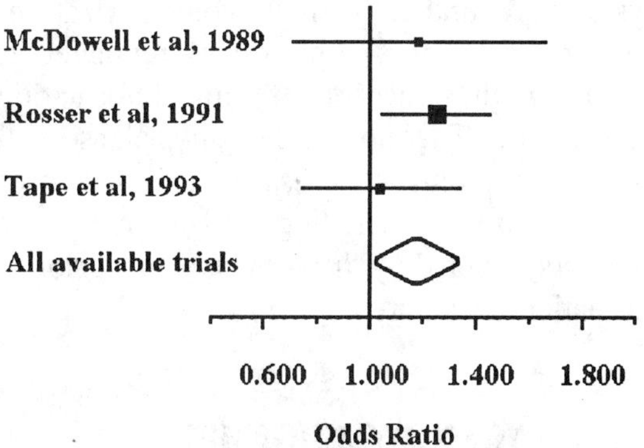

Figure 1 Cervical screening

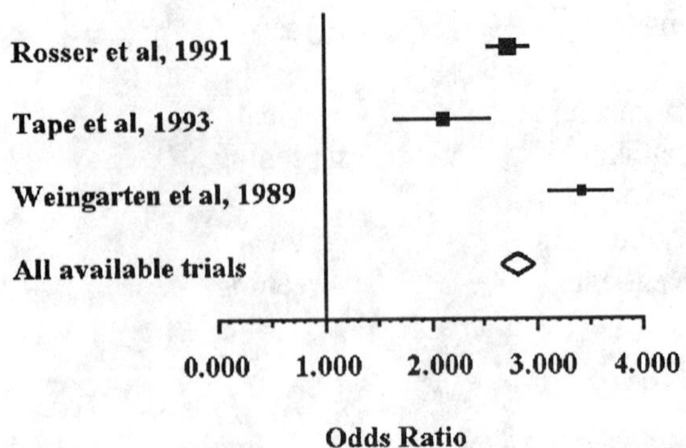

Figure 2 Tetanus immunization

DISCUSSION

It is well-known that reminders represent the most frequently tested information intervention category. Many reminder trials have been conducted. However, when specific interventions are examined, enough evidence to draw a valid conclusion may not be present. By examining the tolerance calculation, the evidence for the use of reminders for tetanus immunization is much stronger than for the use of reminders for cervical cancer screening. The evidence for tetanus immunization is strong enough to indicate that further randomized controlled clinical trials on tetanus immunization reminders would probably be unethical.

The physician reminder intervention is very suitable for computerization. In fact, it would be difficult to effectively administer physician reminders without computerization. The timeliness of the physician reminder is crucial to the success of this information intervention. Therefore, the physicians will require either on-line access to a computer or have a form, including preventive care reminders, printed by the computer just prior to each patient encounter.

ACKNOWLEDGEMENT

This project was supported in part by grant number HS07268 from the Agency for Health Care Policy and Research and in part by a grant from the Research Board of the University of Missouri.

REFERENCES

1. Balas EA, Mitchell JA, Bopp KD, Brown GD, Ewigman BG. The Columbia Registry of Controlled Clinical Computer Trials. In Frisse ME (Ed): Proceedings of the Symposium on Computer Applications in Medical Care, McGraw-Hill, 1992.

2. Yusuf S, Peto R, Lewis J, Collins R, Sleight P. Beta blockade during and after myocardial infarction: an overview of the randomized trials. Prog Cardiovasc Dis 1985;27:335-371.

3. Breslow NE, Day NE. Statistical methods in cancer research: The analysis of case-control studies. Lyon, International Agency for Research on Cancer, 1980.

4. Rosenthal R. The "File Drawer Problem" and tolerance for null results. Psychological Bulletin 1979;86(3):638-641.

5. McDowell I, Newell C, Rosser W. Computerized reminders to encourage cervical screening in family practice. J Fam Pract 1989;28:420-4.

6. Tape TG, Campbell JR. Computerized medical records and preventive health care: success depends on many factors. The American Journal of Medicine 1993;94:619-625.

7. Rosser WW, McDowell I, Newell C. Use of reminders for preventive procedures in family medicine. Can Med Ass J 1991;145(7):807-813.

8. Weingarten MA, Bazel D, Shannon HS. Computerized protocol for preventive medicine: a controlled self-audit in family practice. Family Practice 1989;6:120-4.

Implementation of a Relational Patient Record with Integration of Educational and Reference Information

Christopher Nielson, M.D.
C. Scott Smith, M.D.
David Lee, M.D.
Mark Wang, B.A.

Boise Veterans Affairs Medical Center
Boise, Idaho

Department of Medicine
University of Washington School of Medicine
Seattle, Washington

ABSTRACT

The clinician must identify pertinent diagnostic information and develop appropriate medical management plans in the context of rapidly changing research information, new therapeutic options and expanding diagnostic modalities. To assist in recognition of patterns relevant to diagnostic or therapeutic interventions, the medical record must be presented in a format that emphasizes important data interrelationships. Reference and educational information specifically pertinent to the case being reviewed must be immediately accessible.

A system that presents point of care patient centered clinical information, a summarized patient record, in a relational format with linked reference information has been developed. Data is acquired from the VA patient information database and provided over a PC network. At the time of data transfer, preliminary analysis and reorganization of data is performed such that interrelationships between laboratory, pharmacy and diagnostic information can be rapidly recognized. During data compilation reference and educational information is linked with patient data such that it can be accessed with a mouse click ("hotspot") when the record is subsequently reviewed. The medical record and CD-ROM based reference databases are then made available to users on a PC network in a Windows (tm) environment. Initial experience with the system is very favorable and suggests that evaluation of patient data may be significantly enhanced.

INTRODUCTION

The traditional approach to patient care requires a clinician to seek each item of information necessary for development of diagnostic and management plans. Fortunately, routine visits to the clinical lab, radiology and the record room as well as time consuming searches through a chart are being replaced by a few keystrokes at the computer terminal. However, data organization at the computer frequently mirrors the traditional data seeking pathways. The clinician must seek each laboratory result, medication list or note and pursue a computer path to the single result that is displayed independently from critically related information. Although the computerized medical record has been recognized to be a priority in health care [1], computer-based records are not in common use [2]. If data can be organized to meet the clinician's needs then acceptance and use of computer records may increase. Just as the experienced clinician learns to rapidly move between appropriate sections of a chart, the computer must provide immediate access to all needed information [3].

The DHCP (decentralized hospital computer program) system used by Veterans Affairs hospitals provides a massive amount of patient information but exemplifies the problem. Each laboratory result, medication, X-ray or diagnosis must be sought and viewed independent from related results. The clinician must take several menu driven steps to pursue each potentially related item of information. For example, discovery of a low hematocrit requires a search for data concerning a range of problems such as iron deficiency, renal failure, gastrointestinal bleeding or medication reaction. However, the hematocrit is routinely displayed without the trend of past results or relevant related information such as the serum iron, renal function, past diagnoses or radiology results.

While clinicians are accustomed to the process of searching for each item in the medical database, the process is not efficient and may predispose to errors and increased costs. Clearly the more difficult information is to identify the more likely it is that the data will be overlooked. Conversely, an excess of irrelevant information is similarly detrimental. In the example of a patient with a reduced hematocrit, the trend of several past hematocrits is useful but multiple screens full of daily in hospital hematocrits obscure the longer trend as well as other more important laboratory information. Suboptimal presentation of data is not only frustrating to the clinician but also contributes to inaccurate diagnosis, inappropriate or unnecessary diagnostic procedures and therapeutic errors.

In the current environment of rapidly changing medical information, acquisition of reference and educational information is inefficient and sporadic. At the time and site of patient care in clinic or hospital rooms, needed reference information must be immediately available and very quickly accessible. If the clinician is not aware of needed facts then patient care may be delayed or inappropriate. Lack of access to reference information may induce expensive referral practices.

Optimally, the medical record should be presented such that abnormal results, trends and potential data interrelationships are immediately apparent. Results that are repetitive or of unlikely importance must be available but should be relegated to a second tier of access that does not obscure primary data. Reference and educational information must be immediately available. However, just as unnecessary patient data can obscure important relationships, irrelevant reference and educational information impedes access to needed facts. Thus, a useful medical informatics system should provide initial organization and data links that encourage the clinician to recognize important relationships. It must then facilitate the rapid pursuit of data, references and educational information concerning alternative diagnoses and therapeutic interventions.

METHODS

Given adequate resources nearly any envisioned informatics system could be constructed. However, a system that can be widely implemented requires use of cost effective, easily available components and programming which can interface to a range of data sources. A simple PC network allows for provision of core resources while allowing the marked variation in user interface that is required by different health care providers. PC workstations allow for distributed processing capabilities and provide a cost effective, flexible platform for both data analysis and information presentation.

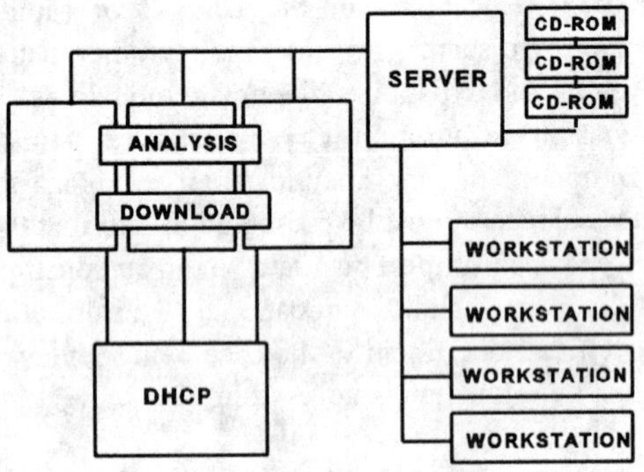

The current project was structured with programming and PCs that provided for four primary functions: 1) input/download, 2) cache, 3) analysis and formatting and 4) user interface. Functions were structured to be performed by parallel PCs, a design that allowed use of inexpensive machines, provided high reliability through redundancy and introduced the flexibility to meet virtually any workload through simple addition of machines. Because even a pause of a few seconds in data access is annoying and not tolerable in a busy patient care situation, it is not feasible to perform any significant degree of run time data analysis or formatting. Therefore, a fundamental characteristic of the project design was that data would be downloaded, analyzed, formatted and linked to reference information prior to user access. Although selected sections and minor variations in the formatted record could be provided in accordance with user needs, required data is maintained in a formatted, crosslinked file that the user can obtain in a virtually instantaneous fashion.

Data Input.

The VA clinical database (DHCP) system is MUMPS based and provides data to terminals throughout the hospital. All medical record information required for this project was available within the DHCP system. Most DHCP input and access functions are adequate. However, limitations of core computer resources, slow asynchronous serial data transfer to terminals and inadequate terminal capabilities eliminated the possibility of using DHCP computers to directly implement the project. However, serial data transfer methods are widely used and provide inexpensive, easily implemented access to many sources of data. Consequently, if the project could be designed to tolerate serial data transfer then the flexibility of the data input interface would be a valuable asset.

Available patient data within the DHCP system at our facility pertinent to the current project included demographics, laboratory, radiology, pathology, pharmacy, discharge diagnosis and progress note information. Up to five years of data was available. Although existing DHCP MUMPS routines were used for some data access, in most cases routines were modified to transfer data in an abbreviated format. A DHCP "update" global was established to identify DHCP records with new laboratory, medication or radiology data. PC download computers access this global to detect which records require updating on the PC network. In addition, all patients scheduled to be seen in a clinic or who are hospitalized have their PC network files updated. Thus, data transfer to the PC network is largely a process "triggered" by activity in DHCP files.

Transfer of five years of data over an asynchronous serial link is time consuming. Therefore, to reduce data transfer but not require a duplication of DHCP storage capabilities, a file cache design was used.

File Cache.

Download PCs access the DHCP update global to identify records that require data download. The PCs then request needed records from DHCP. A new request will include all files available. After data is transferred it is temporarily stored on the PC network in a B tree database. Subsequent data requests specify that only recent data be transferred (to the date of the last database input). Because new data inputs occur in clusters (typically limited to a few days surrounding a clinic visit or hospitalization), after seven days of inactivity the temporary database files are purged. New DHCP data would subsequently induce a complete file transfer. This approach minimizes the frequency of complete record transfer as well as limiting the required PC storage space. Activity of the records of patients scheduled in clinics is anticipated and complete DHCP record downloads are requested during the weekends or nights before a clinic appointment, a process which minimizing the need for complete record transfers during the daytime periods of frequent data input.

Data analysis and formatting.

Analysis PCs (which may be the same as download PCs on a small system) access the B tree database files of each record that has been updated. The database allows rapid access to all fields in the individual medical record facilitating data evaluation. Trends and abnormalities in the data are identified. Data is then organized into a clinically relevant format that emphasizes data interrelationships, and includes links to available reference data. The formatted, summarized record is then stored on the PC network for user access. The record is updated when new data is input to DHCP. Because only information of immediate clinical relevance is kept in this record, the required file space is modest.

Reference and educational resource links.

The network allows CD-ROM database information to be made available on all network PCs. Although these information sources are of major value, access and retrieval of needed information in the busy patient care setting must be very rapid. Optimally, the data that may be required must be anticipated and directly linked to the patient record. Thus, when results such as a low hematocrit are presented, clicking the mouse on the result of interest should provide immediate reference information concerning the differential diagnosis and management of anemia. Furthermore, within that information additional related reference or educational data should be identified and linked.

To meet the requirement for immediately accessible reference data, internal links to windows help files are installed at the time of data analysis and formatting. Microsoft Windows help files are generated in two phases. Initially RTF (rich text format) files are generated and internally cross referenced from locally generated free text and network CD-ROM sources. The RTF files are then compiled and compressed with the MS help file compiler. Very large help files can be generated and efficiently accessed. The prototype reference source includes the several complete texts, over 1000 selected journal references with abstracts and locally generated reference and guideline data. Although the initial cross referencing and generation of RTF files require a dedicated PC work continuously for several days, the complete source compiles to only 15 MB of disk space and specific topics can be accessed with virtually no delay.

Consistent with the philosophical approach to the entire project, information that is specifically relevant to the current record is directly accessible. However, the entire CD-ROM sources are available at the same workstations and more extensive information can be obtained through the standard CD-ROM programs.

Data Access

A standard Windows program is used to access preformatted, reference linked patient record files. Records can be identified by patient name, record number, clinic or hospital location. Searches are performed in a logical sequence that attempts to match patients seen by the clinician or recently treated in clinic and hospital before seeking patients with less active records.

Electronic records maintained on the PC network include demographics, scheduling, laboratory, microbiology, pharmacy, radiology, pathology, discharge diagnoses, admission and discharge summaries, problem lists and clinic notes. Information is presented in color highlighted text that can be reviewed either with standard scrolling, accelerator keys, push-button jumps or hotspot jumps. Laboratory results are grouped in accordance with likely clinical associations. For example, serum iron results appear in proximity to the report of a low hematocrit and hepatitis B results are listed with data concerning liver function tests. The last four results of each test are listed to allow recognition of trends. Abnormal results are displayed in red and recently abnormal or rapidly changing results in pink. Potential drug related abnormalities are highlighted with yellow. Immediate jumps to any section of the record are accomplished with hotkeys or screen pushbuttons.

A double click on any laboratory result or medication brings up a windows help file screen that displays relevant data extracted from network CD-ROM sources. Help records are internally cross referenced with hotspots that facilitate rapid identification and retrieval of needed information.

RESULTS

The objectives of the project were to cost effectively provide efficient medical record and reference information access. All clinical components of the medical record needed to be accessible with no delay so that the clinician could quickly review potentially related data. These goals have been achieved. The system is now fully functional in physician offices, the emergency room, pharmacy, some clinics and at central locations for general use. Expansion to nursing stations, clinics and hospital locations is in progress. Costs of implementation are very modest. Each new location requires only that a PC be used instead of the terminal which would otherwise be required for DHCP access. Terminal functions remain available on all PCs. The serial interface with file cache between the PC network and DHCP computers has been much more effective than initially anticipated. Using only two computers for both download and data analysis, network records remain no more than 15 minutes behind new data even at peak morning hours.

Although the Boise VA hospital is a small 121 bed hospital, outpatient clinics are active with about 90,000 visits yearly. Records of all patients seen within the past year or who have a future appointment are maintained on the PC network. The initial project was established without degradation of network performance on an existing Novell network with a single 1 GB server. The concept of parallel download PCs has been successful with respect to efficiency and reliability. Despite running unattended 24 hours/day system failure has not occurred except as the consequence of an error in a programming upgrade. Even when DHCP computers are disconnected or fail, error detection prevents PC record degradation and download computers automatically reinitiate data transfer when the serial link is restored.

Complete record download, analysis, formatting and reference linking averages just under 60 seconds. Data transfer averages 25 seconds, analysis takes 15 seconds, formatting and linking of records for network use require 10 seconds. The time required for updating database records (file cache hits) is much less.

Record access is very efficient. Because analysis and formatting is performed at the time of data transfer from DHCP, users are able to access records on screen within 0.5 second of a request. The windows GUI interface has been rapidly accepted and appears to be easily learned by most users. Security is provided through a requirement for Novell access and passwords. After five minutes of inactivity a screensaver is activated and a user's network password is required for reentry. Sensitive file access is tracked and reported to the station security officer . Computers in common use locations have the floppy drive disabled and have a modified windows interface that prevents access to any windows controls or programs other than those installed by the system manager.

Although not a focus of this report, the PC network provides many useful capabilities in addition to medical record access. Fourteen CD-ROMs on the network server provide access to multiple commercially available reference sources. CD-ROM functions have been very actively used by the full range of health care providers including physicians, residents, nurses, pharmacists, medical students and research scientists.

CONCLUSION

This pilot project has demonstrated that medical record information can be cost effectively provided in an enhanced format with integration of reference and educational information. Of importance, an efficient, easily implemented approach was utilized and demonstrated to be feasible. Because a modular approach to system design was used, each component can be modified. The serial data interface could be replaced with an ethernet link or the simple Btree database could be replaced with any network database. Data formatting and and reference links can be designed in accordance with specific user requirements.

The point of patient care is the time at which information is most needed and often is an optimal "teachable moment [4]". The clinician's interest is focussed and new information is likely to be remembered in the context of the current case. Clearly, physician education which can be achieved during patient care is efficient. Information including preventive care reminders and suggestions concerning cost effective or otherwise preferred diagnostic and therapeutic alternatives can be effectively integrated with the patient record. The use of computer based information resources in the clinic appears to be accepted by most clinicians as well as patients [5].

Medical care is information intensive in the extreme. Computers can provide massive quantities of data. However, information is of limited value without organization. The more difficult problem which this project has only begun to approach is how to optimally organize and present information which is now available.

References

[1] R.S. Dick, E.B. Steen. The computer-based medical record: an essential technology for health care. National Academy Press, Washington, D.C. 1991.

[2] R.A. Grenes, E.H. Shortliffe. Medical Informatics. An emerging academic discipline and institutional priority. JAMA, 1990; 263:1114-1120.

[3] E. Nygren, P. Henriksson. Reading the medical record. Analysis of physician's ways of reading the medical record. Comput Methods Programs Biomed 39:1-12, 1992.

[4]J.C.Leist, R.E.Kristofco. The changing paradigm for continuing medical education:impact of information on the teachable moment. Bull Med Libr Assoc; 1990; 78:173-179.

[5]J.D. Legler, R. Oates. Patients' reactions to physician use of a computerized medical record system during clinical encounters. J Fam Pract 1993 37:241-244.

Section II

Vocabularies and Nomenclature

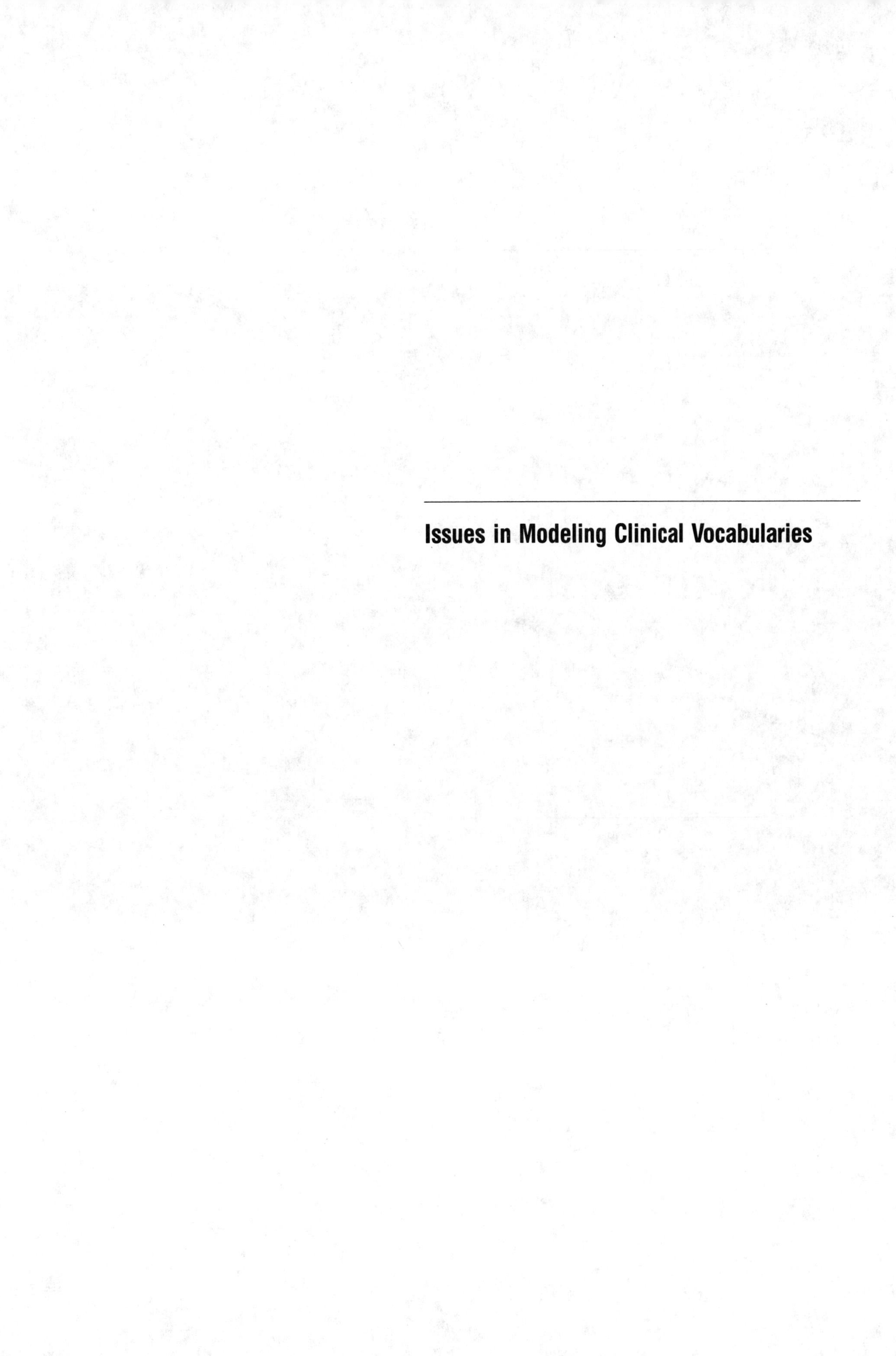

Issues in Modeling Clinical Vocabularies

Coping with Changing Controlled Vocabularies

James J. Cimino, M.D, Paul D. Clayton, Ph.D.
Center for Medical Informatics
Columbia University
New York, New York 10032

For the foreseeable future, controlled medical vocabularies will be in a constant state of development, expansion and refinement. Changes in controlled vocabularies must be reconciled with historical patient information which is coded using those vocabularies and stored in clinical databases. This paper explores the kinds of changes that can occur in controlled vocabularies, including adding terms (simple additions, refinements, redundancy and disambiguation), deleting terms, changing terms (major and minor name changes), and other special situations (obsolescence, discovering redundancy, and precoordination). Examples are drawn from actual changes appearing in the 1993 update to the International Classification of Diseases (ICD9-CM). The methods being used at Columbia-Presbyterian Medical Center to reconcile its Medical Entities Dictionary and its clinical database are discussed.

INTRODUCTION

One of the greatest impediments to the development of electronic medical records is the lack of a high-quality controlled medical vocabulary [1]. A number of private and public research projects are underway to help address this deficiency. An important adjunct to this research is the development of methods for coping with changes in a controlled vocabulary once it becomes relied upon.

An important use of controlled medical vocabularies is the storage of coded patient information in clinical databases. Data stored one day may be difficult to interpret the next day if the vocabulary used to encode it has changed in the interim. One method for dealing with such changes is to maintain an historical database for the vocabulary, such that the original meaning of codes can be resurrected if their storage dates are known. This strategy works well for some purposes, such as batch processing for summary reporting of archived data. However, for systems which require rapid regeneration of information from codes, such as interactive clinical record review or automated decision support, an historical coding system may be impractical. Alternatively, a change in coding could be reflected in the patient data by rewriting records in the database. But this strategy is both impractical, for a large database, and dangerous, since the original meaning of the data could be lost.

The controlled medical vocabulary used in the clinical information system at the Columbia-Presbyterian Medical Center (CPMC) is in a constant state of change. It is used successfully for storing and retrieving patient data, yet it does not rely on an historical format for maintenance. This paper describes the strategy used to retrieve historical data, coded in a changing vocabulary, without losing the meaning of the original data. Examples of vocabulary evolution will be drawn from changes in the *International Classification of Diseases, Ninth Revision, with Clinical Modifications* (ICD9-CM) [2] from the 1992 to the 1993 version.

BACKGROUND

The CPMC clinical information system is coded using the CPMC Medical Entities Dictionary (MED) [3]. The MED consists of a semantic network, based on the Unified Medical Language System (UMLS) [4], with a directional acyclic graph to provide for multiple, coexisting hierarchies. The MED grows in a monotonic manner; that is, concepts are incrementally added and, once added, cannot be removed nor have their *inherent* meaning altered. This is not to say that individual concepts may not change; however, they may only change in ways which clarify or improve their meaning *explicitly*. For example, if a term exists called "glucose test", it might be later changed to "serum glucose test" if and only if the change reflects its true meaning. If the term was previously used to code data which were actually serum test results, then the name change would be allowed. If, on the other hand, the term was used to code data which could reflect either serum or plasma test results, then the name change would be invalid. In this latter case, the original term would be left unchanged (or perhaps changed to "serum or plasma glucose tests") and two new terms ("serum glucose test" and "plasma glucose test") would be added as descendants of the original term.

The MED currently contains over 40,300 terms drawn from a number of sources, including the UMLS, local departmental systems, and ICD9-CM. As each of these sources undergoes changes, the MED must be modified to reflect those changes. On the surface, these changes consist of name changes in existing codes, term deletions, and term additions. If the MED were only used to look up terms in current vocabularies, as one might do with the UMLS when retrieving on-line information or with ICD9-CM when filling out a coding form, simply reflecting these changes in the MED would be adequate. However, when patient data are to be encoded and stored for later retrieval and reconstitution, close attention must be paid to how alterations affect the meaning of the terms. These changes are incorporated into the MED in a systematic way, depending on the type of change involved.

RENAMING TERMS

Changes in controlled vocabularies are often detectable only because the name associated with a unique identifier differs from the name which was present in a previous version. The October 1993 update to ICD9-CM, for example, includes 47 instances of name changes. Such changes are classified as minor (no meaning change) or major (meaning change).

Minor Name Change

Minor name changes are common and (by definition) do not effect term meaning. Sometimes, change is needed to correct a spelling error. For example, in ICD9-CM code 681.10, CELULITIS was changed to CELLULITIS. In other cases, change is enacted to better reflect accepted medical terminology. For example, in code 733.1, PATHOLOGICAL FRACTURE to PATHOLOGIC FRACTURE. In still other cases, change is intended to clarify a term without changing its intended meaning. For example, code 250.11 TYPE I DIABETES MELLITUS WITH KETOACIDOSIS was changed to include the phrase NOT STATED AS UNCONTROLLED.

In cases such as these, the MED concept name is changed. Since the meaning has not changed, the meaning of the data represented by it will not be misrepresented through reconstitution using the new name (for example, by improving the spelling).

Major Name Change

In some cases, the change in a term name corresponds to a true change in its meaning. Occasionally, this might come about due to "code re-use" For example, the code 99.71 was originally assigned to the term MERCURY-ZINC PACEMAKER BATTERY but at some point between 1980 and 1992, the codes was reassigned to THERAPEUTIC PLASMAPHERESIS. More often, however, the change is due to some refinement of meaning which is, nevertheless, a change in meaning. For example, the code 354.4 changed from CAUSALGIA to CAUSALGIA OF UPPER LIMB. In cases such as these, it would be inappropriate to allow a doctor to assign the diagnosis of "causalgia" to a patient in 1992 and then, in 1993, report that the actual diagnosis was "causalgia of upper limb", since the physician might originally have meant "causalgia of lower limb", a term which was not available until 1993.

In the MED, these changes in meaning are treated as if the old terms were deleted and new terms added with the same code. The sections below describe the individual handling of a deletion and an addition.

DELETING TERMS

Terms may be deleted from a vocabulary if the creators of the terminology no longer wish to include the corresponding concept in the domain of the terminology. For example two codes were removed from ICD9-CM in 1993 (e.g., 665.14 RUPTURE OF UTERUS DURING LABOR, POSTPARTUM CONDITION OR COMPLICATION). Presumably, these codes could be reused in some later version.

The deletion of concepts poses problems for systems which have already made some use of them. For example, if a patient was noted to have a particular diagnosis on a particular date, it would be unacceptable to simply delete that fact just because the disease term was removed from the vocabulary. In many cases, however, no changes are needed to the MED. For example, if the laboratory ceases to perform a particular test, the persistence of the term in the MED is harmless - the laboratory system will simply cease to send data about that test. Meanwhile, any previous occurrences of the test remain coded in the patient databases and remain interpretable. In some cases, the term must be flagged in the MED to prevent inappropriate use. For example, in the case of deleted ICD9-CM terms, the ICD9-CM code for the "deleted" term is moved out of the "ICD9-

CODE" attribute field and into the "OLD-ICD9-CODE" attribute field. Thus, as stated above, concepts are not deleted from the MED. This approach provides a means for a data entry program to recognize that the code is no longer usable, while providing a means for interpreting previously stored occurrences.

ADDING TERMS

The periodic addition of terms to a controlled medical vocabulary is required by the evolution of the discipline of medicine. When a new concept is established, such as a new medication, disease or procedure, the creation of a new term is proper and expected. The 1993 ICD9-CM update, for example, included 160 new terms. The appropriate response to a particular concept addition depends on how the new term influences appropriate use of previously existing terms.

Simple Additions

When the new term represents a truly new concept, the proper response is simply to accept it into the vocabulary and use it when appropriate. For example, the addition of the new ICD9-CM code 704.02 TELOGEN EFFLUVIUM does not influence how any of the previously existing codes are used. Therefore, a new concept is added to the MED, corresponding to this new term.

Refinement

In many cases, one or more terms are added to allow greater levels of detail to be specified. For example, the 1992 version of ICD9-CM contained 434.0 CEREBRAL THROMBOSIS. In 1993, the codes 434.00 CEREBRAL THROMBOSIS WITHOUT MENTION OF CEREBRAL INFARCTION and 434.01 CEREBRAL THROMBOSIS WITH CEREBRAL INFARCTION were added. In cases such as these, the new terms can be added as children (in the MED hierarchy) of the existing term.

Redundancy

Sometimes, a code is added which is identical in meaning to an existing term. In ICD9-CM this often occurs in the course of adding refining terms. For example, in 1992 ICD9-CM contained 530.1 ESOPHAGITIS. In 1993, the codes 530.10 UNSPECIFIED ESOPHAGITIS, 530.11 REFLUX ESOPHAGITIS, and 530.19 OTHER ESOPHAGITIS were added. Two of these (530.11 and 530.19) were added easily as refinements. However, the new term 530.10 is synonymous with 530.1.

Adding a new concept to the MED which has the same meaning as an existing concept would introduce undesirable redundancy. Instead, the existing term is given the new code (530.10) and its preexisting code (530.1) is moved to the "OLD-ICD9-CODE" attribute field. In addition, the name of the concept is altered to reflect the new variation.

Disambiguation

If a term in a controlled vocabulary is discovered to have two or more meanings (referred to as "polysemy"), an appropriate response is to disambiguate these meanings by creating a separate term for each. No examples of such disambiguation were found in ICD9-CM updates. However, the UMLS provides several examples of disambiguation. These occur mainly because UMLS developers notice that terms with the same name in different sources may have different meanings in the different sources, or because one UMLS source vocabulary was found to have two meanings for the same term. For example, the original term "Atrium" was subsequently disambiguated into "Heart Atrium" (a body part) and "atrium <2>" (an organic chemical). An important consideration in dealing with disambiguation is to determine whether the unique identifier for the original term can be retained for use with one of the original meanings.

The appropriate response to disambiguation in the MED depends on the meaning of the term from the MED's perspective. In the above example, the MED included "Atrium", but only in its anatomic meaning. In this case, the name was changed to "Heart Atrium" and the existing concept was associated with the appropriate UMLS concept. Since the meaning of the concept was always intended to be anatomical, the name change had no effect on the meaning of the information stored in the patient database. (No concept corresponding to the chemical meaning has been added to the MED.)

There have been no situations to date in which a concept in the MED was found to have multiple meanings such that patient data corresponding to the different meanings might have been stored in the database with the same code. There is no guarantee, however, that this situation will not occur. In such an event, it may be impossible to correct the database by determining which meaning was intended in each occurrence. Instead, some response will be needed in the MED to represent the ambiguity explicitly and prevent its recurrence.

Consider a hypothetical example in which the MED contained the concept "Paget Disease", without specifying whether it was a disease of bone or breast. To correct this situation, it would be necessary to add two new terms "Paget Disease of the Breast" and "Paget Disease of the Bone". The original term could be left with its ambiguous name; however, an alternative would be to rename the term so that the inherent ambiguity is made explicit, such as "Paget Disease, Not Specified as Bone or Breast". Of course, this is a meaningless term, from a clinical point of view; however, since it can't deleted, the new name at least makes the ambiguity explicit.

SPECIAL CASES

CPMC's experience with maintaining the MED, particularly with respect to keeping the ICD9-CM information current, has provided some additional insights into how controlled vocabularies can evolve and how changes can be dealt with in a way that maintains both the monotonicity of the vocabulary and the integrity of stored coded data. The following additional vocabulary modifications, while not found in recent ICD9-CM updates are, nevertheless, likely in the future.

Obsolescence

New knowledge often requires the addition of new terms to a vocabulary; it may also render existing terms obsolete. For example, with advances in virology and immunology, the terms "Infectious Hepatitis" and "Serum Hepatitis" were replaced by "Hepatitis A", "Hepatitis B" and "Non-A, Non-B Viral Hepatitis". This last term has, in turn, been replaced by a further collection of terms.

Although a term such as "Non-A, Non-B Viral Hepatitis" has fallen out of favor, it is not possible to remove it from vocabularies such as the MED. This is because previous patient diagnoses have been coded using the term. Even though we may now be able to differentiate a new patient's condition into Hepatitis C or E, it is generally not possible to go back and determine what a patient had in the past and recode the database. Thus, the "obsolete" concept is still valid and still has valid meaning. It must therefore be retained in the MED. The new terms can be added as refinements to the obsolete term, just as with any refining terms.

Discovering Redundancy

Redundancy is an undesirable condition in any controlled vocabulary; however there is no way to prevent it from occurring. Sometimes it occurs because synonymous terms are added without recognizing their synonymy. In other cases, the true synonymy may only be recognized through subsequent medical advances.

Consider, for example, the AIDS virus. Originally, there were two reported agents: Human T-Cell Lymphoma Virus III (HTLV-III) and Lymphadenopathy-Associated Virus (LAV). Since the original description of these agents, they have been recognized to be identical (now named Human Immunodeficiency Virus-1, or HIV-1). The easiest solution would be to discard one term and save the other, with renaming or addition of synonyms as appropriate. Unfortunately, this would render data coded with the discarded term to be uninterpretable. An alternate solution is to create a class which includes all the redundant terms. The new superclass would be the preferred form and the child terms can have a pointer to that term to indicate its preferred status. Thus, in the above example, HIV-1 would become the superclass for HTLV-III and LAV. When reconstituting the coded data, the preferred name could be obtained and, when retrieving all cases of HIV-1, including a search for all descendant terms would retrieve all appropriate instances of any of the three codes. In this way, the redundancy can at least be made transparent, if not totally eliminated.

Precoordination

One troublesome way which controlled vocabularies evolve is by adding more specific, "precoordinated" terms. For example, coding Type I Diabetes with Hyperosmolarity used to require two "atomic" codes: 250.8 DIABETES WITH OTHER SPECIFIED MANIFESTATION and 276.0 HYPEROSMOLALITY AND/OR HYPERNATREMIA. ICD9-CM now provides a single convenient code (250.23 TYPE I DIABETES WITH HYPEROSMOLARITY). Querying a database which has stored patient diagnoses both ways may produce undesirable results, unless the dual representation is recognized. However, reliably detecting such situations is problematic.

The CPMC clinical database does not yet provide a simple way to query for data which might be coded as atomic, precoordinated or both. However, the MED does provide a facility for assisting with such a process. The UMLS Semantic Net provides for concepts to be related through a has-part/part-of relation. Thus, the MED is capable of including the information that 250.23 TYPE I DIABETES WITH HYPEROSMOLARITY has parts TYPE I DIABETES and HYPEROSMOLARITY. As a result, terms can be given a "molecular" appearance, such that a single precoordinated term can be disassembled into its constituent atomic elements. Similarly, when given a set of atomic terms, the MED can be searched to locate a corresponding precoordination, if one exists. It should therefore be possible to design a database retrieval routine which can take advantage of this feature of the MED in order to cope with multiple codings of the same information.

DISCUSSION

Controlled vocabulary evolution is a fact of life for clinical system developers. Unless care is taken, patient data stored in a compact, useful coded form may become obsolete if they become uninterpretable due to vocabulary changes subsequent to their storage. Rather than wait for change and then attempt to retrofit old data to new codes, it will be imperative for developers of electronic medical record systems to anticipate the types of changes which may occur. This paper proposes an initial formal framework by which vocabulary changes can be classified and addressed.

CPMC has expended considerable effort to develop automated vocabulary maintenance methods. These methods have proved useful for applying changes in source vocabularies to the content of the MED. However, the right method can only be applied when the type of change is well understood. At present, no method exists which can automatically decide the type of change and the appropriate response (e.g., to differentiate between a minor and major name change). Instead, manual review by domain experts is needed. One reason is that vocabulary changes usually do not include information about the reason for the change. Such additional information could enhance vocabulary management, particularly if the information were to be included in a structured, machine-readable format. For example, if each disease term included references to involved body parts, then it might be possible to distinguish a minor name change (say, from PATHOLOGICAL FRACTURE to PATHOLOGIC FRACTURE, where both terms would have a reference to BONE) from a major name change (e.g., the change from CAUSALGIA to CAUSALGIA OF UPPER LIMB, which would entail the addition of new body location information).

The CPMC approach offers a means to retrieve patient information based on concepts of interest. It does not guarantee that retrieval can be done by ICD9-CM code, nor that the original form of the code (e.g., a misspelling) can be reconstructed. Old codes are kept in the MED, but the date of changes are not, nor could the correct old code be determined if the concept's code had been changed more than once. However, if such a reconstruction were needed, it could be handled by including the ICD9-CM code with the MED code in the clinical database at the time of storage or by reviewing the log files of MED changes which will identify when and how concept information was modified.

Additional research in vocabulary maintenance is needed and the lessons learned must be fed back to the developers of controlled vocabularies, such as ICD9-CM. For example, the repercussions of seemingly arbitrary actions such as major name changes and term deletions need to be clarified so that developers will be aware of the needs of the users and users will better understand the intentions of the developers. This paper attempts to define a taxonomy for describing types of vocabulary changes and offers one set of approaches for dealing with them.

Acknowledgments

This work was supported in part the IBM Corporation and the National Library of Medicine.

References

1. United States. General Accounting Office. *Automated Medical Records: Leadership Needed to Expedite Standards Development.* Washington, D.C.: USGAO/IMTEC-93-17; April 1993.
2. United States National Center for Health Statistics. *International Classification of Diseases, Ninth Revision, with Clinical Modifications,* Washington, DC; 1980.
3. Cimino JJ, Clayton PD, Hripcsak G, Johnson SB: Knowledge-based approaches to the maintenance of a large controlled medical terminology. *JAMIA,* 1994; 1(1):35-50.
4. Lindberg DAB, Humphreys BL, McCray AT. The Unified Medical Language System. *Meth Inform Med.* 1993; 32(4):281-291.

Subsumption Principles Underlying Medical Concept Systems and their Formal Reconstruction

Jochen Bernauer, Institute for Medical Informatics, University of Hildesheim, Germany

Conventional medical concept systems represent generic concept relations by hierarchical coding principles. Often, these coding principles constrain the concept system and reduce the potential for automatical derivation of subsumption. Formal reconstruction of medical concept systems is an approach that bases on the conceptual representation of meanings and that allows for the application of formal criteria for subsumption. Those criteria must reflect intuitive principles of subordination which are underlying conventional medical concept systems. Particularly these are: The subordinate concept results (1) from adding a specializing criterion to the superordinate concept, (2) from refining the primary category, or a criterion of the superordinate concept, by a concept that is less general, (3) from adding a partitive criterion to a criterion of the superordinate, (4) from refining a criterion by a concept that is less comprehensive, and finally (5) from coordinating the superordinate concept, or one of its criteria. This paper introduces a formalism called BERNWARD that aims at the formal reconstruction of medical concept systems according to these intuitive principles. The automatical derivation of hierarchical relations is primarily supported by explicit generic and explicit partitive hierarchies of concepts, secondly, by two formal criteria that base on the structure of concept descriptions and explicit hierarchical relations between their elements, namely: formal subsumption and part-sensitive subsumption. Formal subsumption takes only generic relations into account, part-sensitive subsumption additionally regards partive relations between criteria. This approach seems to be flexible enough to cope with unforeseeable effects of partitive criteria on subsumption.

INTRODUCTION

Conventional medical concept systems have the following characteristics: (1) They combine the ordering of concepts with a coding schema which represents concept relations by meaningful codes. (2) Their use presupposes a certain amount of intuitive knowledge [1]. These characteristics limit the services of computer-based concept representations for the following reasons: Often, the structure of the coding scheme is constraining the structure of the concept system, and terminological principles are sacrificed in favour of coding principles. Common phenomena in this respect are: The potential number of hierarchical levels is constrained by hierarchical coding principles, i.e. hierarchical, group sequential or combinatorial codes, with fixed length. Typical compensations are the parallel representation of independent criteria on the same level of subordination, or the introduction of sibling concepts although child concepts were adequate. The potential number of siblings on a particular hierarchical level is restricted by the length of the coding alphabet. This sometimes leads to "artificially" balanced concept formation and ordering. Finally, common hierarchical coding principles support only strict hierarchies. This may be circumvented by assigning several codes to a concept as realized by MeSH, but gives rise to the problem of redundancy and consistency of views [2].

Conventional medical concept systems comprise the following implicit knowledge types. Commonly, they make no difference between generic and partitive relations, sometimes they mix both in a transitive manner. In general, the criteria for subordination are hidden, often they are partitive. This situation is acceptable if the coding schemes are for intuitive use, but is an obstacle for computer-based services. A global effect is the limited potential for automatical subsumption.

Formal subsumption has been investigated in the context of term subsumption languages in the tradition of KL-ONE [3,4]. These languages focus on the formal definition and automatical classification of concepts. In general, they distinguish between definitorial and assertional knowledge and base subsumption strictly on definitorial knowledge.

In contrast to term subsumption languages, the concept representation formalism developed in the GALEN project emphasizes the formation of sensible concepts, instead of classification of already defined ones. The classificator makes no difference between definitorial and assertional knowledge and takes also partitive criteria into account [5,6].

This paper introduces a constrained representation formalism for medical concepts based on conceptual graphs [7] which focuses on the principles of subordination underlying conventional medical concept systems and which aims at their formal reconstruction. Formal criteria for subsumption are given that reflect the intuitive principles of subordination.

PRINCIPLES OF SUBSUMPTION

Subordination in conventional medical concept systems is based on several intuitive principles. They are illustrated by the generic concept ladder of Figure 1, which is in the style of a conventional concept system. In principle, a concept description is assumed to be composed by a base concept and a set of criteria. In the Aristotelean sense of a definition the base concept refers to the primary category which the concept belongs to, and the set of criteria refer to the differentiae, which distinguish the concept from the primary category. (cf. [8])

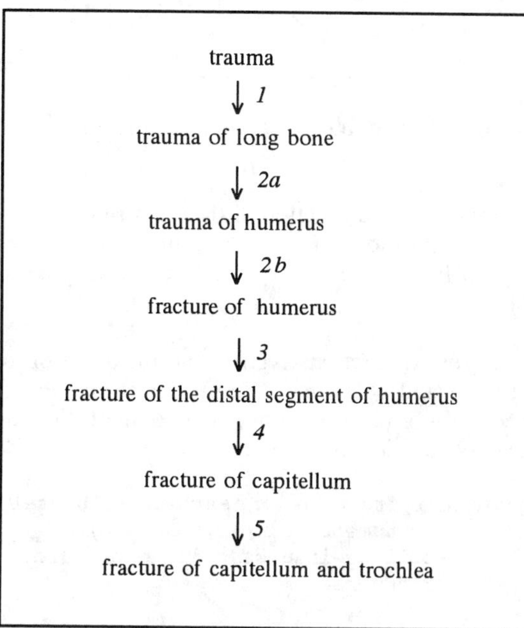

Figure 1: A generic concept ladder presenting different intuitive principles of subordination

Informally, a composite concept description can be superordinate to another concept for any of the following reasons:

Introduction of a specializing criterion
The subordinate description includes a specializing criterion of the base concept (1), or of a criterion (numbering refers to Figure 1), which is not present in the superordinate description.

Generic refinement of a concept element
A criterion (2a), or the base concept (2b) in the superordinate description is more general than one in the subordinate description.

Introduction of a partitive criterion
The subordinate description includes a partitive criterion of a criterion, which is not present in the superordinate description (3).

Partitive refinement of a criterion
A criterion in the superordinate description is more comprehensive than one in the subordinate description (4).

Conjunctive coordination
The primary category or a criterion of the subordinate description is a conjunctive coordination of one in the superordinate description (5). The inverse situation holds for disjunctive coordination (not depicted in Figure 1).

Of these principles the introduction of a specializing criterion and the generic refinement of a concept element are typically realized by the classifier of the languages of the KL-ONE-family [4].

FORMAL RECONSTRUCTION

A model for the formal reconstruction of medical concept systems must be capable for representing the intuitive principles of subordination and must support the automatical classification of concept descriptions by formal subsumption criteria.

Structure of conceptual descriptions

Concept descriptions in BERNWARD (Building Essential concept Representations in Well-Arranged Restricted Domains) are of the following types: primitive, composite, coordinated, negated and defined. A primitive concept description consists of a name of a primitive concept type, and has no formal substructure. A composite concept description is constructed from other concept descriptions by means of concept-forming operators. The structure reflects the definition of the concept and serves for the formal classification of conceptual descriptions. Formally, a composite concept consists of a base concept and a set of criteria, where a criterion consists of a role symbol and a concept description. The base concept reflects the primary category of the concept, the set of criteria reflects its essential characteristics. A composite concept may have one particular criterion, called "partitive criterion", which consists of the symbol designating the part-of-role and a concept description, which is called the "whole" of the composite concept. A coordinated concept description is a set of concept description combined by a logical conjunction (AND, OR), a negated concept description is combined by a negator (NOT). A defined concept description is of composite, coordinated or negated type, that is given a name. It can be used like a primitive type. Concept descriptions can be represented in the conceptual graphs notation [7].

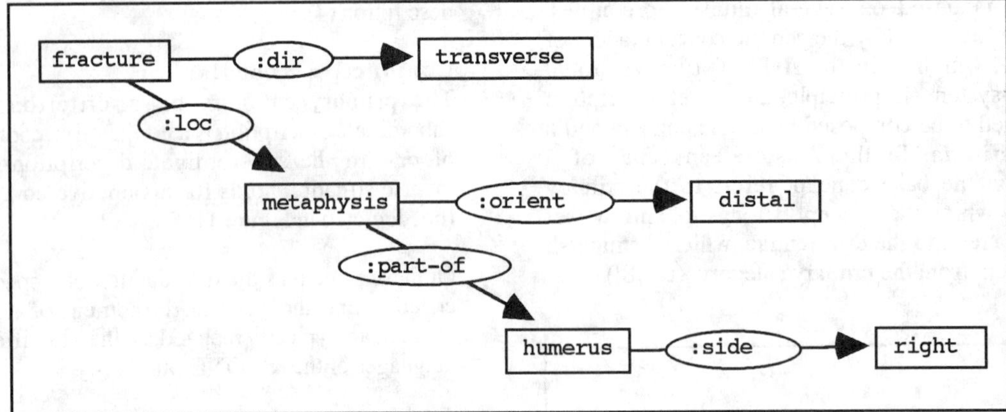

Figure 2: Representation of the concept "transverse fracture of the distal metaphysis of the right humerus"

Figure 2 shows the graphical representation of a fracture type as a composite concept description. Its base concept is "fracture", its criteria are "has direction transverse" and "has location distal metaphysis of right humerus". The concept which is in the latter criterion has the partitive criterion "is part of right humerus". Its whole is "right humerus".

Explicit hierarchical relations

Concept descriptions can be explicitely organized in a generic and a partitive hierarchy. The generic hierarchy (taxonomy) reflects the a priori subordination of concepts because of reasons that are not further relevant. Its ordering relation is designated by <. For example `fracture < trauma` means: a fracture is a trauma. In parallel, the partitive hierarchy (partonomy) reflects the a priori part-whole relation between concepts, which is designated by $<_p$. For example `capitellum` $<_p$ `dist_segment_humerus` means that the capitellum is a part of the distal humerus segment. The relation $<_p$ is supposed to be transitive. This approach is partly in contrast to the results of [9], where six different types of part-whole-relations are identified with potential intransitivity in case of mixing particular types. It is justified by the observation, that firstly the predominant medically related types of part-whole relations are "component/integral whole" and "place/region" ("segment/organ"). Secondly, the transitive mixing of these types is almost intuitively acceptable [10].

Constrained composition of concepts

The formal reconstruction of medical concept systems must realize the intuitive principles of subordination described above. Therefore, BERNWARD provides different types of restrictions that control the formation of subordinate concept descriptions. The function of these restriction types shall be illustrated on reconstructing sections of the AO/ASIF classification of fractures of long bones [11].

Local role restrictions restrict the introduction of sensible and relevant criteria. These are either specifying or partitive. For instance, the following local role restriction

```
lrestr(:dir;fracture_extraarticular_distal_
metaphysis_humerus_simple;fracture):=
        {oblique-inwards,oblique-outwards,
        transverse}
```

restricts the direction of a extra-articular simple fracture of the distal humerus to the concepts "oblique-inwards", "oblique-outwards", and "transverse".

The local role restriction

```
lrestr(:fragm;fracture_extraarticular_
distal_metaphysis_humerus_wedge;wedge):=
        {fragmented,non-fragmented}
```

states that the concept "wedge" in the context of the concept "extra-articular wedge fracture of the distal humerus metaphysis" can be modified by "fragmented" or "non-fragmented".

The local role restriction:

```
lrestr(:part;fracture_long_bone;long_bone):=
        {proximal_segment,diaphysis,
        distal_segment}
```

restricts the introduction of a partitive criterion for "long bone" in the context of "long bone fracture" to the concepts "proximal segment", "diaphysis" and "distal segment".

The generic refinement of concept elements can be restricted by subconcept restrictions. A subconcept restriction defines the set of concept candidates which might used for generic refinement of a concept description. For instance, the subconcept restriction:

```
subrestr(long_bone_fracture;long_bone):=
{humerus,radius,ulna,femur,tibia,fibula}
```

restricts the refinement of the concept "long bone" in the context of "long bone fracture" to "humerus", "radius", "ulna", "femur", "tibia", and "fibula".

In analogy to subconcept restriction, part restrictions define the set of concept candidates, which might be used for partitive refinement. The following part restriction:

```
partrestr(fracture_partial-articular-
distal_humerus_medial-sagittal;
distal_humerus):=
        {medial-trochlea,
        trochlea-grove}
```

means, that for the concept "partial articular fracture of the distal humerus with medial-sagittal direction" the concept "distal humerus" can be refined by the partitive concepts "medial-trochlea", or "trochlea-grove".

Coordination restrictions define which concepts are allowed for coordination with an element of a concept description. For instance, the coordination restriction:

```
coordrestr(fracture_partial-articular_
frontal_capitellum;capitellum):=
        {trochlea}
```

allows the conjunctive coordination of "capitellum" and "trochlea" in the composite description "partial-articular frontal fracture of the capitellum".

Formal subsumption

For conventional medical concept systems automatical classification is restricted to those relations that are represented by hierarchical coding principles. Common obstacles are the inconsistent use of different coding principles, i.e. the mixing of hierarchical, group sequential or combinatorial codes within particular hierarchical ladders, the mixing of generic and partitive relations, or the disregard of hierarchical relationships. The main goal of formal reconstruction of medical concept systems is to allow for the automatical classification of composite concept descriptions. In contrast to conventional coding schemes, concepts are not represented by meaningful codes, but by formal definitions.

The principle of formal subsumption is to derive logical relationships between concept descriptions from their structure and from explicit hierarchical relationships between their elements. Criteria for formal subsumption have been developed for term subsumption languages [4], and for conceptual graphs (canonical formation rules) [7].

A peculiar problem especially for medical concepts is the effect of partitive relations between criteria on subsumption. There are different approaches for coping with this problem. Doyle and Patil [12] suggest to include axioms of the kind "a disease of a part of an organ is a disease of the organ" in the axiomatic component of a terminological representation system, and thus, to deal with the problem outside of formal subsumption. In GRAIL [6] subsumption over partitive criteria is integrated into formal subsumption. There are syntactical means for specifying for a particular role (e.g. "has location") to be refineable along a transitive role (e.g. "is part of"). However, this approach seems to be too general in certain situations, like for instance the following: A scoliosis of the thoracic spine is not a scoliosis of the spine, a revision of the colon is not a revision of the gastro-intestinal system, an avulsion of the humerus apophysis is not an avulsion of the humerus, etc. In these cases pathological conditions regarding body structures do not subsume pathological conditions regarding parts.

The unforeseeable implications of partitive relations between criteria justify the introduction of two separate criteria for formal subsumption and formal part-whole-relation. This allows for the distinction between a formal criterion for subsumption, which disregards partitive relationships between criteria, called "formal subsumption" and a different, which takes also partitive criteria into account, called "part-sensitive subsumption".

A conceptual description c_1 is formally subsumed by a conceptual description c_2, iff the base concept of c_1 is explicitely subsumed by the base concept of c_2 and the criteria set of c_2 is a subset of the criteria set of c_1, and all the concepts of the criteria set of c_2 formally subsume the concepts of the criteria set of c_1. (A formal definition is given in [10].)

A conceptual description c1 represents a formal partitive concept of one represented by the conceptual description c2, iff either c2 is the whole of c1, or the base of c1 is an explicit partitive concept of the base of c2 and the criteria sets of both are equal. (A formal definition is given in [10].)

Part-sensitive subsumption is equal to formal subsumption, but additionally, takes formal part-whole-relations between criteria into account [10].

Figure 3 illustrates the difference between formal subsumption and part-sensitive subsumption.

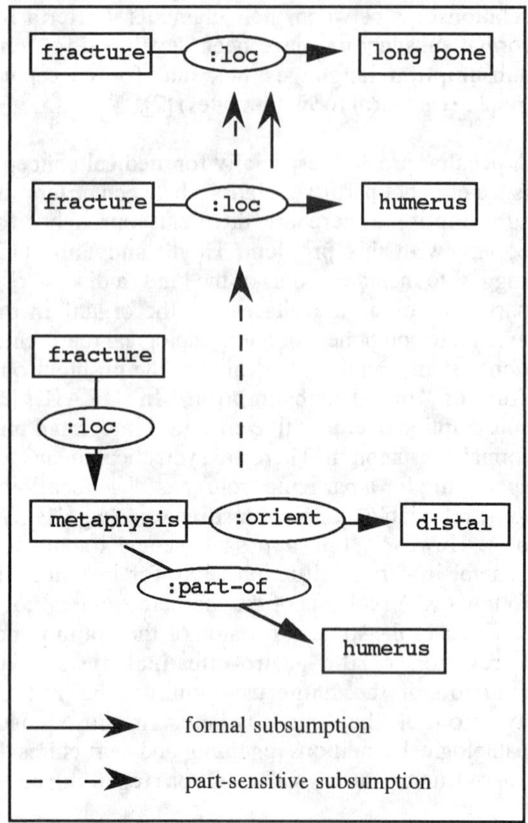

Figure 3: Formal subsumption and part-sensitive subsumption between conceptual descriptions.

SUMMARY

There are several intuitive principles of subordination that are underlying conventional medical concept systems. Some of them involve part-whole relations. A model for the formal reconstruction of medical concept systems has been outlined which considers these principles by mechanisms for constraining subconcept formation. For automatical classification two formal criteria for subsumption are introduced: formal subsumption and part-sensitive subsumption. The latter takes partitive relations between concept forming criteria into account.

REFERENCES

[1] Rossi Mori A., et al. (1993). Model for Representation of Terminologies and Coding Systems in Medicine, in: de Moor G.J.E., McDonald C.J., Noothoven van Goor J., (eds.), Progress in Standardization in Health Care Informatics, IOS Press, 1993; 92-104

[2] Cimino J.J., Hripcsak G., Johnson S.B., Clayton P.D. (1989). Designing an introspective, multipurpose, controlled medical vocabulary. In: Kingsland L.C. (ed.), Proc. 13th Symposium on Computer Applications in Medical Care (SCAMC), McGraw-Hill pp 513-18

[3] Woods W.A., Schmolze J.G. (1992). The KL-ONE family. Computers and Mathematics with Applications, 23; pp 133-177

[4] Woods W.A. (1991). Understanding Subsumption and Taxonomy: A Framework for Progress. In Sowa J.F., (ed.), Principles of Semantic Networks. Morgan Kaufmann Publishers, San Mateo CA, 1991, pp 45-94

[5] Rector A.L., Nowlan W.A., Glowinski A. (1993). Goals for concept representation in the GALEN project. In: Safran C. (ed.), Proc. 17th Symposium on Computer Applications in Medical Care (SCAMC), McGraw-Hill pp 414-418

[6] GALEN: The GRAIL Kernel, Version 1. 1993 GALEN Deliverable 6. The GALEN Consortium.

[7] Sowa J.F. (1984). Conceptual Structures: Information Processing in Mind and Maschine, Addison-Wesley

[8] Campbell K.E., Das A.K., Musen M.A. (1994). A Logical Foundation for Representation of Clinical Data, J Am Med Informatics Assoc. 1:218-232

[9] Winston M.E., Chaffin R., Herrmann D. (1987). A Taxonomy of Part-Whole Relations. Cognitive Science 11: 417-444

[10] Bernauer J., Modelling Formal Subsumption and Part-Whole Relation for Medical Concept Descriptions, European Conference on Artificial Intelligence 94 (ECAI´94), Workshop Parts and Wholes: Conceptual Part-Whole relations and Formal Mereology

[11] Müller M.E., Nazarian S., Koch P., Schatzker J. (1990). The Comprehensive Classification of Fractures of Long Bones. Springer-Verlag

[12] Doyle J., Patil R.S. (1991). Two theses of knowledge representation: language restrictions, taxonomic classification, and the utility of representation services. Art. Intelligence 48; 261-297

Formal Properties of the Metathesaurus®*

Mark S. Tuttle[1], Nels E. Olson[1], Keith E. Campbell, MD[2], David D. Sherertz[1], Stuart J. Nelson, MD[3], William G. Cole, PhD[4]

[1]Lexical Technology, Inc., Alameda, CA; [2]Stanford University, Stanford, CA ; [3]Medical College of Georgia, Augusta, GA; [4]University of Washington, Seattle, WA

The Metathesaurus is a machine-created, human edited and enhanced synthesis of authoritative biomedical terminologies. Its formal properties permit it to be a) exploited by computers, and b) modified and enhanced without compromising that usage. If further constraints were imposed on the existence and identity of Metathesaurus relationships, i.e., if every Metathesaurus concept had a "genus" and a "differentia," then the Metathesaurus could be converted into an "Aristotelian Hierarchy." In this sense, a genus is a concept that classifies another concept, and a differentia is a concept that distinguishes the classified concept from all other concepts in the same class. Since, in principle, these constraints would make the Metathesaurus easier to leverage and maintain computationally, it is interesting to ask to what degree the maintenance and enhancement procedures now in place are producing a Metathesaurus that is also an "Aristotelian Hierarchy." Given a liberal interpretation of the current Metathesaurus schema, the proportion of the Metathesaurus that is "Aristotelian" in each annual version is increasing in spite of dramatic concurrent increases in the number of Metathesaurus concepts.

> *Without formality there is no modifiability nor scalability.[1]*

> *We need formal methods and computer-based tools that can help us with the task [of controlled medical vocabulary construction]. We need research in which controlled vocabulary development is the focus rather than a stepping stone for work on other theories and applications.[2]*

INTRODUCTION

The National Library of Medicine (NLM) Unified Medical Language System® (UMLS®)[3] Metathesaurus is a machine generated and human edited synthesis of authoritative biomedical terminologies that is updated and enhanced annually. Meta-1.0, the first version of the Metathesaurus, was released in 1990, and Meta-1.4, the fifth version, was released in 1994. While the evolution of the form, or *schema*, of the Metathesaurus has slowed, the evolution of *content* has accelerated.

The Schema of the Metathesaurus is Stable

It is the schema of the Metathesaurus that specifies that it is exactly an inter-related set of syntactically homogeneous and semantically unique entries - one entry per concept. Evidence for the current stability of the schema is the fact that the documentation and release format for Meta-1.4, changed only slightly from the documentation and release format for Meta-1.3, continuing a trend begun with the transition from Meta-1.1 to Meta-1.2. A review of the role of "Terminologies," "ATOMS," and "CONCEPTS" in the current Metathesaurus schema appears in **Figure 1**, below.

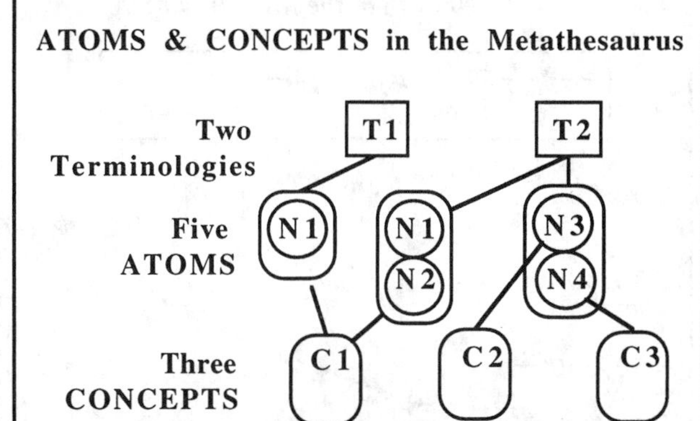

Figure 1 - Two terminologies containing a total of five ATOMS yields three CONCEPTS in the Metathesaurus. Terminology T1 contains a single ATOM, named N1. Terminology T2 contains four ATOMS , namely another instance of N1, and three additional names, N2, N3 and N4. In T2, N2 is a synonym of N1, and N4 is a synonym of N3. From the point of view of the Metathesaurus, T1-N1, and T2-N1,N2 , name CONCEPT C1; N3 names CONCEPT C2; and N4 names CONCEPT C3.

The Content of the Metathesaurus is Increasing

Evidence for the increase in content is displayed in **Figure 2**, below. Since the Metathesaurus grows through the addition of terminologies, one measure of growth is the number of names, or ATOMS, added from each additional terminology. Another measure is the number of new meanings, or CONCEPTS, added to the Metathesaurus by the new names. More precisely, as illustrated in **Figure 1**, we call the occurrence of a name in a terminology an ATOM, and a CONCEPT is an occurrence of a unique named meaning in the Metathesaurus. Thus, both within and between terminologies, more than one ATOM can name the same CONCEPT.

In **Figure 2** the upper line tracks the growth in the number of ATOMS and the lower line the growth in the number of CONCEPTS, in each version of the Metathesaurus. The distance between the two lines represents the degree to which the ATOMS have named the same CONCEPTS.

As implied by **Figure 1**, the Metathesaurus editors are the final arbitrators of whether two ATOMS name the same CONCEPT, or whether they name two different CONCEPTS. On average, the Metathesaurus tends to make fine distinctions, e.g, "Ornithosis" and "Psittacosis" are not synonyms in the Metathesaurus, though they are in some of its constituent terminologies. Further, the Metathesaurus distinguishes "Gentamicins," a "complex of closely related aminoglycoside sulfates ...," from "Gentamicin <1>," a familiar antibiotic, from "Gentamicin <2>," an assay for the antibiotic. Since, fine or not, these distinctions are maintained only in the "Reviewed" portion of the Metathesaurus, "Unreviewed" entries were not counted. A reviewed entry contains only reviewed ATOMS.[4]

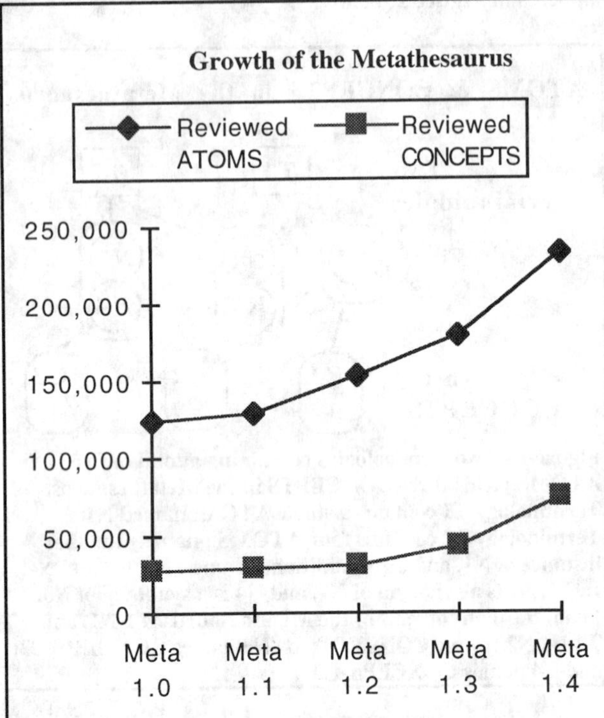

Figure 2 - The number of ATOMS and CONCEPTS in the reviewed portion of the five extant versions of the Metathesaurus: An ATOM is an occurrence of a name in a terminology. A CONCEPT is an occurrence of a unique named meaning in the Metathesaurus. While both ATOMS and CONCEPTS are being added at an accelerating rate, ATOMS are being added faster than CONCEPTS, implying that names are being added faster than meanings.

The Metathesaurus May Be "Converging"

Since, as observed, the Metathesaurus tends to "split" rather than "lump" the concepts named in its constituent terminologies, as with "Ornithosis" and "Psittacosis," it is remarkable that there is preliminary evidence of "convergence." That is, for all four annual transitions displayed in **Figure 2**, the rate at which ATOMS were added exceeded the rate at which CONCEPTS were added; and, for the first and third of the three intervals for which it can be computed, the rate of increase of the rate at which ATOMS were added exceeded the rate of increase of the rate at which CONCEPTS were added.

While we believe that the *non-synonymous* relationships between CONCEPTS in the Metathesaurus are what will make the Metathesaurus the most useful in the long run, the practical importance of any potential "convergence" cannot be overestimated. In Meta-1.4 there are 25 terminologies that partially or fully participate in the reviewed portion of the Metathesaurus. Obviously, each ATOM in each terminology was deemed useful by an authoritative body or it wouldn't have been included. Over the next few years, the number of concepts in the Metathesaurus may double again from the addition of a half-dozen new terminologies alone. If the Metathesaurus continues to show even weak evidence of "convergence" after these additions have been made, then it may mean that there is an "empirical" consensus on what some of the relevant biomedical concepts are, independent of what they are called.

Potential Reasons for "Convergence"

Whether there are such things as intrinsic "concepts" independent of language is a controversy that is more than two millennia old. In brief, the contemporary view can be summed up in two extreme positions. The optimists would assert that any "convergence" of the Metathesaurus would mean that intrinsic "truths" were emerging. The pessimists would assert that we were all just retelling the same "lies," that is we are all influenced by the same dominant scientific paradigm. Complicating the controversy is the fact that both assertions could be true at the same time, though perhaps in different sub-domains. While the Metathesaurus maintenance and enhancement process represents a unique international experiment, one that may shed new light on this old question, the Metathesaurus is a large extant reflection of "where we're at," and it's hard to imagine any future biomedical terminology efforts ignoring this reality. E.g., even to decide that one wants to do something "different," is to acknowledge both its existence and its influence. This position is a variation on the notion of "Neurath's Boat," (after Otto Neurath), namely, "that we are all at sea without a dry dock; all repairs must be made while we are afloat."

Accelerating Growth and Its Impact on Developers

Independent of whether or not the Metathesaurus demonstrates a useful degree of convergence, the observation, from **Figure 2**, that the reviewed portion of the Metathesaurus is growing at an accelerating rate is important for developers. Developers will need to decide if their applications that use the Metathesaurus will "scale" to accommodate the new growth.

But what of the complexity, utility and quality of the Metathesaurus? Are these increasing comparably? And, regardless, how will any new complexity, utility and quality affect existing and emerging applications? Metrics for complexity, utility and quality are still being developed for the still immature notion of large-scale, multi-use, terminology enhancement, but one way to begin to assess each of these notions is with respect to an abstract model. One long-standing model is the "Aristotelian" model of classification.

Aristotelian Classification
In the 4th century B.C., the Greek philosopher and polymath Aristotle invented the earliest known classification system for the biological world. This system, employed and much elaborated upon by "Aristotelian" scientists for more than two millennia after his death, served as the foundation for taxonomy until the mid-19th century when Darwin's *Origin of Species* convinced empiricists that they had to take evolutionary relationships into account for proper classification.

> *The standard Aristotelian definition of a form was by genus and differentia. The genus defined the general kind of thing being described; the differentia gave its special character. . . . The two together made up the definition, which could be used as a name."[5]*

Linnaeus Rationalized Aristotelian Classification
The 18th century Swedish scientist Linnaeus rationalized the Aristotelian taxonomy by being the first to use binomial Latin nomenclature consistently. Thus, in modern Biology, we have as a member of the genus *dissosteira* (grasshopper) the species *Dissosteira longipennis* (long-winged grasshopper), and from the genus *latrodectus* (spider) the species *Latrodectus mactans* (black widow spider).

In these examples, among many thousands, the Aristotelian classification applied to living things leads to lexical definitions, the differentia, which are incorporated in the names of species. Like these Aristotelian species, concepts in the Metathesaurus can often be seen to have hierarchical relationships that can be interpreted as "genera," and other relationships specifying uniquely defining characteristics that can be interpreted as "differentia."

Genera and Differentia May Support Automation
A potentially important hypothesis is that having "genera" and "differentia" are one way to achieve the computational economies of scale that will be required to sustain the use, maintenance, and enhancement of the Metathesaurus.[6] Thus, even though Linnaean classification suffered from the need to create and understand differentia for larger and larger classes, the hypothesis regarding its compatibility with automation may be true. If it is true, then the extent to which the Metathesaurus is "Aristotelian" is of more than purely historical interest.

Why Formality?
The most important reason to have a Metathesaurus with *formal* properties is to support reproducibility. The schema of the current Metathesaurus[7] is formal in the sense that, in principle, it specifies how ATOMS and CONCEPTS can be added to the Metathesaurus by more than one individual. Further, the current schema lays the foundation for comparable experiments to be done using the Metathesaurus. Those who exploit the schema in the same way should expect comparable results.

The problem with formality is that evolution has not equipped us to deal with it very productively. Humans are “formal,” in the sense here, only with difficulty. In addition, whether one believes in the potential power of formality or not, one should keep in mind the problems implicit in the *magnitude* of the numbers appearing in **Figure 2**, and the problems implicit in the scale of the trends to be inferred there, e.g., tradeoffs between formality and tractability per works by C. Cherniak, PhD, on the notion of “undebuggability”[8] and "minimal rationality"[9] and J. Sowa on "local vs. global consistency." However, implicit in the hypothesis that an “Aristotelian” approach is part of the answer is the assumption that human effort will be supported with computational tools.

Naturalistic vs. Experimental Observations
The figures in this paper reflect "naturalistic" observations of the evolution of the Metathesaurus. In brief, there is no notion of "artificially" holding some variables constant while measuring others, as is the case with "experimental observations." Thus, while naturalistic observations do not lend themselves to inferences about causality, they can lead to inferences about correlation.

Why focus on Inter-Concept Relationships?
The remaining results displayed here concern the explicit and implicit relationships between reviewed concepts in the Metathesaurus. In our opinion, these relationships will become the central formal semantics of future versions of the Metathesaurus, independent of the utility of Aristotelian Hierarchies. Relationships will become the dominant representation of meaning because computers can be programmed to manipulate them.

More specifically, one way naming systems specify what their names *mean* is to place those names in a structural context in the naming system. If, as humans, we find these structures semantically impoverished does not mean that they are not useful computationally. In this spirit we explore the past and current state of reviewed inter-concept relationships in the Metathesaurus using a framework adapted, freely, from Aristotle. This framework permitted us to combine years of unilateral and collaborative background study, analysis, and discussion into a single coherent presentation.

THE PROBLEM

Our objective is to determine the degree to which the recent versions of the Metathesaurus represent an "Aristotelian" classification system, given some mappings between the Metathesaurus and "Aristotelian" schemas.

METHODS

As stated, only reviewed concepts, and relationships between reviewed concepts, were analyzed. At present, all *unreviewed* concepts are "Supplementary Chemicals" that are not yet fully Metathesaurus-integrated. Counts were made on the "MR" (Metathesaurus Relational) files. Because of the evolution of the Metathesaurus schema, all counts below were made on the most recent three versions of the Metathesaurus, only. ATOM counts are actually MRSO (Metathesaurus Relational Source) line counts; this ignores a few cases where the same name occurs multiple times in a source without a code. *The fact that Metathesaurus relationships result from separate and combined processes that are themselves axiomatic, lexical, judgmental, principled, and empirical , is ignored.* A more fine-grained analysis would distinguish the *origin* of relationships.

An "exclusive" view of Metathesaurus GENERA would count only "parent" and "broader" relationships as "genera" for a given concept. An "inclusive" view would adds "semantic types" as GENERA, since each type is itself the name of a class in a hierarchy. Thus, since each Metathesaurus concept has one or more semantic types, all Metathesaurus concepts have genera viewed inclusively.

An "exclusive" view of Metathesaurus DIFFERENTIA would count only relationships labeled "other" as a "differentia" for a given concept. While Aristotle's notion of differentia assumes the existence of functions that represent the "essence" of a given form, we assume here that "horizontal" (non-hierarchical) relationships to other concepts are surrogates for such functions. An "inclusive" view would add "definitions," "associated expressions" (ATXs) and "co-occurrences" as DIFFERENTIA, because all could be used by a computer to "differentiate" a Metathesaurus concept from sibling Metathesaurus concepts. Definitions and co-occurrences are assumed to be unique. ATXs do not differentiate concepts unless they are unique, i.e., a few ATXs are identical, currently.

Only the counts for the "inclusive" view of genera and differentia are presented here.

RESULTS

For Meta-1.2, Meta-1.3, and Meta-1.4, and for the "inclusive" definitions, **Figure 3**, below, displays the total number of CONCEPTS - the same data as appears in **Figure 2** - and the number of CONCEPTS with both GENERA and the DIFFERENTIA. The graphs reveal that the degree to which the Metathesaurus is Aristotelian, by our definition, is increasing, though not as fast as the total number of CONCEPTS is increasing.

A refinement of the previous question is to ask it again but only for the 31,064 CONCEPTS common to Meta-1.2, Meta-1.3 and Meta-1.4. That is, for these "sustained" CONCEPTS do the maintenance and enhancement procedures in place increase the degree to which they, alone, are Aristotelian?

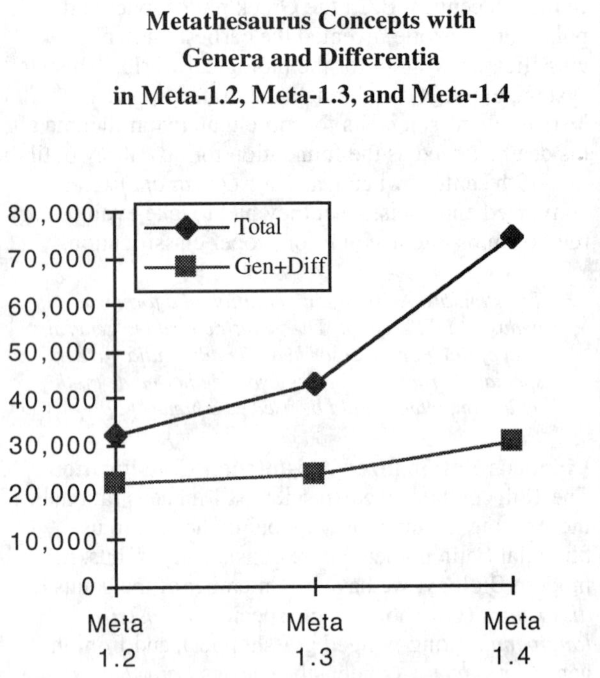

Metathesaurus Concepts with Genera and Differentia in Meta-1.2, Meta-1.3, and Meta-1.4

80,000
70,000
60,000
50,000
40,000
30,000
20,000
10,000
0
Total
Gen+Diff
Meta 1.2
Meta 1.3
Meta 1.4

Figure 3 - The total number of CONCEPTS and the number of CONCEPTS with both GENERA and DIFFERENTIA for the last three versions of the Metathesaurus: The number of concepts with both GENERA and DIFFERENTIA is increasing, though not as fast as the total number of CONCEPTS.

Since all Metathesaurus CONCEPTS have GENERA currently, using our definition, the question reduces to one concerning the growth in DIFFERENTIA. For the 31,064 sustained CONCEPTS, 21,383 had DIFFERENTIA in Meta-1.2; 21,763 had DIFFERENTIA in Meta-1.3; and 22,163 had DIFFERENTIA in Meta-1.4. Thus the increases are 380 and 400 additional CONCEPTS with DIFFERENTIA for the two transitions, about 2% per transition. While these increases are small they are potentially significant because they mean that the Metathesaurus maintenance and enhancement process is "naturally" Aristotelian to a small degree, and that part of the observed effect is due to the terminology integration process and not completely to the degree to which the constituent terminologies are Aristotelian already.

DISCUSSION

Examination of the Metathesaurus creation and editing "experience"[10],[11], relative to the Aristotelian notion of classification sharpens three issues: First, the formal needs and cognitive needs to be fulfilled by the Metathesaurus may prove to be different. Second, *when viewed in the aggregate*, any Metathesaurus "persona" to emerge regarding the addition of relationships has yet to dominate, *numerically*, the effect of whatever relationships come with the constituent naming systems.

And, third, Metathesaurus maintenance procedures will have to address the observation that as naming sources are added, Metathesaurus relationships become more tightly entwined.

The first issue brings to mind an early confrontation between cognitive and computational needs. The first time the PDQ (cancer information database) "terms file" was matched against the names in the Metathesaurus, a large number of matches between PDQ names of the form [<body part> <histologic cancer type>], or equivalent, and Metathesaurus names, were put in a report for the physician responsible for review of the PDQ portion of the Metathesaurus "locator" field. When the compound concept did not already exist in the Metathesaurus, the reviewer tended to approve suggested relationships from the "compound" PDQ concept to the "atomic" Metathesaurus concept for the <histologic cancer type>, and tended to disapprove suggested relationships between the "compound" PDQ term and the "atomic" Metathesaurus <body part> concept. While, formally, this seemed like a loss of information, it makes clinical sense. E.g., once a cancer is diagnosed histologically, notions of body site are less important determiners of management and predictors of outcome. This is the "clinical" (human) need, and the anatomic connections would have been less important, and, potentially cluttering cognitively. Of course the relationships might have been useful computationally, independent of their cognitive utility. E.g., combined with other criteria, information about site associations might be used by some future application. Interestingly, however, one "cognitive" technique employed in definitions, namely the appearance of both genera and differentia there, could be exploitable by future automatic methods were it made explicit. For example, the Metathesaurus definition for "Ornithosis," is ...

> *Infection with CHLAMYDIA PSITTACI, transmitted to man by inhalation of dust-borne contaminated nasal secretions or excreta of infected birds. This infection results in a febrile illness characterized by pneumonitis and systemic manifestations.*

An example of the second issue is the critical enhancement of Meta-1.4, namely the mapping of all 18,000 ICD Preferred Terms to MeSH Concepts or MeSH Expressions, so that given a diagnosis, a user can retrieve potentially relevant literature. The magnitude of Metathesaurus growth is now such that this effort, significant by any other measure, is not visible in this analysis.

Relevant to the third issue, one of us (KEC) is developing methods to reduce the "local update penalty."[12] His view is that "Aristotelian compliance" may prove to be an investment that supports coherent maintenance, i.e., before we know whether it would improve the content of the Metathesaurus directly, it will first become necessary computational overhead rather than a cognitive investment in content.

ACKNOWLEDGMENTS

BL Humphreys, WT Hole, MD, PL Schuyler, AT McCray, PhD and RA Zalutsky, PhD, contributed many years of provocative discussions on the notion of "relationships" in the Metathesaurus, and Humphreys and Hole helped clarify some of the specific observations described here. More than a dozen (1986-94) UMLS Contractor Meetings provided feedback on the emerging utility of the Metathesaurus and the relationship of that utility to its formal properties; JJ Cimino, MD, SM Huff, MD, and a sequence of graduate students at Brigham and Women's Hospital, deserve special mention. CG Chute, MD, DrPH, Y Yang, PhD, began analyzing properties of Metathesaurus relationships soon after the first version appeared. MS Erlbaum, MD, LF Fuller, PhD, O Suarez-Munist, SS Lipow and GT Hsu, , LM Fagan, MD, PhD, RD Acuff, MA Musen, MD, PhD, D Oliver, MD, and RW Carlson, MD, contributed directly or indirectly. C Cherniak, PhD, assisted with a review of many of the relevant issues, and J Thomas, PhD contributed to the exposition.

References

*Partially supported by contracts NLM N001-LM-0-3515 and NCI N44-CO-33071. All "®" are held by the NLM.

[1]. Harbison, K, Presentation at the ARPA DSSA Healthcare Workshop, Vail, Colorado, December, 1993.
[2]. Cimino, JJ, "Controlled Medical Vocabularly Construction: Methods from the Canon Group" (Editorial), *J Am Med Informatics Assoc*. 1994; 1:296-7.
[3]. Lindberg, DAB, Humphreys, BL, McCray, AT, "The Unified Medical Language System," *Methods of Information in Medicine*, 1993; Vol. 32, pp. 281-291.
[4]. UMLS Knowledge Sources Documentation, National Library of Medicine, 5th Experimental Edition, 1994.
[5]. Solomon, Arthur K., "Biological Sciences: Taxonomy," *The New Encyclopedia Britannica - 15th Edition*, Chicago, 1992, pp. 965-75.
[6]. Campbell, KE, "Distributed Development of a Logic-Based Controlled Medical Terminology (Dissertation Proposal)," Stanford University, 1994.
[7]. McCray, AT, Nelson, SJ, "The Semantics of the UMLS Knowledge Sources," *Meth Inf Med*, to appear.
[8]. Cherniak, C, "Undebuggability and Cognitive Science," *Comm ACM*, 31, 1988, pp. 402-412.
[9]. Cherniak, C, *Minimal Rationality*, MIT Press, Cambridge, 1986.
[10]. Tuttle, MS, et al., "Implementing Meta-1: The First Version of the UMLS Metathesaurus," LC Kingsland, ed, *SCAMC*, 1989:494-9.
[11]. Sperzel, WD, et al., "Editing the UMLS Metathesaurus: Review & Enhancement of a Computed Knowledge Source," RA Miller ed, *SCAMC*, 90:136-40.
[12]. Tuttle, MS, et al., "Adding Your Terms and Relationships to the UMLS Metathesaurus," PD Clayton ed, *SCAMC*, McGraw-Hill, New York, 1991, pp. 219-23.

From Terminology to Terminology Services

WA Nowlan* AL Rector§ TW Rush* WD Solomon§
*Medical Products Group, Hewlett-Packard Ltd, Bristol, BS12 6QZ, UK
§Medical Informatics Group, Department of Computer Science, University of Manchester, Manchester M13 9PL, UK.

ABSTRACT

Terminologies have traditionally been considered as static datasets held in books or databases. The GALEN Terminology Server presents a prototype for a new view of terminologies delivered as a set of functions and services provided to other applications. This facilitates their development and integration as part of a strategy for sharing and re-using information and knowledge. The essential features of the Terminology server are the functions which it can perform; questions which it can answer and statements which it can be told. The GALEN Terminology Server supports these operations through a modular architecture and uniform applications programming interface which allows client applications to ignore the internal structure and simply use the Server for terminological, coding, and linguistic functions.

INTRODUCTION: THE IDEA OF A 'TERMINOLOGY SERVER'

The development of 'vocabulary servers' has been mooted by various organisation in both the United States and Europe, but there is no general consensus on what such a server should be and how it should be used. This paper describes one vision of a slightly broader concept — a *Terminology Server* — and the progress towards its realisation in the GALEN[1] project sponsored by the European Union's AIM programme. The Terminology Server is seen as a key component in a broad strategy for developing and integrating clinical and related systems. It provides terminological services to applications, ranging from acting as a repository for vocabularies and lexicons, to the dynamic transformation and encapsulation of complex concepts, to support for sophisticated user interfaces.

Structure versus function

The authors [1-3]and others [4-6] have argued that if computer systems are to play a significant role in clinical care, then concept systems or 'ontologies', formally modelled, which can be manipulated by computer systems, are essential. The requirement to manage those complex concept systems leads to a choice between two options: either every application will itself have to deal with the concept model, or the services will have to be 'subcontracted' to a separate server that is general enough to support a wide variety of applications. GALEN aims to demonstrate the feasibility of the server option. The belief behind GALEN is that a wide range of applications have a common need for formal concept systems, linguistic support, and translations to and from existing coding schemes.

This Terminology Server option leads to a different view of terminologies. Traditionally terminologies have been seen as *static data structures* which could be written down or at least stored in a straight forward database Large schemes such as SNOMED-III, the READ Codes, and ICD-10 all provide one degree or another of prescriptive advice about how the coding system is to be used, but they are defined in terms of the structure rather than the functions performed. The belief within GALEN is that this is no longer adequate and the Terminology Server is described in terms of the *functions* and *services* it delivers to applications through its applications programming interface. These functions will require the manipulation of highly complex conceptual, linguistic and coding structures, but the application is deliberately protected from knowing the detail of these. The Terminology Server provides a high level uniform view of concepts, language, and codes.

Aims of the Terminology Server

The GALEN Terminology Server aims to:

- facilitate the development and integration of systems for patient care that can effectively deal with the detail, complexity, and heterogeneity of clinical information and clinical usage
- mediate between systems to integrate information sources, including conversion between coding schemes, transformation between the conceptual structures of different medical record and database schemata, encapsulation of complex data structures

---

1 General Architecture for Languages Encyclopædias and Nomenclatures in Medicine. The members of the GALEN consortium are: University of Manchester (UK, Coordinator), Hewlett-Packard Ltd (UK), Hôpital Cantonal Universitaire de Genève (Switzerland), Consiglio Nazionale delle Ricerche (Italy), University of Liverpool (UK), Katholieke Universiteit Nijmegen (Netherlands), University of Linköpking (Sweden), The Association of Finnish Local Authorities (Finland), The Finnish Technical Research Centre (Finland), GSF-Medis Institut, (Germany), Conser Systemi Avanzati (Italy)

in forms suitable for storage in relational databases, and linkage of knowledge-based and patient care systems

- provide natural language generation and, eventually, understanding, in multiple languages and facilities to simplify the development of multilingual clinical systems.
- support knowledge editing and acquisition, including the compilation and extension of coding and classification systems, support for the terminological needs of editors for knowledge based systems, and the developers of information systems models and user interface designs.

The server is designed to act as a repository of terminological and linguistic information both as a reference during system development and as a run-time service for existing systems. It is also aimed at supporting information sharing both within and across sites. Sharing and mediation will, of course, be easiest between applications developed using tools linked to the server. However facilities for mapping to pre-existing 'external representations' such as coding systems are provided. As regards the medical content of the server the medium term goal is to achieve collaborative distributed development of the large fund of detailed conceptual knowledge which will be needed to support the next generation of clinical applications.

Defining the functions required to support these applications and an architecture in which such development is feasible has been a major part of the GALEN project. The remainder of this paper describes this functionality, architecture, and briefly the implementation.

A FUNCTIONAL DESCRIPTION OF THE GALEN TERMINOLOGY SERVER

The basic description of the server is simple. Requests are made of the Terminology Server by an application and answers returned. There are three kinds of request: questions it can be asked; statements it can be told; and global checks it can perform. All share a common structure.

Structure of Requests

A request is specified in three parts: a named operation, its input arguments, and the form of the required output(s). The input or output types for the Terminology Server may be any of the forms:

- **Concept references** to entities in the server's own representation. References uniquely identify concept entities and can be either simple (e.g. a number) or compound expressions.
- **Linguistic expressions** in a supported natural language. Linguistic expressions do not, in general, identify internal concepts uniquely, and answers may include information on ambiguities which applications may either deal with themselves or treat as the basis for further questions to the terminology server. In the current implementation, linguistic expressions are only available as an output, but work on more than rudimentary natural language understanding for input is just beginning.
- **External expressions** such as codes from existing coding and classification systems, which have been mapped into the internal representation. An external expression can always identify a unique concept entity, but a concept entity may map to several codes in an external representation, possibly with further information indicating the differences between them, closeness of match, etc.

In general the Terminology Server will accept input objects and produce answers in any of these forms. Any necessary coercion between types is performed internally.

Internal Representation of concept entities: The CORE Model and GRAIL

Internally, the primary representation for concepts is the COncept REference (CORE) model, which is a compositional model expressed in the GALEN Representation and Integration Language (GRAIL) Kernel. The GRAIL Kernel is described in detail elsewhere[1, 7]. It is a strongly constrained compositional formalism. The model contains simple entities and the constraints which govern how these entities can be combined. Hence an indefinitely large number of concepts can be represented using a compact and efficient model. Because of the strong constraints, it is possible to verify whether proposed composite entities are 'sensible' and to generate lists of all 'sensible' compositions involving any given concept entity.

Requests: Things the Terminology Server can be Asked.

All these produce no change in the conceptual knowledge contained within the CORE Model.

What does this reference or expression mean?

- Is this a legal expression, and what is its simplest corresponding concept entity in the CORE Model (e.g. with any redundancies removed)?
- If the expression is legal, how is the corresponding concept entity classified— what more general concept entities subsume it? What more specialised concept entities does it subsume?
- What is known about this concept entity from the CORE Model? What other extrinsic information has been said about this concept entity?

<hasSpecificLocation UrinaryBladder>
This it returns as a simple reference and a French natural language phrase to display to the user. A specific lexical entry is found by the Multilingual Module and hence the Server returns 'cystite'. The user goes on to describe the cystitis in more detail by choosing to say it is *acute*. The Server thus produces

InflammatoryProcess which
<hasSpecificLocation UrinaryBladder
hasChronicity acute>.

This is again returned by the Server as a concept reference and a French phrase 'cystite aiguë'. The application then asks for a corresponding expression in SNOMED and receives via the Code Conversion Module 'D7-21110'. Throughout the interaction the application has simply received sets of pointers, and the user has read natural language phrases.

Requests: Things the Terminology Server can be Told

One of GALEN's major goals it to support local extensions and flexible development within an overall coherent framework provided by the CORE Model. Local sites and applications must therefore be able to add information to the Terminology Server in a number of different ways.

To extend the existing model

- Give new local names to existing or potential concept entities. Adding local names does not increase the range of things which can be expressed by the model, but it can make the model easier to use by simplifying what would otherwise be complex expressions.
- Add new primitive concept entities. The range of primitive concept entities may not include things which are important locally. For example, a surgical system might not include names for all of the surgical instruments used at a particular site.
- Add new statements so that existing attributes and concept entities can be used in new ways. It is often the case that the sanctions in the CORE model are too specific for local use and may have to be extended.
- Add new attributes and associated sanctions so that new things can be said. The range of attributes may not support sufficient detail for local use.

In general, additions of fine detail can performed locally, although central communication allows coordination of the model

To add to the other information sets supported.

- Add or modify the linguistic information
- Add or modify the mappings to an external representation such as a coding system or database schema.
- Add or change editorial information about items
- Add or modify the additional extrinsic information the model.

Information can be added to or modified in any of the data sets related to the linguistic or external representations. It also provides for maintaining editorial and version information about all items stored. If some datasets require special operations — e.g. to cope with special features of coding systems such as the dagger-asterisk structure in ICD-9 — these can be packaged in a standard form and exported through the Server's applications programming interface. In addition, the Server allows applications to store closely related information attached to the terminology structure, e.g. drug information, diagnostic criteria, and triggers to decision support.

Requests: Global Operations on the Model

- Coherence checking
- Managing updates
- Generation of local coding schemes

The Server provides a range of tests on the overall coherence of the model and a range of facilities for managing version control and updates are under development. One important function to potential users is the ability to 'compile out' fixed special purpose coding systems from the CORE model. These are simple coding systems for special purposes, and only contain a subset of the possible concepts and relationships within the CORE model. Nonetheless they are guaranteed to be coherent with the overall system and interchangeable with others using the Terminology Server or systems based on it.

ARCHITECTURE

Internally, the overall task has been modularised into different aspects - conceptual, linguistic, coding, and extrinsic - which are implemented by separate modules within the Terminology Server (figure 1). The Terminology Server combines these modules, adds reference and coercion mechanisms, and exports it's services via the API, to applications. The Terminology Server's reference management makes it easy for external applications to manipulate and store concept entities, for example as part of a patient record system. The Terminology Server's coercion mechanism provides efficient ways of combining multiple module services and relieves applications of needing to know how specific requests are handled. A flexible interface has been developed so that individual modules may 'export' their services, via the API, to external applications, so additional functionality can be made available very quickly.

The 'meaning' of a concept reference is its complete expansion and classification as a concept entity in the CORE Model, including all of the essential characteristics which can be inferred from its definition.

What can be said about this concept entity?

- What statements can sensibly be made about this concept entity? What are its sensible modifiers and relations?
- How can this concept be specialised according to given criteria? — *e.g.* anatomically, functionally, according to clinical indications or effects.
- What are the 'sensible' ways in which this set of concepts can be combined into a single larger concept?

A major function of the Terminology Server is to tell applications what further can be sensibly said about a concept entity — to support a user interface to help clinicians enter the information; to assist a bibliography system refine a query; or to assist a natural language system to disambiguate candidate phrases.

What are the nearest representations to this concept entity in some other representation?

- What are the expressions for this concept entity in a particular external system such as ICD-9? What is the preferred term for this concept entity in that system? If no exact match is possible provide the 'best' matches according to given criteria and supplementary information to assist the application in choosing among them. What information is lost or added in the conversion?
- What are the natural language expressions for this concept in a particular language? What is the preferred form for a particular 'clinical linguistic group'.
- Are these two concept entities derived from two different external representations the same? If not, how do they differ? What information would have to be added or removed from each to make them the same?
- Find all of the expressions in a given external representation which correspond to children of this concept entity, i.e. all of the codes which this concept entity subsumes. This is a particularly important question for information retrieval. It allows the Terminology Server to compensate for the deficiencies in the organisation of external coding systems. For example, forms of heart disease are found in at least five different chapters of ICD-9.

Answers to these questions provide a comprehensive service for translating between the concepts used by various representations — coding systems, database schemata, internal representations of knowledge based systems, simple linguistic 'rubrics', etc.

What is the encapsulated form of this expression?

- Provide a volatile or persistent fixed length reference for this concept entity.
- Encapsulate these concept entities according to a given format for an application as a set of references or a set of external expressions.

These functions provide fixed length 'handles' to complex concepts which can be easily manipulated by applications and relational databases. The application is protected from the problems of potentially unbounded compositional structures.

What other extrinsic information has been attached to this concept besides the indefeasible terminological knowledge?

- Find the most specific information in a given category about a concept entity.
- Find all of the information in a certain category about a concept entity and all of its parents.
- Find all the children of a particular concept entity such that a particular piece of extrinsic information holds.

Strictly speaking, the CORE Model contains only concrete conceptual knowledge which is indefeasible and true 'by definition'. However, a major function of the CORE model is to provide a framework with which to organise other, more general information - *e.g.* concerning drug interactions, clinical procedures, or diagnostic methods. Holding such information and using the conceptual framework to retrieve the most specific information in a certain category is so useful that additional operations are provided to support these functions directly. However the Terminology Server makes no attempt itself to reason with this additional information.

An example

A simple example will illustrate the flow of requests to the Server. The Terminology Server is not itself an end user application but assume a clinical data entry application holds a reference to the concept *UrinaryBladder* as a starting point. During the course of its dialogue with the user the application asks the Server for those attributes concerned with locations that can sensibly apply to this concept, and the possible values for these. One of the replies is

isSpecificLocationOf-InflammatoryProcess.

This is selected by the user who asks to go on and describe the inflammation in more detail. The Server is thus asked to combine the components to give the concept

InflammatoryProcess which

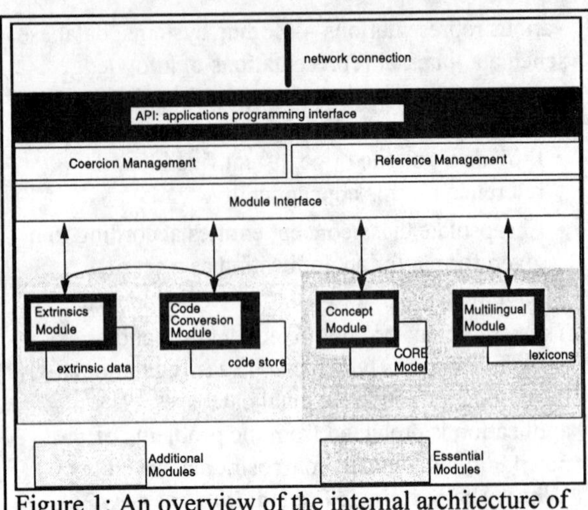

Figure 1: An overview of the internal architecture of the Terminology Server.

The central task of concept modelling is addressed by the 'Concept Module' which interprets the 'Concept Reference' (CORE) Model The CORE Model serves as an *inter lingua* amongst medical nomenclatures, vocabularies, and the terminological aspects of database schemata.

The Multilingual Module provides lexicons and grammatical information for expressing, and eventually understanding, phrases in natural languages. External representations can depend on the Multilingual module to translate the CORE Model expansion of their representation, in addition to any 'official' translation.

The Code Conversion Module maintains the external representations, along with special information related to their structure and browsing, *e.g.* information on the cross referencing in SNOMED or the dagger-asterisk mechanism and exclusions in ICD-9/10. The Code Conversion Module also provides the functionality concerned with resolving ambiguities and conflicts when there is not an immediate one-to-one correspondence between the GALEN CORE Model and the target external representation, for example when the expansion of a term from one external coding system has no direct representation in a different external coding system.

The Extrinsic Information Module provides a repository in which applications or sites can store detailed information about the clinical criteria for using concepts in the Terminology Server. These definitions are appended to the classification structure of the CORE Model but are not part of it.

CURRENT STATUS

All the modules described above have been implemented using Parc Place Smalltalk™ (VisualWorks™) with Sybase™ for database support. Client ends are available in Smalltalk™ and C. The Server is currently being used within the GALEN project to support clinical user interfaces for test ordering in nosocomial infections and entry of arthroscopic findings. Applications to support a knowledge editor for Medical Logic Modules and a Classification Manager for assisting in the development of coding and classification systems are under way. The architecture and interface language have been demonstrated including the ability to operate multiple client application and a server on separate machines linked either by local area networks or across the Internet.

The current applications have allowed an analysis of the functions required which has so far proved robust. The modular architecture provides a smooth means of expansion. Full evaluation must await maturation of the applications, and above all of the demonstration of multiple coherent applications sharing the same server. Even at this early stage the Terminology Server provides a vision of new possibilities - of a shift in emphasis from providing terminology *per se* to providing terminological services.

REFERENCES

1. Rector A, Nowlan W, Glowinski A. Goals for concept representation in the GALEN project. 17th Annual Symposium on Computer Applications in Medical Care (SCAMC-93). McGraw Hill, 1993: 414-18.
2. Rector A, Nowlan W, Kay S. Foundations for an electronic medical record. Meth Inform Med 1991;30:179-86.
3. Rector A, Nowlan W, Kay S. Conceptual knowledge: the core of medical information systems. In: Lun K, Degoulet P, Pierre T, Rienhoff O, (ed). Seventh World Congress on Medical Informatics, MEDINFO-92. Geneva: North-Holland Publishers, 1992: 1420-1426.
4. Evans DA, Cimino J, Hersh WR, Huff SM, Bell DS. Toward a medical concept representation language. J Am Med Informatics Assoc 1994, 1 (3) 207-217.
5. Masarie Jr F, Miller R, Bouhaddou O, Giuse N, Warner H. An interlingua for electronic interchange of medical information: using frames to map between clinical vocabularies. Comp Biomed Res 1991;24(4):379-400.
6. Cimino JC, Hripscak G, Johnson S. Knowledge-based approaches to the maintenance of a large controlled medical terminology. J Am Med Informatics Assoc 1994;1(1):35-50.
7. Rector A, Nowlan W. The GALEN Representation and Integration Language (GRAIL) Kernel. GALEN deliverable 6. (Medical Informatics Group, University of Manchester), 1993.

Methodologies for Coding Clinical Information

An Application of Expert Network to Clinical Classification and MEDLINE Indexing

Yiming Yang
Christopher G. Chute

Section of Medical Information Resources
Mayo Clinic/Foundation
Rochester, Minnesota 55905 USA

ABSTRACT

An effective and efficient learning method, Expert Network (ExpNet), is introduced in this paper. ExpNet predicts the related categories of an arbitrary text based on a search of its nearest neighbors in a set of training texts, and a reasoning from the expert-assigned categories of these neighbors. Evaluations in patient-record text classification and MEDLINE document indexing show a performance of ExpNet in recall and precision comparable to the Linear Least Squares Fit (LLSF) mapping method, and significantly better than other methods tested. We also observed that ExpNet is much more efficient than LLSF in computation. The total training and testing time on the patient-record text collection (6134 texts) was 4 minutes for ExpNet versus 96 minutes for LLSF; on the MEDLINE document collection (2344 documents), the total time was 15 minutes for ExpNet versus 4.6 hours for LLSF. It is evident in this study that human knowledge of text categorization can be statistically learned without expensive computation, and that ExpNet is such a solution.

INTRODUCTION

The task of text categorization is to assign predefined categories to a free text according to its contents. Diagnoses in patient records, for example, need to be assigned to insurance categories for the purpose of billing. Citations in a bibliographic database, as another example, need to be indexed using subject categories for the purpose of retrieval. Manual categorization remains the dominant method in practical databases. MEDLINE, for example, spends over two million dollars each year for indexing new entries (about 350,000 per year) by human indexers [1]. There is thus a strong motivation for automatic or semi-automatic text categorization.

A major problem in automatic text categorization is the large vocabulary differences between free texts and canonical categories. That is, a matching method based on shared words ("word-based matching") in a text and a category description would be ineffective, because related concepts are often expressed by different words. Using terminology thesauri ("thesaurus-based matching") attempts to reduce the vocabulary differences. General-purpose thesauri, however, often do not have a sufficient vocabulary coverage crossing different applications [2] [3] [4]. Statistical learning from human decisions in text categorization is another effort [3] [5] [6] [7], and has shown promising results in solving the vocabulary difference problem. Many statistical approaches, however, have a relatively high computation cost. Our Linear Least Squares Fit (LLSF) mapping method, for example, while showing significant improvements over word-based matching and thesaurus-based matching, has a cubic time complexity for its training, which makes it expensive to apply this method to very large data collections. Bayesian belief networks, as another example, have a similar problem in large applications [7].

What we need is a statistical learning method which is highly effective and does not require intensive training. We have found Expert Network to be such a solution.

METHOD

Expert Network is designed to predict the category or categories of an arbitrary text ("the request") based on previously categorized texts. The basic idea to search "the nearest neighbors" (NNs) of the request in a set of training texts, and to estimate the relevance of a category based on how often this category is assigned to the neighbors. This idea can be traced back to the well known NN classification method which has been studied in pattern recognition for four decades, and used to classify a point in a feature space based on a training sample of previously classified points [8]. The NN approach was later found useful in word pronunciation (to determine the phonemes of a novel word according to the pronunciations of training words) [9] and in text categorization (to categorize Census Bureau documents, for example, according to previously categorized documents) [10] [11]. These applications were generalized in a cognitive paradigm, named Memory-based Reasoning, and characterized by its implementation on

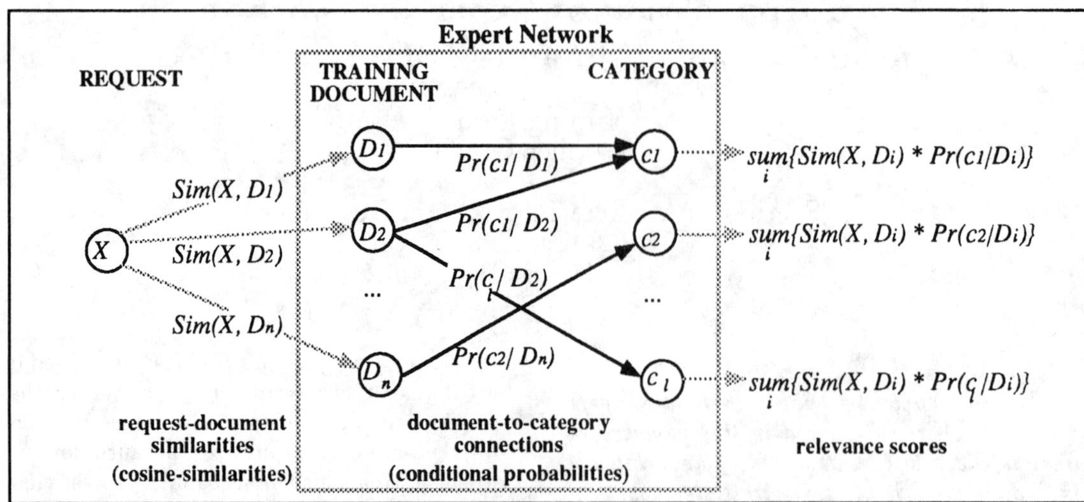

Figure 1. Category ranking via Expert Network.

the Connection Machine parallel computers. Our recent study has further pursued the NN approach in both text categorization and retrieval. We use a network formalism to define the method and to encode the statistical evidence of human decisions: a one-layer network is used for text categorization, and a three-layer network is used for text retrieval [12]. Our focus in this paper is on the effectiveness and the efficiency of ExpNet in clinical classification and MEDLINE indexing. In a separate paper, we describe its practical use in assisting human coding of patient record texts at the Section of Medical Information Resources, Mayo Clinic [13].

The Network

ExpNet is a bipartite network as illustrated in Figure 1. It provides empirical linkages from documents to categories. We use "document" as a generic word for a text which can be the title plus abstract of an article in MEDLINE, or a diagnosis or procedure report in a patient record. A document is treated as a set of weighted words. The input nodes of ExpNet are training documents. The output nodes are the categories of the training documents. The links between documents and categories are weighted using the conditional probabilities of a category being related to a document by human judgment. The conditional probabilities are estimated as the following:

$$P_r(c_k|D_j) \approx \frac{\text{number of times } c_k \text{ is assigned to } D_j}{\text{number of times } D_j \text{ occurs in the sample}}$$

where $D_1, \ldots, D_n$ are unique training documents, and $c_1, \ldots, c_l$ are unique categories. Note that a document may have more than one occurrence in the training sample. Diagnoses in patient records, for example, often repeat. MEDLINE documents, as another example, are unlikely to repeat; however, some may become identical if an aggressive "stoplist" is applied to remove non-informative words. Consequently, the number of times a category is assigned to a document may also be more than one.

Category Ranking

The category ranking via ExpNet consists of two steps. The first step is to compute the similarity between a given document (the request) and each training document, using the conventional "cosine-measure":

$$sim(X,Y) \stackrel{\text{def}}{=} \frac{\sum_{t_i \in (X \cap Y)} x_i \times y_i}{\sqrt{x_1^2 + x_2^2 + x_3^2 + \ldots} \times \sqrt{y_1^2 + y_2^2 + y_3^2 + \ldots}}$$

where

X and Y are two documents;

t_i is the ith word in the document vocabulary;

x_i is the weight of word t_i in X;

y_i is the weight of word t_i in Y.

For word weighting, we adopted the commonly used schemes as options, including binary weights, within-document term frequency (TF), Inverse Document Frequency (IDF), and the combination TF×IDF [14].

After the similarity values of training documents are computed, these values are propagated to the document-to-category links, multiplied by the weights of these links, and summed at the category nodes. This results in a weighted sum of the conditional probabilities, which we use as the estimated relevance score of a category with respect to the request,

$$rel(c_k|X) \approx \sum_{j=1}^{n} sim(X, D_j) \times P_r(c_k|D_j) \qquad (1)$$

Optimization

While using a weighted sum of the conditional probabilities is a reasonable way to estimate the relevance of a category, the question is whether we should count all the training documents as the neighbors of an input document. In other words, should we just count the few nearest neighbors and ignore the remaining ones? Would we gain improvement by doing so? To answer these questions, we tested different choices on n' ($n' \leq n$) where n' is the number of selected NNs. Formula (1) is therefore modified as below,

$$rel(c_k|X) \approx \sum_{D_j \in S} sim(X, D_j) \times P_r(c_k|D_j) \qquad (2)$$

where S is the set of the n' top-ranking documents.

We used a collection of MEDLINE documents for this test (MEDCL in the next section). We arbitrarily picked a quarter (586 documents) of the total (2344 documents) for training, and used the remaining ones (1758 documents) for testing. There was no overlap between the training documents and the testing documents. The NN selection thresholds were set to $n' = 1, 5, 10, 20, 30, ..., 586$. For each value of n' we computed the precision values at recalls of 10%, 20%, ..., 100% and averaged them for a global measure. Figure 2 shows the result curve. The interesting points are:

(1) the poorest result occurred when $n' = 1$;

(2) the best result occurred when $n' = 30$;

(3) for $n' > 30$, the performance slowly decreased and converged to the level of selecting all the documents (n' =586).

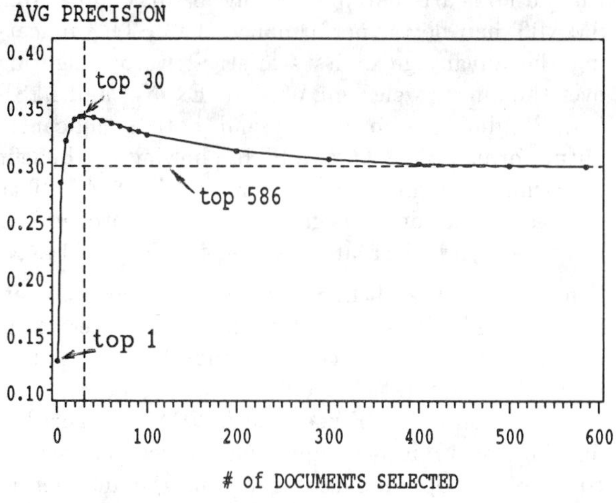

Figure 2. The effect of document selection

These testing results suggest:

(1) the top-ranking document by itself would not give sufficient information about the categories of the request, if there is only a partial match between the request and the top-ranking document;

(2) a few top-ranking documents together are much more informative about the contents (categories) of the request;

(3) after a certain point, counting more documents with lower similarity values only contributes noise.

Note that the above observations are based on the test where the training documents and the testing documents are different. This is typically true for bibliographical documents but not necessarily true for patient-record texts because diagnoses or procedure reports are relatively short and often repeat. Our experiences in patient-record text categorization suggest to use the following rules for NN selection:

(1) choose the top-ranking training document if its similarity score is 1 or "sufficiently" close to 1;

(2) choose the n' top-ranking training documents otherwise.

The parameter n' can be empirically determined. For a patient-record text collection (SURCL in the next section), we found that n'=10 is the best setting; for the MEDLINE documents, around 20 or 30 are the best choices. The point is, the optimal threshold is application dependent, and the choice should be left to application and experiment.

EVALUATION

Two text collections were chosen for evaluation, and three different categorization methods were tested for the comparison with ExpNet.

Data Sets

SURCL: a collection of surgical reports from patient records in the Mayo Clinic archive. About 1.5 million patient records are manually coded each year at Mayo for the purpose of billing and research. From the 1990 surgical reports, we arbitrarily chose a cardiovascular subset which contains 6150 procedure/category pairs. We sorted these pairs by category and split them into odd and even halves. The odd-half was used as the training set, and the even-half was used for testing. The average length of texts was about 9 words; 99.8% of them had a uniquely matched category; the rest had two or three categories. There are 281 categories in the cardiovascular subdomain, the procedure volume of the canonical classification system ICD-9-CM (International Classification of Diseases, 9th Revision, Clinical Modifications).

MEDCL: a collection of MEDLINE documents. This data set was originally designed for an evaluation of the Boolean search of MEDLINE retrieval [15], and has been used for evaluations of other retrieval and categorization systems [1] [3] [4]. The categories of the documents were assigned by MEDLINE index-

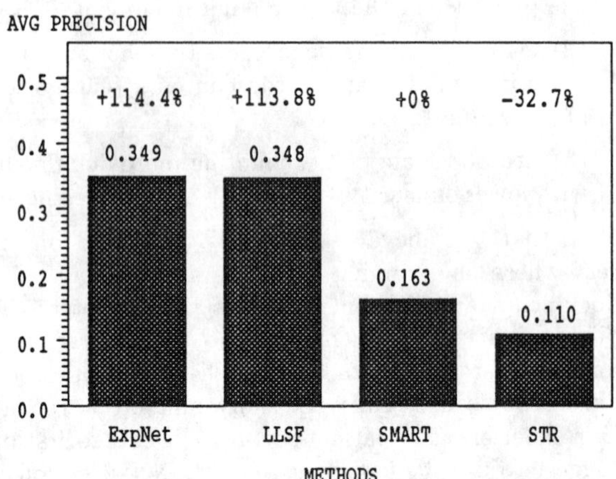

Figure 3. Different methods on MEDCL

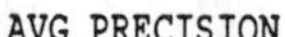

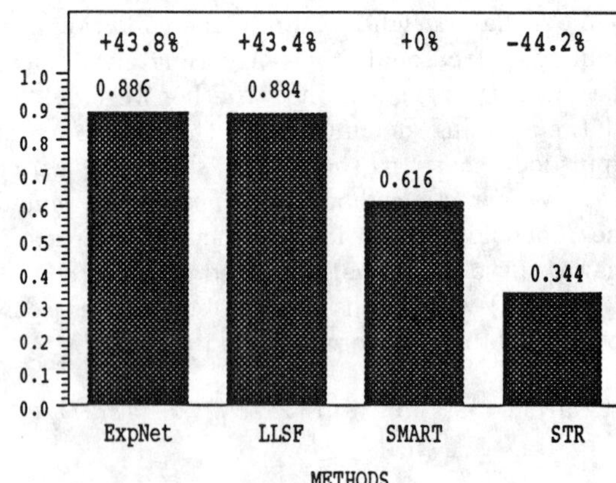

Figure 4. Different methods on SURCL

ers; about 17 categories per document on average, and 4020 unique categories in total. The average number of words per document was 168. We arbitrarily used a quarter of the documents for training, and the remaining ones for testing.

A preprocessing was applied to these texts or documents to remove punctuation and numbers, and to change uppercase letters to lowercase; neither stemming nor removal of noise words was applied. The parameter n' in ExpNet was set to 10 for SURCL, and 30 for MEDCL.

Methods for Comparison with ExpNet

LLSF, a statistical learning method which uses the same kind of training data as used in ExpNet, that is, a training sample of manually categorized documents. LLSF computes a mapping function from a document space to weighted combinations of categories. This function guarantees the globally minimized squares error in the mapping.

STR (STRing matching) is our implementation of a category ranking method based on shared words. STR represents documents using free words in the documents, and categories using the words in their canonical descriptions. Binary word weights are used for either case. The cosine-similarity between a document and a category is used as the relevance score of the category.

SMART, developed by Salton's group [2], is one of the most representative retrieval systems. SMART provides a word-based matching mechanism and allows the use of statistical word weights. We use the SMART software to test the effects of statistical weights on word-based matching. Relevance feedback is not used because it is not applicable [3]. Documents and categories in the tests of SMART are represented in the same way as in STR, except the binary word weights are replaced by the statistical word weights of SMART. The default parameter settings were used in the tests, including word weighting options TF ("nnn" in the SMART nomenclature) and TF×IDF ("atc"). We will refer to the better result (using TF×IDF) among these two choices in the comparison of SMART with other methods. No claim is made that this result is the best possible for SMART.

Results

Figures 3 and 4 show the testing results on MEDCL and SURCL. All the methods had a better result on SURCL than their performance on MEDCL, indicating that the former was an easier task than the latter. Nevertheless, the relative differences between the methods are more interesting in this comparison. SMART had better performance than STR, indicating the advantage of its statistical word weighting over the binary weighting of STR. ExpNet and LLSF had a similar performance, and both significantly outperformed SMART and STR, showing the benefit of learning human knowledge. By setting SMART as the base of the comparison, the relative improvements of ExpNet and LLSF are between 43.4% and 114.4%.

While ExpNet and LLSF were almost equally effective (under the condition that parameter n' in ExpNet was properly chosen), they differed significantly in computational efficiency. Our current implementation of LLSF uses the LINPACK algorithm for singular value decomposition, which has a time complexity approximately cubic in the number of training documents [6]. In ExpNet, on the other hand, the major computation is to find the nearest neighbors of a request in the training documents. Such a computation can be done in time approximately linear in the number of training documents [12]. The training of LLSF on MEDCL, for example, took about 2.25 hours of CPU time on a SUN SPARCstation 10, while the training of ExpNet took only 16 seconds. The testing (categorization) was 5 seconds per document for LLSF and 0.4 seconds per document for ExpNet. Counting the total time including training and testing as a global measure, the computation on MEDCL took 4.6 hours in LLSF but only 15 minutes in ExpNet. On the SURCL set, as another example, the total time was 96 minutes in LLSF and only 4 minutes in ExpNet.

DISCUSSION

To summarize this paper, a major problem in automatic text categorization is the large vocabulary gap between free text and canonical categories. The vocabulary gap makes the matching methods based on shared words unavoidably ineffective. ExpNet, with its capability of learning from human categorization decisions, solves this problem effectively and efficiently.

The effectiveness and efficiency come from the intelligent use of lexical similarity. ExpNet uses lexical similarity to allocate a request to a neighborhood of training documents where human assigned connections to the related categories are available. The lexical similarity scores of training documents also provide a means to weight and integrate local estimates into a global measure. Since ExpNet does not break training documents into individual words, no assumption of independence among words is made or used in category ranking. Such a use of training documents also keeps the computation of ExpNet much simpler than other statistical learning methods. In LLSF and Bayesian belief networks, for example, the word-category connections have to be made explicitly in their models, which requires intensive computation for the learning.

In conclusion, the simplicity of the model, the effective use of human knowledge, and the efficient computation together make ExpNet a preferable solution to pursue for text categorization. A potential problem we have not focused on in this paper is the real-time response of ExpNet. Since it requires an on-line search of the NNs, the computation must be done in a few seconds. This would be a computational bottleneck when the training sample is very large. Employing parallel computing or distributed computing over multiple computers through networking remains the focus of our future research.

Acknowledgement

We would like to thank Dr. Kent Bailey for fruitful discussions about the original idea, and Geoffrey Atkin for programming. This work is supported in part by NIH grants LM-07041, LM-05416, and AR30582.

References

1. Hersh WR, Haynes RB. Evaluation of SAPHIRE: an automated approach to indexing and retrieving medical literature. *Proc 15th Ann Symp Comp Applic Med Care* 1991; 15:808–812

2. Salton G. Development in Automatic Text Retrieval. *Science* 1991; 253:974-980

3. Yang Y, Chute CG. An example-based mapping method for text categorization and retrieval. ACM Transaction on Information Systems 1994; in press

4. Yang Y, Chute CG. Words or Concepts: the Features of Indexing Units and their Optimal Use in Information Retrieval. *Proc 17th Ann Symp Comp Applic Med Care* 1993; 17:685–689

5. Fuhr N, Hartmann S, Lustig G, et al. AIR/X - a rule-based multistage indexing systems for large subject fields. *Proceedings of the RIAO'91* 1991; 606-623

6. Yang Y, Chute CG. A Linear Least Squares Fit mapping method for information retrieval from natural language texts. *Proc 14th International Conference on Computational Linguistics* 1992; 447–453

7. Tzeras K, Hartmann S. Automatic indexing based on Bayesian inference networks. *Proc 16th Ann Int ACM SIGIR Conference on Research and Development in Information Retrieval* 1993; 22–34

8. Dasarathy BV, Ed. Nearest Neighbor (NN) Norms: NN Pattern Classification Techniques, IEEE Computer Society Press, 1990.

9. Stanfill C, Waltz D. Toward Memory-based Reasoning. *Comm. ACM*, 1986; 29, 1213–1228

10. Creecy RH, Masand BM, Smith SJ, Waltz DL. Trading MIPS and memory for knowledge engineering: classifying census returns on the Connection Machine. *Comm. ACM*, 1992; 35, 48-63.

11. Masand B., Linoff G., Waltz D. Classifying News Stories using Memory Based Reasoning. *15th Ann Int ACM SIGIR Conference on Research and Development in Information Retrieval* 1992; 59-64

12. Yang Y. Expert Network: Effective and Efficient Learning from Human Decisions in Text Categorization and Retrieval. *17th Ann Int ACM SIGIR Conference on Research and Development in Information Retrieval*, 1994; 13–22

13. Chute CG, Yang Y, Buntrock J. An evaluation of computer-assisted clinical classification algorithms. *18th Ann Symp Comp Applic Med Care* 1994, in press.

14. Salton G. *Automatic Text Processing: The Transformation, Analysis, and Retrieval of Information by Computer.* Addison-Wesley, Reading, Pennsylvania, 1989

15. Haynes R, McKibbon K, Walker C, Ryan N, Fitzgerald D, Ramsden M. Online access to MEDLINE in clinical settings. *Ann. Int. Med.* 1990; 112:78–84

An Evaluation of Computer Assisted Clinical Classification Algorithms

Christopher G. Chute
Yiming Yang
James Buntrock

Section of Medical Information Resources
Mayo Clinic/Foundation
Rochester, MN

The Mayo Clinic has a long tradition of indexing patient records in high resolution and volume. Several algorithms have been developed which promise to help human coders in the classification process. We evaluate variations on code browsers and free text indexing systems with respect to their speed and error rates in our production environment. The more sophisticated indexing systems save measurable time in the coding process, but suffer from incompleteness which requires a back-up system or human verification. Expert Network does the best job of rank ordering clinical text, potentially enabling the creation of thresholds for the pass through of computer coded data without human review.

INTRODUCTION

Interest in Health Care Reform has highlighted the need for well organized indicies to clinical information. Manual classification of diagnoses, procedures, and findings remains the standard method for creating these indicies, although "auto-coder" technology has been introduced to harness computer assistance to the task. Most computer assisted tools today attempt to navigate the user to a correct code using hierarchical menus. Few attempt to pattern match natural language entries from a health provider to a target coding system, such as ICD-9-CM or SNOMED-3.

The Mayo Foundation has maintained careful indicies to its "master sheet" summarization of findings and diagnoses upon dismissal since 1909 [1]. The clinical classifications have changed over time, but today involve a highly extended derivative of HICDA-2 [2]. numbering 29,762 discreet rubrics. The Section of Medical Information Resources at Mayo is operationally responsible for this coding, and expends over $1.4 million annually in the effort. The resolution and purpose of the master sheet entries has been incompatible with the reimbursement needs of business office coding, and therefore this specialized coding for research retrieval has been done in parallel.

We have developed several techniques for statistically based information retrieval, and have applied them to the free text phrase classification problem [3][4][5][6]. We have also developed a workstation application to assist our coding personnel in the classification process, so that we can code more clinical data with the same or fewer resources. In this paper, we outline our preliminary experience with alternative techniques for pattern matching free text diagnoses, and the process we are using to continuously improve our machine assisted classification tools.

METHODS

This evaluation was conducted on inpatient and outpatient summary diagnoses entered on Mayo Clinic's "Master Sheet;" these are typically 3-10 words of descriptive free-text. The Section of Medical Information Resources codes over 1.3 million diagnoses and findings from the paper based summary master sheet entries of the Mayo medical record annually. After more than a year of prototyping, X-terminal workstations were installed on the desks of all master sheet coders to improve speed and precision of coding. In anticipation of an on-line master sheet by 1995, coders type the master sheet text into a window of the coding application. This text is spell checked against a locally developed lexicon of 107,000 master sheet words and variants, using a proprietary fuzzy match algorithm (Proximity Scan P2 Library, Proximity Technology, Ft. Lauderdale, FL), however the human coders may accept terms not known by the lexicon.

For our evaluation, we employed five algorithms for matching the natural language text strings from the master sheet to the 29,762 codes in our locally extended version of HICDA-2; these include:

- Exact Browse - This method employs an exact string match on shared words and terms between the text string of the HICDA-2 codes and the master sheet entry, supplemented by browsing words entered by the coder.
- Fuzzy Browse - As exact browse, but string matching can be partial. String closeness is ranked by the Proximity Scan software.

• Hashed Index - Master sheet words are normalized to match the lexical variants and spelling of the local lexicon, and then matched to the HICDA-2 coding system. Matches are ranked by the number of word strings that match the coding system entry terms.
• Least Squares Fit - A statistically based technique that learns associations between text phrases and their humanly assigned classification[4][5] . This technique is very computationally intensive, and is therefore solved in parts. For the 49,262 training set pairs used in this evaluation, 24 sub-set matrices were independently solved and later merged.
• Expert Network - A new approach that avoids the cubic computational complexity of Least Squares Fit, invoking a linear learning pattern.[6][7]. For this evaluation, 235,422 training pairs form the knowledge base. No problem sub-division was required, obviating a sub-set merge.

For each of these five techniques, approximately 1,000 master sheet entries were randomly chosen for coding. Trained personnel used clinical coding workstation software, specially developed for this evaluation, that invoked only one of the algorithms. A subsequent review by a supervisor edited the work, correcting oversights attributable to the software or human error. Supervisor judgment at this step included what constituted a codable master sheet clinical finding (as opposed to an administrative notation); this contributed to the variable number of verified items among the evaluated techniques in the final tally. The master sheet entries used to evaluate each coding system were not identical to save costs, but were drawn from the same source pool and are functionally equivalent.

The project software also tracked wall clock timing information, separating master sheet term typing time from coding time. Since electronic transfer of master sheet text is imminent at Mayo, we discounted the contribution of entry typing .

To provide comparable statistics, the three algorithms (not browsers) that returned a rank ordered list of matches were restricted to the top 40 matches found. Statistics compiled for each algorithm include the number of text strings coded, the resulting number of codes generated (allowing multiple codes per text), the percent of verified codes not included among the top 40 matches, average time to code in seconds, percent of initial codes corrected by the supervisor verification (codes with error), and the average rank order of the correct code among the 40 matches returned (based on last code in the event of multiple codes needed).

All processing was done on text in real time, with results ranked results (for the non-browsers) returned to the coder in under three seconds. We are striving for sub-second response time, but the human delay in review and confirmation of the best code in this computer assisted coding scenario overwhelms machine time contributions for now. Average rank statistics were computed after the correct answers were validated by the supervisor reviewer; the statistics were computed only for the 83% of texts which had a single correct code.

RESULTS

Table 1 shows the evaluation statistics of the five systems.

Number of Texts: each system uses a different testing set, and the sizes of these sets are similar but not exactly the same.

Number of Codes: the majority (83%) of our DXs had

Method	Number of Texts	Number of Codes	Candidate Codes Passed to Coders		Codes Not Found
Exact Browse	904	1112	unlimited		0.18%
Fuzzy Browse	1000	1224	unlimited		0.49%
Hashed Index	1197	1444	40		26%
Least Squares Fit	1025	1252	40		11%
Expert Network	1077	1340	40		16%
	Average Precision	Average Recall	Average Rank	Coding Error	Avg Time to Code
Exact Browse	–	–	–	5.1%	59 sec
Fuzzy Browse	–	–	–	5.0%	46 sec
Hashed Index	60%	72%	4.94	3.0%	24 sec
Least Squares Fit	45%	88%	4.63	8.8%	23 sec
Expert Network	83%	81%	1.63	2.5%	34 sec

Table 1. Performance of 5 computer assisted classification algorithms. See text for explanation of statistics.

exactly one correct code, the remaining DXs have 2-6 correct codes.

Candidate Codes Passed to Coders: the browsers allow a coder unlimited inquiry; the classifiers (Hashed Index, Least Squares Fit and Expert Network), on the other hand, return 40 top-ranking candidate categories for each text to the coder to choose.

Codes not Found: For the classifiers, the percentage of missed codes simply means the correct codes which are not included in the 40 top-ranking candidates. Browser figures reflect percent overlooked.

Average Time to Code: this includes system response, the time the coder checks through candidate categories returned by the system, and the coding decision. In case the correct code is not in the candidate list, the coder makes the decision based on knowledge.

Coding Error: the error rate of humans when using one of our systems to assist the coding. The error rate using manual methods is 7% on average.

Average Precision: defined as the ratio of the number of codes found and correct divided by the number of codes found. For each text, we computed a precision value at each position in the ranked candidate list where a correct code is found. If a text has more than one correct codes, then it can have more than one precision value; we average these values into a single measure for this text. The precisions of individual texts are further averaged for a global measure of a method. For the browsers, no such information was available to compute the precisions.

Average Recall: defined as the ratio of the number of codes found and correct divided by the number of correct codes. For the classifiers, we computed a recall for each text at the end (the 40th position) of the ranked candidate list, and then averaged the recalls of all texts for a global measure of a method. For the browsers, no such information was available.

Average Rank: the average rank of a correct code in the 40 element candidate list. It gives intuitive idea about how well a system does if all DXs have one correct code. In such a case, the best possible average rank is 1, and the smaller the average rank, the better the system. However, the average rank is problematic for DXs which have more than one correct code. For example, suppose the DXs have exactly two correct codes, then the best possible average rank is 1.5 (assuming the correct codes appear in the 1st and 2nd positions on the ranked list), but not 1 (assuming one correct code is found in the 1st position but the other correct code is simply missed)! Therefore, in this statistic, we only counted the DXs (83% of the total) which had only one code.

The table summarizes the statistics generated in our evaluation. Each technique was tested with a comparable number of input texts, and generated a similar number of resulting codes. The browser techniques had very few codes not found in the initial pass (not presented), by the nature of freely navigating browsers. The index and ranking algorithms were restricted to 40 possible matches in their returning window, which in this evaluation allowed between 11% to 26% correct codes to be overlooked.

The browser techniques took nearly twice as long, on average, to code a given text phrase. Expert Network took somewhat longer than the other indexing methods, due in part to its larger knowledge base of nearly one quarter million data pairs. Least Squares Fit was the fastest technique, but this does not account for the several hours of SPARC 10 time needed to compute the intervening matrices.

Least Squares Fit returned correct answers that, on average, were five or six lines from the top on the rank ordered list returned by the algorithm. Error rates for this system were also the highest (8.8%), perhaps due to the relative burying of correct answers further down the list. Despite these problems, Least Squares Fit tended to have the lowest rate of failure (11%) to include the correct answer among the restricted set of 40 potential matches returned for human review.

Expert Network tended to do the best at correctly ranking validated responses among the codes it did find. This appears to correlate with the error rate found in review that required correction (2.5%). It was intermediate in failure to return correct codes (16%). Time performance of Expert Network was better than the browsers, but worst among the indexing methods.

The browsers were slow and generated an intermediate number of errors. An average rank statistics has no meaning, since the browsers allowed coders to look among all 29,762 codes rather than a rank ordered list of 40 potential matches.

DISCUSSION

This evaluation shows that indexing algorithms can be faster and generate fewer errors than coding system browsers. Intelligent (fuzzy matching) browsers are faster than simple string browsers, and intelligent algorithms are faster still. For the time being however, a sufficient number of correct codes are missed altogether that human review and confirmation is required to ensure high fidelity coding.

The fastest system, Least Squares Fit (LSF), also had the highest rate of human error and a precision significantly lower than Expert Network and Hashed Index. The low precision is probably due to an improper decomposition of the problem. That is, our current algorithm is not efficient enough to handle the large training sample used in this evaluation, so we split the training sample (about 50000 DXs) into subsets of 24 subdomains of the ICD-9-CM categories. We computed an LSF solution for each subset, and use these local solutions to estimate category scores in each subdomain. In principle, these local scores ("local evidences") should be used in combination with "global evidences", i.e. the likelihood estimates of a text as a concept under each subdomain. We have a method under development to integrate these two kinds of evidences [4]; however, for the time being, we only used local evidences in LSF for this evaluation. Such a temporary arrangement unavoidably introduced local biases in category ranking, and evidently caused the significant decrease of the precision (in our previous tests on smaller data sets where the training samples were not split, LSF had the precisions similar to Expert Network [6] [7]). The recall, on the other hand, is higher than the other systems.

The question is, how much does the precision (and recall) of a system effect the quality and cost of human coding in an interactive computer assisted coding environment? In Table 1, we observe a strong correlation between the low precision of LSF and the high rate of human errors; on the other hand, no such correlation is evident between precision and coding time. A low precision means that correct codes have relatively high ranks in the candidate list brought to the coder. That is, the coder has to check through many alternatives until a correct code is found. Since experienced coders are fast in checking through candidates, as long as the correct codes are included in the 40 top-ranking candidate list, their relative low ranks did not seem to slow down the coding speed by much. On the other hand, if a correct code is missed in the candidate list, it takes a much longer time for the coder to figure out the code. This means that the recall among the 40 top-ranking candidate list is probably more important than the precision from the view point of coding speed. LSF had the highest recall and also the fastest response time (about 1 second per query), all together it made the coding time by humans the shortest.

The cause of the high human errors may or may not be the low precision of LSF. It is possible that a coder would be confused by the low ranked alternatives in a candidate list. If this is true, then a precision enhancement would solve the problem. Our present work in sparse matrix algorithms and parallel computing, may significantly reduce the number of training subsets; by combining local and global evidencies in a "split-merge" method, we expect a substantial improvement in precision, and possibly in error rate. Another potential reason for human error would be the "scrambled" mixture of candidates, i.e. adjacent codes in the candidate list can be totally different concepts, and this may be very disorienting for coders. A solution for this problem is to improve the representation of the candidates, e.g. instead of giving a ranked list of codes, grouping the codes by concepts and laying out the grouped codes for coders to review.

Expert Network shows the precision and lowest error rate, approaching the point of permitting computers to indicate correct codes without human review. This evaluation did not exploit the information contained in the similarity matching scores which are integral to Least Squares Fit and Expert Network. Future work must establish if there are threshold values which will permit the confident acceptance of computer matches, without further human review or editing. Passing only 10-15% of such codes in this way would imply millions of dollars in savings to the health care industry in reduced coding costs.

Several limitations exist in this work. Most notably, the evaluations were not conducted on identical subsets of data. Our experience indicates that system performance is consistent over similar data types, somewhat attenuating this concern. Our alternative was to create a standard dataset with standard answers. However, the training effect of coding this dataset using the same coding personnel would have been large and confounded the evaluation of algorithms later in the sequence. While we could have used different persons, we reasoned that the variation in source material was smaller than the variation in coder consistency with these experimental techniques. We therefore opted to use different source material to enable us to use a consistent panel of human coders.

The generalizability of these findings is also not tested. We restricted this testing to our high volume production coding in the Section of Medical Information Resources, because that is where we targeted the development and early implementation of the system. However, the target coding space is an idiosyncratic adaptation of HICDA-2, which is much larger and more specific than ICD-9-CM, and architecturally unrelated (non-axial) to SNOMED. As we broaden the implementation of our coding algorithms in the Mayo environment, we will be able to test how consistently these findings apply to alternative coding systems.

We have demonstrated that Computer Assisted Coding workstation tools save time in a production coding environment for a large, tabular coding system. Several algorithms make few errors, and Expert Network generates average rankings statistics that create substantial interest in threshold value research for complete automation of parts of the coding system.

ACKNOWLEDGMENTS

Supported in part by NIH grants LM05416, LM07041, and AR30582. We thank Geoffrey Atkin for computer support and Karen Elias for manuscript assistance. We specially thank Lorraine Fiksdal, Joan Wooner, and the medical indexing staff for their efforts and patience.

REFERENCES

[1] Kurland LT, Molgaard CA. The patient record in epidemiology. *Scientific American* 1981;245(4):54-63.

[2] HICDA-2, Hospital Adaptation of ICDA, 2nd Edition. Ann Arbor, MI: Commission on Professional and Hospital Activities, 1968.

[3] Chute CG, Yang Y. An evaluation of concept based Latent Semantic Indexing for Clinical Information Retrieval. *Proceedings of the 16th Annual Symposium on Computer Applications in Medical Care (SCAMC 92)* 1992;16:639-43.

4] Yang Y, Chute CG. A Linear Least Squares Fit Method for Terminology Mapping. *Proceedings of Fifteenth International Conference on Computational Linguistics (COLING 92)*, 1992;II:447-53.

[5] Yang Y, Chute CG. An application of least squares fit mapping to clinical classification. *Proceedings of the 16th Annual Symposium on Computer Applications in Medical Care (SCAMC 92)* 1992;16:460-4.

[6] Yang Y . Expert Network: Combining Word-based Matching and Human Experiences in Text Categorization and Retrieval. *Proc 17th Ann Int ACM SIGIR Conference on Research and Development in Information Retrieval* (SIGIR94), in press.

[7] Yang Y, Chute CG. An application of Expert Network to Clinical Classification and MEDLINE Indexing. *Proceedings of the 18th Annual Symposium on Computer Applications in Medical Care* 1994, submitted.

[8] Yang Y, Chute CG. An application of least squares fit mapping to text information retrieval. *Proc 16th Ann Int ACM SIGIR Conference on Research and Development in Information Retrieval (SIGIR 93)* 1993;281-90.

A Computational Model of Information Retrieval with UMLS

Jean-Jacques Robert, M.S., Michel Joubert, Ph.D., Laurent Nal, M.S., Marius Fieschi, M.D., Ph.D.
CERTIM. Faculté de Médecine.
Boulevard Pierre Dramard. F-13326 Marseille Cedex 15. France

A high level representation of data would clarify the complex collection of medical concepts, terms and relationships derived from standard classifications that the Unified Medical Language System contains. A conceptual model is described which represents the data structure. A second objective of this conceptual model is to provide users with the capability to build queries to information databases as easily as possible on the basis of this data structure. The methods used to build this model are semantic networks and conceptual graphs. The object-oriented computational model which implements this conceptual model is detailed. It reuses part of the generic C++ classes of the National Institutes of Health library. New classes are added to this library to implement the needed functionalities.

1. INTRODUCTION

The Unified Medical Language System (UMLS) is a major project of the U.S. National Library of Medicine [8]. Three main components constitute the UMLS data structure: the so-called Metathesaurus (Meta-1) [13], the Semantic Network [9] and the Information Sources Map [10]. The UMLS is a complex collection of medical concepts, terms and relationships derived from standard classifications [5]. To optimally benefit from the rich resources the UMLS provides, researchers and developers must understand its structure and data relationships. Four successive versions have been delivered to date. Among them, the third version of the Metathesaurus [16] presented a simpler schema than the previous versions. Nevertheless, as noticed by authors, a high level representation of data would clarify the Metathesaurus and Semantic Network contents and potential applications [15].

The fixed objective is to help users in formulating queries to information databases as naturally as possible. To achieve this goal, it is necessary to give them the ability to operate the closeness link between their view of concepts they use and the representation of these concepts in computer systems. The principle we adopt is to build a logical and conceptual interface between users' applications and information databases. In a previous work, we proposed to build a conceptual model for information retrieval with UMLS [6]. This model, based on conceptual graphs [12] and semantic networks [14], provides the ability to express declarative knowledge relevant to medical concepts and the relationships which link them to each other. The exploitation of the conceptual model results in a query translated by a graph which is further matched to data graphs derived from information databases. This model, we will present briefly in section 2, is conceived to assist end-users to query large information databases. It has been used experimentally to query patients records [7] and is currently being experimented with documents databases. The object-oriented computational model which implements this conceptual model is presented in section 3.

2. THE CONCEPTUAL MODEL

In the following we will only be concerned with the Metathesaurus and the Semantic Network of UMLS. The core concepts which have been isolated in Meta-1 are connected to generic types of concepts in the Semantic Network. These types are interconnected by semantic relationships. The data structure of Meta-1 is based on hierarchies and associations. The association relationship links a given term to related terms and to a preferred term. The hierarchy structures the preferred terms into more generic terms and more specific ones. This hierarchical relationship divides Meta-1 into several so-called microthesauri, according to a local specificity of concepts. The presence of these microthesauri translates the various contexts in which a medical concept can be viewed.

A first objective of the conceptual model is to represent this data structure. We organise the above elements according to the diagram of figure 1 conceived for semantic networks exploitation [11]. When applied to the UMLS components, this structure shows the three following levels:

- the core concepts identified in Meta-1 constitute the lowest level,
- the upper level is the ontology of types of concepts which constitutes the basis of the UMLS Semantic Network,
- the intermediary level is constituted by views which represent microthesauri in Meta-1.

0195-4210/94/$5.00 © 1994 AMIA, Inc.

A given concept may have various instances in different views. For instance, an aneurysm can be either viewed as an acquired abnormality -thus, connected to this related type of concept- or as a congenital abnormality -thus, connected to this latter type. Congenital abnormality and acquired abnormality are two distinct types in the UMLS Semantic Network. Semantic relationships, which are not represented in figure 1, are set between types of concepts to translate the UMLS Semantic Network totally.

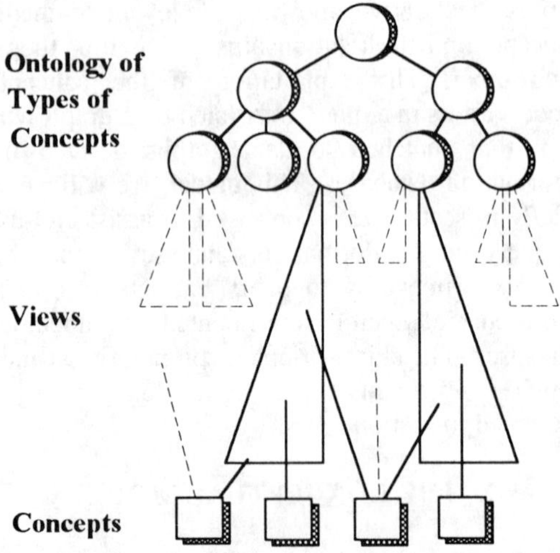

Figure 1: Organisation of concepts in views connected to the ontology of types

A second objective of the conceptual model is to provide users with the capability to build conceptual graphs which involve instances of concepts in views interconnected by instances of semantic relationships inherited from the Semantic Network. These graphs are built at the intermediate level of figure 1. Since the semantic relationships set between types are inherited neither by the concepts nor by their instances automatically, the Semantic Network must be considered as a frame knowledge which describe valid associations and not as an expert knowledge base which should describe relevant associations. For instance, a coronary aneurysm cannot be diagnosed by every diagnostic procedure, but, when viewed as a cardiovascular disease, it can be diagnosed by some (but, not every) cardiovascular diagnostic procedure, such as an angiography. Valid conceptual graphs are built under the control of the Semantic Network. The end-users determine the medical relevance of these graphs. The figure 2 shows the building of an elementary conceptual graph. If the type A (e.g., Diagnostic Procedure) is linked to the type B (e.g., Disease or Syndrome) by the means of the semantic relationship R_1 (e.g., diagnoses), then instances of concepts a (e.g., Angiography) and b (e.g., Coronary Arteriosclerosis) in their respective views V_1 (e.g., Cardiovascular Diagnosis) and V_2 (e.g., Cardiovascular Diseases) may be linked by an instance of the above relationship R_1. Valid operations on conceptual graphs - such as join, restriction and projection - allow the users to build complex graphs which translate full sentences such as "treatment by angioplasty of coronary diseases diagnosed by angiography" [7,12]. This is illustrated in figure 2 by a join of the above graph with a second elementary graph on the same b linked in this latter by R_2 (e.g., treated by) with c (e.g., Angioplasty), issued from C (Therapeutic Procedure), viewed in V_3 as a Cardiovascular Therapeutic Procedure.

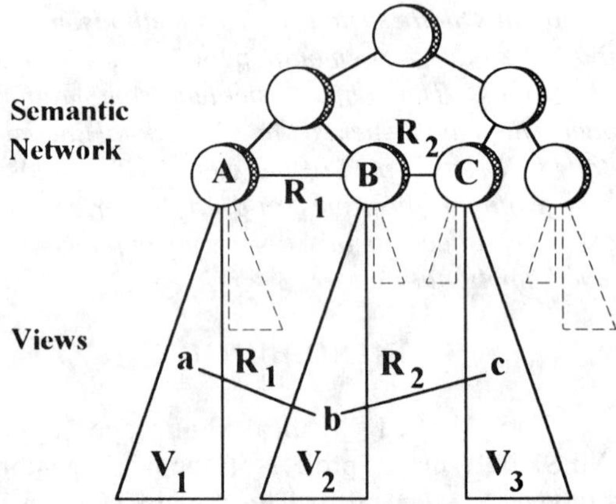

Figure 2: Building a conceptual graph from the Semantic Network

A typical exploitation of the model when building a conceptual graph is as follows:

- select a concept
- select a view on this concept: the related type is then selected automatically,
- select a relationship involving this type: the destination type is selected automatically,
- select a view connected to this latter type,
- select an instance of a concept in this view.

This sequence of operations builds an elementary conceptual graph which links two nodes, the two selected instances of concepts, by the means of an edge, the instance of the selected semantic relationship. Iterations of such a sequence allow the building of more complex connected graphs (each node is linked to another node, at least) which involve several instances of concepts linked by various relationships.

Records in an information database are patients records or bibliographical references, for instance. Fields are identified in information records which contain codes or key-words which index the records. A conceptual graph represents a user's focus or interest in an information database, i.e. a query to this database which translates a full sentence as exemplified above. Such a graph expresses a generic query which is satisfied by coded or indexed data in an information database which

- either matches the nodes exactly,
- or is the code of a descendant of a node in the relevant view.

For instance, if a patient record contains the coded data which expresses that (s)he has been treated by a transluminal angioplasty for a coronary arterio-sclerosis diagnosed by a coronary angiography, the previous query is satisfied, since transluminal angioplasty, coronary arteriosclerosis and coronary angiography are descendants of angioplasty, coronary diseases and angiography in their respective views.

The conceptual model unifies the representation of the Semantic Network and the conceptual graphs by the means of (weakly) connected graphs [4]. In this way, conceptual graphs appear as specializations of the graphs at the semantic level, since they have the same structure and the former graphs are obtained from the latter ones in replacing types nodes by concepts instances nodes.

3. THE COMPUTATIONAL MODEL

The objects involved in the conceptual model are complex. They are concepts, instances of concepts, types of concepts, semantic relationships, graphs, and so on. Powerful tools are needed to design and implement them. Object-orientation allows capabilities to design computer programs [2] which store and treat complex data [1]. Object-oriented programming languages provide the facility to define hierarchies of classes of objects in which the subclasses inherit the properties of their ancestor classes automatically. Objects have the properties of the classes of which they are instances. So, the classes constitute a model for the instantiated objects. The current success of object-programming languages leads developers to create powerful libraries of generic classes of objects. The National Institutes of Health (NIH) Library of Classes [3], implemented in C++ language, provides a large set of hierarchically structured classes. This library contains generic classes of objects such as "list", "ordered list", "set", "dictionary", and so on, which can be reused with benefit. The NIH library of classes is partly represented in figure 3.

A graph is designed as a set of 3-uples: two nodes and the directed relationship which links them. In our case, we needed to implement classes such as:

- "concept", instantiated by concepts or types of concepts,
- "relationship", instantiated by semantic relationships both in conceptual graphs and in semantic networks,
- "tree", instantiated both by the ontology of types and by concepts instances structured in views,
- "graph unit", instantiated by graphs nodes designed as 3-uples,
- "graph", instantiated both by semantic networks and by a conceptual graphs,

and their related procedures among which are the valid operations on graphs. So, we specialized the hierarchy of classes of the NIH library in such way that these new classes benefit from the already defined properties. For instance, since a procedure is defined in the class "set" which verifies that an instantiated set does not contain duplicated elements, to make the class "graph" a subclass of the class "set" entails that the former class inherits this property. Figure 3 presents the hierarchy of classes we implemented. It shows a part of the NIH library we reused and how we implemented new classes as subclasses in it. We can remark that the classes "concept" and "relationship" are new classes directly attached as subclasses of the root class "object", when "node", "tree" and "graph" are attached to classes in the hierarchy and thus benefit from the inheritance.

- Object - Root of the NIH library of classes
  - **Concept** - Unique representation of a concept
  - **Relationship** - Semantic relationship
  - Collection - Abstract class for collections
    - ArrayOb - Array of objects references
      - **GraphUnit** - 3-uple graph unit
    - Set - Collection of non duplicated objects
      - Dictionary - Set of associations
        - IdentDict - Dictionary
      - **Graph** - Set of graph units
      - **Tree** - Tree of objects references
  - Iterator - Collection iterator
  - Link - Abstract class of links for linked lists
    - LinkOb - Link with an object reference
    - LookUpKey - Dictionaries associations
      - Assoc - Association of references

Figure 3: Part of the computational hierarchy of classes. Bold names refer to the classes added into the NIH library

The first time a concept is referenced, an object which instanciates it is created in memory. The selected view of this concept is also instantiated by the means of tree-structured references to the related instantiated concepts. When a relationship links two instantiated concepts, it is also instantiated. A graph unit is created which references the two concepts and the relationship instances. According to this structure, when a graph is created, it is instantiated as a set of instances of units. In this way, no object is duplicated in memory. Duplication is avoided by the use of references to objects identified internally by the object-oriented mechanism. Such a computational instanciation process is summarised by figure 4 which details instances of the concerned objects with an example. It shows the instanciation of the graph which translates the previous query "treatment by angioplasty of coronary diseases diagnosed by angiography".

Users queries are instantiated by the means of graphs after a navigation in UMLS components as described previously. When an information database is queried, data graphs issued from individual records are also instantiated according to the data model the Semantic Network provides. The query graph is successively compared to the individual data graphs by the means of a matching process which implements an operation on graphs named "projection" [12]. This process verifies that the query, or a specialization of it, as described above, is a subset of the individual data graph.

The software we developed in C++ implements the above computational model. The UMLS data (the Semantic Network and Meta-1 components), excluding the chemical data, have been imported from the relational format delivered by the NLM [16] into the Oracle relational database system which allows easy communications with C and C++ programs.

4. DISCUSSION

Efficiency in information retrieval requires all the most integrated system as the information is complex in form and type. The main problem the users encounter is to express queries when the semantics of the domain does not explicitly appear in the information database. This problem is increased by the diversity of the methods to

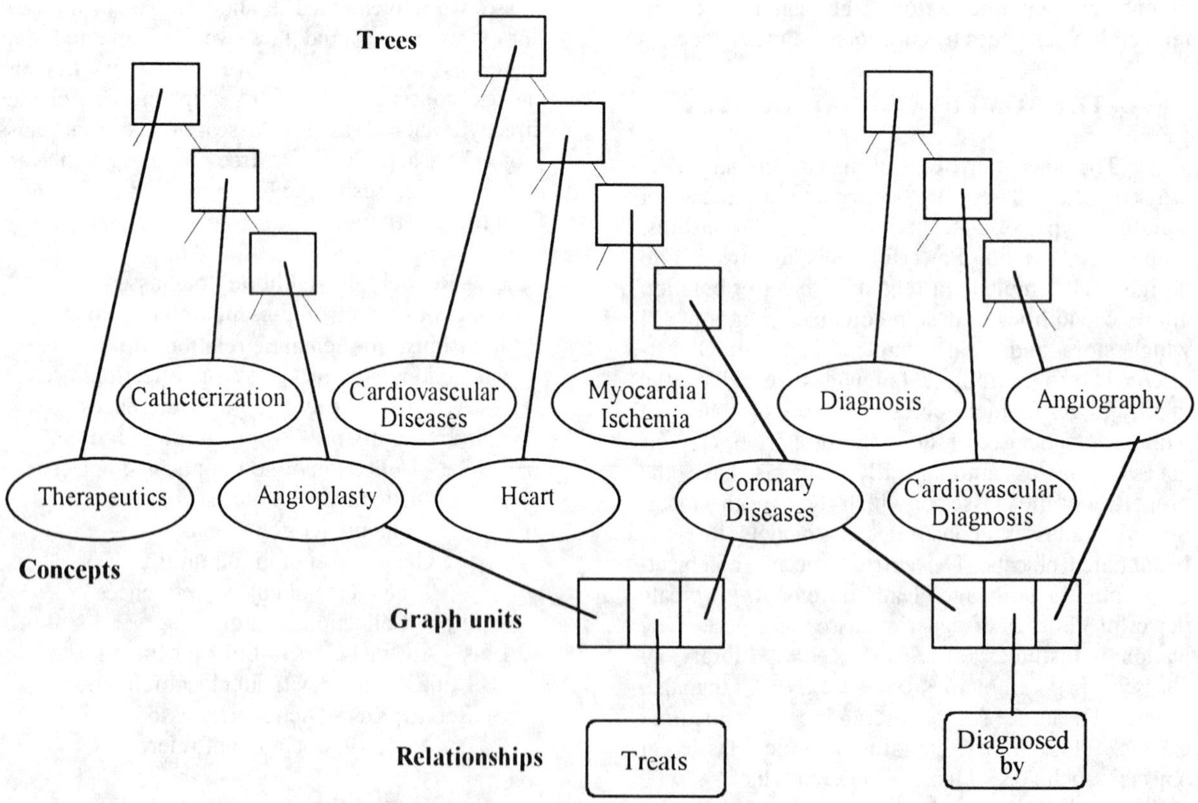

Figure 4: An example of instantiated graph

implement these systems where representation and storage are commonly proprietary even if they offer a high level of query language. We did have an approach, based on the current results of the UMLS project, which mixes the usage of both key-words coming from a standardized vocabulary (Meta-1) and core concepts isolated from it. The Semantic Network of UMLS structures, by the means of semantic relationships, the types of concepts to which the core concepts of Meta-1 are connected. The fixed goal is to help users in formulating queries to information servers as easy as possible. Thus, the semantic approach is significant as well because, using knowledge of the domain, it is able to represent part of the meaning though associations between the concerned concepts.

After we have represented the conceptual model by the means of conceptual graphs and operations on these graphs, it was necessary to select powerful tools to implement it. Object-orientation is a suitable approach to design such systems and permitted us to define the generic classes of the computational model to implement. The C++ language and the library of classes developed by the NIH are efficient supports for implementation. This kind of implementation is general enough to be done with other object-oriented languages and databases. Promising experiments have been done with patients records databases. Complementary experiments with documents databases are underway currently and should conclude to the efficiency of this conceptual approach and the suitability of the developed software. We hope that our object-oriented conceptual and computational modelling of UMLS components will be helpful for designers concerned with information science, and especially for other UMLS users and developers.

ACKNOWLEDGEMENTS

This work has been partially founded by the French Ministry of Education. We thank the U.S. National Library of Medicine which graciously furnished us the UMLS data.

REFERENCES

[1] R.G.G. Cattell. Object Data Management: object-oriented and extended relational database systems. Addisson Wesley; 1991.

[2] P. Coad, E. Yourdon. Object-Oriented Design. Prentice-Hall, 1991.

[3] K. Gorlen, S. Orlow, P. Plexico. Data Abstraction and Object-Oriented Programming in C++. John Wiley & Sons, 1991.

[4] F. Harary. Graph Theory. Addison Wesley, 1971.

[5] B.L. Humphreys, D.A.B. Lindberg. Building the Unified Medical Language System. Proc. 13rd SCAMC. L.C. Kingland editor. IEEE Computer Society Press, 1989: 475-480.

[6] M. Joubert, M. Fieschi, J-J. Robert. A Conceptual Model for Information Retrieval with UMLS. Proc. 17th SCAMC. C. Safran editor. McGraw-Hill, 1993: 715-719.

[7] M. Joubert, M. Fieschi, J-J. Robert, A.G. Tafazzoli. Users Conceptual Views on Medical Information Databases. Int. J. Biomed. Comput. In press.

[8] D.A.B. Lindberg, B.L. Humphreys, A.T. McRay. The Unified Medical Language System. Methods of Information in Medicine 32, 1993: 281-291.

[9] A.T. McRay. The UMLS Semantic Network. Proc. 13rd SCAMC. L.C. Kingland editor. IEEE Computer Society Press, 1989: 503-507.

[10] D.R. Masys, B.L. Humphreys. Structure and Function of the UMLS Information Sources Map. Proc. MEDINFO 92. K.C. Lun, P. Degoulet, T.E. Piemme, O. Rienhoff editors. North-Holland, 1992: 1528-1521.

[11] L. Shastri. Why Semantic Networks? In: Principles of Semantic Networks: Exploration in the representation of knowledge. J.F. Sowa editor. Morgan Kaufmann, 1991: 109-136.

[12] J.F. Sowa. Conceptual Structures: information processing in mind and machine. Addison Wesley, 1984.

[13] M.S. Tuttle, D.D. Sheretz, M.S. Erlbaum, N.E. Olson, S.J. Nelson. Implemeting Meta-1: the first version of the UMLS metathesaurus. Proc. 13rd SCAMC. L.C. Kingland editor. IEEE Computer Society Press, 1989: 483-487.

[14] W.A. Woods. Understanding Subsumption and Taxonomy: a framework for progress. In: Principles of Semantic Networks: exploration in the representation of knowledge. J.F. Sowa editor. Morgan Kaufmann, 1991: 45-94.

[15] Y. Yang, C.G. Chute. A Schematic Analysis of the Unified Medical Language System. Proc. 16th SCAMC. M.E. Frisse editor. McGraw-Hill, 1992: 204-208.

[16] UMLS Knowledge Sources, 4th Experimental Edition. National Library of Medicine, 1993.

Using Digrams to Map Controlled Medical Vocabularies

Roberto A. Rocha, MD and Stanley M. Huff, MD
Department of Medical Informatics, University of Utah 84112

A program for matching between controlled medical vocabularies has been developed which adopts methods used in the domain of Information Retrieval. This program combines a stemmer based on fragments of words (digrams) with a similarity function. The proposed stemmer did not require any knowledge about word-formation rules and helped the identification of several kinds of word variants. The adopted similarity function assigned the highest score to the best candidate match in 99.0% of the cases.

INTRODUCTION

Several controlled medical vocabularies (CMVs) are currently available. However, they usually cover diverse domains with uneven scopes and objectives [1]. The absence of an accepted "standard" method for representing medical concepts, and the need to translate clinical data to existent CMVs has made computerized vocabulary mapping an active area of medical informatics research [2-7].

In our site, several projects require some form of vocabulary matching, ranging from the integration of clinical systems [8,9], to our participation in the Unified Medical Language System (UMLS) project [10,11]. In addition, our research in the area of medical data representation and controlled medical vocabularies has directed many of our efforts toward an automated vocabulary translation method [6,12].

The problem of automated mapping ("translating") between CMVs can be approached in two different ways. One method is known as lexical matching, or "string matching", where the goal is to try to identify similarities among the strings (words and phrases) used in both source and target vocabularies [5,7]. The other method is know as conceptual matching, where instead of comparing words and phrases, the process tries to identify similarities between concepts ("meanings") [3,4,6].

Ideally, both methods should be combined. For example, lexical matching methods could be used to refine the output of a conceptual matching application. In theory, conceptual matching should produce better results, but for small and well-defined domains its complexity may not be justifiable.

The methods applied to vocabulary matching are closely related to the methods utilized in the area of Information Retrieval (IR). IR systems look for similarities between queries and collections of documents [13], while vocabulary matching systems seek similarities between source vocabularies and target vocabularies. We could say, for instance, that each source term is a "query" against the "collection" of target terms. In addition, the use of "meanings" versus "strings" to retrieve information is an active area of research in IR [13,14].

Our intention in this paper is to describe how we adapted IR methods to the area of vocabulary translation. The experiments described here examine lexical matching as a potential technique to create mappings between vocabularies.

METHODS

Matching Algorithm

Initially, we adapted a stemming technique known as n-gram [15]. The n-gram method decomposes terms into sets of adjacent characters. These sets of characters can be of any length. Based on the experience of Adamson and Boreham [16], we decided to used pairs of adjacent characters, called "digrams" or 2-grams. Table 1 presents some examples of words with their respective digrams.

Table 1 - Examples of words and their digrams.

id	*word*	*unique digrams*
1	dyspnea	dy, ys, sp, pn, ne, ea
2	dyspneic	dy, ys, sp, pn, ne, ei, ic
3	dypsnea	dy, yp, ps, sn, ne, ea
4	dysp	dy, ys, sp
5	dyspepsia	dy, ys, sp, pe, ep, ps, si, ia

In addition to the digram method, we adopted a similarity scoring method known as "Dice's Similarity Coefficient" (D_{st}) [13]. D_{st} is defined as:

$$D_{st} = \frac{2 \times M}{S + T}$$

where S is the number of unique elements of the source term, T is the number of unique elements of the target term, and M is the number of unique elements common to both source and target.

Several variations in word morphology and orthography are known to decrease the efficiency of any lexical matching algorithm [13,15,16]. In Table

2, we present some examples of how digrams and Dice's coefficient help the identification of word variations, like the ones displayed in Table 1.

The combination of the digram stemming method and Dice's similarity coefficient was the matching algorithm used for this project.

Table 2 - Using Dice's coefficient to calculate similarities between words.
(Refer to Table 1 for decoding the ids)

Variant form	*Comparison (id vs. id)*	D_{st}
derivation	2 vs. 1	0.77
misspelling	3 vs. 1	0.50
truncation	4 vs. 1	0.67
truncation	4 vs. 5	0.54
(unrelated)	5 vs. 1	0.43

Matching Process

In addition to the matching algorithm, we implemented routines to "normalize" both source and target terms. These routines were applied as pre-matching processes. The normalization steps are summarized in Table 3.

Table 3 - Steps used to normalize terms

Original term: *"Thyroid Function Study :Serum :Quantitative - TSH or Thyroid Stimulating Hormone - MIU/ML"*
Step 1 - Remove punctuation, special characters, and numbers: *"Thyroid Function Study Serum Quantitative TSH or Thyroid Stimulating Hormone MIU ML"*
Step 2 - Lower case all characters: *"thyroid function study serum quantitative tsh or thyroid stimulating hormone miu ml"*
Step 3 - Remove duplicate words: *"thyroid function study serum quantitative tsh or stimulating hormone miu ml"*
Step 4 - Remove stop words: *"thyroid function study serum quantitative tsh stimulating hormone miu ml"*
Step 5 - Sort words in ascending order: *"function hormone miu ml quantitative serum stimulating study thyroid tsh"*

Following the normalization process, a word index was created so that a given word pointed to one or more terms where it occurred. A unique word list was then created by extracting only distinct words from the word index. Finally, a "digram index" was obtained from the word list. The digram index was very similar to the word index, but having the words replaced by their respective digrams. Table 4 has examples of entries found in these ancillary files. All ancillary files were loaded into a relational database.

In order to observe the interactions between the digram method and Dice's similarity coefficient, three matching strategies were implemented: 1) *No-digram strategy*: the digram method was not used, only the original source term words were matched; 2) *Standard-digram strategy*: the digram method was used to identify words similar only to those present in the source term and not found in the target vocabulary; and 3) *Full-digram strategy*: the digram method was used to identify words similar to all those present in the source term.

Experiments

Two experiments were conducted to evaluate our approach to lexical matching. The first experiment was designed to determine how useful a similarity score like Dice's coefficient is in ranking the best candidate mappings. The matching strategy used for this first experiment was the standard-digram strategy.

Table 4 - Examples of the entries found in the target vocabulary indexes.

Normalized terms with numeric identifiers: *"chest pain / 25575", "chronic pain / 133595"*
Word index entries: *"chest / 25575 / 2", "chronic / 133595 / 2", "pain / 25575 / 2", "pain / 133595 / 2"*
Word list entries: *"chest / 1269", "chronic / 145", "pain / 489"*
Digram index entries: *"pa / 489 / 3", "ai / 489 / 3", "in / 489 / 3"*

For this first experiment, we obtained a large set of commonly used PTXT [17] codes to match against the UMLS Metathesaurus version 1.3 (Meta 1.3) [18]. PTXT is challenging to match because it has many peculiarities of a vocabulary supporting a complex information system. These peculiarities are usually format-related (i.e., abbreviations, truncations, misspellings, etc.), or content-related (i.e., daily-use clinical terminology, protocol-oriented terms, etc.).

The initial set of PTXT codes represented a variety of domains, including laboratory, radiology, discharge diagnosis, nurse charting, etc. This source file was called "PTXT-mixed". From PTXT-mixed we isolated codes corresponding to prescribed drugs, generating a second source file called "PTXT-drugs".

Considering the actual sources and coverage of Meta 1.3, we expected fewer format-related intricacies. However, because Meta 1.3 makes the distinction between strings and their underlying concepts, it can easily mislead a lexical matching method.

Also during this first experiment, we normalized the PTXT-drugs file using a "specialized" filtering routine. This special routine removed units, drug concentrations, and drug presentation forms, leaving only the chemical name and the brand name.

The second experiment was designed to evaluate whether digrams improved the recognition of variant forms, and we used all three matching strategies. The source terms were chest x-ray descriptions from the Iliad data dictionary [19]. The file with these terms was called "Iliad-cxr", and the target vocabulary was again Meta 1.3.

Knowing the differences in granularity between Iliad and Meta [6], we modified Dice's coefficient to handle one-to-many matches. In this case, we added a new search condition to select all terms from Meta 1.3 having the total number of words identical to the number of shared words, i.e., forcing T and M to be equal (see Dice's formula).

The output of the first and the second experiments was reviewed by the authors. A simple tool was used to display the source term and the candidate target terms. For the first experiment, only a *single best match* was selected, usually disregarding modifiers or explicit contexts found in the PTXT terms. For the second experiment, either *a single best match or a combination of matches* was selected. Also during the second experiment, all candidate Meta 1.3 terms were presented to the reviewer with their respective semantic types, helping the identification of the most appropriate concepts and not simply the matching string forms.

RESULTS

First Experiment

The results of the first experiment are presented in two parts: matching PTXT-mixed to Meta 1.3, and matching PTXT-drugs to Meta 1.3.

Matching PTXT-mixed to Meta 1.3: The file PTXT-mixed had 2,671 entries. Normalizing PTXT-mixed, we obtained 2,530 unique terms.

All the terms in English from the Meta 1.3 were used as the target vocabulary, corresponding to 255,742 entries. After normalization, we obtained 200,730 unique terms. From these unique terms, we generated the word index with 578,526 entries, the word list with 91,029 entries, and the digram index with 823,649 entries.

The time required to identify all candidate mappings for a given source term was variable. When extensive searches against the digram index were necessary, the matching process usually took a couple of minutes. However, searches against the word list and the word index usually took just a few seconds.

After completing the matching process, an average of 170.85 candidate target terms per source term were obtained. The results of the manual review, grouped by Dice's coefficient, are summarized in Table 5.

Out of the 831 matches obtained, in 823 (99.0%) cases the matched term had the highest Dice's coefficient, and in 8 (1.0%) cases, the matched term did not have the highest Dice's score.

Table 5 - Summary of the review of the first experiment (PTXT-mixed to Meta 1.3).

Dice's coefficient range	*Match (%)*	*No Match (%)*
Perfect score: 1.0	219 (26.3)	129 (7.0)
High score: from 0.8 to 0.99	42 (5.1)	58 (3.1)
Medium score: from 0.6 to 0.79	161 (19.4)	518 (28.2)
Low score: from 0.0 to 0.59	409 (49.2)	1135 (61.7)
Total	831 (31.1)	1840 (68.9)

Matching PTXT-drugs to Meta 1.3: The file called PTXT-drugs had 1,142 entries. Normalizing PTXT-drugs with the *standard method* generated the same number of unique terms. Normalizing it with the *special method* generated 970 unique terms.

After running the matching process, for those terms normalized with the special routine, we obtained an average of 36.35 candidate target terms per source term. The results of the manual review, grouped by Dice's coefficient, are summarized in Table 6. Table 7 summarizes the performance of Dice's coefficient for the matched terms.

Second Experiment

The file called Iliad-cxr had 238 entries. After normalizing these terms, we obtained the same number of unique terms. The results of the matching processes are summarized in Table 8.

DISCUSSION

The results of our first experiment demonstrate the usefulness of Dice's similarity coefficient, despite its simplicity. Although we identified only 31.1% of matches between PTXT-mixed and Meta 1.3, Dice's coefficient ranked the best match with the highest score on 99.0% of the cases. Similar performance in ranking the best match was observed between PTXT-drugs and Meta 1.3 (99.2%, 98.7%).

Table 6 - Summary of the review of the first experiment (PTXT-drugs to Meta 1.3).

	PTXT-drugs (standard filter)		*PTXT-drugs (special filter)*	
Dice's coefficient range	*Match (%)*	*No Match (%)*	*Match (%)*	*No Match (%)*
Perfect score: 1.0	14 (2.6)	4 (0.6)	264 (28.7)	56 (25.0)
High score: from 0.8 to 0.99	17 (3.2)	3 (0.5)	54 (5.9)	9 (4.0)
Medium score: from 0.6 to 0.79	101 (19.0)	59 (9.7)	491 (53.5)	90 (40.2)
Low score: from 0.0 to 0.59	400 (75.2)	544 (89.2)	109 (11.9)	69 (30.8)
Total	532 (46.6)	610 (53.4)	918 (80.4)	224 (19.6)

Dice's coefficient was in some cases mislead by the normalization process, and by the digram method. High scores end up being assigned to terms that did not match, ranging from 0.5% to 25.0%. Using less generic filters and limiting the domains of the target vocabulary, we will certainly improve precision.

Table 7 - Matched terms and the value of their Dice's coefficients (PTXT-drugs to Meta 1.3).

	Highest D_{st} (%)	*Not highest D_{st} (%)*
standard filter	528 (99.2%)	4 (0.8%)
specialized filter	906 (98.7%)	12 (1.3%)

In addition to ranking unrelated concepts as good candidates for a match, Dice's coefficient was also responsible for hiding candidate matching terms. This effect was obvious when the percentage of matches between PTXT-drugs and Meta 1.3 almost doubled (from 46.6% to 80.4%) after we applied the special filter. This filter improved the precision of the matching process, reducing the average number of candidate target terms per source term from 170.85 to 36.35. The normalization process also helped to reduce the redundancy of both source and target vocabularies. However, the practice of using "aggressive" filters may not be indicated when format-related details are important.

The second experiment has demonstrated that the digram method can improve the recall of the matching process. We observed an increase in the number of candidate target terms per source term, from 39.70 to 54.67. The full-digram strategy produced a slightly higher average number of target terms per match, reflecting the improvement in recall.

The differences in granularity between Iliad-cxr and Meta 1.3, combined with the adaptation of Dice's coefficient to handle one-to-many matches, produced low average Dice's coefficients. However, despite this effort, many "modifiers" present in the Iliad vocabulary were not available in the Meta 1.3 vocabulary, making almost all matches incomplete. These problems were reflected in the performance of the full-digram strategy, which identified only four additional concepts not revealed by the other two strategies (56 versus 54 and 50).

Reviewing the candidate Meta 1.3 terms with their semantic types attached, helped the identification of important deficiencies of the lexical matching process. Fifty-six concepts were correctly identified because they were either nonambiguous (such as disease names and body parts), or because only a single meaning of the string was present. In other cases, the opposite occurred, i.e., the exact same string was present, but with an inappropriate meaning. For instance, words like "opacity", "abnormality", and "inflation" were perfect string matches, but their meanings in Meta 1.3 did not correspond to their meanings in the Iliad-cxr terms.

Overall, the combination of a n-gram stemmer with a similarity coefficient was a good choice for a general purpose lexical matching tool. The digram algorithm did not require any knowledge about word-formation rules, and did not rely upon the existence of affix dictionaries. An additional benefit of digram

	No-digram strategy	Standard-digram strategy	Full-digram strategy
1. Average number of candidate target terms per source term	39.70	45.17	54.67
2. Average Dice's coefficient of the candidate target terms	0.34	0.34	0.35
3. Average number of target terms per match	3.17	3.17	3.41
4. Total number of concepts identified	50	54	56
5. Total number of concepts identified only by this method	0	2	4

Table 8 - Summary of the results of the second experiment.

stemmers is their applicability in detecting spelling problems [13], and their usefulness in multilingual environments. Dice's coefficient was very simple to implement and has shown its potential as well.

The lexical matching system described here was successful, and it will help the maintenance of our local systems [12]. Future plans include a study to compare this method with InterMatch [6].

Acknowledgment

Roberto A. Rocha is supported by a scholarship from the National Council for Scientific and Technological Development (CNPq), Secretary for Science and Technology, Brazil. This project was partially supported by grant number 1 R03 HS 08053-01 from the Agency for Health Care Policy and Research.

Reference

[1] Evans, DA, Cimino, JJ, Hersh, WR, Huff, SM, Bell, DS (for the Canon Group). Toward a Medical-concept Representation Language. *JAMIA* 1(3):207-17, 1994.

[2] Wingert F. Medical Linguistics: Automated Indexing into SNOMED. *CRC Critical Reviews in Medical Informatics* 1(4): 335-403, 1987.

[3] Masarie FE, Miller RA, Bouhaddou O, Giuse NB, Warner, HR. An Interlingua for Electronic Interchange of Medical Information: Using Frames to Map between Clinical Vocabularies. *Computers and Biomedical Research* 24: 379-400, 1991.

[4] Cimino JJ, Barnett GO. Automated Translation Between Medical Terminologies Using Semantic Definitions. *MD Computing* 7(2): 104-109, 1990.

[5] Sherertz DD, Tuttle MS, Blois MS, Erlbaum MS. Intervocabulary Mapping within the UMLS: The Role of Lexical Matching. *Proc. of the 12th Symposium on Comp. Applic. in Medical Care*, 201-206, 1988.

[6] Rocha RA, Rocha BHSC, Huff SM. Automated Translation Between Medical Vocabularies Using a Frame-Based Interlingua. *Proc. of the 17th Symposium on Comp. Applic. in Medical Care*, 690-694, 1993.

[7] Sherertz DD, Tuttle MS, Olson NE, Erlbaum MS, Nelson SJ. Lexical Mapping in the UMLS Metathesaurus. *Proc. of the 13th Symposium on Comp. Applic. in Medical Care*, 494-499, 1989.

[8] Gibson, R, Haug, P. Linking the Computerized Severity Index (CSI) to Coded Patient Findings in the HELP System Patient Database. *Proc. of the 17th Symposium on Comp. Applic. in Medical Care*, 673-77, 1993.

[9] Wong ET, Pryor TA, Huff SM, Haug PJ, Warner, HR. Interfacing a Stand-Alone Diagnostic Expert System with a Hospital Information System. *Computers and Biomedical Research* 27: 116-129, 1994.

[10] Huff SM, Warner HR. A Comparison of Meta-1 and HELP Terms: Implications for Clinical Data. *Proc. of the 14th Symposium on Comp. Applic. in Medical Care*, 166-169, 1990.

[11] Bouhaddou O, Warner H, Huff S, Bray B. Sorenson D, Dougherty N. Evaluating How the UML Meta1.1 Covers Disease Information Contained in a Diagnostic Expert System (Iliad). *Abstract presented at the 1993 AMIA Spring Congress*, St. Louis, May 9-12.

[12] Rocha RA, Huff SM, Haug PJ. Implementing a Controlled Medical Vocabulary Server. *Abstract presented at the 1994 AMIA Spring Congress*, San Francisco, May 4-7.

[13] Salton, G. *Automatic Text Processing - The Transformation, Analysis, and Retrieval of Information by Computer*. Addision-Wesley Publishing Co., 1989.

[14] Yang Y, Chute CG. Words or Concepts: the Features of Indexing Units and their Optimal Use in Information Retrieval. *Proc. of the 17th Symposium on Comp. Applic. in Medical Care*, 685-689, 1993.

[15] Frakes WB, Baeza-Yates R, eds. *Information Retrieval - Data Structures & Algorithms*. Prentice Hall, 1992.

[16] Adamson GW, Boreham J. The Use of an Association Measure Based on Character Structure to Identify Semantically Related Pairs of Words and Document Titles. *Information Storage and Retrieval*, 10(7-8):253-260, 1974.

[17] Kuperman GJ, Gardner RM, Pryor TA. *HELP: A Dynamic Hospital Information System*. Springer-Verlag, 1991.

[18] Lindberg, DAB, Humphreys, BL, McCray, AT. The Unified Medical Language System. *Methods of Information in Medicine*, 32(4):281-91, 1993

[19] Warner HR, Haug P, Lincoln M, Warner H Jr, Sorenson D, Fan C. Iliad as an Expert Consultant to Teach Differential Diagnosis. *Proc. of the 12th Symposium on Comp. Applic. in Medical Care*, 371-376, 1988.

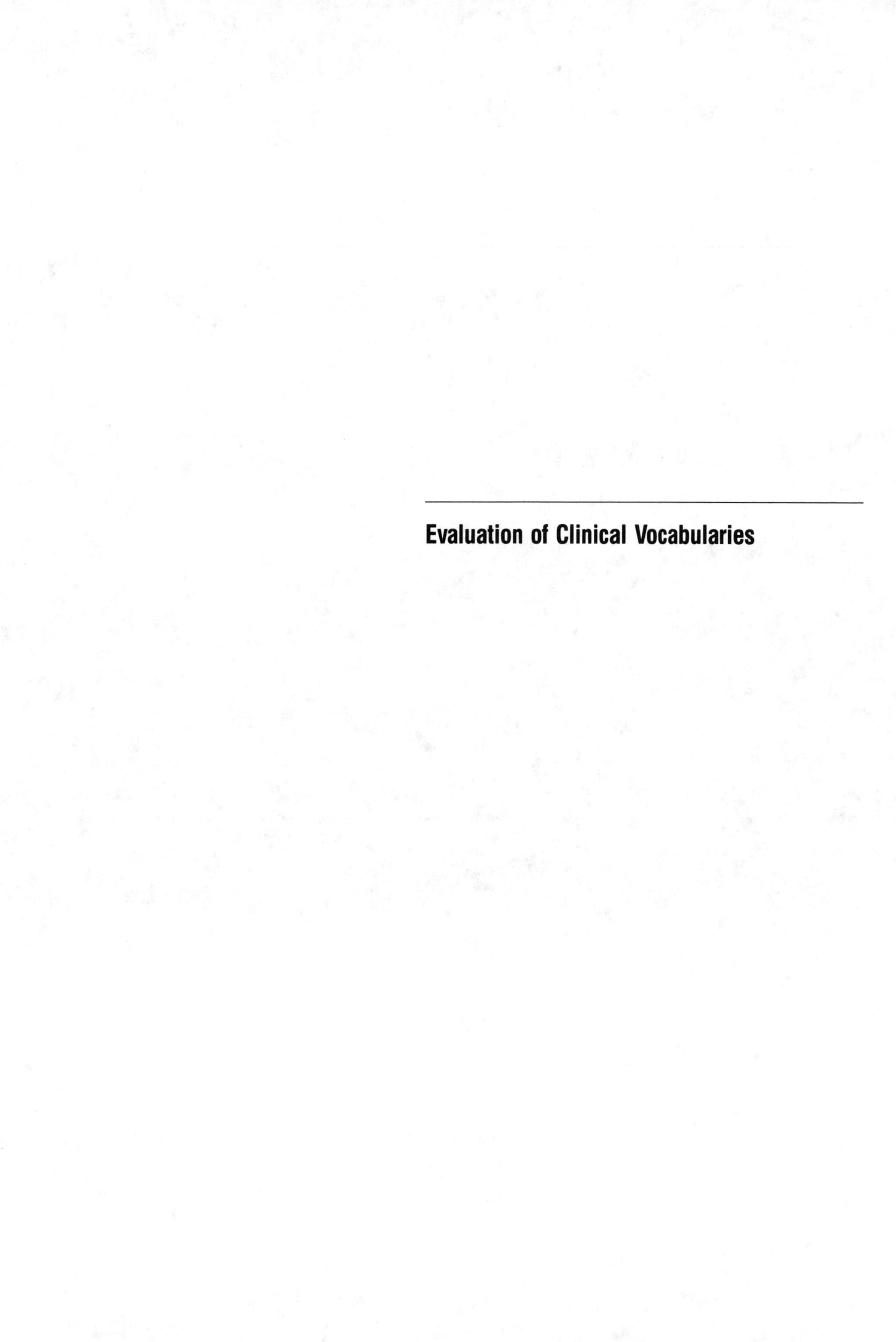

Evaluation of Clinical Vocabularies

Extraction of SNOMED Concepts from Medical Record Texts

Diane E. Oliver, MD and Russ B. Altman, MD, PhD
Section on Medical Informatics
Stanford University School of Medicine
Stanford, CA 94305
oliver@camis.stanford.edu, altman@camis.stanford.edu

ABSTRACT

Clinicians have traditionally documented patient data using natural language text. With the increasing prevalence of computer systems in health care, an increasing amount of medical record text will be stored electronically. However, for such textual documents to be indexed, shared, and processed adequately by computers, it will be important to be able to identify concepts in the documents using a common medical terminology. Automated methods for extracting concepts in a standard terminology would enhance retrieval and analysis of medical record data. This paper discusses a method for extracting concepts from medical record documents using the medical terminology SNOMED-III (Systematized Nomenclature of Human and Veterinary Medicine, Version III). The technique employs a linear least squares fit that maps training set phrases to SNOMED concepts. This mapping can be used for unknown text inputs in the same domain as the training set to predict SNOMED concepts that are contained in the document. We have implemented the method in the domain of congestive heart failure for history and physical exam texts. Our system has a reasonable response time. We tested the system over a range of thresholds. The system performed with 90% sensitivity and 83% specificity at the lowest threshold, and 42% sensitivity and 99.9% specificity at the highest threshold.

INTRODUCTION

Although computers show much promise for improving storage and access of medical records, retrieval and analysis will be difficult if records are stored as natural language text with inadequate indexing and processing to establish semantic content. Major barriers in the effort toward the development of a computer-based patient record in medical care are the lack of a standardized medical terminology and the ability to code medical record text using such a standard. Clinicians do use a constrained vocabulary in their patient records, but like natural language, there is still a fair amount of variability in how they might express ideas in writing. Clinicians cannot be expected to learn a standardized vocabulary and will either require guidance for data entry through a structured computer interface, or text written by clinicians will have to be analyzed automatically for concepts in a common vocabulary.

In this paper, we propose a method for automated mapping of natural language text in medical record documents to concepts in a controlled medical terminology. The method is based on using a training set of "free text to terminology" mappings using a linear least squares fit (LLSF) and singular value decomposition (SVD) technique. The medical terminology selected for this task is SNOMED-III (Systematized Nomenclature of Human and Veterinary Medicine) [1], although our method is relevant to any terminology. SNOMED is a medical terminology developed by the College of American Pathology that aims to cover broad areas in clinical medicine. It includes terms for anatomy, morphology, signs and symptoms, living organisms, drugs, occupations, devices and activities associated with disease, social context, diagnoses, procedures, and modifiers.

There are a number of potential uses for automated extraction of controlled terminology concepts from medical record text documents. First, if patient data are stored electronically in text format and the volume of data is large for a given patient, searching through a patient's record can be simplified if the data is indexed using a controlled terminology. Second, if queries are to be made across a population of patients in a database made up of textual documents, retrieval can be enhanced if the content of the texts is based on a standardized terminology. Queries across patient populations and often across different databases are important for research on practice patterns, retrospective clinical studies, linking of costs to processes of care, and identification of patients who are eligible to be included in clinical trial protocols. Third, decision support systems that are based on the common controlled terminology could trigger alerts or recommendations on patients whose textual medical records contained the relevant content. Finally, this method could be used to compare the value of one

0195-4210/94/$5.00

terminology to another by looking at the performance of each terminology when applied to the same set of data.

Yang and Chute [2, 3] used a linear least squares fit approach to map physician-recorded diagnoses to ICD-9-CM codes [4]. Our method follows a similar approach, but rather than trying to identify the single most likely code for an input text, we map an input text to a group of relevant SNOMED codes that collectively represent the content of the input text. Yang and Chute found the LLSF method to be superior to string matching, statistical weighting, and latent semantic indexing in their application domain.

METHODS

The methodology described here and implemented in our system is an LLSF approach. The mapping learns a linear function that maps texts to SNOMED concepts on a training set of data. It then can predict SNOMED terms for unknown input texts.

Data were collected for the training set from a set of 21 medical record hospital admission summaries of patients diagnosed with congestive heart failure. Phrases that were deemed of medical importance for patients with congestive heart failure and that could be represented in SNOMED were selected from these documents by a person who has experience in the practice of medicine as well as in the use of SNOMED. Phrases were selected from the chief complaint, history of present illness, and physical examination sections of the medical record. In the physical examination, only lung, heart, and extremity examinations were included.

Each text phrase was matched with one or more SNOMED concepts. The training set data, which consists of the text phrases and their corresponding SNOMED concepts, is stored in two matrices: Matrix **A** contains data on the words in the training set text phrases, and matrix **B** contains data on the SNOMED terms selected as equivalent in meaning to concepts in the training set phrases. A total of 197 training set phrases were included. The number of distinct words in the union of all the words in the training set is 365. The number of distinct SNOMED terms in the union of all the SNOMED terms selected for the training set is 139. Characteristics of matrices **A** and **B** are described below.

Matrix **A**

(1) There are 197 columns with one column for each text phrase.
(2) There are 365 rows with one row for each word that is found one or more times in the training set.
(3) An entry $\mathbf{A}_{ij}$ is set to 1 if word i is found in phrase j.
(4) An entry $\mathbf{A}_{ij}$ is set to 0 if word i is not found in phrase j.

Matrix **B**

(1) There are 197 columns with one column for each text phrase.
(2) There are 139 rows with one row for each SNOMED term that is found one or more times in the training set.
(3) An entry $\mathbf{B}_{ij}$ is set to 1 if SNOMED term i is relevant to phrase j.
(4) An entry $\mathbf{B}_{ij}$ is set to 0 if SNOMED term i is not relevant to phrase j.

Using a linear least squares fit for the data, a mapping matrix **W** was calculated that optimally solves the equation **WA** = **B**. Then for an unknown input vector, **a**,

$$\mathbf{Wa} = \mathbf{b} \quad (1)$$

where the predicted output values are in vector **b**.

Since solving for **W** does not always yield an exact solution, the goal is to find an appropriate **W** that minimizes the error in **WA** - **B**. A measure of this error is the sum of the squares of the entries in matrix **E** = **WA** - **B**. That is, if **E** = **WA** - **B** is an $m \times k$ matrix, then the value to minimize is

$$\sum_{i=1}^{k} \sum_{j=1}^{m} \mathbf{E}_{ij}^2 \quad (2)$$

where $\mathbf{E}_{ij}$ is the *ith* row and *jth* column of matrix **E**.

A commonly used method for solving a linear least squares fit problem is based on a matrix factorization technique known as singular value decomposition (SVD) [5]. For an $n \times k$ matrix **A** and an $m \times k$ matrix **B**, the computation for an LLSF for **WA** = **B** is as follows:

Compute the SVD of matrix **A**. That is, determine **U**, **S**, and **V** such that $\mathbf{A} = \mathbf{USV}^{\mathbf{T}}$. **A** is the $n \times k$ matrix being decomposed, **U** is an $n \times p$ orthogonal matrix, S is a $p \times p$ diagonal matrix with all positive values on the diagonal, and $\mathbf{V}^{\mathbf{T}}$ is a $p \times k$ orthogonal matrix where $\mathbf{V}^{\mathbf{T}}$ is the transpose of **V**. Since **U** and $\mathbf{V}^{\mathbf{T}}$ are orthogonal, they can be multiplied by their transposes to yield the identity matrix. This fact is used in the following sequence of matrix manipulations to find an equation for **W**.

$$A = USV^T \quad (3)$$
$$WA = B \quad (4)$$
$$WUSV^T = B \quad (5)$$
$$W = BVS^{-1}U^T \quad (6)$$

where S^{-1} is the inverse of **S** and U^T is the transpose of **U**.

Therefore, the SVD approach allows us to calculate a matrix **W** that solves the linear least squares fit problem **WA = B**. The resulting matrix **W** is $m \times n$. In the training set, there are k text phrases, n distinct words, and m distinct SNOMED terms.

$$\underset{m \times n}{\mathbf{W}} \times \underset{n \times k}{\mathbf{A}} = \underset{m \times k}{\mathbf{B}} \quad (7)$$

We used a published algorithm [5] for determining the SVD of a matrix **A**. We then calculated the mapping matrix **W** using equation (6) above.

The purpose of calculating the mapping matrix **W** is that it can be multiplied by an unknown vector **a** to get a corresponding vector **b** where **a** is a column vector indicating words in an input text phrase and **b** is an output column vector indicating the relevance of SNOMED concepts. The vector **a** is similar to a column in matrix **A** from the training set. It consists of 1s and 0s that indicate which words are in the text. Vector **b** is similar to a column in matrix **B** from the training set. However, it does not consist only of 1s an 0s. Instead, it consists of values between 0 and 1 where each calculated value gives an indication of how relevant the corresponding SNOMED concept is to the input text phrase. The closer a value is to 1, the more relevant the SNOMED concept is, and the closer a value is to 0, the less relevant the SNOMED concept is.

In order for the user to decide whether a SNOMED concept is relevant to the input text or not given the calculated value between 0 and 1, a threshold needs to be specified. For a given threshold, all SNOMED concepts whose values are greater than or equal to the threshold are said to be relevant, and all SNOMED concepts whose values are less than the threshold are said to be irrelevant to the input text.

The system is implemented in Macintosh Common Lisp (MCL). The calculation of matrix **W** is computationally intensive and only needs to be performed once; the SVD calculation was done on an HP720 and took two CPU minutes.

EVALUATION

To evaluate our methods, we ran the program with 116 sentences taken from hospital admission history and physical examinations for five patients admitted with congestive heart failure. Two of the patients were hospitalized at Stanford University Hospital, and three were hospitalized at Palo Alto Veterans Administration Hospital.

The unit chosen for a single text input was a sentence. In the five history and physical examinations, there were a total of 116 sentences. We ran the program on each of the 116 sentences and compared the SNOMED codes selected by the program with those selected by a human encoder, who was used as a de facto gold standard.

For each of the 116 sentences, the program was run with varying values of threshold. The threshold range was from .1 to .9 in increments of .1. Each SNOMED code selected or not selected at a given threshold for a given sentence was determined to be a true positive, a false positive, a true negative, or a false negative. From these data, sensitivities and specificities were determined. This was done in two ways: One method was to calculate sensitivity (sensitivity = TP / (TP + FN)) and specificity (specificity = TN / (TN + FP)) for each sentence at a given threshold and then average the values over all the sentences. This resulted in an average sensitivity and average specificity for each threshold. The other technique was to count the total true positives and false negatives for all the sentences at a given threshold and calculate an overall sensitivity. Similarly, the true negatives and false positives for all the sentences at a given threshold were counted and an overall specificity was calculated .

The sensitivity and specificity determined for each threshold provided data for plotting a receiver operating characteristic (ROC) curve.

RESULTS

The program successfully extracted SNOMED concepts from input text data, with greater sensitivity at lower thresholds and greater specificity at higher thresholds. The two methods for calculating sensitivities and specificities gave very similar results.

Sample output at varying thresholds for an input sentence taken from a patient history is shown in Fig. 1. Also shown are the number of true positives, false positives, true negatives, and false negatives associated with each threshold.

Test input sentence:
"He describes this as a knot developing in his chest that was constant along with shortness of breath."

Output for threshold .2:

"Chest pain, NOS"	"F-37000"
"Dyspnea, NOS"	"F-20040"
"Hydrochlorothiazide"	"C-72260"
"Lasix Tablets"	"C-C1C6E"
"Lower extremity, NOS"	"T-D9000"
"Mild"	"G-A001"
"Negative for"	"G-A201"

TP=2 FP=5 TN=132 FN=0

Output for threshold .5:

"Chest pain, NOS"	"F-37000"
"Dyspnea, NOS"	"F-20040"

TP=2 FP=0 TN=137 FN=0

Output for threshold .8:

"Dyspnea, NOS"	"F-20040"

TP=1 FP=0 TN=137 FN=1

Fig. 1 Sample Output

In this sample, the expert determined that the correct responses were "Chest pain, NOS" and "Dyspnea, NOS." Each SNOMED concept that was output by the program was either a true positive or a false positive. There were a total of 139 SNOMED concepts known to the program. Every SNOMED concept that was correctly excluded in the output of the program was a true negative, and every SNOMED concept that was missed by the program was a false negative.

The results from the entire data set are shown in Fig. 2, showing performance as a function of threshold. TPR signifies true positive rate (sensitivity) and FPR signifies false positive rate (1 - specificity). The "AVG" data refers to the first method of calculating average sensitivities and specificities. The "TOTAL" data refers to the second method of determining the total number of true positives, false positives, true negatives, and false negatives, and calculating overall sensitivities and specificities from the totals. The ROC curve for the average data is shown in Fig. 3.

Threshold	AVG TPR	AVG FPR
0.1	0.8932	0.0732
0.2	0.8824	0.0336
0.3	0.8457	0.0175
0.4	0.7971	0.0098
0.5	0.7633	0.0055
0.6	0.6830	0.0028
0.7	0.6460	0.0020
0.8	0.5567	0.0011
0.9	0.4657	0.0013

Threshold	TOTAL TPR	TOTAL FPR
0.1	0.9094	0.0730
0.2	0.8960	0.0336
0.3	0.8418	0.0175
0.4	0.8040	0.0097
0.5	0.7703	0.0054
0.6	0.6993	0.0028
0.7	0.6463	0.0020
0.8	0.5495	0.0011
0.9	0.4261	0.0013

Fig. 2
Performance as a Function of Threshold

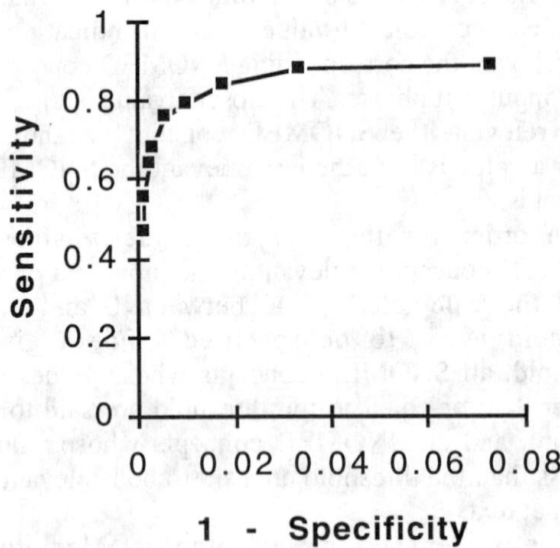

Fig. 3 ROC Curve (Average Data)

DISCUSSION

This program demonstrates that a linear least squares fit approach can be used to automatically assign SNOMED codes to arbitrary natural language text when appropriate training set data have been used to create the mapping function. Yang and Chute [1, 2] demonstrated that the LLSF approach was successful for assigning ICD-9-CM codes to natural language input. Our work differs in that we were attempting to map as many SNOMED codes as were relevant to the entire text of a history and physical examination. In addition, they used a cosine measure to assess similarity between an output result and an ICD-9-CM code, whereas we implemented a threshold model.

The program was trained to extract SNOMED codes from natural language text in history and physical exams for patients with congestive heart failure. When tested, the program was able to assign SNOMED codes for sentences that were relevant to congestive heart failure and that contained concepts similar to those found in the training set. There may be some situations in which a high sensitivity is more important than a high specificity or vice versa. The preferred threshold then would depend on the requirements of the application.

We are now testing several ways in which we could modify the methods to improve performance. For example, we might store all sentences or clauses from the documents in the columns of matrix A rather than phrases that were selected by a physician as medically relevant. Similarly, we could keep our test documents the same but change the method of running the program on test documents by making each unknown input a paragraph rather than a sentence.

The evaluation performed for this study assessed the ability of the program to meet the performance level set by the physician who encoded the training set and provided the gold standard codes for the evaluation. Thus, it evaluated the validity of the method for reproducing the performance of a single encoder. It did not evaluate the degree to which that encoder was a valid gold standard.

Further evaluation should assess the ability of the program to meet the expectations of a group of physicians who have their own particular biases and no prior information about the program. This would be a measure of the knowledge stored in the system as well as an evaluation of the method. In addition, further work could focus on expanding the domain to include patients with other conditions besides congestive heart failure. One might create separate mapping matrices for different diagnoses and patient complaints. A patient's medical record document could then be processed by applying the appropriate matrices, in sequence, for each of the patient's diagnoses or major complaints. Another option would be to store training data on multiple domains all in the same matrix, but scaling may be a problem as the matrices expand greatly in size and computations become more complex.

In conclusion, the LLSF and SVD approach may be a useful technique for automatic extraction of standardized vocabulary concepts from medical record text documents. This study suggests that it is useful for a small domain. Further work using larger training sets would be required to determine the utility of this approach in larger domains.

ACKNOWLEDGEMENTS

Computing facilities were provided for this work by the Center for Advanced Medical Informatics at Stanford, which is supported by NLM grant LM05305. Dr. Oliver is supported by AHCPR training grant HS 00028. Dr. Altman is supported by NIH grant LM05652 and the Culpeper Foundation.

REFERENCES

1. Cote RA, Rothwell DJ, Palotay JL, Beckett RS, Brochu L. The Systematized Nomenclature of Human and Veterinary Medicine, SNOMED International, College of American Pathologists, Northfield, IL, 1993.

2. Yang Y, Chute CG. An application of least squares fit mapping to clinical classification. Proceedings of the 16th Annual Sumposium on Computer Applications in Medical Care, 1992, pp. 460-464.

3. Yang Y, Chute CG. A linear least squares fit mapping method for information retrieval from natural language texts. Proceedings of the 14th International Conference on computational Linguistics-92, Nantes, Aug. 23-28, 1992, 447-453.

4. International Classification of Diseases, 9th Revision, Clinical Modification, Fourth Edition. Practice Management Information Corporation, Los Angeles, CA, 1993.

5. Forsythe GE, Malcolm MA, Moler CG. Computer Methods for Mathematical Computations. Prentice-Hall, Inc. Englewood Cliffs, NJ, 1977.

Can SNOMED International Represent Patients' Perceptions of Health-Related Problems for the Computer-Based Patient Record?

Suzanne Bakken Henry, RN, DNSc and William L. Holzemer, RN, PhD, FAAN
School of Nursing, University of California, San Francisco, California

As the United States moves towards a computer-based patient record, there is much discussion related to the contents of such a record and the manner in which the data elements will be represented. Recent health care reform has emphasized the need for increased patient involvement in health care decision making, however, there has been little discussion about including the patient perspective in the computer-based patient record. Using an existing data set of 201 patients who were hospitalized for Pneumocystis carinii pneumonia, this study examined the ability of SNOMED International to represent patients' perceptions of health-related problems. The majority of concepts used by patients to describe health-related problems could be matched with existing SNOMED terms. The addition of the social context module as an adjunct to existing terminologies of medical diagnoses, NANDA diagnoses, and signs/symptoms provided additional matching terms. Patient goals did not match existing SNOMED terms. The findings of this study suggest that SNOMED International has the potential to adequately represent patients' perceptions of health-related problems for the computer-based patient record. Additional studies are needed that will examine the extent to which patients' perceptions of health-related problems are already documented in the patient record by healthcare providers. The utility of patients' perceptions of health-related problems in the prediction of patient outcomes must also be analyzed.

INTRODUCTION

The Institute of Medicine report on the computer-based patient record identified the standardization of health care vocabularies as a prerequisite for the patient record of the future and recommended a collaborative effort towards establishing a composite clinical data dictionary [1]. In addition, the report identifies a patient problem list and the systematic measurement and recording of patient's health status and functional level as attributes of computer-based patient records. While a few studies have tested the ability of existing vocabularies to represent medical or nursing concepts in the patient record [2-5], no studies were located that focused on the terms used by patients to describe their health-related problems.

Patient Perceptions

The significance of patient perceptions of health-related problems has been identified by several authors. Reiser [6] stressed the importance of making the experience of individuals with illness significant features of health care practice, education, research, and policy. Longo [7] proposed a new model for examination of practice variation that includes "patient practice style variation". He stated that "studies of outcomes must take advantage of what is known about patient problem perception, problem status measurement (by contrast with health status assessment), patient satisfaction, sick role and illness behavior in a life style context, and characteristics and dimensions of disease as experienced through the eyes of patients" (p. YS83).

SNOMED International

SNOMED International [8] is a compilation of nomenclatures that classifies patient findings into eleven modules or taxonomies: 1) *topography* - anatomic terms (12,385 records); 2) *morphology* - changes found in cells, tissues, and organs (4,991 records); 3) *living organisms* - bacteria and viruses (24,265 records); 4) *chemicals, drugs, and biological products* - drugs, chemicals, and plant products (14,075 records); 5) *function* - signs and symptoms (16,352 records); 6) *occupation* - terms to describe occupations (1,886 records); 7) *diagnosis* - diagnostic terms used in clinical medicine (23,623 records); 8) *procedure* -

administrative, therapeutic, and diagnostic procedures (27,033 records); 9) *physical agents, forces, and activities* - devices and activities commonly associated with disease (1,355 records); 10) *social context* - social conditions and relationships of importance in medicine (433 records); and 11) *general* - syntactic linkages and qualifiers (1,176 records). Nomenclatures in SNOMED include ICD-9-CM [9], DSM-III-R [10], Current Procedural Terminology [11], and North American Nursing Diagnosis Association Taxonomy 1 [12].

Evaluation Studies

Three studies were located which tested a version of SNOMED with data from the patient record. Chute et al. [2] conducted an empirical evaluation of concept capture for 675 surgical diagnoses using three medical nomenclatures, the UMLS Metathesaurus, ICD-9-CM, and SNOMED II. Concept match scores were assigned for the natural language terms and for the base concepts (main concept stripped of modifiers) using a semi-automated coding tool based on lexical matching. The eight category nominal concept scores ranged from complete to poor match based on hierarchical classification relationships. For example, a broad match corresponds to a hierarchical parent concept. SNOMED II consistently outperformed the other two classification systems due to the atomic nature of its terms, however, none of the three systems captured more than 60% of the clinical terms. Campbell et al. [3] evaluated the clinical utility of Meta 1.1, which included SNOMED II, to describe the process of ambulatory care related to management of hypertension based on 2,500 progress notes from the COSTAR ambulatory care system. The progress note terms were matched into UMLS semantic types based on machine-assisted, manual review of clinical concepts. Matches for clinical concepts were: subjective, 68%; objective, 20%; assessment, 75%, plan, 64%, and overall, 58%. Henry et al. [4] examined the feasibility of SNOMED III to represent nursing concepts. Forty-four percent of the terms recorded by the nurse were direct matches with one SNOMED III term. These were primarily NANDA diagnoses and single signs or symptoms. Two SNOMED III terms were required to represent 10% of the nursing terms charted. More than two SNOMED III terms were needed to match the terms used by nurses in 130 instances. Overall, 69% of the terms recorded by nurses were matched by using one or more SNOMED III terms. The addition of the NANDA Taxonomy I classification scheme to SNOMED III provided exact matches for the nursing diagnoses in the data set in these analyses. However, NANDA terms alone were not sufficient to represent the broad variety of terms recorded by nurses in the nursing care plan and in the nurses' progress notes/flowsheet. Other SNOMED III terms were direct matches for the signs and symptoms recorded by the nurses to describe patient problems. Using NANDA terms alone provided matches for 30% of the patient problems described. The inclusion of other SNOMED III terms and combinations of SNOMED III terms increased the percent of matches to 69%.

METHODS

Research Question

The question addressed in this descriptive study is: Can SNOMED International terms represent patients' perceptions of health-related problems?

Sample

The data source for the patients' descriptions of health-related problems was more than 600 patient interviews conducted as part of a larger study examining the quality of nursing care of persons living with AIDS (PLWAs) hospitalized for *Pneumocystis carinii* pneumonia. Each patient was asked to identify his three or four major problems in interviews that were conducted during hospitalization and at three and six months post-hospitalization. The total number of unique text strings used to describe problems was 1259.

Procedure

All patient problems were entered verbatim into a relational database. Each problem was placed into one of the following categories: medical diagnosis, nursing diagnosis, sign/symptom, patient goal, or other. Matches were manually identified by the investigators by locating the SNOMED International term that most closely matched the main concept in the patient's description of the health-related problem rather than the natural language terms. For instance, the patient statement "Fear about what is going on" was coded as fear, and the patient statement "throwing up alot" was coded as emesis/vomiting (F-52770).

RESULTS

As shown in Table 1, patients most frequently used sign/symptom terms (45%) to describe their problems with medical and NANDA diagnoses accounting for another 15% of the descriptions.

Table 1. Number of Problems by Category

Category	N	%
Medical Diagnosis	116	9
NANDA Diagnosis	77	6
Sign/Symptom	569	45
Patient Goal	89	7
Other	408	32

Problems described in sign/symptom, medical diagnosis, and NANDA terms can be represented by SNOMED International terms from a variety of modules including diagnoses, function, morphology, and living organisms (See Table 2). Descriptions of medical diagnoses such as CMV retinitis and *Pneumocystis carinii* pneumonia (PCP) require two terms joined by a relational modifier from the general module of SNOMED International. Some disease states are represented by terms from the morphology axis, ie. Kaposi's sarcoma (KS). Terms expressed as NANDA diagnoses and signs/symptoms primarily match with terms from the function module.

Table 2. Examples of Matching Terms

Concepts	SNOMED Terms
AIDS	DE-36310 - *AIDS, NOS*
CMV retinitis	DA-71020 - *Retinitis* G-C001 - *Due to* L-36500 - *Cytomegalovirus, NOS*
PCP	D2-50140 - *Pneumonia, NOS* G-C001 - *Due to* L-50F00 - *Pneumocystis carinii*
KS	M-91403 - *Kaposi's sarcoma*
SOB	F-20040 - *Dyspnea/shortness of breath*
Fever	F-03003 - *Increased body temperature/fever*
Boredom	F-92610 - *Boredom*
Memory deficit	F-0B180N - *Uncompensated short term memory deficit*
Anxiety	F-0B320N - *Anxiety*

Some of the problems classified as Other in the taxonomy coding scheme in the study can be represented by SNOMED terms from the social context. Examples of these terms are shown in Table 3.

Additional patient descriptions of problems classified as Other and not matched with SNOMED terms related to "dealing" with the system in areas such as disability and insurance forms or general complaints about the hospital such as noise level or food quality.

Problems described as patient goals were unable to be classified with SNOMED terms. Examples include "being more conscious of what my body's telling me", "building up strength so I can get back to work", and "eating without throwing up".

CONCLUSIONS

The majority of concepts used by patients to describe their health-related problems were

Table 3. Social Context Terms

S-11030	Celibacy, NOS
S-32030	Cigarette smoker, NOS
S-00040	Cultural deprivation
S-20500	Adjusting to work situation
S-30050	Disturbance in life pattern associated with community
S-30020	Disturbance in life pattern associated with family
S-30040	Disturbance in life pattern associated with recreation
S-30030	Disturbance in life pattern associated with work
S-30010	Disturbance in life pattern, NOS
S-20400	Economic problem
S-20480	Housing problem
S-50330	Poor
S-00070	Psychosocial deprivation
S-00030	Social isolation
S-00100	Unemployment

matched with existing SNOMED terms. The addition of the social context module as an adjunct to existing terminologies of medical diagnoses, NANDA diagnoses, and signs/symptoms provided additional matching terms. Patient goals did not match existing SNOMED terms.

The findings of this study suggest that SNOMED International has the potential to adequately represent patients' perceptions of health-related problems for the computer-based patient record. Additional studies are needed that will examine the extent to which patients' perceptions of health-related problems are already documented in the patient record by healthcare providers. The utility of patients' perceptions of health-related problems in the prediction of patient outcomes must also be analyzed.

REFERENCES

[1] Institute of Medicine. The computer-based patient record: An essential technology for health care. Washington, DC: National Academy Press, 1991.

[2] Chute CG, Atkin GE, Ihrke DM. An empirical evaluation of concept capture by clinical classifications. In: Lun KC, Degoulet P, Piemme TE, Riehoff O, eds. MedInfo92. Geneva, Switzerland: North-Holland, 1992:1469-1474.

[3] Campbell JR. The clinical utility of META: An analysis for hypertension. In: M Frisse ed. Proceedings of the Fifteenth Annual Symposium on Computer Applications in Medical Care. New York: McGraw-Hill, 1992:397-401.

[4] Henry SB, Holzemer WL, Reilly CA, Campbell KE. Terms used by nurses to describe patient problems: Can SNOMED III represent nursing concepts in the patient record? JAMIA 1994;1:61-74.

[5] Henry SB, Reilly CA, Miller TJ, Holzemer WL. Coding of nursing interventions using Iowa Nursing Intervention Classification and Current Procedural Terminology terms: A pilot study. 1994 Spring Congress of the American Medical Informatics Association, 89.

[6] Reiser SJ. The era of the patient: Using the experience of illness in shaping the missions of health care. JAMA 1993;269:1012-1017.

[7] Longo DR. Patient practice variation: A call for research. Med Care 1993;31:YS81-85.

[8] Cote' RA, Rothwell DJ, Palotay JL, Beckett RS. SNOMED International. Northfield, IL: College of American Pathologists, 1993.

[9] International classification of disease - clinical modification, 9th Revision. Salt Lake City, UT: Med-Index, 1992.

[10] American Psychological Association. Diagnostic and statistical manual of mental disorders. Washington, DC: 1992.

[11] American Medical Association. Physician's current procedural terminology. Chicago: American Medical Association, 1991.

[12] Kim MJ, McFarland G, McLane A. A pocket guide to nursing diagnosis (3rd ed). St. Louis: CV Mosby, 1989.

A SNOMED Analysis of Three Years' Accessioned Cases (40,124) of a Surgical Pathology Department: Implications for Pathology-Based Demographic Studies

Jules J. Berman, Ph.D., M.D., G. William Moore, M.D., Ph.D., William H. Donnelly, M.D., James K. Massey, M.S.E.E. and Brian Craig
Veterans Administration Medical Center, University of Maryland School of Medicine, The Johns Hopkins Medical Institutions, Baltimore, MD; Shands Hospital and University of Florida, Gainesville, FL

ABSTRACT

Pathology departments devote considerable energy toward indexing diagnoses. To date, there have been no detailed tabulations of the results of these efforts. We have thoroughly analyzed three years' surgical pathology reports (40,124) generated for 29,127 different patients from the University of Florida at Gainesville between Jan 1, 1990, and December 31, 1992. 64,921 SNOMED code entries (averaging 1.6 codes per specimen and 1.4 specimens per patient) were accounted for by 1,998 distinct SNOMED morphologies. A mere 21 entities accounted for 50% of the morphology code occurrences. 265 entities accounted for 90% of the morphology code occurrences, indicating that the diagnostic efforts of pathology departments are contained within a small fraction of the many thousands of morphologic entities available in the SNOMED nomenclature. One of the key problems in using SNOMED data collected from surgical pathology reports is the redundancy of lesions reported for single patients (i.e., a patient's disease may be coded on more than one specimen from the patient, leading to false conclusions regarding the incidence of disease in the population). In this study, redundant SNOMED data was removed by eliminating repeat morphology/topography pairs whenever they occur for a single patient. SNOMED data can be stratified on the basis of age and sex (data fields included on every surgical pathology report). This analysis represents the first published analysis of SNOMED data from a large pathology service, and demonstrates how SNOMED data can be compiled in a form that preserves patient privacy.

INTRODUCTION

Before the advent of computerized laboratory information systems, pathologists were severely limited in the way they could obtain information related to the scope of their activities. Paper filing systems permitted pathologists to review the reports issued for a specific patient, but there was no practical way of summarizing data collected from many different patients. In the past, when pathologists were asked to comment on the incidence or age distribution of a lesion, at best they might quote a published statistic (from a report reflecting the experience of another hospital in another geographic and social environment) or offer a vague recollection from their own experience, such as, "I've seen half a dozen of these things, and they seem to occur in older people".

Despite the fact that modern pathology information systems all index reports under retrievable and universally recognized diagnostic codes (e.g., the International Classification of Disease (ICD)[1], or the Systematized Nomenclature of Medicine (SNOMED))[2], few services take the step of analyzing their own surgical pathology data. The reason for this is simple. Just like paper filing systems, modern laboratory information systems are only designed to answer queries related to a particular patient or diagnostic category. No laboratory information system supports unrestrained queries relating all report data fields and all diagnostic categories for all patients. Such an undertaking would consume considerable computational resources of the institution, would require additional programming effort and would provide a service of no direct clinical necessity to any specific patient.

Perhaps the most telling indicator of the difficulties associated with analyzing surgical pathology databases resides in the absence of published reports of organized global data summaries encompassing all the diagnostic entities encountered in the catchment population. The lack of such studies underscores the failure of pathology departments to satisfy the intended goals of indexed coding. According to Cote and Robboy, current systems of disease nomenclature and classification are directly descended from earlier classifications (beginning with the London Bills of Mortality in the early 1700's) created to determine the prevalence of diseases in a population [3]. Cote and Robboy, both principals in the development of SNOMED, suggest that a coding system should serve the needs of the entire health care system and provide data for epidemiologic studies and medical audit [3].

We have analyzed three years' SNOMED coded data obtained from a general hospital in Florida, eliminating diagnostic redundancies in the database and stratifying data based on age. This study addresses several important issues: 1) it demonstrates that the obstacles that must be overcome when preparing a database summary from raw data retrieved from the electronic files of a laboratory information system; 2) it offers a sample database to illustrate the values and limitations of SNOMED data and serves as a baseline for comparison with databases from other pathology services; and 3) it provides a way of preparing a complete demographic profile of the pathology received in a large hospital.

0195–4210/94/$5.00

MATERIALS AND METHODS

We examined data from 40,124 cases accessioned at the Shands Hospital, Gainesville, FL, between January 1, 1990, and December 31, 1992, inclusive. From these, there were 29,127 patients with complete demographics and 304 patients with incompletely coded reports, for a total of 28,823 patients with complete reports. Shands Hospital is a general teaching hospital for the University of Florida College of Medicine in Gainesville, Florida, which covers all major areas of medicine and surgery. Consultation cases were primarily referrals for oncology patients.

Approximately 90% of cases were coded by pathology residents, the remainder by faculty members. All coders participated in a two-hour tutorial course on SNOMED coding, taught by one of us (WHD). All coding was performed by referring to publications of the College of American Pathologists (CAP) that list the SNOMED codes [2], sometimes referred to as SNOMED-II, currently the most widely used edition of SNOMED. As a rule, each accession received one topography code and one morphology code per specimen. Redundant coding (assigning more than one morphology code to a specimen) was performed only for special cases, such as unusual tumors. On a daily basis, the pathologist enters terms into the various SNOMED fields. Although six SNOMED axes are accessible to the pathologist, the axes used at Shands Hospital are topography, morphology and procedure. From our own collected experience and from discussions with other pathologists, we feel that this is a very typical way of preparing SNOMED data. About 30 minutes was devoted each day to coding reports.

The computer used for the present study was an IBM PC/AT-compatible computer programmed with American National Standard M (ISO 11456 previously MUMPS), and the public-domain File Manager (FileMan) database management system of the United States Department of Veterans Affairs, used routinely in 169 VA medical centers [4]. Reports were obtained as a raw ASCII file of the M global variable that contained all the textual material and data fields for every surgical pathology report downloaded from the mainframe computer at the Shands Hospital, and containing the complete text of surgical pathology reports obtained between January 1, 1990, and December 31, 1992. The entire contents of each report, including patient demographics, date and time of accessioning and signout, specimen source, gross description, final microscopic diagnosis, pathologist's identification, and manually-entered SNOMED codes, were passed into the ASCII file, a total of 24 Megabytes. All routines were written with MGlobal (Houston, TX) M.

RESULTS

The distribution frequency of patients by age is shown in Table 1. The average age of patients who contributed tissue to surgical pathology was 35.8 years. The ability to stratify the ages of the population is extremely important, as it permits comparison of the data to other data sets for which the age distributions of the individuals are known (i.e. age adjustment).

TABLE 1. AGE DISTRIBUTION OF PATIENTS CONTRIBUTING SURGICAL PATHOLOGY MATERIAL

0-10 years old	3,096
10-20 years old	2,596
20-30 years old	5,038
30-40 years old	4,578
40-50 years old	3,301
50-60 years old	2,881
60-70 years old	3,958
70-80 years old	2,971
80-90 years old	665
>90 years old	43

One of the most difficult problems in extracting epidemiologically useful data from a SNOMED database is data redundancy. For instance, a single patient may have many basal cell carcinomas of the skin removed from various skin sites. A simple count of coded specimens may provide a false impression of the prevalence of basal cell carcinoma in the population. For epidemiologic purposes, the total number of people with basal cell carcinoma would, in general, be more useful than the total number of basal cell carcinoma specimens. The frequency distributions of the number of specimens submitted per patient is shown in Table 2.

Among the patients who had tissue submitted to pathology, there were, on average, 1.37 specimens per patient. The greatest number of specimens submitted for any patient in the 3-year study period was 21.

The total number of morphology codes in the database is 64,921. Redundant codes for patients were eliminated by preparing a list of all of the topography and morphology codes for each patient and eliminating topography-morphology pairs that shared the same first two digits of their morphology codes. The reason for matching only the first two digit-pairs was to allow for differences among pathologists in their choice of a morphology code (i.e., idiosyncratic differences in the last three digits). Considering the example of basal cell carcinomas in the patient population, the tumors may all have different topography codes (skin of face T02120, skin of neck T02300, skin of forearm T02630, etc.) and they may have different morphology codes (basal cell carcinoma M80903, morphea type basal cell carcinoma M80923, basosquamous carcinoma M80943) But for this example, any of the topography/morphology code-pair permutations deriving from the different topography and morphology listings will have the same pair of 2-digit leading strings (in this case T02/M80). Using matches in the first 2 digits of topography/morphology code pairs effectively catches most redundancies due to coding idiosyncracy. Code idiosyncracy is a commonly occurring phenomenon [5]. It occurs when the same lesion is coded differently by different coders (e.g. one coder's basal cell carcinoma is another coder's basosquamous carcinoma). After elimination of redundancies (defined as two or more topography/morphology pairs identical to the first 2 digits of code) there were a total of 58,712 topography/morphology pairs. The ability to perform this elimination reliably is an essential step in SNOMED database interpretation.

TABLE 2. FREQUENCY DISTRIBUTION, NUMBER OF SPECIMENS SUBMITTED PER PATIENT

Specimens submitted	number of patients with the specified number of submitted specimens
1	22206
2	4378
3	1318
4	462
5	186
6	90
7	56
8	18
9	20
10	19
11	16
12	10
13	6
14	13
15	4
16	9
17	4
18	1
19	3
20	3
21	1
TOTAL	28,823

An interesting finding was that a very small number of morphologic entities account for the majority of morphology and topography codes. As shown in Tables 3 and 4, the 'median morphology code' (i.e. the 50-percentile morphology code representing the halfway point in the morphology code ranking) for manual coding occurs at rank 21. This means that at least 50% of all morphology codes are covered by the 21 most frequent (i.e., highest-ranking) diagnoses. 90% of all manual morphology codes are covered by the 265 most frequent diagnoses.

Table 4 shows a distribution of the 21 most common morphologies and their occurrences, ranked in descending frequency of occurrence, and accounting for 50% of all diagnoses made in the period of study. Non-diagnostic and non-specific morphologic codes account for the bulk of the high-frequency morphologies (e.g. normal tissue, no evidence of malignancy, inflammation).

TABLE 3. SUMMARY OF CODED MORPHOLOGIES FOR 40,124 SPECIMENS ACCESSIONED BETWEEN JAN 1, 1990 AND DEC 31, 1992

Total number of morphology codes	64,921
Number of disease entities accounting for 50% of the coded morphologies	21
Number of disease entities accounting for 90% of the coded morphologies	265
Number of disease entities accounting for 100% of the coded morphologies	1998
Average number of coded morphologies per accessioned specimen	1.6
Entities coded only once in the accession period	865

TABLE 4. LIST OF 21 ENTITIES ACCOUNTING FOR 50% OF ALL MORPHOLOGY CODES

	Number of cases
Normal tissue morphology	8712
Acute and chronic inflammation	2797
Chronic inflammation	2542
No evidence of malignancy	1774
Acute inflammation	1745
Adenocarcinoma	1441
Condyloma acuminatum	1315
Squamous cell carcinoma	1314
Protein Deposition	1193
Fibrosis	1063
Inflammation	968
Necrosis	882
Basal cell hyperplasia	871
Calcium deposition	864
Edema	716
Mild dysplasia	658
Products of conception	628
Proliferative Endometrium	588
Ulcer	587
Severe dysplasia	550

As shown in Table 5, the 'median topography code' (i.e. the 50-percentile morphology code representing the halfway point in the morphology code ranking) for manual coding occurs at rank 24. This means that at least 50% of all manual morphology codes are covered by the 24 most frequent (i.e., highest-ranking) topographic locations. 90% of all topography codes are covered by the 213 most frequent sites.

TABLE 5. SUMMARY OF CODED TOPOGRAPHIES FOR 40,124 SPECIMENS ACCESSIONED BETWEEN JAN 1, 1990 AND DEC 31, 1992

Total number of topography codes	64,921
Number of anatomic sites accounting for 50% of the coded topographies	24
Number of anatomic sites accounting for 90% of the coded topographies	213
Number of anatomic sites occurring once only	933
Number of anatomic sites accounting for 100% of the coded topographies	1554
Average number of coded topographies per accessioned specimen	1.6
Number of uniquely coded entities (entities coded only once in the accession period)	621

The distribution frequencies for any topographic code or for any leading string of topographic code could be assessed by age or by sex or both. Table 6 is an example of the age distribution of all pancreatic neoplastic lesions encountered in the 3 year period of study. A pancreas topography code was considered to be any topographic code that began with the two-digit numeric string 59... This would capture T59000, Pancreas N.O.S. (not otherwise specified), as well as head of pancreas (T59100), pancreatic duct (T59010), etc. Just as Table 6 demonstrates the age distribution for all pancreatic lesions, a similar distribution could be achieved for lesions of any specified morphology code or leading numeric string of morphologic codes. All pancreatic neoplastic morphology codes were accounted for by 8 sets of 2-digit leading strings (M80, M81, M82, M83, M84, M88, M89 and M93). A table could be compiled that lists the age/sex distribution for all lesions of all topographic sites, but a single topographic site was selected due to limitations of space.

TABLE 6. DISTRIBUTION FREQUENCY OF ALL PANCREATIC NEOPLASTIC LESIONS BY AGE

<10	0
10 - 19	1
20 - 29	3
30 - 39	4
40 - 49	8
50 - 59	4
60 - 69	16
70 - 79	11
80 - 89	1
> 90	0

DISCUSSION

A pathologist's understanding of the incidence of diseases is determined by how often a lesion is encountered. This frame of reference is inherently biased and can lead to misleading impressions. For instance, in the 3-year database of the Shands Hospital, there were 415 hernia sacs and 26 cases of hemorrhoids. Hemorrhoids occur much more frequently than inguinal hernias, but a pathologist's experience would indicate otherwise. Actually, surgery is almost always performed for inguinal hernias, whereas patients with hemorrhoids seldom seek surgical relief. Thus, we should not use a surgical pathology database to determine the relative incidences of diagnosis or treatment may not involve surgery. Surgical pathology databases are good sources of data pertaining to lesions that must have biopsy confirmation or surgical treatment. We can probably get a reasonably good idea of the incidence of clinically-detected hernias in the patient population, because 1) a hernia repair is a general surgical procedure performed at virtually every medical center (i.e., patients do not cluster toward a few facilities that specialize in hernia repair); 2) a procedure is performed on the majority of patients with an inguinal hernia; and 3) tissue is received on almost every hernia repair.

Another error that results from estimating disease incidence by frequency of encounter relates to the multiplicity of biopsies associated with a disease process in a single patient. For instance, a single patient with chronic lymphocytic leukemia (CLL) may, over a period of several years, have the SNOMED morphology for CLL entered when a blood smear is assessed, when a lymph node is biopsied, when a skin infiltrate is sampled, when a spleen is removed, etc. For this reason, any analysis of disease frequencies must be able to represent data in a form where repeat morphologies for a patient are eliminated. In this study, redundant specimens for a patient were eliminated by searching for repeated topography/morphology code-pairs listed for a patient. However, this solution to the problem of specimen redundancy has its own drawbacks and may not be appropriate for all types of studies. For instance, patients may develop separate lesions of the same morphologic type over a period of time (e.g., bilateral breast cancer), and an epidemiologist interested in this phenomenon may need to account for both tumors in a valid analysis of the incidence of cancers occurring in a population. Partly as a result of these difficulties, commercial laboratory information systems do not lend themselves to direct epidemiologic analysis, and database queries must be carefully designed to produce useful results.

In an effort to insure that diagnoses can be retrieved from databases, a variety of coding systems have been developed, all with the intention of categorizing disease entities as a unique number. Thus, a renal cell carcinoma, which may appear on a report as renal cell adenocarcinoma, hypernephroma, clear cell carcinoma, kidney carcinoma, kidney adenocarcinoma, adenocarcinoma of kidney or even as Grawitz tumor, can all be coded under the same, unique morphology and topography codes. Reports written in English, French, German, or any language, may all use the same code numbers to index their reports. Unfortunately, coding efforts may vary greatly in their accuracy. The reliability of indexed data related to diagnosis has received very little discussion in the medical literature. Hall and Lemoine, in one of the few available studies, found errors in more than 10% of indexed codes [5]. Currently, many pathology departments have employed automatic coding software and thus relieved themselves from the time-consuming burden of manual coding. In a recent study, we have shown that accurate automatic coding can only be achieved by monitoring the quality of the coded output and adding appropriate changes in the code look-up dictionary and in the manner that reports are written [6]. Furthermore, automatic coding can potentially produce databases with codes chosen in a uniform and predictable way optimized to support epidemiologic studies [6].

In the current study, the Shands Hospital laboratory information system was used only as the source of raw data files, not as a database engine supporting queries. Commercial laboratory information systems cannot budget their computational resources (the amount of computer time required to respond to a query) to perform in-depth database analyses. It is our observation that departments desiring full query access to their databases must acquire a devoted database application and then query their raw database file with their own programs written in a database specific language or a generalized database language (e.g., SQL, System Query Language).

Using routines written in the M programming environment, we have shown that it SNOMED databases can be fully analyzed, that the problem of code redundancy can be overcome, and that data relating the frequency of SNOMED morphology and topography entries according to patient demographics (age and sex) can be performed. SNOMED databases are one of the fastest growing and comprehensive medical databases, in that all U.S. hosptitals seeking accreditation by the College of American Pathologists or the Joint Commission for Accreditation of Healthcare Organizations must index all surgical pathology cases. In the last decade, most of the medical centers that had previously indexed their cases using card filing systems, have switched to electronic coding. SNOMED (specifically SNOMED version II) is, in our estimation, the most commonly used surgical pathology indexing system. A formidable amount of SNOMED data is accruing daily, and it would be a terrible waste if these data were not shared and analyzed. Unlike tumor registry data, which only provide cancer statistics, the SNOMED databases produced by surgical pathology departments cover every aspect of medicine. Prepared in the manner described in this study, SNOMED data can be tabulated as listings of topography and morphology codes, devoid of patient identifiers. Each record in a distributable database might consist of: 1) a unique patient identifier number that can be linked to a specific patient name by the contributing medical center only; 2) a list of topography and morphology code-pairs that describe all the different lesions biopsied for the patient exclusive of lesion redundancies; 3) the date of birth of the patient and 4) the sex of the patient.

REFERENCES

[1]. The International Classification of Diseases, 9th Revision: ICD-9CM, Second Edition, U.S. Department of Health and Human Services, Public Health Service, Health Care Financing Administration, U.S. Government Printing Office, 1980.

[2]. College of American Pathologists. Systematized nomenclature of medicine (SNOMED). College of American Pathologists, Skokie, 1976.

[3]. Cote RA, Robboy S: Progress in Medical Information Management: systematized nomenclature of medicine (SNOMED). JAMA 243:756, 1980

[4]. Davis R.G. FileMan: A User Manual. National Association of VA Physicians, Bethesda, 1987

[5]. Hall P.A., Lemoine N.R. Comparison of manual data coding errors in two hospitals. J Clin Pathol 39:622, 1986

[6]. Moore GW, Berman JJ: Performance analysis of manual and automated Systematized Nomenclature of Medicine (SNOMED) coding. Am J Clin Pathol 101:253, 1994

Acceptability of Unified Medical Language System Terms as Substitute for Natural Language General Medicine Clinic Diagnoses

Kevin M. Rosenberg, MD
David B. Coultas, MD
Department of Internal Medicine
University of New Mexico

ABSTRACT

The acceptability of using the Unified Medical Language System (UMLS) concept phrases to substitute for physicians' diagnosis statements was investigated. Physician diagnosis statements recorded in the University of New Mexico's General Medicine Clinic were input into a computer program that automatically finds the best matching UMLS concept phrases. The computer program written in C++ integrates UMLS searching and browsing with a graphical user interface. Five attending physicians in the Department of Internal Medicine rated the acceptability of the UMLS concept phrase as a substitute for the original physician statement. One hundred and ninety-five patients' notes were examined with 447 diagnosis statements recorded of which 271 statements were unique. Attending physicians rated their satisfaction with the automated UMLS substitutes on a scale of 1 (extremely dissatisfied) to 5 (extremely satisfied). Intrarater (mean 0.94) and interrater correlations (mean 0.75) were high. The mean rating was 4.0 (quite satisfied). Most (73%) of the substitution were satisfactory (rating of 4 or 5), 16% were neutral (rating of 3), and 21% were unsatisfactory (rating of 1 or 2). A review of the substitutions showed a frequent lack of clinical modifier terms in UMLS as has been previously described. Comparison to a previous study shows the broader term coverage of UMLS to be a more acceptable source of diagnosis codes than using International Classification of Diseases revision 9 alone. These results suggest that UMLS can be an effective tool for coding unconstrained physician diagnoses.

INTRODUCTION

The use of an computerized patient record (CPR) has many theoretical advantages over the customary paper record [1]. These include improvement in medical record availability and retrieval, legibility, organization, and linkage and integration with other users and institutions [2]. Currently, there are technical and standardization limitations to implementing a CPR system. One of the more difficult issues is balancing the expressive power of natural language and the computing efficiency of encoded concept phrases [3]. A robust CPR will need to implement both natural language and encoded concept phrases [4,5] and be able to convert one to the other.

Development of a database of the contents of all medical nomenclatures is a long-term project of the National Library of Medicine. This database, the Unified Medical Language System (UMLS), though still not comprehensive, is in its fourth experimental version. This version of the UMLS contains over 279,000 concept phrases from twenty-one sources, including all of the International Classification of Disease Revision 9 with Clinical Modifiers (ICD9-CM). The purpose of this study was to examine the feasibility and acceptability of using UMLS for automated coding of natural language physician diagnosis statements written in general medicine clinic records.

METHODS

Medical records of 195 patients whose last names began with A through M seen in the University of New Mexico Hospital's General Medicine Clinic during May 1993 were reviewed by KR. All diagnosis statements recorded in the general medicine clinic notes were directly entered into a master file -- the diagnosis statements file. These diagnoses were recorded by medical students, residents, physician assistants, and attendings. Records with illegible or no diagnoses were counted, but not used in further analyses. Words and phrases that modified a diagnosis were included in the statement, but phrases relating to diagnostic and therapeutic plans were not included. Spelling errors found in the diagnosis statement file were corrected.

A computer program, the UMLS Search Engine (USE), was written by KR to find, score, and display the best-matching concepts in UMLS for a

0195-4210/94/$5.00

physician's diagnosis written in a medical record. In addition to finding the best matching concept phrases in UMLS, the USE program integrates browsing of UMLS. This includes viewing UMLS concept phrases; sorting the concepts by concept name, concept identifier, semantic type, and source; displaying and selecting relatives of a concept; displaying concept definitions; and calculating statistics on UMLS as a whole and on selected records. The program was written for the Microsoft Windows and Windows NT operating system using Microsoft's 32-bit C++ compiler. The program implements a windowed graphical user interface and uses multiple colors and fonts are used to organize information. The program was developed and executed on an Intel 80486 CPU running at 66MHz with 16MB of RAM and 800MB of disk space.

The UMLS files were compiled from ASCII text into a binary format suitable for the computing needs of this project. Non-English terms were discarded during the compilation. Raima's Object Manager Library was used to provide object-oriented access to the UMLS data. Both relational (keyed) and network (hierarchical) indices were used. Raima's Object Manager managed all indices except for the UMLS word index (MRWD). Moderate tolerance to spelling errors in the terminus of a word was achieved by writing a customized binary tree algorithm to search this file.

The module of the USE program that finds and scores the best-matching concept phrases in UMLS was termed the *autocoder*. The autocoder developed for this project uses a combination of phrase stemming and word matching. The autocoder:

1. Recursively stems a list of search phrases using multi-word morphologic and semantic substitution from the diagnosis statement.

For example, the input phrase "*decr. k*" generates 5 search phrases: *"decr. k", "decr. potassium", "decreased k", "decreased potassium", and "hypokalemia"*

2. Selects all concept phrases in UMLS that have words contained in the list of search phrases

For each word in the search phrases, the word index is search via the spelling-error tolerant binary tree. This lookup method is tolerant of substitution and transposition errors in the terminus of a word but is not tolerant of errors in the beginning of a word or of insertion and deletion errors.

3. Scores each search phrase against the diagnosis statement.

Each word in a search phrase is compared to each word in the UMLS phrase. The highest scoring word match is identified and its score is added to the phrase-match score, and the matched words are marked as used. After all possible words have been matched, a penalty is assigned for unmatchable words. The score is adjusted based on the closeness of word order in the two phrases. In all operations, a semantic weight is used, giving linking words (e.g., *the, with, for*) less weight than clinical modifiers (e.g., *mild, increased, possible*) which in turn are given less weight than all other words.

4. Outputs the search phrases in descending score order.

To create the ratings file used in this study, the number of initial letters in a diagnosis word that had to exactly match a word in the word index was set to three. Two letter substitution errors were tolerated per word. Two dictionaries were created to support the autocoder's functions. These are the semantic dictionary that provides the semantic weighting used in phrase scoring and the substitution dictionary used to stem search phrases.

The qualitative effectiveness of the autocoder was assessed by a semi-automated review of the autocoder's final output. A match was rated as sub-optimal when the autocoder did not select, in KR's judgment, the best match from UMLS.

The diagnosis statements recorded from the notes were input into the USE program. The USE program outputs a ratings file containing the original diagnosis statements and the best match from UMLS. Five attending physicians in the Department of Medicine rated the acceptability of each match on a scale of zero to five. The instructions and scoring system were replicated from the methodology of a similar study by Payne [6] with one modification: A rating of zero was added to indicate that the rater had *"no guess"* about the meaning of the diagnosis statement. Intrarater reliability was assessed using ten random diagnosis statements that were presented twice within the ratings file.

Statistics on the raters' scores were calculated with StatView version 4.0 on an Apple Macintosh IIci. Intrarater reliability was assessed using Pearson's product-moment correlation of the ratings given to the duplicated diagnosis statements. Preliminary review of the ratings data showed the distribution of ratings to be non-normal, necessitating the use of non-parametric tests. The linearity of interrater correlations was estimated using Pearson's product-moment correlations. Inferences regarding the differences in mean ratings between reviewers were performed using the Wilcoxon rank-order statistic, a non-parametric statistic for comparing two groups of paired measurements [7]. The 10 most frequent diagnoses documented were collated manually by KR.

RESULTS

Of 195 patients identified, there were an average of 2.3 diagnosis per patient corresponding to 447 valid diagnosis statements. Five (0.9%) diagnosis statements were illegible and two (0.4%) of the clinic notes lacked an diagnosis. Of the 447 available diagnosis, 271 (60%) were unique. The 10 most frequent diagnoses recorded in clinic notes were comprised entirely of chronic diseases (table 1).

Table 1: Most common diagnoses

Diagnosis Group	Count	% of Total
Hypertension	56	20.7%
Diabetes Mellitus	47	17.3%
Asthma/COPD	18	6.6%
Arthritis	15	5.5%
Hypothyroidism	12	4.4%
Hyperlipidemia	11	4.1%
Coronary Artery Disease	10	3.7%
Depression	10	3.7%
Obesity	8	3.0%
Gastroesophageal Reflux	7	2.6%

The ratings file contained 271 unique diagnosis statements and required 153 minutes to create or an average of 21 seconds per statement. Of the 271 unique statements, 123 (45%) matched phrases from ICD9-CM. Of the 148 (55%) non-ICD9-CM phrases matched, 74 (50%) could be automatically mapped to ICD9-CM codes using the concept equivalence information contained within UMLS. Thus, 222 (82%) of the UMLS matches have ICD9-CM codes. The majority, 174 (64%), of the matches had a UMLS semantic type of *"Disease or Syndrome"*. UMLS preferred terms were matched for 221 (82%) statements. The morphologic substitution dictionary generated phrases that accounted for 123 (45%) of the matches, and the original diagnosis statement matched 148 (55%). For the 271 unique diagnosis statements, 210 (77%) unique UMLS concepts were identified.

All raters used a score of zero for some matches with a mean of 8.4 zero's assigned per rater (range 2 to 17). Overall, 27 (10%) of the diagnosis statements received a score of zero from at least one rater. For these 27 diagnosis statements, an average of 1.6 raters (31%) rated them a zero. The mean rating for these 27 statements was 2.1. Two (0.7%) diagnosis statements (each was only a three letter abbreviation) were rated as zero by all five attendings. Items rated as a zero by any rater were excluded from further analyses.

Overall, ratings were high (table 2) with a mean of 4.0 (SD = 1.4) and a median of 5 and the individual average ratings ranging from 3.9 to 4.3. In general, intrarater agreement was higher than interrater agreement. Intrarater correlations ranged from 0.86 to 0.98, with a mean of 0.94. Interrater correlations ranged from 0.67 to 0.81, with a mean of 0.75. Wilcoxon signed-rank tests showed one rater who rated significantly more highly than any of the other four raters; otherwise, the raters show similar ratings. Examples of ratings are seen in table 3.

Table 2: Rating Frequency

Rating	Count	Percent of non-zero ratings
5	771	58.5%
4	191	14.5%
3	75	5.7%
2	166	12.6%
1	115	3.0%
0	42	N/A

Table 3: Sample substitutions for given ratings

	Physician Diagnosis	UMLS Substitute
5	myofascial pain	myofascial pain syndrome
5	sz's	seizures
4	passed kidney stone	Kidney stone
3	decr hct probably beta thalassemia	beta-Thalassemia
3	r/o cad	Coronary Artery Disease
2	sinus drainage	drainage
1	feet with prominent MTP	Metatarsal
1	incr fecal number, ? etiology	fecal impaction
0	had	HAD-glucuronide

Based on a semi-automated review of matches by KR, 19 (7%) diagnoses statements were sub-optimally matched to UMLS phrases. The mean and median ratings by the five raters for these matches judged sub-optimal by KR were 2.0. When these sub-optimal matches were removed from the analysis, the overall mean rating increased from 4.0 to 4.2. The majority (58%) of these diagnosis statements contained five or more words and had a modifying phrase. To correct these sub-optimal matches, four types of modifications needed to improve a future autocoder were identified and tallied: 1) adjusting word weighting based on word size; 2) additions to the morphologic substitution dictionary; 3) multi-word (phrase) semantic weighting as opposed the current implementation single word semantic weighting, e.g., the phrase *steroid dependent* would be weighted as a clinical modifier; and, 4) natural language parsing (interpretation) and semantic matching. This would add tolerance of multiclause diagnosis. Table 4 summarizes the modifications needed to correct these sub-optimal matches and the frequency with which these were encountered.

Table 4: Possible Modifications to Autocoder

Modification	Count
Adjust single-word semantic weight	1
Adjust multi-word semantic weight	1
Morphologic substitution additions	5
Natural language parsing	12

DISCUSSION

Attending physicians in internal medicine rated 73% of the matches from UMLS as satisfactory (ratings of 4 or 5), with a mean rating of 4.0 (quite satisfied) and a median rating of 5 (extremely satisfied). Of all the matches, 21% were considered unsatisfactory (ratings of 2 or 1). A neutral rating (3) was used the least (16%) indicating little ambivalence toward the rating method.

Several potential limitations must be considered in the interpretation of these results. The major limitations include the heterogeneous sources and quality of diagnosis statements, failure to assess the USE program tolerance for spelling errors, and imperfections of autocoder matching. The clinic diagnosis were obtained from persons with a wide range of experience, ranging from medical students to attending physicians. However, this diverse group may best represent the challenges that a "real-word" system would encounter. Another challenge for a practical system is spelling errors. Though the USE program is designed to be moderately tolerant of spelling errors, this tolerance was not assessed since all spelling errors were corrected by KR. A limitation which may impact the results of this study is the autocoder's failure to chose the best UMLS concept phrase for 7% of the diagnosis statements. Eliminating the sub-optimal matches boosted the mean rating by 0.2 points to a rating of 4.2.

To reduce these sub-optimal matches, four modifications in the autocoder were identified. Two of these modifications (adjusting word weights and additions to the morphologic substitution dictionary) are simple and would assist the autocoder in 6 (31%) of the sub-optimal matches. Twelve (63%) of the sub-optimal matches would require the addition of full natural language parsing (NLP) and matching of semantics. Implementation of NLP and semantic matching requires the autocoder to be knowledgeable in English syntax, semantics, and idioms [8]. NLP involves interpretation of the grammatical structure of the sentence and is analogous to "diagramming of sentences". Semantic matching involves scoring the concordance of meaning for two "diagrammed sentences". Two methods described that are suitable for this task are conceptual graphing and sub-language analysis [9,10.11]. In either case, natural language is often vague even for human interpreters. This is clearly illustrated by 27 (10%) of the diagnosis statements where at least one rater stated that they had no guess at all about the meaning of the diagnosis statement.

A systematic analysis of low rating scores was not performed. However, an informal review suggested that a UMLS frequently lacked clinical modifier terms, which has been described by others [12]. Clinical modifier terms have been added to the next version of UMLS (release 5). To utilize these modifier terms will require a fundementally different approach where the coding of a diagnoses is created from a semantic graph of component concepts. This approach would work best using a single, consistant nomenclature like SNOMED rather than UMLS's collection of nomenclatures.

To improve searching speed, a hashing method like the Soundex [13] algorithm could be used instead of the binary tree to search the word index. The Soundex algorithm was devised to correct for typical errors when an English name is given verbally. In this application, though, errors are written and most medical words are Latin or Greek. The effectiveness of Soundex in tolerating spelling errors in medical documents was analyzed and reported to be low, ranging from 52% to 63% specificity [14,15,16].

The findings of this study, compared with a similar study by Payne and coworkers[6], showed a higher satisfaction with UMLS phrases as opposed to using only ICD9 phrases. Payne and coworkers reported a mean satisfaction rating of 3.0 (neutral) when using ICD9 to substitute for ambulatory care problem list phrases. An important feature of Payne's results is that large proportion of problem list phrases (41%) could not be converted to ICD9 concepts and weren't rated. Of course, there are many uncontrolled biases comparing these studies. However, given the much larger term coverage, UMLS would be expected to give more acceptable substitutes.

CONCLUSIONS

UMLS most often has extremely satisfactory substitutes for general medicine clinic diagnosis. This suggests that UMLS can be an effective tool for encoding uncontrolled physician diagnosis.. These results and comparison with the findings of Payne and coworkers suggests that UMLS is a superior method for encoding ambulatory care diagnoses than ICD9 alone. Further improvements in UMLS encodings may be accomplished by adding natural language understanding to the autocoder.

Reference

[1]. Dick RS, Steen EB. The Computer-Based Patient Record: An Essential Technology for Health Care. National Academy Press, Washington, DC, 1991.

[2]. Hall H, Rosenberg KM. The Institute of Medicine Abstract on Computer-Based Patient Record Development. Presentation to the UNM Dept. of Medicine Research Seminar. May 1992.

[3]. Hersh WR, Hickam DH, Leone TJ. Words, Concepts, or Both: Optimal Indexing Units for Automated Information Retrieval. *Proceedings of the Annual Symposium on Computer Applications in Medical Care.* 644-648(1992).

[4]. Clark AS, Shea S. Developing a controlled vocabulary for the Columbia-Presbyterian Medical Center outpatient clinical information system. *Proceedings of the Annual Symposium of Applications in Medical Care*, 654-7 (1992).

[5]. Stead WH, Wiederhold G, Gardner R, et al. Database systems for computer-based patient records. Aspects of the Computer-based Patient Record. Springer-Verlag, New York, NY (1992), pp 83-98.

[6]. Payne TH, Murphy GR, Salazar AA. How well does ICD9 represent phrases used in the medical record problem list? *Proceedings of the Annual Symposium on Computer Applications in Medical Care*, 205-209 (1992).

[7]. Hirsh RP, Riegelman RK. Statistical First Aid: Interpretation of Health Research Data. Blackwell Scientific Publications, Cambridge, MA.

[8]. Sowa R. Conceptual Structures. IBM Press, 1986.

[9]. Campbell KE, Musen MA. Representation of clinical data using SNOMED III and conceptual graphs. *Proceedings of the Annual Symposium of Applications in Medical Care,* 354-58 (1991).

[10]. Bernauer J. Conceptual graphs as an operational model for descriptive findings. *Proceedings of the Annual Symposium on Computer Applications in Medical Care*, 214-223 (1991).

[11]. Johnson SB, Gottfried M. Sublanguage analysis as a basic for controlled medical vocabulary. *Proceedings of the Annual Symposium on Computer Applications in Medicare Care*, 519-523 (1989).

[12]. Friedman C. The UMLS Coverage of Clinical Radiology. *Proceedings of the Annual Symposium on Computer Applications in Medical Care*, 309-313 (1992).

[13]. Knuth DE. The Art of Computer Programming. Vol 3, Addison-Wesley, Reading, MA, 1973.

[14]. Joseph DM, Wong RL. Correct of misspellings and typographical errors in a free-text medical English information storage and retrieval system. *Method. Inform. Med.* **18**(4), 228-234 (1978).

[15]. Greenfield RH. An experiment to measure the performances of phonetic key compression techniques. *Method. Inform. Med.* **16**, 230-233, (1977).

[16]. Goehring R. Identification of patients in medical databases – Soundex codes verses match code. *Method. Med. Inform.* **10**(1), 27-34, (1985).

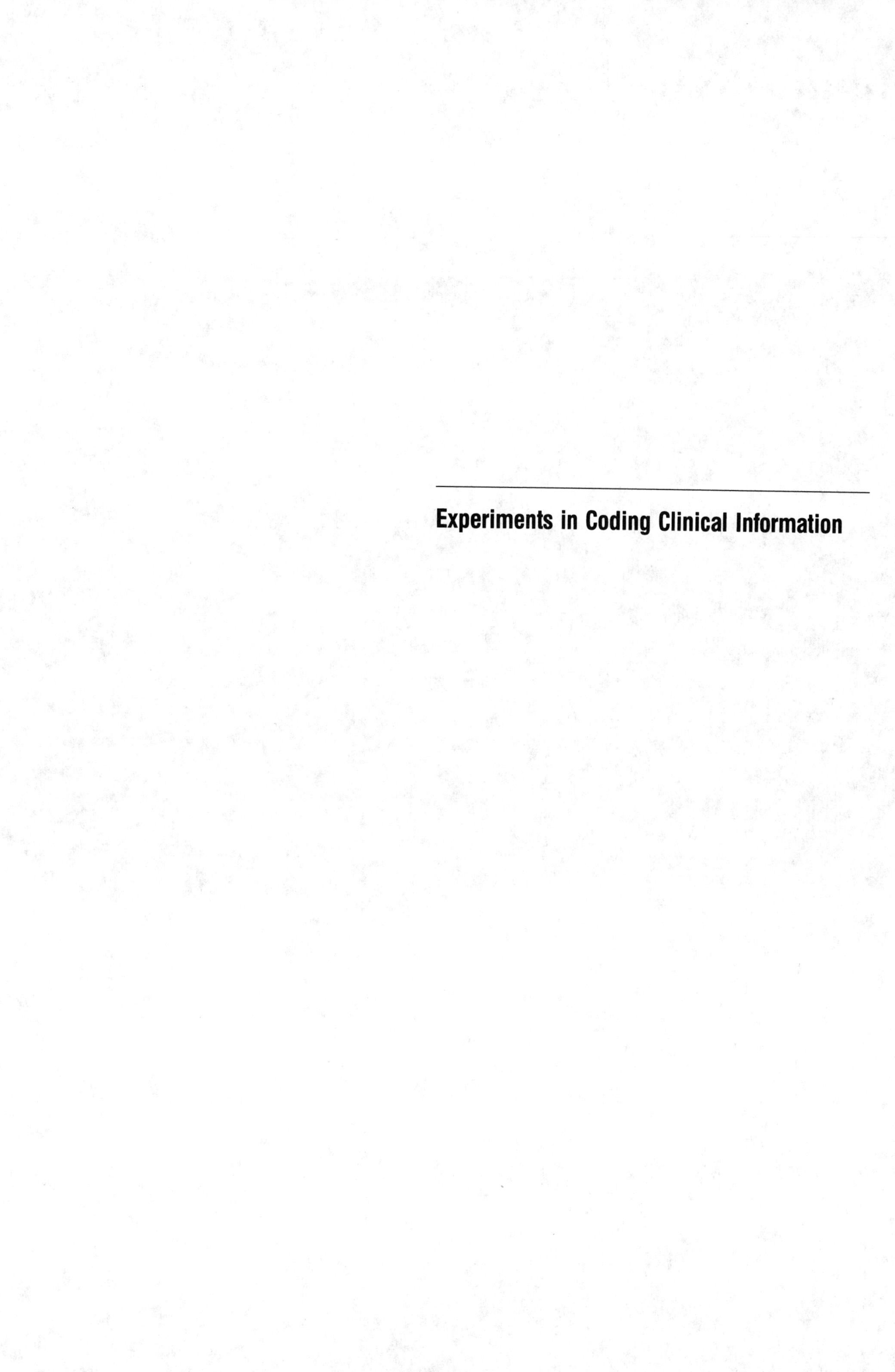

Experiments in Coding Clinical Information

A Comparison of Four Schemes for Codification of Problem Lists

James R. Campbell M.D., University of Nebraska Medical Center, Omaha NE
Thomas H. Payne M.D., Group Health Cooperative of Puget Sound, Seattle, WA

ABSTRACT

We set out to evaluate the completeness of four major coding schemes in representation of the patient problem list: the Unified Medical Language System (UMLS, 4th edition), the Systematized Nomenclature of Medicine (SNOMED International), the Read coding system (version 2), and the International Classification of Diseases (9th Clinical Modification)(ICD-9-CM). We gathered 400 problems from patient records at primary care sites in Omaha and Seattle. Matching these against the best description found in each of the coding schemes, we asked five medical faculty reviewers to rate the matches on a five-point Likert scale assessing their satisfaction with the results. For the four schemes, we computed the following rates of dissatisfaction, satisfaction, and average scores:

	Unsatisfactory	*Satisfactory*	*Average*
UMLS	*.22*	*.65*	*3.92*
SNOMED	*.24*	*.60*	*3.57*
READ	*.38*	*.38*	*2.99*
ICD-9-CM	*.42*	*.37*	*2.85*

From this analysis, we conclude that UMLS and SNOMED performed substantially better in capturing the clinical content of the problem lists than READ or ICD-9-CM. No scheme could be considered comprehensive. Depending on the goal of systems developers, UMLS and SNOMED may offer different, and complementary, advantages.

INTRODUCTION

The 1991 publication by the Institute of Medicine (IOM)[1] has set the goals and defined the agenda for this decade of computerized patient record (CPR) development. Critical issues for research into CPR design include data standards for content and clinical vocabulary. Criteria for selection of the best schemes or strategies are not a matter of general agreement nor have comprehensive studies been done to define those attributes which best guarantee utility of a proposed data standard.

A definition of the CPR content and vocabulary must begin, practically speaking, with studies of the data recorded in current paper record systems. Virtually all published studies[2-5] have focused on limited clinical realms, and on one or two coding schemes. Recent work accomplished by the Codes and Structures work group of the Computerized Patient Record Institute (CPRI)[6] has added meaningful information to the discussion of a core data scheme. This study evaluated eight major coding systems, comparing them against the content of clinical documents garnered from four medical centers. The best schemes emerging from this evaluation were the Systematized Nomenclature of Medicine (SNOMED International)[7,8] and the Unified Medical Language System (UMLS, 4th edition)[9,10] of the National Library of Medicine. One limitation of this study was the exclusion of tabular or flow-charted source material, much of which is critical to the content of the patient record.

Probably the best studied and most useful feature of medical records is the problem list [11,12]. Established as a required feature of hospital records by the Joint Committee for the Accreditation of Hospitals (JCAHO), it has been shown to improve coordination of care, assure follow-up of patient concerns, and better organize record keeping. Nonetheless, problem lists were excluded from the CPRI study which only evaluated textual data.

We were concerned that such a short-coming should be corrected, and decided to evaluate the problem coding capability of the best of the coding schemes studied by the CPRI. We limited our project to those schemes that were best oriented toward diagnostic findings. These included SNOMED, UMLS, the READ coding scheme (version 2)[13] employed by the National Health Service of the United Kingdom, and the International Classification of Diseases (9th Clinical Modification)(ICD-9-CM). As a part of planning projects in our respective institutions, this served the further purpose of refining our plans for local CPR implementation.

METHODS

In order to prepare a study that would be geographically representative, we obtained medical records material from the University of Nebraska Medical Center (UNMC) Internal Medicine clinics, and from the Primary Care clinics of the Group Health Cooperative of Puget Sound (GHC). A list of candidate problems taken from medical records at each institution was assembled. The 200 most frequent problems found in COSTAR®[14] records at UNMC were identified by record query. Charts were pulled by convenience sample from pediatric records at GHC clinics. The first 200 problems found in these records were added to the list. From the total of 400 candidates, duplicate items were eliminated and ambiguous terms were clarified by chart review. This yielded a study sample of 359 problems taken from adult and pediatric medicine at the two institutions.

We matched the study sample against the four major coding schemes using textual references and coding browsers. In some cases, no reasonable match for the concept could be found in the coding scheme using the most liberal clinical judgement. These items were scored zero. In some cases exact lexical matches were found. These were scored as five points. All items for each coding scheme with "near matches" were assembled on a study sheet, comparing the source problem and the nearest coding match. The sheets were prepared using the published terminology of the coding scheme, with no attempt at ordering or clarification of terminology. For example, the problem "back pain" was displayed opposite the four coding schemes as in figure 1.

Five university faculty from the two institutions, all users of the problem oriented record, were asked to rate each match using the five point Likert scale listed in figure 1. This was based upon previous work at GHC and was designed to reflect their satisfaction with the coded representation of the original problem.

The results of the five evaluations were collated and frequency statistics were computed for match scores. Average acceptability scores were computed for each coding scheme. A review of this summary made it clear that modifying words used in the publication of each scheme had an impact on the faculty evaluation. For example, phrases including words such as "unspecified" and "NOS" were scored lower by faculty physicians, even when the conceptual content was otherwise exact. We did a second lexical analysis by stripping these words from the codes. For example, we converted "BACK, NOS; PAIN, NOS" to "BACK PAIN." We then recomputed the frequency of exact matches for each scheme using this revised code list.

```
BACK PAIN   1 2 3 4 5     BACK, NOS; PAIN, NOS         (SNOMED)
                          BACKACHE                     (READ)
                          BACK PAIN                    (UMLS)
                          BACK ACHE UNSPECIFIED        (ICD-9-CM)

1=EXTREMELY DISSATISFIED
2=QUITE DISSATISFIED
3=NEUTRAL, NOT SATISFIED BUT NO OBJECTION
4=QUITE SATISFIED
5=EXTREMELY SATISFIED
```

Figure 1

RESULTS

From the original list of 400 problems, 359 remained after duplications and ambiguous terms were discarded. Misprints on coding sheets caused one or two terms to be ignored in the final analysis of each scheme. Table 1 summarizes the frequency of scores assigned to each scheme by the five faculty evaluators. The column at far right is the average acceptability score for all problems and all evaluators.

A review of the scores assigned to each concept made it clear that our presentation biased the faculty against schemes which used coding parlance such as "NOS." On the other hand, a programmer might choose to implement those schemes having stripped such repetitive terms from the vocabulary presented to users of the computerized record. Table 2 summarizes the exact matches for each scheme as they were taken from their published source (baseline). The far right column of table 2 summarizes the exact match score after stripping terms such as "NOS" and "unspecified" and reanalyzing for exact matches ignoring punctuation and lexical order.

DISCUSSION

For a coding scheme to be useful in development of a CPR, it must be comprehensive, multi-disciplinary, concise, provide meaningful taxonomic relationships, be linguistically representative, and should support useful links to administrative and knowledge schemes. The purpose of this project was to evaluate the completeness of four candidate coding schemes relative to the conceptual content of the problem list at our institutions. We chose schemes that performed well in other evaluations (SNOMED, UMLS, READ), or are in common use in the United States (ICD-9-CM).

The accuracy of a coded representation of a clinical concept may be judged in a variety of ways, but we chose to echo the coded output to senior clinicians and asked them to compare the results to those originally recorded. The lexical method we used to prepare the evaluation may have created a bias against schemes which are conceptually and taxonomically oriented. This same method may have favored those that are linguistically based. The frequency of exact

Table 1
Scoring Frequency and Average Scores by Scheme

	0	1	2	3	4	5	Average
UMLS	.00	.08	.14	.14	.07	.58	3.92
SNOMED	.02	.15	.07	.16	.20	.40	3.57
READ	.03	.14	.21	.23	.24	.15	2.99
ICD-9-CM	.01	.21	.20	.22	.11	.26	2.85

Table 2 Matches at Baseline and After Stripping of Modifiers

	Baseline	Modifiers stripped
	Exact match	Exact match
UMLS	.52	.52
SNOMED	.10	.38
READ	.13	.21
ICD-9-CM	.09	.10

matching with UMLS relative to all other schemes may be an example of this bias. This should be kept in mind when evaluating the results.

Reviewing the summary statistics makes it clear that UMLS is a well developed and reasonably complete scheme with some obvious advantages for problem list encoding. If a system developer is interested in populating a data dictionary, and establishing links to systems such as ICD-9-CM, MESH and SNOMED, then UMLS will provide many benefits by virtue of its cross-references. If the developer is further interested in a gateway from the problem list to the medical literature, then UMLS is the only choice. That is the purpose for which it was designed.

On the other hand, the internal structuring of UMLS is primarily semantic, which may support natural language processing but is not helpful for deducing relationships between concepts that may be important for decision support. SNOMED is designed to support such a taxonomy, and is also cross referenced into ICD-9-CM, International Classification of Diseases for Oncology (ICD-O), and American Hospital Formulary (AHFS) coding schemes. The multi-axial features of the scheme are especially helpful to avoid an explosion of the number of coding elements when faced with adding new terms with common features. Based upon work done by the Major Codes group of the CPRI, SNOMED is also much more complete outside of the domain of diagnoses, making it a more suitable candidate if the system developer is interested in a coded problem list with meaningful relationships to other coded portions of the CPR. Nonetheless, a systems developer who chooses SNOMED must be prepared to build a clinician term vocabulary, an effort in itself that requires substantial work.

Comparing the cumulative frequencies of unsatisfactory matches by coding scheme (scores 0-2), it is clear that the READ and ICD-9-CM schemes perform much more poorly for problem coding. They showed 38% and 42% unsatisfactory matches respectively, approximately twice the rate for either UMLS or SNOMED. This performance generally mirrors a weaker showing by these schemes in other CPR domains[6].

In summary, the systems developer of a CPR has many choices to make when choosing standard coding schemes. Based upon this evaluation of problem encoding, both UMLS and SNOMED are more complete than alternative systems. Depending upon the goals of the project, UMLS will offer advantages for systems that wish to employ natural language processing and literature links. If the goal is an integrated, comprehensive coded record with decision support features, SNOMED is more attractive.

Reference

[1]. Dick RS, Steen EB, eds. The Computer-Based Patient Record: An Essential Technology for Health Care. 1991; Institute of Medicine, National Academy of Sciences

[2]. Henry SB, Campbell KE, and Holzemer WL. Representation of Nursing Terms for the Description of Patient Problems Using SNOMED III. Annu Symp Comput Appl Med Care 1993; In press

[3]. Zielstorff RD, Cimino C, Barnett GO, et al. Representation of Nursing Terminology in the UML Metathesaurus: A Pilot Study. Proc Annu Symp Comput Appl Med Care. 1992; 354-348

[4]. Campbell JR, Kallenberg GA, Sherrick RC. The Clinical Utility of META: An Analysis for Hypertension. Proc Annu Symp Comp Appl Med Care 1992; 397-401

[5]. Payne TH, Martin DR. How Useful is the UMLS Metathesaurus in Developing a Controlled Vocabulary for an Automated Problem List? Proc Annu Symp Comput Appl Med Care. 1993; 705-709

[6]. Chute CG, Cohn S, Campbell JR, Campbell KE, Oliver DE and the CPRI Major Codes Workgroup. The Adequacy of Existing Clinical Classifications: Content Coverage. Submitted for publication

[7]. Cote RA, Rothwell DJ, Palotay JL, Beckett RS, Brochu L, eds. The Systematized Nomenclature of Human and Veterinary Medicine: SNOMED International. 1993, College of American Pathologists

[8]. Cad RA; Robboy S. Progress in Medical Information Management. Systematized Nomenclature of Medicine (SNOMED). JAMA 1980; 243(8):756-762

[9]. Lindberg DAB, Humphreys BL, McCray AT. The Unified Medical Language System. Meth Inform Med 1993; 32:281-291

[10]. Lindberg DAB, Humphreys BL, McCray AT. Yearbook of Medical Informatics. "The Unified Medical Language System" 1993; 41-51

[11]. Weed,L. Medical Records that Guide and Teach. NEJM 1968; 278:593-600

[12]. Weed L. The Problem Oriented record as a Basic Tool in Medical Education, Patient Care and Research. Ann Clin Res 1971; 3(3):131-4

[13]. Read Codes File Structure Version 3: Overview and Technical Description. Woodgate, Leicestershire, UK: NHS Centre for Coding and Classification, 1993

[14]. Computer Stored Ambulatory Record. Research Digest Report of NCHSR Grant HS-00240. Barnett GO. United States DHHS Publication HRA 76-3145, National Center for Health Services Research, 1976

A Simple Approach to Physician Entry of Patient Problem List

Harm J. Scherpbier, M.D.[1], Richard S. Abrams, M.D.[2], David H. Roth[1], Jennifer J.B. Hail[2]

[1] SMS, Malvern, Pennsylvania

[2] Rose Medical Center, Denver, Colorado

ABSTRACT

The patient's problem list is one of the key components of the electronic medical record. Besides the immediate benefits of using the patient problem list for medical records coding and creation of discharge documentation, a coded problem list is a prerequisite of patient management, clinical decision support and research. The ICD9 coding system that is the current standard for coding diagnoses and procedures is not conducive to physician usage. In this paper we describe a simple system that provides physicians with a quick and easy method to enter and maintain a patient's problem list. Physicians can use their own terminology. ICD9 codes are included where possible, but free text is allowed. The system strikes a balance between capturing a fully coded patient problem list and encouraging usage by a wide physician user group.

INTRODUCTION

Previous studies have shown that the ICD9 coding system and the English descriptions in ICD9 do not meet physicians' needs for maintaining a patient problem list[1,2]. Yet, despite its shortcomings to express a clinically accurate problem list, ICD9 remains the coding system of choice in many institutions because of reimbursement and billing. We set out to create a system that gives physicians freedom of expression in entering the patient problem list while maintaining the link to ICD9 codes.

The system described here was developed at Rose Medical Center (RMC), a 420-bed acute care facility with 1,100 physicians in Denver, Colorado. RMC is part of a health care network that includes primary care sites, outpatient surgery facilities and a home health care network. It is a teaching hospital affiliated with the University of Colorado Health Sciences Center. RMC uses an IBM mainframe based HIS with a PC-based Graphical User Interface on the physicians' desktops. The electronic medical record presently contains data from lab, nursing, radiology, transcription, pharmacy, as well as financial data.

The problem list system is part of a larger set of functions that assist physicians in the discharge of patients. Besides entering the patient's problem list, the physician can build discharge prescriptions on-line starting with the patient's current inpatient medications. The system also assists the physician in filling out the appropriate discharge forms (nursing home transfer forms, home health care forms, etc.). Although this system began as part of the discharge functions, it has evolved to become part of the admission functions. Besides speeding up chart completion, the computer-based problem list plays an important role in the communication between clinicians.

SYSTEM REQUIREMENTS

To encourage physicians to enter the patient's problem list, we set out to design a system that would meet the following requirements:

1. Provide physicians with a short picklist of frequently used diagnoses[3].
2. Allow physicians to add, change and delete diagnoses on the picklist without the assistance of Information Systems staff.
3. Allow physicians to use their own terminology[1, 2, 4].
4. Provide a link between physicians' personalized descriptions and ICD9 codes.

To satisfy requirement 1, we needed to define a short picklist. The standard screen size in the Clinical Information System can easily accommodate 36 selection items. We studied which percentage of discharge diagnoses used by physicians during one year would be covered by 36 diagnoses. Figure 1 shows that 36 diagnoses covered 73.4% of discharges for the group of internists at Rose Medical Center between March 1, 1993, and March 1, 1994. For an individual member of this group, 36 diagnoses covered 99.3% of discharges during the same period. For the department of General Surgery, the same group vs. individual comparison does not show the same increase of coverage for the individual: coverage for the group is 67.4%, for the individual 64.9%.

clustering by body location does not have the same effect in Internal Medicine that it has in General Surgery, it does increase the coverage. With the introduction of two diagnosis clusters (Diabetes and Myocardial Infarction), 99.3% of discharges are covered by 29 diagnoses, compared to 36 without clustering.

These results show that a short picklist needs to rely on individualization and clustering to get a good rate of coverage. We added the following two items to the other four requirements for the system:

5. Individuals can build and maintain a personalized list of frequently used diagnoses, without the intervention of Information Systems staff.
6. The system supports clustering of diagnoses, allowing for a second level of selection of body site for a given diagnosis.

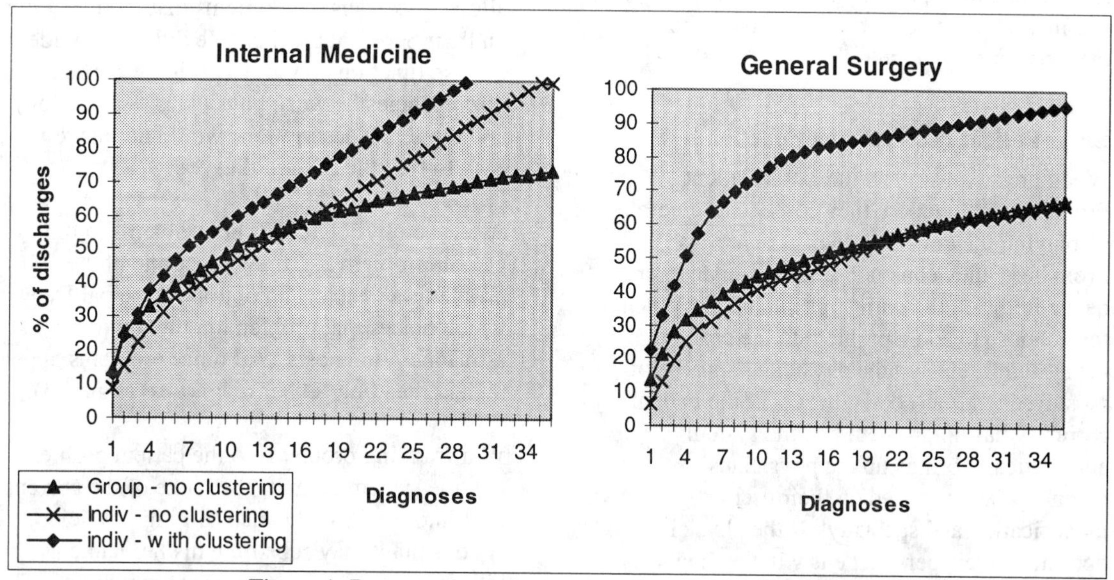

Figure 1: Percentage of discharges covered by 36 diagnoses.

One of the reasons that the coverage for General Surgery is lower than for Internal Medicine is the fact that ICD9 codes are different if the same disease occurs in a different location in the body. Since Internal Medicine focuses more on systemic diseases, the effect of location on the number of ICD9 codes used is smaller. To increase the coverage of 36 diagnoses for General Surgery, we introduced the concept of clustering. By using diagnosis clusters, we can count all hernias as one diagnosis group rather than one for each different site. Similarly, one can combine all benign neoplasms, malignant neoplasms, cellulitis, intestinal obstructions, etc. Clusters not only serve to increase the number of diagnoses covered, they also help organize the picklist in a logical manner, following the physicians' pattern of thought.

Figure 1 demonstrates the effect of clustering in General Surgery. Thirty-six diagnoses for an individual surgeon covered 95.3% of discharges in the period covered. Although the effect of

DESIGN

The system is designed around two profiles. The first profile, the Diagnosis Profile, contains a set of 36 diagnoses, each with a slot for the ICD9 code, and a pointer to a cluster of subclassifications. The second profile, the Subclassification Profile, contains clusters of diagnoses. There is no limit to the number of subclassifications for a diagnosis cluster.

Physicians can create and maintain their personal copy of the diagnosis profile without Information Systems staff assistance, using functions described below. The sub-classification profile is standard across the institution and maintained by Information Systems personnel.

The same structure is maintained for procedures. Each physician can have a personalized list of diagnoses and a list of procedures. Since the design and the functions for the diagnosis profile and the procedure profile are the same, here we will describe the diagnosis profile only.

Enter Patient Problem List Function

When physicians select the Enter Patient Problem List function, they come to a screen displaying the current patient problem list. From here, they can choose to add, change or delete items on the patient problem list. When they choose to add a problem to the problem list, the system brings up the physicians' profile of most frequently used diagnoses. If the patient currently has no problem list, the system automatically brings up the physicians' diagnosis profile based on their user identification and specialty. If the physician does not have a personal entry in the diagnosis profile, the system displays the set of frequently used diagnoses for the physician's specialty.

From the physician's diagnosis profile, they can select one or more items and add them to the patient's problem list (figure 2). If a selected item is a clustered diagnosis, the system displays all members in that cluster. The physician can select one or more cluster members from the subclassification profile to add to the patient's problem list.

Once the selected items are added to the patient's problem list, the physician has the option to accept the new patient problem list. They can also manually add additional diagnoses or problems using free text. Although free text selections are not ICD9 coded, they allow physicians to add items that did not occur on their personal profile. We did not provide a browse function on the ICD9 file, because the discrepancies between physicians' terminology and the ICD9 descriptions would not make it easy to find the desired diagnosis.

After the physician adds all problems to the patient problem list, they select one of the problems and select an option 'Principal Dx,' which places that problem on the top of the list as primary diagnosis. All other problems appear under a heading 'Other diagnoses' (figure 3).

While adding problems to the patient problem list, the system defaults the name of the current user into a column labeled 'billing physician.' A consultant may substitute his/her name as billing physician on appropriate diagnoses. This helps avoid situations where two physicians bill Medicare patients for the same diagnosis and only one of them receives reimbursement.

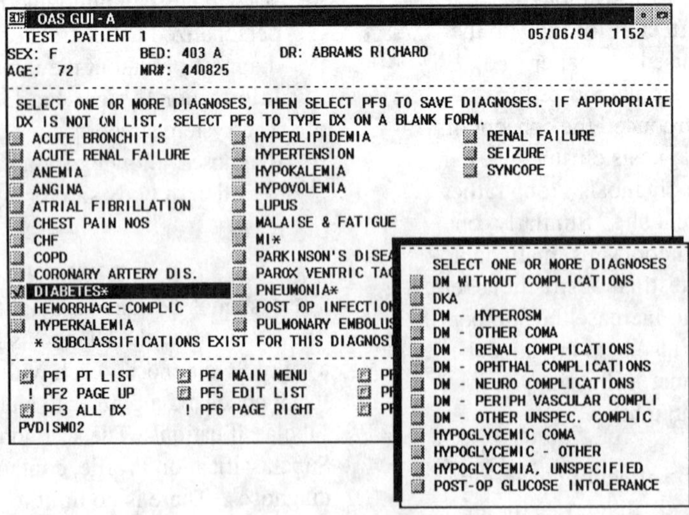

Figure 2: Diagnosis Profile Selection Screen. Insert: Subclassification selection for diagnosis cluster 'Diabetes.'

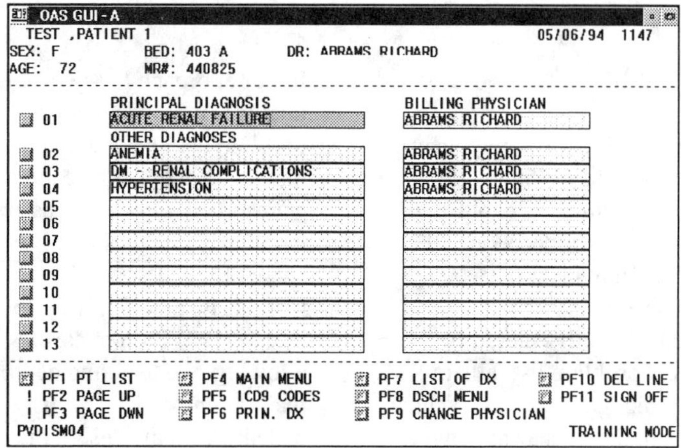

Figure 3: Patient Problem List - Editing Screen.

Medical Records coders review and complete the physician entered patient problem list during the patient's stay. They add any complicating and comorbid conditions, and enter the estimated length of stay for each of the patient's diagnoses. When necessary, coders communicate with physicians by phone, E-mail or paper mail.

Personalize List

Physicians can create a personal copy of the set of frequently used diagnoses by copying the specialty list. Once they have created a personal copy, they can delete existing items, change the description of existing items, or add new items. When adding new items, one can choose an option to enter the ICD9 code for the new item. It is recommended that physicians enter the ICD9 code to facilitate the concurrent coding by Medical Records staff. Physicians can sort their list alphabetically or leave the list as entered.

Edit List

Once users have created a personal list, they will automatically see their own list when entering a patient problem list. At any time, physicians can edit their personal list, using the same functions to add or delete items, or to change the description of existing items. For example, physicians prefer to use the term "FUO" (Fever of Unknown Origin) over the ICD9 description "Pyrexia of undetermined etiology."

The system can be set up to prohibit deletion of entire diagnosis clusters without assistance of Information Systems personnel.

EXPERIENCES

The system described here has been in use by a number of physicians since March 1994. One of the main benefits of the system is the addition of the problem list as essential component of the electronic medical record. The problem list facilitates communication among physicians, consultants, nurses and others treating the patient, and makes them less dependent on the manual medical record.

The second important benefit, and the incentive to the physician to enter the problem list, is the automatic creation of discharge documentation. The discharge forms include the patient problem list as entered by the physician and supplemented by medical records coders. The ability for medical records staff to complete the coding during the patient's stay, without searching for elusive charts, speeds up chart completion and reduces the number of cases involving patient diagnoses that the medical records coder needs to consult with the physician about. This in turn shortens the billing cycle.

Because of the option to add billing physician to the patient problem list, the system helps avoid rejection of reimbursement by Medicare if multiple physicians bill under the same diagnosis.

We are in the process of measuring physician compliance, usage of the option to individualize the picklist, and effects of the computer problem list on chart completion.

DISCUSSION

A coded patient problem list is a key component of the electronic medical record. Whiting-O'Keefe *et al* identify the dilemma of capturing clinical data as the foundation for decision support and research [5]. They identify two types of data capture problems: data from ancillary systems and data directly entered by the clinician. The patient problem list falls in this second category. Although physicians value a computer-based problem list, it is a challenge to get a large number of physicians to enter it into the computer [4]. The system described here aims to provide physicians with a quick and easy method to enter a patient's problem list. The purpose is to achieve short-term benefits, such as improved physician communication, quicker chart completion and the automatic creation of discharge documentation, as well as to achieve the long-term goal to provide source data for clinical decision support and research.

To circumvent some of the problems associated with physicians' use of the ICD9 coding system, we created a buffer structure that allows physicians to use their own terminology and still maintain the link to an ICD9 code where possible. We provided physicians with a short picklist of frequently used diagnoses, and demonstrated that such a list can cover the majority of diagnoses used by personalizing the list and allowing users to cluster certain diagnoses into groups.

Franco *et al* describe a different method to present the physician with a short picklist when entering the patient problem list [6]. They use an expert system to base the short selection list on patient data rather than on physician characteristics. Deriving the problem list with an expert system from patient data has strong appeal in a finite domain with sufficient structured data. In a wider domain, where the essential patient data is not available at all or not in computer readable form, one has to rely on physician charateristics to create a short picklist. The expert system approach may be applied to code complicating and comorbid conditions during the patient's hospital stay, when sufficient structured data is available.

In our approach to the problem list, the primary goal was to have physicians enter the patient problem list in a quick and easy way. Getting this list coded was a secondary goal. In order to get as many physicians as possible to participate in entering the problem list, we incorporated some of the lessons McDonald learned: "Free text has its place", and "Do the easiest things first" [7]. Wilton makes a strong case for allowing free text, and demonstrates the value of maintaining a problem list even if it's not fully coded[2]. In the design of our system we traded off a fully coded problem list that would be used by a minority of physicians against a problem list that may include free text but is conducive to physician usage. Rather than creating the ideal coding system, we've created a way to make the current, unsatisfactory system work better. We realize that the next step is to create a fully coded patient problem list that would be used by all physicians for all patients. To paraphrase Voltaire, we have taken the simple approach: "Don't let the best be the enemy of the good."

References

[1]. Payne TH, Murphy GR, Salazar AA: How well does ICD9 represent phrases used in the medical record problem list? Proc 16th Ann Symp Comput Applic Med Care 1992; 654-657.
[2]. Wilton R: Non-categorical Problem Lists in a Primary-Care Information System. Proc 15th Ann Symp Comput Applic Med Care 1991; 823-827.
[3]. Ingersoll S, Personett JD: A Simplified Approach to the Ambulatory Care Diagnostic Summary List. QRB 1990; 16:127-129.
[4]. Safran C, Rury C, Rind DM, Taylor WC: Outpatient Medical Records for a Teaching Hospital: Beginning of the Physician-Computer Dialogue. Proc 15th Ann Symp Comput Applic Med Care 1991; 114-118.
[5]. Whiting-O'Keefe QE, Whiting A, Henke J: The STOR Clinical Information System. MD Comput 1988; 5(5); 8-21.
[6]. Franco A, Farr FL, King JD, Clark JS, Haug PJ: "NEONATE"- An Expert Application for the "HELP" System: Comparison of the Computer's and the Physician's Problem List. J Med Syst 1990; 14(5); 297-306.
[7]. McDonald CJ, Tierney WM, Overhage MJ, Martin DK, Wilson GA: The Regenstrief Medical Record System: 20 Years of Experience in Hospitals, Clinics, and Neighborhood Health Centers. MD Comput 1992; 9(5); 206-217.

Mapping Clinically Useful Terminology to a Controlled Medical Vocabulary

Randolph C. Barrows Jr., MD, James J. Cimino, MD, Paul D. Clayton, Ph.D.
Center for Medical Informatics
Columbia University
New York, NY 10032

We have mapped clinically used diagnostic terms from a legacy ambulatory care system to the separate controlled vocabulary of our central clinical information system. The methodology combines elements of lexical and morphologic text matching techniques, followed by manual physician review. Results of the automated matching algorithm before and after partial manual review are presented. The results of this effort will permit the migration of coded clinical data from one system to another. Output from the system after the term review process will be fed back to the target vocabulary via automated and semi-automated means to improve its clinical utility.

INTRODUCTION

The Columbia-Presbyterian Medical Center (CPMC) has a dataset including coded clinical diagnoses and medications pertaining to ambulatory patients that was captured from primary care practitioners using the outpatient Clinical Profile system [1]. The base set of terms in the system dictionary, from which providers choose diagnoses, came from the Systematized Nomenclature of Medicine (SNOMED), but users of the system are free to define new terms as needed, and have frequently done so. New dictionary terms are assigned a unique code by the system, which is used to reference the term in the database. This system uses a hierarchical database and is isolated from the CPMC Clinical Information System (CIS) with its relational database and decision support capabilities [2].

Ongoing work at CPMC aims to develop a clinical system for ambulatory care that functions as part of the CIS and uses the central patient database with its own controlled medical vocabulary and data dictionary called the Medical Entities Dictionary (MED) [3]. In order to prevent the loss of clinical information to users of the new system, and redundant data entry efforts on the part of health care providers, it is desirable to map coded terms from the outpatient Clinical Profile system to coded entities in the MED and migrate patient data from the Clinical Profile system into the CIS. Manual mapping is feasible but time consuming for a medical domain expert, even given the presence of reasonable tools for browsing the target vocabulary. It would presumably, however, have the highest degree of accuracy.

METHODS

Given the importance of accurately representing real data on real patients, the approach taken is that of an initial enhanced lexical matching algorithm followed by manual review of the match results by a medical domain expert.

The match algorithm utilizes a unix-based implementation of the MED that is maintained to be concurrent with the CIS version. The MED is conceptually organized as a semantic network of about 35,000 medical entities. Each entity has a unique numerical identifier ("medcode") and a number of term attributes ("slots"). Some slots, such as SUBCLASS-OF, are link attributes (have medcodes as values), and other slots, such as the NAME and SYNONYM slots, are literal attributes (have string values). Some slots, such as SYNONYM, may have multiple uniquely-valued instances. For example, medcode 9624 is a SUBCLASS-OF 9623 ("Disease of Upper Respiratory Tract"), has a NAME value of "Acute Upper Respiratory Infection", has a SYNONYM value of "Acute URI", and another SYNONYM value of "Common Cold". Development efforts (by Dr. Barry Allen and Nilesh Desai) in the Center for Medical Informatics have resulted in an implementation of the MED that is optimized for speed of queries and compactness of representation, and resides in shared-memory on an IBM RS/6000. A library interface allows complex queries to be performed on the contents of the MED from application programs, and a command line interface, a menu-driven interface, and an X Window graphical browser have been developed as well.

0195-4210/94/$5.00 © 1994 AMIA, Inc.

The match algorithm is dependent upon preprocessing information from the MED available as part of the unix implementation. In preprocessing, all string-valued slots of all MED entities are tokenized. Each token (a word or term fragment separated by non-alphanumeric characters) is indexed to the medcodes of the entities in which it is found to occur in some string-valued slot, and redundant token occurrences are eliminated. Also available in preprocessed form is a set of Word Groups (WG), consisting of groups of medically synonymous tokens that were originally obtained from lexical variants and synonyms in the Unified Medical Language System (UMLS). The base set includes medical morphemes such as "hepatic" = "liver" = "livers" in one set, and "cardiac" = "heart" = "hearts" in another, and was enhanced based on deficiencies noted after manual review and algorithmic use.

In the matching algorithm, a term from the Clinical Profile system is tokenized, and each token is mapped to a WG (which has the index token as a member). Each member of a WG maps to 0 or more medcodes where the member token occurs in some string valued slot. The union of the medcodes associated with each WG member comprises a set of MED entities, each of which might contain a conceptual match for the token in some literal-valued slot. Such a set of medcodes is determined for each token comprising the Clinical Profile term, and the intersection of these sets is then taken to yield a solution set of possible MED matches for the Clinical Profile term. If this solution set is empty, the intersection is relaxed so that, of n sets of medcodes, one for each of the n tokens comprising a Clinical Profile term, any medcode need only be common to n-1 of the sets, rather than all n, for inclusion in the solution set. If only a single medcode exists in the solution set, that match is returned as a "SOLO"; otherwise the MED entities in the solution set are ranked in order of their likeness to the Clinical Profile term according to the Longest Common Substring (LCS) algorithm [4]. An LCS scoring is performed between the Clinical Profile term and the NAME slot, as well as each SYNONYM instance, of each MED entity in the match solution set.

Results of the automated match are output to a file, and another program is run to analyze the results and generate a statistical characterization. The output of the automated match is reviewed manually by a clinical vocabulary domain expert (RCB and Dr. Olveen Carrasquillo). The manual review process identifies five types of matches: true positive matches (in which the algorithm proposes a correct match); true negative matches (in which the algorithm correctly identifies that no accurate match exists); false negative matches (in which the algorithm falsely states that no accurate match exists in the MED); false positive matches in which the algorithmically proposed match is not accurate, but another MED term exists which is an accurate match; and false positive matches in which the algorithmically proposed match is not accurate, and no accurate match exists in the MED. Another program is then run on the reviewed file and it generates 3 output files: one file maps the code of each successfully matched Clinical Profile term to a MED code; another file maps each unmatched Clinical Profile term (no accurate MED match exists after manual review) to the closest more general concept that can be identified in the MED; and a third file maps newly identified synonyms (Clinical Profile terms judged as useful by the reviewer) to existing MED terms.

RESULTS

Clinical profile terms were divided into two groups: those SNOMED-derived terms actually used to describe patients, and those user-defined terms actually used to describe patients. Unused dictionary terms were not matched. An LCS match value of 0.75 or greater was used to identify possible matches between Clinical Profile terms and Med terms. This number was chosen heuristically as a reasonable cutoff, based on earlier matching work which showed no improvement in the sensitivity of the match below this level, but significantly less specificity. The algorithm matched 65% (674/1045) of the SNOMED-derived Clinical Profile terms to at least one MED term (371 failed to match at an LCS cutoff of 0.75). Thirty seven percent (387/1045) of these terms matched to only a single MED entity, including 15% (159/1045) that matched "SOLO". Ninety seven percent of the terms that matched (647/674) did so to fewer than 10 MED terms, but one term matched to 48 MED terms. Thirty percent of the terms matched "exactly" (each was either a "SOLO" match or matched with a perfect LCS score of 1.00). Of SNOMED-derived terms with more than one potential match (after Term Group intersection), 81% (421/515) matched to the NAME of a MED entity, and 19% matched via SYNONYM instances.

The algorithm matched 51% (631/1225) of the user-defined terms to at least one MED term. Thirty one percent (377/1225) matched to a single MED term. Of user-defined terms that matched, 97% (613/631) matched to fewer than 10 MED terms, and 1 term matched to 31 MED entities. Twenty five percent of the terms matched "exactly", as defined above. Of user-defined terms with more than 1 potential match, 77% (348/453) matched to the NAME of a MED entity, and 23% to a SYNONYM instance.

Examples of match results and reviewer actions follow. In the first example, the Clinical Profile term matched "SOLO" (uniquely), so no LCS scoring was invoked. Here the reviewer need do nothing.

SRC|D0121001|ERYSIPELAS|
TARG|6458|L|Erysipelas|SOLO

In a second example, the term matched perfectly (LCS score == 1) to one MED entity, and with 81% agreement to another MED entity (the textual qualifier NOS --"Not Otherwise Specified" was removed in preprocessing). Here a reviewer need only delete the second, less exact, match.

SRC|D0102001|VENEREAL DISEASE, NOS|
TARG|6828|P|Venereal Disease|1.000
TARG|6984|P|Other ICD9 Venereal Disease|0.815

In the third example, the term matched with a high degree of accuracy to a very different appearing MED term via one of its synonyms. It also matched with lesser accuracy to the NAME of another MED term, and to another synonym (but only the NAME of the MED entity is displayed). Here a reviewer need only verify the accuracy of the top match, and delete the less accurate matches.

SRC|D0131001|GONORRHEA|
TARG|6929|S|Acute Gonococcal Infection of Lower Genitourinary Tract|0.909
TARG|6946|P|Chronic Gonorrhea|0.794
TARG|6929|S|Acute Gonococcal Infection of Lower Genitourinary Tract|0.750

In a fourth example, the term does not match with good agreement to any MED term (LCS score < 0.75), but the closest 10 matches according to LCS scoring are listed.

SRC|D0525001|HEPATITIS DISEASE OR SYNDROME|
PROB|no matches >= 0.750
POOR|33838|P|Hepatitis D (Delta Agent)|0.683
POOR|14747|P|Hepatitis|0.650
POOR|14750|P|Hepatitis in Viral Disease|0.629
POOR|6706|P|Hepatitis A|0.621
POOR|6709|P|Hepatitis B|0.621
POOR|33837|P|Hepatitis C|0.621
POOR|33839|P|Hepatitis E|0.621
POOR|14751|P|Hepatitis in Nonviral Infectious Disease|0.508
POOR|6701|P|Viral Hepatitis|0.483
POOR|6720|P|Mumps Hepatitis|0.483

Here a reviewer notes that the MED term "Hepatitis" in the list of sub-threshold matches is actually the appropriate conceptual match, and labels the algorithmic match as an FN (False Negative) while indicating the correct match and deleting unused alternatives:

SRC|D0525001|HEPATITIS DISEASE OR SYNDROME|
FN|14747|P|Hepatitis|0.65

In the following example, the Clinical Profile term matches with above-threshold agreement to a MED term, but this a false positive match due to lexical similarities:

SRC|D0521001|VIRAL HEPATITIS, TYPE A|
TARG|6701|P|Viral Hepatitis|0.826

In this case, the correct matching entity had to be identified by manual search and browsing of the MED, so the algorithmically suggested match is labeled as an FP (False Positive), and the correct (COR) match subsequently listed. In addition, the reviewer indicated that the Clinical Profile term should be added as a synonym to the MED term:

SRC|D0521001|VIRAL HEPATITIS, TYPE A|
FP|6701|P|Viral Hepatitis|0.83
COR|6706|M|Hepatitis A
ADDSYN

In a final example, the term was an algorithmically false positive match, and after manual review it was determined that no conceptually accurate match exists in the MED. However, the closest more general term was identified and listed in the NOMATCH line:

SRC|D2262001|HYPERPARATHYROIDISM, PRIMARY|
FP|3322|P|Hyperparathyroidism|0.839
NOMATCH|3322|Hyperparathyroidism|0.839

Algorithmic matches for the 1045 SNOMED-derived terms have been manually reviewed and edited as indicated in the preceding paragraphs. The edited version was then processed to generate the final match output and related files including performance statistics. Algorithm performance is as follows:

403 TP + 103 FN + 73 FP(match found) = 579 matches

285 TN + 181 FP(no match found) = 466 no-matches

With the current MED content, the best the matching algorithm could have done was to match 55% (579/1045) of Clinical Profile terms. It actually matched 39% (403/1045) of the terms, or 403 of 579 possible matches for a match recall of 70%. It was accurate in 403 of 657 (403+73+181) algorithmic matches for a match precision of 61%. Forty five percent (466/1045) of Clinical Profile terms could not be matched to the MED. The algorithm correctly identified 285 of 466 possible no-matches for a no-match recall of 61%, and was accurate in 285 of 388 (285+103) algorithmic no-matches for a no-match precision of 73%. In all, the algorithm correctly classified 688 (403+285), or 66%, of the 1045 terms.

DISCUSSION

The matching algorithm described above performs with reasonable recall and precision compared to other standard techniques[5] in the 1045 clinically used SNOMED-derived terms. It is likely that the algorithm would perform slightly less well on the collection of user-defined terms that has yet to be reviewed, just based on the automated analysis of that match.

The algorithmic mapping saves considerable time for medical domain experts who are ultimately responsible for the equivalency of medical concepts expressed in the two separate vernaculars used to represent patient states. The manual review process provides for maximal accuracy and permits statistical reporting on the accuracy of the automated match compared to "gold standard" experts. This process has proved to be, as expected, the principle bottleneck due to limited person-power and (until recently) adequate vocabulary browsing tools.

The immediate value of this work is two fold. First it will allow coded patient data to be migrated from one clinical information system to another despite complete disparity in their respective data dictionaries. Second, it provides valuable feedback to the MED regarding deficiencies and possible improvements that can be made toward the support of ambulatory patient care activities.. This is an important aim at CPMC, where there is strong interest in creating a truly useful controlled clinical vocabulary for electronic medical record systems and decision support. Output from the described system lists newly identified synonyms that can be automatically incorporated into the MED. The 45% of instances where target MED concepts are missing and new entities need to be defined in the MED will require some non-automated effort, but these instances are valuable increments towards constructing a general and clinically useful vocabulary for the storage of coded patient data.

Future directions of this work include comparing the results experimentally with other mapping techniques. Current methods for mapping text phrases that represent medical concepts include lexical techniques, such as the string matching techniques used by UMLS developers [6]; morphologic text analysis [7]; statistical techniques [8]; and semantic indexing [9,10]. In addition, a novel least squares fit mapping technique using large collections of human-assigned matches as training sets has been reported to outperform other available methods [5].

Although the MED is conceptually organized as a semantic network of medical entities, terms from the Clinical Profile have no associated structure, so semantic mapping techniques were not employed. However, much of the term-content for diagnoses and procedures in the MED was derived from ICD9 [11], so the post-review results reported above approximate those expected in a mapping of 1045 SNOMED terms to ICD9. This suggests that another interesting experiment would be to utilize the UMLS metathesaurus to translate SNOMED-derived Clinical Profile terms to ICD9, and then map these into the MED via the ICD9 code (which is retained as another term attribute, or slot, in the MED). Also, initial efforts toward implementing a statistical n-gram algorithm (considers occurrence of 2 letter "2-gram" sequences, 3 letter "3-gram" sequences, etc.) to accomplish the same mapping task are nearly completed, and there is interest in implementing the least squares fit mapping technique as reported by Yang.

References

1. Shea S, Clark AS, Clayton PD. Columbia-Presbyterian Medical Center Integrated Academic Information Management System (IAIMS) outpatient clinical information system implemented in a faculty general medicine practice. *Proceedings of the 14th SCAMC*, Washington, DC, 1990; 730-734.
2. Hripcsak G, Clayton PD, Cimino JJ, Johnson SB, Friedman C. Medical decision support at Columbia-Presbyterian Medical Center. IMIA Working Conference on Software Engineering in Medical Informatics, Amsterdam, Netherlands, 1990.
3. Cimino JJ, Clayton PD, Hripcsak G, Johnson SB. Knowledge-based approaches to the maintenance of a large controlled medical terminology. *JAMIA* 1994; 1(1):35-50.
4. Friedman C, Sidelli R. Tolerating spelling errors during patient validation. *Comput Biomed Research* (October 1992); 25(5):486-509.
5. Yang Y, Chute C. An application of least squares fit mapping to clinical classification. *Proceedings of the 16th SCAMC*, Baltimore, MD. McGraw-Hill, Inc., 1992; 460-464.
6. Sheretz DD, Tuttle MS, Olson NE Erlbaum MD, Nelson JS. Lexical mapping in the UMLS Metathesaurus. *Proceedings of the 13th SCAMC*, Washington, DC, 1989; 494-99.
7. Wingert F. An indexing system for SNOMED. *Meth Inform Med* 1986; 25:22-30.
8. Kimbrell RE. Searching for text? Send an n-gram. *Byte* (May 1988):297-312.
9. Cimino JJ, Barnett GO. Automated translation between medical terminologies using semantic definitions. MD Computing 1990; 7(2):104-9.
10. Chute CG, Yang Y, Evans DA. Latent semantic indexing of medical diagnoses using UMLS semantic structures. *Proceedings of the 15th SCAMC*, Washington, DC, 1991; 185-189.
11. Cimino JJ, Barrows RC, Allen BA. Adapting ICD9-CM for clinical decision support. (abstract) American Medical Informatics Association Spring Congress, 1992.

Evaluation of UltraSTAR: Performance of a Collaborative Structured Data Entry System

Douglas S. Bell, M.D.
Robert A. Greenes, M.D., Ph.D.

Harvard Medical School, Division of Health Sciences and Technology, and Department of Radiology, Decision Systems Group, Brigham and Women's Hospital, Boston, Massachusetts

The UltraSTAR structured data entry system is now in routine use for reporting ultrasound studies at Brigham and Women's Hospital, having been used for 3722 reports in its first ten months of service. Reports entered through GUI-based forms are uploaded via HL7 to a radiology information system and distributed through a hospital network. UltraSTAR introduces collaborative reporting, in which nonmedical and medical staff collaborate to produce a single report for each patient visit.

Performance of UltraSTAR was measured as user satisfaction, data entry time, report completeness, free text annotation rate, and referring-physician satisfaction with reports. Results show high satisfaction with UltraSTAR among radiologists and acceptance of the system among ultrasound technicians. Data entry times averaged 5.3 minutes per report. UltraSTAR reports were slightly more complete than comparable narrative reports. Free text annotations were needed in only 25.2% of all UltraSTAR reports. Referring physicians were neutral to slightly positive toward UltraSTAR's outline-format reports.

UltraSTAR is successful at structured data entry despite somewhat long reporting times. Its success can be attributed to efficiencies from collaborative reporting and from integration with existing information systems. UltraSTAR shows that the advantages of structured data entry can outweigh its difficulties even before problems of data entry time and concept representation are solved.

INTRODUCTION

Clinical observations in a computer-based patient record may be acquired as natural language or through structured data entry. Natural language offers flexibility of expression, but summarizing natural language data requires a human encoder or automated natural-language processing (NLP). Although progress is being made in NLP [1], concepts abstracted by NLP still carry a degree of uncertainty. Structured data entry, defined here as recording observations by selecting concepts directly from a standard concept set, offers several potential advantages. Standardized observational data acquired directly from the clinician would lower the cost and increase the certainty of data summaries. Data gathered through structured data entry may also be more complete than comparable natural language records, as demonstrated in the domain of endoscopy [2]. Finally, the structured data entry process may be more directly integrated with decision support, as demonstrated by Ivory and T-Helper [3].

Attempts to implement structured data entry have had a long history. The earliest efforts used paper forms [4], or touch-sensitive screens [5, 6], but never achieved routine use. A structured data entry system implemented on a general medical ward was rejected after considerable investment [7]. Efforts in narrower subdomains have achieved more lasting use [2, 8-13], but data abstraction has remained difficult and systems have in general not been successful outside the institutions where they were developed. These efforts illustrate that challenges to structured data entry remain to be addressed. Interface techniques are needed to minimize data entry time, concept structures need to flexibly match the clinician's documentation requirements, and data entered must be integrated with existing information systems. UltraSTAR (Ultrasound STructured Attribute Reporting) was developed to address these challenges while meeting immediate needs for efficiency in report generation. In so doing, UltraSTAR introduced "collaborative reporting," in which observations and interpretations are obtained from multiple sources to comprise a single report. In the ultrasound domain, the collaboration is among technologist and radiologist. In other clinical domains, the collaboration could include nurses, physicians at different levels of training, patients, and even expert systems.

METHODS

Software

Design and Implementation. The UltraSTAR system provides structured data entry for ultrasound

0195-4210/94/$5.00

results, with preliminary reports generated by ultrasound technologists (sonographers) being later edited and signed by attending radiologists in lieu of dictation. The original design of the system has been published [14], but its main features are briefly reviewed here. Concepts are selected using checkboxes and radio buttons arranged in small forms that are displayed in overlapping windows. Any report may be saved as a template and later reused to start a new report that is then edited for the new patient. Reports are printed in an outline format that mirrors UltraSTAR's concept hierarchy (Figure 1).

UltraSTAR is implemented in SuperCard™ for the Apple Macintosh (Apple Computer, Inc., Cupertino, CA), with external functions written in Think C. (Symantec Corp, Cupertino, CA). Network communications with IDXrad (a radiology information system of IDX Corp, Burlington, Vermont) handle user identification and security, patient demographic queries, and uploading of signed reports using HL7 [15] messages. Pending reports are stored as individual Macintosh files and may be located on any Macintosh volume on the same AppleTalk network, with UltraSTAR maintaining the indices and file locks appropriate for a distributed database. When a report is signed and sent to IDXrad, its coded content is also stored on the Macintosh in a flat file for later statistical analysis.

The system is installed on four Macintosh workstations connected to IDXrad by Ethernet, using the DECnet protocol.

Figure 1

UltraSTAR reports follow a fixed, outline format.

BRIGHAM AND WOMEN'S HOSPITAL
Preliminary Report of Radiologic Procedure

Patient Name: TEST, TEST
Patient Age: 100Y Sex:
Medical record #: 000 00 00 0
Date of procedure: 4/26/94
Accession #: 123

```
INDICATIONS
    This pelvic ultrasound exam is performed to check follicular
      size.

FINDINGS
    Uterus
        Endometrium
            multilayered
            thickness: 5.8 mm
    Right Adnexa
        Ovary
            Simple Cyst(s)
                Few (2-4)  5-11 mm simple cysts
                2 Measured simple cysts
                    12 x 23, 22 x 25 mm
    Left Adnexa
        Ovary
            Non-simple Cyst(s)
                size(s): 15 x 12 x18 mm
                echogenic
```

Concept Authoring. UltraSTAR's knowledge base consists of a hierarchy of increasingly detailed concepts, each with attributes that govern its display and reporting. Each button or field in a data-entry form corresponds to a unique concept in the knowledge base. Each valid concept-modifier combination is represented in the knowledge base by a new unique concept. An authoring interface has been added to UltraSTAR that allows a domain expert to add, edit, and retire concepts from use (Figure 2).

Figure 2

UltraSTAR's concept authoring module provides a single interface for adding and retiring concepts, changing their layout on data-entry forms, and editing their attributes.

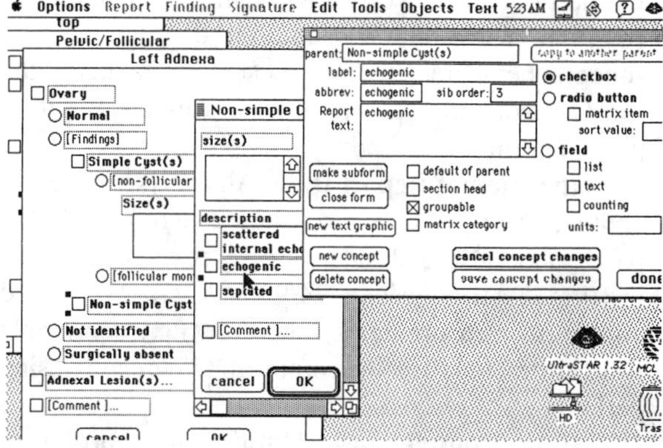

Evaluation

Sonographer and Radiologist Survey. A three-part paper questionnaire was administered to the sonographers and attending radiologists who had used UltraSTAR.

Part one of the questionnaire consisted of items that we designed for this study. These included 7 items that used a Likert-scale response (a five-point scale with 1 representing "strongly agree," 3 representing "neutral," and 5 representing "strongly disagree") to evaluate users' overall satisfaction with UltraSTAR. Because these items were previously untested, they were evaluated using methods outlined in [16]. Items that had the best covariance were formed into a mean satisfaction scale. (Scores on this scale are obtained by taking the mean of an individual's Likert-scale responses, after reversing the responses to negatively-worded items.) This scale was then evaluated with Cronbach's alpha and confirmatory factor analysis.

Part two of the questionnaire consisted of 23 items testing satisfaction with specific user interface features of UltraSTAR. These items were taken from the 26-item Questionnaire on User Interface Satisfaction (QUIS 5.0), an instrument developed and validated at the University of Maryland [17]. We deleted two items from the QUIS that were not applicable to our system and one that had poor reliability in original testing of the QUIS.

Part three of the questionnaire was a control for part two. The same 23 QUIS items were applied to evaluate the user interface of OBUS, an obstetrical calculation and reporting program that is also used by both sonographers and radiologists in the Ultrasound Department.

Data Entry Time. For every reporting sesion, UltraSTAR logs the amount of time taken from report opening to report closing. Data was extracted from the UltraSTAR session log using the perl scripting language [18]. To validate the data entry times that UltraSTAR logs, we manually timed 15 reporting sessions, recording the amount of time from a sonographer's first sitting down at the computer to the time the sonographer was able to walk away with a printed preliminary report.

Extraction of Report Data. All analyses of report content were performed on the 3254 reports (3235 pelvic and 19 scrotal) that were generated and signed in UltraSTAR between 5/24/93 and 3/15/94. Coded concepts, measurements, and free text comments were abstracted from the corpus of 3254 reports using perl.

Report Completeness. UltraSTAR reports were compared with narrative reports for content of data elements considered essential to pelvic ultrasound reporting. Seventy-one "follicular monitoring" pelvic ultrasound reports were sampled from reports dictated and transcribed into IDXrad between 5/1/93 and 7/8/93. (Reports were occasionally dictated after 5/24/93 during times of patient overload or when UltraSTAR was undergoing repair.) Content was abstracted from narrative reports by manual review. Content was abstracted from the 2222 "follicular monitoring" exams among the full corpus of 3235 UltraSTAR pelvic ultrasound reports using perl, as described above.

Referring-Physician Satisfaction with Outline Reports. A paper questionnarie consisting of 16 items was constructed to evaluate attitudes toward outline-format UltraSTAR reports as compared with dictated narrative reports. Questionnaires were given serial numbers that enabled identification of nonresponders. Forms were distributed along with a cover letter that promised anonymity, to the 12 gynecologists who were the primary recipients of UltraSTAR reports. A second copy of the form was distributed to nonresponders after two weeks. Survey evaluation was performed as described above.

Statistical Analyses. Ninty-five percent confidence intervals (95% CI) were based on the *t* distribution for variables that appeared normally distributed on normal-quantile plots. Calculations of mean, standard deviation (SD), Pearson's correlation coefficient (r), Pearson's χ^2-test, analysis of variance (ANOVA), Cronbach's alpha, and factor analysis, were performed using Stata (Stata Corp, College Station, Texas).

RESULTS

System Use

During the first 10 months of routine use (6/1/93 to 4/1/94) 3722 ultrasound reports have been generated using UltraSTAR. As UltraSTAR use has expanded to scrotal ultrasound and pelvic ultrasound on nonfertility patients, monthly volume has increased, with 730 reports generated during 3/94. At an estimated in-house transcription cost of $1.16 per report, UltraSTAR is now potentially saving the Radiology Department $847 per month.

Sonographer and Radiologist Survey

User satisfaction scale: Testing. Our questionnaire was returned by 9 of 15 sonographers and 4 of 6 attending radiologists who are currently active users of UltraSTAR. Five Likert-scale questions, shown in Table 1, form a reliable scale (Cronbach's alpha = 0.79, based on our sample of 13 responses). Factor analysis shows that one primary factor accounts for most of the variation in the responses to these five questions. We consider this factor to be the users' overall satisfaction with the UltraSTAR system and its effect on their work.

Table 1
Items forming the user satisfaction scale.

Items
I enjoy using UltraSTAR.
UltraSTAR makes my work more difficult.
I would like to see more exam types reported with UltraSTAR.
With UltraSTAR, I feel good that my work doesn't have to be repeated.
I preferred the previous system of handwritten preliminary reports.

User satisfaction scale: Results. Sonographers were relatively neutral toward UltraSTAR, giving a mean satisfaction score of 2.9 (95% CI: 2.5–3.3), where 3 is neutral, 1 is strongly positive, and 5 is strongly negative. Attending radiologists were positive toward the system, giving a mean satisfaction score of 1.8 (95% CI 0.6–3.0).

QUIS 5.0: Results. Table 2 shows the mean responses of all users for each subscale of the Questionnaire on User Interface Satisfaction (QUIS) [17]. It also shows mean responses on the individual QUIS items for which UltraSTAR scored the best and the worst. For comparison, mean responses are shown for our users' evaluation of OBUS, along with the responses originally published in the valiation of the QUIS against DOS and WordPerfect.

Table 2
User interface satisfaction, as measured by QUIS 5.0. Each item is scored on a scale from 0 (most negative) to 9 (most positive). (Ultra=UltraSTAR, WP=WordPerfect)

QUIS subscale	Ultra	OBUS	DOS	WP
Learning	6.5	7.1	4.9	6.9
Terms and System Information	6.5	7.5	4.1	4.6
System Output	5.1	7.6	6.2	7.2
System Characteristics	4.5	6.7	5.2	7.0
QUIS item				
Learning to operate the system	7.4	7.7	3.6	5.1
Consistent use of terms throughout the system	6.8	7.4	6.4	7.5
System Speed	4.2	5.5	5.3	6.8
Error Messages	3.3	5.2	3.5	5.8

Data Entry Time

The mean of all data entry times logged by UltraSTAR for initial report generation by sonographers was 3.75 minutes (SD 2.28 min). The mean number of concepts in a report was 19 (SD 4.0). Data entry times correlated weakly with the number of concepts in a report (r = 0.37).

Fifteen manually-recorded overall session times correlated linearly with the data entry times logged for the same sessions by UltraSTAR (r = 0.92), but overall session times were 1.55 minutes longer (95% CI 0.84–2.27 min). Thus, the mean overall reporting time has been approximately 5.3 minutes per report.

Significant variation existed among individual sonographers (*P*<.001, ANOVA), but Figure 3 shows that considerable variance remains within each individual's data entry times.

Report Completeness

Table 3 shows completion rates for information that should be in every pelvic ultrasound report. All 2222 follicular monitoring ultrasound exams in our corpus of signed UltraSTAR reports are compared with a sample of 71 narrative reports of the same exam type.

Proportion of Free Text

Of the 3254 pelvic and scrotal ultrasound reports studied, 820 (25.2%) contained at least one free text annotation. The 200 text comments modifying the uterus were examined and categorized. Forty three comments (22%) described an echogenic or hypoechoic focus or area within the uterus, using fairly stereotypical descriptors. Thirty four comments (17%) described free fluid in the cervical canal, a location not included in UltraSTAR's concept set. Twenty eight (14%) comments made comparisons with findings from a previous study. Nine comments (5%) were inappropriate in that they could have been expressed using the UltreSTAR concept set alone. The remaining 86 comments (43%) were classified as miscellaneous, most being used less than five times. Almost none of these, however, were so idiosyncratic that they would require natural language.

Figure 3
Variation in data entry times for individual sonographers. Box plots are shown for individual sonographers, arranged by the total number of reports generated by each person.

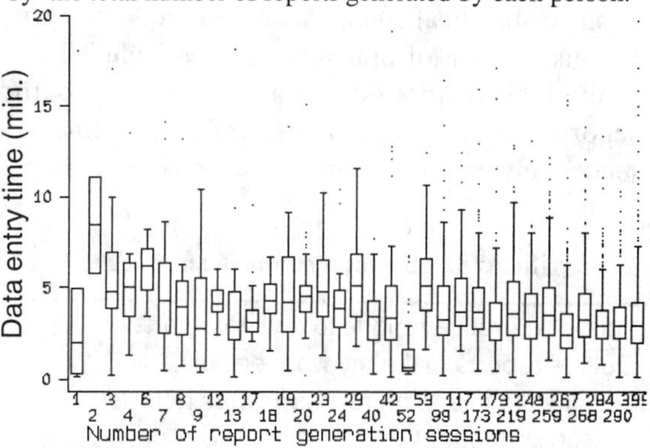

Table 3
Completion rates of UltraSTAR reports vs. narrative reports for six essential data elements in follicular monitoring ultrasound exams.
(*: significant difference, *P*<.001, Pearson's χ^2-test)

	Completion Rate	
Data element	UltraSTAR	Narrative
Uterus (any description, including "normal")	100.0%*	95.8%*
Endometrial thickness	99.5%*	95.8%*
Right adnexa (any description)	99.9%	100.0%
Rt. ovary simple cysts (or "no simple cysts")	94.0%	93.0%
Left adnexa (any description)	99.9%*	98.6%*
Lt. ovary simple cysts (or "no simple cysts")	92.8%	91.5%

Referring-Physician Satisfaction with Outline Reports

Scale testing. Of the 12 gynecologists who have been the primary recipients of UltraSTAR reports, 11 returned our survey after one round of re-surveying nonresponders. Of the 16 questions administered, the four Likert-scale questions shown in Table 4 produced the most reliable responses. A summary preference scale constructed from these four items shows good internal consistency in our sample of 11 responses (Cronbach's alpha = 0.81). Factor analysis shows that one primary factor accounts for most of the variation in the responses to these four questions. This factor may be considered to be the reciepients' preference for outline reports over narrative reports.

Survey results. The mean score on our preference scale for the 11 gynecologists responding was 2.75 (95% CI 2.24–3.26), thus showing a trend toward preference for outline reports that did not achieve statistical significance. Figure 4 shows that the distribution of preference scores included some individuals with a strong preference for outline reports, some who were neutral, and some who moderately preferred narrative reports.

Table 4
Items forming the report preference scale.

I prefer narrative reports to outline reports.
Outline reports make my work easier.
I would like to see more exam types reported in outline format.
Given a choice of ultrasound facilities, I would refer patients to one that returns outline reports.

Figure 4
Histogram of preference scores from survey of referring physicians. A score of 1 indicates strong preference for UltraSTAR ourline-format reports; 3 indicates neutrality, and 5 indicates strong preference for narrative reports.

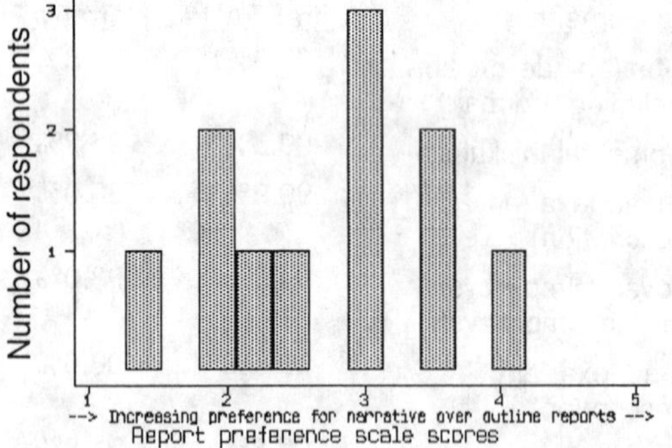

DISCUSSION

This study shows that structured data entry can be implemented and evaluated in a real patient care environment. Our evaluation further shows that structured data entry can provide high quality reports and user satisfacion even though problems of concept representation and data entry time remain to be solved.

Report quality is measured in this study by referring physician satisfaction with reports and by report completeness. UltraSTAR is unique among structured data entry systems in its generation of structured, outline-format reports. Referring physician satisfaction with these reports was measured by a survey scale on which a score of 1 indicates strong preference for outline reports, 3 indicates neutrality, and 5 indicates strong preference for outline reports. Referring physicians did not show unanimous preference for our outline reports over narrative reports. We can conclude, however, that on average narrative reports are not preferred over outline reports, since the 95% confidence interval of the mean preference score result excludes any preference stronger than 3.26. Further work is warranted toward improving the clarity of outline reports as judged by those reading them. Optimal report format might also be studied objectively by measuring reading speed and comprehension for alternate formats.

Report completeness was somewhat higher for UltraSTAR reports than for dictated reports in three of six data elements considered essential for pelvic ultrasound reports. Although these differences were statistically significant they may not be clinically significant, as completion rates were high in both samples. This comparison looked only at the simplest (and most common) type of pelvic ultrasound exam. Examining completion rates for more complicated exams may reveal larger differences. UltraSTAR does not force the user to complete any data element, so any enhancement of completeness it causes is probably due to a reminder effect of having relevant concepts presented. This reminder effect was not strong enough, however, for UltraSTAR to reproduce the 100% completeness rate found by Kuhn in structured endoscopy reporting [2].

An important measure of UltraSTAR's success is the high level of satisfaction found in our survey of attending radiologists. Our sample of four responding radiologists is quite small, however. It will be important to continue to monitor attending satisfaction as the use of structured data entry broadens.

Although our surveys of users and referring physicians showed enough reliability to support conclusions in this study, neither survey can be considered thoroughly tested, each having been used on less than 15 individuals. There is need for further development of methods for evaluating satisfaction with and effectiveness of medical information systems.

Two features of UltraSTAR—collaborative reporting and integration with an existing information system via HL7—are unique among structured data entry systems and may account for much of UltraSTAR's success. Collaborative reporting allows each participant in patient care to contribute to a single report documenting a single patient study. This collaboration stands in contrast to the usual clinical documentation, in which each health care worker documents observations and interpretations separately, and often redundantly. UltraSTAR's HL7 link to the radiology departmental information system allows UltraSTAR reports to substitute for dictation.

UltraSTAR's mean overall reporting time of 5.25 minutes per report and its modest scores on the QUIS indicate room for optimization in the user interface. Speed issues that could be addressed include heavy Ethernet traffic, slow printing, suboptimal layout of data-entry forms, and the interpreted execution of our code in SuperCard. Meanwhile, the neutral overall satisfaction lavels among sonographers indicate that UltraSTAR's user interface is at least tolerable.

UltraSTAR's concept set was complete enough to report 75% of the exams in this domain without further text annotations. Preliminary examination of text annotations shows that the majority would be amenable to coverage in an expanded concept set. We also find that text comments were very seldom used inappropriately when content should have been expressed using the controlled concept set. These results indicate the success of UltraSTAR's hybridization of structured data entry with free text annotations. Further investigation will follow the proportion of reports using free text as the concept set is improved. This improvement is occurring in both the content and the structure of the concept set. Expansion of content is being prioritized by standardizing expression of the most frequent free text annotations. Work on the structure of our concept set focuses on moving our content to a semantic network model [19] and on general methods for building and using such models in structured data entry [20].

The UltraSTAR concept set has additionally demonstrated that structured reporting requires more detail than is typically present in existing controlled vocabularies[21]. The UMLS Metathesaurus [22] contained exact matches for 14% of UltraSTAR's concept set, while SNOMED [23] contained 23% and ACR codes [24] contained 19%. UltraSTAR's concept set is therefore being contributed to the UMLS Metathesaurus.

UltraSTAR's success has resulted in a growing body of routine patient data that *consists of* standardized codes, rather than being coded after the fact by a third party. Perhaps the most important avenue of future investigation will be in structuring systems to acquire routine patient data in a way that will maximally contribute to medical knowledge and the practice of evidence-based medicne [25]. To avoid biased outcomes data, such systems may need to incorporate randomization into routine patient care in areas of diagnostic and theraputic uncertainty.

ACKNOWLEDGMENTS

I am grateful for the support of the National Library of Medicine, through grants LM 07037 and 07092, and contract 04572.

REFERENCES

1. Sager N, Lyman M, Bucknall C, Nhan H, Tick LJ. Natural Language Processing and the Representation of Clinical Data. *J Am Med Inform Assoc* 1994;1:142–60.

2. Kuhn K, Gaus W, Wechsler JG, et al. Structured reporting of medical findings: Evaluation of a System in Gastroenterology. *Methods Inf Med* 1992;31:268–74.

3. Campbell KE, Wieckert K, Fagan LM, Musen MA. A computer-based tool for generation of progress notes. In: Safran C, ed. *Proceedings of the Seventeenth Annual Symposium on Computer Applications in Medical Care.* New York: McGraw-Hill, 1993: 284–8.

4. Hall P, Mellner C, Danielsson T. J5—A data processing system for medical information. *Methods Inf Med* 1967;6:1–6.

5. Greenes RA, Barnett GO, Klein SW, Robbins A, Prior R. Recording, retrieval and review of medical data by physician-computer interaction. *NEJM* 1970;282(Feb. 5):307–15.

6. Pendergrass HP, Greenes RA, Barnett GO, Poitras JW, Pappalardo AN, Marble CW. An on-line computer facility for systematized input of radiology reports. *Radiology* 1969;92(4):709–13.

7. Fischer PJ, Stratmann WC, Lundsgarrde HP. User reaction to PROMIS: Issues related to acceptability of medical innovations. *Proceedings of the Fourth Annual Symposium on Computer Applications in Medical Care.* Los Angeles: IEEE Computer Society Press, 1980: 1722–30.

8. Leeming BW, Simon M, Jackson JD, Horowitz GL, Bleich HL. Advances in Radiologic Reporting with Computerized Language Information Processing (CLIP). *Radiology* 1979;133:349–53.

9. Wheeler PS, Simborg DW, Gitlin JN. The Johns Hopkins Radiology Reporting System. *Radiology* 1976;119:315–9.

10. Greenes RA. OBUS: A microcomputer system for measurement, calculation, reporting, and retrieval of obstetric ultrasound examinations. *Radiology* 1982;144:879–83.

11. Gouveia-Oliviera A, Raposo VD, Salgado NC, Almeida I, Nobre-Leitao C, Galvao de Melo F. Longitudinal comparative study on the influence of computers on reporting of clinical data. *Endoscopy* 1991;23:334–7.

12. Bernauer J, Gumrich K, Kutz S, Lindner P, Pretschner DP. An interactive report generator for bone scan studies. In: Clayton P, ed. *Proceedings of the Fifteenth Annual Symposium on Computer Applications in Medical Care (SCAMC).* New York: McGraw-Hill, 1991: 858–60.

13. Kuhn K, Zemmler T, Reichert M, Heinlein C, Roesner D. Structured data collection and knowledge-based user guidance for abdominal ultrasound reporting. In: Safran C, ed. *Proceedings of the Seventeenth Annual Symposium on Computer Applications in Medical Care.* New York: McGraw-Hill, 1993: 311–5.

14. Bell DS, Greenes RA, Doubilet PD. Form-based clinical input from a structured vocabulary: Initial application in ultrasound reporting. In: Frisse M, ed. *Proceedings of the Sixteenth Annual Symposium on Computer Applications in Medical Care.* New York: McGraw-Hill, 1992: 789–91.

15. HL7. Health Level Seven. In: 900 Victors Way, Ann Arbor, MI.

16. DeVellis RF. *Scale Development: Theory and Applications.*Newbury Park: Sage Publications, 1991:121. (Bickman L, Rog D, ed. Applied Social Research Methods; vol 26).

17. Chin JP, Diehl VA, Norman KL. Development of an instrument measuring user satisfaction of the human-computer interface. *Proceedings of CHI'88, Human Factors in Computing Systems.* New York: Association for Computing Machinery, 1988: 213–8.

18. Wall L, Schwartz RL. *Programming perl.* Sebastopol, Calif.: O'Reilly & Associates, 1990.

19. Bell DS, Greenes RA. Building a semantic network for radiologic records. In: Kahn M, ed. *Proceedings of the 1993 Spring Congress of the American Medical Informatics Association.* Bethesda, Md.: American Medical Informatics Association, 1993: 58.

20. Bell DS, Pattison-Gordon E, Greenes RA. Experiments in concept modeling for radiographic image reports. *J Am Med Inform Assoc* 1994;1(3):249–62.

21. Bell DS, Greenes RA. Comparison of the UltraSTAR Concept Set with Meta-1, SNOMED, and ACR codes. Decision Systems Group Technical Report DSG-93-03, 1993.

22. Lindberg DAB, Humphreys BL, McCray AT. The Unified Medical Language System. In: van Bemmel J, McCray A, ed. *Yearbook of Medical Informatics 1993: Sharing Knowledge and Information.* Stuttgart: Schattauer, 1993: 41–51.

23. Cote RA, Rothwell DJ, Beckette R, Palotay J, ed. *SNOMED International.* Chicago: College of American Pathologists, 1993.

24. American College of Radiology. *Index for Radiological Diagnoses.*Reston, Virginia: American College of Radiology, 1986.

25. Evidence-Based Medicine Working Group. Evidence-based medicine: A new approach to teaching the practice of medicine. *JAMA* 1992;268:2420–5.

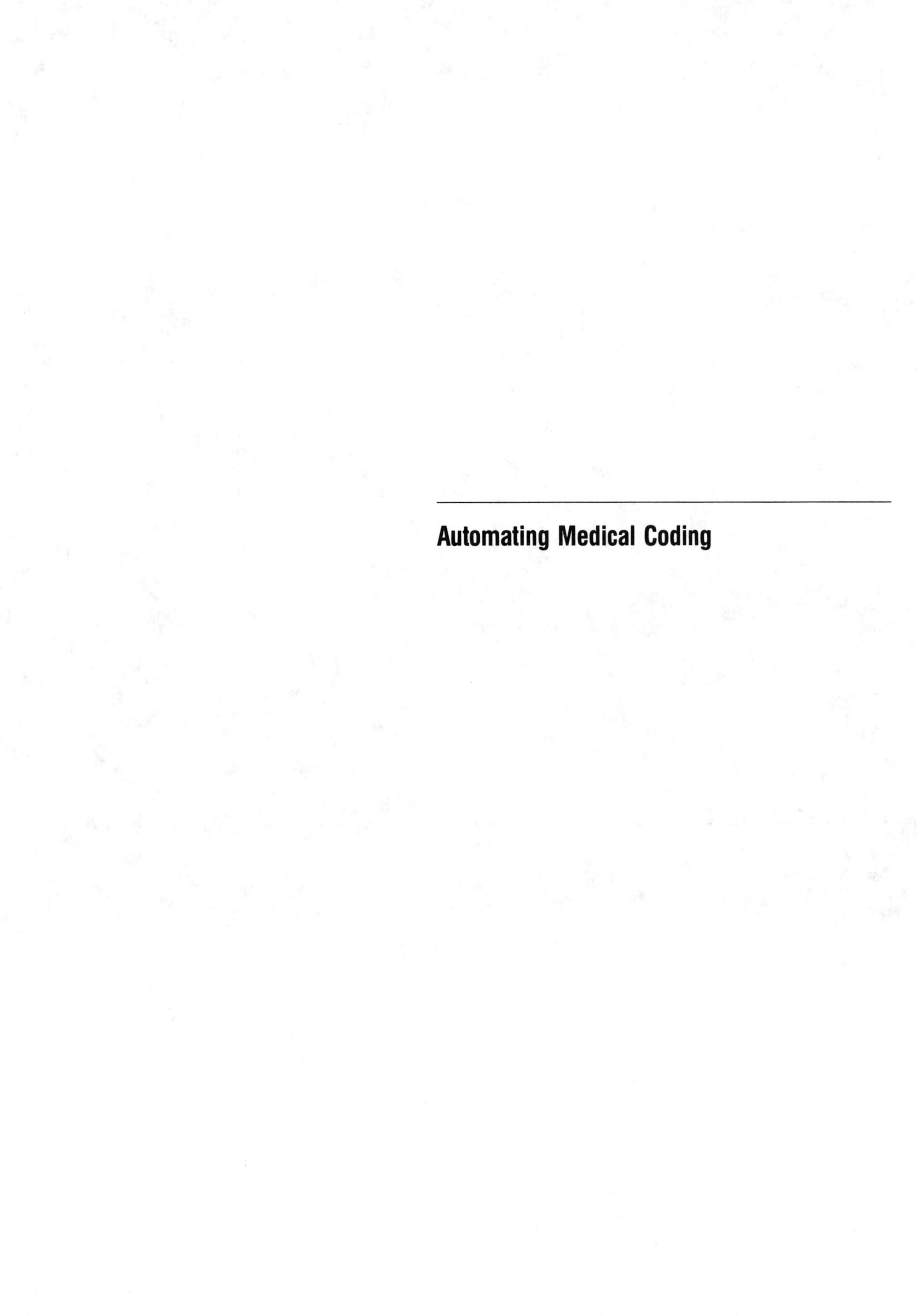

Automating Medical Coding

Automatic SNOMED Coding

G. William Moore, M.D., Ph.D., and Jules J. Berman, Ph.D., M.D.

Departments of Pathology, Baltimore VA Medical Center, University of Maryland School of Medicine, and The Johns Hopkins Medical Institutions, Baltimore, Maryland

ABSTRACT

Medical coding has become an important new industry that has originated from the field of medical informatics. Automatic coding of specimens has emerged as a way of relieving hospitals from the cost of paying professional coders and for achieving uniform coding for all specimens. Unfortunately, automatic coding, like manual coding, has numerous pitfalls. Further, the coding algorithms employed by manufacturers of automatic coders are typically proprietary. We have developed a method for automatic coding of pathology reports. Using this public domain autocoder, we have previously demonstrated that automatic SNOMED coding was superior to manual coding in several measurable categories, including the overall number of codes generated and the number of distinct code entities provided. In this report, we describe an algorithm that executes this strategy in the M-Technology environment.

INTRODUCTION

Medical coding has become an industry in its own right. Some hospitals employ professional coders trained to list diagnoses in a manner that supports linkage to reimbursable diagnosis-related groups (DRGs). Inaccurate diagnostic coding may cause a report to be uncountable, irretrievable, or unreimbursable. In the future, coded databases, stripped of patient identifiers and collected from many contributing health care services, may assist epidemiologists in tracking the spread of diseases, identifying areas of special risk, and providing reliable quantitative information for developing national health care policies. All these activities require accurately coded databases (i.e., databases that contain all the codes for all the specimens collected by a pathology department). However, the ability of any pathology department to obtain an accurately coded database is far from trivial.

In one of the few studies addressing the difficulties in coding, Hall and Lemoine [1] found errors in more than 10% of cases. They divided manual coding errors into five types: (1) Factually correct but unhelpful codes (e.g., coding all benign lesions as `negative for tumor'); (2) Inconsistent codes (coding `dysplasia' on Monday and `atypia' on Tuesday); (3) Idiosyncratic codes (using a mnemonic for a lesion, often inscrutable to other people); (4) Entry errors (e.g., entering `lipoma' when one intends to enter `lymphoma'); (5) Incomplete coding due to impatience or laziness.

In our experience, the way that coding is performed varies considerably depending upon the intended use of the codes. For instance, some pathologists attempt to choose the single best code for a given specimen. Other pathologists code a single case under multiple related morphologic or topographic terms to insure the success of some future search. For example, a single vocal cord lesion may be given all the following morphologies and their corresponding codes: cytologic atypia, precancer, dysplasia, carcinoma in situ, squamous carcinoma. The topography code may be listed as larynx, neck, vocal cord, and even respiratory tract. In addition, when the diagnosis of a specimen is equivocal, the pathologist may code for all the possible diagnoses in the histopathologic differential, even when those diagnoses may be mutually exclusive (i.e., reactive atypia and invasive carcinoma). An epidemiologist trying to determine the respective incidences of vocal cord dysplasia and vocal cord carcinoma may be perplexed by the many code listings for a single biopsy specimen. Vendors and pathologists are left on their own to choose a coding strategy, from the two extremes of coding: 1) a single best fit diagnosis or 2) coding all the related terms for a given lesion. This question will have greater relevance when administrators and epidemiologists attempt to collect and use coded databases.

Considering the enormous resources devoted to manual coding, as well as the inescapable introduction of human error into the collected data, the incentives for automatic diagnostic coding are obvious. A variety of software systems that perform automatic coding (`autocoders') are commercially available. Unfortunately, the algorithms, source code and even the basic coding strategies of proprietary systems lie outside the public domain, and have not been scrutinized in the informatics literature. The Systematized Nomenclature of Medicine (SNOMED) is a widely-used coding system in pathology departments [2,3]. In a recent publication, we have compared the performance of a non-commercial (public domain) SNOMED autocoder against the performance of manual coders [4]. We found that fully automatic SNOMED coding is a practical alternative to manual SNOMED coding, and that automatic SNOMED coding was superior to manual coding in several measurable categories, including the overall number of codes generated and the number of distinct code entities provided. We describe here the techniques we have used in automatic coding and the problems that may arise when coding surgical pathology reports.

MATERIAL AND METHODS

Manual Coding. Manual coding was performed by three board-certified anatomic pathologists at the Baltimore VA Medical Center. Nearly all cases were assigned one topography and one morphology code. The other axes of SNOMED (etiology, function, procedure, disease, occupation) were usually ignored.

Automatic Coding. Reports were obtained as a raw global ASCII file downloaded from the mainframe computer at the Baltimore VA Medical Center. The entire contents of each report, including patient demographics, date and time of accessioning and signout, specimen source, gross description, final microscopic diagnosis, pathologist's identification, and manually-entered SNOMED codes, were passed into an ASCII file, a total of 21,168,261 bytes. The full text of the `specimen source' and `final microscopic diagnosis' for each case served as source text for the SNOMED autocoder. All numerals, punctuation marks, and barrier words (see below) were removed from the source-text, as well as all letter-strings shorter than 3 letters, except for: `no', `os' (=`bone' or `left eye'), `od' (=`right eye'), `eg' (=`esophago-gastric'), and `ge' (=`gastro-esophageal'), to produced a REDUCED REPORT, as shown in the following examples. The manual/autocoder discrepancies in these examples are typical of our experience.

EXAMPLE 1:
ORIGINAL REPORT:
SPECIMEN: 1. TOE.
DIAGNOSIS: 1. BONE WITH HYPERTROPHY AND GOUTY TOPHUS.

REDUCED REPORT:
toe bone hypertrophy gouty tophus

MANUAL CODES:	AUTOMATIC CODES:
TY9800 TOE	TY9800 TOE
	T1X500 BONE
M71000 HYPERTROPHY	M71000 HYPERTROPHY
M55070 TOPHUS	M55070 TOPHUS

EXAMPLE 2:
ORIGINAL REPORT:
SPECIMEN: 1. PUNCH BIOPSY RIGHT GROIN.
DIAGNOSIS: 1. CHANGES CONSISTENT WITH MILD, SUBACUTE DERMATITIS.
COMMENT. THERE IS HYPERKERATOSIS, FOCAL PARAKERATOSIS WITH CRUST FORMATION, ACANTHOSIS, MILD SPONGIOSIS, AND MILD UPPER DERMAL PERIVASCULAR CHRONIC INFLAMMATION. PAS STAIN IS NEGATIVE FOR FUNGI. PSORIASIS AND KAPOSI'S SARCOMA ARE NOT LIKELY, AND THERE IS INSUFFICIENT SPONGIOSIS FOR A DIAGNOSIS OF SEBORRHEIC DERMATITIS.

REDUCED REPORT:
right groin subacute dermatitis hyperkeratosis parakeratosis crust formation acanthosis spongiosis dermal perivascular chronic inflammation negative fungi psoriasis kaposi sarcoma not spongiosis seborrheic dermatitis.

MANUAL CODES:	AUTOMATIC CODES:
T01000 SKIN	T01000 SKIN
	TY9800 INGUIN. REGION
M43000 CHRON. INFLAM.	M36380 CRUST
	M72600 HYPERKERAT.
	M42000 SUBAC. INFLAM.
	M43000 CHRON. INFLAM.
	M30490 FUNGUS BALL
	M74030 PARAKERAT.
	M36500 EDEMA
	M48840 PSORIASIS
	M91403 KAPOSI'S SARC.
	M48820 SEBORR. DERM.

EXAMPLE 3:
ORIGINAL REPORT:
SPECIMEN: 1. LENS OD.
DIAGNOSIS: 1. CATARACT (GROSS DESCRIPTION ONLY).

REDUCED REPORT:
lens od cataract

MANUAL CODES:	AUTOMATIC CODES:
TXX700 LENS, NOS	TXX756 LENS, RIGHT
M51100 CATARACT	M51100 CATARACT
	TXX700 LENS, NOS

EXAMPLE 4:
ORIGINAL REPORT:
SPECIMEN: 1. RIGHT PROSTATE BIOPSY.

2. LEFT PROSTATE BIOPSY.
DIAGNOSIS: 1, 2. BENIGN STROMAL AND GLANDULAR HYPERPLASIA.

REDUCED REPORT:
prostate prostate benign stromal glandular hyperplasia

MANUAL CODES:	AUTOMATIC CODES:
T77100 PROSTATE	T77100 PROSTATE
	M09450 NO MALIGN.
M72000 HYPERPLASIA	M72400 STR. GL.HYP.

EXAMPLE 5:

ORIGINAL REPORT:
SPECIMEN: 1. PUNCH BIOPSY FOREHEAD.
DIAGNOSIS: 1. ACTINIC KERATOSIS.

REDUCED REPORT:
forehead actinic keratosis

MANUAL CODES:	AUTOMATIC CODES:
T01000 SKIN	T01000 SKIN
	T10110 FOREHEAD
M72850 ACT.KERAT.	M72850 ACT. KERAT.

In our SNOMED autocoder, a word-sequence of arbitrary length in each pathology report is pointed to a one-or-more SNOMED codes in the dictionary. Each SNOMED code is repeatedly enriched with additional synonyms, using the 'barrier word method', as described below. In this manner, nearly every significant term in the three years of reports issued by our department could be captured and pointed to an appropriate SNOMED code in a timely fashion. This approach requires one person to function as a 'dictionary policeman' within the department, but is repaid by a very low level of false negatives.

Automatic coding of free-text diagnoses into SNOMED codes was performed on TRANSOFT, a table-driven public-domain computer translation shell, written in M or HyperPAD [5,6]. TRANSOFT is designed for translation between any two languages using the Roman alphabet. The M source code is available through Internet [7]. TRANSOFT is embedded in the File Manager (FileMan), the core database management and program development environment of the Decentralized Hospital Computer Program of the U. S. Department of Veterans Affairs [8]. The user supplies the dictionary and a grammar in the augmented transition network style, which is common to many computer translators [9]. Input is through the FileMan user interface or through an ASCII word processor. The user controls the behavior of the translator through externalized language-specific information and generic program code. TRANSOFT prototype translators have been constructed between English and several languages, simply by changing the FileMan databases [5].

Barrier Word Method. The 'barrier word method' is a computer method for extracting multiple-word terms from a free-text document. All punctuation-marks, numerals, articles, prepositions, and common adjectives and verbs are called 'barrier words' (alternatively, 'stop words'). In addition, each large source document in a particular subject area will have its own, idiosyncratic set of barrier words, which become apparent after repetitive application of the barrier word method to that document. For example, the the following report, the barrier-words are shown in lower-case and the remaining, main-words are shown in upper-case:

specimen: 1 . biopsy APPENDIX .
2 . biopsy CECUM .
3 . biopsy HEPATIC FLEXURE .
diagnosis: 1 . COLONIC MUCOSA with rare CRYPT ABSCESS and CRYPTITIS .
2 . COLONIC MUCOSA with focal ULCERATION , FIBRINOPURULENT MATERIAL , and GRANULATION TISSUE .
3 . COLONIC MUCOSA with mild EDEMA and rare NEUTROPHILS .
comment: findings are consistent with mild INFLAMMATORY BOWEL DISEASE .

barrier words:	MAIN WORDS:
specimen	APPENDIX
biopsy	CECUM
diagnosis	HEPATIC
with	FLEXURE
rare	COLONIC
and	MUCOSA
with	CRYPT
focal	ABSCESS
and	CRYPTITIS
with.....	COLONIC.....

It is apparent from this short excerpt that many multiple-word-sequences of main words that appear between two consecutive barrier words constitute a technical term that might possibly be pointed to a SNOMED code, as follows:

MULTIPLE-WORD TERMS:
HEPATIC FLEXURE
COLONIC MUCOSA
CRYPT ABSCESS
COLONIC MUCOSA
FIBRINOPURULENT MATERIAL
GRANULATION TISSUE
COLONIC MUCOSA
INFLAMMATORY BOWEL DISEASE

False-negative and False-positive rates. A `false-negative case' is one to which a correct code for a major diagnosis has not been assigned. A `false-positive case' is one to which an incorrect code for a major diagnosis has been assigned. The `false-negative rate' is the proportion of false-negative cases among all cases. The `false-positive rate' is the proportion of false-positive cases among all cases. In principle, false-negative and false-positive rates may be obtained both for manual coding as well as for the various methods of autocoding. Unfortunately, obtaining these rates requires that each case be examined by a human coding expert, and the correct codes determined for that case. From this set of `true positive' codes, a computer program can determine whether a particular case has been correctly assigned by manual or various automated methods. Most pathology laboratories cannot devote the human resources necessary to determine the exact set of true-positive codes for their caseloads.

For retrieval problems, the most important information is the false-negative rate for the autocoder. This is the proportion of cases in which the autocoder fails to assign a correct code needed for retrieval. If the autocoder has, say, a 10% false-negative rate, this means that, on average, 10% of cases desired in a particular retrieval request will not be recovered. The false-positive rate, namely the proportion of unwanted cases that will be recovered, can be regarded as a nuisance-factor, which only becomes important if it is very large. For example, when one performs a MEDLINE literature search, one typically detects numerous unwanted citations; but these can easily be bypassed at a glance. The desired citations which are not detected (false-negatives) is the more vexing aspect of a literature search.

For the present investigation, we assumed initially that the manual coding for each case contained no false-negatives for major diagnoses. That is, we assumed that the major sense of the case was always captured manually. We then reviewed every case in which a major diagnosis from manual coding had been missed by the autocoder. The list of `major missed diagnoses' was obtained as follows: First, we assembled a list of `minor diagnoses', such as `M09450 NO EVIDENCE OF MALIGNANCY', `M00100 NORMAL TISSUE MORPHOLOGY, NOS', as well as non-specific inflammation, such as `M41000 INFLAMMATION, ACUTE, NOS', `M43000 INFLAMMATION, CHRONIC, NOS', etc. A minor diagnosis in the manual coding was not required to find a match in the autocoder diagnoses. Second, a list of near-synonyms was assembled, such as `M81400 ADENOMA' near-synonym for `M82110 TUBULAR ADENOMA'. A major diagnosis in the manual coding was considered matched if its near-synonym appeared in the autocoder diagnoses. Finally, a match was only required in the first three digits of the SNOMED-code (where the first digit is either `M' or `T'). Thus, `M72000 HYPERPLASIA' was considered a match for `M72400 HYPERPLASIA, GLANDULAR AND STROMAL'.

RESULTS AND DISCUSSION

A total of 9,353 cases was examined over the 33-month duration of the study [4]. In the first pass of the autocoder, 463 (5%) discrepant cases were detected, in which a major diagnosis in the manual coding had been missed by the autocoder. A final set of true-positive diagnoses were assigned to the initially discrepant cases, and the cases were passed through the autocoder again. In this second pass, there was a missing, major, true-positive diagnosis in only 44 (0.5%) cases.

The nomenclature for automatic coding is somewhat vague. The term `computer-assisted coding' has been used to refer to a variety of distinctly different activities. Our impression is that the term `computer-assisted coding' describes a system where the person entering data is prompted by the computer to enter the name of a topographic site or morphologic entity. The computer then points to a matching entry, if any, in the SNOMED file. If there is a match, then the computer reports the code number assigned to the matching file entry. If there is no match, then the user is prompted to enter another morphologic diagnosis or topography. It is our experience that most pathologists regard this form of coding as `manual' coding, since the pathologist must manually re-enter the specimen source and final microscopic diagnoses for every specimen. This system is faster than searching for diagnoses in the SNOMED books, but is not as fast as having the computer extract codes from the free text report. We use the term `automatic coding' to describe systems in which the computer does all of the work of coding, with no user interaction.

Confusion with these aspects of SNOMED coding is reflected in the complex strategy that we finally settled upon for comparing manual coding to results of the autocoder. First, we assembled a list of `minor diagnoses', such as `M09450 NO EVIDENCE OF MALIGNANCY', which were not required to find a match among the autocoder diagnoses. Second, a list of near-synonyms was assembled, such as `M81400 ADENOMA' near-synonym for `M82110 TUBULAR ADENOMA', in which the manual coding was considered matched if its near-synonym appeared among the autocoder diagnoses. Third, a match was only required in the first three digits of the SNOMED-code, so that, say, `M72000 HYPERPLASIA' was considered a match for `M72400 HYPERPLASIA, GLANDULAR AND STROMAL'. Finally, we found it necessary to have a `dictionary policeman', who reviewed all new encounters with previously unused phrases occurring in our natural language text file, and pointed these phrases to appropriate SNOMED codes. Without these conditions, the performance of the autocoder would have been appreciably worse. This experience suggests that many departments which employ autocoders will have significant deterioration in performance, unless the autocoders are continually updated.

Remarkably, this automatic SNOMED coding strategy resulted in only 0.5% missed major SNOMED codes by the autocoder as compared to the spell-corrected manual codes. The missed major codes were the result of complex syntax in the source text stream, which would require a sophisticated parsing algorithm [5]. This result suggests that perfect orthography in the source text and vigilant dictionary maintenance are sufficient to achieve highly accurate coding. Complex parsing algorithms, available in computer translators such as TRANSOFT, could not be expected to increase coding accuracy to an appreciable extent.

Currently, coding in pathology departments is done primarily so that reports of a certain lesion or location can be recovered by the pathologist. In the near future, coding activities may relate more closely to broader questions of regional, national, and international importance. Once uses of coded reports become prioritized, and an optimal coding dictionary can be chosen. Additionally, coding algorithms can be designed to minimize errors based on the intended uses of the codes.

REFERENCES

1. Hall PA, Lemoine NR. Comparison of manual data coding errors in two hospitals. J Clin Pathol 1986;39:622-626.
2. College of American Pathologists. Systematized nomenclature of medicine (SNOMED), College of American Pathologists, Skokie, 1976
3. Cote RA, Robboy S. Progress in Medical Information Management: systematized nomenclature of medicine (SNOMED). JAMA 1980; 243:756-762.
4. Moore GW, Berman JJ: Performance analysis of manual and automated systematized nomenclature of medicine (SNOMED) coding. Am J Clin Pathol 1994; 101:253-256.
5. Moore GW, Wakai I, Satomura Y, Giere W. TRANSOFT: Medical translation expert system. Artif Intell Med 1989;1:149-157.
6. Moore GW, Berman JJ. Object-oriented English-to-SNOMED translator using TRANSOFT+HyperPAD. 15th Annual Symposium on Computer Applications in Medical care. 1991; 15:973-975, Washington, DC.
7. TRANSOFT source code (in the M language, ISO standard 11456) may be obtained through anonymous ftp at nctucca.edu.tw, pathname /misc/medicine/transoft, filename trs.zip. Fax inquiries to: 1-410-433-6324.
8. Davis RG: FileMan: A User Manual. National Association of VA Physicians, Bethesda, 1987.
9. Woods W: Transition network grammars for natural language analysis. Commun Assn Comp Mach 1970;13:591-606.
10. Moore GW, Miller RE and Hutchins GM. Indexing by MeSH titles of natural language pathology phrases identified on first encounter using the barrier word method. In: Computerized Natural Medical Language Processing for Knowledge Engineering, JR Scherrer, RA Cote and SH Mandil (eds.), Elsevier Science Publishers, North-Holland, pp 29-39, 1989

Automatic Encoding into SNOMED III: A Preliminary Investigation

Naomi Sager [1], Margaret Lyman [2], Ngô Thanh Nhàn [1], Leo J. Tick [2]

[1] Courant Institute of Mathematical Sciences, New York University, New York, NY 10012

[2] New York University Medical Center, New York, NY 10016

ABSTRACT

The Linguistic String Project (LSP) medical language processing (MLP) system converts narrative clinical reports into database tables of patient data. A procedure for mapping the output of the LSP MLP system into SNOMED III codes was developed. Preliminary results and further requirements are discussed.

INTRODUCTION

As part of the movement toward a computer-based patient record, CPR [1] (or electronic medical record system, EMRS [2]), increased attention is being paid to lexical issues: the development of the Unified Medical Language System (UMLS) [3]; the release of a much expanded version of SNOMED (SNOMED International, or SNOMED III) [4] and exploration of its use to represent clinical data [5]; new methods for maintaining controlled vocabularies [6]; integration of medical knowledge bases via an "interlingua" [7]; and the use of medical language processing (MLP) to extract clinical information from free-text patient documents [8, 9, 10], or to automatically index patient documents according to an established code [11, 12].

This paper describes initial work in using the LSP MLP system [10, 13] as the first component of an encoder that produces SNOMED III codes from free-text clinical documents. This activity seemed especially timely in light of AMIA's position paper of April 20, 1993 that named SNOMED III the "Preferred Code System" for Diagnoses (along with ICD9 which it includes); for Symptoms and Findings + Modifiers; for Anatomic location; and for Microbes and etiologies [14].

MANUAL ENCODING IN CPRI EXERCISES

To begin, we examined the results of manual SNOMED III coding that was performed for the Computer-based Patient Record Institute (CPRI) in 2 Exercises, each involving 10 case reports [15]. In the Exercises, Medical Concepts and their instantiations were manually determined from narrative case reports, which were then manually coded into a number of standard terminologies.

It was striking to observe that the medical semantic categories developed by LSP for processing clinical text were extremely similar to the Medical Concepts developed in the Exercises as a step toward manual coding. This is illustrated in Fig.1, where on the left is a list of the Medical Concepts with examples that occurred in the CPRI Exercise 1 data, and on the right the corresponding linguistic categories of the LSP MLP system. For brevity, Medical Concepts with less than 3 occurrences in the Exercise 1 data are not included in Fig. 1; the words fitted reasonably into other Medical Concepts used in the Exercises.

In the CPRI Exercises the path from patient document to code was via Medical Concepts:

Text → Medical Concepts → Coded Text

The similarity of LSP categories to Medical Concepts suggested a similar path for automatic encoding:

Text → LSP MLP System → Coded Text

To explore this possibility, an algorithm was devised (still quite preliminary) to map the output of the LSP MLP system into SNOMED III. We used texts from the CPRI Exercise 1 as input so that the results obtained by the LSP procedure could be compared with the SNOMED III codes that had been assigned manually to the texts as part of the Exercise.

MLP IN THE LSP SYSTEM

Figure 2 shows findings retrieved from the relational database table obtained from the MLP output for one case report (014A) in the CPRI Excercise 1 data. Each row contains one medical fact statement, with the words placed in semantically labeled fields. The SID field contains the sentence identifier. A sentence may contain more than one medical fact statement; the ROW field contains the row number of the medical fact statement within that sentence. The symbol # marks a "break point" between words in a given field that were separated in the sentence. Fields not queried

FIGURE 1 - MEDICAL CONCEPTS AND CORRESPONDING LINGUISTIC CATEGORIES

MEDICAL CONCEPTS (CPRI Exercises)		LINGUISTIC CATEGORIES (LSP dictionary classes, or LSP-computed if starred)	
Diagnosis	*cancer, hypertension, anemia*	DIAG	*adenoma, diabetes, tumor, malaria*
Symptoms	*nausea, diaphoresis, discomfort*	INDIC	*abnormal, cramping, warmth*
Qualitative	*soft, vague, asymmetric, standard*	DESCR	*acinar, inactive, shotty, red*
Qualitative	*tiny shotty, within normal limits*	NORMAL	*uneventful, well, rational*
Anatomy	*thigh, ovary, hop, acetabulum*	PTPART	*decidua, ileum, sacral, ramus*
Topology	*left, superficial, bilaterally*	PTAREA	*adjacent, edge, left, ventral*
Functional Status	*normally active, appetite, oral intake*	PTFUNC	*ambulate, eat, heal, pulse*
Severity	*excessive, severe, markedly*	AMT	*impressive, mild, rare, scant*
Stage	*stage 1C, benign, 2+*	QUANT*	
Grade	*grade 2-3, grade 2, benign*	QUANT*	
Extent	*Clark's level 2, 0/3 lymph nodes*	QUANT*	
Quantitative	*.84 mm, 1.5 cm long, 5-8, 2 units*	QUANT*	
Diagnostic Exam	*Holter monitor, tilt table test,*	TXPROC	*xray, biopsy, scan, ultrasound*
Laboratory Name	*CBC, creatinine, hemoglobin, TIBC*	TXVAR	*acetone, electrolyte, FEP, WBC*
Therapeutic Procedures	*open reduction, pinning, D&C*	TTCHIR	*shunt, wired, ablation, shortened*
Treatments	*darvocet, irradiation, ibuprofen,*	TTMED	*heparin, lasix, immunization*
Treatments	*splint, Pavlik harness*	TTCOMP	*bandage, cane, catheter, mask*
Disposition	*poor prognosis, observation*	TTGEN	*care, admission, workup, visit*
Negation	*negative, without evidence of*	NEG	*absence, never, not, unable*
Reliability	*question of, rule out, possible*	MODAL	*feel, hope, likely, maybe, claim*
Chronicity	*history of, chronic, recurrent*	TMPER	*briefly, persist, sustain, usual*
Time	*nocturnal, four years, recent,*	TMLOC	*childhood, last, earlier, hence*
Time	*present for 2 years duration*	TIME*	
Physical Finding**			
motion limited, positive pivot shifts, skin folds asymmetric, visceromegaly, healing of vaginal cuff, neck supple, bleeding at biopsy site		Physiological function or anatomic site examined + Result	
internal rotation, respirations, heart rate, BP, hip motion, abduction, external rotation, flexion, range of motion, extremities		Physiological function or anatomic site examined	
prominent, nodes, incision, lymphadenopathy, less developed		Result	

* The LSP system recognizes quantitative phrases syntactically, and similarly for time expressions involving quantities (*3 days post op*).

** All examples of Physical Finding are from CPRI data, classed here into 3 groups that correspond to the LSP representation as (1) subject and predicate of a Physical Finding statement type, (2) subject only, (3) predicate only.

in the retrieval of Fig. 2 include treatment, patient management, laboratory findings and neutral descriptors, e.g. RED in sentence 14A.1.08 (Fig. 3).

The language processing causes modifiers that apply to several findings to be "distributed" so that each of the findings carries the modifier (e.g. all the negated findings in Fig. 2). Rows number 6 and 7 of SID=014A.1.02 in Fig. 2 show the effect of an unresolved syntactic ambiguity: SIGMOID CANCER AND HYPERTENSION → SIGMOID CANCER AND [SIGMOID] HYPERTENSION, in the same way as JOINT SWELLING AND REDNESS → JOINT SWELLING AND [JOINT] REDNESS. A knowledge base that identifies body parts in relation to classes of diagnoses and symptoms would resolve the ambiguity in this case.

FIGURE 2 - RETRIEVAL OF POSITIVE AND NEGATIVE FINDINGS FROM CASE 014A SENTENCES 1-20

SID	ROW	SIGN-SYMPTOM OR DIAG	BODY PART OR BODY FUNCTION	QUANT	TIME WORDS
014A.1.01	1	PAINFUL # RASH #	RIGHT # FACIAL # INVOLVING THE EYE		
014A.1.02	3	CORONARY ARTERY DISEASE			A PAST MEDICAL HISTORY
014A.1.02	6	# CANCER #	SIGMOID		A PAST MEDICAL HISTORY
014A.1.02	7	# HYPERTENSION #	SIGMOID		A PAST MEDICAL HISTORY
014A.1.03	1	PAINFUL RASH	DEVELOPED		APPROXIMATELY 6 DAYS P
014A.1.03	2	BLISTERS	ON THE RIGHT SIDE OF HIS FOREHEAD		
014A.1.03	3	REDNESS	ON THE RIGHT SIDE OF HIS FOREHEAD		
014A.1.03	4	REDNESS	ON THE RIGHT SIDE OF HIS # SCALP #		
014A.1.03	5	BLISTERS	ON THE RIGHT SIDE OF HIS # SCALP #		
014A.1.05	2	PAIN			
014A.1.07	1	WORSENED			GRADUALLY # OVER APPRO
014A.1.08	1	WAS SWOLLEN	RIGHT EYE #		
014A.1.08	2	WAS SWOLLEN	SURROUNDING TISSUE #		
014A.1.08	7	DIFFICULTY	VISION		
014A.1.09	2	POOR	INTAKE		
014A.1.10	4	HERPES ZOSTER		V1 DISTRIBUTION	
014A.1.11A	3	CONJUNCTIVITIS		SOME	
014A.1.13	1	HAD WORSENED	EYE		SINCE THEN
014A.1.13	3	PAINFUL	TEARING	INCREASED # VERY #	
014A.1.13	4	SWELLING			
014A.1.16A	2	PAIN			
014A.1.19	2	BE DISORIENTED			
014A.1.19	4	FEBRILE			

SID	ROW	SIGN-SYMPTOM OR DIAG	BODY PART OR BODY FUNCTION	TIME WORDS	NEGATION
014A.1.11B	1	INVOLVEMENT	CORNEAL		NO
014A.1.17	1	ASSOCIATED HEADACHE			NO
014A.1.17	2	ASSOCIATED # LOSS OF CONSCIOUS			NO
014A.1.17	3	ASSOCIATED # INJURY #	HEAD		NO
014A.1.17	4	ASSOCIATED # PAIN #	CHEST		NO
014A.1.17	5	ASSOCIATED # SHORTNESS OF BREATH	CHEST		NO
014A.1.20	1	SHINGLES	EYE	HISTORY	NO
014A.1.20	2	SHINGLES	# TO THE # FACE #	HISTORY	NO
014A.1.20	3	# OTHER INJURIES #	EYE	HISTORY	NO
014A.1.20	4	# OTHER INJURIES #	# TO THE # FACE #	HISTORY	NO

AUTOMATIC ENCODING USING MLP

Figures 3, 4, 5 and 6 contain results of the automatic encoding for sentences 08, 10, 11 and 20 of the text of report 014A. Part A contains the CPRI Exercise 1 data. Part B shows the results of the LSP automatic encoding.

The input to the encoding algorithm consists of the words in a row of the relational database (excluding the TIME field for now). Four types of search are employed. "Full search" constructs a text string of all the words in the row in their order of occurrence in the sentence, and searches SNOMED strings for a complete or partial match. "Field search" does the same for each nonempty field in the row. "Text flow break search" does the same for the substrings within a field (strings set off by break marks "#"). Finally, as a last resort, "Single word search" treats every word individually.

The "best match" is the set of codes that covers the most words in the least number of codes (Wingert strategy [16]). However, by displaying all the non-null results of searches, as is done in Figs. 3-6, including those that cover the same word string by different codings (Fig. 3, Part B, Row 1), the automatic encoder also functions as a means of discovering alternative codings within SNOMED.

DISCUSSION OF PRELIMINARY RESULTS

Because the encoding algorithm is at a preliminary stage of development, no attempt has been made to compare automatic vs. manual codings quantitatively. A fully developed encoder will require auxiliary knowledge about word relations (synonomy, hyponomy, hypernomy), methods for treating inflectional differences (singular/plural, adjective/noun, etc.), analysis of compound medical words into semantic roots [17] and a representation of correspondences (*cardi* ↔ *heart*). This experiment used an ad hoc synonym list for all term equivalences. For some word relations, SNOMED itself, while the target of encoding, is also a tool. Synonomous variants are often included under the same code number. The text word SWOLLEN in Fig. 3 was manually coded to M-02570 Swelling, NOS, the preferred term (class 01). However, 5 other terms with the same numerical code are Bulge, Tumefaction, Tumescence, Swollen, Bulging, having other class numbers. The value of bringing together variants under one code number is seen in Figs. 4 and 6. In Fig. 4 (text sentence 10) we learn of the diagnosis Herpes Zoster (DE-32400), and ten sentences later the report of no history of Shingles (DE-32400).

An important feature of the method used is that each individual medical fact statement within a complex sentence is encoded as a unit. This is especially

FIGURE 3 - ENCODING OUTPUT, SENTENCE 8

014A.1.08 THE RIGHT EYE, PARTICULARLY THE SURROUNDING TISSUE, WAS SWOLLEN, RED, AND TEARING AND HE HAD DIFFICULTY WITH HIS VISION.

A. CPRI Exercise 1 Data
Medical Concept

<Symptoms>	swollen
<Symptoms>	red
<Anatomy>	eye
<Topology>	right
<Symptoms>	difficulty with vision
<Symptoms>	tearing

Manual SNOMED Coding from Medical Concepts

M-02570	01	Swelling, NOS
M-04040	01	Red color
T-AA000	01	Eye, NOS
G-A100	01	Right
DA-74900	02	Decreased vision, NOS
T-AA970	01	Tears

B. Automatic Encoding from MLP Output

Row 1:	T-AA010	01Right eye
	G-A100	01Right
	T-AA000	01Eye, NOS I C69.9
	M-02570	05Swollen
Row 2	G-A125	02Surrounding
	T-D0050	02Tissue, NOS
	M-02570	05Swollen
Row 4:	T-AA010	01Right eye
	T-AA970	01Tears
	G-A100	01Right
	T-AA000	01Eye, NOS I C69.9
Row 6:	T-AA970	01Tears
	G-A125	02Surrounding
	T-D0050	02Tissue, NOS
Row 7:	F-F0000	01Vision, NOS

---

important when a sentence contains both positive and negative findings (Fig. 5).

A final point regarding Fig. 4, where the difference between manual coding and automatic coding for the text *V1 distribution* is striking. Whereas the manual coder recognized that *V1 distribution* referred to the Ophthalmic division of the fifth cranial nerve, SNOMED code T-A8210, the automatic encoder matched the text *V1* with SNOMED V1 under "TNM classification of malignant tumors after operation". Further, the MLP system placed V1 DISTRIBUTION in the QUANT, not BODYPART, field, which only shows that mathematicians and linguists should not be let loose on clinical vocabulary without proper medical supervision.

FIGURE 4 - ENCODING OUTPUT, SENTENCE 10

014A.1.10 HE WAS EVALUATED AT THE EMERGENCY ROOM HERE AND FELT TO HAVE HERPES ZOSTER OF THE V1 DISTRIBUTION .

A. CPRI Exercise 1 Data
Medical Concept

<Diagnosis>	herpes zoster
<Anatomy>	V1 distribution

Manual SNOMED Coding from Medical Concepts

DE-32400	01	Herpes zoster, NOS
T-A8210	02	Ophthalmic division of fifth cranial nerve

B. Automatic Encoding from MLP Output

Row 4:	DE-32400	01Herpes zoster, NOS I (L-36401) I 053.9
	G-F231	01V1

FIGURE 5 -ENCODING OUTPUT - SENTENCE 11

014A.1.11 HE HAD BEEN SEEN BY OPHTHALMOLOGY AND THEY ALSO THOUGHT THAT THERE WAS SOME ASSOCIATED CONJUNCTIVITIS BUT NO CORNEAL INVOLVEMENT .

A. CPRI Exercise 1 Data
Medical Concept

<Diagnosis>	conjunctivitis
<Negation>	no
<Anatomy>	corneal involvement

Manual SNOMED Coding from Medical Concepts

DA-75605	01	Conjunctivitis, NOS
G-A201	01	Negative
G-A658	02	Not involving
T-AA200	01	Cornea, NOS

B. Automatic Encoding from MLP Output

Row 3:	DA-75605	01Conjunctivitis, NOS I 372.30
	G-A606	01Some
Row 1:	G-A657	02Involving
	T-AA200	01Cornea, NOS I C69.1
	G-A201	01Negative

FIGURE 6 - ENCODING OUTPUT, SENTENCE 20

014A.1.20 THE PATIENT HAS NO HISTORY OF SHINGLES OR OTHER INJURIES TO THE EYE OR FACE.

A. CPRI Exercise 1 Data
Medical Concept

<Diagnosis> shingles
<Diagnosis> injuries
<Anatomy> eye
<Anatomy> face
<Negation> no

Manual SNOMED Coding from Medical Concepts

DE-32400	02	Shingles
M-10000	01	Injury, NOS
T-AA000	01	Eye, NOS
T-D1200	01	Face, NOS
G-A201	01	Negative

B. Automatic Encoding from MLP Output

Row 1:	DE-32400	02Shingles I (L-36401) I 053.9
	T-AA000	01Eye, NOS I C69.9
	G-A201	01Negative
Row 2:	DE-32400	02Shingles I (L-36401) I 053.9
	T-D1200	01Face, NOS I C76.0
	G-A201	01Negative
Row 3:	T-AA000	01Eye, NOS I C69.9
	G-A201	01Negative
	G-A609	01Other
	M-10000	01Injury, NOS I 959.-
Row 4:	T-D1200	01Face, NOS I C76.0
	G-A201	01Negative
	G-A609	01Other
	M-10000	01Injury, NOS I 959.-

References

[1] Dick RS, Steen EB, eds. *The Computer-Based Patient Record. An Essential Technology for Health Care.* Wash DC: Nat'l Acad. Press, 1991.

[2] RFA: Applied Research Relevant to an Electronic Medical Record. *NIH Guide for Grants and Contracts*, Vol 23:5, Feb 4, 1994, pp 5-8.

[3] Humphreys BL, Lindberg DAB. The UMLS Project:: a distributed experiment in improving access to biomedical information. North-Holland, Amsterdam: *MEDINFO 1992*;265-8.

[4] Coté RA, Rothwell DJ, Beckette R, Palotay J, eds. *SNOMED International.* Northfield, IL: College of American Pathologists, 1993.

[5] Campbell KE, Das AK, Musen MA. A logical foundation for representation of clinical data. *J Am Med Informatics Assoc.* 1994;1:218-232.

[6] Cimino JJ, Clayton PD, Hripcsak G, Johnson SB. Knowledge-based approaches to the maintenance of a large controlled medical terminology. *JAMIA.* 1994;1:35-50.

[7] Masarie FE, Miller RA, Bouhaddou O, Giuse NB, Warner HR. An Interlingua for electronic interchange of medical information: using frames to map between clinical vocabularies. *Comput Biomed Res* 1991;24:379-400.

[8] Zingmond D, Lenert LA. Monitoring free-text data using medical language processing. *Comput Biomed Res.* 1993;26:467-81.

[9] Friedman C, Alderson PO, Austin JH, Cimino JJ, Johnson SB. A general natural-language text processor for clinical radiology. *JAMIA.* 1994;1:161-74.

[10] Sager N, Lyman M, Bucknall C, Nhàn N, Tick LJ. Natural language processing and the representation of clinical data. *JAMIA.* 1994;1:142-60.

[11] Satomura Y, Do Amaral MB. Automated diagnostic indexing by natural language processing. *Med Inf (Lond)* 1992;17:149-63.

[12] Sager N, Lyman M, Nhàn NT, Tick LJ. Medical Language Processing: Applications to Patient Data Representation and Automatic Encoding. *Meth Inform Med*, to be published.

[13] Sager N, Friedman C, Lyman MS. *Medical Language Processing: Computer Management of Narrative Data.* Addison-Wesley, 1987.

[14] Board of Directors of the American Medical Informatics Association. Position Paper: Standards for Medical Identifiers, Codes and Messages Needed to Create an Efficient Computer-Stored Medical Record. *J Am Med Informatics Assoc.* 1994;1:1-7.

[15] Case histories and concept identification obtained from Computer-based Patient Record Institute (CPRI) exercises presented at *Annual Symposium on Computer Applications in Medical Care*, Wash DC, Nov 1993.

[16] Wingert F. An Indexing System for SNOMED. *Meth Inform Med.* 1986;25:22-30.

[17] Wingert F. Morphologic Analysis of Compound Words. *Meth Inform Med.* 1985; 24:155-62.

Lexical Methods for Managing Variation in Biomedical Terminologies

Alexa T. McCray, Suresh Srinivasan, Allen C. Browne

National Library of Medicine
Bethesda, Maryland

ABSTRACT

Access to biomedical terminologies is hampered by the high degree of variability inherent in natural language terms and in the terminologies themselves. The lexicon, lexical programs, databases, and indexes included with the 1994 release of the UMLS® Knowledge Sources are designed to help users manage this variability. We describe these resources and illustrate their flexibility and usefulness in providing enhanced access to data in the UMLS Metathesaurus®.

INTRODUCTION

There is a great deal of lexical variation in the vocabulary of a natural language. This variation may be rule-governed, or it may be quite idiosyncratic. The variation may be morphological, that is, it relates different forms of the same lexical item through inflection or derivation, or the variation may be simply orthographic, that is, it relates different spellings of the same lexical item. Morphological variation is fairly well understood and is described in several standard references (e.g., [1-3]), and orthographic variation is generally studied either from the point of view of spelling errors or from the point of view of variant spellings in particular dialects [4-6].

The development of methods for capturing lexical variation in computerized systems is, however, a difficult problem because of the wide range of possible variations and the possibility for seemingly unconstrained combinations of these variations. The development of so-called stemming algorithms and spelling error detection algorithms has been the subject of some research (see, for example, [7-8]).

The availability of the UMLS knowledge sources [9], and especially its Metathesaurus, has led to a number of experiments involving automated lexical matching methods, either as part of the development process [10], or for the purpose of comparing the Metathesaurus content with some other vocabulary (e.g., [11-12]), or in order to identify Metathesaurus concepts in free text (e.g., [13]). Each of these experiments has used lexical methods that have some similarity to the others, but that also differ in a variety of ways.

The 1994 release of the UMLS knowledge sources includes a fourth knowledge source, the SPECIALIST™ lexicon, together with a set of lexical programs. The lexicon has been developed in the context of the authors' work in biomedical language processing [14]. The lexical programs generate a range of variations for English lexical items and should be useful for recognizing and thereby abstracting away from lexical variation in biomedical terminologies and texts.

SPECIALIST LEXICON

The SPECIALIST lexicon is an English language lexicon containing many biomedical terms. The lexicon entry for each word or term records syntactic, morphological, and orthographic information. Lexical entries may be single or multi-word terms. Entries which share their base form and spelling variants, if any, are collected into a single lexical record. The base form is the uninflected form of the lexical item; the singular form in the case of a noun, the infinitive form in the case of a verb, and the positive form in the case of an adjective or adverb. Currently the lexicon contains some 60,000 records, with approximately 120,000 forms. Lexical information includes syntactic category, inflectional variation (e.g., singular and plural for nouns, the conjugations of verbs, the positive, comparative, and superlative for adjectives and adverbs), and allowable complementation patterns (i.e., the objects and other arguments that verbs, nouns, and adjectives can take).

Lexical items are selected for coding from a variety of sources. These include data from MEDLINE® citation records, terms in the Dorland's Illustrated Medical dictionary, the 10,000 most frequent words listed in the American Heritage Word Frequency book and the 2,000 lexical items used in the controlled definitions of Longman's Dictionary of Contemporary

English. Lexical records are created using a lexicon building tool called Lextool. Lextool is a menu based system that accepts as input either a file of lexical items or lexical items entered at the keyboard. Lextool is supported by an underlying lexical grammar that constrains the information that can be entered for lexical items of a particular syntactic category and also serves to validate the information that has been encoded. A variety of reference sources is used in coding the lexical records. These include dictionaries of general English (primarily learner's dictionaries), medical dictionaries, and data derived from actual usage of the lexical items in MEDLINE.

The SPECIALIST lexicon is distributed in both unit record and relational table format. The unit record format is a frame structure consisting of slots and fillers. The slots are the basic lexical attributes, such as syntactic category, variants, complements, etc. The fillers express the possible values of those attributes for that particular lexical item. The relational table format expresses the same information in ten tables. These tables have been created so as to maximize their usefulness for different types of applications. For example, there is one table that contains only agreement and inflection information, another for complementation patterns, a table for spelling variants, and another table for abbreviations and acronyms and their fully expanded forms.

The lexicon is also available for lookup and browsing on a World Wide Web server. The URL for the server is http://wwwetb.nlm.nih.gov/. The lexicon can be found under the Information Technologies/Natural Language Systems Program menu items.

LEXICAL PROGRAMS

The lexical variant programs are written in C and use data from the SPECIALIST lexicon as they compute the different forms of lexical items. The lexical programs consist of several different modules that can be combined in a variety of ways to generate variants. For example, users may be interested in seeing only the singular or plural of an input term. In that case, they would choose the inflection option. Or, they may be interested in running their terms against a stop word list and also ignoring word order so as to maximize their chances of finding related terms in a particular vocabulary or text. In this case, they would choose the stopword removal and word sorting options.

The programs allow for a good deal of flexibility in matching one term to another. The basic principle that is involved in using the programs is that any manipulation of a (source) input term or terms must involve the same manipulation of the target terms. For example, if users want to see if terms in their particular vocabulary (source) are found in the Metathesaurus (target), and if they want to find those terms regardless of whether they appear there in the singular or plural or whether they are in upper or lower case, then they would transform the source vocabulary using the lowercasing and inflectional options and, importantly, they would do the same for the Metathesaurus terminology.

Normalization Routines

Since some users will prefer to use a method that does not involve additional processing of the Metathesaurus data, a normalization program ("norm") together with a normalized string index of all Metathesaurus terminology is included with the UMLS Knowledge Sources. The norm program is essentially one set of lexical variant options. The normalization process involves splitting a string into its constituent words, lower-casing each word, converting each word to its base form, ignoring punctuation, and sorting the words in a multi-word term into alphabetic order. This means that when matching a normalized string in a source vocabulary to the Metathesaurus normalized string index, alphabetic case, inflectional variation, punctuation, and word order are ignored in the comparison.

Some examples of the normalization process using the 1994 Metathesaurus terminology as the target vocabulary and a list of terms provided by J. Vries as the source vocabulary are discussed below. The source vocabulary terms are from the University of Pittsburgh MARS system (see [15] for some discussion of this system), and originally did not readily map to Metathesaurus terms. The examples serve to illustrate the normalization process.

The source term "abdominal binder" does not exist in that exact form in the Metathesaurus. The two forms "Binders, Abdominal" and "Abdominal Binders" do, however, exist. The normalized index entry for both of these forms is "abdominal binder", and, thus, the term is found. The source term "battery" maps to the term "Batteries" in the Metathesaurus because "battery" is the normalized form of the Metathesaurus term. And, "eye-patch" maps to the terms "Patches, Eye", and "Eye Patches" because all are normalized to "eye patch". In these cases, the general English inflectional pluralization rules (add "s", convert "y" to "ies", and add "es" to words ending in "ch, sh, s, or x") have been recognized as part of the normalization process. In addition, word order and alphabetic case have been ignored.

The following two examples illustrate that the normalization routines recognize Greco-Latin inflectional variation. The source term "nasal cannula" is not found in the Metathesaurus, but its plural "Cannulae, Nasal" is found and is mapped through normalization to "nasal cannula". The source term "elbow prosthesis" maps to "Prostheses, Elbow" through normalization. Irregular plurals are also handled by the normalizer, if the information is stored in the SPECIALIST lexicon. This allows the source term "gamma knife" to map to the Metathesaurus term "Gamma Knives". The source term "blood type" is also not found in the Metathesaurus, but its inflectional variant "Blood Typing" is found through normalization.

Some examples of word order variation are shown in the next two examples. As noted above, the normalization routines ignore word order in multi-word terms, since they alphabetize the words in source and target terms. The normalized form of the source term "introducer catheter" is "catheter introducer", as are the normalized forms of the Metathesaurus terms to which it maps: "Catheter Introducers" and Introducers, Catheter". Ignoring word order may in some cases lead to the well-known "venetian blind", "blind venetian" phenomenon. That is, if two terms that vary only with regard to word order and that have different meanings do exist in the target vocabularly, both will be retrieved through the normalization routines. When using the normalization routines in unconstrained contexts, such as free text, it is wise to review the results for cases where concepts might fall together. Review of the Metathesaurus terminology, however, has yielded very few of these types of examples. Since word order is highly variable in the Metathesaurus vocabularies, there appears to be significant benefit in abstracting away from it.

The source term "meckel diverticulectomy" does not exist in that form in the Metathesaurus, but two genitive (possessive) forms do: "Diverticulectomy, Meckel's" and "Meckel's diverticulectomy". In this case, ignoring punctuation and ignoring sequences smaller than two characters (i.e., "s") give the normalized form "diverticulectomy meckel" for both source and target terms. The option "remove genitive markers" of the lexical variant generation programs, which will be discussed below, would give the same result.

With the 1993 release of the UMLS knowledge sources, an index of all the words in the Metathesaurus was provided. The 1994 release again contains a word index, and it also contains a normalized word index in which all the words have been normalized according to the routines discussed above. In some cases, use of the normalized word index will provide additional terminology of interest. For example, if the user were interested in finding all terms in the Metathesaurus that include the word "suture", using the simple word index would yield the following, among others: "Suture", "Closure by suture", "Cranial Suture", "Suture granuloma", "Suture Technic", and "suture line care". The use of the normalized word index would yield all those terms as well as terms such as the following: "Suturing" and "Congenital ossification of sutures", since "suturing" and "sutures" are both normalized to "suture".

Lexical Variant Generation

In some cases, the normalization routines may not give the desired results. This may be because the source vocabulary or text has certain characteristics that are not accounted for by normalization, or it may be because the user would like to be more "aggressive" in the matching routines (that is, by accepting greater variation, with the hope that there will be some correct matches). In this case, the user may decide to use some of the other options that are provided as part of the lexical variant generation (lvg) programs. For example, the lvg stopword option removes highly frequent common words such as "of, and, with, for, in, by", etc. Using this option together with the word order option would, for example, match the term "splenic artery aneurysm" to the Metathesaurus term "Aneurysm of splenic artery".

Use of the lvg derivational morphology module allows the user to find closely related terms that may not have the same syntactic category, but that are usefully related nonetheless. For example, if the source vocabulary or text includes the adjective "hyperplastic", using the derivational option will map this to the noun "Hyperplasia", which is a Metathesaurus term. Nominalizations (noun forms of verbs or adjectives) are prevalent in the biomedical vocabulary. Often a medical dictionary will list only the nominalization and will not list the verb or adjective form. When mapping terms from free text to the Metathesaurus, it might prove fruitful to use the derivational module of lvg to identify such variants. For example, verbs such as "aspirate", "consume", and "deceive" would map to the nominalized Metathesaurus terms "Aspiration", "Consumption", and "Deception", respectively. Analogously, the adjectives "bacterial", "endometrial", and "ganglial" would map to the Metathesaurus nouns "Bacteria", "Endometrium", and "Ganglia", respectively.

The morphology modules of lvg are based on a rule and fact paradigm designed to capture the morphological relations between terms. Rather than analyzing words into morphemes and describing morphological relations in terms of morphemes and their meanings, the program captures common morphological relations. Derivational and inflectional morphology are both handled by a set of rules (with any exceptions noted) and associated facts. Derivational morphology deals with the alternations between lexical items that often involve a change in syntactic category, or part of speech. For example, "malaria" and "malarial" are related through derivational morphology. "Malarial" is the adjectival form of the noun "malaria". This relationship is captured in the form of a heuristic rule stating that nouns ending in "-a" often correspond to adjectives ending in "-al". Rules are recorded in a relational format of the form: "suffix 1| syntactic category 1| suffix 2| syntactic category 2". This rule states that a term of syntactic category 1 ending in suffix 1, may be morphologically related to another term of syntactic category 2 ending in suffix 2. The rule for "malarial" and "malaria" has the form: "al|adj|a|noun". Rules are symmetric, e.g., "al|adj|a|noun" is equivalent to "a|noun|al|adj". Derivational variation is rule-governed to some extent, but some alternations are more productive than others. The effectiveness of these rules is increased by recording for each rule a list of known exceptions. For example, "aura" and "aural" are not related (they mean different things) and are, therefore listed as known exceptions to the rule "al|adj|a|noun". Exceptions to rules have been discovered empirically by comparing words from various machine readable sources, including the Unix system dictionary, Dorland's Illustrated Medical Dictionary, and the Oxford Advanced Learner's Dictionary.

Not all instances of derivationally related words are productive enough to be usefully stated as rules. Particular instances of morphologically related words are recorded as facts in a similar format to the rules. Examples of facts used by the derivational module are: the adjective "presidential" related to the noun "president", the adjective "tyrosinate" related to the noun "tyrosine", and the noun "column" related to the adjective "columnar".

The inflectional rules and facts are similar to the derivational rules and facts with appropriate changes. For example, nouns ending in "us" often have plurals in "i" as in "focus" and "foci". This inflectional fact is also recorded in terms of a heuristic rule stating that singular nouns ending in "us" may have plurals ending in "i". This rule is like the derivational rules discussed above except that an additional field indicates the inflection that the suffix signals. Most of the inflectional rules are derived from the inflectional classes used by the SPECIALIST lexicon. The rule just mentioned is part of the Greco-Latin (glreg) inflectional class in the lexicon. Just as with derivational rules, known exceptions may be listed with the rule.

LEXICAL DATABASES

Three databases that may be useful for some developers have also been provided. The first (dm.db) is a file that contains some 10,000 pairs of known derivational variants. The rules and facts used by the derivational morphology module have been drawn from this file. The file relates pairs of words that are derivationally related and gives their syntactic categories. Sample terms that are listed there are:

pharyngeal (adj)|pharynx (noun)
disabled (adj)|disability (noun)
comply (verb)|compliance (noun)
blastogenic (adj)|blastogenesis (noun)
transparent (adj)|transparency (noun)
dosage (noun)|dose (noun)

A second database of closely related terms that mean the same thing, but may sometimes differ in syntactic category is provided in the sm.db file. These closely related terms, currently approximately 2,500 pairs, have been drawn from a variety of sources including medical dictionaries and may or may not be represented in the Metathesaurus. If one of the terms in the pair is in the Metathesaurus, but the other is not, then this file may serve to provide additional entry points into that knowledge source. Some examples from the file are:

false paralysis (noun)|pseudoparalysis (noun)
asphyxiation (noun)|suffocation (noun)
ablate (verb)|remove (verb)
pneumal (adj)|lungs (noun)

hepatocellular (adj)|liver cells (noun)
nasal (adj)|nose (noun)
digital (adj) / finger (noun)

The third database contains about 4,000 pairs of spelling variants. These have been extracted from the SPECIALIST lexicon. These may also serve as additional entry points into the Metathesaurus if one of the items in the pair is in the Metathesaurus, but the other is not. Some examples from the file (sp.db) are:

linoleic acid (noun)|linolic acid (noun)
amebicidal (adj)|amebacidal (adj)
leukocyte (noun)|leucocyte (noun)
haematocrit (noun)|hematocrit (noun)
nanogramme (noun)|nanogram (noun)
fibre (noun)|fiber (noun)

CONCLUSION

The lexical methods described above offer a variety of techniques for the management of lexical variation in biomedical terminologies and texts. The indexes provide standard ways to access the UMLS Metathesaurus, and the lexical programs and databases provide users with the flexibility to design their own access methods. Future releases of the UMLS knowledge sources should involve growth and improvement of these resources, particularly as they are used in a variety of applications.

REFERENCES

1. Bauer L. English Word Formation. Cambridge: Cambridge University Press, 1983; 311 pages.

2. Marchand H. The Categories and Types of Present-Day English Word-Formation. Munich: C.H. Beck, 1969; 545 pages.

3. Quirk R, Greenbaum S, Leech G, Svartvik J. A Comprehensive Grammar of the English Language. London: Longman Group Limited, 1985; 1515-1585.

4. Benson M, Benson E, Ilson R. Lexicographic Description of English. Studies in Language Companion Series, 1986; Volume 14:14-18,169-174.

5. Emery DW. Variant Spellings in Modern American Dictionaries. National Council of Teachers of English, 1973; 130 pages.

6. Dirckx JH. The Language of Medicine, its Evolution, Structure, and Dynamics. Hagerstown: Harper & Row Publishers, 1976; 170 pages.

7. Peterson JL. Computer programs for detecting and correcting spelling errors. Communications of the ACM 1980;23(12):676-687.

8. Porter MF. An algorithm for suffix stripping. Programming 1980;14:130-137.

9. Lindberg DAB, Humphreys BL, McCray AT. The Unified Medical Language System. Methods of Information in Medicine 1993;32:281-91.

10. Sherertz DD, Tuttle MS, Blois MS, Erlbaum MS. Intervocabulary mapping within the UMLS: the role of lexical matching. In: Greenes RA, ed. Proceedings of the 12th annual symposium on computer applications in medical care. Los Angeles: IEEE Computer Society, 1988;201-206.

11. Huff SM, Warner HR. A comparison of Meta-1 and HELP terms: Implications for clinical data. In: Miller RA, ed. Proceedings of the 14th annual symposium on computer applications in medical care. Los Angeles: IEEE Computer Society, 1990;166-169.

12. Cimino JJ. Representation of Clinical Laboratory Terminology in the Unified Medical Language System. In: Clayton PD, ed. Proceedings of the 15th annual symposium on computer applications in medical care. New York: McGraw Hill, 1991;199-203.

13. Miller RA, Gieszczykiewicz FM, Vries JK, Cooper GF. CHARTLINE: Providing bibliographic references relevant to patient charts using the UMLS Metathesaurus knowledge sources. In: Frisse ME, ed. Proceedings of the 16th annual symposium on computer applications in medical care. New York: McGraw Hill, 1992;86-90.

14. McCray AT, Sponsler JL, Brylawski B, Browne AC. The role of lexical knowledge in biomedical text understanding. In: Stead W, ed. Proceedings of the 11th annual symposium on computer applications in medical care. Los Angeles: IEEE Computer Society Press, 1987;103-107.

15. Vries JK, Marshalek B, D'Abarno JC, Yount RJ, Dunner LL. An automated indexing system utilizing semantic net expansion. Computers and Biomedical Research 1992; 25:153-167.

Ambiguity Resolution while Mapping Free Text to the UMLS Metathesaurus

Thomas C. Rindflesch and Alan R. Aronson
National Library of Medicine
Bethesda, MD 20894

We propose a method for resolving ambiguities encountered when mapping free text to the UMLS® Metathesaurus.® Much of the research in medical informatics involves the manipulation of free text. The Metathesaurus contains extensive information which supports solutions to problems encountered while processing such text. After discussing the process of mapping free text to the Metathesaurus and describing the ambiguities which are often the result of such mapping, we provide examples of rules designed to eliminate mapping ambiguities. These rules refer to the context in which the ambiguity occurs and crucially depend on semantic types obtained from the Metathesaurus. We have conducted a preliminary test of the methodology and the results obtained indicate that the rules successfully resolve ambiguity around 80% of the time.

INTRODUCTION

As automated methods in medical informatics mature, researchers are increasingly addressing the problems inherent in manipulating free text. Due to the complexity of natural language, such processing poses a particular challenge to system developers. The Unified Medical Language System® (UMLS) ([1]) provides extensive support for processing natural language.

Several studies ([2], [3], and [4], for example) discuss projects which exploit the UMLS Metathesaurus in natural language processing. In addition to its value for such research, [1] summarizes research using UMLS for a variety of purposes involving the manipulation of text, including information retrieval, indexing, and data creation applications.

In order to effectively use the information contained in the 4th (1993) Experimental Edition of the Metathesaurus it is first necessary to map the text being processed to Metathesaurus concepts. Many researchers have proposed various methods for such mapping. (The early projects map to the MeSH® vocabulary, but the principles involved are identical to those involved in mapping to the Metathesaurus.) Some examples are [5] (mapping to MeSH), [6] (mapping to MeSH), [7], [8], [9], [10], [11], and [12].

Regardless of the method used for mapping to the Metathesaurus, ambiguous mappings result. Such mappings, which occur when a text phrase maps correctly to more than one Metathesaurus concept, have to be resolved before further processing can be reliably pursued. In this paper, after discussing the process of mapping free text to Metathesaurus concepts and elucidating the resulting ambiguity, we describe a pilot study which investigates an approach to resolving such ambiguity.

MAPPING PHRASES IN FREE TEXT TO THE UMLS METATHESAURUS

An example of a general and robust algorithm for mapping to a controlled vocabulary is described in [6]. This algorithm has a number of characteristics which ensure that the concepts identified accurately represent the source text. The algorithm first identifies noun phrases in the input text and then maps to concepts within each noun phrase. It further produces morphological variants, and deals with various kinds of partial matches, including permutation of words, synonymy, intervening unimportant words, partial matches, and complex matches.

We have developed a program for mapping free text to the Metathesaurus which has most of the desirable characteristics found in [6], but which differs considerably in implementation and in our treatment of partial and complex matches. Our program, which is described in more detail in [4], first identifies simple noun phrases in free text. This syntactic analysis relies on the SPECIALIST lexicon ([13]) and the Xerox Part-of-Speech Tagger ([14]). The following examples demonstrate the crucial characteristics of our mapping program as it identifies Metathesaurus concepts for each noun phrase.

We employ intensive variant generation, which, in addition to accommodating purely string-based variants, such as upper and lower case distinctions and inflectional variants, establishes a relationship between variants based on derivational morphology, synonymy, and abbreviation. For example, although the term *renal transplant* does not occur in the Metathesaurus, our variant generation determines that *renal* is a synonym of *kidney* and thus the text *renal transplant* maps to the Metathesaurus term "KIDNEY TRANSPLANT", one of the terms for the concept "Kidney Transplantation". Similarly, *thermogram* is not in the Metathesaurus; however, morphological variant generation allows this term to map to "Thermography". Finally, our treatment of abbreviations and acronyms allows us to map *ICU* to "Intensive Care Unit".

We also allow complex matches, in which more than one Metathesaurus concept represents the text of a noun phrase. For example, the noun phrase in (1a) maps to the Metathesaurus concepts (1b) and (1c).

(1) a. digoxin overdose

b. "Digoxin"

c. "Overdose"

It should be noted that the mapping algorithm does not itself specify the relationship between the Metathesaurus concepts in a complex match; further processing is required to determine the relationship between concepts in complex matches.

For those cases in which only part of the noun phrase has a mapping to the Metathesaurus, we distinguish between instances in which the head is involved in mapping (2), and those in which it is not (3). (The head of a noun phrase is the rightmost noun in the structure.)

(2) a. liquid crystal thermography

b. "Thermography"

(3) a. cochlear implant subjects

b. "Cochlear Implant"

A further sub-type of partial match involves a mapping to Metathesaurus concepts which do not contiguously cover the text of the noun phrase, as in (4).

(4) a. adjuvant-induced arthritis

b. "Arthritis, Adjuvant"

(5) illustrates the problem of ambiguous terms in the Metathesaurus. The noun phrase in (5a) has a complete mapping to the Metathesaurus as indicated in (5b-d). However, *dialysis* maps to the two concepts shown, where the corresponding semantic types are given in brackets to indicate the two meanings of *dialysis*.

(5) a. lymph dialysis

b. "Lymph"

c. "Dialysis <1>" ['Natural Phenomenon or Process']

d. "Dialysis <2>" ['Therapeutic or Preventive Procedure']

AMBIGUOUS MAPPINGS

Regardless of the effectiveness of the algorithm employed for mapping free text to concepts in the Metathesaurus, ambiguities will result. Ambiguous mappings to the Metathesaurus fall into two general categories: those caused by variant generation (this may be due to morphological variants, synonyms, or abbreviations), and those caused by ambiguity inherent in a Metathesaurus concept itself, as illustrated in (5) above.

With regard to variant generation, morphology together with synonymy conspire to produce multiple mappings which must be resolved in a particular context. For example, these phenomena cause the word *fundamental* to map infelicitously to the Metathesaurus concepts "Foundation" (with semantic type 'Organization') and "base" (with semantic type "Inorganic Chemical"). Abbreviations cause particular problems due to the fact that they often have several expansions, none of which are semantically related to each other. For example, the single letter *c* matches Metathesaurus concepts including: "Carbon", "Complement", Cytidine", and "Cytosine".

Ambiguous words and phrases are distinguished in the Metathesaurus either by integers in angled brackets or by a note in parentheses. The ambiguous word *dialysis,* for example, is represented by the preferred term "Dialysis <1>", which has semantic type 'Natural Phenomenon or Process' and by the preferred term "Dialysis <2>", which has semantic type 'Therapeutic or Preventive Procedure'. *Inhibition* is represented as "Inhibition (Psychology)" with semantic type 'Mental Process' and as "Inhibition <2>" with semantic type 'Molecular Function'.

Ambiguities, of whatever type, have to be resolved if the Metathesaurus concepts obtained by the mapping algorithm are to accurately support further processing of the input text. We have decided to first address the type of ambiguity which is due to ambiguous concepts in the Metathesaurus itself. The technique being developed can then serve as the basis for resolving ambiguity due to variant generation. (Also see [2] for an example of ambiguity resolution in the context of a natural language processing system.)

AMBIGUITY RESOLUTION

The type of ambiguity exemplified by ambiguous Metathesaurus concepts is often referred to as word sense ambiguity. The general principle which supports the resolution of this ambiguity is the notion that a particular sense of a term occurs in a definable textual context. Beginning with [15] a number of researchers in computational linguistics have proposed various systems for exploiting contextual information for the purposes of word sense disambiguation (for example [16], [17], and [18]). We would like to take advantage of the insights these systems offer with regard to the general approach to word sense disambiguation, especially with regard to what kinds of information can contribute to the disambiguation and the general ways in which this information can be exploited.

A further consideration is how much context has to be specified for effective ambiguity resolution. That is, the context might be the sentence in which the word occurs, or it might be the paragraph, or it might be some larger text unit, for example the entire document in which the ambiguous term occurs.

As a pilot study, we have implemented a word sense disambiguation algorithm in a Prolog program and have tested it on the NLM Test Collection ([19]). Our system has been influenced in particular by [18]; however, in this prototype system, we limit the context used for disambiguation to that occurring in the sentence in which the ambiguous term occurs. Within this context, the rules which resolve ambiguity may refer either to the presence of patterns of particular words or to patterns of UMLS semantic types associated with the Metathesaurus concepts which constitute the mapping of the sentence in which the ambiguous term occurs. Either of these pattern types may be defined as occurring in a particular syntactic structure. In the discussion that follows we provide examples of the process of ambiguity resolution using partial, informal statements of the rules involved.

The disambiguation process is driven by rules which are associated with semantic types. Each semantic type has associated with it a disambiguation rule which specifies the evidence that supports selection of this semantic type. Upon selection of a semantic type, ambiguity is resolved in that the Metathesaurus concept associated with that type is selected and the other candidates are rejected. An important characteristic of the entire approach is that it is probabilistic; the successful application of a rule in favor of a particular semantic type indicates that there is a certain likelihood that the ambiguity should be resolved in favor of that semantic type, but the determination is not categorical.

As an example of the application of the disambiguation rules first note that *immunology* ambiguously maps to the Metathesaurus concepts shown in (6).

(6) a. "immunology <1>" ['Biologic Function']

b. "Immunology <2>" ['Biomedical Occupation or Discipline']

c. "Immunology <3>" ['Laboratory Procedure']

One of the rules for the semantic type 'Laboratory Procedure' is:

(7) Evidence in favor of 'Laboratory Procedure':

One of the following list of words occurs to the right of the ambiguous concept: classify, indicate, procedure, reveal, show, analysis, experiment, finding, method, technique.

In the text given in (8), rule (7) applies to select semantic type 'Laboratory Procedure' and its associated concept "Immunology <3>" since the word *analysis* follows the word in the text which is involved in the mapping ambiguity. (In this and the following examples, the textual material which is involved in a mapping ambiguity is underlined, and the textual context which contributes to the resolution of the ambiguity is given in bold type.)

(8) Immunological **analysis** of the released fibronectin indicated that LTA was the only surface component which could be detected as a soluble complex with the released fibronectin.

The following rule describes some of the evidence which supports selection of the type 'Biologic Function'. (Reference to a semantic type in a rule is to be interpreted as also referring to all the children of that semantic type in the UMLS Semantic Network.)

(9) Evidence in favor of 'Biologic Function':

A prepositional phrase occurs to the right of the ambiguous concept, the preposition is *in* or *of*, and the head of the object of the preposition maps to a concept which has the semantic types 'Plant' or 'Animal'. The prepositional phrase occurs "close" to the ambiguous concept but need not be immediately contiguous.

OR

A phrase which maps to a concept having the semantic type 'Disease or Syndrome' occurs to the right of the ambiguous concept.

In the following examples, rule (9) chooses the correct mapping for *immunology.* In both (10) and (11) this is the concept "immunology <1>", which has the semantic type 'Biologic Function'. In (10) the ambiguous term is followed by one which has the semantic type 'Animal'. In (11) the contextual evidence supporting selection of 'Biologic Function' is a term having the semantic type 'Disease or Syndrome'.

(10) The immunological responses **of owl monkeys** to L. b. panamensis were similar in many respects to those observed in humans with localized cutaneous leishmaniasis.

(11) This nonhuman primate model should be useful for future studies involving the immunology and chemotherapy of **cutaneous leishmaniasis**.

There is a general principle that if the evidence which could support a particular semantic type does not in fact occur in the text, then that semantic type is disfavored and the alternatives are favored. *Imipramine* (as shown in (12)) is one of the Metathesaurus terms which belong to the ambiguity class having one semantic type 'Laboratory Procedure', and one or more additional semantic types which are children of 'Substance' in the Semantic Network.

(12) a. "Imipramine <1>" ['Organic Chemical', 'Pharmacologic Substance']

b. "Imipramine <2>" ['Laboratory Procedure']

In examples (13) and (14), although the rule for 'Laboratory Procedure' has a chance to apply (since that semantic type occurs associated with one of the possible mappings), there is no evidence to support selection of 'Laboratory Procedure'. Thus, this semantic type is eliminated in favor of the alternative semantic types ('Organic Chemical' and 'Pharmacologic Substance') and "Imipramine <1>" is selected to resolve the ambiguity.

(13) Moreover, imipramine, an inhibitor of protein kinase C, had little effect.

(14) Fluoxetine has overall therapeutic efficacy comparable with imipramine, amitriptyline and doxepin in patients with unipolar depression treated for 5 to 6 weeks, although it may be less effective than tricyclic antidepressants in relieving sleep disorders in depressed patients.

Additional rules might enhance the evidence in support of either 'Organic Chemical' or 'Pharmacologic Substance' but could not contradict the elimination of 'Laboratory Procedure'. Alternatively, after the elimination of 'Laboratory Procedure', it could be the case that there is also no evidence to support either 'Organic Chemical' or 'Pharmacologic Substance'. In such a case the ambiguity must be left unresolved.

TESTING THE METHODOLOGY

In order to determine the viability of our general approach to ambiguity resolution, we conducted a pilot study limited to instances of *immunology* in the NLM Test Collection. We extracted 110 sentences containing instances of morphological variants of *immunology.* As noted above *immunology* maps ambiguously to three Metathesaurus concepts, which have semantic types 'Biologic Function' ("Immunology <1>"), 'Biomedical Occupation or Discipline' ("Immunology <2>"), and 'Laboratory Procedure' ("Immunology <3>"). This experiment thus tests the viability of the rules relevant to these three semantic types.

Our disambiguation rules resolved 86 of the 110 instances correctly (78.2%). The program resolved *immunology* to 'Biologic Function' ("Immunology <1>") 95 times, 75 of which were correct (78.9%). Four instances were resolved to 'Biomedical Occupation or Discipline' ("Immunology <2>"), two of which were correct; and eleven instances were resolved to 'Laboratory Procedure' ("Immunology <3>"), nine of which were correct (81.8%).

CONCLUSION

In conclusion, we would like to suggest that the methodology for ambiguity resolution which we propose can make a significant contribution to increased precision in an information retrieval system. Additional research which we have recently conducted supports this conclusion. As noted earlier this methodology is part of a general algorithm for mapping free text to the UMLS Metathesaurus. In [20] we describe an experiment to test our general mapping algorithm with regard to retrieval effectiveness.

In that study we report that our mapping algorithm chooses the correct Metathesaurus concept around 90% of the time, without word sense disambiguation. Document retrieval conducted on the basis of that mapping resulted in about 60% average precision.

Since incorrect mappings detract from precision and since a significant number of the incorrect mappings are due to ambiguity, resolving ambiguity will contribute to increased precision. Given that the work described in this paper suggests that our method for resolving ambiguous mappings is effective around 80% of the time, we feel that this method shows considerable promise for continued research aimed at increasing precision in information retrieval systems.

References

1. Lindberg DAB, Humphreys BL and McCray AT. "The Unified Medical Language System." *Methods of Information in Medicine* 32:281-291, 1993.

2. Johnson SB, Aguirre A, Peng P and Cimino J. "Interpreting natural language queries using the UMLS." In Safran C (ed.) *Proceedings of the 17th Annual SCAMC*, 294-298, 1993.

3. McCray AT, Aronson AR, Browne AC, Rindflesch TC, Razi A and Srinivasan S. "UMLS knowledge for biomedical language processing." *Bulletin of the Medical Library Association* 81:184-194.

4. Rindflesch TC and Aronson AR. "Semantic processing in information retrieval." In Safran C (ed.) *Proceedings of the 17th Annual SCAMC*, 611-615, 1993.

5. Moore GW, Hutchins GM, Boitnott JK, Miller RE and Polacsek RA. "Word root translations of 45,564 autopsy reports in MeSH titles." In Stead WW (ed.) *Proceedings of the 11th Annual SCAMC*, 128-132, 1987.

6. Elkin PL, Cimino JJ, Lowe HJ, Aronow DB, Payne TH, Pincetl PS and Barnett GO. "Mapping to MeSH: The art of trapping MeSH equivalence from within narrative text." In Greenes RA (ed) *Proceedings of the 12th Annual SCAMC*, 185-190, 1988.

7. Canfield K, Bray B, Huff S and Warner H. "Database capture of natural language echocardiographic reports: a Unified Medical Language approach." In Kingsland LC, III (ed.) *Proceedings of the 13th Annual SCAMC*, 559-563, 1989.

8. Chute CG, Yang Y, Tuttle MS, Sherertz DD, Olson NE and Erlbaum MS. "A preliminary evaluation of the UMLS Metathesaurus for patient record classification." In Miller RA (ed.) *Proceedings of the 14th Annual SCAMC*,161-165, 1990.

9. Hersh WR, Hickam DD and Leone TJ. "Words, concepts, or both: Optimal indexing units for automated information retrieval." Frisse ME (ed.) *Proceedings of the 16th Annual SCAMC*, 644-648, 1992.

10. Lin R, Lenert L, Middleton B and Shiffman S. "A free-text processing system to capture physical findings: Canonical phrase identification system (CAPIS)." In Clayton PD (ed) *Proceedings of the 15th Annual SCAMC*, 168-172, 1991.

11. Wagner MM. "An automatic indexing method for medical documents." In Clayton PD (ed.) *Proceedings of the 15th Annual SCAMC*, 1011-1017, 1992.

12. Miller RA, Gieszczykiewicz FM, Vries JK and Cooper GF. "CHARTLINE: Providing bibliographic references relevant to patient charts using the UMLS Metathesaurus knowledge sources." In Frisse ME (ed.) *Proceedings of the 16th Annual SCAMC*, 86-90, 1992.

13. Browne AC, McCray AT and Srinivasan S. *The SPECIALIST Lexicon*. National Library of Medicine, Report No. NLM-LHC-93-01 (available from NTIS, Springfield VA: PB93-217248), 1993.

14. Cutting D, Kupiec J, Pedersen J and Sibun P. "A practical part-of-speech tagger." In *Proceedings of the Third Conference on Applied Natural Language Processing*, 1992.

15. Wilks YA. "An artificial intelligence approach to machine translation." In Schank RC and Colby KM (eds) *Computer Models of Thought and Language*, 114-151. San Francisco: W. H. Freeman and Co., 1973.

16. Hirst GJ. *Semantic interpretation against ambiguity.* Brown University Doctoral dissertation, 1984.

17. Stallard D. "The logical analysis of lexical ambiguity." In *Proceedings of the 25th Annual Meeting of the Association for Computational Linguistics*, 179-185, 1987.

18. McCroy SW. "Using multiple knowledge sources for word sense disambiguation." *Computational Linguistics* 18:1-30, 1992.

19. Schuyler PL, McCray AT and Schoolman HM. "A test collection for experimentation in bibliographic retrieval." Barber B, Cao D, Qin D and Wagner G (eds.) *MEDINFO 89*, Amsterdam: North-Holland, 810-912, 1989.

20. Aronson AR, Rindflesch TC, Browne AC. "Exploiting a large thesaurus for information retrieval." Proceedings of RIAO-94, to appear.

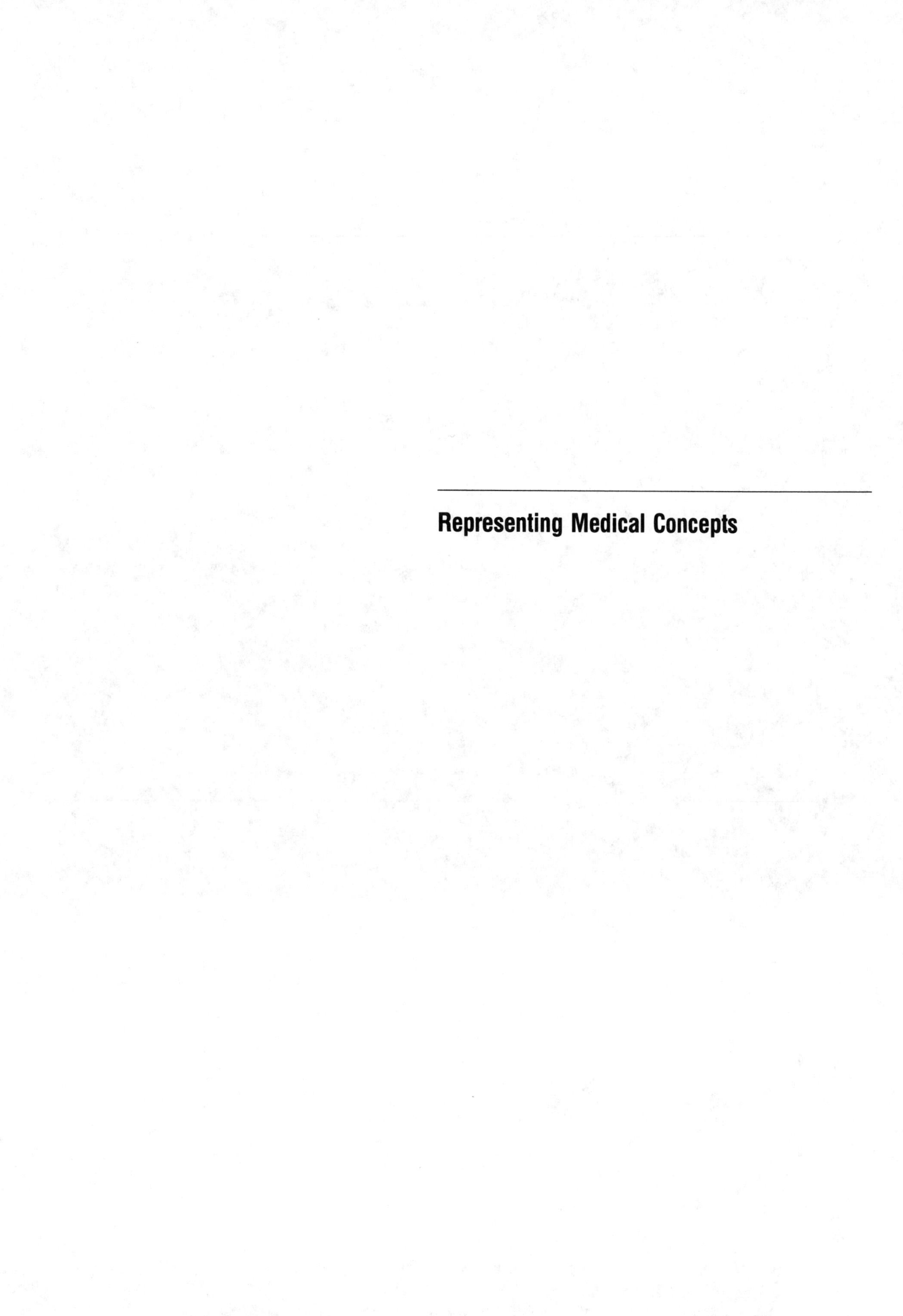

Representing Medical Concepts

A Natural Language Understanding System Combining Syntactic and Semantic Techniques

Peter Haug, Spence Koehler, Lee Min Lau, Ping Wang, Roberto Rocha, and Stan Huff
Department of Medical Informatics, LDS Hospital, Primary Children's Medical Center, and the University of Utah, Salt Lake City, Utah

A large proportion of the medical record currently available in computerized medical information systems is in the form of free text reports. While the accessibility of this source of data is improved through inclusion in the computerized record, it remains unavailable for automated decision support, medical research, and management of medical delivery systems. Natural language understanding systems (NLUS) designed to encode free text reports represent one approach to making this information available for these uses. Below we describe an experimental NLUS designed to parse the reports of chest radiographs and store the clinical data extracted in a medical data base.

INTRODUCTION

The last decade has witnessed a growing awareness of the usefulness of computers in medical care. With this awareness has come increasing pressure to capture and store clinical data in computerized medical records systems. Several groups have reported significant accomplishments in developing a computerized medical record both in the inpatient and outpatient settings [1,2,3].

One of the central challenges in this process is that of capturing clinical data in a form that serves the needs of a variety of different information consumers. The first of these consumers are the physicians, nurses, and therapists that provide day to day care for the patient. Ease and speed of access are the principal goals of this group, but a characteristic of growing importance to these information users is the ability to drive medical decision support from the information in the data base.

A second group of consumers are medical researchers. These information users expect clinical data to be stored in a form that will support investigation into the science of medicine and health care delivery.

A third, and an increasingly important group of medical data users are the people who administer health care systems. They expect to use the information available in attempts to modify the ratio of benefits to costs in medical care delivery systems. To serve their needs clinical data must be collected in a way that supports quality assurance initiatives, health care planning, and computer administered protocols to help standardize the health care product.

These groups are joined by the federal government as well as other third party payers in a desire for more and better data with which to monitor health care in the United States.

The needs and goals of these information consumers are best served by data that is stored in a carefully encoded form defined in a controlled medical vocabulary (CMV). A variety of CMVs have been developed and various groups are promoting an effort to define the essential terminology for a medical vocabulary as well as the basic characteristics of clinical data storage on a national basis [4,5].

Unfortunately, a large proportion of the information that finds its way into the medical record consists of free text data. This includes highly relevant information in reports of the history and physical examination, accounts of x-ray examinations, pathology reports, the narrative descriptions of surgical interventions and other invasive procedures, and the condensed description of hospitalization contained in the discharge summary. To fill the needs of the groups mentioned above this data must be encoded secondarily.

Several groups have evaluated techniques for automatically encoding textual documents from the medical record. The Linguistic String Project has developed a series of tools for analyzing medical text [6,7]. Gabrielli has described a system for encoding discharge summaries for quality assurance [8].

X-ray reports appear to have a special appeal. Two groups have developed systems whose focus is the radiologists' report of the chest x-ray. Zingmond has applied a semantic encoding tool to these reports to recognize abnormalities that should receive follow-up [9] and Friedman has studied techniques for encoding interpretations found in these reports [10].

We have been using a semantic parser for five years to encode salient features from the reports of chest radiographs [11,12]. While the accuracy of this system is far from perfect, the results have been adequate to support a computerized expert system for screening nosocomial infections [13]. At present, we are actively involved in the development of an experimental natural language understanding system (NLUS) designed to answer a set of questions concerning the synergistic relationship between semantic and syntactic parsing techniques.

A NLUS whose goal is to read medical text and to extract and encode the clinical data embedded in this text has one basic requirement. This requirement is a model of the data representation into which the encoded data will be stored. A data model serves to provide both a target for the parsing process and to identify and circumscribe the set of concepts which will be managed by the NLUS system. We have chosen to use a controlled medical vocabulary and set of data structures known as the event definition model [14] as the target for a new medical parser. To this we have added a syntactic parser based on an augmented transition network grammar [15] and a semantic grammar managed as a Bayesian network [16]. These constituents are described below.

EVENT DEFINITIONS

The event definition data model consists of a dictionary whose purpose is to define not only the medical lexicon used in the data base, but also to specify salient structural components of the data base. Slots are defined and their relationships to each other and to objects called event definitions (ED) are cataloged. The extended dictionary in which this occurs is referred to as the master object index (MOI).

Specific medical facts are recorded using the event definitions themselves. These structured multi-slot objects provide the basic framework in which atomic concepts defined in the MOI are integrated into complex concepts adequate to represent instances of clinical data or events. Figure 1 shows an instantiated event definition, drawn from the realm of chest radiology. This example representing the medical event documented in the sentence, *"A hazy opacity is seen in the right upper lobe."* The goal of the NLUS engine described below is to parse sentences like this one, to properly instantiate event definitions, and to store these event definitions in a general purpose medical data base. The process is controlled by a syntactic parser.

Finding Event:** ***Localized Infiltrate
- ***State:** ***Present***
  - **Presence Marker:** ***demonstrates***
- ***Finding Unit:** ***Poorly-marginated opacity (infiltrate)***
  - **Finding:** ***opacity***
  - **Finding Modifier:** ***hazy***
  - ***Severity:** ***null***
- ***Anatomic Unit:** ***Right upper lobe***
  - ***Link Unit:** ***Involving***
    - **Anatomic Location Link:** ***in***
  - **Anatomic Location:** ***lobe***
  - **Sidedness Modifier:** ***right***
  - **Superior/Inferior Modifier:** ***upper***
- ***Change Unit:** ***null***

Figure 1: An instantiated event from a chest x-ray report. The slots indicated with a * are higher-level concepts found in a controlled medical vocabulary. The other slots are holders for words from the sentence. "Null" slots at the word level are not shown.

SYNTACTIC TECHNIQUE

The NLUS developed for this experiment is based on a set of augmented transition network (ATN) grammars [15] and a lexicon derived from the Specialist Lexicon developed at the National Library of Medicine [17]. This lexicon has been augmented with a group of multi-word phrases representing frequently seen combinations with standard meanings (i.e. "consistent with", "no significant"). A small list of synonyms is used to replace words that represent a combination of concepts with the specific concepts (i.e. "cardiomegally" = "enlargement of the heart").

The ATN grammars are used in a cascaded fashion. A first grammar is applied to constraint the syntactic identity of the individual words of a sentence. The syntactic classification of a word is constrained to a single category based on the syntactic categories of its neighboring elements. For example, the word “project” could be classified as a noun or as a verb. Given the two words “the project”, the classification would be constrained to noun since “project” follows the article “the”. Given the two elements “will project”, the classification would be constrained to verb since it follows a verb auxiliary.

The goal in this stage of syntactic classification is to find a single syntactic interpretation for each word which is mutually consistent with the categories of its neighbors and to determine which groups of words can be additionally categorized as higher level syntactic elements such as noun phrases. These groups of words will be referred to as constituents of the sentence. Note that for some sentences multiple syntactic interpretations may be possible.

Upon successfully recognizing a constituent, the NLUS collects the words comprising that constituent and bundles them as a single element. This element is classified using the appropriate higher-level syntactic category (noun-phrase, prepositional-phrase, etc.). Constituent grammars that use these phrase level syntactic assignments can then be applied until the sentence is completely categorized. The resulting structure has a one to one correspondence with a syntactic parse tree.

Ordering the application of constituent constraining ATNs is itself accomplished by an ATN with a constituent application grammar. This concept is similar to that of a cascaded ATN where the output of one ATN becomes the input of another.

A final step in the process of syntactic analysis is a transformational step aimed at producing a set of structures that match the needs of the semantic grammar. The principal goal here is to accurately associate those components of the sentence that, when combined, completely specify the clinical events represented in the sentence. The principal target of the transformations are the conjunctions found in these reports. The results are groups of syntactically categorized words and phrases divided into subsets (sentence fragments) likely to represent semantically meaningful utterances.

SEMANTIC APPROACH

The semantic knowledge used by this NLUS is stored and applied in the form of a Bayesian Network [16]. Figure 2 shows one of the experimental networks which we have used in testing. It is designed to represent the subset of information in a chest x-ray report used to indicate the abnormalities which have been seen on the film. Each of the nodes in the network represents a specific slot from the event definition. Leaf nodes provide place holders for individual words or phrases from the x-ray report. The intermediate and root nodes are associated with slots for higher level concepts defined in the MOI.

We use the Bayesian network representation in two ways. First, the structure of the network is used to indicate the relationship between the words from the sentence and the concepts associated with these words. For instance, the network in figure 2 indicates that an **Anatomic Unit** can be represented by words from the **Anatomic Location, Anatomic Location Modifier, Sidedness,** and **Inferior/ Superior** nodes plus a concept from the **Link Unit** node. Relationships among sets of concepts are also captured within the network. Each node has a restricted set of words or concepts which it can represent. This, combined with the network structure, allows the parser to restrict slot fillers to the limited set that can be used to express the concepts native to chest radiology.

Second, the probabilistic behavior of the network tends to further restrict word and concept assignments within the slots to those that are semantically meaningful. For example, the leaf nodes associated with the **Finding Unit** node could be successfully filled with words from the fragment, "*a hazy infiltrate*" and the words from the fragment "*of the right heart*" could fill the word nodes under **Anatomic Unit**, but the network would give a zero probability if both sets of leaf nodes were instantiated together. This would simply indicate that the finding "*a hazy infiltrate of the right heart*" should be considered semantically unacceptable. Similar behavior exists within the subtrees. The network would reject "*inferior cardiac enlargement*" because the combination of "inferior" with "cardiac" does not produce a meaningful probability for any concept in the **Anatomic Unit** node.

The semantics embedded in the Bayesian networks are invoked at the beginning of the parse of each sentence to set expectations for the syntactic parser and at the end of the syntactic analysis to test the set of slot instantiations which have been produced. Typically a group of possible instantiations are proposed by the syntactic processor and the best of these is chosen by the semantic grammar.

We are developing individual Bayesian networks to represent the semantics of each of the event types seen in chest radiology. In addition to the

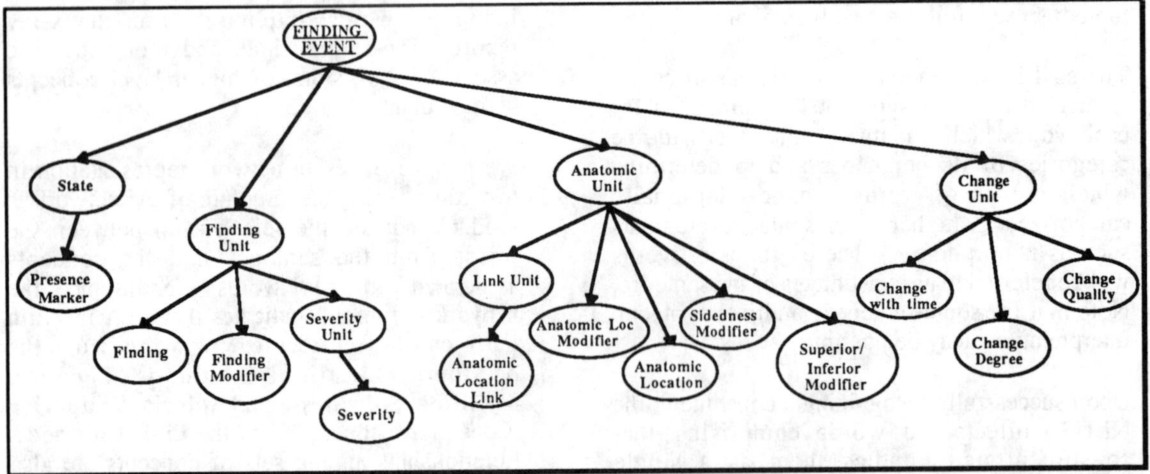

Figure 2: A simplified Bayesian network representing the semantics involved in sentences from chest x-ray reports describing findings.

networks for Findings, we have a network representing pathophysiologic interpretations (principally diseases) as well as a network for the various tubes and other hardware frequently described in radiologist examinations. The semantic and syntactic approaches which have been developed can clearly compliment each other even more effectively if proper ways of linking them can be developed. This is a subject which we are currently exploring.

We are developing this system through a series of small formative studies designed to focus our attention on the complexities of the syntactic-semantic relationship. To test progress we feed individual sentences into the parser and examine the ability of the system to recognize the key top level concept as well as the group of level two concepts that are associated with this key concept. In the example in figure 1 the key concept is the **Finding Event** and the second level concepts are the **State,** the **Finding Unit,** the **Anatomic Unit,** and the **Change Unit**.

RESULTS

In an analysis of ten chest x-ray reports collected sequentially from the HELP hospital information system, we found 50 sentences. Thirty-one of these sentences contained a total of 42 relevant key concepts. Nineteen expressed information outside of the realm of pathologic findings. The system correctly recognized the primary concept in 34 of the 42 cases (81%). Of 168 second level concepts, the system recognized 133 (79%).

The system's greatest current failing is a tendency to find concepts in sentences where they are not present. In this set of reports it generated 18 erroneous conceptual groupings. However, all but one were in sentences that dealt with the presence of various tubes, elements of patient history, and details of the radiologic procedure itself. We will soon begin testing with multiple Bayesian networks, each covering a different set of these concepts. As we begin using frameworks capable of encoding these other forms of conceptual abstraction, we expect a decrease in the frequency of these concept assignment errors.

DISCUSSION

The value of clinical data, accurately encoded using a CMV, has been demonstrated multiple times. In order to encode the medical data currently collected in a text-based form, system designers can attempt to replace natural language centered tools with structured interfaces designed to capture coded clinical information directly. The success of these interfaces has been limited in the past, particularly when the physician is the primary data source. The alternative is to supply tools capable of taking unstructured textual information, extracting salient facts, and encoding them.

The accuracy seen in the experiments described above does not yet match that of the semantic parser which we have been using. This tool has demonstrated a true positive rate of 87%-90% for chest x-ray findings similar to those in this study[12]. Unfortunately, this application has proven difficulty to maintain and cannot currently support the types of semantic and syntactic extensions which we wish to test. Because it was designed principally to explore a set of semantic theories, re configuring it to include syntactic knowledge and to properly integrate the syntax and semantics would be difficult.

The experimental system described above is fully configurable. Both its syntactic and its semantic knowledge are stored separate from the program and can be altered to match the needs of other types of medical free text. We intend to use this feature to provide access to coded data from other natural language documents in the medical record.

Our experience with the nosocomial infection monitor has led us to design several new applications that depend on encoded free text. The first of these is a system for computer-assisted antibiotic ordering. It uses information extracted from the chest x-ray report to determine the character and duration of pulmonary infections. It is currently being tested in our intensive care units.

The second new application is a system for determining the problem that brought each patient to the hospital. This information is entered as free text at the time of admission and is later encoded by the Medical Records Department. In order to expedite medical decision support we are planning to parse and encode this data at the time of admission.

The ultimate goal of this development effort is to allow computing systems full access to text-based medical information. Creation of robust NLUSs will bring us a step closer to medical information systems that can act as full participants in the process of health care delivery.

* This publication was supported in part by grant number 5 R01 LM05323 from the National Library of Medicine.

References

1. McDonald CJ, Tierney WM, Overhage JM, Martin DK, Wilson GA. The regenstrief medical record system: 20 years of experience in hospitals, clinics, and neighborhood health centers. MD Computing (1992); 9:206-217.
2. Kuperman GJ, Gardner RM, Pryor TA. *HELP: A Dynamic Hospital Information System.* 1991 Springer-Verlag, New York.
3. Clayton PD, Anderson RK, Hill C, McCormack M. An initial assessment of the integrated academic information system (IAIMS) at Columbia Presbyterian Medical Center. Proceedings of the Fifteenth Annual Symposium on Computer Applications in Medical Care. (1991): 109-113.
4. Committee on Improveing the Patient Record, Institute of Medicine. *The Computer-Based Patient Record.* Ed. Dick RS, Steen EB. National Academic Press, Washington, D.C., 1991.
5. Board of Directors of the American Medical Informatics Association. Standards for Medical Identifiers, Codes and Messages Needed to Create an Efficient Computer-Stored Medical Record. American Medical Informatics Association JAMIA 1994; 1:1-7.
6. Sager N, Friedman C, Lyman MS. *Medical Language Processing: Computer Management of Narrative Data.* Addison-Wesley, Menlo Park, CA (1987).
7. Sager N, Margaret L, Bucknall C, Nhan N, Tick LJ. Natural language processing and the representation of clinical data. JAMIA (1994); 1:142-160.
8. Gabrielli ER. Computer assisted assessment of patient care in the hospital. J Med Syst(1988); 12:135.
9. Zingmond D, Lenert LA. Monitoring free-text data using medical language processing. Comp Biomed Res 1993; 26:467-481.
10. Friedman C, Alderson PO, Austin JHM, Cimino JJ, Johnson SB. A general natural-language text processor for clinical radiology. JAMIA 1994; 1:161-174.
11. Ranum DL, Haug PJ. Knowledge based understanding of radiology text. In: Greenes RA, ed. Proceedings of the Twelfth Annual Symposium on Computer Applications in Medical Care. (1988): 141-145.
12. Haug PJ, Ranum DL, and Frederick PR. Computerized Extraction of Coded Findings from Free-Text Radiology Reports. Radiology (1990); 174:543-548.
13. Evans RS, Gardner RM, Bush AH, Burke JP, Jacobsen JA, Larsen RA, Meier FA, Warner HR. Development of a computerized infectious disease monitor (CIDM). Comput Biomed Res (1985) 18:103-113.
14. Huff S. Medical Data Dictionary for Decision Support Applications. Proceedings: Eleventh Annual Symposium on Computer Applications in Medical Care (1987); pp 310-317.
15. Woods WA. Transition Network Grammars for Natural Language Analysis. Communications of the ACM (1970); 13:591-606.
16. Pearl J. *Probabilistic Reasoning in Intelligent Systems: Networks of Plausible Inference.* Morgan Kaufman, San Mateo, CA, 1988.
17. McCray A. Personal communication.

MD Concept: A Model for Integrating Medical Knowledge

Yves Lévesque MD*◊; A. Robert LeBlanc, PhD◊; Michel Maksud, MSc*
◊ Institut de Génie Biomédical, Université de Montréal, Montréal, CANADA
* Développement Purkinje Inc., 7333 place des Roseraies, suite 401,
Anjou, Qc, CANADA, H1M 2X6

ABSTRACT

Many integrated clinical information systems depend on large knowledge bases containing dictionary of terms as well as specific information about each term and the relationships between terms. We propose a knowledge base model called MD Concept which is based on a semantic network and uses an object-oriented paradigm and relational tables. A prototype has been developed which integrates the Unified Medical Language System (UMLS) with other databases including the Systematized Nomenclature of Medicine (SNOMED II), the Diagnostic and Statistical Manual of Mental Disorders (DSM-IIIR) and a pharmaceutical database. We demonstrate how a user can easily navigate in this knowledge world using a browser .

INTRODUCTION

Health professionals deal with information: They need access to knowledge in the medical field [1], to data about particular patients (medical records) and they need to make links between the two [2]. To be more useful, all these information systems should be integrated [3,4]. Terminology is a key factor for integrating these systems [5]. Many terminologies are currently in use but none is adequate for all purposes [6,7]. Many of these terminologies, in particular the *Systematized Nomenclature of Medicine* (SNOMED III) [8] and the *Unified Medical Language System* (UMLS) [7], have evolved from simple lists of terms and codes to knowledge representation systems. Such systems make it possible to integrate clinical tools such as computerized medical record systems, decision support systems, and information retrieval systems. They could help information systems to show "intelligent" behavior.

We propose a model for integrating this knowledge in a comprehensive knowledge base called MD Concept. A prototype has been developed to explore the model. UMLS Knowledge Sources [9] were used as the core of the knowledge base.

OBJECTIVES

Ideally, a knowledge base such as MD Concept should contain a multilingual terminology covering all of medicine along with information on the terms and concepts represented, for example synonyms, translations, the codes for various other systems of classification and nomenclature (*eg* CPT), definitions, hierarchical (taxonomic) and other semantic information, linguistic (lexical, syntactic) information, and so on. There should also be data specific to the type or class of the term; for example, along with a particular commercial drug should be stored information about its ingredients and their concentrations; indications and contraindications; side effects; manufacturer; dispensing information, and so on.

A user should be able to consult the knowledge base to get answers to questions such as: What is Cushing's disease? What are its symptoms or its treatment? What is its ICD-9CM code? Another question might be, what diseases affecting the meninges are caused by a virus?

A knowledge base should confer some "intelligence" on information systems. For example, if a clinician were to ask the computerized medical record if his patient has heart disease, the system should know that myocardial infarction *is a* heart disease so as to report that the patient has a myocardial infarction. Linguistic information can also enable the system to understand queries and generate reports in a more "natural" language.

THE MODEL

We use the ANSI/SPARK Model [10] to describe our knowledge base architecture. This architecture is divided in three levels: the external level (user view), the conceptual level (application view), and internal level (physical model).

The External Level: semantic network

The external level is the *user view* of the knowledge base, how the user understands it and interacts with it. Following Gabrieli [11] and Rector, Nowlan and Kay [12], our model can be represented as a *semantic network* [13] in which elements of information (nodes) are linked together by relations (arcs).

Elements, or nodes, include words or groups of words, texts, numbers, images, sounds, etc. Most of the elements in MD Concept represent *concepts*. A concept is an abstraction; it is something which has meaning all by itself. For example, symptoms such as earache, diseases such as measles, treatments, lab tests, etc. are all concepts. As in the UMLS model [14], a concept typically will be represented by several different synonyms, or *terms*, possibly in more than one language. A *term* is defined as a word or a group of words representing a concept. As

0195-4210/94/$5.00 © 1994 AMIA, Inc.

examples, "Sexually transmitted disease", "STD", "Venereal disease", "Maladie transmissible sexuellement", "Maladie vénérienne" are the terms representing the concept of a disease that is transmitted by sexual contact. Each concept has a *preferred term* in each language.

A term can have a number of *lexical variations* (called *strings* in UMLS) that are minor variations of that term caused by singular-plural forms, order of words, etc. "Venereal Diseases", "Venereal, disease", "Disease, venereal ", "Diseases, venereal" are lexical variations of the same term. Each term has a *preferred lexical variation*.

In our model, the above semantic structure is actualized by assigning each element to a *class*, such as CONCEPT, TERM, LEXICAL VARIATION, CODE, etc. As in the UMLS, each element in the class CONCEPT is further subclassified into one or more *semantic types*, such as DISEASE, BACTERIA, HORMONE, TISSUE, etc. For example, the concept "Insulin" has two semantic types: HORMONE and PHARMACOLOGICAL SUBSTANCE. It is important to note that semantic types are themselves concepts.

A **relation** is a link between two elements (*table 1*). Relations are bidirectional: if myocardial infarction *has as a symptom* chest pain, then chest pain *is a symptom of* myocardial infarction. Most relations are heritable: if myocardial infarction *is a* heart disease and a heart disease *has as a site* heart, then we can conclude, if nothing else is specified, that myocardial infarction *has as a site* the heart.

The types of relations which can exist between any two concepts are determined by the semantic types of the two concepts; for example, "BACTERIA *causes* DISEASE" is possible, but "BACTERIA *causes* HORMONE" is not possible.

The Conceptual Level: the Object Oriented Model

The conceptual level represents knowledge as viewed by software applications. We use the object-oriented model [15]. Elements correspond to *objects* of a class and relations correspond to *methods* (sub-programs or functions) to find related elements.

There is an object class for each class of elements: TERM, CONCEPT, LEXICAL VARIATION, CODE, etc. These classes derive from the virtual class ELEMENT. Semantic type concepts derive from the CONCEPT class.

All elements have a *label* (a name). An element of the CONCEPT class has as its label the PREFERRED TERM for that concept. An element of the TERM class has the PREFERRED LEXICAL VARIATION as its label. For the LEXICAL VARIATION class, the label is simply the words for the lexical variation.

ELEMENT	RELATION	ELEMENT
myocardial infarction	is a	heart disease
myocardial infarction	ICD-9 code	410
myocardial infarction	has symptom	chest pain
chest pain	is a symptom of	myocardial infarction
venereal disease	is synonymous with	sexually transmitted disease

Table 1: Examples of elements and relations

For the CODE class, a concatenation of the source and the code (*eg* "ICD-9CM 412.34") forms the label.

Each class has its own data members (attributes): elements from the CONCEPT class have an ID, a preferred French term, a preferred English term, one or more semantic types, a syntactic category, etc. Elements from the TERM class have an identifier (ID), a language, a concept, a lexical tag, etc.

An object class includes *methods*, or programs, which define the relations between elements of that class and elements belonging to other classes. Methods can be quite simple, *eg* table lookup, but can also be very complex, including the capacity to make deductions. For example, suppose we want to know the site for the element "Myocardial infarction" (class CONCEPT). We would activate the method *has as a site* to search for a related element. If the method cannot find an element using this relation, it would next try to find elements using the relation *is a*. If it finds any (in our example, the method would come up with "heart disease"), it then recursively searches for the relation *has as a site* (it would find the element "heart"). The method can then infer that "myocardial infarction" *has as a site* "the heart".

This deduction of new knowledge uses primarily *is a* relations, but in some cases, the *is part of* relation provides more information. For example, to find diseases that "*have as a site* the heart", one should also look for diseases that *have as a site* part of the heart (myocardium, left ventricle, etc.)

Knowledge bases differ from simple data bases in this capacity to infer new information [16]. However, the user must be told that the knowledge was obtained by inference and how it was inferred.

As defined in the object oriented model, methods can be *overloaded*. So, in a class derived from a superclass, the method of the derived class can replace the method of the superclass. See [15] for a more complete description of the object oriented model.

The Internal Level: the Relational Model

The internal level represents how the knowledge base is physically stored in files. The relational model [10] is well suited to this task. Information is stored into and retrieved from relational tables using methods.

THE PROTOTYPE

A prototype was developed to explore the model. Borland C++ 3.1 and Object Window Library (OWL 1.0) were used to create a Windows 3.1 application running on an Intel486 DX2/66 microcomputer. The database is accessed via IS, a locally developed library of programs for managing indexed sequential files. Two modules have been implemented to date: MD Concept Integrator and MD Concept Browser.

MD Concept Integrator

The integrator can input files from multiple sources and output an integrated relational database. For the prototype, we integrated databases from UMLS, SNOMED II [17], DSM-IIIR [18], and a pharmaceutical database derived from the Canadian Drug Identification Code and monographs from the University of British Columbia Drug and Poison Information Center [19].

The process was as follows: first, using UMLS Knowledge Sources (meta 1.3, April 1993 [9]), the integrator set up relational tables containing 152,444 concepts, 202,000 terms, 279,238 lexical variations, 680,345 semantic relations, 52,085 concept definitions, 311,046 codes, and many of their attributes. Our data base differs from UMLS in that lexical variations, terms and concepts are placed into separate normalized tables .

Second, using SNOMED codes already present in UMLS and the SNOMED II bilingual database, we added 11,814 SNOMED II French terms and their lexical variations. We used the SNOMED code (*termcode)* and *the* English term (*enomen)* to find an English lexical variation. We tried to find an existing French term and lexical variation equivalent to the SNOMED French term (*fnomen).* If we did not find one, we added the term and/or the lexical variation. We did not add new concept. Translation relations were also created between French and English terms. The SNOMED *reference* field was used to add semantic relations (*has location, is associated with, cause*, etc) between concepts. Employing similar methods, we added french terms and translation relations from a bilingual DSM-IIIR database.

Finally, from the pharmacological database, 5,432 commercial drug names with their ingredients, codes, dose, manufacturer, form and route of administration were added as new concepts (of the new semantic type "Commercial Medication"), terms and lexical variations. Relations to 336 medication monographs and 14,318 pharmacological interactions between medications were integrated. New relations *have ingredient, made by, form, route, monograph, interact with* were created to link these commercial medications into the UMLS and SNOMED data.

The complete MD Concept knowledge base consists of approximately 230 megabytes of relational data files.

MD Concept Browser

The browser allows a user to find a particular element in the semantic network and to browse from one element to another using relations. There are two ways to access an element: with key words or with a code (Fig. 1), either gives rise to a lexical variation. The lexical variation can be used to access the term for the concept (*ie* the concept itself). From here, relations can be used to find the related concept, other terms (synonyms), terms in other languages, and all their lexical variations. For any term, one can look up codes (*e.g.* DSM-IIIR, SNOMED, ICD-9CM). It is possible to navigate to other concepts using any of the semantic relations defined for that concept.

Some relations are actually combinations of several relations. For example, as seen in Fig. 1, the user can go from a keyword directly to the concept (keyword →lexical variation→term→concept). If the *codes* relation for a concept are requested, all codes for all lexical variations for all terms for that concept will be found.

A simple generic *Elements-Relations-Messages* dialog box (Fig. 2) is used for browsing. It contains two lists and a message field. The *Element List* shows the element labels for any class. When one element is selected, the *Relation List* shows all relations defined for the class and the semantic type of that element. When the user selects one relation, the browser shows the new elements either in the *Message Field* (for a simple text element) or in a new overlapping *Elements-Relations-Messages* dialog box. The *Message Field* is also used to show a definition for the relation or the path that MD Concept used to infer some relations (as in the "Myocardial infarction *has as a site* heart" example). The caption on each

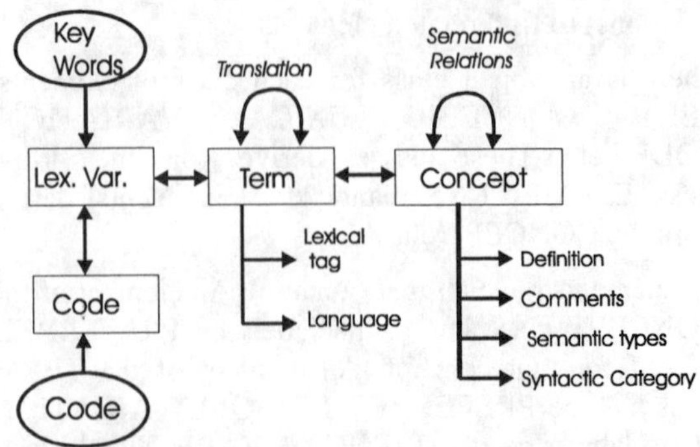

Fig 1: Browsing in the semantic network

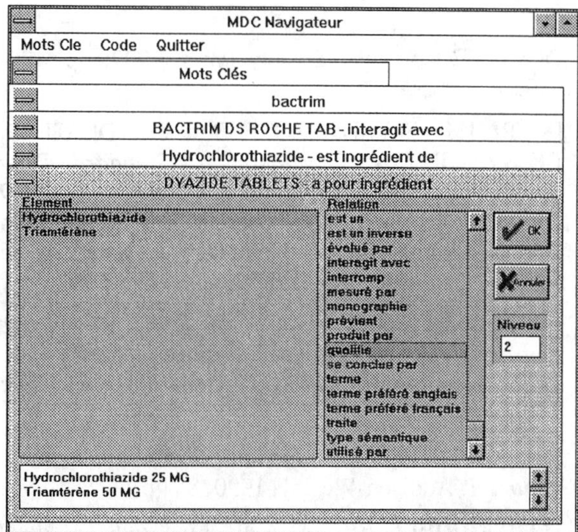

Fig. 2: MD Concept browser with overlappec *Elements-Relations-Messages* dialog boxes

overlapping dialog box shows the elements and the relations chosen by the user. A specialized dialog box displays the monograph text for pharmacological ingredients of a medication.

Fig. 2 shows a series of overlapped *Elements-Relations-Messages* dialog boxes. The caption bars of each window show the path followed by the user: starting with the keyword *bactrim,* MD Concept found 5 concepts (*ie* it found 5 lexical variations containing the word bactrim); then the terms for each of these variations, and finally the concepts for these terms (timing: less than 2 seconds).

The next caption bar shows that the user then selected the element *"BACTRIM DS ROCHE TAB"* and the relation *"interagit avec" (interacts with).* The system located 21 elements. Out of these, the user selected element *"Hydrochlorothiazide"* and the relation *"est ingrédient de" (is ingredient of)* to get 43 commercial medications (timing: 2 seconds). Finally, the element *"DYAZIDE TABLETS"* and the relation *"a pour ingredient" (has ingredient)were chosen.* The topmost Element List shows the two ingredients of *DYAZIDE TABLET* (timing: less than 1 second). The Message Field shows concentrations for these ingredients.

In summary: *bactrim is a keyword of the concept BACTRIM DS ROCHE TAB that interacts with Hydrochlorothyazide that is an ingredient of DIAZIDE TABLETS that has for ingredient Hydrochlorothiazide 25 MG and Triamterene 50 MG.*

The relational model gives fast access to knowledge. The response time was surprisingly good, considering the size of the database (230 megabytes): 1.1 million words in 300,000 lexical variations, hundreds of thousands of relations, etc.

DISCUSSION

MD Concept extends the UMLS model in three ways: with a simplified user interface for browsing in the knowledge base, with a mechanism for inferring new knowledge, and with additional content.

At the user level (external level), a semantic network appears to be a simple but effective way to represent knowledge. Compared to other browsers like *Metacard* or *COACH* [9] used with the UMLS, MD Concept uses a generic *"Elements-Relations-Messages"* dialog box to navigate in his knowledge base. While this generic dialog box is simple to use and is adequate for general browsing, a series of specialized user interfaces would be useful for regular use of the knowledge base in certain domains.

The methods of the object model facilitate the representation of inheritance of knowledge and the inference of new knowledge. As this inference process can lead to erroneous conclusions (e.g. with ICD-9 codes), the user must always be told how the information was inferred.

We found that it is possible for a personal computer to handle a large knowledge base.

We added some content to the UMLS: french terms with diacritical marks and upper-lower case; new, clinically useful semantic relations; and a pharmaceutical database. The inclusion of medication data demonstrates that MD Concept can be more than a terminological knowledge base and that different types of knowledge can be added using all the codes and lexical variations provided by the UMLS.

The UMLS was of great help in this project. Because it integrates several knowledge sources it formed an ideal core for MD Concept. Unfortunately, the UMLS is still an experimental project and it contains many inconsistencies; for example, many *is a* relations are defined as *unspecified hierarchical relations* and many clinically important semantic relations are missing. SNOMED II was useful in adding these important semantic relations, in particular *location of* and *cause*. But these relations (*reference* field) are not always explicit between elements of different axes. SNOMED also provides many important French terms with diacritical marks. The UMLS includes many French terms but they are in capital letters without marks.

CONCLUSIONS

MD Concept is a prototype and its content has not been tested extensively. Our objective was to evaluate the possibility of integrating existing knowledge sources into a large usable knowledge base. We found that:

- semantic networks and a generic *Elements-Relations-Messages* dialog box can be used to represent and browse into a wide variety of knowledge;
- methods are useful for implementing knowledge inheritance;
- the UMLS is useful as the core of a terminological knowledge base and that other type of knowledge can be added to the UMLS;
- a large knowledge base containing hundreds of thousands of terms and much additional information can be implemented on a microcomputer.

REFERENCES

[1] LEAO BdF, MANTOVANI, ROSSI FRI, ZIELINSKY P. *Incorporating knowledge to databases - a solution to complex domains.* in: Frise M, ed., Proceedings of the 16th annual symposium on computer application in medical care. Washington DC: McGraw Hill, 1992; pp. 234-238

[2] WEED LL et al. *Representation of medical knowledge and PROMIS* in Proceedings of the second Annual Symposium in Computer Applications in Medical Care, 1978; pp. 368-400.

[3] LINNARSSON R, WIGERTZ, O. *The Data Dictionary- A controlled Vocabulary for Integrating Clinical Databases and Medical Knowledge Bases.* Methods of information in medicine 28(1989); pp. 78-85.

[4] TIMMERS T, van MULLIGEN, EM, van den HEUVEL F. *Integration of an Object Knowledge Base into a Medical Workstation.* in: Clayton P.D., ed., Proceedings of the 15th annual symposium on computer application in medical care. New York: McGraw Hill, 1991; pp. 654-658.

[5] RECTOR AL, NOWLAN WA, KAY S. *Conceptual Knowledge: the core of medical information systems.* in LUN, K.C. et al, ed., MEDINFO 92. North-Holland: Elsevier Science Publishers; 1992; pp. 1420-1426.

[6] CIMINO JJ, BARNET GO. *Automated translation between Medical Terminologies using Semantic Definitions.* MD Computing Vol. 7 No 2 1990; pp. 104-109.

[7] HUMPREYS BL. *Building the Unified Medical Language System.* in: Kingsland LC III, ed. Proceedings of the thirteenth annual symposium on computer application in medical care. Washington DC: IEEE Computer Society Press, 1989; pp. 475-479.

[8] ROTHWELL DJ, COTE RA, CORDEAU JP, BOISVERT MA. *Developing a Standard Data Structure for Medical Language - The SNOMED Proposal.* In SAFRAN, Charles, ed. Seventeenth Annual Symposium on Computer Applications in Medical Care. McGraw Hill 1994; pp. 695-699.

[9] National Library of Medicine. *UMLS Knowledge Sources, 4th experimental Edition- April 1993 Documentation and CD-ROM.* Bethesda MA, 1993; 157p.

[10] DATE CJ. *An Introduction to Database Systems, volume 1.* Addison-Wesley, 1990; 854 p.

[11] GABRIELI ER. *A New Electronic Medical Nomenclature.* Journal of medical systems. Vol. 13 No 6 1989; pp. 355-373.

[12] RECTOR AL, NOWLAN WA, KAY S. *Unifying medical information using an architecture based on descriptions.* in: Miller, Randolf A., ed. Proceedings of the fourteenth annual symposium on computer application in medical care. Los Alamitos, CA: IEEE Computer Society Press, 1990; pp. 190-194.

[13] SOWA JF. *Semantic Networks.* in SHAPIRO, Stuart C. Encyclopedia of Artificial Intelligence. New York, Wiley, 1992; p 1493-1511

[14] TUTTLE MS, SPERZEL WD, OLSON NE, ERLBAUM, MS, et al. *The Homogenisation of the Metathesaurus Schema and Distribution Format,* in: Frise M, ed., Proceedings of the 16th annual symposium on computer application in medical care. Washington DC: McGraw Hill, 1992; pp. 299-303

[15] BOOCH G. *Object Oriented Design with Applications.* Redwood City, CA. Benjamin/Cummings 1991; 580p.

[16] TOURETZKY DS. *Inheritance Hierarchy* in SHAPIRO, Stuart C. Encyclopedia of Artificial Intelligence. New York, Wiley, 1992; pp. 690-701.

[17] COTE RA. *SNOMED: Systematized Nomenclature of Medicine.* Second edition. College of American Pathologist. Skokie, Il. 1979- 1982.

[18] American Psychiatric Association. *Diagnostic and Statistical Manual of mental Disorders.* Third Edition, Revised (DSM-III-R). Washington D.C. American Psychiatric Association, 1987.

[19] LEATHEM AM, CADARIO BJ. *Drug Information Reference* third edition. Vancouver B.C. Drug And Poison Information Center.1993. 1518 p.

An Empirical Investigation into the Conceptual Structure of Chest Radiograph Findings

Edward Pattison-Gordon, MS
Robert A. Greenes, MD, PhD

Decision Systems Group, Harvard Medical School, Brigham and Women's Hospital
Boston, Massachusetts

A method of investigating the conceptual structure of findings is presented, in which: 1) finding statements are extracted manually from free text, 2) the main concepts in each finding are manually identified and classified, and 3) the resulting sets of classes are examined for insights into finding structure. This study applies the method to chest radiograph reports. Although the subjects of the findings studied fall into seven classes, the same conceptual structure can be used for most of them.

INTRODUCTION

Today's health-care system requires the processing and analysis of patient data not only for the purpose of providing medical care, but also for monitoring the quality of that care, seeking compensation for its provision, and performing research so that it may be improved. Increasing portions of the patient record are available electronically, but the full potential of computer processing of patient data will not be realized until the contents of the electronic medical record can be analyzed by computer. Although this is relatively easy when the data are numeric, such as laboratory results, most physician notes are free text. Two approaches have been explored for handling free text patient data [1]. One approach is to use natural language understanding techniques to try to interpret textual information [2]; the other approach uses structured data entry to capture information in a format that is already interpretable by computer [3, 4, 5, 6]. Both approaches, however, depend on a conceptual model of the information that is explicitly stated as well as underlying knowledge.

Knowledge representation has long been a focus of artificial intelligence, where such formalisms as semantic nets [7], frames [8], and conceptual graphs [9] have been introduced. These systems attempt to provide, in one form or another, ways to construct and use conceptual models. Such models identify concepts and define relationships between them.

We have previously observed that there are two complementary ways to set about modeling concepts and their relations, *top-down* and *bottom-up* [10], and in an earlier effort used the top-down approach to model findings [11]. This paper uses a bottom-up approach to test the following hypothesis:

> Hypothesis. Different types of findings occur in chest radiograph reports, depending upon a finding's subject. That is, their conceptual structures differ by at least one of the following:
> - the sets of relations used;
> - the values allowed for a relation.

This work was carried out as part of our participation in both the National Library of Medicine's Unified Medical Language System© project [12] and in the Canon group's efforts to create a multi-purpose model of chest radiograph findings [13]. It also extends our previous modeling efforts [14]. In this study, finding statements in free text chest radiograph reports were examined. Previous studies have looked at sentences [15], terms [16], and noun phrases [17] to determine conceptual structure.

METHODS

Chest radiograph reports, findings, and main concepts were entered into an object oriented database, Mainstay's Phyla™ for the Apple® Macintosh® computer, (a relational database, however, would be sufficient). The database sorting and retrieval functions supported the analysis of finding conceptual structure.

Reports and Sentences

Eighteen chest radiograph reports were used in the study. These reports had been previously selected for conceptual modeling by the Canon group [13] because of their intermediate length and because of the challenges they posed to modeling.

The reports were entered into the database with each sentence as a separate entry. To preserve context, the complete report was entered including, for example, headings (*e.g.*, "Description," "Impression"), which were entered as separate sentences. Figure 1 shows sample sentences from the reports.

Findings

In order to determine finding conceptual structure, it was necessary to collect all of the information

0195-4210/94/$5.00 © 1994 AMIA, Inc.

CPMC17.01. AP PORTABLE CHEST X-RAY
OHSU12.02. There is coarsening of the interstitial lung markings which are most marked in the lung bases bilaterally.
BWH39.04. There are a few scattered small nodular opacities that are not clearly vascular in origin, possibly representing granulomata.
LDS64.10. There is no evidence of pneumothorax.

Figure 1. Sample sentences from the eighteen chest radiograph reports. Sentence IDs are report IDs—the characters and digits to the left of the first period—followed by the number of the sentence in the report.

provided for each finding from the natural language sentences in the reports. This was done manually, for two reasons. First, because there is not a one-to-one correspondence between sentences and findings in the reports. That is, some sentences contain no findings, others several. Information about the same finding may also be presented in multiple sentences. In addition to headings, sentences without findings include sentences that describe the reason for the radiographic study (*e.g.*, "rule out sepsis and renal failure"), that provide clinical information about the patient (*e.g.*, "pre-op cataract"), that describe the imaging procedure (*e.g.*, sentence CPMC17.01 in Figure 1), that present "information concerning technique" [16] (*e.g.*, "comparison is made to prior PA and lateral chest #1, dated 7 October 1988"), and sentences with "patient management issues" [cf. 16] (*e.g.*, "follow-up film in 6-8 weeks to rule out progression is recommended, if clinically indicated").

Second, when multiple findings are contained in the same sentence, information about one finding may be intermixed with information about the other findings. Multiple findings occur in a sentence when independent findings are joined with "and" (*e.g.*, "the costophrenic angles are clear *and* the domes of the diaphragm are smooth") or when findings that have some item of information in common (*e.g.*, location) are combined so that the information is only stated once (*e.g.*, "again noted is relative elevation and eventration of the left hemidiaphragm"). Multiple findings are also placed in the same sentence when one finding is inferred from the other, linked by words expressing the radiologist's certainty of the inference (*e.g.*, sentence BWH39.04 in Figure 1).

For each finding, the words used to express it in the reports were collected as a statement of the finding. Articles and verbs that did not contribute to the information content of the finding were omitted. For example, "the" was omitted from "the left lung", but "a" was kept in "a pleural effusion" because it specifies the number of effusions (one). Figure 2 gives examples of finding statements.

Usually, identifying findings within a sentence was straightforward but, occasionally, it was difficult. For example, how many findings are in sentence OHSU12.02, shown in Figure 1? Two were chosen (see Figure 2) because the sentence makes two slightly different statements: one about the interstitial lung markings generally and the other particularly about those at the lung bases.

The finding statements were reviewed as a collection, to see if similar findings had been treated consistently, and corrections made. Ultimately, 234 findings were identified in the eighteen reports. Sixteen finding statements were found to be identical—word for word—to other finding statements. They were not removed from subsequent analysis, however, because they are simply more instances of their finding types.

Concepts: Identification and Classification
The main concepts in each finding were identified and classified. Typically, main concepts were the nouns in noun phrases. Although the modifiers in a noun phrase may also represent concepts, they often reflect the conceptual structure of the noun concept, not that of the finding as a whole. For example, consider the noun "opacities" in Finding BWH39.04.01 (Figure 2). The modifiers "a few," "small," and "scattered" specify quantity, size, and distribution, respectively, of the opacity. Thus a model of "opacity" should include these attributes.

OHSU12.02.01. coarsening of interstitial lung markings
OHSU12.02.02. [coarsening of interstitial lung markings] most marked in lung bases bilaterally
BWH39.04.01. a few scattered small nodular opacities
BWH39.04.02. not clearly vascular [opacities] (BWH39.04.01)
BWH39.04.03. possibly granulomata (BWH39.04.01)
LDS64.10.01. no evidence of pneumothorax

Figure 2. Findings from the sample sentences in Figure 1. (Note the first sentence had no findings.) Square brackets indicate text that appeared only once in the original sentence, but was copied into more than one finding. Parentheses enclose references to other findings; here, findings from which the referencing finding was inferred. Finding IDs are sentence IDs plus the number of the finding in the sentence.

Exceptions to this rule were made for modifiers belonging to one of the classes to which main concepts were assigned. In this case, the modifier was assigned to the class and not kept with the noun. "Pleural," in "pleural effusion," for example, was not left as a modifier of effusion but assigned to Body Location (see below).

Concept classification was done manually. Each main concept was examined in turn and grouped with other concepts based on the role it played in the finding (*e.g.*, location, certainty, negation). When the role of a concept was the finding's subject, the concept was further classified with similar subjects (*e.g.*, medical device, medical procedure, pathologic process or entity). New classes were introduced as needed. Classification was reviewed for consistency by examining the members of the resulting classes for concepts that seemed out of place.

In all, thirteen classes were used: X-ray Image Feature (opacity, density, silhouette), X-ray Image View (AP, PA, lateral), Body Location[1] (lung, lobe, heart), Pathologic Process or Entity (effusion, nodule, atelectasis, lung cancer), Physiologic Process (pregnancy, *i.e.*, normal processes), Medical Device (surgical clip, sternotomy wire), Medical Procedure[2] (lobectomy, cardiac transplant), Body Substance (fluid), Comparison Result[3] (new, again, persistent), Inference Certainty[4] (probably, consistent with, less likely), Relationship to Other Finding (related to, due to), Attribute-Value (enlarged, normal, distended, elevated), and Negation (no radiographic evidence).

Attribute-Value is a special class, created because attributes and values for a main concept were often not expressed as modifiers of the main concept. Instead, the attributes and values occurred in other parts of the sentence. In finding OHSU12.02.01, in Figure 2, for example, "coarsening" is not part of the prepositional phrase containing the noun. Such words were classified as Attribute-Value to see if they differed from those modifiers that had been expressed in the concepts' noun phrases. Figure 3 shows an example of concept identification and classification.

[1]Body Location corresponds to Friedman's "body part" and "body part region" modifier classes [16].
[2]Medical Device and Medical Procedure together correspond to Friedman's second "broad informational unit" [cf. 16].
[3]Comparison Result corresponds to Friedman's third broad informational unit and her "change" modifier class [cf. 16].
[4]Inference Certainty roughly corresponds to Friedman's "certainty" modifier class, although negation is treated separately in this study [cf. 16].

Concept	Class
coarsening, most marked	Attribute-Value
interstitial lung markings	X-ray Image Feature
lung bases bilaterally	Body Location

Figure 3. Classification of the main concepts in finding OHSU12.02.02. The resulting set of classes—Attribute-Value, X-ray Image Feature, Body Location—reflects the finding's conceptual structure.

ANALYSIS

To determine finding conceptual structure, the classes to which all of a finding's main concepts had been assigned were taken together, as a set, and properties of these *class sets* were examined. 48 distinct class sets were found among the 234 findings.

Co-occurrence of the 13 classes within the 48 class sets was tabulated. Table 1 shows which classes co-occurred with each other at least once. Sorting the table by the number of classes with which each class co-occurred reveals that five classes never co-occur: Body Substance, Medical Device, Medical Procedure, Pathologic Process or Entity, and X-ray Image Feature. (Physiologic Process also did not co-occur with the other five classes but, because there was only one finding with a concept in this class, it was dropped from further analysis.) The concepts in these mutually exclusive classes had filled the subject role in the findings.

Sorting the 48 class sets according to which of the mutually exclusive classes occurred in them revealed the existence of class sets that did not contain any of the mutually exclusive classes. These class sets fell into two groups: 1) a single class set containing just the class Comparison Result (*i.e.*, findings, like "no change," that summarize comparing the current study with a previous one); and 2) five class sets whose only common feature—besides the absence of the mutually exclusive classes—was the presence of the class Body Location (*i.e.*, findings that describe organs, body parts, and regions as in "continued fullness of AP window"). These class sets represent two additional finding subjects.

An examination of each of the groups of class sets with the same mutually-exclusive class, shows the mutually exclusive class in various combinations with the remaining, non-mutually exclusive, classes. Reasons for this variability may be, for example, the inappropriateness of a role in some contexts (e.g., of Comparison Result when the finding is from the only study) or the omission of details by the radiologist. For the sake of a simpler model, and because a need for this level of detail had not been established, each

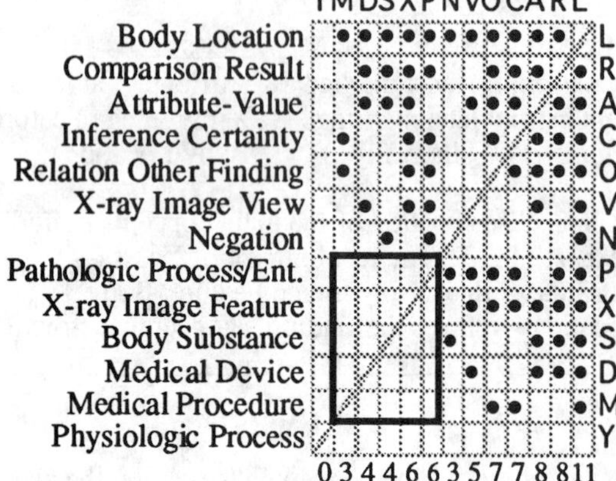

	Y	M	D	S	X	P	N	V	O	C	A	R	L	
Body Location		•	•	•	•	•	•	•	•	•	•	•		L
Comparison Result			•	•	•	•			•	•	•		•	R
Attribute-Value			•	•	•			•	•	•		•	•	A
Inference Certainty		•			•	•			•		•	•	•	C
Relation Other Finding		•			•	•				•	•	•	•	O
X-ray Image View			•		•	•					•		•	V
Negation				•		•							•	N
Pathologic Process/Ent.							•	•	•	•		•	•	P
X-ray Image Feature								•	•	•	•	•	•	X
Body Substance							•				•	•	•	S
Medical Device								•			•	•	•	D
Medical Procedure									•	•			•	M
Physiologic Process														Y
	0	3	4	4	6	6	3	5	7	7	8	8	11	

Table 1. Examining class co-occurrence in class sets reveals a group of mutually exclusive classes; that is, classes that tend to co-occur with the other classes within the class sets, but never with each other (outlined area). Dots indicate two classes that co-occur in at least one class set. The columns were originally ordered by the total number of classes with which classes co-occur (shown across the bottom). Negation and X-ray Image View have been moved in order to group the mutually exclusive classes together. Information below the diagonal is redundant, but is shown in order to make the table easier to read.

group of class sets with the same subject was replaced with a single class created from their union. Table 2 shows the resulting seven class sets.

Attribute usage was analyzed in two ways: 1) within the same finding type, the modifiers in noun phrases were compared with those that occurred elsewhere in the finding statement and, consequently, had been assigned to the class Attribute-Value; and 2) between finding types, concepts that had been classified as Attribute-Value in one finding type were compared against those classified as Attribute-Value in the other finding types.

RESULTS

Relations. A conceptual model of a finding type can be constructed from its class set by representing each class in the set and the finding itself with a concept, then creating relations from the finding concept to each of the class concepts. Because the seven class sets each have a different set of classes, each finding type will have a different set of relations, which is one of the criteria for distinguishing between types. These results are not sufficient, however, to require that a model of chest radiograph findings contain seven finding types. Because of the variability in which classes co-occur with a mutually exclusive class among the findings in the reports and the relatively small number of findings studied, it cannot be concluded that all such co-occurrences have been observed. Examination of additional reports might show, for example, findings in which Medical Device co-occurs with Inference Certainty, or in which Body Location—in the absence of the mutually exclusive classes—co-occurs with X-ray Image View. The more such co-occurrences there are, the more the seven finding types will tend to have the same set of relations. This trend can continue potentially until the only differences between the finding types are the relations to the concepts that represent the mutually exclusive classes themselves. This may not be sufficient grounds to maintain distinct finding types in some applications, especially because a single relation, has_subject, say, could be used to relate a more generic finding type to a concept composed of all of the mutually exclusive classes. A compelling reason for preserving distinct finding types, even if they all had the same set of relations, would be if relation values were different for some finding types.

Relation Values. Of the potential relations—those to Body Location, Comparison Result, Attribute-Value, Inference Certainty, Relationship to Other Finding,

	M	D	S	X	P	R	L	
Body Location	•	•	•	•	•		•	L
Comparison Result		•	•	•	•	•	•	R
Attribute-Value		•	•	•			•	
Inference Certainty	•			•	•		•	
Relation Other Finding	•			•	•		•	
X-ray Image View		•		•	•			
Negation			•		•			
Pathologic Process/Ent.					•			P
X-ray Image Feature				•				X
Body Substance			•					S
Medical Device		•						D
Medical Procedure	•							M
	M	D	S	X	P	R	L	

Table 2. The class sets created from the union of class sets with the same mutually exclusive class. Also shown is the class set containing only Comparison Result and the class set created from the union of those sets that contain the class Body Location but don't contain any of the mutually exclusive classes. Dots show membership of a class (rows) in a set (columns). Sets are labeled with the class that characterizes them: a mutually exclusive class, Comparison Result, or Body Location.

X-ray Image View, and Negation—the only one whose values clearly vary depending on finding type is Attribute-Value. Many attribute/values are particular to specific concepts (*e.g.*, blunting – costophrenic angle, coarsening – interstitial lung markings), but this has implications for modeling those concepts, not findings. For the class Body Location, however, it was observed that modifiers in concepts' noun phrases were used to modify the location (*e.g.*, bilateral, basilar, superior, area in), whereas co-occurring concepts classified as Attribute-Value were used to describe condition or state (*e.g.*, blunted, clear, distended, tortuous). This suggests that a Body Location finding should be modeled with a relation for those attribute/values describing condition and the body locations should be modeled with relations for detailing location.

CONCLUSION

An empirical method of determining the conceptual structure of clinical findings, based on the analysis of finding statements expressed in free text, has been presented. Focusing on the entire statement of individual findings makes it possible to determine concept class co-occurrence within findings and, thus, finding structure.

Although the findings studied can be classified into seven groups based on each finding's subject, it was discovered that it may be possible to represent most of the finding classes using the same set of relations. These results needs to be verified with additional chest x-ray findings and studies need be made to determine the applicability of the model to other domains (e.g. mammogram and ultrasound findings).

ACKNOWLEDGMENTS

This work was supported in part by contract LM04572 from the National Library of Medicine. David Wormuth, MD, Charles Kahn, MD, and Douglas Bell , MD, provided additional medical expertise.

Reference

[1] Sager N, Lyman M, Bucknall C, Nhan N, Tick LJ. Natural language process and the representation of clinical data. J Am Med Informatics Assoc. 1994;1(2):142-160.

[2] Friedman C, Alderson PO, Austin JHM, Cimino JJ, Johnson SB. A general natural-language text Roesner D. Structured data collection and processor for clinical radiology. J Am Med Informatics Assoc. 1994;1(2):161-174.

[3] Bell DS, Greenes RA, Doubilet P. Form-based clinical input from a structured vocabulary: Initial application in ultrasound reporting. In: *Proceedings - 16th SCAMC*. New York: McGraw-Hill, 1992.

[4] Kuhn K, Zemmler T, Reichert M, Heinlein C, knowledge-based user guidance for abdominal ultrasound reporting. In: *Proceedings - 17th SCAMC*. New York: McGraw-Hill, 1993.

[5] Fischer PJ, Stratmann WC, Lundsgarrde HP. User reaction to PROMIS: Issues related to acceptability of medical innovations. In: *Proceedings - 4th SCAMC*. Los Angeles: IEEE Computer Society Press, 1980.

[6] Rector AL, Nowlan WA, Kay S. Foundations for an electronic medical record. Methods Inf Med 1991;30:179-86.

[7] Mac Randal D. Semantic networks. In: Ringland GA and Duce DA, eds. *Approaches to Knowledge Representation: An Introduction*. Letchworth, England: Research Studies Press Ltd, 1988.

[8] Minsky M. A framework for representing knowledge. In: Brachman RJ and Levesque HJ, eds. *Readings in Knowledge Representation*. Los Altos, CA: Morgan Kaufmann, 1985.

[9] Sowa JF. *Conceptual Structures: Information Processing in Mind and Machine*. Reading, MA: Addison-Wesley, 1984.

[10] Barr CE, Komorowski HJ, Pattison-Gordon E, Greenes RA. Conceptual modeling for the Unified Medical Language System. In: *Proceedings - 12th SCAMC*. IEEE Computer Society Press, 1988.

[11] Greenes RA, McClure RC, Pattison-Gordon E, Sato L. The Findings-Diagnosis Continuum: Implications for image descriptions and clinical databases. In: *Proceedings - 16th SCAMC*. New York: McGraw-Hill, 1992.

[12] Lindberg DAB, Humphreys BL, McCray AT. The Unified Medical Language System. In: *1993 Yearbook of Medical Informatics*. Internat. Medical Informatics Assoc., the Netherlands, 1993:41-51.

[13] Evans DA, Cimino JJ, *et. al*. Position statement: Toward a medical concept representation language. J. Am Med Informatics Assoc. 1994;1(3):207-217.

[14] Bell DS, Pattison-Gordon E, Greenes RA. Experiments in Concept Modeling for Radiographic Image Reports. J Am Med Informatics Assoc. 1994;1(3):249-262.

[15] Johnson SB, Gottfried M. Sublanguage analysis as a basis for a controlled medical vocabulary. In: *Proceedings - 13th SCAMC*. 1989.

[16] Friedman C. The UMLS coverage of clinical radiology. In: *Proceedings - 16th SCAMC*. New York: McGraw-Hill, 1992.

[17] Evans DA, Hersh WR. *CXR Reports: Model and Analysis*. Technical Report, Laboratory for Computational Linguistics, CMU, 1994.

UVAL-MED a Universal Visual Associative Language for Medicine

[1]Benjamin Preiss; [2]Vincent Échavé; [3]Sandra Forster Preiss and [4]Marc Kaltenbach

Departments of [1]Biochemistry and [2]Surgery,
Faculty of Medicine, Université de Sherbrooke,
Sherbrooke (Québec), Canada,
[3]130, Howard Street, Sherbrooke (Québec), Canada
[4]Department of Management and Information Sciences,
Bishop's University,
Lennoxville (Québec), Canada.
Email : bpreiss@vm1.si.usherb.ca

Abstract

We describe UVAL-MED, a Universal visual associative language for medicine, and propose its use in combination with diagnostic reasoning and decision support systems. When fully developed, our system will automatically translate SNOMED terms to UVAL-MED terms. Grammar and syntax for UVAL-MED are defined and its features as a language-independent tool are discussed. The percieved advantages of our graphical language for rapid integration of knowledge and the assessment of developing situations could thus facilitate decision making.

Introduction

This paper describes UVAL-MED and proposes it for use in medicine as an application of a general approach. In this approach expert knowledge is visualized through "pictures" of mental models assumed to be held by domain experts. UVAL-MED is directly derived from the Concept Graphics described earlier [1-3]. In this paper rules of grammar and syntax are defined to allow the generative assembly of concepts and data at different levels of complexity from visual primitives. When fully developed, the UVAL-MED based system will be capable of automatically translating SNOMED III [4, 5, 19] terms into UVAL-MED terms. The system will thus provide information in a highly ergonomic form that can be read and manipulated by both computers and humans almost regardless of the original language of the data. Questions of the design of graphical representations and their effectiveness have been addressed, among others by Fitter and Green [6], McKinlay [7], Chernoff [8] and more recently by Cole [9]. UVAL-MED incorporates, in a more explicit context, at least four of the five principles proposed by Fitter and Green [6]: **relevance**, providing the useful information, **representation**, of both meaning and underlying processes, structures **restricted** to correct expert knowledge in a **revisable** form. Concept Graphics as used in UVAL-MED incorporate the major advantages of Chernoff faces [8] while avoiding their disadvantages [3]. Cole [9] has defined the terms **integrality** and **meaningfulness** for graphical data displays. A part of this paper discusses the desirability of these qualities in different types of graphical data displays. Wang et al. [3] described an intelligent interface for a diagnostic expert system based on Concept Graphics. In this paper, we discuss the perceived advantages of the use of UVAL-MED as an alternative representation for the **Diagnostic Units** and **Diagnostically-Operative Causal graphs** (DOC graphs) developed by Jang [10,11].

UVAL-MED grammar and syntax

UVAL-MED is directly derived from the Concept Graphics described earlier [1-3]. Here, the rational basis for the design of the graphics is reinforced and their use is extended to display, when requested, **causality, conditional causality** and **enablement** [12]. Two subcategories for graphics are defined: Situation Graphics and Process Graphics.

1. Primitive icons represent their meaning either explicitly in shape and color (the heart, the brain), as a metaphore of their meaning (Alcoholism: a hand holding a wine glass) or in a few cases, an invented symbol that must be learned (pain).

2. New concepts are generated by combining primitive icons [2].
3. Concept Graphics in UVAL-MED are assemblies of composite or primitive icons that are displayed together in a square of uniform size. Neither shape nor size of individual icons is standardized. They are determined by considerations of comprehension and design. Wherever possible, the same icon will occur at the same size and place in the square. Concept Graphics folow the principle of connectedness [6,13]. Icons simply occur together in the same square to define the context of a situation.
4. In UVAL-MED Concept Graphics can be displayed in a causally connected mode. Causal, enabling or non causal relations are made explicit, based on the arrow types of Rieger [12].
5. In UVAL-MED primitive or composite icons with their modifiers, time references etc, are highligted as a unit upon request and explained.
6. Diagnostic solutions produced by an expert system will be displayed in UVAL-MED as graphics in progressively distant planes (in perspective) with their attached diminishing probabilities. Two or more co-occuring diseases will be in the same plane. One would then click each proposed disease to obtain its typical time sequence, displayed as a series of graphics with a time scale. One would display the diagnostic problem at hand on the same screen for comparison.

A graphical representation language for integration and assessment of knowledge

Our earlier work [1] has demonstrated that second year medical students briefly exposed to Concept Graphics in nephrology, in addition to text of equivalent information content, performed significantly better on a subsequent quiz than controls exposed to text alone. The advantage appeared with questions requiring correlation of a number of diagnostic elements, not for memorization of a single fact. A significant advantage was also found in the listing of two pathognomonic criteria for the nephritic syndrome. A more complete study is currently under way involving 4th year medical students and residents in surgery. We believe that graphical representation can enhance the ability of the user to integrate knowledge acquired through reading and other means and to integrate rapidly developing or new situations based on prior domain knowledge. Graphics would help "connect" with possibly dormant prior knowledge and could thus facilitate decision making.

Some examples of the graphical language

In Figure 1. a textbook description of acute cholecystitis is represented. Note the cause-effect arrow. Cause: the common bile duct is blocked by stones. Effect: jaundice.

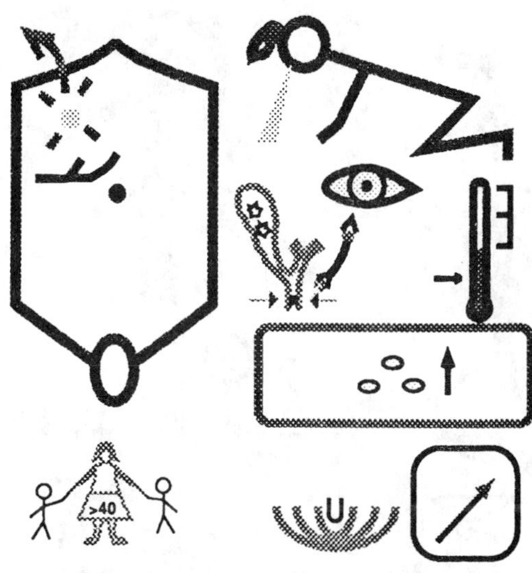

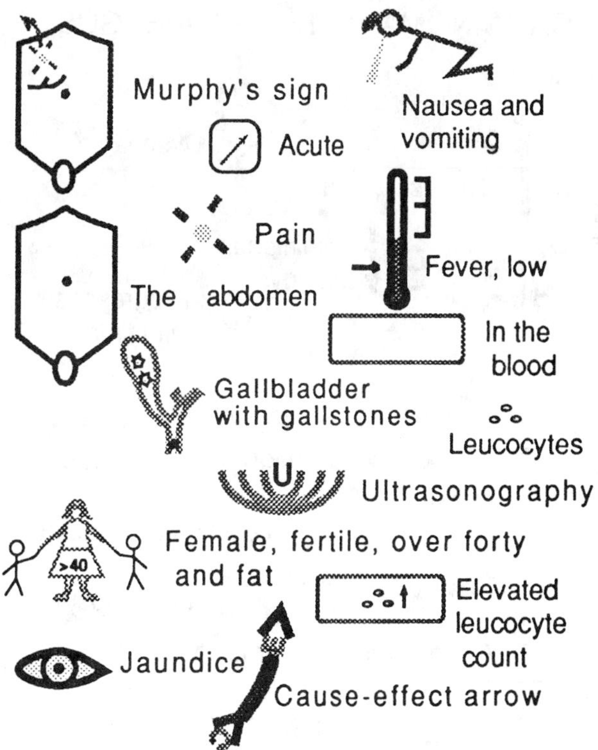

FIGURE 1

Figure 2. represents a textbook description of cancer of the esophagus. Note here the notation that the cancer can occur anywhere within the esophagus in contrast with a situation where a specific location is indicated.

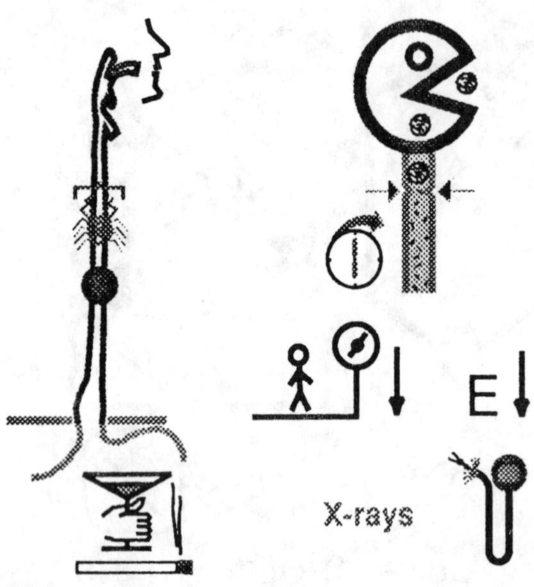

CARCINOMA OF THE ESOPHAGUS

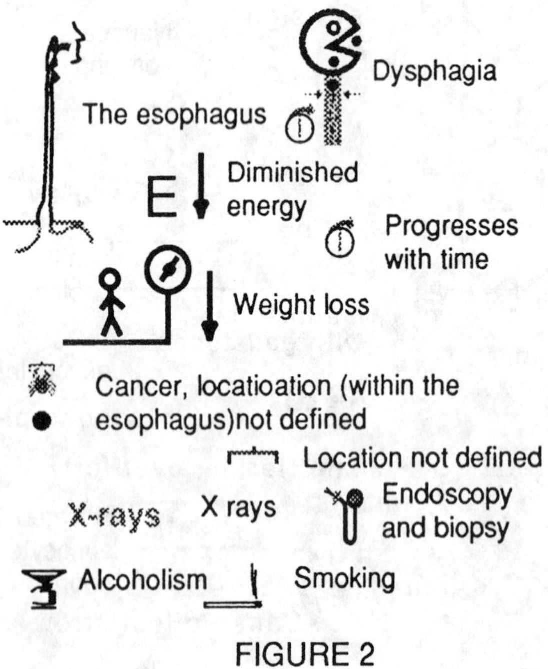

FIGURE 2

UVAL-MED, expert mental models and situated cognition

We propose that users of UVAL-MED or other model-based associative languages would gain advantages in the construction of their own correct mental models of knowledge and of situations requiring a decision. Johnson-Laird and Shafir [14] and Legrenzi et al. [15] advance the hypothesis that both reasoning and decision making depend on the construction of mental models. Future work will be needed to compare possible benefits of our approach with other forms of knowledge and data representation.

Integrality and meaning

Cole [16] has proposed two principles of graphical data display as fundamentally significant criteria. These are **integrality** and **meaningfulness**.

Cole [16] has compared his elegant displays of mechanical ventilation data of ICU patients with Concept Graphics, among others. He has concluded that while the metaphor graphics describing mechanical ventilation data are both high in **integrality** and in **meaningfulness**, Concept Graphics are high in **meaningfulness** and low in **integrality**. Integrality here is described as a quality that allows immediate recognition of a pattern and in which any changes to that pattern would be clearly understood as changes in the real world. This works very well when the graphic display has only one type of shape, a rectangle in Cole's example, assuming a number of meaningful roles.

It seems relevant to ask whether displays of high integrality would be predominantly processed automatically [17, 18]. If this possibility is considered plausible, we may advance the hypothesis that displays of low integrality but high in meaning as well as relatively high in the number of variables under consideration could be treated by controlled search and controlled processing [17], at least when first encountered. Is high integrality a "good" quality for a graphic display? We argue that the answer would depend on the use for which the display has been designed. That is, where one should look for integrality and where it may have negative effects. Shiffrin and Schneider [18] have shown that subjects trained to process images automatically, expecting certain categories of symbols in the same role, perform very poorly when the roles are switched.

The Concept Graphics should be considered as a set in order to discern patterns that help learning and processing. The analysis of a single member of our general surgery set done by Cole [16] lead to the conclusion that Concept Graphics have low integrality, because the multiple shapes of the component icons do not amount to a single salient pattern or overall shape. "Are there emergent features, features that exist when all elements are present and take on certain values, but would disappear if any individual element were to disappear?" [16]. Encoded information, to be useful, must be precisely organized in order to be read. This assumes an even greater importance when one moves away from natural language to perhaps more powerful but less familiar forms of expression such as graphic displays. Concept Graphics should be looked at as assemblies of their component parts before they are seen as a whole pattern. As the reader of a sentence in a paragraph assembles in his or her mind the elements expressed in words, the reader of a Concept Graphic should "put together" the separate elements of the "story" the graphic is telling and then also memorize, we hope without too much effort, the overall shape of the graphic for future reference. We propose that **integrality** should be sought in the component icons of Concept Graphics in order to facilitate search and comprehension of the overall meaning. The component icons such as the thermometer metaphor can be compared to the **radicals** in Chinese characters which often give the reader a clear message on the context of the complete character and help situate its exact meaning even if one were not previously familiar with the character. It would perhaps be easy to conclude that the 5000 chinese characters the native speakers of chinese possess have low integrality. This leads to the question of training in the use of Concept Graphics. Recognition of icons and graphics is not immediate and does require some training or practice. The UVAL-MED based system will translate automatically medical terms (SNOMED III terms) to their graphic equivalents. The graphics will also translate to natural language definitions upon request. A novice user should be able to train with little effort, we hope, while using the system.

UVAL-MED as a language-independent semantic code

SNOMED [19] is designed to allow translation of its terms into any language and multilingual versions of it are emerging. The need for a further development of auxiliary dictionaries, structured in a language-independant form on the basis of semantic analysis of medical information, has been addressed by do Amaral and Satomura [20]. We propose that UVAL-MED can be implemented as an **interlingua** that can situate the user at a glance regarding a medical situation, its past course and ramifications. We propse UVAL-MED as a companion to SNOMED with the capacity to express semantic units of different degrees of complexity and at different levels of abstraction, according to need. In order to implement automatic translation of assemblies of SNOMED terms into UVAL-MED representations it will be necessary to adopt the approach developed by Campbell and Musen [5]. These authors used conceptual graph theory to provide SNOMED III with a standard syntax. The example given in [5] "Substernal chest pain with radiation to left jaw and to left arm" can be readily assembled and visualized in UVAL-MED. A more elaborate treatment of this subject will appear elsewhere.

UVAL-MED representations in an intelligent interface for diagnostic and decision support systems

We chose HYDI, a recent hybrid system for the diagnosis of multiple disorders [11] for a discussion of the perceived advantages to users through alternative representations in UVAL-MED. "An optimal diagnostic unit is an instantiated causal graph, with a single elemental disorder root, such that the causal explanation identified by the graph can be immediately inferred to be the most likely causal explanation for all the findings in the graph" [11]. We propose that, at least in the context of simulation for learning and training purposes, an explicit visual representation of such **diagnostic units** in the form of causally linked Situation Graphics would enhance understanding and integration of medical knowledge. Situation Graphics are Concept Graphics containing only surface features of a medical situation without process explanations or statistical data on susceptible patient groups etc. We also propose that descriptions of underlying processes (Process Graphics when only a process is described) can enhance understanding and integration of the proper sets of symptoms and signs specific to a medical situation. Similarly, at higher levels of complexity, we believe that explicit visual displays in UVAL-MED could be advantageous as alternative representations of **Diagnostically-Operative Causal graphs**

(DOCgraphs), the form in which solved medical problems are stored in HYDI [11].

Acknowledgement

We want to thank Dr. Roger A. Côté for his continued encouragement and for many helpful discussions. We are grateful to Mme Sylvie St-Laurent for expert word processing.

References

[1] Preiss, B., Black, R., Caron, C. and Shapcott, D. Graphic summaries of expert knowledge for the medical curriculum I. An experiment in second year nephrology. *Meth Inform Med* 31;1992:303-309.

[2] Preiss, B., Kaltenbach, M., Zanazaka, J. and Echavé, V. Concept Graphics: A language for medical knowledge. In *The sixteenth Annual SCAMC*, Baltimore MD:McGraw-Hill 515-519.

[3] Wang, S., El Ayeb, B., Échavé, V. and Preiss, B. An intelligent interactive simulator of clinical reasoning in general surgery. *Proceedings of the Seventeenth Annual SCAMC*, Washington DC: McGraw-Hill. 1993;419-423.

[4] Côté, R.A. and Rothwell D.J. Optimizing the structure of a standard vocabulary: The SNOMED model. In Miller, R.A. (ed). *Proceeding of the Fourteenth Annual SCAMC*, Washington DC:1990;181-184.

[5] Campbell, K.E. and Musen, M. Representation of clinical data using SNOMED III and conceptual graphs. *Proceedings of the sixteenth annual SCAMC*, Baltimore, MD:McGraw-Hill 1992;354-358.

[6] Fitter, M. and Green, T.R.G. When do diagrams make good computer languages? *Int. J. Man-Machine Studies*, 1979;11:235-261.

[7] Mackinlay, J. Automating the design of graphical presentations of relational information. *ACM Transactions on Graphics* 1986;2:110-141.

[8] Chernoff, H. The use of faces to represent points in k-dimentional space graphically. *J. Am Stat Assoc* 1973;68:361-368.

[9] Cole, W. Integrality and meaning: Essential and orthogonal dimensions of graphical data display. *Proceedings of the Seventeenth Annual SCAMC*, Washington DC: McGraw Hill. 1993;404-408.

[10] Jang, Y. A hybrid system for diagnosing multiple disorders. *Seventeenth SCMAC*:1993;454-460.

[11] Jang, Y. HYDI: A hybrid system with feedback for diagnosing multiple disorders. Ph.D. dissertation, Technical Report MIT/LCS/TR-576, Massachussetts Institute of Technology, Cambridge MA; October 1993.

[12] Rieger, C. The commonsense algorithm as a basis for computer models of human memory, inference, belief and contextual language comprehension. Technical report 373, Department of Computer Science, University of Maryland. May 1975.

[13] Harel, D. On visual formalisms. *Communications of the ACM*. 1988;31:514-530.

[14] Johnson-Laird, P.N., and Shafir, E. The interaction between reasoning and decision making: an introduction. *Cognition*. 1993;49:1-9.

[15] Legrenzi, P., Girotto, V., and Johnson-Laird, P.N. Focussing in reasoning and decision making. *Cognition*. 1993;49:37-66.

[16] Cole, W. Integrality and meaning. Essential and orthogonal dimensions of graphical data display. *Seventeenth Annual SCAMC*. 1993;404-408.

[17] Schneider, W. and Shiffrin, R.M. Controlled and automatic human information processing : I. Detection, search and attention. *Psychological Review*. 1977;**84**:1-66.

[18] Shiffrin R.M. and Schneider, W. controlled and automatic human information processing II. Perceptual learning, automatic attending and a general theory. *Psychological Review*, 1977;**84**:127-190.

[19] R.A. Côté ed. *Systematized Nomemclature of Medicine - SNOMED International*. Skokie, Illinois. College of American Pathologists, 1993.

[20] do Amaral, M.B. and Satomura, Y. Multilingual applications: Processing natural languages at Chiba University Hospital. *M. Computing*. 1993;1:6-14.

Section III

Database Methods: Support for Administration

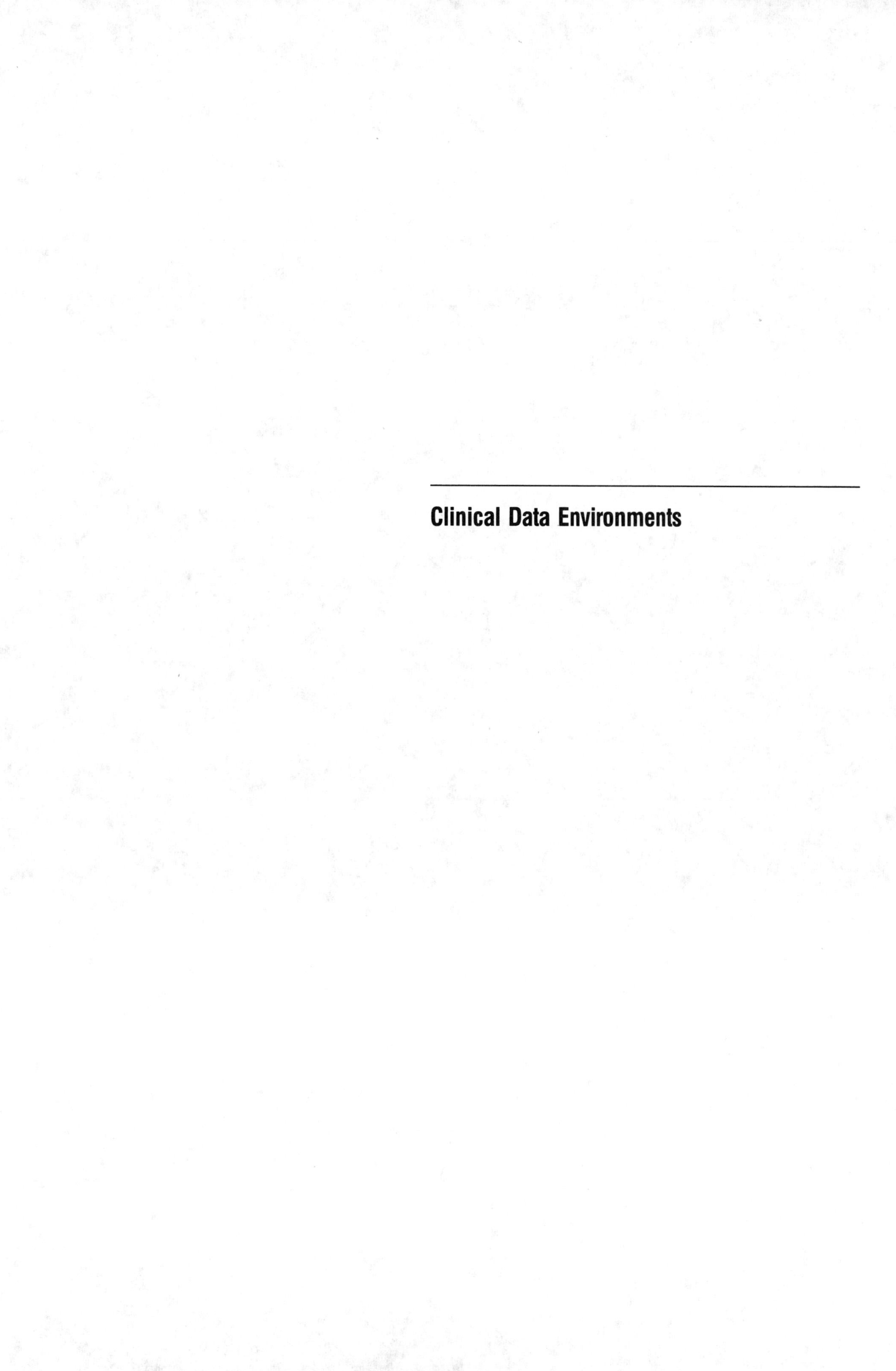

Clinical Data Environments

HELP The Next Generation: A new Client-Server Architecture

Stanley M. Huff, M.D.[1,2], Peter J. Haug, M.D.[1,2], Lane E. Stevens, M.S.[2], Robert C. Dupont[3], T. Allan Pryor, PH.D.[1,2]

[1]Department of Medical Informatics, University of Utah
Salt Lake City, UT 84113
[2]Information Systems, Intermountain Health Care Inc.
Salt Lake City, UT 84111-1486
[3]Health Information Systems, 3M Health Care
Murray, UT 84157-0900

A new client-server based system which is centered around a lifetime data repository (LDR) is under construction. The goal of the new system is to maintain the patient centered decision support aspects of the existing HELP system while providing an open architecture that supports faster application development and allows execution of applications to be distributed across many computers. These goals are achieved by implementing the system with software components that are commercially available or by adhering to national and international standards for software integration. Keys to successful integration include the use of MS-DOS@, OS/2#, and UNIX§ as operating systems, Microsoft OLE 2.0 as a standard interface to the clinical database, the use of TUXEDO as a transaction/communication manager, and the use of ORACLE¶ RDBMS as the underlying database management system.*

INTRODUCTION

The HELP system has been an important part of patient care within Intermountain Health Care (IHC) for the past 20 years [1]. The system was designed with the goal of improving patient care and reducing patient costs by using the computer as a patient-centered decision support system integrated with the clinical care of the patient. The system was specifically designed to be used by physicians, nurses, and other clinicians at the bedside and at the nursing station for data entry, data analysis, and display. The system has been very successful in meeting its goals for improving patient care, as well as facilitating clinical research [2,3].

Over the years the HELP system has evolved new programs, new data structures, and new terminology as needed to keep up with the changing functional requirements. However, a new system is now being created (as a cooperative venture between IHC and 3M Health Information Systems) to meet the demands of a changing social/political climate in the health care environment and to take advantage of technological advances in both hardware and software development. The new system is not just a recreation of the HELP system using new technology, but includes a whole new philosophy of system architecture and approach. Before describing the new system it is important to first outline some of the specific goals of the new design philosophy.

- Ambulatory care is playing an ever increasing role in medical care and the outpatient environment provides many of the events and follow-up data that allow the determination of the long term outcomes of medical therapy.
- There is a need to integrate health plan coverage, scheduling, billing, and referral services across both inpatient and outpatient facilities within an enterprise.
- The increased complexity of protocol and alert logic that the HELP system performs creates a need for distributed processing.
- Some compute intensive applications like voice recognition and natural language processing tend to overload our current system.
- The development of high performance/low-cost workstations makes distribution of processing feasible.
- A faster software development cycle that uses standard languages and software development tools is a necessity in order to keep up with ever increasing application needs.
- The need to incorporate increasing amounts of textual information in the system, and the ability to do *ad hoc* queries based on word co-occurrence within a document.
- The need to enhance the HELP vocabulary (called PTXT for Pointer to TeXT), including the support of synonyms and homonyms, increased depth of the hierarchy, support of multiple hierarchical views, and support of a more formal definition of how

---

* HELP is a registered trademark of 3M Corporation.
@ MS-DOS, MS Windows, Windows NT, OLE, Word, Excel and Visual Basic are trademarks of Microsoft Corporation.
# OS/2 and IBM are registered trademarks of International Business Machines Corporation.
§ UNIX and TUXEDO are registered trademarks.
¶ ORACLE is a registered trademark of Oracle Corporation.

atomic codes are combined to make meaningful records in the database.
- Modern database management systems provide levels of data integrity, security, and internal consistency. It is desirable to use these tools as provided by commercial vendors rather than create and maintain these processes internally.

In the midst of describing the requirements for the new system there are a set of fundamental design considerations that were the foundation of the HELP system and that continue to be valid today. The new system incorporates these time tested assumptions. Specifically, the new system is patient centered and optimized for use by clinicians as an integrated part of direct patient care. This includes data entry at the point of care. Secondly, we are convinced that the best and most cost effective patient care requires the integration of alerts, protocols, and other decision support applications in the system. Thirdly, an essential component of the system is a well defined, comprehensive, coded patient database. Finally, the system must provide for the administrative activities of patient care (scheduling, billing, data security, administrative decision support, etc.) along with the patient care and clinical research aspects of the system.

SYSTEM ARCHITECTURE

The new system is currently under construction and applies an open system approach [4] to the system architecture. The elements of the overall software architecture are diagrammed in Figure 1, and individual aspects of the system are described in the following sections.

Client Environment

The client part of the system has been left as open as possible so that many application development strategies can be employed. Clients may exist on an IBM PC with Microsoft Windows or OS/2, a Macintosh§ , or a UNIX workstation. Three layers of software participate in the functions provided by a client: the application presentation layer, the business logic layer, and the communication layer.

The presentation layer provides the actual interface to the user. It presents and collects data from the user. This layer can be a GUI (Graphical User Interface), forms based, character oriented, or pen-based. The business logic layer enforces presentation and collection rules and supports application specific logic and navigation. Visual Basic was chosen as the language of choice for our first applications , but Visual C++ and Power Builder are equally supported.

The communication layer gives the client the ability to communicate with the transport component of the system to request services. We have chosen

§ Macintosh is a registered trademark of Apple Computer, Inc.

Client
Hardware:
IBM PC, Mac, Unix WS
Operating System:
OS2, Windows, Unix

Presentation Layer
GUI, Forms, Character, Pen-based

Business Logic Layer
Visual Basic, Visual C++, Power Builder
OLE 2.0

Communications Layer
ATMI API
Tuxedo/WS

Communication Protocols
TCP/IP
SNA
LU6.2

Server
Hardware:
RISC Server, Mini, Mainframe
Operating System:
Unix, Gaurdian, Others

Communications Layer
ATMI API
Tuxedo

Business Logic Layer
C, C++

Database Layer
ANSI SQL
ORACLE RDBMS

Figure 1: A summary of the client and server software layers.

TUXEDO, a commercially available UNIX-based transaction manager [5] to provide this function. A component of TUXEDO called TUXEDO/WS resides on the client while a matching counterpart of TUXEDO resides in the server. The Application Program Interface (API) to TUXEDO is ATMI (Application Transaction Manager Interface) which is a superset of the XATMI standard [6]. XATMI is supported by the X/OPEN group as one of three standard APIs for open systems.

A further constraint placed on the communication layer is a requirement that clients access the clinical database using Microsoft Object Linking and Embedding (OLE 2.0) standard [7]. OLE 2.0 is an application interoperability standard that is being integrated into all Microsoft products, including operating systems (MS Windows and Windows NT), and applications (Word, Excel, etc.). The goal of providing access to the clinical database via OLE objects is two fold. First, the OLE objects can be accessed by any OLE enabled application such as Excel or Access. Secondly, since the database and data transfer mechanisms are hidden from the application programmer, he/she can use the properties and methods of the OLE objects without worrying about changes to the structure of the underlying database files.

The first clients are applications that manage clinical data in the outpatient setting. These applications are the most urgent since the current HELP system has a good set of programs for the hospital or inpatient setting.

Server Environment

Servers in the new system may exist on mainframes, minicomputers, or UNIX-based RISC machines. Our initial servers are UNIX-based RISC machines. As in the client environment, the servers consist of three software layers: the communication layer, the business logic layer, and the database layer.

The communication layer in the server is provided by TUXEDO and is the complementary part of the same product that was described for the client environment. The server part of TUXEDO provides two important functions. First, it handles communication protocol support for TCP/IP, SNA, LU6.2, etc. Second, it provides a transaction monitoring service. This service maps a service request to the correct server and balances the load among servers. With hundreds of concurrent requests for the same service, this layer allows multiple copies of the same server to respond to requests and then distributes the requests appropriately.

The business logic layer supports application specific logic and accesses the database. We have chosen "C" and "C++" as the programming languages for the business logic layer.

The final layer of the server architecture is the database layer which includes the database files themselves and an API to access the database. For the initial UNIX-based servers the ORACLE RDBMS product has been selected. The API to ORACLE from the business logic layer is ANSI standard SQL (Structured Query Language) for most tables, while the "text database" capabilities of ORACLE will be used for manipulation and retrieval of full-text documents in the remaining tables.

Some of the most important services provided by the UNIX-based servers are described below, along with a description of the structure of some of the tables that exist in the clinical database. Figure 2 depicts an example of how a working system might be configured and the types of clients and servers that exist in the system.

Security

An essential aspect of the new architecture is preventing unauthorized persons from reading or modifying the clinical database. The security services are used by both clients and database servers to prevent unauthorized access. Where possible these services are built on the underlying security capabilities of ORACLE. The most important piece of the security system is the logon method which provides for positive identification of the user. The initial logon method provides for authentication by eliciting a secret password from the

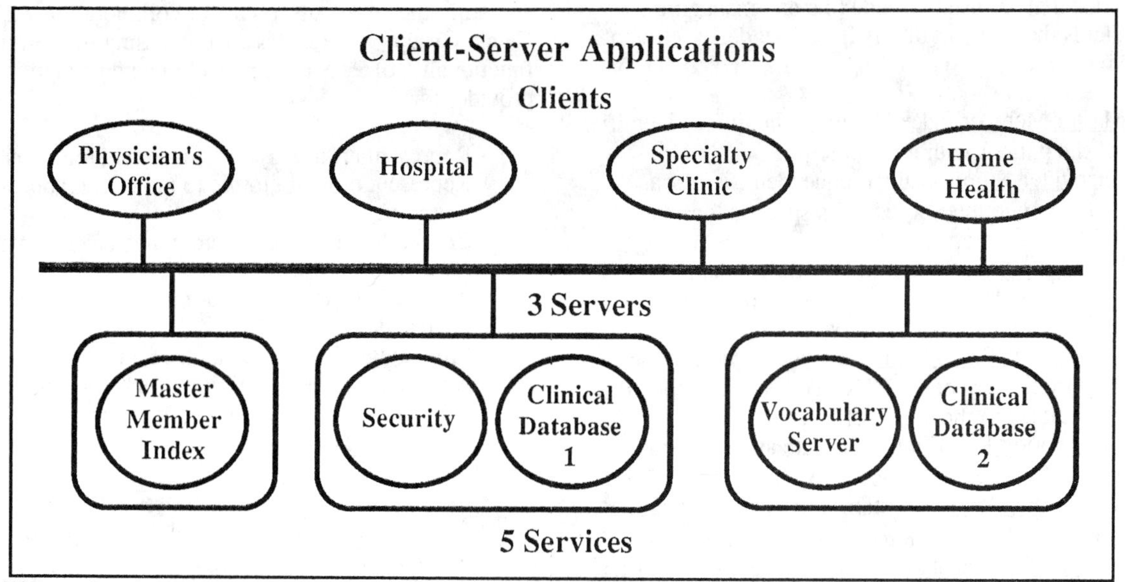

Figure 2: An example configuration of the system showing clients and servers attached to a wide area network. Only one client per facility is shown, but there would typically be several clients per facility. There may be one or more services provided by a server depending on the load balancing requirements.

user. Following identification of the user, services are invoked which indicate the functions and data tables that the user can access. Multiple levels of security are provided, with the first phase of security allowing restriction of access based on which data tables a user can read and modify. Future levels of security will be added as the client applications become more sophisticated and include restrictions based on columns within tables and on values within columns.

Patient Identification

A second essential part of the clinical database is the Master Member Index (MMI). The goal of the MMI is to provide an index of all patients or members of the health care enterprise. The MMI provides the following services:

- Establish an enterprise-wide member identifier that crosses both inpatient and outpatient settings.
- Establish a context-specific member identifier for each location within an enterprise.
- Provide search capabilities that link a member with all records in the LDR.
- Provide storage of member demographic information.
- Provide a log (audit trail) of changes to member names and demographic information.
- Provide facilities to detect and merge duplicate member records.

Patient Database

Nearly all clinical data will initially be stored in a single table, though this table will ultimately span more than one CPU. The table structure can be divided into two segments. The first portion of the table consists of fields that identify the patient that the data belongs to and other fields that are used for indexing and managing the data. Fields that are part of this fixed "header" section of the table include:

- Master Member Index Number - the unique identifier of the patient within the enterprise.
- Encounter Number - the unique identifier for a patient encounter or visit at a specific location within the enterprise.
- Event Identifier - a link to the clinical data dictionary that describes the structure and content of the data that is in the data portion of the record.
- Data Class, Type, and Field Code - a link to the first three parts of the PTXT codes that encode the data that is in the data portion of the record.
- Observation Date/Time - the date and time that the clinical observation was made.
- Store Date/Time - a system time stamp indicating when the data was stored in the database.
- Source of Information - indicates the user identifier or internal process identifier of the person or process that recorded the clinical data.
- Audit Information - several fields that are used in combination to create an audit trail of deletes and modifications to records in the database.

The second part of the table is a single relational field of variable length that contains the actual clinical data. The contents of this field are a packed PTXT string, similar in structure to the current PTXT strings used in the HELP system.

The patient data table, with its fixed relational portion and its packed PTXT string portion, is an intermediate step in the further evolution of the structure of the LDR. The exact next step is unknown, but two possible scenarios have been considered. The first option would be to evolve to a truly relational form where all the data is represented in normalized tables, possible table names would be Coagulation, Complete Blood Count, Blood Chemistry, etc. A second option would be to evolve to an Object Oriented Database (OODB). The innate structure of clinical data invites an object oriented approach, but these systems are not yet as stable as relational database platforms. The advantage of either of these models over the initial model described above is that they could be manipulated and viewed by off-the-shelf software solutions.

PTXT/Vocabulary/Data Dictionary

One of the key elements in the new architecture is an object oriented structure for the clinical vocabulary (clinical data dictionary). The new capabilities are implemented in a series of files that are too complex to present in this overview article. Many of the characteristics of the vocabulary are inherited from PTXT, but others are an adaptation of the Unified Medical Language System (UMLS) Metathesaurus structures [8] and still others are outgrowths of collaboration with the Canon Group [9]. Besides encompassing the current functionality of PTXT the new clinical data dictionary provides for:

- Representation of synonyms and homonyms.
- Representation of atomic to molecular concept mappings.
- Cross referencing of different medical encoding systems.
- Addition of site-specific terms for centrally defined concepts.
- Multi-lingual representation of concepts.
- A place to record a definition for each concept.
- A "string dictionary" that defines the component PTXT codes that can be legally combined into a valid PTXT string (record).
- Multiple hierarchical views of a given concept.
- A semantic network for non-hierarchical concept relationships.
- A link between selection lists used in client applications and the codes that are used to represent the clinical data in the database.

• Mechanisms for auditing and managing changes made to the terms in the dictionary.

Decision Support Services

Alerting and execution of other decision support logic is supported from both the client and server environments. Application and context specific rules that require foreground execution will be accessed in the client via an OLE object. System wide types of alerts and logic will be executed by the database server in response to the addition or modification of data in the database (i.e. data driven), or time driven based on elapsed time in the server.

DISCUSSION

We are not the first group to propose or build a client-server system for patient data management [10, 11]. Indeed, due to the prevalence of low cost clinical workstations most new patient care applications could be considered as client-server. What makes our experience somewhat unique is that we are migrating to a new architecture from a well established and successful existing system. The problems that this creates are much more difficult than creating a new system from scratch. A major part of our design must include plans for moving nearly 15 years of patient data from existing hardware and software to a new platform. Additionally, hundreds of user applications that operate against the old database must also be rewritten. Since neither the data transfer nor the application rewrites will happen instantaneously we have created a plan for coordinated use of both databases as work progresses. The migration plan is summarized below.

When the new MMI services are completed, a central MMI database will be loaded with our past and current patients and existing HELP system software will be modified to access the central database for MMI services instead of reading local files. A prerequisite for this change will be the reconciliation and merging of all duplicate patient identifiers.

A second major transition will occur when the clinical database services are available. At this point clinical data from existing HELP systems will be loaded into the new LDR. We currently have about 8 gigabytes of data that will need to be loaded. However, existing HELP systems in the hospitals will continue to operate against their own local databases. The data drive mechanism of the system will be used to cause any new data to be written to both the local HELP database and the new LDR. Because the data will exist redundantly in both databases, old HELP applications can continue to run while new versions are rewritten that access the new database directly. One reason that the packed PTXT strings from the old system were retained in the new architecture was to allow new and old applications to more easily coexist during what may be a rather long transition period. Also, further research is needed to test that any further evolution of the patient database can provide the same hierarchical inferencing functions as the current string structure while maintaining adequate performance.

In parallel with the activity taking place in the hospitals, outpatient clinics and physicians offices within IHC will begin using MMI services for identifying patients and the LDR for storage of ambulatory data. The outpatient activity will grow in volume as the available outpatient applications grow in number and sophistication.

In conclusion, we are optimistic about our new architecture. However, its success is by no means assured. Some potential problems include unacceptable response time of the new more atomic database, downtime or unreliability of the network servers, overload of the network due to greatly increased network traffic, and problems orchestrating the interfaces between the many commercial software packages that we are using. We hope to be able to report findings based on use of the new architecture in the near future.

Reference

[1] Warner HR, Olmsted CM, Rutherford BD. HELP - a program for medical decision making. *Comput Biomed Res* 1972;5:65-74.

[2] Kuperman GJ, Gardner RM, Pryor TA. *HELP: A Dynamic Hospital Information System*, Springer-Verlag, New York.

[3] Pryor TA. The HELP medical record system. *M.D. Computing* 1988; 5:22-33.

[4] Zimmermann H. OSI reference model - the ISO model of architecture for open systems interconnection. *IEEE Trans Commun* 1980; 28:425-32.

[5] TUXEDO. Novell Inc., 122 East 1700 South, Provo, Utah, 84606, USA.

[6] XATMI. Design Principles for Vendor-Independent OLTP Applications. Tandem Computers, Cupertino, California, 95014-2599, USA.

[7] Brockschmidt K. Inside OLE 2. Microsoft Press, Redmond, Washington.

[8] Lindberg DAB, Humphreys BL, McCray AT. The Unified Medical Language System. *Methods of Information in Medicine* 1993; 32:281-91.

[9] Evans DA, Cimino JJ, Huff SM, Hersh WR. Position statement: Toward a medical concept representation language. *Jour Amer Med Inform Assoc* 1994; In Press.

[10] Van Mulligen EM, Timmers T, Van Bemmel JH. A new architecture for integration of heterogeneous software components. *Methods of Information in Medicine* 1993; 32:292-301.

[11] Chueh HC, Barnett GO. Client-server, distributed database strategies in a health-care record system for a homeless population. *Jour Amer Med Inform Assoc* 1994; 1:186-98.

Report on the Clinical Workstation and Clinical Data Repository Utilization at UNC Hospitals

J. E. Hammond[1], R. G. Berger[2], T. S. Carey[3], S. M. Fakhry[4], R. Rutledge[4],
J. P. Kichak[5], T. J. Cleveland[5], M. J. Dempsey[5], N. M. Tsongalis[5] & C. F. Ayscue[5]
Departments of Medicine,[2,3] Pathology[1] & Surgery[4], School of Medicine,
University of North Carolina, Information Services Division[5],
UNC Hospitals, Chapel Hill, NC 27514

Abstract

On December 1, 1993, we implemented version 2.1 of the Clinical Workstation-Clinical Data Repository application in the Ambulatory Care Center. This version of the workstation allowed access of laboratory data from the clinical data repository that had been populated by a real-time HL7 interface between the Clinical Data Repository and the Laboratory Information System. This implementation completed a major part of the Clinical Workstation project. Also in December, we implemented a security system that records the date and time, user logon code, clinical workstation functions used, and the patient medical record number on whom data were displayed. In addition to the security function, this system has proven to be a valuable tool in evaluating the utilization of the clinical workstation and is the source of the data presented in this paper.

Introduction

Over the last few years the term physician workstation has appeared in the the medical informatics literature and as with many new concepts, this term has been applied loosely. Safran has suggested that these workstations must be patient centered; the interface must be uniform and data acquisition must be addressed at the system level (1). Current literature on the subject of workstations range from the theoretical (2,3) to demonstaration projects in education (4) or to limited patient care areas (5).

The large scale Clinical Workstation (CWS) project at UNC Hospitals is an effort to improve information management for healthcare providers. The Clinical Workstation and Clinical Data Repository (CDR) project began in 1991 (6). In 1993, we reported on the evolution of the CWS from the prototype to the production version 2.1 that included access to laboratory data from the CDR (7). Progress has continued and version 3 of the CWS is currently in production and version 4 is under development. Version 3 of the CWS has an icon based user interface with more consistency in displays between functions.

The CWS was designed to achieve four basic goals. The first goal was to give the physician user the illusion that the data was obtained from a single integrated information system while that system is being built over the next few years. The second goal was to make it possible for departmental information systems in the Hospital to evolve without requiring retraining of all physician users when these systems changed. The third goal was to develop a Clinical Data Repository using IBM's Relational Database Manager DB2 that would store radiology results, clinical and anatomic pathology results, discharge summaries, op-notes and clinic notes. The fourth goal was to develop HL7 interfaces between departmental systems, where this standard was supported, or locally develop Application Program to Program Communications (APPC) using the LU 6.2 standard when necessary. The purpose of this paper is to report the utilization of CWS/CDR in the ambulatory care setting.

Hardware, Software and Network Environment

The CWS is an IBM PS/2, model 77 with 12 mbytes of RAM running the IBM OS/2 version 2.1 operating system. Access to the UNC Hospital IBM ES9000 computer and the School of Medicine's distributed computing environment is provided via token ring network and the OS/2 Communications Manager, and TCP/IP v1.1 (IBM Corp., Armonk, NY). The CWS application is written in EASEL version 2.0 (Easel Corp., Burlington, MA) programming language with some C language communication subroutines. The Easel Workbench tool set provides a functionally rich environment for the development of the CWS. Routers (Cisco Systems, Menlo Park, CA) are used to bridge between the token ring network in the Hospital and the ethernet in the School of Medicine.

Laboratory data is transferred from the Laboratory Information System (LIS) (CHC, Houston, TX) to the CDR via an HL7 real-time interface. Radiology data (CHC, Houston, TX) and anatomic pathology data are currently moved from the radiology information system and LIS, respectively, to the CDR by daily tape transfers. This tape transfer system is temporary until the HL7 interface is completed for this text based data.

Clinic notes, operative notes and discharge summaries are transferred from the Hospital's dictation system (Softmed Systems, Bethesda, MD) via an internally developed (APPC) program using the LU 6.2 protocol. Access from the physician's office to the transcription system is provided either via the token ring network of the Hospital or the ethernet system of the School of Medicine, depending on the location of the office.

CWS Version 3 Enhancements

The major enhancements introduced in version 3 of the CWS include an icon based interface to supplement the menu bar interface that was used in version 2.1. In addition, the interface was made more uniform between the various display functions. For example, laboratory data, clinic encounters, and patient reports are all presented as cascading windows. Figure 1 below shows the initial icon based screen displayed to the user.

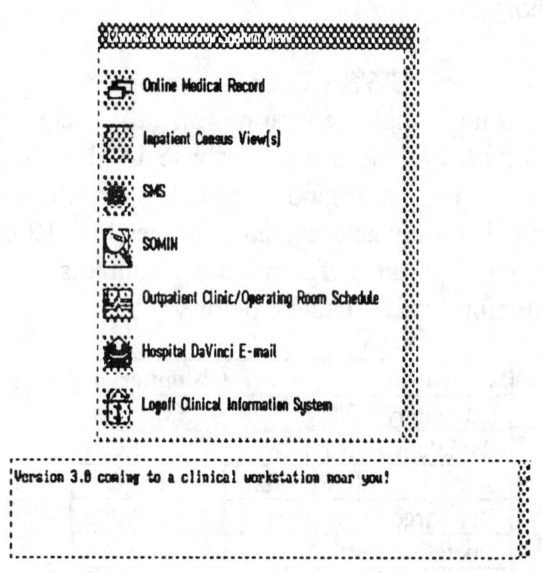

Figure 1. Initial icon based function screen.

From this screen it is possible to: use the CDR via the On-line Medical Record icon; use the inpatient view of the workstation via the Inpatient Census View icon; initiate a 3270 terminal session for SMS functions via the SMS icon; access the School of Medicine Information Network via the SOMIN icon; access the outpatient clinic and operating room scheduling system via its icon; read email via the DaVinci Email icon; and finally log off, using the log off icon. Once in the on-line medical record system navigation is via icons for major components of the system such as general information, medications, clinic visits, laboratory data and patient reports. This increased consistency in the user interface has made it easier to navigate through the different components of the CWS application.

In addition version 3 supports the ability to print any data to network printers associated with each workstations and fax data to approved recipients via a fax server. The fax capability is expected to enhance our ability to provide referring physicians with discharge summaries and other information generated on their patients while in our hospital.

CWS/CDR Utilization

The implementation of the clinical pathology laboratory database in the CDR and its corresponding CWS display application was completed November, 1993. Clinical Data Repository contents are summarized in Table 1 below.

Data Type	Number
Laboratory Tests	5,000,000
Radiology Reports	431,000
Anatomic Path Reports	145,000
Discharge Summaries	70,000
Operative Notes	40,000
Clinic Notes	23,000

Table 1 Contents of the CDR as of 5/1/94.

The CWS clinical laboratory display application was placed in routine operation on December 1, 1993. The implementation of the laboratory display function represented the completion of a major goal in CWS/CDR project.

Also, implemented on December 1, was a security sub-system that records all user actions each time the CWS is used. The security system records the date and time of use; user name, physician identification number if a physician, CWS workstation function used and patient's medical record number. The security system has also allowed us to generate data to monitor the utilization of the CWS. The data from the security system was downloaded from the DB2 relational database in the IBM ES9000 to a PC and analyzed using Paradox for Windows version 4.5.

The major functions summarized in Table 2 below include: the total number of visits **(Visits)** in the Ambulatory Care Center (ACC) where the majority of the forty-eight CWS are installed; Select Patient function **(Sel Pt)** that must be used each time patient data is displayed; Laboratory Display Folder **(Lab)** that must be used each time laboratory data is displayed; display of physician outpatient appointments **(Appts)**; display of patient medications **(Meds)**; display of discharge summary reports **(DCS Rept)**; display of radiology text reports **(Rad Rept)**; and the display of operative notes **(Op Note)**.

The number of patient records accessed via the CWS has climbed from 1,948 in December to 4,104 in April. This represents a 211% increase in use of the CWS in five months. The number of requests for laboratory data has grown from 690 or 35% of the patients selected in December to 2,460 or 60% of the patients selected in April. The increase in laboratory data display is most likely related to increased data in the CDR. Approximately, 25,000 results are transferred per day from the LIS to the CDR. Further, it should be noted that a major increase in workstation utilization (123%) occurred between March and April. The increase utilization between March and April was not due to increased patient volume in the ACC since in this interval the number of clinic visits decreased from 14,130 in March to 11,310 in April. During the month of March 1994, version 3 of the

CWS with the new icon based interface was installed in the ACC. It is possible that the increase in utilization of the CWS that occurred between March and April is due in part because of improved user interface.

Function	Dec	Jan	Feb	Mar	Apr
Visits x 10^{-1}	1077	1148	1184	1413	1131
Sel Pt	1948	2524	2131	3319	4104
Lab	690	885	810	1701	2460
Appts	270	345	243	406	352
Meds	268	262	234	394	490
DCS Rept	167	240	132	219	276
Rad Rept	114	185	239	302	426
Op Note	39	33	45	58	79
Somin	180	208	175	97	125

Table 2 Summary of frequency of use of the major CWS functions and monthly patient visits in the ACC.

In addition to growth in utilization of laboratory data, access to Radiology reports grew from 114 in December to 426 in April or a 373 % increase in utilization. Access to information on medications grew from 268 in December to 490 in April or a 183 % increase in utilization. The SOMIN system is principally used to access the local MedLine database that covers the medical literature from 1985 to the present and is maintained by the Office of Information System in the School of Medicine and Health Science Library.

The data from the security system also allowed us to determine who was using the CWS. All physicians at UNC Hospitals are assigned a unique five digit identification number that is recorded in the security system database. Non-physicians have no such number and zero is placed in the physician number field in the security system database. Based on the physician number field it is very easy to separate the physicians from the non-physician users. Non-physicians users of the CWS include nursing staff, medical students, pharmacy staff, medical secretaries, etc. The users of the CWS are shown in Table 3 above.

User	Dec	Jan	Feb	Mar	Apr
Physicians	88	89	87	109	123
Staff	26	41	48	61	49
Total	114	130	135	170	172

Table 3 Shows the number of Physician and non-physician users of the CWS between December 1993 and April 1994.

From the data in Table 3 it is apparent that the number of physician users has increased from 88 in December, to 123 in April, representing an increase of 140%. The greatest increase in physician use occurred in the months of March and April. Again, the increase in physician use between March and April can not be explained by increase in patient volume since patient volume in the ACC actually decreased in this interval. It is possible that this increase in use was related to the improved user interface. Non-physician staff use was less predictable but could have possibly decreased because of greater use of the CWS by the physicians themselves.

Phy Users	Dec	Jan	Feb	Mar	Apr
Med Fac	29	32	32	37	40
Surg Fac	9	7	7	8	6
Other Fac	10	10	9	10	14
Fac Total	48	49	48	55	60
Med HS	25	23	27	29	30
Surg HS	3	2	1	6	8
Other HS	12	15	11	19	25
HS Total	40	40	39	54	63

Table 4 CWS physician users by medical specialty and position on faculty (Fac) or House Staff (HS).

Although the total number of physician users were small it was possible to break physician user down by medical specialty. Table 4 above shows a distribution of physician users by specialty. As might be expected the top two users of the CWS were internal medicine and surgery. The other medical specialties group was comprised of pediatrics, dermatology, family medicine, emergency medicine, radiation oncology, ob/gyn, and orthopedics. The data shows a progressive increase in CWS utilization in both Faculty and House Staff and that both groups appear to be equal users of the CWS at the present time.

Future CWS/CDR Enhancements

The next major advance in the CWS/CDR project will occur in July, 1994, when one hundred fifty-five Clinical Workstations will become operational on the inpatient services of UNC Hospitals. The major display interface will be the same as in the outpatient version but the user will enter the inpatient application via the Inpatient Census View icon shown in Figure 1. The implementation of the CWS in the inpatient environment will give UNC Hospitals a uniform method for the display of patient care data for all health care providers in the Hospital. In addition to the inpatient system a remote dial-in version of the CWS has been completed and is being field tested by a group of physicians on the CWS development team.

Currently, the SMS order entry system is being installed at UNC Hospitals. This order entry system will provide the transaction processing system for the order module of the CWS that is planned for version 4. Future work will concentrate on creating data structures that will support acquiring data directly from the physician-patient encounter. Such structured data will allow the creation of an order entry function for the CWS that will support direct physician use and provide medical alerts based on institutional patient care rules.

Much has been accomplished at UNC Hospitals in a relatively short period of time but clearly, the next phase of the CWS/CDR development will be the most critical for achieving maximum utility of this information system. We will continue to use the data from the security system to monitor use of the CWS/CDR and, upon completion of the inpatient version, develop tools for monitoring user satisfaction with the information system.

References

1. Safran, Charles, Defining Clinical 'workstation', *Int J Biomed Comp*, **34**, pp 261-265, 1994.

2. C.G., Cesnik, B., and van Bemmel, J.H., Medical Data and Knowledge Management by Integrated Medical Workstations: Summary and Recommedations, Chute, *Int J Biomed Comp*, **34**, pp175-183, 1994.

3. Grams, R., et al, Earthbound Applications for NASA's Physician's Workstation, *J Med Syst*, 17:6, pp 353-361, 1994.

4. Litt, H.I. and Loosk, J.W., Digital Patient Records and the Medical Desktop, *Proc Annu Symp Comput Appl Med Care*, pp 555-559, 1992.

5. Connelly, DP, et al, Physician Use of an NICU Laboratory Reporting System, *Proc Annu Symp Comput Appl Med Care,* pp 8-12, 1993.

6. Hammond, J.E., Berger, R.G., Carey, T.S., Rutledge, R., Cleveland, T.J., Kirchak, J.P., and Ayscue, C.F., Making the Transition from Information Systems of the 1970's to Medical Information Systems of the 1990's: The Role of the Physician's Workstation, *J Med Sys*, **15**:3, pp. 257-267, 1991.

7. Hammond, J.E., Berger, R.G., Carey, T.S., Rutledge, R., Cleveland, T.J., Kirchak, J.P., Dempsey, M. J., Tsongalis, N. M. and Ayscue, C.F., Progress Report on the Clinical Workstation and Clinical Data Repository at UNC Hospitals, *Proc Annu Symp Comput Appl Med Care,* pp 243-247, 1993.

Accessing The Columbia Clinical Repository

Stephen B. Johnson, Ph.D., George Hripcsak, M.D.,
Joan Chen, M.S., Paul Clayton, Ph.D.

Center for Medical Informatics
Columbia Presbyterian Medical Center
New York, NY 10032

The Columbia Clinical Repository is the foundation of the Clinical Information System at the Columbia Presbyterian Medical Center (CPMC). The Repository is implemented as a relational database on an IBM mainframe, using a generic design that employs a small number of tables. Client applications on remote platforms send and receive data through Database Access Modules (DAMs), which support the HL7 protocol, while applications on the mainframe manipulate data through DAMs supporting a locally defined "query template". Implementation using static (compiled) SQL is compared to dynamic (ad hoc) SQL in terms of efficiency and flexibility.

INTRODUCTION

Clinical databases are the foundation of clinical information systems. Systems such as HELP [1], TMR [2], RMRS [3], and STOR [4] have revealed many important issues about the management of clinical data and the ways in which clinical applications need to access that data. The Columbia Clinical Repository benefitted greatly from the experience of these systems, particularly the HELP system. In a manner similar to these other systems, The Repository is designed to:

• support transactions for one patient at a time, in an efficient manner;

• store controlled vocabulary (data elements) as defined in the Medical Entities Dictionary (MED) [5];

• enable Medical Logic Modules (MLMs) to monitor patient events as they occur in the CIS and notify health care personnel as necessary [6].

The Repository is interesting in that it is implemented as a relational database using a generic design that employs a very small number of tables [7]. This approach allows new data elements to be stored in the database simply by defining them in the MED, rather than adding new columns to tables. This model is similar to a relational model developed independently for the HELP system [8]; however, unlike the HELP relational design, the Repository tables are normalized. The relational design is generated from a conceptual schema (expressed in the Entity-Relation formalism) which is based on a model of clinical events [9].

Additional information about the Repository is maintained in a "metadatabase" [10], a relational database that contains the MED, the collection of Medical Logic Modules, and information about how messages (data transactions) are routed to ancillary systems. One of the most important consequences of representing the MED in a relational form is that patient data can be queried by a class of medical entity in an efficient manner. For example, one can query whether a patient has any drug order in the class "antibiotics", without having to explicitly specify each such medication.

The Repository is intended to serve as a complete electronic medical record, and has the ability to store both in-patient and out-patient data in a longitudinal manner (spanning all encounters with the hospital). The coded data that is currently available includes demographics, laboratory results, and pharmacy orders. There is also a great wealth of narrative clinical data (radiology, pathology, cardiology, operative reports, discharge summaries, etc.).

The most challenging issue confronting the developers of the Repository is providing access to clinical data both for applications running on the same platform (e.g., the Event Monitor that executes Medical Logic Modules), and for client applications making requests from other platforms on the network. The remainder of the paper describes the different techniques used to provide access to

0195-4210/94/$5.00 © 1994 AMIA, Inc.

data, and discusses the advantages and disadvantages of the various approaches.

METHODS

The Columbia Clinical Repository is implemented on an IBM mainframe using the DB2 database management system. Clinical applications running locally on the same platform (under the CICS system) include a home-grown results review application and the Event Monitor. Applications on remote platforms include ancillary systems uploading clinical data (laboratory, pharmacy, cardiology, radiology, pathology, etc.), a primary care information system, and a resident sign-out system.

DB2 provides two forms of SQL for accessing tables: static SQL and dynamic SQL. Static SQL is used when a program containing SQL is compiled: the SQL statements are parsed, a plan of access is determined for each statement (e.g., what indexes will be used), and the SQL is replaced by appropriate procedure calls. Dynamic SQL is invoked when a program passes a SQL statement (represented as a string) to DB2 at execution time: the statement is parsed and a plan of access is determined "on the fly". This method incurs some overhead, since the DB2 catalogue (itself a DB2 database) must be queried by the DBMS to determine the best means of access.

SQL cannot be embedded directly in Medical Logic Modules and compiled into static SQL because they are executed by an interpreter (in our implementation). A similar limitation exists for the results review application which was developed using IBM's PCS/ADS system. We also do not currently possess the database and network software that would enable applications on other platforms to use static SQL that is bound to DB2 tables on the mainframe.

A satisfactory solution to these obstacles was reached through development of Data Access Modules (DAMs). These are mainframe programs, written in the PL/I language that can issue static SQL. On the mainframe, the Event Monitor interpreter and the results review application can call a DAM, pass parameters to specify a database request, and then receive data back through other parameters.

Remote applications cannot call mainframe DAMs directly, but instead make use of a utility that resides on an intermediate UNIX machine (an IBM RS 6000). This utility acts as a "clinical data mediator", carrying out the communication with the mainframe DAMs through IBM's Advanced Program to Program Communications (APPC) network protocol.

Since SQL could not be used as the standard of access, a suitable interface had to be defined. For mainframe applications, which need to query the Repository, a generic "query template" was developed as the interface between these applications and each of the DAMs [11]. When invoked, a DAM examines the parameters of the query template and chooses from a fixed set of static SQL statements to carry out the query. Data retrieved by the DAM is passed back through the template.

Data exchange standards were considered essential for applications residing on other platforms, and Health Level 7 (HL7) was chosen as the protocol. For mainframe applications, the query template was preferred over HL7 as it is somewhat simpler for application developers and MLM authors to understand.

The functions performed by data access modules can be summarized as follows:

1. Request Handling: the data request message submitted by the client process is parsed, and the various parameters in the message are checked for validity.

2. Data Conversion: data elements in the request message are translated into a standard coded form as defined by the MED.

3. Database Operations: the SQL statements required to update or query the database are executed.

4. Notification: the Event Monitor is notified about the type of database action that just

occurred. MLMs may get triggered as a result of a database update.

5. Response Generation: a response message is generated indicating whether the request has been carried out successfully or not, and any data retrieved from the database is returned as part of the response.

Adding new features to data access modules can be time consuming. To enable developers building applications on remote platforms to query the Repository more directly, a DAM was made available that supports dynamic SQL. This DAM works in a similar manner to those described above, except that the client application passes a SQL statement embedded in an HL7 message. The SQL statement is executed dynamically by DB2, and the results are returned to the client application in an HL7 format.

Some extensions to the HL7 standard were required by added "Z" segments to the HL7 message: a "ZQL" segment is passed along with standard HL7 segments for a query. In the response, a "ZMH" segment returns the number of rows retrieved, the number of database columns of which the data is composed, and the names of the columns. The data itself is returned in multiple "ZMO" segments, which each item of data (a cell of a relational table) occupying one segment.

RESULTS

Timing studies of the production system showed that review of laboratory data using a mainframe program takes 0.375 seconds per transaction (total elapsed time), on average. This is similar to the average elapsed time of 0.195 seconds previously obtained for queries executed by MLMs [12]. Upload of laboratory data requires 0.685 seconds per transaction (elapsed time), on average.

Queries submitted by remote applications were also compared. Pharmacy orders and laboratory results for a specified patients were retrieved, using the DAM that executes static SQL, and the DAM that uses dynamic SQL. The average elapsed times in seconds were as follows:

	Dynamic	**Static**
Order	1.58	0.98
Result	0.97	0.81

These results suggest that dynamic SQL is only slightly more expensive than static. It is interesting to note that the lab query was faster, despite involving a relational join.

DISCUSSION

HL7 is a useful standard of access for applications residing on platforms remote from the mainframe. The chief benefit of this architecture is that client applications are made independent of the implementation of the Clinical Repository. As a result, application programmers do not have to use SQL, or understand the design of the relational database.

Application developers also benefit from the other services provided by DAMs. They can use the data elements with which they are familiar, since the DAM performs the conversions. In addition, the DAM automatically notifies the Event Monitor, freeing applications from this responsibility.

Finally, the architecture enables the implementation of the Repository to be changed, (e.g., to an object-oriented DBMS), with a minimal impact on applications.

HL7 has been found to be best suited for interfaces to ancillaries that are well understood, and that do not have changing requirements, such as routine uploads and downloads. The syntax is very cumbersome for human users, e.g., developers of review programs, and authors of MLMs.

The query templates developed for mainframe applications, such as the Event Monitor, are clinically oriented, and have a marginally better syntax than HL7 for users. However, this interface is not a standard, and requires that a second set of DAMs be maintained in addition to the HL7 DAMs.

The biggest drawback in both these approaches is the software maintenance of the DAMs that interpret the client request (HL7 messages or query template) and then execute the appropriate SQL. This is consistent with the earlier finding that data access is the most costly aspect of developing Medical Logic Modules, in terms of coding, maintenance, and execution time [12].

A large part of this maintenance burden is due to the inflexibility of static SQL. In DB2 SQL, a table cannot be expressed using a variable, thus a separate SQL statement must be coded for each table in the database, and for each useful join (when information must be combined from two tables). While the number of tables is small, and the possible joins very limited, the DAMs are still rather complex.

Another limitation concerns the use of lists. For example, the client may wish to retrieve values for a given list of observations. Since DB2 does not permit the use of an array as a host variable, the list must be coded as a collection of individual host variables:

```
:LISTLEN = 0 OR <column> IN (:VAR1,
:VAR2, ..., :VARN)
```

The maximum list size (N) must be determined ahead of time, and dummy values must be placed in unused variables if less than N items are requested. The test (LISTLEN = 0) must be used to insure that the condition is true when the list is empty.

While dynamic SQL is less efficient, it has the advantage of great flexibility. A skilled user can perform any desired database transaction. This method requires that the user possess complete knowledge of the design of the relational tables in the Repository. While the generic design has provided efficient access, it has proven to be difficult for users to understand.

An interesting consequence of the generic design of the Repository is that certain common queries are much simpler (and more efficient) to express in a procedural manner than using SQL alone. For example, the most frequently used form of clinical query requests the most recent N values of a given observation (e.g., the last 3 serum sodium levels). While it is possible to express this in SQL, the query is extremely complex and inefficient.

The use of procedural code permits a simple (and efficient) solution: the transaction need only retrieve N rows meeting the criteria (perform just N fetches). This is easily accomplished by embedding the SQL query within procedural code containing a loop executed N times:

```
EXEC SQL
DECLARE c CURSOR FOR
SELECT ...
FROM ...
WHERE ...

EXEC SQL OPEN c;

DO FOR I = 1 TO N;
        FETCH c INTO :structure
        [Add data from structure to
        response]
END;

EXEC SQL close c;
```

The generic design also makes certain views of clinical data very difficult to express in SQL. For example, laboratory tests (e.g., levels of sodium, potassium, and chloride) are not stored as individual columns of a table. To construct a view of lab values with test names as columns requires an SQL statement with as many joins as there are tests. However, the view can easily be constructed by a DAM, using a procedural loop like the one show above.

CONCLUSION

The database component of any Clinical Information System will need to provide access to clinical applications residing on the same platform and on remote platforms as hospital computing environments become increasingly distributed. The approach taken at Columbia has been to encapsulate important types of queries in Data Access Modules, which insulate clients from the database structure, provide efficient access to data, and construct views of data that are too costly to define using SQL by itself.

These modules are effective for routine uploads and downloads but are complex and hard to modify to meet the needs of application developers in a timely manner.

These findings indicate an important direction for further study: data access modules supporting dynamic SQL are appropriate when a high level, flexible means of accessing data is required (e.g., in developing Medical Logic Modules). However, these DAMs must support a view of the database which users can easily understand, and provide those temporal operations that are not easily expressed in SQL (e.g., "the 3 most recent values of ...").

Acknowledgements

Support for this project was provided by the IBM Corporation.

References

[1] Pryor TA. The HELP medical record system. MD Computing, 1988;5(5):22-33.

[2] Stead WW, Hammond WE. Computer-Based Medical Records: The Centerpiece of MD Computing, 1988;5(5):48-62.

[3] McDonald CJ, Blevins L, Tierney WM, Martin DK. The Regenstrief Medical Record. MD Computing, 1988;5(5):34-47.

[4] Whiting-O'Keefe QE, Whiting A, Henke J. The STOR Clinical Information System MD Computing, 1988;5(5):34-47.

[5] Cimino JJ, Hripcsak G, Johnson SB, Clayton PD. Designing an introspective, multi-purpose controlled medical vocabulary. In: Kingsland LC, editor. Proceedings of the Thirteenth Annual Symposium on Computer Applications in Medical Care; 1989 November 5-8; Washington. Washington: IEEE Computer Society Press, 1989:513-518.

[6] George Hripcsak, James J. Cimino, Stephen B. Johnson, Paul D. Clayton. The Columbia-Presbyterian Medical Center decision-support system as a model for implementing the Arden Syntax. In: Clayton PD, editor. Proceedings of the Fifteenth Annual Symposium on Computer Applications in Medical Care; 1991 Nov 17-20; Washington, D.C. New York: IEEE Computer Society Press, 1991: ?.

[7] Friedman C, Hripcsak G, Johnson SB, Cimino JJ, Clayton PD. A generalized relational scheme for an integrated clinical patient database. In: Miller RA, editor. Proceedings of the Fourteenth Annual Symposium on Computer Applications in Medical Care; 1990 November 4-7; Washington. Washington: IEEE Computer Society Press, 1990: 335-339.

[8] Huff SM, Berthelsen CL, Pryor TA, Dudley AS. Evaluation of an SQL model of the HELP patient database. In: Clayton PD, editor. Proceedings of the Fifteenth Annual Symposium on Computer Applications in Medical Care; 1991 November 17-20; Washington. New York: McGraw Hill, 1992:386-90.

[9] Johnson SB, Friedman C, Cimino JJ, Hripcsak G, Clayton PD. Conceptual data model for a central patient database. In: Clayton PD, editor. Proceedings of the Fifteenth Annual Symposium on Computer Applications in Medical Care; 1991 November 17-20; Washington. New York: McGraw Hill, 1992: 381-385.

[10] Johnson SB, Cimino JJ, Friedman C, Hripcsak G, Clayton PD. Using metadata to integrate medical knowledge in a clinical information system. In: Miller RA, editor. Proceedings of the Fourteenth Annual Symposium on Computer Applications in Medical Care; 1990 November 4-7; Washington. Washington: IEEE Computer Society Press, 1990: 340-344.

[11] Hripcsak G, Johnson SB, Sideli RV, Clayton PD. Using Data Access Modules for Legacy Databases. Accessing the electronic medical record using HL7. In: Rindfleisch TC, editor. Proceedings of the 1994 AMIA Spring Congress; 1994 May 4-7; San Francisco. Washington, D.C.: AMIA, 1994.

[12] Hripcsak G, Johnson SB, Clayton PD. Desperately Seeking Data: Knowledge Base-Database Links. In: Safran C, ed. Proceedings of the Seventeenth Annual Symposium on Computer Applications in Medical Care, 1993 Oct 3-Nov 3; Washington (DC). New York: McGraw Hill, 1993:639-42.

Using a Computerized Patient Record to Reengineer an Outpatient Clinic

Stephen M. Borowitz, M.D.
University of Virginia Health Sciences Center, Charlottesville, Virginia, 22908

ABSTRACT

By employing process flow analysis and work redesign techniques during the design and implementation of a computerized patient record in the pediatric outpatient clinics at the University of Virginia Health Sciences Center, we have developed a database of clinical observations while simultaneously shortening the time that patients spend waiting in the pediatric clinics and decreasing the number of support staff employed within the clinics.

Like most other large medical institutions, the University of Virginia has a long history of administrative and financial computing systems, however our first entry into the realm of clinical computing didn't begin until five years ago when the institution installed a computerized electronic physician order entry and communication system. The implementation of this system was a very painful process, but the system is now deeply ingrained in the institutional culture [1]. While there were some altruistic motives for developing this system, the biggest single reason for its development was anticipated cost-savings. While the system has resulted in many benefits ranging from faster order processing to a dramatic decline in medication errors, the overall cost savings have been small. This is not a unique experience. As a whole, information technology has generated neither tremendous cost savings nor substantial gains in productivity [2,3]. In those organizations that have realized significant benefits from the adoption of information systems, this success has only been achieved when the system has been designed to serve process requirements, and the organization has focused on the implementation and post-implementation management of the information system to insure its adoption and proper use [4,5].

When we reviewed the development and implementation of our order entry and communication system, we found that in many circumstances the system seemed to create more rather than less work. This was a direct consequence of computerizing old ways of doing business, and as such, actually adding more steps to existing processes [6]. Therefore, before implementing a computerized patient record in the Department of Pediatrics at the University of Virginia we performed a comprehensive assessment of current practices. Management Information Systems graduate students from the McIntire School of Commerce at the University of Virginia reviewed work and information flow in the outpatient clinics.

Rather than being a seamless operation, the delivery of patient care was a composite of three discrete and distinct enterprises: 1) patient registration and its associated documentation; 2) the delivery of care and its associated documentation; and 3) patient billing and its associated documentation. While these three processes related to one another, they often proceeded in parallel as well as opposing directions. Moreover, these three enterprises were managed by three distinct groups of people. The end result of this division of labor was a series of extremely complex and convoluted processes. As an example, ***figure 1*** depicts outpatient billing and registration at the beginning of our assessment. While computers have been incorporated in many places, they have not been used to integrate the process, but rather to dis-integrate it.

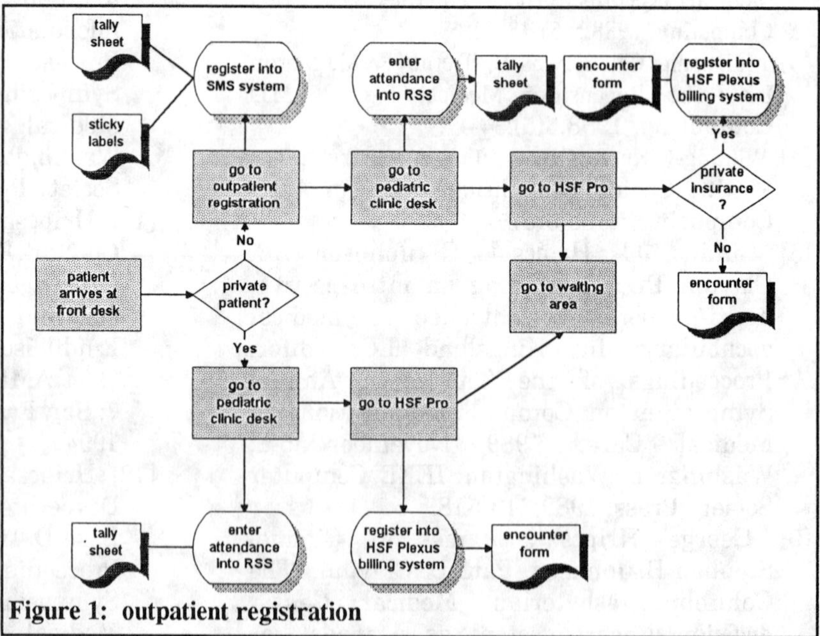

Figure 1: outpatient registration

Ideally, patient care should be an iterative process with needed documentation as well as billing and administrative information being an outgrowth of the delivery of care. We have tried to use the Lifetime Clinical Record (LCR) as a means of redesigning work and information flow in our outpatient clinics while simultaneously capturing clinical information.

At its very best, a patient encounter in all outpatient settings should be very simple. The patient arrives, he or she is escorted to an examination room, the physician, already armed with all the information he or she needs, visits with the patient, delivers whatever care is appropriate, and the patient leaves. In the process of delivering care, information should be automatically collected and routed to the appropriate resources, and the needed documentation generated. For such an encounter to occur, there must be complete integration of billing and administrative functions with the actual delivery of care as well as with the documentation processes. We employed process redesign to streamline the outpatient registration process and integrate it into the delivery of patient care (*figure 2*). With the new system, when a patient is registered

```
                    PEDIATRIC ATTENDANCE DISPLAY

   MED REC      PATIENT NAME          RESOURCE      APPT    REGS    INRM
   -------      ------------          --------      ----    ----    ----
 1 XXXXXXX XXXXXX ,XXXXXXX XXXX   PULMONARY DRS  09:30   09:11   09:16
 2 XXXXXXX XXXXXX ,XXXXXXXXX XX   RA GOMEZ       09:30   09:02   09:39
 3 XXXXXXX XXXXXXX ,XXXXX XXX     RA GOMEZ       09:30   08:13   09:47
 4 XXXXXXX XXXXXXXX ,XXXXX        WL CLARKE      09:30   10:12   10:22
 5 XXXXXXX XXXXXX XX ,XXXX XXXX   PW HEYMANN     09:30
 6 XXXXXXX XXXXXX, XXXXXX XXXX    RA GOMEZ       10:00
 7 XXXXXXX XXXXXX ,XXXXX XXXX     RA GOMEZ       10:00   09:52   10:10
 8 XXXXXXX XXXXXXX ,XXXX XXXXX    PW HEYMANN     10:00   09:50
 9 XXXXXXX XXXXXX ,XXXXXXX XXXX   PW HEYMANN     10:00   09:35
10 XXXXXXX XXXX ,XXXXXXXX XXXXX   PULMONARY DRS  10:15   09:55   10:28
11 XXXXXXX XXXX XX ,XXXXXXX XXX   RA GOMEZ       10:30   09:56   10:08
12 XXXXXXX XXXX ,XXXXXX XXXXX     WL CLARKE      10:30
13 XXXXXXX XXXXXXXX ,XXXXXXX XX   PULMONARY DRS  10:30   10:31   10:50
14 XXXXXXX XXXXX ,XXX X           RA GOMEZ       10:30   10:10   11:19

__ <------ SELECT ITEM, PRESS ENTER TO COMPLETE SELECTION
```

Figure 3: waiting room status screen

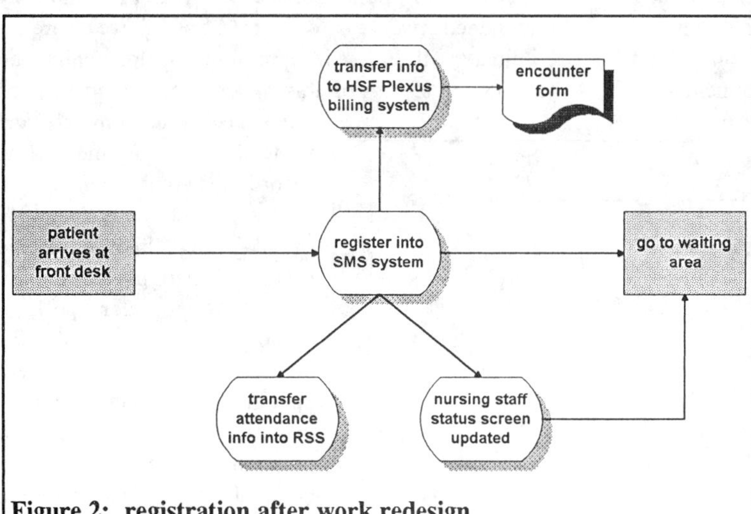

Figure 2: registration after work redesign

at the front desk of one of the pediatric clinics, the nursing staff are immediately notified on a status screen that the patient is in the waiting room, as well as the time of the patient's appointment and the time the patient arrived to be seen (*figure 3*). By entering vital signs and growth parameters directly into the clinical database, nursing staff automatically notifies physicians that the patient is in a room and ready to be seen, as well as the time the patient arrived in the room.

This relatively simple process redesign enabled the development of a database of clinical observations that previously were not accessible to providers while simultaneously shortening the time that patients spend waiting in the pediatric clinics. On average, every patient visit has been shortened by fifteen minutes. While most of this time has been shaved from registration and waiting room time, there has also been a decrease in the amount of time patients spend waiting in exam rooms. The end result has been a substantial decrease in the cycle time associated with a patient visit thus allowing more patients to be seen in the same number of examination rooms. Moreover, the information system has improved the efficiency of nursing staff. Before implementation, approximately 60% of nursing time in the outpatient setting was spent performing clerical functions. By streamlining the visit process, we have decreased the amount of paper documentation the nursing staff are required to generate. Patient flow through the clinics has been significantly improved, parents are more satisfied, and we have been able to eliminate one full-time nursing position.

Data retrieval from the LCR is very straight-forward and widely accessible. Terminals are available throughout all inpatient and outpatient units in the medical center, and the system can be easily accessed across the university-wide ethernet as well as remotely by modem. This provides faculty, housestaff, students, and referring physicians ready access to the system from their offices and their homes. The LCR has been integrated into the medical center wide computerized appointment scheduling system, as well as the electronic mail system. Many terminals also have direct access to the health sciences center library's card catalog,

```
                      PATIENT VERIFICATION                      04/23/94  1832

      SEX: F  DOB: 11/19/1990  MRN: XXXXXXX
  RACE: W  M/S: S                                        SSN: XXX-XX-XXXX
---------------------------------------------------------------------------------
    DEMOGRAPHIC DATA                    |    ****** LCR PEDS CLINIC MENU ******
ADDRESS:     XXX PEACOCK DRIVE          |     ! 01 VITAL SIGNS GROWTH DATA ENTRY
ADDRESS2:                               |     ! 02 VIEW PEDIATRIC FLOWSHEET
CITY:        CHARLOTTESVILLE            |     ! 03 VIEW FLOWSHEET OPTIONS
STATE:       VA  DISTRICT CODE:    1    |     ! 04 CORRECT PEDIATRIC OBSERVATIONS
ZIP CODE:    XXXXX                      |     ! 05 VIEW CASE HISTORY
PHONE:       XXX-XXX-XXXX               |    ****** LCR IMMUNIZATION MENU ******
COUNTRY:                                |     ! 06 IMMUNIZATION DATA ENTRY
NEAREST RELATIVE                        |     ! 07 VIEW IMMUNIZATION RECORD
LAST NAME:  XXXXXXXX                    |     ! 08 CORRECT IMMUNIZATION DATA
FIRST NAME: XXXXXXXX XXXX               |     ! 09 PRINT IMMUNIZATION RECORD
REL TO PAT:   M                         |
PHONE:         XXX-XXX-XXXX             |     ! 10 VIEW OLPR DOCUMENTS
                                        |                 ENTER SELECTION  __
---------------------------------------------------------------------------------
  ! (PF11) SIGNOFF                          (PF17) RECORD PATIENT IN ROOM TIME
  ! (PF14) RETURN TO PT LOCATE MAIN MENU    (PF18) RECORD PATIENT DEPARTURE TIME
                                            (PF16) SEND PATIENT DATA TO LCR
```

Figure 4: LCR retrieval screen

MEDLINE®, and a number of other full-text and bibliographic databases.

To retrieve patient information from LCR, the desired patient is identified by name, hospital number, or social security number and the provider is presented with a short list of retrieval options (***figure 4***). The level of access is regulated by linking menu options to provider identification. All coded information has been entered into a flowsheet which currently includes a history of medical encounters, diagnoses, vital signs, growth data, immunization information, and all laboratory results (***figure 5***). The system also includes a powerful search function that allows clinicians to search for particular data elements rather than forcing them to browse through the entire worksheet.

```
  PATIENT RESULTS DISPLAY              SELECT A SET                04/23/94  1835
NAME: XXXXXXXXXXXXXXXXXXX
-----------------------------------------------------------------PAGE   1 OF   2
  ? 1  PED FLOWSHEET
  ? 2    PED VS
  ? 3    PED GROWTH
  ? 4    ADM SET
  ? 5    LAB - PEDIATRICS SET
  ? 6      CBC PROFILE
  ? 7      CHEM DEPT SET
  ? 8        ARTERIAL BLOOD GAS
  ? 9        ELECTROLYTES (WHOLE BLOOD)
  ? 10       ENZYME PROFILE
  ? 11       LIPID PANEL
  ? 12       REABSORBED PHOSPHORUS
  ? 13       URIC ACID CLEAR
  ? 14       UREA NITROGEN CLR
  ? 15       CHEM/IMM/OTHER
--------------------------------------------- KEY IN A NUMBER __ AND PRESS ENTER
  !(PF14) RETURN TO PT MENU             ! PF8 MAX
  !(PF15) DISPLAY OPTIONS               ! PF6 UP
                                        ! PF7 DOWN
                                        ! PF9 MAX
```

Figure 5: LCR flowsheet

Transcribed text, including discharge summaries, operative reports, radiology reports and selected consultation reports and outpatient notes, is linked to an encounter history. This affords clinicians the ability to reconstruct a narrative of the patient's record at any workstation.

We have tried to use similar techniques in the development of a regional immunization database for Central Virginia. Nowhere is the failing of the paper patient record more apparent than with childhood immunizations. Childhood immunizations are among the most cost effective of health interventions. It has been estimated that for every dollar spent on childhood immunizations, we save $14 down the line [7]. Despite the fact that virtually all children in this country are completely immunized by the time they enter school at age five, only 50-60% are completely immunized by age two [8]. It is during the first two years that children are at greatest risk for many of the diseases we are trying to prevent with immunizations. Without any changes in patient behavior, we could increase the rate of completely immunized two-year olds to 85% if we were to eliminate all missed opportunities for childhood vaccination [9]. For this to happen, providers need quick access to complete and up-to-date immunization records for all children.

Since more than 40% of all young children receive their vaccinations from more than one provider [10], a computerized immunization database must be patient specific rather than institution specific. That is, each child must have his or her own complete immunization record which includes all immunizations administered regardless of whether those immunizations have been administered at a single geographic site, or many different sites.

Since the immunization database is shared among many providers, each with their own unique information management system, and therefore each with their own unique patient identification system, a master index has been created which associates all the different patient identifiers with a specific child. This allows providers to query and update the database using the patient identifier associated with their own current information management system.

With our current paper-based system, there are many obstacles to immunizing a child. First, a complete immunization record must be available and accessible, then the record must be reviewed, consent obtained, and finally the immunization administered. Not surprisingly, there is a great deal of paper work associated with this process (*figure 6*). By integrating the immunization database with the registration and billing systems, we have eliminated a number of the potential stumbling blocks for immunizing children, and essentially forced providers to consider immunization at every opportunity. At the same time we have managed to eliminate much of the nursing and clerical paperwork associated with the administration of immunizations (*figure 7*).

The immunization database allows providers at any site quick and easily obtainable immunization records on-line for any child within Central Virginia. By mapping immunization information to a simple one page grid, caregivers can quickly determine a child's immunization history and administer appropriate immunizations to bring that child "up to date". Current immunization recommendations can be retrieved with a keystroke. Data entry screens have been designed to improve workflow so that all necessary information is captured on-line. This results in significantly less paper work and the ability to retrieve information enhanced. As the database evolves, it will provide decision support in the form of actively advising the provider of all vaccinations currently due a patient, identify true versus false contraindications for the administration of immunizations, and provide new information about immunization practices at the point of use. With further development, the system will also be able to assist in the reminder process, identifying children who are due for immunizations, and automatically generating reminder letters.

In summary, a computerized patient record can improve the delivery of health care by providing health care professionals with better and faster access to clinical data of higher quality. There are no longer significant technological barriers to the development and implementation of a computerized patient record, but rather, there are substantial behavioral, administrative, and political barriers. In order for the health care industry to realize substantial cost savings and gains in overall productivity with computerization, we cannot simply computerize our current paper-based medical record. Computerizing existing processes adds more steps to existing work flow, and as such, decreases

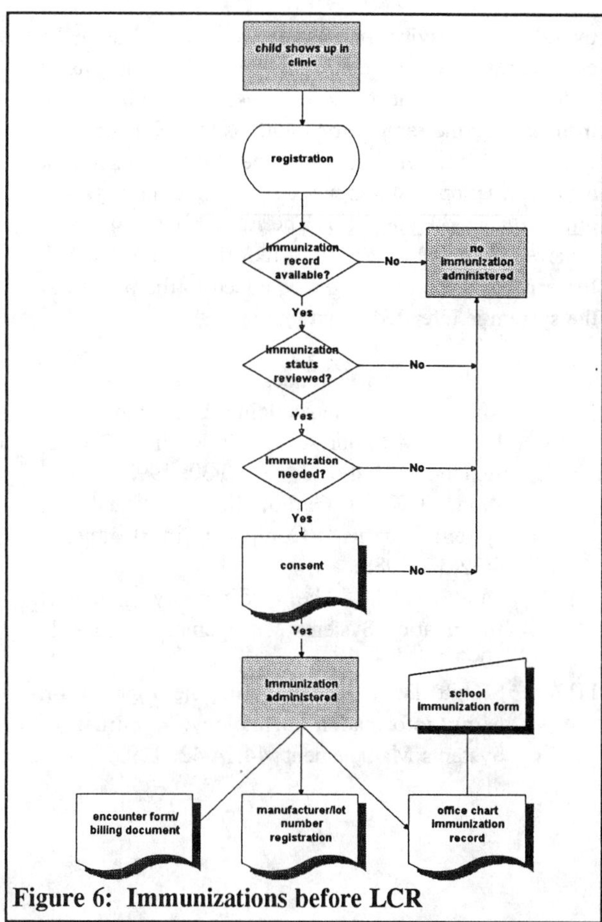

Figure 6: Immunizations before LCR

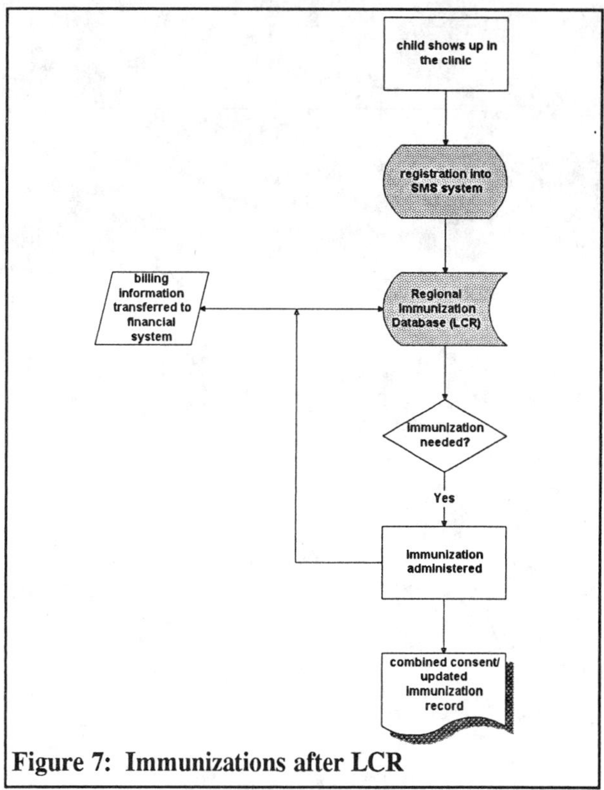

Figure 7: Immunizations after LCR

overall productivity and increases costs. Rather, a computerized patient record must be used as a means of redesigning current work processes and eliminating many ad hoc and temporary solutions that have become institutionalized over time. The over-riding principle of any information system must be **"capture information once, and at the source".** The further data capture is removed from where it is collected, the greater the risk for error and the more work is added to the processes the system is intended to automate.

References

[1] Massaro, T. Introducing Physician Order Entry at a Major Academic Medical Center. Academic Medicine 68: 20-30, 1993.

[2] Zinn, T.K., DiGiulio, L.W. Actualizing system benefits. Computers in Healthcare 9:32-34. 1988.

[3] Due, R.T. The productivity paradox. Information Systems Management 10:68-71, 1993.

[4] Schnitt, D.L. Reengineering the organization using information technology. Journal of Systems Management 44:14-42, 1993.

[5] King, W.R., Raghunathan, T.S. How strategic is information systems planning. Datamation 22:133-140, 1987.

[6] Hammer, M., Champy, J. Reengineering the Corporation. Harper Collins Publishers, Inc., New York, 1993.

[7] White, C.C., Kaplan, J.P., Orenstein, W.A. Benefits, risks, and costs of immunization for measles, mumps, and rubella. Am. J. Public Health 75:735-744, 1985.

[8] Shalala, D.E. Giving pediatric immunizations the priority they deserve. JAMA 269:1844-1845, 1993.

[9] Szilagyi, P.G., Rodewald, L.E., Humiston, S.G. Missed opportunities for childhood vaccination in office practices and the effect on vaccination status. Pediatrics 91:1-7, 1993.

[10] Blumen, L. Proposal for a National Immunization Tracking System. Centers for Disease Control 1993.

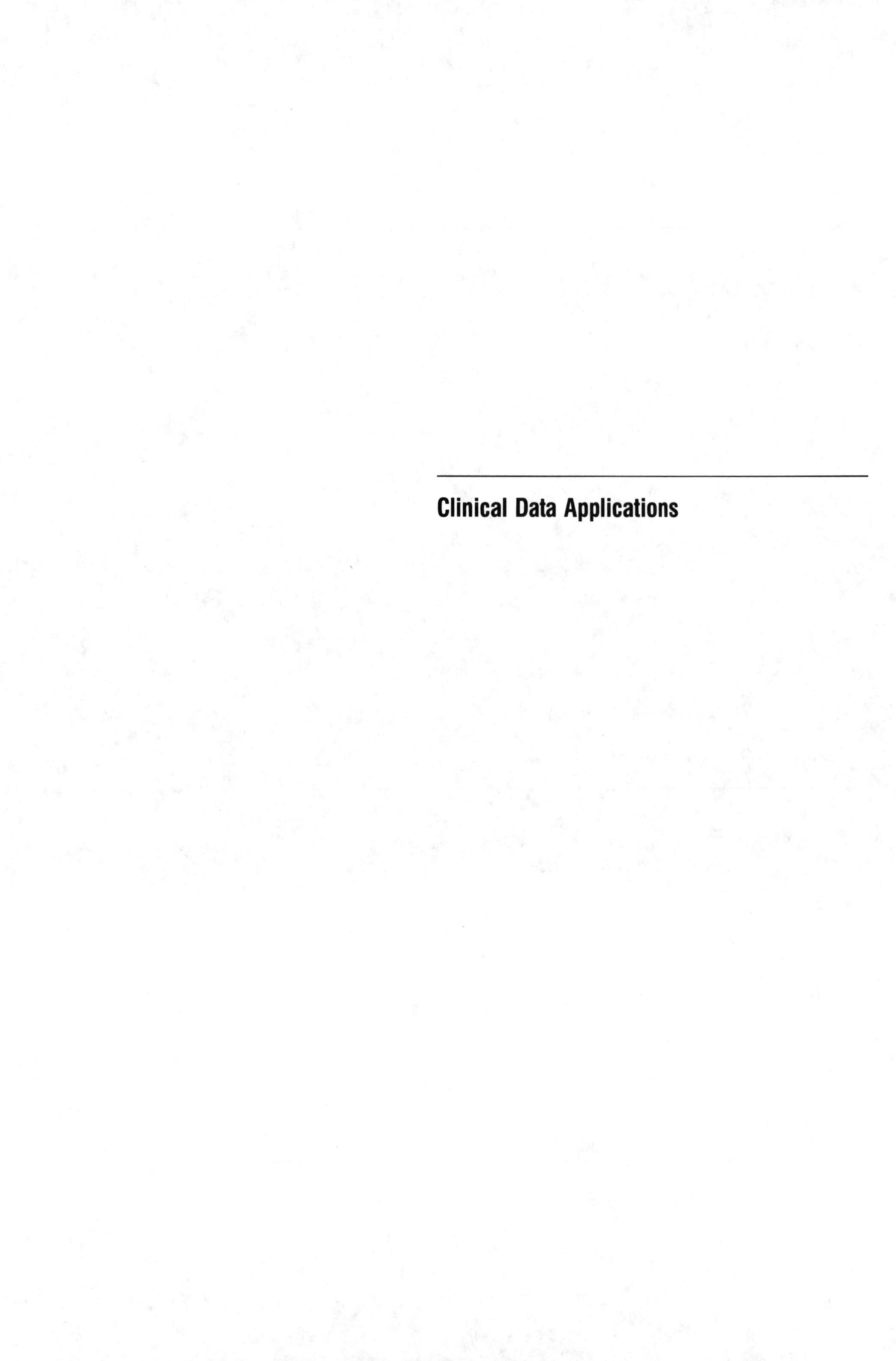

Clinical Data Applications

Information Engineering for Molecular Diagnostics

James M. Sorace , M.D., Michele Ritondo, M.S., Kip Canfield Ph.D.
Department of Pathology and Laboratory Medicine, Baltimore VAMC,
Department of Pathology at The University of Maryland and
The Laboratory for Health Care Informatics at The University of Maryland Baltimore County

ABSTRACT

Clinical laboratories are beginning to apply the recent advances in molecular biology to the testing of patient samples. The emerging field of Molecular Diagnostics will require a new Molecular Diagnostics Laboratory Information System which handles the data types, samples and test methods found in this field. The system must be very flexible in regards to supporting ad-hoc queries. The requirements which are shaping the developments in this field are reviewed and a data model developed. Several queries which demonstrate the data models ability to support the information needs of this area have been developed and run. These results demonstrate the ability of the purposed data model to meet the current and projected needs of this rapidly expanding field.

INTRODUCTION

Molecular Diagnostics (MD) is a new family of techniques which will greatly increase the type and amount of information generated on clinical samples. MD is currently enjoying considerable success in two major areas. The first is the area of Clinical Microbiology, which involves the detection and characterization of infectious agents [1]. Both the diagnosis for therapeutic purposes, and characterization of the pathogen for epidemiological purposes are important. Interest in this data is greatly increasing due to the rapid rise of antibiotic resistance and the spread of new diseases. The second area is in the field of Anatomic Pathology, in which molecular techniques are being used to characterize infectious agents directly from tissue samples, the molecular changes underlying malignancy, and the determination of malignant cellular lineage [2].

Despite intense interest in informatics support for molecular biology, none of the current databases are principally designed to support clinical research in this field [3,4]. In order to address this issue we are developing a data model for a Molecular Diagnostic Laboratory Information System (MDLIS). The database resulting from this model allows for rapid searching and retrieval of information for clinical, research, and epidemiological needs. While numerous databases and software systems exist for biological sequence comparisons, key elements for an MDLIS are lacking. These elements fall into three main areas. First there is the need to actually manage and store the work flow of the laboratory. This includes keeping track of tests ordered, inventorying DNA extractions, and archiving test result data. Secondly, the system needs to be able to support a very broad range of potential queries. For example, the species of the bacterial isolate and its antibiotic resistance, the microscopic diagnosis and morphology/topography codes of a tumor, or the sequence of the PCR primers used to generate the result, may all be relevant information. Thirdly, there is a large communication need in this area. Laboratories will need to share data, methods, and new discoveries regarding the genetic changes regarding diseases states.

REQUIREMENTS ANALYSIS

MD data has several unique requirements in database design. For example, several entities not typically found in hospital laboratory information systems must be stored and manipulated. These include sequence data, and molecular weight data (MWD). In MWD molecules are separated by size using gel electrophoresis (the presence or absence of a specific band is detected), and the molecular weight of the resulting band is then calculated. In addition, MWD is unique in that different interpretations of the same data type can be generated by differing assays. For example, both a restriction enzyme digest of a bacterial isolate and the PCR amplification of a bacterial gene produce MWD. However in the first case, the test will produce multiple bands while in the second case the test will produce a single band. In some cases, tests can be multiplexed so that a single assay can produce multiple molecular weight bands, each representing a different target molecule. Besides MWD, sequence data can be generated. A sequence mutation can involve point mutations, deletions, or insertions.

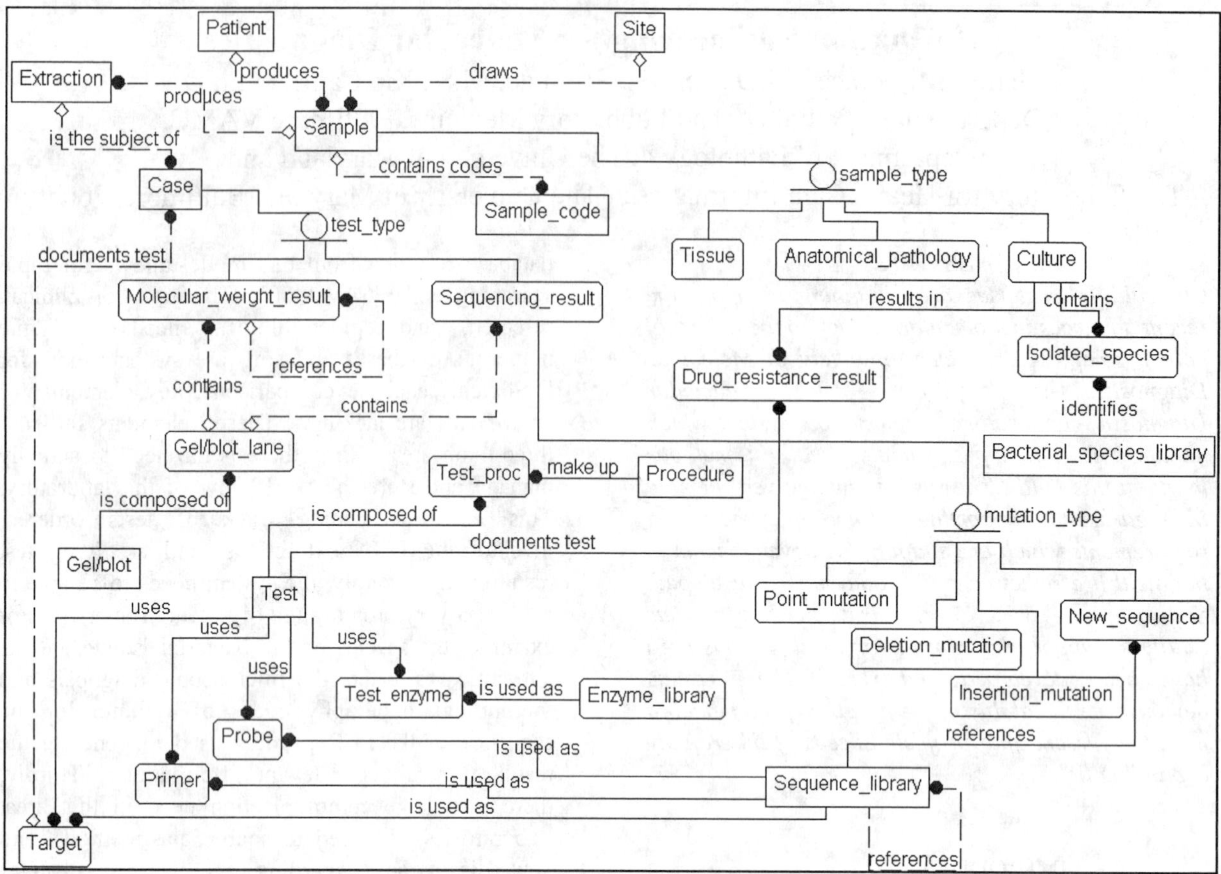

igure 1: Data model for Molecular Diagnostics.

MD also has a more complex specimen work flow than most other areas of the clinical laboratory [5]. Nucleic acid (DNA or RNA) must first be extracted from the sample. These extracts are then inventoried and serve as the starting material for additional tests. The sources of the samples themselves are very diverse. Tests may be run on specimens received directly from patients (blood, amniotic fluid etc.), from surgical pathology samples which have been processed for histological examination, or from bacterial cultures which have already been isolated by the microbiology laboratory. Thus the nucleic acid extract must be linked to a detailed record of the sample's history. The nature of the target sequence present in the extract is also broad. Tests may be run to detect alleles present in the normal population, the presence of mutations and translocations found in a tumor, the pulse field electrophoresis pattern of an entire bacterial genome, or the presence of an antibiotic resistance plasmid in a microbiology isolate.

MD will also have very significant communication requirements. Laboratories will need to share data , methods, and new discoveries regarding the mutations found in disease states. These issues will only increase as data from the human genome project becomes available and the number of genetic test increases. Also current goals of the human genome project include increasing the rate of DNA sequencing methods. When these methods are applied to clinical microbiology samples with the inherent genomic variability of bacterial and viral isolates, the number of comparisons which need to be made between laboratories will increase. This type of communication can best be insured if the databases use a common data model or a subset of a common data model [6]. Such a data model can also form the basis of specialized repository databases for the molecular diagnostics community. It is also important to supply adequate links to currently available databases like GenBank, so that the database can be readily cross-referenced.

METHODS

In order to begin to develop software which will meet

the needs as outlined above, our group has performed a detailed requirements analysis, including the fields of anatomic pathology and clinical microbiology. Several iterations of model building (including data entry trials) resulted in the data model displayed in figure 1. This entity-level model is relational. It can generate SQL to create the relational database in that each entity is a table, there are no many-to-many relationships, and there are no ternary (or higher) relationships (a complete text version of the model is available by anonymous file ftp from 130.85.105.8). The model has several features relevant to the issues discussed, and outlines a rational guide towards future growth.

First, patient samples can be subgrouped as either tissue, anatomic pathology, or clinical microbiology samples in a one-patient-to-many-samples relationship. Entities covering these possibilities contain information unique to each specimen source. In the case of culture (clinical microbiology) samples, additional tables are present which allow the entry of antibiotic resistance and strain-isolated data. Thus it is possible to retrieve data based on queries searching for this important information. This structure also clearly separates results which could otherwise be misinterpreted. A tissue biopsy with appropriate PCR testing may reveal a mixed pattern of infection , while the microbiology sample may only contain a single isolate which had a growth advantage under the laboratory culture conditions. Anatomic pathology samples can be searched for under morphology/topography codes or ICD-9 codes, and by tracking the sample's surgical pathology number, other forms of information (microscopic images of tissue samples, links to the patients medical record) found in the hospital's information system can be retrieved.

We have developed a Test library, and a Sequence library which acts as the data dictionary for the data model. Each test can be linked to the target, probe, primer and enzyme tables as appropriate. A test is given a unique Test_ID and it is linked in a one-to-many relationship with a procedure library. The procedure entity provides a field for the classification of the procedure (e.g., extraction, pulse field electrophoresis etc.), and a memo field describing the method. This allows each test to be defined as an ordered set of procedures and assures the laboratory staff a modular procedure library.

Perhaps the most challenging aspect of MD informatics lies in the archiving and interpretation of the laboratory results. The Case entity links the nucleic acid sample being tested to the test being performed and the test target sequence (thus supporting multiplexed assays with more than one target sequence). Results of each unique case can then be recovered under the Molecular_weight_result or Sequence_result entities. These sections of the data model contains sequence, and MWD data types. Support is also available for the entry of text results were appropriate. Given the complexities of the MWD, the database designer faces the prospect of numerous entities optimized for each potential combination of data, or a single entity which is more comprehensive. The model described here implements the latter choice. Each band in the Molecular_weight_result table has its molecular weight, and intensity recorded, is assigned to the gel and lane in which it was detected and linked via its Case_ID to the Test_ID and Sample_ID used to generate it. A case can have many such bands related to it, and the bands can be in one lane of one gel or widely dispersed over many gel/lane combinations.. Gel images can also be stored and recalled when appropriate.

The Case entity also links to the Sequence_result entity. Sequence mutations are then stored in specific entities for point mutations, deletions, insertions, or new sequences. The tables support the entry of mutations in a variety of formats including the codon which is involved and the nature (substitution, frame shift etc.) of the change. Again the results can also be linked to the Sequence_library, allowing the target sequence to be quickly recovered for comparison.

The Sequence_library contains several types of information. First, it contains the actual sequences of the targets, probes, and primers specified in the test library, and it can also store new sequences generated by laboratory testing. By including entries for the GenBank number, and the Genome Database number, other databases can be quickly cross-referenced. Other relevant information such as the bacterial species/target protein and genomic locus, can be stored. This table is heavily cross-referenced throughout the database with links to the target, primer, and probe tables. The actual sequence of the nucleic acid can be stored in this table, enabling rapid access to state-of-the-art sequence search and comparison algorithms.

TABLE 1

Output for query 1; see text for details.

GEL NUMBER	LANE NUMBER	SEQUENCE #	TEST ID	SAMPLE ID	CASE ID
1	6	1	1	3172	5
1	7	1	1	3774	6
2	2	1	1	3530	8

TABLE 2

Output for query 2; see text for details.

SEQUENCE #	CASE ID	CODON	FROM	TO	EXON	A.A. FROM	A.A. TO
2	WXYZ100	286	GAA	AAA	8	Glu	Lys
2	WXYZ110	273	CGT	CAT	8	Arg	His
2	WXYZ131	282	CGG	GGG	8	Arg	Gly
2	WXYZ135	273	CGT	CAT	8	Arg	His
2	WXYZ140	269	AGC	CGC	8	Ser	Arg
2	WXYZ600	271	GAG	AAG	8	Glu	Lys
2	WXYZ80	282	CGG	TGG	8	Arg	Trp
2	WXYZ356	273	CGT	CAT	8	Arg	His
2	WXYZ22	280	AGA	AAA	8	Arg	Lys
2	WXYZ177	282	CGG	TGG	8	Arg	Trp
2	WXYZ484	275	TGT	TCT	8	Cys	Ser

TABLE 3

Output for query 3; see text for details.

SEQUENCE #	CASE ID	EXON	CODON DELETED
2	WXYZ11	5	157
2	WXYZ12	5	158
2	WXYZ14	5	159

QUERY SUPPORT

Given the data model as outlined above, it is important to demonstrate its ability to support a wide range of scientifically and clinically relevant ad hoc queries. This is especially true given the extensive communications needs which will develop in this field. We performed a trial using a Microsoft ACCESS implementation of the data model. This is currently implemented on a stand-alone PC. Data was entered from several sources. First, Hepatitis C PCR test result data, bacterial restriction fragment length polymorphism, and antibiotic resistance data were entered from the Molecular Diagnostics Laboratory at the Baltimore VA Medical Center (MDVA). Point mutation data for P53 oncogene mutations from Breast Cancers obtained from the Armed Forces Institute of Pathology (AFIP) were also entered. Based on the current and projected needs of the field we developed 20 queries which include:

(1) Be able to assist in epidemiological research by searching for restriction enzyme patterns of bacterial pathogens. This allows for comparisons of species isolated between laboratories. An example of this type of query is shown in Table 1, This query searches the database for all samples which have a specified number of bands within a defined molecular weight range for a given test and target sequence. In this instance the database has been searched for all Hha1 digest (Test_ID =1) of all Streptococcus Agalactae gb B genomes (Sequence_number = 1) which have 3 bands present in the 6,000-to-15,000 molecular weight range. In this query the Sample, Extraction, and Molecular-weight-result entities were linked

(2) Retrieve all the samples with a given point mutation in a given codon range in a given sequence. Table 2 illustrates the output of such a query searching for point mutations between codons 250 and 290 of the p53 oncogene (Sequence_number=2). The nucleic acid sequence of the normal and mutated codon and the resulting

amino acid change are also presented, as is the Case_ID and the involved exon.
(3) Summarize all the known deletion mutations of a given sequence. This was done for the P53 ocogene. Table 3 shows the output of such a query , which presents the involved exon, and the deleted codon.

Both queries 2 and 3 involved linking the Case and Sequencing_result entities with either the Point-mutation or Deletion_mutation entites.

DISCUSSION AND CONCLUSIONS

MD will significantly change both the practice of medicine and the information system requirements for the clinical laboratory. We have presented a data model for discussion that meets several of these requirements. These requirements can be grouped into 2 basic categories: communication and content.

First, a standard data model after refinement and user trials allows an infrastructure to support communications in the rapidly growing field of MD. The common fields and structure of the model simplify data sharing and database querying. Data sharing is made possible because the content and structure of the database model standard is understood by all users. Furthermore, simple database scripts allow users to import and export data over a network. This feature allows the development of intelligent software agents to support and manage the creation and update of research repositories that receive data from many sites. We are now implementing a trial of this technology for a research repository.

Query from multiple sites is also simplified by a standard data model. Not only the data but also supporting data dictionaries can be transferred over networks using the same database script methodology. These scripts are text files containing the SQL statements necessary to perform the desired actions on the target database. The SQL statements can be wrapped in a language/protocol such as Knowledge Query and Manipulation Language (KQML) [7] to supply the transport and per formatives for use on an network using intellegent agents. The creation and sharing of useful user interfaces is also simplified with a standard data model as the programmer is freed from worrying about data structures and compatibility. Querying of repositories could accomplish such tasks such as the geographic distribution of mutations. This type of query has already proven important as a P53 codon 249 mutation in hepatocellulare carcinoma is associated with environmental exposure to aflatoxin B1 [8]. The ability to search for mutation distribution based on patient zipcode might aid in this type of query. Without a common data model these and other types of queries are hindered.

Finally, the content of this data model explicitly defines our vision of what the needed requirements are for this field. This allows others in the field to respond to and improve this model with additions and deletions. Such a dialog is essential to standards initiation and only possible in a published forum.

ACKNOWLEDGMENTS

The authors thank Jack H. Lichy, M.D., Ph.D., and Jeffery K. Taubenberger, M.D., Ph.D., of the AFIP and Judy J. Johnson, Ph.D. of the BVAMC for sharing their data. We also thank Lawrence Brown, M.D. for help in preparing this manuscript. This material is based in part upon work supported under a National Science Foundation Graduate Research Fellowship.

REFERENCES

[1] J. Veralovic et. al, DNA-Based identification and epidemologic typing of bacterial pathogens. Archives of Pathology and Laboratory Medicine 117: 1088-1090, 1993.

[2] J. Rowely et. al, The clinical application of new DNA diagnostic technology on the management of cancer patients. JAMA 270: 2331-2337, 1993.

[3] H. Bilosky, C. Burks, The GenBank genetic sequence data bank. Nucleic Acid Research ,16: 1861-1863, 1988.

[4] P. Pearson, The GDB human genome database. Nucleic Acid Research 20: sup 2201-2206, 1992.

[5] B. McCreedy, T. Calloway, Laboratory Design and Work Flow, in Diagnostic Molecular Biology: Principle and Applications, D. Persing et. al eds., American Society for Microbiology. Washington DC, 1993.

[6] K. Canfield et. al, The standard data model approach to patient record transfer, TR Ihi-ifsm-umbc-jan-1994.

.[7] Finin T., et al., Specification of the KQML Agent-Communication Language. Technical report EIT TR 92-04, Enterprise Integration Technologies, Palo Alto, Ca, 1992.

[8] C. Harris, p53: At the crossroads of molecular carcinogenesis and risk assessment. Science 262:1980-1981, 1994.

A Clinical Database as a Component of a Diagnostic Hematology Workstation

Lawrence W. Diamond, Vladimir G. Mishka, Apollo H. Seal, and Doyen T. Nguyen
Pathology Institute, University of Cologne, Germany

A clinical database was designed as part of a comprehensive workstation for diagnostic laboratory hematology. The database stores coded findings pertinent to hematologic disorders including inherited abnormalities, previous surgery, malignancies, current therapy, and laboratory test results. The workstation includes knowledge-based systems for peripheral blood analysis, flow cytometry studies, and bone marrow morphology. The peripheral blood system renders an interpretive report based on data from a complete blood count with manual review of a blood smear by a technologist. The flow cytometry module interprets the immunophenotyping and DNA content results, and correlates them with the clinical findings and the peripheral blood data. The bone marrow system bases its report on all of the available information including the morphologic review of the bone marrow specimen by a physician, the peripheral blood data, immunophenotype, and clinical/laboratory findings. Before generating an interpretive report, each of the knowledge-based systems automatically searches the clinical database for specific information pertinent to the findings in the case. Since the workstation must function in situations where access to distributed databases is not feasible or not yet practical, a data entry module with a graphical user interface has been created.

INTRODUCTION

Knowledge-based systems for decision support in medical diagnosis and therapy need access to the same clinical and laboratory data that a physician would use in working-up a patient. If the decision support modules are part of a hospital information system interfaced to a laboratory computer as in the HELP system [1], access to existing on-line information is facilitated. The extensive work being done on electronic patient records [2] and open architectures for distributed databases [3] will ultimately improve access to the needed clinical information. In the meantime, there is still a role for local databases integrated into workstations designed for interpretive reporting, education, and clinical research.

We have designed a hematology workstation [4] with knowledge-based systems for peripheral blood interpretation [5], flow cytometry (FCM) immunophenotyping and DNA content analysis [6], and bone marrow morphology [7]. The three modules communicate with each other by means of a set of relational databases [8]. Each of the systems modifies its report based on the interpretation stored in the respective databases by the other modules. The patient database has been designed to include coded information relevant to hematologic disorders from the clinical history, physical examination, radiology reports, and laboratory tests outside of hematology. In this paper, we describe the design of this database and the role it plays in the hematology workstation.

KNOWLEDGE-BASED SYSTEMS

The workstation is interfaced to state-of-the-art hematology analyzers such as the Coulter STKS and ONYX. The STKS is a high performance analyzer with five-part automated leukocyte differentials suitable for processing several hundred to several thousand complete blood counts (CBCs) each day. The ONYX has automated three-part differentials and is intended for mid-range laboratories with a moderate volume. The workstation is being tested on two hardware platforms, one for STKS sites and one for ONYX laboratories. The computer at the STKS test sites is an NEC Image 466es (486-DX2 66 MHz) with 20 MB of RAM and a 540 MB hard disk drive running Windows NT (Microsoft Corporation, Redmond, WA). The ONYX sites are using an Intel 486sx-25MHz computer with 8 MB of RAM and a 170 MB hard disk drive running Windows 3.1. The knowledge-based systems have been programmed with Turbo Pascal for Windows,

0195-4210/94/$5.00 © 1994 AMIA, Inc.

version 1.5, and the database components have been designed with Paradox Engine, version 3.01 (Borland International, Scotts Valley, CA). All knowledge engineering and computer programming have been carried out by a trained hematopathologist.

The three knowledge-based systems have been described in detail previously [4-8]. Briefly, the peripheral blood system, known as Professor Petrushka, interprets the hemogram data downloaded across the interface from the hematology analyzer [5]. In order to maintain just one version of Petrushka, the database components for peripheral blood specimen results must be the same for both the STKS systems (which download five-part leukocyte differentials and complex three-dimensional scatterplots) and the ONYX systems (which download three-part differentials and simple one-parameter histograms). The databases are identical for the two systems with the exception of the names of the database fields which hold the graphics (binary large object fields). At startup, Petrushka checks the name of one of the graphics fields in the database and automatically configures itself to display the appropriate screens for a STKS or ONYX system. Professor Petrushka determines the predominant pattern of the hemogram parameters, and, if the preparation of a peripheral blood smear is indicated, recommends a specific approach to the review of the smear. A technologist enters red blood cell morphology with a mouse. The workstation keyboard also functions as a differential counter for doing manual leukocyte differentials. Petrushka's final interpretation takes into account the data entered by the user, pertinent clinical information and laboratory test results retrieved from the clinical database, and the results of previous CBC specimens. The interpretive reports include the predominant pattern of the peripheral blood data, a differential diagnosis, any features which indicate a more specific diagnosis, and recommendations for additional clinical history and laboratory tests which may be helpful in making a final diagnosis. If, for example, a reticulocyte count is indicated, the database is checked for reticulocyte results. If none are found, Petrushka recommends an absolute reticulocyte count. If the results are already posted to the database, Petrushka interprets the reticulocyte count in light of the rest of the CBC findings.

The FCM system, Professor Fidelio, interprets the immunologic data in leukemias/lymphomas from a panel of up to 37 antibodies, and DNA content data including cell size by light scatter, DNA index (a measure of DNA ploidy) and the percentage of cells in the S-phase of the cell cycle [6]. The system is also used for T-cell subset analysis and follow-up in AIDS patients. Patient-specific clinical data stored in the database, such as a previous history of chronic myeloid leukemia, are used to modify the interpretation of the results. For example, immunologic findings which are otherwise compatible with a diagnosis of acute lymphoid leukemia, are indicative of a blast crisis of chronic myeloid leukemia when the Philadelphia chromosome was documented by previous cytogenetic studies.

When a patient identification number is entered into Professor Belmonte [7], the module for bone marrow morphology, the program searches the peripheral blood specimen database for any recent results and uses them to remind the physician of any additional studies to be performed on the bone marrow specimen, such as FCM immunophenotyping and cytogenetics. Using Belmonte's graphical user interface, a physician enters the qualitative morphologic findings and the bone marrow differential. The program then summarizes the peripheral blood findings and checks the FCM and patient databases for specific information before writing an interpretive report. For example, in a patient with acute leukemia, the diagnosis of an acute myelomonocytic leukemia (AML-M4) requires either a positive stain for non-specific esterase (a monocyte marker) in bone marrow blasts or an increased lysozyme in the serum or urine. If the non-specific esterase stain was negative or not done, and the bone marrow findings are otherwise suggestive of AML-M4, Belmonte will check the database for the lysozyme results in order to establish the diagnosis. If, in this example, no lysozyme results are available, the system will not subtype the acute myeloid leukemia but will append a comment to the report indicating the need for this test.

DATABASE DESIGN

The patient database for clinical findings and laboratory test results has been specifically designed for speed and integration into the hematology workstation. It is intended to capture only those findings which are appropriate to diagnostic hematology. No attempt has been made to capture all of the history, physical examination findings, radiology results, or laboratory test results appropriate for all of internal medicine. The fields in the patient database are listed in Table 1. The last nine fields listed in the table contain the coded information for specific pieces of clinical and laboratory data. The information is coded in strings of characters. Fields 7-14 each contain space for 16 alphanumeric characters. The last field, laboratory tests, contains 24 alphanumeric characters. Unused spaces at the end of the strings have been reserved for future expansion, when other data relevant to hematologic diseases are added to the medical repertoire.

Table 1
Patient Database Fields

1. Patient Identification Number
2. Name
3. Sex
4. Date of Birth
5. Date of Data Entry
6. Race
7. Inherited diseases
8. Social History
9. Previous Surgery
10. Current Drug Administration
11. Cancer History
12. Autoimmune Diseases
13. Physical Examination/Radiology
14. Laboratory Tests for Impaired Immunity
15. General Laboratory Tests

The medical data is coded into the strings by allowing each character in the string to represent one piece of information. Unknown or missing data is represented by a blank space. A negative finding is represented by a '0' (zero). Positive findings are represented by other ASCII characters. For example, lymphoproliferative disorders are coded in the fourth character of the cancer history field. The codes for lymphoproliferative disorders and their meaning are listed in Table 2.

Using this scheme, retrieval of various types of information is very efficient. For instance, Professor Petrushka may need to know if a patient is currently on chemotherapy as an explanation for pancytopenia. If this information is missing, the interpretive report may contain a comment to check for this possibility. In this case, the system needs only to retrieve the drug history string using the patient's identification (medical record) number as the key field, and check if the twelfth character is "less than" zero, equal to zero or "greater than" zero. If it is less than zero, then it must be a blank space which means that the information is missing and the comment should be appended. If the character is zero, then the patient is not on chemotherapy and a different explanation must account for the pancytopenia. The finding that the character is greater than zero confirms chemotherapy as the cause of the pancytopenia. The combination of chemotherapeutic agents being administered is contained in the value of the character, but Petrushka will not bother to decode that information unless it is necessary to the generation of the interpretive report.

Table 2
Codes for Lymphoproliferative Disorders

'Blank'	Missing Data
0.	No evidence of disease
1.	Lymphoproliferative Disorder, NOS
2.	Chronic Lymphocytic Leukemia
3.	Prolymphocytic Leukemia
4.	Hairy Cell Leukemia
5.	Multiple Myeloma
6.	Waldenstrom's Macroglobulinemia
7.	Adult T-cell Leukemia/Lymphoma
8.	Large Granular Lymphocytosis
9.	Mycosis Fungoides/Sezary Syndrome
A.	Plasmacytoma

NOS: Not otherwise specified

The value of many types of medical information is time dependent. A patient who has just had a bone marrow transplant is an example. The critical information needed to interpret CBC and bone marrow findings properly depends on the length of time since the transplant was performed. The length of time post transplant is coded in six intervals ranging from less than one week to greater than two months. The knowledge-based systems (Petrushka and Belmonte) check the date of the clinical data and compare it to the date of the specimen, re-calculating the information contained in the database, if necessary. If a patient was one week post transplant when the patient database was last updated, and a week has elapsed between the date stamped in the database entry and the date of the specimen, the programs will interpret the findings in light of the knowledge that the patient is now two weeks post transplant.

In addition, in this scheme of data encoding, unused characters can be reserved to keep track of time. For example, in a patient who has been treated with combination chemotherapy and radiotherapy for Hodgkin's disease, and who subsequently develops an acute myeloid leukemia, it is important to know the interval of time between the start of therapy and the onset of leukemia, in order to determine if the leukemia is therapy related. The time factor can be stored in the database by a cumulative counter which keeps track of the number of days since the start of therapy (in hexadecimal notation) in four characters of the string. The counter is started at '0000' at the time when current chemotherapy is noted in the patient record. The database program adds to the counter the number of days which have elapsed when the record is subsequently updated. This same scheme can be used to time laboratory results and 'discard' them from influencing the interpretation after they have 'expired'.

In order to allow for the possibility of manual entry of clinical data, a Windows program with a graphical user interface was developed to store the coded information (Figure 1). With the exception of the medical record number, no typing is required to enter data.

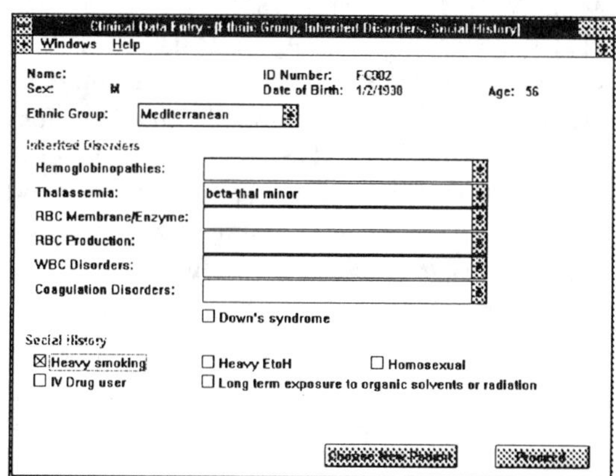

Figure 1. First Screen for Manual Data Entry

DISCUSSION

In the design of a comprehensive workstation for diagnostic laboratory hematology, we have decided to keep track of relevant patient-specific clinical and laboratory information. The power of an intelligent computer system lies in its knowledge base. Therefore, the design of our clinical database has been influenced by our knowledge of the practice of laboratory hematology. At present, we have limited ourselves to a single patient clinical record. Although this may be viewed as a weakness by some database developers, much of the information we keep track of, such as inherited diseases, malignancies, or surgery are effectively mapped to a patient in a single record. As has been described above, we have also taken into consideration methods which will allow us to keep track of time for specific items within the context of our database design.

Our approach is best suited to diagnosis. We acknowledge that systems designed primarily for supporting therapy, like ONCOCIN, are likely to need a different database design based on a time-oriented model of reasoning, with multiple records for the same patient [9].

Miller and Maserie have utilized an elegant and efficient algorithm for the QMR relationships function by taking advantage of compiled bitmapped data structures [10]. Our clinical database strings can be thought of as "byte-mapped" structures which allow for fast and efficient use of positive, negative, or missing clinical information by our knowledge-based systems.

Although our clinical database is specific to our applications, the principles used in the design may be useful to other researchers developing real-world diagnostic systems which must be capable of existing in both highly networked hospitals (with access to distributed databases), and small satellite facilities without current access to electronic medical records.

Two of the most important issues that have been identified as necessary features for a knowledge-based system to function beyond the author's laboratory and really be used in medical practice are: (1) Working with patient data contained in the medical record; and (2) Integration into the daily routine of medical practice [11]. Our knowledge-based systems are designed with both of these goals in mind. Our clinical database represents a medical record of hematology data which is scanned by each of our modules as they generate an interpretive report. The systems modify the report to reflect the clinical and laboratory data. In addition, when a case is interpreted by the bone marrow system, important diagnoses are posted back to the database to keep the record up-to-date.

For integration into the hematology laboratory environment, our workstation is designed to be used on-line for interpretive reporting and clinical research in addition to education. We have carefully followed the established protocols for system development with respect to design, prototyping, human-computer interface issues, and in-house validation of the knowledge base [12].

The workstation has now progressed to the phase of large scale outside evaluation at many laboratories in multiple countries. The first outside evaluations took place at the University of Florida and M.D. Anderson Cancer Center in late 1993. The workstation was installed (April 1994) as an ONYX site at Scott and White Hospital and Clinics, Temple Texas, a tertiary medical center with 18 satellite laboratories. In June 1994, systems were installed at both the University of Cincinnati, and MDS Laboratories in Toronto, Canada (a reference laboratory processing 3000 CBCs per day). Three sites in the United Kingdom, Addenbrookes Hospital, (Cambridge), St. Thomas Hospital (London), and St. James Hospital (Dublin) have agreed to become test sites with installations planned at the end of 1994.

At the large medical centers, the next phase of development will be interfaces/networking to existing hospital and laboratory information systems for automatic retrieval and processing of the information which is stored in our patient database. In addition, at MDS laboratories, work is underway to integrate the workstation into their state-of-the-art computer-controlled laboratory robotics system.

Each of the test sites has been impressed with the initial performance of the workstation. Currently, the manual data entry module is being used to enter clinical information. As clinical data is collected and reviewed, it is used to increase the number of clinical scenarios recognized by the knowledge-based systems.

References

[1] Nelson BD, Gardner RM. Decision support for concurrent utilization review using a HELP-embedded expert system. *SCAMC*, 1993;17:176-182.

[2] Rind DM, Safran C. Real and imagined barriers to an electronic medical record. *SCAMC*, 1993;17:74-78.

[3] Chueh HC, Barnett GO. Client-server distributed database strategies in a healthcare record system for a homeless population. *SCAMC*, 1993:17:119-124.

[4] Nguyen DT, Diamond LW. The concept of a computer workstation for laboratory haematology. *Aust J Med Sci*, 1993;14:71-75.

[5] Nguyen DT, Diamond LW, Priolet G, Sultan C. A decision support system for diagnostic consultation in laboratory hematology. *MEDINFO*, 1992;7:591-595.

[6] Diamond LW, Nguyen DT, Jouault H, Imbert M. Evaluation of a knowledge-based system for interpreting flow cytometric immunophenotyping data. *MIE*, 1993;11:124-128.

[7] Nguyen DT, Cherubino P, Tamino PB, Diamond LW. Computer-assisted bone marrow interpretation: A pattern approach. *MIE*, 1993;11:119-123.

[8] Diamond LW, Nguyen DT. Communication between expert systems in haematology. In: *Current Perspectives in Healthcare Computing*: BJHC Books, 1993:111-119.

[9] Kahn MG, Fagan LM, Tu S. Extensions to the time-oriented database model to support temporal reasoning in medical expert systems. *Meth Inform Med*, 1991;30:4-14.

[10] Miller RA, Maserie FE Jr. The Quick Medical Reference (QMR) relationships function: Description and evaluation of a simple efficient multiple diagnoses algorithm. *MEDINFO*, 1992;7:512-518.

[11] de Zegher I, Venot A, de Rosis F. The five commandments of KBS to be used in daily clinical practice. In: *Knowledge and Decisions in Health Telematics*: IOS Press, 1994:132-138.

[12] Shortliffe EH. Clinical decision-support systems. In: *Medical Informatics: Computer applications in health care*: Addison-Wesley, 1990:466-502.

Multiple Imputation as a Missing Data Machine

Jaap Brand[1,2], Stef van Buuren[2], Erik M. van Mulligen[1,3], Teun Timmers[1], Edzard Gelsema[1]
[1]Dept. of Medical Informatics, Erasmus University Rotterdam, The Netherlands
[2]Dept. of Statistics, TNO Prevention and Health, Leiden, The Netherlands
[3]University Hospital Dijkzigt, Rotterdam, The Netherlands

This paper deals with problems concerning missing data in clinical databases. After signalling some shortcomings of popular solutions to incomplete data problems, we outline the concepts behind multiple imputation. Multiple imputation is a statistically sound method for handling incomplete data. Application of multiple imputation requires a lot of work and not every user is able to do this. A transparent implementation of multiple imputation is necessary. Such an implementation is possible in the HERMES medical workstation. A remaining problem is to find proper imputations.

INTRODUCTION

The occurrence of missing data is a pervasive problem in clinical data analysis. Missing data can have many causes: respondents may be unwilling to fill in all items in a questionnaire, equipment can become defective, loss to follow up, and so on. Problems that are associated with incomplete data are: (1) cases with missing data may differ systematically from complete cases so that the sample is no longer representative. (2) less information is gathered than was intended, resulting in decreased power in statistical testing, and (3) many conventional statistical methods for complete data are not applicable anymore. Despite great effort that may have gone into collecting data, incomplete data are a fact of life.

In practice there are several methods to tackle the missing data problem. However, most of these methods have serious disadvantages. Three popular methods are:

(1) The deletion of incomplete cases. Simplicity is the main advantage of this method. However, an important disadvantage of this method is the potential loss of costly collected data. Moreover, estimators may be strongly biased, when incomplete cases differ systematically from complete cases.

(2) The development of adapted statistical methods for a postulated missing data mechanism. A theoretically elegant method is the Expected Maximalistion (EM) algorithm [1]. In this method, an explicitly defined missing data mechanism is combined with the selected sample model into a likelihood function. The parameters of the sample model are estimated with maximum likelihood. When the postulated missing data mechanism is correct, the results derived with EM are valid. However this method requires much statistical expertise and often specialised computer programs are required. Moreover EM is sometimes mathematically intractable.

(3) Completion filling in reasonable values for the missing data. An important advantage of this method is that after filling in the missing data, conventional methods for analyzing complete data can be applied. However, the disadvantages of this method are that it results in too small confidence intervals and correlations that are strongly biased, caused by the fact that the values filled in, are treated automatically as if they were known.

Clearly there is a need for an easy, generally applicable and statistically sound method. Such an method is multiple imputation as proposed by Rubin [2]. Multiple imputation is a very promising method and is the state of the art [3].

In this paper, we outline the general idea behind multiple imputation. Next we discuss the problem of implementing multiple imputation in a transparent way and propose how this problem can be solved by implementing multiple imputation in the HERMES medical workstation. Finally we discuss the remaining difficulties with multiple imputation, which still require research.

MULTIPLE IMPUTATION

The main goals of multiple imputation are taking into account the uncertainty about the missing data in a proper way and application of existing statistically methods for complete data. This can be done by filling in each missing value m times ($m>=2$), resulting in m completed data sets. When the fraction of missing information is modest, $m=5$ is sufficient [4]. The completed data sets are analyzed separately with the requested complete data method. Finally the m intermediate results are combined into one result. The flow of operations is illustrated in Figure 1.

The uncertainty about the missing data is reflected by the mutual variation between the imputed data sets. Little mutual variation between the imputed data sets means that there is little uncertainty about the missing data while much mutual variation between the imputed data sets means that there is much uncertainty about the missing data. Proper imputations can be obtained by drawing the values to impute Y^*_{mis} from the predictive distribution $P(Y_{mis} | Y_{obs}, R)$, R being the response indicator and Y_{mis} and Y_{obs} respectively the missing and observed part of the data Y.

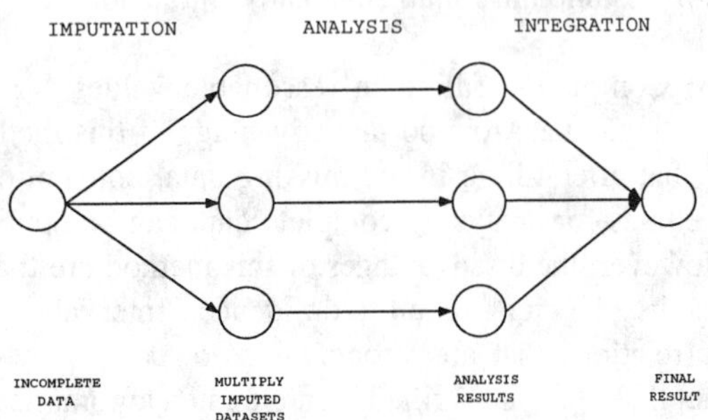

Figure 1. *Schematic representation of multiple imputation with m = 3*

The combination of the *m* intermediate results into one result can be performed by simple and sound procedures. The final parameter estimations are derived by averaging the intermediate parameter estimates. The uncertainty reflected by the variance between the imputations is taken into account by the final estimations of the variances and the p-values. The following three sources of uncertainty are taken into account: (1) the sample variation, (2) the missing data mechanism, and (3) the finite number of imputations used. The finite number of imputations is also a source of uncertainty, because from repeated application of the multiple imputation algorithm, different final results are obtained.

Application of multiple imputation requires much work for the user. For instance when a user applies multiple imputation to linear regression, he has to find *m* proper imputations for the incomplete data. The *m* completed data sets have to be analyzed separately with a statistical package like BMDP or SPSS. The *m* different intermediate results the user have to be combined into one result, with explicit formulas. Not every user is able to do this.

TRANSPARENT IMPLEMENTATION

To make multiple imputation applicable to a large group of users, multiple imputation has to be implemented in a transparent way, so that users can apply multiple imputation automatically. For a transparent implementation, the following is required:

- An imputator.
- Complete data analysis software (BMDP or SPSS).
- Filtering of the output, belonging to the complete data analysis.
- Pooling of the parameter estimators.
- An environment to integrate the modules.

Such an environment is the HERMES medical workstation [5]. The HERMES workstation is described below.

The design of the HERMES medical workstation accommodates the need to integrate different medical databases and software packages into a workstation. Its main goal is to offer the clinical user a friendly and transparent access to medical data and an easy use of existing software packages like BMDP, SPSS, WingZ and Harvard Graphics. The graphical user interface within HERMES has been developed with OSF/Motif and X11 and UIMX on a Hewlett Packard 9000/700 series workstation.

The architecture of the HERMES medical workstation is client-server based. Different applications in the HERMES environment can communicate with each other as client and server with a specially developed message language. A client, usually a graphical task-oriented user interface sends a request to a server which contains the functionality to solve the request. The results are sent back to the client. An application can act both as a client and as a server.

The communication between a client and a server is indirect, via a broker or a router. The broker uses a database to search the proper server that can handle the request. The broker database can be edited to add new servers. When alternative services have been defined in the database for a request, the broker can automatically select the most appropriate server.

The main advantages of the HERMES environment for the application programmer are: (1) Abstraction of the complexity of a program by division of the program into different modules. HERMES allows integration of these modules. (2) The possibility of using existing software, by encapsulating it with plugs into HERMES. Such a plug bridges between the

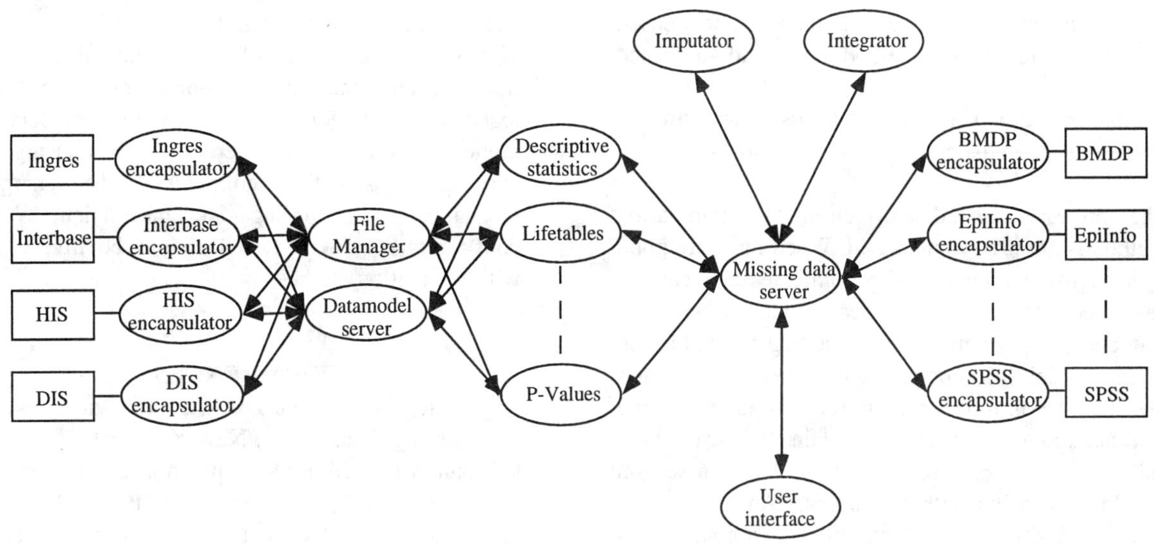

Figure 2. *Schematic representation of a client-server architecture for multiple imputation*

HERMES message language and the specific input and output formats of the application.This makes it possible to incorporate complete data analysis as required for transparent implementation of multiple imputation. How multiple imputation can be implemented transparently in HERMES is illustrated in Figure 2.

The missing data server receives the request from the statistical client and detects missing data. If no data are missing, the request is directly forwarded to the statistical service and the result is returned to statistical client. If data are missing, for each of the *m* completed data files generated by the imputator service the missing data service sends a request to the statistical service. Finally, all results are combined by the integrator service into one result and returned to the statistical client.

DISCUSSION

Multiple imputation is a promising method to solve the problems with missing data. It is possible to implement multiple imputation in a transparent way. The HERMES medical workstation is a suitable environment for this. A remaining difficulty is the derivation of the predictive distribution from which the imputations have to be drawn. The derivation takes the missing data mechanism and the sampling mechanism into account. In the literature there are three disjunct classes of missing data mechanisms.

There are two ways to take the sampling mechanism into account: model based and an data driven. In model based multiple imputation a statistical model (for instance the multivariate normal distribution), is used for the derivation of the predictive distribution. The concept of data driven imputation is to find an imputation that preserves the structure in the data as well as the uncertainty about this structure [6]. For instance, when in an incomplete data set two variables have an approximately quadratic relationship, the same variables should preserve this relationship after completing with a data driven imputation method.

The data driven imputation method has several advantages compared to model based imputation methods. Some advantages are:

- for different statistical methods for complete data,

the same imputation method can be used.

- a data driven imputation method does not force the conclusions of subsequent analysis into a particular direction, a principle which is very important in statistics. If the data does not fit the assumed statistical model well, application of a model based multiple imputation method may lead to biased estimates.
- this method is very suitable for users with limited training in statistics.

The application of a data driven multiple imputation method is not always indicated. When there are good reasons to assume that the complete data can be described well by a statistical model, it is more suitable to apply a multiple imputation method based on this model, than applying a data driven imputation method. An intuitive reason for this is that using external knowledge such as a certain statistical model leads to more precise inferences. This assertion should be verified with simulation. Another reason is that by a simple model, model based imputation is much faster than data driven imputation.

Finally, a real data driven imputation algorithm is probably a utopia. Each imputation method always requires weak assumptions about the sampling mechanism. The idea of data driven imputation should be used on a gradual scale: an imputation method A is more data driven than another imputation method B when the sampling model used for method B is included in the sampling model used for method A.

To select the proper multiple imputation method and number of imputations *m*, especially for users with a limited training in statistics it is necessary to build in a selector in the missing data server, to come algorithmically to appropriate choices. The selector tests for each multiple imputations method a number of constraints and selects from the methods satisfying the constraints the most appropriate one. Constraints to be tested are for instance: The type of data, the number of variables, the percentage of missing data and some statistics concerning the sampling mechanism and missing data mechanism. Which constraints are to be tested should be investigated with simulation studies.

REFERENCES

[1] Little RJA, Rubin DB. Statistical analysis with missing data. Wiley, New York, 1987

[2] Rubin DB. Multiple imputation for nonresponse in surveys. Wiley, New York, 1987

[3] Tukey JW. Mixture modelling versus selection modelling with non-ignorable respons. In: Drawing Inferences from Self-Selected Samples. Springer-Verlag, New York, 1986

[4] Rubin DB. Multiple imputation in health - care data bases: an overview and some applications. Statistics in medicine. 1991;10:585-98

[5] Van Mulligen EM, Timmers T, van Bemmel JH. A new architecture for integration of heterogeneous software components. In: Methods of Information in Medicine, 1993:292-301

[6] Van Buuren S, Van Rijckevorsel JLA, Rubin DB. Multiple imputation by splines. In: Bulletin of the International Statistical Institute, Contributed Papers II, 1993:503-4

Representative Charting of Vital Signs in an Intensive Care Unit

Thomas A. Oniki, MS, Terry P. Clemmer, MD, LDS Hospital Department of Critical Care,
Reed M. Gardner, PhD, LDS Hospital/University of Utah Department of Medical Informatics,
and Kyle V. Johnson, LDS Hospital Department of Medical Informatics.

ABSTRACT

An automatic vital signs charting system had been operational in the intensive care units of our hospital for over 10 years, but the system was susceptible to non-representative transients in the data. A median selection rule was implemented to make the system less susceptible to transients. After implementation of the median rule, we examined (1) the agreement of the resulting medians and the values that would have been reported using the previous "real-time" system and (2) the frequency of occurrence of "out-of-range" values for each system. The median value system was found to improve the representativeness of the recorded data. Improved representativeness will enhance the usefulness of reports, but more importantly will enable us to use the resulting data as inputs to computerized practice protocols and other computerized decision support applications.

INTRODUCTION

Patients in the intensive care unit (ICU) and in surgery present a monitoring paradox. On one hand, their condition calls for frequent and timely vital sign reporting. On the other hand, their condition also requires constant vigilance by the caregiver (a nurse, anesthesiologist, respiratory therapist, etc.). Unfortunately, it is difficult for a caregiver to be both a frequent, timely vital signs charter and a constant, careful observer. What most often occurs is that both the charting and the vigilance suffer -- the charting is not always timely or frequent when the caregiver attends to other duties, and the vigilance is sometimes intruded upon when the caregiver attends to charting. Automated charting of vital signs presents a solution to the paradox. Automated charting has been observed to improve timeliness, accuracy, legibility, and completeness of the patient record in anesthesia [1-3] and similar benefits are expected in the ICU [4].

Automatic charting must not only be frequent and timely, but of course must also be accurate. Simply sampling a patient monitor's output at regular intervals allows for the possibility that a transient event may occur at the sampling time. The result is the acquisition of non-representative data. "Non-representative" will be defined herein as not accurately depicting the parameter's central tendency during a given period. A non-representative value need not be non-physiological (i.e., caused by some problem in the monitoring process such as flushing the catheter, drawing blood, etc.). A non-representative value may in fact be an accurate representation of a true, albeit fleeting, physiological state. However, we assume that the goal of an automatic charting system is *routine* charting, not *exception* charting. *Routine* charting periodically reports physiological parameters to illustrate relatively long-term trends. *Exception* charting, on the other hand, involves detecting and recording specific, clinically important events that can sometimes be very short-lived.

Reports that search the database and decision support applications that use the data as inputs can be rendered untrustworthy by non-representative data. A solution to the problem of non-representative data is to chart a measure of central tendency instead of the actual value. In the ICUs at LDS Hospital in Salt Lake City, we have implemented a vital signs charting system that automatically charts median values every 15 minutes.

METHODS

For over 20 years, clinicians at LDS Hospital have used the Health Evaluation through Logical Processing (HELP) clinical information system [5]. The main feature of the HELP system is a centralized patient database located on a Tandem mainframe computer. The database receives inputs from many departments and ancillary services throughout the hospital. Automatic monitoring of vital signs in the ICUs is one of those many inputs..

Each ICU has a Charles River Data Systems minicomputer that receives data from Marquette patient monitors. "C"-based software on the minicomputer originally sampled the patient monitors in "real-time" every 15 minutes, on the quarter hour. Systolic, diastolic, and mean arterial blood pressures; heart rates; and core temperatures were the five parameters included in the sampling. The sampled data were then transferred to the patient database on

0195-4210/94/$5.00

the Tandem/HELP System.

The system provided timely data but was vulnerable to non-representative transients, even though the patient monitor itself performed some filtering before the minicomputer sampled its output [6]. In turn, the 24-hour Rounds Report was especially sensitive to non-representative data. The Rounds Report selected a patient's minimum and maximum blood pressure values from the past 24-hours. If just one extremely high or low non-representative value occurred during the 24 hours, it would be selected as the high or low. Instead, physicians in the unit wanted to see the minimums and maximums from "routine reporting" data, disregarding minimums and maximums of episodic events.

Furthermore, and more importantly, non-representative data were preventing us from using automatically collected blood pressure values in computerized decision support applications. APACHE acuity scoring had existed in computerized form for several years, but had fallen into disuse largely because of unreliability in its blood pressure input values. Also, LDS Hospital investigators were developing computerized protocols designed to standardize medical care. Protocol developers at the hospital have observed that an important requirement for computerized protocols is accurate, timely data [7,8]. Thus, reliable, automatic blood pressure data acquisition and charting was a fundamental building block of our medical informatics efforts in the ICU.

To ameliorate the problem of non-representative data, a new automatic recording scheme was devised. The "pilot" unit to implement the scheme was LDS Hospital's Shock/Trauma/Respiratory Intensive Care Unit (STRICU). The unit is a level 1 regional trauma referral center that employs four attending MD intensivists. It treats critically ill trauma, respiratory, multisystem organ failure, and postoperative liver transplantation patients. The unit provides treatment for one to two patients per registered nurse and has 24-hour physician coverage. Eighty to ninety percent of STRICU patients have arterial lines, permitting continuous vital signs monitoring.

The software on the unit's minicomputer was modified to sample the five vital signs from the Marquette monitor every three minutes instead of every 15 minutes. Every three minutes was the practical sampling limit imposed by polling the 12 rooms in the ICU. The minicomputer software was further modified to select a median every quarter hour for each of the five sampled parameters. Medians were selected from the most recent 15 minutes of collected data. On every quarter hour, the *medians* were transmitted to the HELP patient database instead of the actual, "real-time" values.

To evaluate the new system, files containing both the quarter-hour medians and the actual real-time values were kept on the minicomputer in July and August of 1993. The median values calculated on the quarter-hour were compared with the actual values occurring at the quarter-hour (the values that would have been recorded by the "real-time" system). We assumed that in most cases, there should be close agreement between the 15-minute median and the actual quarter-hour value. Cases in which there was a large disparity between the median and the actual value (> 30 mm Hg for blood pressures or > 30 beats per minute for heart rate) were examined individually to determine if the median was a representative value for the given time period.

"Out-of-range" values were also addressed. Data values were considered to be "out-of-range" according to criteria set forth by hospital physicians. The criteria are listed in Table I. "Out-of-range" temperature values were not found to be a problem and therefore were not considered in the comparison. Mean arterial pressures were not compared since they are a function of systolic and diastolic pressures.

The frequency of occurrence of "out-of-range" data under the "real-time" automatic system was compared with the frequency of occurrence under the median system. Until recently, nurses also routinely charted blood pressures and heart rate manually in the HELP system. Therefore, the frequency of occurrence of "out-of-range" data entered manually by nurses was also compared.

Table I. Definitions of "out-of-range" values for systolic and diastolic pressure and heart rate.

Parameter	Out-of-range definition
Systolic Pressure	<90 or > 220 mm Hg
Diastolic Pressure	<30 or >140 mm Hg
Heart Rate	<20 or >200 bpm

To find "out-of-range" values generated by the "real-time" automatic system, the HELP patient database was searched from July 29, 1993 to August 8, 1993. To find "out-of-range" values generated by the median system, the database was searched from August 31, 1993 to September 10, 1993. To find "out-of-range" values generated by nurse charting, the database was searched from June 12, 1993 to August 24, 1993. The search interval for manually-charted data was larger than for automatically-charted data because nurses only charted every 2 hours, as opposed to the automatic systems which charted every 15 minutes. A larger search interval was necessary to obtain a comparable sample size.

Two-tailed chi-squared tests were performed to detect statistically significant differences in the rates of out-of-range data between the old, the new, and the manual systems taken two at a time. In those cases where the value of any cell was 0 or the values in more than one cell were less than 5, two-tailed Fisher's Exact tests were performed instead.

RESULTS

Comparison of Medians and "Real-Time" Values

One hundred and seventy-five hours of data were collected from 28 STRICU patients. The data contained 702 quarter-hour median calculation times. The largest dataset contained 48 median calculation times, the smallest contained one, and the average per dataset was 21.9 calculation times.

The data allowed 698 comparisons between median systolic pressures and the actual "real-time" systolics recorded on the quarter-hour, 697 comparisons between median diastolics and "real-time" diastolics, and 696 comparisons between median mean arterial pressures and "real-time" means pressures. The numbers of comparisons were different for the various parameters and did not equal 702 because of occasional "missing" data in the datafiles. "Missing" datpoints resulted when errors occurred while writing to the minicomputer datafiles, when the Marquette monitor did not report values at quarter-hour times, and when medians were not calculated because fewer than three datapoints had been received during the previous 15 minutes. The results of the blood pressure and heart rate comparisons are shown in Table II. The comparison for temperature revealed that all 154 median temperatures compared were within 0.1 degree Celsius of the actual temperature sampled on the quarter hour.

Out-of-Range Values

The results of the Chi-squared and Fisher's tests are presented in Tables III through V.

DISCUSSION

The median system was found to report values that were usually in agreement with what was charted under the "real-time" system. In those cases where there were large differences, the median system reported a representative value while disregarding short-term transients. Figure 1 shows an example of a large discrepancy between values reported by the "real-time" and median systems. At 20:30, the systolic pressure value reported by the "real-time" system was 252 mm Hg. At 20:33, the reported systolic was 267 mm Hg. Also at 20:30 and 20:33, the diastolic pressures reported by the "real-time" system were 195 mm Hg and 210 mm Hg, respectively. All these values were almost surely artifactual. The median system at 20:30 reported a value of 119 mm Hg for systolic pressure and 69 mm

Table II. Discrepancies between values recorded by the "real-time" recording system and values recorded by the median recording system.

Parameter	Discrepancy (mm Hg or beats per minute)									
	0-10	11-20	21-30	31-40	41-50	51-60	61-70	71-80	81-90	91+
Systolic (698 total)	606 (86.8%)	59 (8.5%)	17 (2.4%)	5 (0.7%)	5 (0.7%)	4 (0.6%)	0 (0.0%)	0 (0.0%)	0 (0.0%)	2 (0.3%)
Diastolic (697 total)	649 (93.1%)	33 (4.7%)	7 (1.0%)	1 (0.1%)	2 (0.3%)	1 (0.1%)	1 (0.1%)	1 (0.1%)	0 (0.0%)	2 (0.3%)
Mean (696 total)	641 (92.1%)	35 (5.0%)	8 (1.1%)	6 (0.8%)	3 (0.4%)	0 (0.0%)	1 (0.1%)	1 (0.1%)	0 (0.0%)	2 (0.3%)
Heart Rate (813 total)	772 (95.0%)	27 (3.3%)	10 (1.2%)	3 (0.4%)	0 (0.0%)	1 (0.1%)	0 (0.0%)	0 (0.0%)	0 (0.0%)	0 (0.0%)

Table III. Out of range values in the "real-time" system v. in the median system.

Parameter	Out of Range Values/Total Values (%) "Real-Time" System	Median System	Statistically Significant?
Systolic Pressure	71/6528 (1.09%)	23/6531 (0.35%)	yes (p=0.000001)
Diastolic Pressure	21/6528 (0.32%)	0/6520 (0.00%)	yes (p<0.000001)
Heart Rate	1/7720 (0.01%)	1/7037 (0.01%)	no (p>0.95)

Table IV. Out-of-range values in the median system v. in manual charting.

Parameter	Out of Range Values/Total Values (%) Nurse Charting	Median System	Statistically Significant?
Systolic Pressure	87/6561 (1.33%)	23/6531 (0.35%)	yes (p<0.000001)
Diastolic Pressure	27/6552 (0.41%)	0/6520 (0.00%)	yes (p<0.000001)
Heart Rate	44/5197 (0.85%)	1/7037 (0.01%)	yes (p<0.000001)

Table V. Out-of-range values in the "real-time" system v. in manual charting.

Parameter	Out of Range Values/Total Values (%) Nurse Charting	"Real-Time" System	Statistically Significant?
Systolic Pressure	87/6561 (1.33%)	71/6528 (1.09%)	no (p=0.2425)
Diastolic Pressure	27/6552 (0.41%)	21/6528 (0.32%)	no (p=0.4775)
Heart Rate	44/5197 (0.85%)	1/7720 (0.01%)	yes (p<0.000001)

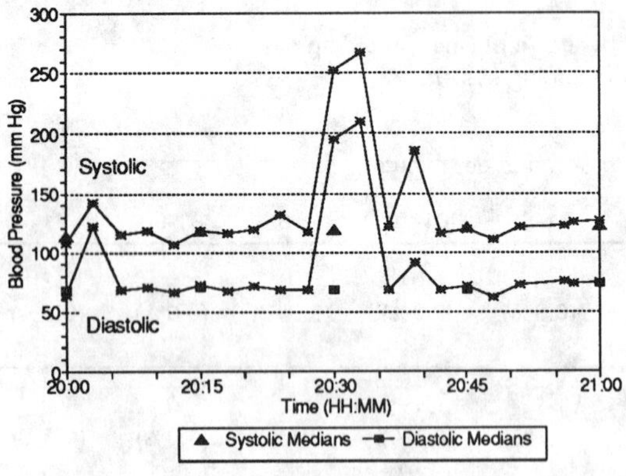

Figure 1. First example of a large discrepancy between medians and actual values. The "real-time" values at 20:30 are obviously artifacts.

Hg for diastolic pressure, which are much more reasonable values.

Figure 2 illustrates another large discrepancy between the two systems. At 11:45, the "real-time" system reported a systolic pressure of 245 mm Hg and a diastolic of 95 mm Hg. Again, these values were most likely artifactual. The median system reported values of 120 mm Hg for systolic pressure and 72 mm Hg for diastolic.

Figure 2 also illustrates a more problematic discrepancy, however. At 12:00, the systolic pressure reported by the "real-time" system was 181 mm Hg while the diastolic was 107 mm Hg. These values are high, but not in the physiologically impossible range. It is possible that they represent a true physiological event. Nevertheless, the median system in essence ignored them, reporting a systolic of 127 mm Hg and a diastolic of 77 mm Hg. This example may be perceived as a shortcoming of the system, unless the system's intended purpose is remembered. The system was designed to perform routine reporting, not exception charting. In other words, the exclusion of events such as the one at 12:00 is deliberate. Documentation of events falls under the jurisdiction of another reporting scheme (presently, manual charting). Admittedly, differentiating between a routine reporting system and an exception charting system requires the difficult demarcation of when a transient episode becomes sustained enough to be considered a trend. By choosing 15 minutes as the median width, we have implicitly made that demarcation.

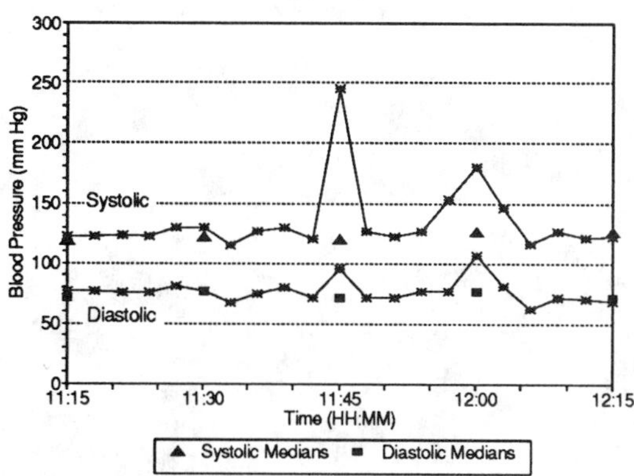

Figure 2. Second example of a large discrepancy between medians and actual values. The "real-time" values at 11:45 are probably artifacts, but the values at 12:00 may be real. Nevertheless, the medians report representative values for the 15 minute time periods.

The median system resulted in a statistically significant reduction in out-of-range systolic and diastolic pressures compared to both the "real-time" system and the nurses' manual charting. Even though the frequency of out-of-range values was not large before implementation of the median system, even a small frequency was enough to cause spurious data in the 24-hour Rounds Reports. Anecdotal evidence suggests that physicians are more satisfied with Rounds Report values since implementation of the median system. The system was implemented in LDS Hospital's other Intensive Care Units in October of 1993. Real-time values are no longer stored.

We expect that the most important gains resulting from the median system are yet to be realized. More accurate and representative data in the Rounds Report is an important accomplishment, but even more important are the expected benefits of being able to use the automatic monitoring data as inputs to other computerized applications. Now that blood pressures are more reliable, the hospital's computerized APACHE system has received renewed attention. Also, we are presently developing a protocol for the administration of sedatives and paralytics. We hope to be able to use automatically recorded blood pressures as an input to the protocol's decisions. In short, the benefits achieved by improving the representativeness of automatically charted vital signs emerge not just in a printout of a report today but in the freedom it allows us to pursue other more ambitious goals in the future.

References

1. Edsall DW, Deshane P, Giles C, Dick D, Sloan B, Farrow J. Computerized patient anesthesia records. Less time and better quality than manually produced records. J Clin Anesth 1993; 5:2750-283.

2. Cook RI, McDonald JS, Nunziata E. Differences between handwritten and automatic blood pressure records. Anesthesiology 1989; 71:385-90.

3. Lerou JGC, Dirksen R, Daele MV, Nijhuis GMM, Crul JF. Automated charting of physiological variables in anesthesia: A quantitative comparison of automated versus handwritten anesthesia records. J Clin Monit 1988; 4:37-47.

4. Gardner RM, Hawley WH, East TD, Oniki TA, Young HFW. Real time data acquisition: Recommendations for the Medical Information Bus (MIB). Intl J Clin Monit Comput 1992; 8:251-258.

5. Kuperman GJ, Gardner RM, Pryor TA. HELP: A dynamic hospital information system. Springer-Verlag Inc, New York, NY, 1991.

6. Gardner RM, Monis SM, Oehler P. Monitoring direct blood pressure: Algorithm enhancements. IEEE Computers in Cardiology 1986; 13:607-610.

7. East TD, Henderson S, Morris AH, Gardner RM. Implementation issues and challenges for computerized clinical protocols for management of mechanical ventilation in ARDS patients. Symp Comp Appl Med Care (SCAMC) 1989; 13:583-587.

8. Henderson S, East TD, Morris AH, Gardner RM. Performance evaluation of computerized clinical protocols for management of arterial hypoxemia in ARDS patients. Proceedings of the Thirteenth Annual Symp Comp Appl Med Care (SCAMC) 1989; 13:588-592.

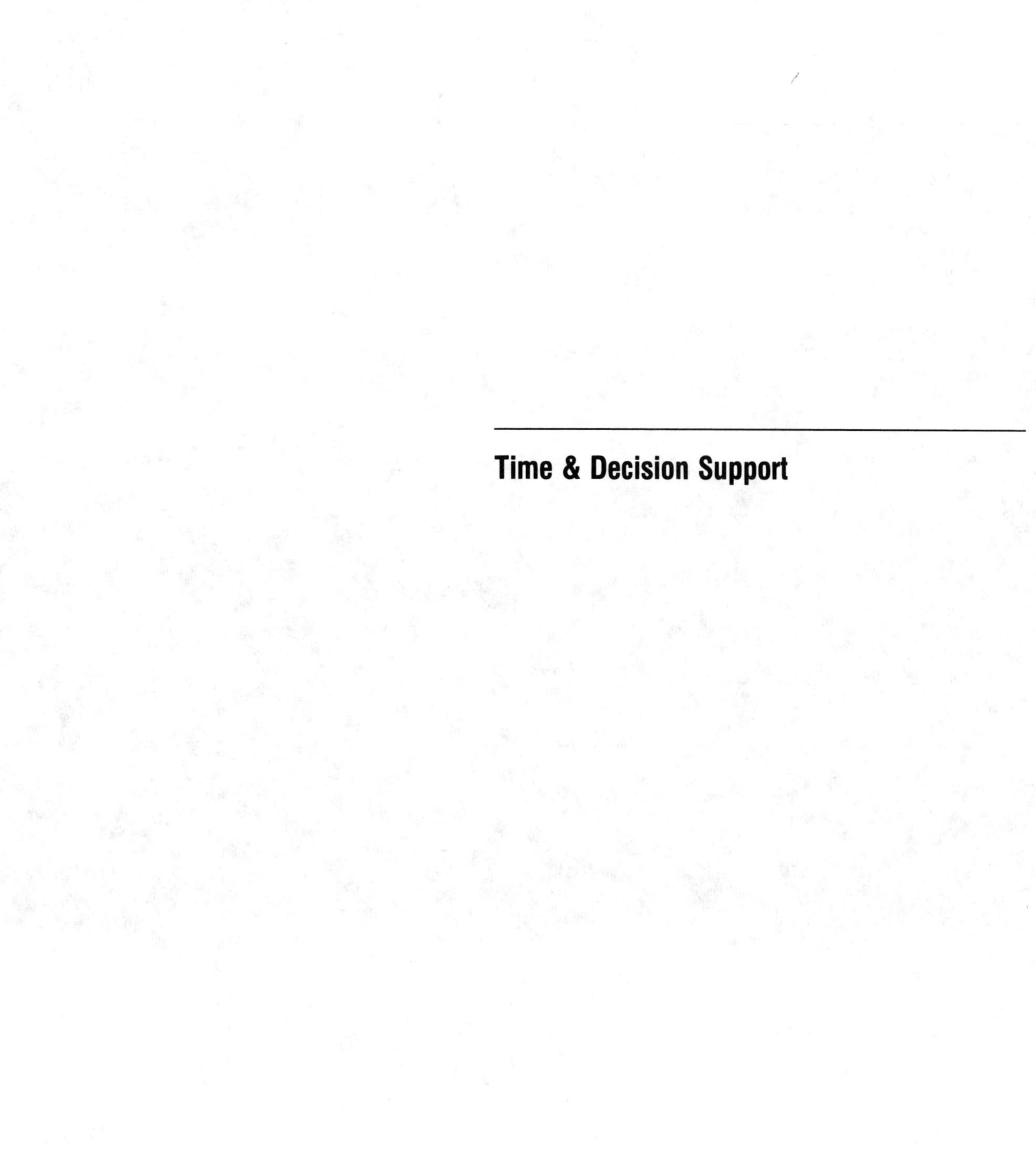

Time & Decision Support

MODELING PAST, CURRENT, AND FUTURE TIME IN MEDICAL DATABASES*

Vram Kouramajian†
Office of the Vice President
for Research & Information Systems
Rice University
P. O. Box 1892, Houston, Texas 77251
vram@rice.edu

Jerry Fowler
Medical Informatics &
Computing Research Program
Baylor College of Medicine
Houston, Texas 77030
gfowler@bcm.tmc.edu

ABSTRACT

Recent research has focused on increasing the power of medical information systems by incorporating time into the database system. A problem with much of this research is that it fails to differentiate between historical time and future time. The concept of bitemporal lifespan presented in this paper overcomes this deficiency. Bitemporal lifespan supports the concepts of valid time and transaction time and allows the integration of past, current, and future information in a unified model.

The concept of bitemporal lifespan is presented within the framework of the Extended Entity-Relationship model. This model permits the characterization of temporal properties of entities, relationships, and attributes. Bitemporal constraints are defined that must hold between entities forming "isa" hierarchies and between entities and relationships. Finally, bitemporal extensions are presented for database query languages in order to provide natural high-level operators for bitemporal query expressions.

INTRODUCTION

Humans naturally describe data in terms of time. Medical data are replete with temporal attributes, including diagnosis, prognosis, orders, duration of treatment, and appointment schedules. Modeling *temporal reality* with relational or object-oriented models leads to awkward modeling and unfriendly query languages. What is needed is a database system that uniformly integrates past, current, and future information in a single model.

Temporal databases preserve the complete history of the "Universe of Discourse;" that is, they follow the *non deletion* rule of data. This permits users to query the current state of the database, as well as past states, and even states that are planned for the future. Clinical patient records systems are a natural application of temporal databases due to the need for complete recall of patient history for clinical, legal, and research reasons [4, 9, 10]. Recent years have witnessed an increase in research on temporal databases [8, 12, 14]. (Excellent glossaries on temporal database concepts can be found in [1, 13]).

A problem with most research in temporal databases is inability to differentiate between historical time and future time. This is especially important for medical information systems where physicians frequently deal with future events such as testing and treatments, and modifications are frequently made to patient treatment schedules based on new information [9, 10]. Historical time is the time that an event *happened* in the real world. Future time is the time an event is scheduled or predicted to happen in the future. Campbell *et al.* [2] observe that expressing time as an interval is necessary to capture uncertainty in medical data. However, intervals alone cannot distinguish the past from the future. The differing semantics of historical time and future time should be reflected in the data model. The goal of this work is to introduce a temporal data model that uniformly integrates past, current, and future information.

A major contribution of this work is the development of the concept of *Bitemporal Lifespan,* which unites two main temporal concepts: valid time and transaction time. This new abstraction allows the integration of past, current, and future information in a unified model. We correlate bitemporal events with terms in English grammar to make the relationships between valid time and transaction time clear. We extend the Extended Entity-Relationship (*EER*) model by using bitemporal lifespans, and we introduce a natural temporal query language over bitemporal regions. We believe that it is more natural to specify temporal data and queries in a conceptual, entity-oriented data model than in a tuple-oriented, relational data model.

This work is an extension to our previous research in the area of temporal conceptual models and query languages [5], where a framework that differentiates between temporal and non-temporal objects was introduced. Here we propose a temporal *EER* conceptual model that distinguishes between the concepts of historical time and future time. Our model allows us to characterize the temporal properties of entities, relationships, and attributes. We also define temporal constraints that must hold between entities forming *isa* hierarchies and between entities and relation-

*Partially supported by National Library of Medicine Grant Number 1T15LM07093-02 and Texas Higher Education Coordinating Board–Advanced Technology Program.

†Current Affiliation: Department of Computer Science, The Wichita State University, Wichita, Kansas 67260, Email: vram@cs.twsu.edu.

0195-4210/94/$5.00 © 1994 AMIA, Inc.

ships. Finally, we propose bitemporal extensions for database query languages that provide natural high–level operators for bitemporal query expressions. For the sake of familiarity, we present these extensions in terms of *SQL*.

TIME ABSTRACTION

Representation of Clock Time

To represent *clock time*, let T be a countably infinite set of totally ordered discrete points in time, or *chronons*. A *time interval*, denoted by $[t_s, t_e]$, is defined to be a set of consecutive chronons; that is, the totally ordered set $\{t_s, t_{s+1}, \ldots, t_{e-1}, t_e\} \subset T$. We call t_s the *start time* and t_e the *end time* of the time interval.

Temporal granularity, the distance between two consecutive chronons, is application–dependent, and can be chosen as month, day, hour, minute, second, or any other suitable time unit. A single discrete chronon t is represented as an interval $[t, t]$, or simply $[t]$.

For historical databases, the domain of a valid time attribute is a time interval $[t_0, now]$, where t_0 represents the starting time of the database mini–world application, and *now* is the current time, which is continuously expanding. In a (general) temporal database, the valid time interval expands to cover the range $(t_{-\infty}, t_{+\infty})$, where values greater than *now* represent future data. In this case, the reference point t_0 is still employed, and negative subscripts are used to represent chronons that precede t_0.

Interval representation has an important shortcoming. Since the set of all intervals in T is not closed under set operations, Gadia and Yeung [7] suggested the concept of temporal elements. A *temporal element*, denoted as TE, is a finite union of time intervals, denoted by $\{I_1, I_2, \ldots, I_n\}$, where I_i is an interval in T. Union, intersection, and difference operations on temporal elements are easily defined. In addition, set comparison predicates of two temporal elements using $=, \neq, \supseteq, \supset, \subseteq$, and $\subset$ are also easily defined.

Bitemporal Lifespan

The *lifespan* of a database object is the time interval over which the object is defined. There are two types of lifespan, each of which is expressed in terms of clock time.

1. **Valid Time Lifespan:** The valid time lifespan of a database object is a temporal attribute that defines the clock time interval during which the object is deemed to be valid within the Universe of Discourse.

2. **Transaction Time Lifespan:** The transaction time lifespan of a database object refers to the clock time of timestamps associated with updates to the object by the database application.

Valid time lifespan refers to historical or predicted events, and can be determined by users of the system. Transaction time lifespan is associated with the recording of those events in clock time, and is determined solely by the system itself.

A *bitemporal lifespan* subsumes both valid time lifespan and transaction time lifespan. We represent

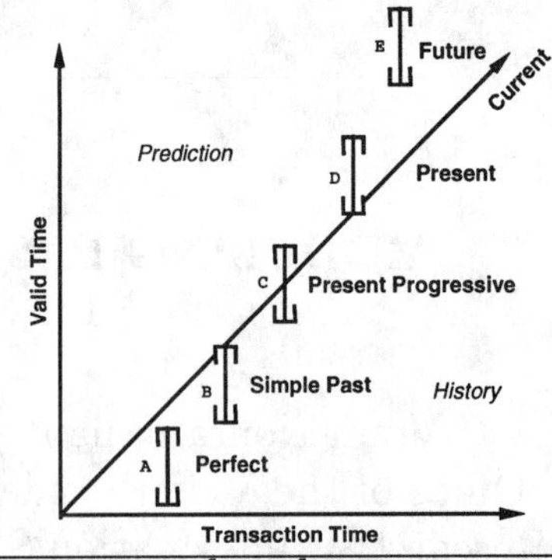

$VT = [t_1, t_2]; TT = t_3$				
Future	Present	Present Progressive	Simple Past	Perfect
$t_3 < t_1$	$t_3 = t_1$	$t_3 > t_1 \vee$ $t_3 < t_2$	$t_3 = t_2$	$t_3 > t_2$

Figure 1: Various Ways of Combining Valid Time with Transaction Time

a bitemporal lifespan BL as a finite set of tuples $BL = \langle VT, TT \rangle$, where VT is a temporal element in $(-\infty, +\infty)$ and TT is a time point in $[0, now]$. A *bitemporal chronon*, denoted by bc, is a point in the two–dimensional space $VT \times TT$; that is, $bc = \langle t_1, t_2 \rangle, t_1 \in VT, t_2 \in TT$. Our representation of bitemporal lifespans allows us to model past, current, and future information in a unified manner.

Figure 1 shows the relationships between valid time and transaction time. The line marked "current" is the line where valid time and transaction time share the same clock time; that is, an event e was recorded at the same time the event occurred. To the right of this line is historical recording, in which an event is entered into the database *after* it occurred. To the left of this line lie predictions of the future, in which an event is entered into the database *before* it occurs. It is natural to describe these relations in terms of grammatical verb tense. Object A in Figure 1 is a historical fact recorded after its occurrence, and corresponds to the perfect tense: "The patient has had a previous pregnancy." Object B represents simple past tense. An event has just occurred, but is no longer active: "A drug was administered." Objects C and D both reflect present tense, because they indicate events recorded during the interval in which they are valid. Object C corresponds to present progressive tense, because it represents an ongoing activity, such as the course of a disease: "The patient is being treated for genital herpes." Object D corresponds to simple present tense: "We begin treatment now." Object E reflects the future. An event is recorded in the database before its occurrence: "The patient will return for an appointment next Tuesday."

THE BITEMPORAL DATA MODEL

The *EER* model has been extensively used in database design applications [3, 6]. In this section, we introduce extensions to the *EER* model that capture temporal data. For brevity, we assume familiarity with the basic concepts of the *EER* model and *EER* diagrams [3, 6], so that we may simply specify the novel concepts of the Bitemporal *EER* model.

Bitemporal Entities

An entity type is a set of entities of the same type; that is, entities that share the same attributes. Entities represent objects in the mini–world situation that is being modeled. Each entity type E_i has a set of attributes A_{i1}, A_{i2}, ..., A_{in}, and each attribute A_{ij} is associated with a domain of values $dom(A_{ij})$.

In the bitemporal *EER* model, each entity e of entity type E is associated with a bitemporal lifespan $BL(e)$ that defines the time during which e is valid.

Example 1: Figure 2 shows a fragmentary *EER* schema for a health care database, which includes the entity types *PATIENT*, *PHYSICIAN*, and *TEST*. A particular *PATIENT* entity may have a bitemporal lifespan $\{\langle[1/1/92, 1/2/93], 1/25/93\rangle, \langle[11/3/93, 2/5/94], 2/5/94\rangle\}$; this means that this patient was treated during the periods $[1/1/92, 1/2/93]$ and $[11/3/93, 2/5/94]$, and that this information was registered in the database at $1/25/93$ and $2/5/94$.

Bitemporal Assignment

The *bitemporal assignment* of each attribute A_i of an entity e, denoted as $A_i(e)$, is a partial function $A_i(e) : BL(e) \rightarrow dom(A)$. (This is similar to the idea of *temporal assignment* where the domain of a partial function is a temporal element [GaYe88].) We use $BL(A_i(e))$ to denote the subset of $BL(e)$ in which $A_i(e)$ is defined. The value of A_i during the time $BL(e) - BL(A_i(e))$ is undefined.

Example 2: Consider the database described by the schema in Figure 2. For simplicity, *day* is used as the temporal granularity. A particular *PATIENT* entity e_1 and a particular *PHYSICIAN* entity e_2 may have the following bitemporal attribute values:

$Name(e_1) = \{ \langle[9/1/75, now], 1/15/94\rangle \rightarrow \textit{Jane Doe} \}$
$UID(e_1) = \{ \langle[1/15/94, now], 1/15/94\rangle \rightarrow 123456789 \}$
$Sex(e_1) = \{ \langle[9/1/75, now], 1/15/94\rangle \rightarrow \textit{Female} \}$
$Problem(e_1) = \{ \langle[1/15/94, 1/16/94], 1/15/94\rangle \rightarrow \{ \textit{Suspicion of Pregnancy} \}, \langle[12/1/93, 8/1/94], 1/16/94\rangle \rightarrow \{ \textit{Pregnancy} \} \}$
$Name(e_2) = \{ \langle[9/1/60, now], 1/15/90\rangle \rightarrow \textit{Yaa Dufie} \}$
$UID(e_2) = \{ \langle[1/15/90, now], 1/15/90\rangle \rightarrow 987654321 \}$
$Office(e_2) = \{ \langle[1/15/90, now], 1/15/90\rangle \rightarrow \{ \textit{BCM \#315, BCM \#1015} \} \}$
$Specialty(e_2) = \{ \langle[1/15/90, now], 1/15/90\rangle \rightarrow \textit{Gynecology} \}$

Bitemporal Attributes and Keys

In our model, each entity has a system–defined, non–temporal, unique, immutable *SURROGATE* attribute (or "UID") whose value is not visible to users. In addition, several types of bitemporal attributes exist:

1. **Bitemporal Single–Valued Attribute:** A bitemporal single–valued attribute has at most a single atomic value for each entity at each bitemporal instant *bc*.

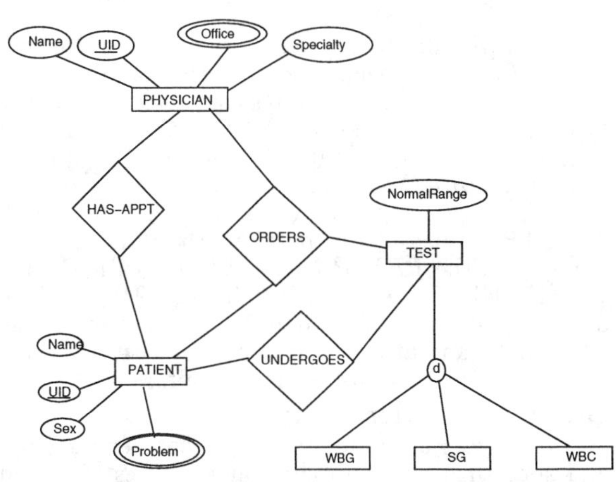

Figure 2: A Schema Fragment

2. **Bitemporal Multi–Valued Attribute:** A bitemporal multi-valued attribute can have more than one value for an entity at a given bitemporal instant *bc*; hence, its domain is the power set $P(V)$ of some simple domain V. For instance, in Figure 2, *Problem* is a multi–valued attribute since a patient may have more than one problem concurrently. *Office* is likewise multi–valued.

3. **Bitemporal Composite Attribute:** A bitemporal composite attribute is a list of several component bitemporal attributes, and its value for each entity at bitemporal instant *bc* is a concatenation of the values of its components.

4. **Key Attribute:** A (simple or composite) attribute A is a key attribute of an entity type E if at any bitemporal instant *bc*, no two entities in E have the same value for A. We allow the update of a key attribute since each entity is uniquely identified by its *SURROGATE*. For instance, the attribute *UID* of entity Type *PATIENT* in Figure 2 is a key attribute since it uniquely identifies a particular patient.

Bitemporal Relationships

A *relationship type* R of degree n has n participating entity types $E_1, E_2, ..., E_n$. Each *relationship instance* r in R is an n–tuple $r = \langle e_1, e_2, \ldots, e_n\rangle$ where each $e_i \in E_i$. In our model, each relationship instance r is associated with a bitemporal lifespan $BL(r)$. The constraint is that $BL(r)$ must be a subset of the intersection of the bitemporal lifespans of the entities $e_1, e_2, \ldots, e_n$ that participate in r. That is, $BL(r) \subseteq (BL(e_1) \cap BL(e_2) \cap \ldots \cap BL(e_n))$. This is because for the relationship instance to exist at some bitemporal instant *bc*, all the entities participating in that relationship instance must also exist at *bc*.

Relationship attributes are treated similarly to entity attributes; the bitemporal value $A_i(r)$ of each simple attribute A_i of r is a partial function (bitemporal assignment) $A_i(r) : BL(r) \rightarrow dom(A_i)$ and $BL(A_i(r)) \subseteq BL(r)$.

Example 3: In Figure 2, the relationship type *HAS_APPT* represents the fact that a patient has an appointment with a physician; the relationship type *ORDERS* represents the fact that a physician orders a test for a patient; and the relationship type *UNDERGOES* represents the fact that a patient undergoes a test. To Example 2, let us add a *HAS_APPT* instance r between the *PATIENT* entity e_1 and the *PHYSICIAN* entity e_2, with $BL(r) = \{\langle[1/15/94], 1/15/94\rangle, \langle[1/16/94], 1/15/94\rangle\}$; this indicates that the patient had a walk–in appointment on 1/15/94 and at that time a second visit was scheduled for 1/16/94 to discuss test results.

Bitemporal Hierarchies

Subclasses can be used to represent generalization and specialization hierarchies and lattices [6]. Membership of entities in a subclass can either be specified via a predicate or categorized explicitly by the user. In the former case, we have a *predicate-defined subclass*, where each entity in the superclass that satisfies a defining predicate will be a member of the subclass. In the latter case, the user *explicitly* partitions entities from the superclass into categorical subclasses.

An entity e of a superclass C will belong to a predicate–defined subclass SC at all bitemporal instants where the predicate evaluates to true. For a user defined subclass, the user will specify the bitemporal instants at which an entity e belonging to the superclass C will also belong to the subclass SC. In either case, the entity will have a bitemporal lifespan $BL(e/SC)$ that specifies the bitemporal instants at which it is a member of the subclass SC. The constraint $BL(e/SC) \subseteq BL(e/C)$ must always hold.

Example 4: Figure 2 shows an example of three subclasses: *WBG* (*Whole Blood Glucose*), *SG* (*Serum Glucose*), and *WBC* (*White Blood Count*) of the *TEST* entity type. The symbol d in Figure 2 indicates that the subclasses *WBG*, *SG*, and *WBC* are always bitemporally disjoint.

THE BITEMPORAL ALGEBRA

To allow for bitemporal constructs in queries, we define the concepts of bitemporal boolean expressions, bitemporal selection conditions, and bitemporal projections.

Bitemporal Boolean Expression

A bitemporal boolean expression is a conditional expression on the attributes and relationships of an entity. A bitemporal boolean condition c_t, when applied to an entity e at a given transaction time point t, evaluates to { *TRUE, FALSE, UNKNOWN* }.

Example 5: The boolean expression (Problem = "Pregnancy")$_{1/16/94}$ for the *PATIENT* entity e_1 given in Example 2 results in:

{ [12/1/93, 8/1/94] → *TRUE*,
[9/1/75, 11/30/93] ∪ [8/2/94, *now*] → *FALSE*,
other-times → *UNKNOWN*}

However, (Problem = "Pregnancy")$_{1/1/94}$ results in:

{ [9/1/75, *now*] → *FALSE*,
other-times → *UNKNOWN*}

True_Time

The true_time of a boolean expression $[\![c_t]\!]$ at a given transaction time point t, evaluates to a *temporal element* for each entity e. The temporal element is the time for which the condition is *TRUE* for e.

Example 6: The true_time of the boolean condition in example 5 evaluated at the transaction time point 1/16/94 is { [12/1/93, 8/1/94] }.

Bitemporal Selection Condition

A bitemporal selection condition compares two true_time expressions (i.e. temporal elements) using the set comparison operators $=, \neq, \supseteq, \supset, \subseteq$, and $\subset$. When applied to an entity type, it evaluates to those entities that satisfy the bitemporal selection condition.

Example 7: Consider the following bitemporal selection condition applied to the *PATIENT* entity type of Figure 2:

$$[\![\text{(HAS\_APPT = "Yaa Dufie")}_{1/15/94}]\!] \supseteq [1/1/94, now]$$

This selects the *entire history*, as registered in the database on 1/15/94, of all patients who had appointments with Yaa Dufie between 1/1/94 and the present.

Bitemporal Projection

A bitemporal projection TE_t of a bitemporal entity e over a temporal element TE at transaction time t, is evaluated in two steps: (1) rollback to the transaction time t and (2) restrict the data displayed for the entity e to the temporal element TE. (This operation is similar to the when operator introduced in [GaYe88] for clock time periods.)

Example 8: The bitemporal projection of bitemporal *PATIENT* entity e_1 of Example 2 over the temporal element {[2/15/94, *now*]} at the transaction time point 2/15/94 results in:

Name(e_1) = { [2/15/94, *now*] → *Jane Doe* }
UID(e_1) = { [2/15/94, *now*] → 123456789 }
Sex(e_1) = { [2/15/94, *now*] → *Female* }
Problem(e_1) = { [2/15/94, *now*] → {*Pregnancy*} }

THE BITEMPORAL QUERY LANGUAGE

In non–temporal databases, a query will typically select certain entities based on boolean predicates that involve attribute values of the entity and of related entities, and then display certain attributes or relationships of each of the selected entities. In a bitemporal database, selection criteria may be based not only on attribute values but also on bitemporal conditions. In addition, once an entity is selected, a user may wish to display the complete history (bitemporal assignment) of some of its attributes or relationships, or to limit the displayed values to a certain time interval.

Our bitemporal algebra can be used to specify temporal queries by extending the *SQL* database language [6]. The bitemporal extensions are illustrated through examples (A number of important bitemporal query constructs, such as bitemporal aggregates, are omitted for brevity).

Example 9: Consider the query to retrieve as of 1/1/92 (transaction time) the name and office number of all pediatricians in the clinic on 1/1/88 (valid time):

SELECT ⟨ Name, Office⟩ : $[1/1/88]_{1/1/92}$
FROM PHYSICIAN
WHERE $[\![$(PHYSICIAN.Specialty = "Pediatric")$_{1/1/92}]\!]$ $\supseteq$ [1/1/88]

It is important to distinguish between the effects of the bitemporal construct used in the SELECT–clause and that in the WHERE–clause. The WHERE–clause evaluates entities based on the state of the database on 1/1/92. It is still necessary to specify the bitemporal projection $[1/1/88]_{1/1/92}$ again in the SELECT–clause in order to obtain the information registered on 1/1/92 rather than the current information.

Example 10: Consider the query to retrieve the current name and office number of all physicians who saw the patient "Jon Smith" during the time period [1/1/88, 4/5/92] as registered in the database on 5/5/92:

SELECT ⟨Name, Office⟩
FROM PHYSICIAN
WHERE $[\![$(PHYSICIAN.HAS_APPT.PATIENT.Name = "Jon Smith")$_{5/5/92}]\!]$ $\supseteq$ [1/1/88, 4/5/92]

To deal with bitemporal data, we need bitemporal query functions not found in traditional databases [11]. The functions *FI* (first instant) and *LI* (last instant) return the first and last time points, respectively, when applied to a temporal element. Other functions we will use are the *VTIME* and *TTIME* functions in the *SELECT* clause, which retrieve the valid time and transaction time of each selected entity respectively.

Example 11: To retrieve the interval during which "Yaa Dufie" was on the staff as of 1/1/94, we write:

SELECT ⟨VTIME⟩
FROM PHYSICIAN
WHERE PHYSICIAN.Name = "Yaa Dufie"

CONCLUSIONS

In this paper, we presented a bitemporal extension to the *EER* model that uniformly supports past, current, and future times. The concept of bitemporal lifespan of an entity or a relationship instance was defined. The bitemporal properties of entities, relationships, and attributes were characterized. Bitemporal constraints that must hold between entities forming *isa* hierarchies as well as between entities and relationships were defined. We also presented the concepts of bitemporal selection conditions and bitemporal projections, and showed how these bitemporal constructs can be used to extend the *SQL* database language.

We believe that the use of the bitemporal *ER* model will provide greater power in the expression of medical queries. We hope to prototype a bitemporal *DBMS* that addresses important implementation issues like bitemporal indexing structures and query optimization. However, temporal databases will not become ubiquitous unless they are able to provide *human–centric* user interfaces over terabytes of temporal data. Needless to say, this is an immensely challenging area worth exploring.

References

[1] K. Al-Taha, R. Snodgrass, and M. Soo. Bibliography on spatiotemporal databases. *ACM SIGMOD Record*, 22(1), March 1993.

[2] K. Campbell, A. Das, and M. Musen. A logical foundation for the representation of clinical data. *Journal of the American Medical Informatics Association*, 1(3), May/June 1994.

[3] P. Chen. The entity–relationship model — towards a unified view of data. *ACM Transactions on Database Systems*, 1(1), March 1976.

[4] A. Das, S. Tu, G. Purcell, and M. Musen. An extended sql for temporal data management in clinical decision-support systems. In *Symposium on Computer Applications in Medical Care*, November 1992.

[5] R. Elmasri and V. Kouramajian. A temporal query language for a conceptual model. In N. Adam and B. Bhargava, editors, *Advanced Database Systems, Lecture Notes in Computer Science*, volume 759. Springer–Verlag, December 1993.

[6] R. Elmasri and S. Navathe. *Fundamentals of Database Systems, 2nd Edition.* Benjamin/Cummings, 1994.

[7] S. Gadia and C. Yeung. A generalized model for a temporal relational database. In *ACM SIGMOD International Conference on Management of Data*, June 1988.

[8] C. Jensen et al. A consensus glossary of temporal database concepts. *ACM SIGMOD Record*, 23(1), March 1994.

[9] M. Kahn, L. Fagan, and S. Tu. Extensions to the time–oriented database model to support temporal reasoning in medical expert systems. In *Methods of Information in Medicine*, 1991.

[10] Y. Shahar, S. Tu, and M. Musen. Temporal–abstraction mechanisms in management of clinical protocols. In *Symposium on Computer Applications in Medical Care*, November 1992.

[11] R. Snodgrass. The temporal query language *TQUEL*. *ACM Transactions on Database Systems*, 12(2), June 1987.

[12] R. Snodgrass, editor. *International Workshop on an Infrastructure for Temporal Databases*, June 1993.

[13] M. Soo. Bibliography on temporal databases. *ACM SIGMOD Record*, 20(1), March 1991.

[14] A. Tansel, J. Clifford, S. Gadia, S. Jajodia, A. Segev, and R. Snodgrass, editors. *Temporal Databases: Theory, Design and Implementation.* Benjamin/Cummings, 1993.

A Temporal-Abstraction Mediator for Protocol-Based Decision-Support Systems

Amar K. Das, Yuval Shahar, Samson W. Tu, and Mark A. Musen

Section on Medical Informatics
Stanford University School of Medicine
Stanford, California 94305-5479
(das@camis.stanford.edu)

ABSTRACT

The inability of many clinical decision-support applications to integrate with existing databases limits the wide-scale deployment of such systems. To overcome this obstacle, we have designed a data-interpretation module that can be embedded in a general architecture for protocol-based reasoning and that can support the fundamental task of detecting temporal abstractions. We have developed this software module by coupling two existing systems — RÉSUMÉ and Chronus — that provide complementary temporal-abstraction techniques at the application and the database levels, respectively. Their encapsulation into a single module thus can resolve the temporal queries of protocol planners with the domain-specific knowledge needed for the temporal-abstraction task and with primary time-stamped data stored in autonomous clinical databases. We show that other computer methods for the detection of temporal abstractions do not scale up to the data- and knowledge-intensive environments of protocol-based decision-support systems.

1. THE TEMPORAL-ABSTRACTION TASK FOR PROTOCOL-BASED DECISION SUPPORT

Many health-care institutions would like to bring applicable clinical protocols to the attention of providers via decision-support systems that automatically examine patient data stored in legacy databases. Since the planning of medical therapies is highly time dependent, an essential task in predicating protocol advice is the detection of clinically relevant **temporal abstractions** from patient data. For example, a health-care provider should modify the standard dose of AZT for a patient if, *after starting treatment according to a California Cooperative Treatment Group protocol (CCTG-522), the patient experiences a second episode of moderate anemia that has persisted for more than 2 weeks.* The clinical condition of anemia is defined explicitly by the CCTG-522 protocol based on ranges of hemoglobin values.

If we analyze the condition, we notice that carrying out this temporal-abstraction task actually requires several subtasks. For example, the inference of hemoglobin-test results into abstract states (e.g., "moderate" or "severe" anemia) requires the use of protocol-defined thresholds; the interpretation of hemoglobin values depends on the context (e.g., the AZT arm of the CCTG-522 protocol) in which the measurement occurred; and the aggregation of abstractions during certain defined intervals (e.g., the second episode of anemia that occurred after the start of therapy) is based on temporal-pattern matching.

Database-query languages (e.g., SQL) do not currently have the ability to satisfy all these subtasks of temporal abstractions on electronically stored patient data. To overcome this obstacle, most developers of protocol-based decision-support programs have either (1) extended the data-abstraction capabilities of databases or (2) provided data-management techniques within the knowledge-based system. In this paper, we argue that implementing temporal-abstraction methods with either of these approaches alone does not permit the seamless integration of decision-support systems with legacy databases. We discuss two systems — RÉSUMÉ and Chronus — that support complementary aspects of the temporal-abstractions task at the application and the database levels, respectively. We indicate that the coupling of these systems, however, requires the system developer to specify the coordination of the two systems. To resolve this problem, we describe a novel software module (based on mediator technology) that integrates logically the temporal-abstraction mechanisms of RÉSUMÉ and Chronus.

2. DATABASE AND KNOWLEDGE-BASED APPROACHES TO THE TEMPORAL-ABSTRACTION TASK

Database-management systems and knowledge-based systems both support the goal of processing data. Yet, their perspectives on data processing historically have been divergent [1]. Database-management systems have been concerned primarily with giving multiple users access to large sets of consistent, permanent data on secondary-storage devices, whereas knowledge-based systems have provided a single application the ability to derive logical consequences from a comparatively smaller number of memory-resident facts. Database-management systems can serve as the central data repository of clinical information system, but they do not provide applications utilities for extracting information not explicitly stored in the database. The developers of knowledge-based systems, on the other hand, have traditionally designed decision-support programs on isolated, single-user machines; the underlying software typically does not support reliable data storage.

Because database-management and knowledge-based systems can provide complementary types of clinical data processing, the integration of such systems should be a prerequisite for a decision-support architecture that can query temporal abstractions from data in clinical databases. Most computer-based methods for temporal abstraction, however, do not support such an architecture. Some temporal-abstraction methods (e.g., VM [2] and TrenDx [3]) allow neither higher-level applications (e.g., protocol planner) to query results nor lower-level data sources (e.g., databases) to provide input.

Several developers of protocol planners have attempted to extend existing database-management systems with inference capabilities for temporal abstractions. This approach ensures that the output of any data abstraction can be stored back in the database in a manner consistent with primary data; the programming facilities of database-management systems, however, do not support the complex reasoning methods required by the temporal-abstraction task. For example, a database-management system that incorporates the Arden Syntax [4] — a procedural method for supporting clinical algorithms in a variety of databases — can alert a health-care provider about the occurrence of a simple temporal condition (e.g., a significantly low hemoglobin value). Although this abstraction result can be placed into the central database, the expressiveness of the Arden Syntax limits the method's ability to provide a protocol planner more complex subtasks of temporal abstractions (e.g., finding the second occurrence of an interval of anemia that has persisted for more than 2 weeks).

Another approach to the implementation of the temporal-abstraction task is to incorporate both data-management and temporal-inference techniques within the knowledge-based system that performs the protocol planning. This type of architecture ensures that knowledge and data are readily available to the temporal-abstraction method from a reliable, consistent source, but such an approach does not permit the temporal-abstraction method to make dynamic queries to existing databases in legacy systems. For example, in the ONCOCIN system [5], the problem-solving method for chemotherapy planning, the temporal-abstraction program for determining a patient's reaction to past chemotherapies, and the data structures for the time-stamped clinical data were written in LISP code. In this decision-support system, the temporal-abstraction method was entirely dependent on the user's entry of data into the internal data structures. To overcome the limitations of approaches that use exclusively database or knowledge-based methods, we have instead developed generic methods that can use domain-specific temporal-abstraction knowledge, and that can provide access to temporal data stored in existing databases.

3. THE RÉSUMÉ AND THE CHRONUS TEMPORAL-ABSTRACTION MODULES

In designing the T-HELPER system [6] — an advice system for protocol-based care of patients who have HIV disease — we have attempted to avoid the problems of previous approaches by creating modular temporal-abstraction components. Consequently, we have used emerging industry wide standards (such as UNIX, C, and SQL) as the basis of our system. To separate the domain knowledge of a protocol planner from the data-access methods of underlying database-management systems, we have also have created a pair of temporal-abstraction modules, the **RÉSUMÉ** system [7] and the **Chronus** system [8], which we have developed in the CLIPS production-rule system and a C-based interface to a Sybase relational database, respectively.

RÉSUMÉ and Chronus provide complementary types of temporal deductions over patient data. RÉSUMÉ uses protocol-specific knowledge to extract from primitive data (in its fact base) high-level summaries of a patient's condition over time (such as the inference of hemoglobin values into "low" states), whereas Chronus provides a general SQL-based data-access language to make temporal queries (such as the ordinal ordering of values within a defined time period) on data stored in relational databases. RÉSUMÉ, unlike Chronus, does not support queries over multiple patients or queries consisting of complex temporal patterns; Chronus, unlike RÉSUMÉ, does not support the identification of intervals that are not stored explicitly in the database. With the complementary actions of these systems, we can support at the application or the database levels the temporal-abstraction subtasks that are the most appropriate for that level.

The flexibility of our dual system does, however, impose a constraint on the developer of the protocol planner: She is responsible for specifying the coordination of the systems for each application. For example, to determine the second episode of moderate anemia after the start of treatment, the developer must first specify the loading of time-stamped hemoglobin values from the database (via Chronus) into the memory-resident fact base of the RÉSUMÉ system. This loading requires a set of *mapping rules* to translate data between the database schema and the fact-base representation. The RÉSUMÉ system then creates anemia abstractions in the clinical context specified by the protocol planner (e.g., the treatment of patients according to a clinical-trial protocol), and the results are saved into the database. Using the query language of the Chronus system, the developer must finally specify a temporal-aggregation query that determines the number of anemia intervals that are stored in the database. Because this integration method requires manual coordination, the system developer must define, for each temporal-abstraction condition, the procedural knowledge necessary to implement the temporal-abstraction task with the RÉSUMÉ and the Chronus systems.

4. THE TZOLKIN TEMPORAL-ABSTRACTION MEDIATOR

To remove the need for manual coordination, we are developing a single system, called **Tzolkin,**[†] that can process automatically queries from different protocol-planning applications and that can make temporal abstractions as needed. Such a system is termed a *mediator*, because it serves as a middle layer between the user-oriented processing of applications and the data-manipulation methods of database systems [9]. A distinguishing feature of the mediator approach to integration is the latter's ability to use encoded knowledge about data to create more abstract information for higher-layer applications. In Section 4.1, we describe the types of encoded knowledge required by the Tzolkin mediator to perform the temporal-abstraction task; in Section 4.2, we discuss the query language that is the interface to the mediator and the query-evaluation strategy that specifies the coordination between the RÉSUMÉ and the Chronus components.

[†] Tzolkin is the Mayan term for the Sun Stone, which served as an accurate representation of calendar time.

4.1 The Knowledge-Based Method

In the design of a temporal-abstraction mediator, we have developed a knowledge-based method [10] that decomposes the temporal-abstraction task into five specific subtasks: (1) temporal-context restriction, (2) vertical temporal inference, (3) horizontal temporal inference, (4) temporal interpolation, and (5) temporal-pattern matching. The first four subtasks are supported by four corresponding problem-solving mechanisms in the RÉSUMÉ program, whereas the last subtask is provided by the Chronus program. To implement these subtasks in a domain-independent manner, we have defined explicitly the knowledge requirements needed by the mechanisms. Using the domain model in the protocol planner and domain-specific knowledge from a domain expert, a system designer can instantiate the knowledge requirements in the knowledge-base representation (*ontology*). In addition to these ontologies, the knowledge base of the mediator contains mapping rules (as described in Section 3). By unifying the temporal-abstraction mechanisms of the RÉSUMÉ and Chronus programs into a single method, we ensure consistency and compatibility of the temporal-abstraction knowledge that is used by both components.

4.2 The Query-Evaluation Strategy

All interactions among the protocol planner, the temporal-abstraction mediator, and the clinical database occurs through message passing of queries and data. For the query language of the clinical database, we require an SQL interface. For the query language of Tzolkin, we have made extensions to the TimeLine SQL (TLSQL) language of Chronus [11] to create **SQLA** (SQL for Abstractions). The following SQLA statement, for example, determines if, in the context of AZT arm of the CCTG-522 protocol, an individual with patient identification 2997 had a second episode of moderate anemia that has occurred after the start of AZT therapy:

```
CONTEXT  CCTG_522_AZT_arm
SELECT   SECOND state_abs.parameter
FROM     state_abs, medication
WHERE    state_abs.parameter =
         "anemia" AND
         state_abs.value =
         "moderate" AND
         medication.drug_name =
         "AZT" AND state_abs.pid =
         medication.pid AND
         state_abs.pid = 2997
WHEN     state_abs.start_time
         AFTER medication.start_time
```

As does TLSQL, SQLA adds temporal extensions (such as the `CONTEXT` and `WHEN` clauses) to the standard SQL syntax.

To implement such queries in Tzolkin, we have defined a **query-evaluation mechanism** that uses the ontology in the knowledge base to determine the domain-specific elements of a query that are needed to process the query. Depending on which temporal-abstraction mechanisms are needed to implement the query, the query-evaluation mechanism also finds the most appropriate query-evaluation strategy. The query-evaluation component inputs the procedural knowledge of the strategy into a **system-control structure** that coordinates the actions of the RÉSUMÉ and the Chronus components.

We have analyzed the integration methods currently required by our dual temporal-abstraction systems, and have identified several evaluation strategies that are needed for the mediator. The example SQLA query requires a strategy that interweaves the temporal-abstractions mechanisms of the RÉSUMÉ and the Chronus components as follows:

1. Using the mapping rules, Chronus loads data from the clinical database into the fact base of the RÉSUMÉ component. (The knowledge base provides information about the scope of the primitive data required for temporal abstractions.)
2. RÉSUMÉ restricts its deduction capabilities to the clinical context specified in the query, and undertakes the required mechanisms for temporal abstraction on the data in the fact base. (The evaluation strategy does not fix the order of the mechanisms in RÉSUMÉ, since the mechanisms iterate alternately on the data and on any intermediate results.)
3. The Chronus component then performs set-based temporal-pattern matching on the resulting temporal abstractions in the fact base.

In essence, the system-control structure automates the coordination that was undertaken previously by the system developer.

5. DISCUSSION

In this paper, we have described a mediator system that protocol planners can query to identify automatically time-related abstractions from primary data in legacy databases. Our novel software module is based on a formal knowledge-based method that decomposes the temporal-abstraction task into five subtasks, each of which is implemented by a specific mechanism in either the RÉSUMÉ or the Chronus components of the mediator. By encapsulating these two components into a novel system that can mediate queries from the protocol planner to the clinical database, we have avoided the problems of most previous approaches, which either supported complex temporal deductions within the database system or provided data-management techniques within the protocol planner.

In contrast to most systems for temporal abstraction, the M-HTP system [12] does provide separate data-access and temporal-deduction components within a decision-support architecture. Unlike our approach, however, the database-access method is supported within an interface to the database-management system, and the temporal-abstraction method is part of the knowledge-based protocol planner. When the M-HTP system acquires patient data from the external database, the database-interface must first translate data from the database schema to the representation in the reasoning methods. Then, the protocol planner performs temporal-abstractions on the data, and stores the results internally in a temporal network.

In contrast to the M-HTP system, we argue that the temporal-abstraction method in Tzolkin is transferable to different decision-support systems for three reasons. First, in our system, we need only to specify the mapping rules to translate data between the data representations of planner and of the database. In the M-HTP system, this mapping information is internalized by the database interface, and is not transparent to the temporal-abstraction method. Second, our temporal-abstraction mechanisms are domain independent, and require only encoded domain-specific knowledge to implement the temporal-abstraction task for the protocol planner. The knowledge for creating temporal abstractions in the M-HTP system, on the other hand, is not separate from the knowledge needed for the problem-solving method of the protocol planner. Third, in our system, the developers of protocol planners do not need to specify the technical and administrative knowledge necessary to implement the temporal-abstraction task; the query-evaluation mechanism and the mapping rules generate automatically this information. To reimplement in another architecture the temporal-abstraction component of the M-HTP system, however, the system developer might have to change the internal codes of the database interface and of the protocol planner.

Because the mediator approach to the temporal-abstraction method is novel, it raises new issues for programs that interpret clinical data. For example, the mediator's evaluation of queries is a hybrid method of both rule-based and database algorithms for pattern matching languages (from the CLIPS expert-system shell and the relational database system); thus, we cannot easily determine a general time complexity for the Tzolkin system. In the generation of a query-evaluation strategy, however, we recognize that we can optimize certain complex queries (such as temporal abstractions from multiple patients) by processing data concurrently at the mediator and database level.

Our approach also raises the issue of the defeasibility of the temporal-abstractions that we create. The RÉSUMÉ program uses a truth-maintenance system that can permit all temporal abstractions to be withdrawn from the fact base in the face of new, contradictory data; however, neither our previous dual-system architecture nor our current mediator architecture ensures that data entered into the database are similarly entered into the fact base. To avoid this problem, we can make all abstraction results sent to the protocol planner contingent on the content of the clinical database at the time the query is evaluated by the mediator. Data that are deleted or added to the database after temporal reasoning has begun will not affect the results of the abstraction process, and the results will not be saved between queries.

We are currently implementing the Tzolkin system, and are investigating the most appropriate solutions to the issues of optimization and nonmonotonicity. In this paper, we have established the necessity of such a general software module, and have indicated that the mechanisms of the RÉSUMÉ and Chronus components are sufficient to provide the functionality of a temporal-abstraction mediator.

ACKNOWLEDGMENTS

We thank L. Dupré for her editorial assistance. This work has been supported in part by grant HS06330 from the Agency for Health Policy and Research, and by grants LM05208 and LM07033 from the National Library of Medicine. Computing facilities were provided by the CAMIS Resource, LM05305. Dr. Musen is a recipient of an NSF Young Investigator Award.

REFERENCES

1. Rundensteiner, E.A. The role of AI in databases versus the role of database theory in AI: An opinion. In Meersman, R.A., Shi, Z., and Kung, C. (eds), *Artificial Intelligence in Databases and Information Systems.* North-Holland: Amsterdam, 1990, pp. 233–252.
2. Fagan, L.M. *Representing Time-Dependent Relations in a Clinical Setting.* Ph.D. Thesis, Computer Science Department, Stanford University, Stanford, CA, 1980.
3. Haimovitz, I.J., and Kohane, I.S. Automated trend detection with alternate temporal hypotheses. *Proceedings of the Thirteenth International Joint Conference on Artificial Intelligence.* Chambrey, France. R. Bajcsy (ed), Morgan Kaufmann. 1993, pp. 146–151.
4. Hripcsak, G., Clayton, P.D., Pryor, T.A., Haug, P., Wigertz, O.B., and van der Lei, J. The Arden syntax for medical logic modules. *Proceedings of the Fourteenth Annual Symposium on Computer Applications in Medical Care.* Washington, DC. R.A. Miller (ed), IEEE Computer Society Press. 1990, pp. 200–204.
5. Kahn, M.G., Fagan, L.M., and Tu, S. Extensions to the Time-Oriented Database model to support temporal reasoning in medical expert systems. *Methods of Information in Medicine* 30:4–14, 1991.
6. Musen, M.A., Carlson, C.W., Fagan, L.M., Deresinski, S.C., and Shortliffe, E.H. T-HELPER: Automated support for community-based clinical research. *Proceedings of the Sixteenth Annual Symposium on Computer Applications in Medical Care.* Baltimore, MD. M.E. Frisse (ed), McGraw-Hill. 1992, pp. 719–723.
7. Shahar, Y., and Musen, M.A. RÉSUMÉ: A temporal-abstraction system for patient monitoring. *Computers and Biomedical Research* 26:255–273, 1992.
8. Das, A.K., and Musen, M.A. A temporal query system for protocol-directed decision support. *Methods of Information in Medicine* (in press).
9. Wiederhold, G. Mediators in the architecture of future information systems. *IEEE Computer* 25:38–50, 1992.
10. Shahar, Y., Das, A.K., Tu, S.W., Kraemer, F.B., and Musen, M.A. Knowledge-based temporal abstraction for diabetic monitoring. *Proceedings of the Eighteenth Annual Symposium on Computer Applications in Medical Care.* (in press).
11. Das, A.K., Tu, S.W., Purcell, G.P., and Musen, M.A. An extended SQL for temporal data management in clinical decision-support systems. *Proceedings of the Sixteenth Annual Symposium on Computer Applications in Medical Care.* Baltimore, M.D. M.E. Frisse (ed), McGraw-Hill. 1992, pp. 128–132.
12. Larizza, C., Moglia, A., and Stefanelli, M. M-HTP: A system for monitoring heart transplant patients. *Artificial Intelligence in Medicine* 4:111–126, 1992.

Towards a Standard Query Model for Sharing Decision-Support Applications

Walter Sujansky, Russ Altman, M.D., Ph.D.

Section on Medical Informatics, MSOB x215
Stanford University Medical School, Stanford, CA 94305
sujansky@camis.stanford.edu, altman@camis.stanford.edu

ABSTRACT

Many clinical decision-support applications are created in a centralized manner, but distributed widely for local use. When such applications include queries to electronic patient databases, the queries must be translated to conform to local database specifications. Because no well-defined standard model of clinical data exists, the translation process is ad hoc, costly, and error-prone. In this paper, we propose an abstract formalism, called the Standard Query Model Framework, for specifying a standard clinical data model and for supporting the automated and reliable translation of queries that appear in shared decision-support applications. We present the components of this framework, discuss their desirable features, and describe a prototype that we have developed for relational patient databases. We also highlight the outstanding research issues relevant to our approach.

INTRODUCTION

Although the medical informatics research community has devoted decades of work towards developing computerized decision-support tools, clinicians use relatively few clinical decision-support (CDS) applications today. Multiple technical and sociological reasons exist for this. Among the technical reasons are (1) the lack of integration of most CDS applications with existing clinical databases, which requires clinicians to re-enter into CDS applications many patient-specific data that are already recorded elsewhere, and (2) the diversity with which existing patient databases represent and retrieve data, which requires developers to customize or rewrite CDS applications that access databases if they wish to share these applications across provider sites. These technical obstacles create a trade-off with respect to deploying and using CDS applications: Applications that relieve users from re-entering patient data by automatically querying clinical databases must include low-level specifications regarding the implementation and the organization of those databases; these specifications vary significantly among existing clinical databases, so that the sharing of such applications across provider sites entails the extensive, complex, and error-prone translation of the database queries in the applications.

If significant heterogeneity among clinical databases persists, one can overcome this trade-off best by *automating* the translation of queries at specific database sites. Automation will allow CDS applications that access patient databases to be shared among provider sites without labor-intensive and error-prone manual customization. We envision a general framework for automating query translation, called the *Standard Query Model Framework*, that consists of the following components:

1. A standard reference schema of clinical data, with respect to which developers of CDS applications can formulate database queries in a site-independent way

2. A formal mapping language, which provider sites can use to represent the correspondence between their local database implementations and the site-independent reference schema

3. A translating compiler, which uses the mappings specified at each site to translate automatically the queries that appear in shared CDS applications to semantically equivalent queries that conform to the local database implementation.

In this paper, we propose a set of desiderata for the components of the standard query model framework, and we present an experimental prototype designed to fulfill the desiderata with respect to relational database implementations. Sections 2 and 3 describe how the heterogeneity of clinical databases currently inhibits the sharing of CDS applications and why past research to overcome database heterogeneity has not yielded an adequate solution. Section 4 presents the general components of the standard query model framework and discusses the desirable features of these components. Section 5 describes the design of TransFER, our prototype implementation, and Section 6 lists several research issues that must be addressed before the standard query model framework can be practically realized.

QUERY MODEL HETEROGENEITY

The benefits of integrating CDS applications with clinical databases has been recognized for many years. In 1974, Shortliffe noted that integrating the MYCIN expert system with hospital information systems would allow more powerful rules to be added to the MYCIN knowledge base "without generating annoying questions for the physician" [1]. Recently, the Institute of Medicine's Committee on Clinical Practice Guidelines recommended the incorporation of practice guidelines into clinical information systems [2].

Despite these observations, there currently exist few CDS applications that are integrated with clinical databases. The heterogeneity of clinical databases makes it difficult for most institutions to integrate their local databases with CDS applications that have been developed elsewhere; the complexity of CDS applications makes it infeasible for most institutions to build their own applications, tailored to local database specifications. Medical informatics researchers can promote the wide-spread deployment of integrated CDS applications either by (1) enabling institutions to develop their own site-specific CDS applications, (2) standardizing every aspect of clinical databases, or (3) developing practical methods to "bridge" the heterogeneity of clinical database implementations. We believe that the latter approach will prove the most effective

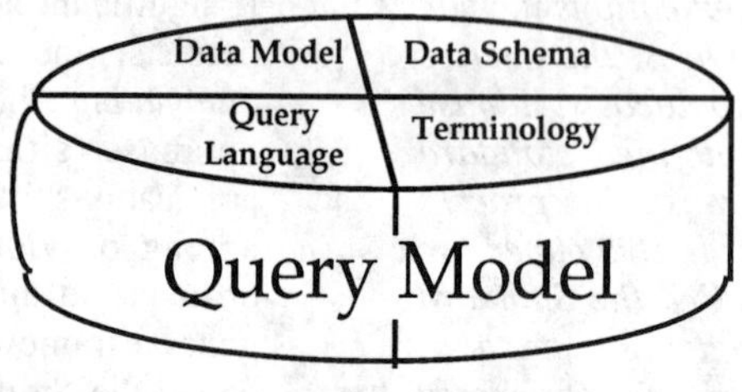

Figure 1. The components of a query model: The data model, the database schema, the query language, and the domain terminology

In the context of sharing CDS applications, bridging database heterogeneity entails resolving the differences between the *query model* that an application assumes and the *query model* that an operational clinical database provides. A query model [3] is the model of data representation and data retrieval that defines the interface between an application and a database. Specifically, a query model (see Figure 1) defines the abstract data model, the database schema, the query language, and the domain terminology that a database implements. Applications that interface to a database must specify queries in a manner that is consistent with the database's query model. Developers cannot currently write queries in CDS applications that will correctly retrieve data from arbitrary clinical databases because the query models of most clinical databases vary significantly [4]. Research to date has yielded no sound, economical, and generalized method to bridge query model heterogeneity so that CDS applications may be shared across provider sites.

PREVIOUS WORK

Researchers have pursued two general strategies for resolving heterogeneity between the query models of applications and databases: data translation and query translation. Data translation entails the transformation of *data* from the varied representations in which they may be collected to a common representation in which they can be accessed by CDS applications. Query translation entails the transformation of *queries* that appear in CDS applications into equivalent queries that are consistent with and can be executed directly against varied data representations.

Manual data translation, a technique used by certain clinical research databases [5], requires that medical records personnel manually abstract primary patient records into a common format that is subsequently uploaded into a centralized databank. The costs and delay of this method are generally prohibitive for routine decision-support. Automated data translation entails the algorithmic conversion of data directly to a common representation [6], or to an "interchange" format (such as HL7 [7]) that is subsequently translated to a common representation. Although automating data translation reduces the costs and delays of transforming data, the duplicate storage of data in the original and the common format increases the costs of operating an information system and compromises data integrity.

Query translation is preferable to data translation because no data need be duplicated and no delay is introduced before data is available to CDS applications. The Arden syntax, a standard and ostensibly portable knowledge-representation language for medical decision logic [4] requires *manual* query translation to share CDS applications. Under the Arden model, local database programmers translate manually each query that appears in a shared Arden program. The Arden syntax, however, includes few standard constructs for formulating database queries and no formal model of clinical data. In short, the Arden syntax specifies no standard query model. Because the representation of queries in the Arden model is, therefore, informal and because existing clinical databases are complex and highly variable, considerable effort may be required to understand and to faithfully translate Arden programs when they are customized to local database environments [8] [9]. A codeveloper of the Arden syntax remarked upon this difficulty after a recent experiment in sharing Arden programs:

> "Although standards for representing clinical decision logic can be of great assistance in sharing the work of many, sharing may be delayed until common standards exist not only in the description of the logic, but in all aspects of the medical information system" [8].

This observation underscores the need to combine and expand current research in standardizing clinical data structures and clinical data terminology [10] to encompasses the development of a unified standard query model. A standard and well-defined query model is a necessary component of any technology for automating reliably the translation of database queries that appear in shared CDS applications. The automated and sound translation of queries will reduce significantly the costs, the delays, and the errors currently associated with sharing CDS applications. We define the *standard query model framework* as the research paradigm concerned with specifying a standard query model and with developing techniques to automatically translate queries based on this model.

THE STANDARD QUERY MODEL FRAMEWORK

The key component of the standard query model framework is a site-independent reference schema of clinical information that is specified using a **semantic data model**. The reference schema formally denotes the types of entities, the valid relationships among entities, and the terms used to denote entities in the domain of clinical medicine. Developers of CDS applications formulate all database queries with respect to this reference schema using a high-level query language. Provider sites use a **mapping language** to encode a set of mappings between the standard query model and their local query model. A **translating compiler** available at each site uses the mappings to translate the site-independent queries that appear in CDS applications to semantically equivalent local queries. The framework that we propose is graphically depicted in Figure 2. The advantage of this framework with respect to ad hoc methods is that it enables the systematic specification of mappings between a well-defined standard query model and a "target" database implementation; the translating compiler subsequently uses the mappings to translate an arbitrary number of queries automatically (eliminating the manual effort required to customize each query), and the translating compiler applies the same set of mappings to each query translation (ensuring that each query is translated consistently). We have identified design criteria for each component of the framework.

1. The **semantic data model** (SDM) [11] used to specify the reference schema must be sufficiently expressive, abstract, and well-defined. The SDM must represent all of the objects, properties of objects, and relationships among objects that typically appear in clinical information systems. For example, the standard relational model is not sufficiently expressive because it cannot explicitly represent associations among objects that are stored in separate relations. Also, the constructs of the SDM model must be sufficiently abstract to subsume the various ways in which data may be modeled in implemented databases. For example, the entity–relationship model [12] is not sufficiently abstract because it forces the reference schema to specify whether certain associations are modeled as relational attributes or as relational joins, a site-specific modeling decision. Lastly, the SDM must have formal semantics so that the meaning of the reference schema is unambiguous. To realize the benefits of a site-independent reference schema, the query language associated with the SDM must be equally expressive, abstract, and well-defined

2. The **mapping language** must be declarative. Declarative specifications facilitate the inspection, validation, and maintenance of encoded knowledge [13]. We believe that the specification and the management of mappings between query models will be complex and will require the assistance of computational tools. A declarative and formal language for the representation of mappings is a prerequisite for the development of such tools. Mappings specified as programs encoded in C or MUMPS are not amenable to automated inspection and validation.

3. The **translating compiler** must conserve the semantics of the mappings and must generate efficient queries. The compiler must apply the encoded mappings in such a way that if the individual mappings are correct, the query translation *in toto* will be correct. Because performance is an important consideration for applications that provide real-time decision support, sacrificing query efficiency in order to automate query translation is not a feasible trade-off.

THE TRANSFER METHODOLOGY

We have developed a prototype of the standard query model framework, called TransFER [3], that automatically translates queries to target

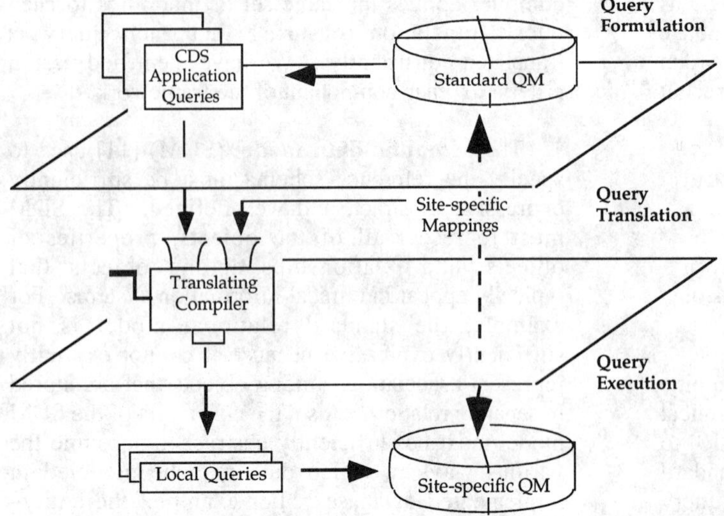

Figure 2. The standard query model framework. CDS application queries are formulated with respect to the standard query model ("Standard QM") using the high-level query language. No knowledge of any site-specific query model ("Site-specific QM") nor the query translation method is required at this level. A translating compiler performs the query translation based on encoded mappings that specify the correspondence between the standard query model and the relevant site-specific query model. The translated queries are semantically equivalent and can be executed by the local database.

heterogeneous relational databases. The TransFER methodology comprises four elements:

- A novel semantic data model, called FER (Functional Entity-Relationship model) for encoding site-independent clinical database schemas
- A query language, called ReFER, that corresponds to the FER data model and that allows users to specify data retrieval requests with respect to a FER schema
- A mapping language, called ERA (Extended Relational Algebra), that is based on the relational algebra [14] and that allows the constructs of an abstract FER schema to be mapped formally to equivalent constructs of a site-specific relational database schema
- A query-translation module, called TransFER, which applies ERA mappings to automatically translate ReFER queries into corresponding site-specific queries

Data Model and Query Language

The FER data model is designed to be sufficiently general to subsume diverse clinical database implementations. FER combines the semantic data modeling features of the entity–relationship (ER) data model [12] and the functional data model [15] to remedy the deficiencies of each model with respect to generality and expressiveness. The ER model distinguishes between attributes and relationships, so that ER schemas commit to a particular relational representation that, in fact, may vary among implemented databases. The functional model restricts the information that may be represented regarding associations among database objects; specifically, the model has no provisions for representing the attributes of functions, a capability that we have found useful for modeling the temporal semantics of legacy databases.

A sample clinical database schema encoded in the FER data model is illustrated in Figure 3. The schema illustrates the following modeling constructs of the FER data model:

Entity Types denote and describe *sets of objects* in the domain of discourse. For example, Patient and Name are entity types.

Entities denote *individual objects* in the domain of discourse. For example, Mr. Doe is an entity of the Patient and the Person entity types.

Relationship Types denote and describe *sets of associations* among members of entity types (that is, among entities). For example, the relationship type MD-Patient describes a set of associations between members of the Physician and the Patient entity types. Each binary relationship type defines a pair of directed functions, called Relationship Functions, that are used in ReFER queries to traverse the relationship type.

Relationships denote *instances of associations* among entities. For example, the tuple <Dr. Bob, Mr. Doe> denotes an instance of the MD-Patient relationship type.

IS-A Connections denote the generalization relationship between pairs of entity types. The semantics of IS-A connections imply set subsumption and relationship inheritance.

This minimal and abstract set of modeling constructs allows FER schemas to subsume query model

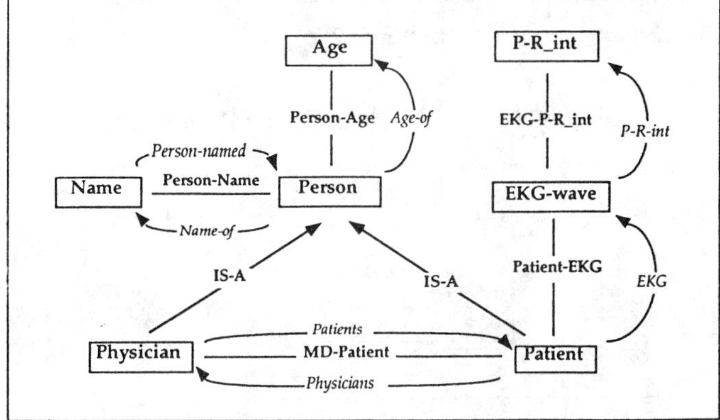

Figure 3. A sample FER schema. Boxes denote entity types; lines annotated with bold-faced text denote relationship types; arrows annotated with italicized text denote relationship functions; arrows annotated by IS-A labels denote IS-A connections. The schema conceptually represents a domain of discourse in which persons have names and ages, patients and physicians are subtypes of persons, patients may be associated with physicians, patients may have EKG test results, and EKG waves may have P-R intervals (clinically relevant features of EKGs). Two relational implementations of this conceptual schema appear in Figure 4.

heterogeneity among relational databases. For example, Figure 4 shows two different relational database schemas representing the domain of discourse encoded in Figure 3. Note that the schemas vary in several respects, including the identifiers used to denote certain entity types (`Doctor` versus `Physician`); whether data is stored or derived (`P-R-int` is explicitly stored in Schema 2 but must be derived from the value of `EKG` in Schema 1); and the representation of type hierarchies (the entity subtypes Patient and Physician are represented in different tables in Schema 1, but are included in the same table in Schema 2, distinguished by values of the `Type` attribute). Despite the representational heterogeneity of schemas 1 and 2, the FER schema in Figure 3 accurately denotes the *conceptual* contents of both schemas.

The syntax and semantics of the ReFER query language are based on the domain calculus [16] and derive their features from declarative query languages developed for the functional data model [15] and the ER data model [17]. The salient feature of the ReFER language is that it combines *declarative* and *functional* representations of query semantics, which allows queries to be expressed at an abstract level when the queries are formulated in CDS applications and later translated to the appropriate low-level operations when the queries are executed by specific clinical databases. For example, the following ReFER query retrieves the names of all patients with an EKG that has a P-R interval greater than 0.25:

name-of(pt) | (pt : Patient) AND
P-R-int(EKG(pt)) > 0.25

Note that the association between an EKG and its P-R interval is expressed as an invocation of the abstract function P-R-int() rather than as a join expression, a SQL select operation, or a foreign-function call. The representation of associations at this level of abstraction allows an association to be computed using whatever operations are indicated by the query models of existing clinical databases. The knowledge of which operations are required for specific clinical databases is represented locally using an extended relational algebra (ERA) mapping language.

Mapping Language and Query Translation

The ERA mapping language is based on the operators of the relational algebra: SELECTION, PROJECTION, CARTESIAN PRODUCT, UNION, and DIFFERENCE [14]. We have enhanced the basic relational algebra with syntactic and semantic constructs that increase its power to resolve representational heterogeneities among relational databases [3]. A mapping between the standard query model (for example, the FER schema in Figure 3) and a specific relational database implementation (Schema 1 or 2 in Figure 4) is defined by *assigning an ERA expression to each construct that appears in the FER schema.* The ERA expression represents the same semantics as the corresponding FER construct but is valid with respect to the relevant relational schema. For example, the entity type `Patient` and the relationship function `Name-of` from the FER schema of Figure 3 are assigned the following schema-specific ERA expressions.

Patient
(Schema 1) `Patient`
(Schema 2) SELECT [`Type = "PT"`] (`Person`)
Name-of (<arg>)
(Schema 1) PROJECT [`Name`] (<arg ERA>)
(Schema 2) PROJECT [`PName`] (<arg ERA>)

Note that the mappings for the FER construct Patient are distinct because schema 1 and schema 2 model the type hierarchy `Person–Patient–Physician` differently, and the mappings for the FER construct Name-of are distinct because the relational attribute `"Name"` appears in Schema 1 whereas the attribute `"PName"` appears in Schema 2. "<arg ERA>" denotes the ERA expression assigned to the *argument*

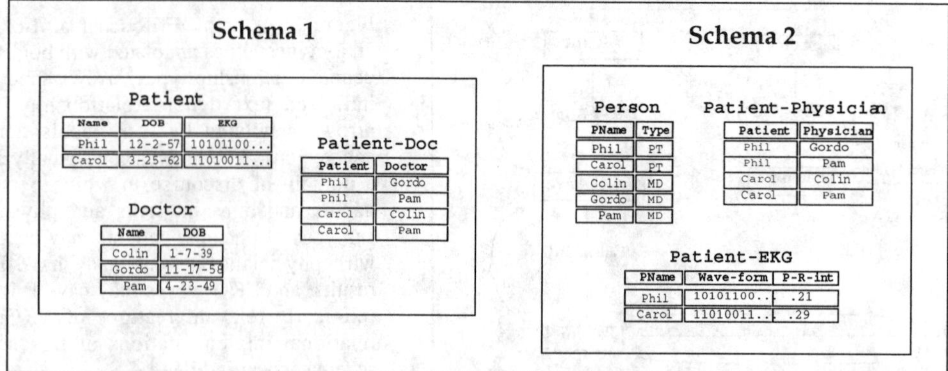

Figure 4. Two relational schemas representing heterogeneous implementations of the conceptual schema in Figure 3. Differences include the naming of entity types (Doctor versus Physician), the use of deroved versus stored attributes (P-R interval), and the representation of type hierarchies (Person–Patient–Physician).

of the Name-of relationship function in a specific query.

The translating compiler translates ReFER queries by composing the ERA mapping expressions that correspond to each construct appearing in the query (applying formal composition rules specified in [3]). For example, to translate the ReFER query

Name-of (pt) | (pt : Patient)

the compiler composes the ERA expressions corresponding to the Name-of construct and the Patient construct for the local schema. The result is a single schema-specific ERA expression that is semantically equivalent to the input ReFER query:

(Schema 1) PROJECT [Name] (Patient)
(Schema 2) PROJECT [PName] (
SELECT [Type = "PT"] (Person))

The TransFER compiler subsequently modifies the expression, if necessary, to improve efficiency. The mathematically formalized semantics of relational algebra allow ERA expressions to be optimized in a sound and automated fashion. The compiler completes the translation by transcribing the resulting ERA expression to the dialect of SQL appropriate for the local relational DBMS (Oracle, Sybase, etc.).

We believe that the FER data model, the ReFER query language, the ERA mapping language, and the TransFER compiler fulfill the design criteria we have outlined for the standard query model framework. We currently are evaluating TransFER formally to test this hypothesis [18]. To meet the design criteria, we have constrained the TransFER methodology to accomodate relational databases only. This constraint allows us to take advantage of relational theory in defining the declarative semantics of the mapping language, in verifying the correctness of the translation process, and in optimizing the query expressions generated by the compiler. Although this constraint prevents clinical database sites that do not use relational technology from taking full advantage of the TransFER methodology, these sites still may benefit from the standard query model framework that we have defined: Non-relational sites will be able to customize CDS applications more consistently and more reliably (using existing methods) when the database queries that appear in CDS applications are encoded using the well-defined syntax and semantics of the standard FER schema and the ReFER query language. In any case, non-relational database sites will be no worse off than they are currently. At the same time, the significant and increasing number of clinical database sites that have relational interfaces will benefit substantially from the sound, efficient, and automated query translation that the TransFER methodology provides.

RESEARCH DIRECTIONS

Although the model we have developed is a sound foundation upon which to build a standard query model for sharing decision-support applications, at least three important research issues must be addressed before the standard query model framework can be practically useful: the incorporation of a standard medical terminology, the definition of sound temporal semantics, and the specification of a useful but finite reference schema of clinical data.

A prominent and difficult aspect of query model heterogeneity is the heterogeneity of medical terminologies. The framework we envision must include both a standard medical terminology as a seamless part of the standard query model and a powerful and sound method to automatically resolve differences between the standard terminology and the terminologies of legacy databases. Knowledge-based methods for representing and translating medical terms [19] are most likely to yield abstract, declarative, and well-defined representations (that is, representations consistent with the desiderata of the standard query model framework).

Because the temporal aspects of clinical data and clinical queries are of paramount importance, the standard query model framework must include well-defined temporal constructs, as well as methods to map these constructs to the heterogeneous representations of temporal semantics in existing clinical databases. Das has defined a formal temporal semantics for relational clinical databases and a set of relational operators to resolve temporal heterogeneities among legacy databases [20]. We are currently investigating the application of these results to augment the TransFER methodology with temporal semantics and with the capability to resolve temporal heterogeneity.

The reference schema of clinical data must be sufficiently rich to support the data retrieval needs of many CDS applications, yet sufficiently general to subsume the data retrieval capabilities of most clinical databases. In defining such a schema, it may be useful to consider the design criteria enunciated by Gruber for the specification of shared domain ontologies [21]. Shared domain ontologies and reference database schemas are similar in content and in purpose: the conceptual representation of information to support the sharing of applications.

References

1. Shortliffe, E.H. *Mycin: A Rule-based Computer Program for Advising Physicians Regarding Antimicrobial Therapy Selection*. Ph.D. thesis, Stanford University, 1974.
2. Field, M.J. and K.N. Lohr, editors. *Guidelines for Clinical Practice*. Washington, D.C.: National Academy Press, 1992.
3. Sujansky, W. *An Extended Relational Algebra for Bridging Representational Heterogeneity among Relational Databases*. Technical Report KSL-94-08, Section on Medical Informatics, Stanford University, 1994.
4. Hripcsak, G., et al., The Arden Syntax for Medical Logic Modules, in *Proceedings of the Symposium on Computer Applications in Medical Care,* R. Miller, Ed. Washington, D.C., 1990, pp. 200-204.
5. Weyl, Stephen, et. al., A Modular Self-describing Clinical Database System. *Computers in Biomedical Research.*, 8:279, 1975.
6. Marrs, K.A., et al. Unifying heterogeneous distributed clinical data in a relational database, in *Proceedings of the Symposium on Computer Applications in Medical Care,* C. Safran, Ed. New York, 1994, pp. 655-648.
7. HL7 Working Group. *Health Level 7 Interface Standard Version 2.1*. Philadelphia, 1989.
8. Pryor, T.A. and G. Hripcsak, Sharing MLMs: An experiment between Columbia-Presbyterian and LDS Hospital, in *Proceedings of the Symposium on Computer Applications in Medical Care,* C. Safran, Ed. New York, 1994, pp. 399-403.
9. Hripcsak, G., Desperately seeking data: Knowledge base-database links, in *Proceedings of the Symposium on Computer Applications in Medical Care,* C. Safran, Ed. *ibid*., pp. 639-643.
10. Board of Directors of AMIA. Standards for medical identifiers, codes, and messages needed to create an efficient computer-stored medical record. *Journal of the American Medical Informatics Association.* 1:1, 1994.
11. Peckham, J. and F. Maryanski. Semantic Data Models. *ACM Computing Surveys*. 20(3): 153, 1988.
12. Chen, P.P.-S., The Entity-Relationship Model—Toward a Unified View of Data. *Transactions on Database Systems.* 1(1):9, 1976.
13. Genesereth, M.R. and N.J. Nilsson, *Logical Foundations of Artificial Intelligence*. Los Altos, CA: Morgan Kaufmann, 1987.
14. Codd, E.F., Relational completeness of data base sublanguages, in *Data Base Systems,* R. Rustin, Editor. New York: Prentice-Hall, 1972.
15. Shipman, D., The functional data model and the data language DAPLEX. *ACM Transactions on Database Systems. 6*(1): 140, 1981.
16. Pirotte, A., High Level Data Base Query Languages, in *Logic and Data Bases,* H. Gallaire and J. Minker, Editors. Plenum Press, 1978.
17. Hohenstein, U. and M. Gogolla. A calculus for an extended entity-relationship model, *in Proceedings of the Seventh International Conference on Entity-Relationship Approach.*. Rome: Elsevier Science Publishing, Inc., 1989.
18. Sujansky, W and Altman, R.A., *Bridging the Representational Heterogeneity of Clinical Databases*. Technical Report KSL-94-07, Section on Medical Informatics, Stanford University, 1994.
19. Cimino, J.J. et. al., Knowledge-based approaches to the maintenance of a large controlled medical terminology. *Journal of the American Medical Informatics Association.* 1:35, 1994.
20. Das, A.K, et. al., A temporal-abstraction mediator for protocol-based decision support. Technical Report KSL-94-44, Section on Medical Informatics, Stanford University, 1994.
21. Gruber, T.R., *Toward Principles for the Design of Ontologies Used for Knowledge Sharing*, Technical Report KSL-93-04, Knowledge Systems Laboratory, Stanford University, 1993.

An Automated Computerized Severity Index

Richard F. Gibson, M.D. and Peter J. Haug, M.D.
Department of Medical Informatics, LDS Hospital/University of Utah, Salt Lake City, Utah

The Computerized Severity Index (CSI) is a commercially available scoring system for hospital inpatients. Trained abstractors review the patient's paper medical record and enter the diagnoses and relevant physiological attributes. The HELP (Health Evaluation through Logical Processing) System at LDS Hospital stores patient data in discrete codes. This paper describes the development of an automatic interface between the standalone, personal-computer-based severity system and the mainframe-based hospital information system. The interface scores patient severity without the need for manual chart review. Severity scores from the automated and manual methods were identical for 70% of 222 general medical patients scored retrospectively. An evaluation of the causes for differing scores between the two methods is presented.

INTRODUCTION

Severity of illness indices are intriguing because they attempt to quantify the intangible feeling that providers have about the seriousness of their patients' illnesses. The long term goal of the authors is to completely automate one such index, the Computerized Severity Index (CSI), as an application in the HELP System using the LDS Hospital patient database. A prior abstract summarized the correlation between the data elements needed by CSI and the data elements defined in the HELP System [1]. A previous paper examined the proportion of 1356 patients with electronic data elements needed for CSI scoring [2].

We have developed an electronic interface between CSI and the HELP System which produces CSI scores without manual paper chart review. The dominant characteristic of the interface is the implementation of logic to correlate the atomic detail of patient data in the HELP System with the abstract concepts required by CSI.

SEVERITY INDICES

Severity of illness indices for hospitalized patients have been studied for more than 10 years. Such indices have been used to predict mortality [3-5], and explain variation in cost and length of stay among patients with similar diagnoses [5-7]. Severity of illness indices have also been used in quality assurance activities [8], and could be used to stratify patients entering clinical trials.

Two severity systems other than CSI use clinical data (as opposed to discharge abstract data) to calculate severity. Both systems use the same clinical data regardless of diagnoses. APACHE III (Acute Physiology and Chronic Health Evaluation) evaluates age, 7 comorbid conditions, and 17 physiologic variables recorded in the patient's chart. Although largely used to predict mortality for patients in the intensive care unit (ICU) [4], APACHE III has been used to explain variation in ICU length of stay [9], and APACHE II was used to explain variation in resource use [6].

MedisGroups (Medical Illness Severity Grouping System) assigns a score (0 to 3) to 250 key clinical findings (KCFs) abstracted from the medical chart. The overall admission score (0 to 4) is computed from the KCF scores. A mid-stay score is also derived using modified KCFs [10]. MedisGroups has been used to predict hospital charges [11] and mortality [12].

There are no literature reports of automatic data collection and score calculation for these two severity systems.

COMPUTERIZED SEVERITY INDEX (CSI)

CSI was developed by Susan Horn, Ph.D., and 200 nurses and physicians at The Johns Hopkins University and Hospital. CSI maps each of the approximately 12,000 ICD-9-CM diagnoses to one of 833 disease groups [13]. Each disease group is comprised of 4-50 indicators: physiological patient attributes such as vital signs, physical exam findings, and diagnostic studies. With rare exceptions, CSI uses no treatment or intervention facts in calculating severity. Severity scores from 1 to 4 are calculated for each indicator, for each disease group, and for the patient overall. A score of 1 indicates normal or mildly abnormal findings. A score of 4 indicates catastrophic or life-threatening signs or symptoms.

Closely related ICD-9-CM diagnoses, such as the various types of bacterial pneumonia, are mapped to the same disease group. A given patient may have 1 to 12 or more disease groups used, depending on the number and independence of the diagnoses. Different indicators are used for each

Table 1: Some Pneumonia Indicators

Temperature	Lowest systolic blood pressure
Dyspnea	Highest white blood cell count
Cyanosis	Lowest oxygen level
Rales on lung exam	Chest X-ray findings

disease group, depending on the disease. A partial listing of the indicators for the pneumonia disease group is given in Table 1.

Each indicator is assigned a score from 1 to 4 based on the severity of the patient attribute. The score given to the same indicator may vary from disease group to disease group. For example, a temperature of 39°C may be a Score 3 in leukemia, but it is only a Score 2 in pneumonia. Table 2 shows two indicators for the pneumonia disease group.

The lower score of the two highest indicator scores determines the score of the disease group. Each indicator can be used only once per patient regardless of the number of the patient's disease groups using that indicator.

In manually scoring a hospitalization, a trained abstractor enters the diagnoses into the computer. The CSI program presents a list of indicators for all the disease groups suggested by the diagnoses. The abstractor then reviews the chart and notes the most extreme patient attributes relating to the indicators. The abstractor then chooses the level of each indicator. For descriptive indicators such as dyspnea (shortness of breath), the abstractor chooses the appropriate menu item. For numerical findings such as lowest systolic blood pressure, the abstractor enters the actual value of the attribute. After completion of the data entry, the computer calculates the severity score for each disease group, and for the patient overall. CSI is typically scored for Admission, Maximum, and Discharge. The Admission and Discharge periods are usually 24 hours after admission and before discharge, respectively. The Maximum score represents the contribution of the highest score of each indicator at any time during the hospitalization without regard to whether the indicators reached their highest scores concurrently. CSI can be tailored to calculate a score for any additional period, such as for admission or discharge from the ICU.

CSI is written in Advanced Revelation for

Table 2: Indicator Scoring for Pneumonia

	Dyspnea	Lowest Systolic BP
Score 1	no dyspnea	> 89
Score 2	dyspnea on exertion	80 - 89
Score 3	dyspnea at rest	61 - 79
Score 4	periods of apnea	< 61

standalone or networked IBM-compatible personal computers (PCs). Abstractors require 15-30 minutes to review the chart and enter the data, depending on the length and complexity of the hospitalization.

THE HELP SYSTEM

Elements of the HELP System have been under development at LDS Hospital, a 520-bed tertiary care center in Salt Lake City, since 1967 [14,15]. HELP provides an integrated, computerized environment for use and development of clinical, administrative, and financial modules. An integrated expert system tool is used to support medical decision making.

HELP uses a hierarchical, numerically-based coding scheme to represent medical terms. Drug names, laboratory tests, diagnoses, admission-discharge-transfer data, physical exam findings, and nursing care plans and actions are all represented by 8-byte codes called PTXT (pronounced "P-text", for Pointer-to-TeXT) defined in a comprehensive data dictionary. There are almost no PTXT codes for patient findings observed by physicians. Despite efforts to restrict new entries and discard unused PTXT codes, there are medical terms linked to more than one PTXT code, and medical events sometimes represented by a single PTXT code and sometimes by a cluster of PTXT codes.

The HELP System runs on a cluster of Tandem mainframes using a proprietary language. Patient data are compacted into "packed strings" which are stored on the permanent media in non-relational format by patient number and data class (the top level of the dictionary hierarchy). One thousand PCs connect with the Tandem via fiber and Ethernet.

THE HELP TO CSI INTERFACE

At present, the automated CSI system uses 4 steps which are manually started. (1) A C program runs on the mainframe and collects into an ASCII file all data that could possibly be used by CSI. After retrieving demographic data, admission and discharge times, and all ICD-9-CM diagnoses, the program collects multiple lines of a fixed format: a PTXT code, a data value (such as the actual blood pressure), and a timestamp. (2) The ASCII file is then transferred from the Tandem to a PC. (3) An interface program, written in Advanced Revelation, then sorts and analyzes the PTXT codes, and stores the most extreme indicator values in the CSI tables.

Table 3: Observed Scores of 222 Test Cases

Auto	Manual CSI Score				
Score	1	2	3	4	
1	74	21	3	1	99
2	7	30	8	5	50
3	0	6	17	10	33
4	0	2	3	35	40
	81	59	31	51	222

(4) The user then enters the regular CSI application program which calculates the severity score.

Nurses enter their observations into the HELP System patient database by choosing menu items and then applying a timestamp. They record the patient findings in an atomic fashion, one finding at a time, such as "chest pain at 1530h". HELP stores this event as 3 PTXT codes: pain, location (anterior chest), pain intensity (on a scale of 1 to 10), and a timestamp. CSI calculates severity scores based on more abstract concepts such as "recurrent severe chest pain". The interface program encodes the logic to map between the atomic PTXT codes and the abstract CSI concepts. In the above example, CSI looks for a pain code, an anterior chest location code, an intensity code with a data value of 7-10, and then checks all three codes for the same timestamp. If CSI can find 4 or more of these code clusters in a 24-hour period then the indicator is considered satisfied at a score of 4.

Medical judgment was necessary to equate the different vocabularies of the two database systems. There are no PTXT codes to represent many of the CSI indicators, but PTXT codes do exist for most of the common indicators (such as temperature and white blood cell count) used in many of the disease groups [1,2].

METHODS

The manual version of CSI has been in use for 2 years at LDS Hospital. In 1993-4 CSI coders manually scored the charts of 2000 patients with pressure sores for use in another clinical study. Of those 2000 charts, a convenience set of 352 was used to develop and test the automatic interface: 130 cases in the training set and 222 cases in the test set. (The most recently scored 352 cases were chosen because the CSI scoring engine has been modified since 1993 and we wanted to avoid scoring discrepancies due to different versions of the CSI software.) For the 130 patients in the training set, an iterative process involved automatically scoring 5 patients, examining the differences in the automated and manual scores, modifying the interface, and then scoring 5 more cases. The instrument was then frozen and used to obtain automated CSI scores on the test set.

In this formative study, no attempt was made to obtain a representative sample of LDS Hospital discharges or to control for diagnosis, hospital division, or length of stay. However, the patients in the pressure sore study exhibited a wide range of medical and surgical diagnoses and all hospital divisions with HELP nurse charting were represented. There is no HELP nurse charting on the rehabilitation, psychiatric, or obstetric wards, and these patients were excluded from study.

The 2 independent variables in this study are the automated and manual CSI scoring methods. The dependent variable is the CSI score. Interrater agreement was measured using the Kappa statistic [16], weighted Kappa [16], intraclass correlation [17], and Finn's intraclass correlation [17]. For weighted Kappa weights we used the square of the difference between CSI scores $(\text{automated-manual})^2$.

RESULTS

Table 3 shows the scores of the 222 test set patients. The observed agreement was 70.3% (156 of 222). The Kappa statistic was $\kappa=.584$ ($p<.001$). Weighted Kappa was $\kappa_W=.823$. The intraclass correlation coefficient was $R_I=.951$ ($p<.001$). Finn's adjusted intraclass correlation was $r_F=.813$.

Figure 1 shows how the automated scores compared to the manual CSI scores. Figure 2 displays the distribution of cases grouped by manual CSI score. Figure 3 shows agreement classified by manual CSI score.

Only the training set was examined case-by-case to determine the reason for differing scores. In the 16 cases (12% of the 130 training cases) where the automatic score was higher than the manual score, there were 8 instances of manual coder error (mostly overlooking a data element). There were 7 instances when a patient finding fell into a post-operative "window". For example, CSI coders ignore hematuria for 48 hours after bladder surgery, but this logic has not yet been encoded into the automated CSI. There were 2 cases where the manual coder exercised judgment in ignoring what appeared to be artifactually low blood pressures. Such logic has not yet been encoded into the electronic interface. There were 2 cases where portions of the laboratory studies and vital signs had not been printed for the summary-to-date report in the paper chart so the manual coders did not find the

Figure 1: Agreement of 222 Test Set Cases

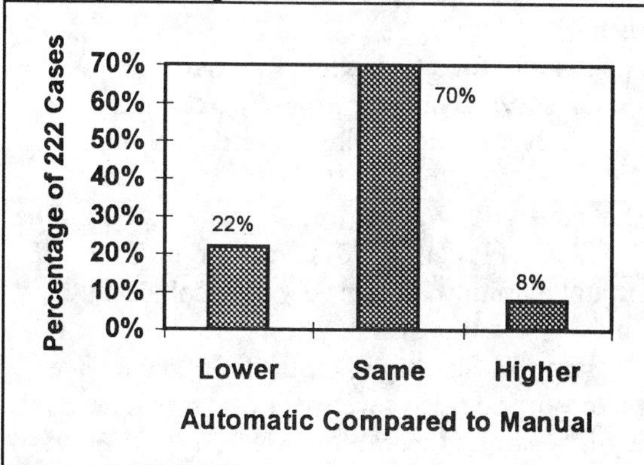

abnormal indicators. Some patients exhibited more than one reason for differing scores. If the 8 cases of coder error are removed from the "high" category, the observed agreement of automated and manual scores rises from 73% to 79% (103 of 130 cases).

Examination of the 19 cases (15% of 130 training cases) where the automated score was lower than the manual score revealed 13 instances where PTXT codes do not exist for the indicator (for example, the number of lower extremity fractures). There were 9 cases where existing PTXT codes were not used by the nursing staff. There were 2 cases with a manual coder error. Only one instance was found where the indicator was derived from physician dictation ("swollen prostate") and thereby missed by automated CSI (no PTXT code). Some cases had more than one reason for the difference in scores. Table 4 highlights the causes of disagreement between automated and manual CSI.

Although the test set cases with unlike scores were not examined, it is likely that the causes for differing automated and manual scores were the same for the test and training sets. The distribution of cases by CSI score was similar, as was the observed agreement between automated and manual

Figure 2: Distribution of 222 Test Set Cases

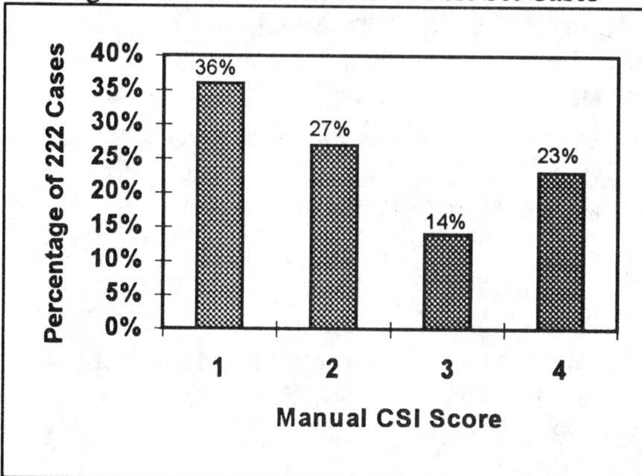

Figure 3: Agreement of 222 Test Set Cases

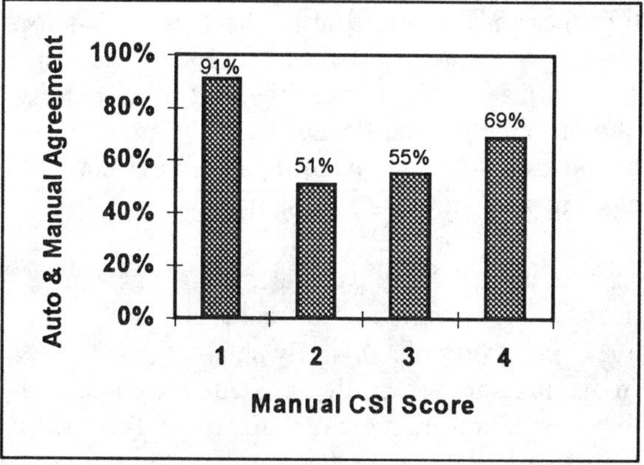

scores (73% in the training set, 70% in the test set).

DISCUSSION

Automated CSI scoring resulted in scores both higher and lower than manual scoring. An advantage of an electronic interface is the avoidance of data collection errors inherent in manual review of complex cases, responsible for half of the higher automated scores in the training set. Most of the remaining higher automated scores were due to patient findings in the post-operative window. Our next task is to modify the automated CSI interface to ignore patient findings in the post-operative window.

After successful encoding of the post-operative window, there is promise that the automated CSI score could become a *minimum* CSI score. That is, the manual score would never be lower than the automated score. If necessary, manual coders could then perform a brief, directed search for indicators known to have no corresponding PTXT codes.

This study demonstrates that manual coders found some patient attributes not yet computerized in the HELP System. Most of these attributes could be collected by nurses if the HELP System menus were modified. Other attributes were computerized, but,

Table 4: Causes of Auto vs. Manual Disagreement

Causes for auto CSI to be higher than manual:

- automated CSI had no post-op window
- manual coder error
- manual coder rejected artifactual data
- paper chart incomplete

Causes for auto CSI to be lower than manual:

- PTXT codes do not exist for patient finding
- nurses did not use existing PTXT code
- manual coder error

in some cases, were not used by the nurses. At the time these patients were hospitalized, the ICU nurses did not have access to the same detailed assessment and charting PTXT items on their menus as did the nurses on the general floors. As of November 1993, all nurses on units served by the HELP System charting application use the same menus.

From prior experience with manual CSI scoring, about 70% of patients in a large general hospital have maximum CSI scores of 1 or 2, and 30% have scores of 3 or 4. By obtaining the test set from a pressure sore study, the study sample tended to be biased toward more ill patients and those with longer length of stays. This is reflected in the 37% of test set patients with manual CSI scores of 3 or 4.

Further study of automated CSI scoring will involve larger sample sizes. Correlation of automated and manual scores will be controlled for hospital division, length of stay, and the Major Diagnostic Group of the principal diagnosis. Examination of more cases where the automated scores are low could suggest additions to the HELP System computerized nurse charting.

CONCLUSION

It appears that a detailed clinical patient database such as the HELP System can drive an automated severity of illness index in areas of the hospital served by the nurse charting system. Significant challenges remain in encoding logic used by manual abstractors to ignore inappropriate data values and expected abnormal patient findings. As the HELP System and other hospital information systems add coded clinical data, automated CSI scoring can be expected to improve.

ACKNOWLEDGMENTS

This publication was supported by grant number F37 LM00012 from the National Library of Medicine. Its contents are solely the responsibility of the authors and do not necessarily represent the official views of the National Library of Medicine. The authors are indebted to Blair C. James for his programming assistance.

Reference

[1]. Gibson RF, Haug PJ, Horn SD, Gardner RM. Linking Computerized Severity Index (CSI) with the HELP System patient database. Abstract, Spring Congress, AMIA, 1993.

[2]. Gibson R, Haug P. Linking the Computerized Severity Index (CSI) to coded patient findings in the HELP System patient database. SCAMC 17:673-7, 1993.

[3]. Alemi F, Rice J, Hankins R. Predicting in-hospital survival of myocardial infarction: a comparative study of various severity measures. Med Care 28(9):762-75, 1990.

[4]. Knaus WA, Wagner DP, Draper EA, et al. The APACHE III Prognostic System: risk prediction of hospital mortality for critically ill hospitalized adults. Chest 100(6):1619-36, 1991.

[5]. Horn SD, Sharkey PD, Buckle JM, et al. The relationship between severity of illness and hospital length of stay and mortality. Med Care 29(4):305-17, 1991.

[6]. Thomas JW, Ashcraft MLF. Measuring severity of illness: six severity systems and their ability to explain cost variations. Inquiry 28(1):39-55, 1991.

[7]. Averill RF, McGuire TE, Manning BE, et al. A study of the relationship between severity of illness and hospital cost in New Jersey hospitals. Health Services Research 27(5):587-604, 1992.

[8]. Iezzoni LI. Using severity information for quality assessment: a review of three cases by five severity measures. QRB 15(12):376-82, 1989.

[9]. Knaus WA, Wagner DP, Zimmerman JE, Draper EA. Variations in mortality and length of stay in intensive care units. Ann Int Med 118(10):753-61, 1993.

[10]. Iezzoni LI. A primer on MedisGroups. PA Med 92(1):28-33, 1989.

[11]. Iezzoni LI, Ash AS, Coffman GA, Moskowitz MA. Admission and mid-stay MedisGroup scores as predictors of hospitalization charges. Med Care 29(3):210-20, 1991.

[12]. Iezzoni LI, Ash AS, Coffman G, Moskowitz MA. Admission and mid-stay MedisGroups scores as predictors of death within 30 days of hospital admission. Am J Pub Health 81(1):74-8, 1991.

[13]. Iezzoni LI, Daley J. A description and clinical assessment of the Computerized Severity Index. Qual Rev Bull 18(2):44-52, 1992.

[14]. Pryor TA, Gardner RM, Clayton PD, Warner HR. The HELP System. J Med Syst 7(2):87-102, 1983.0

[15]. Kuperman GJ, Gardner RM, Pryor TA. HELP: A Dynamic Hospital Information System. Springer-Verlag, New York, NY, 1991.

[16]. Maclure M, Willett WC. Misinterpretation and misuse of the Kappa statistic. Amer J Epidem 126(2):161-9, 1987.

[17]. Whitehurst GJ. Interrater agreement for journal manuscript reviews. Amer Psychologist 39(1):22-8, 1984.

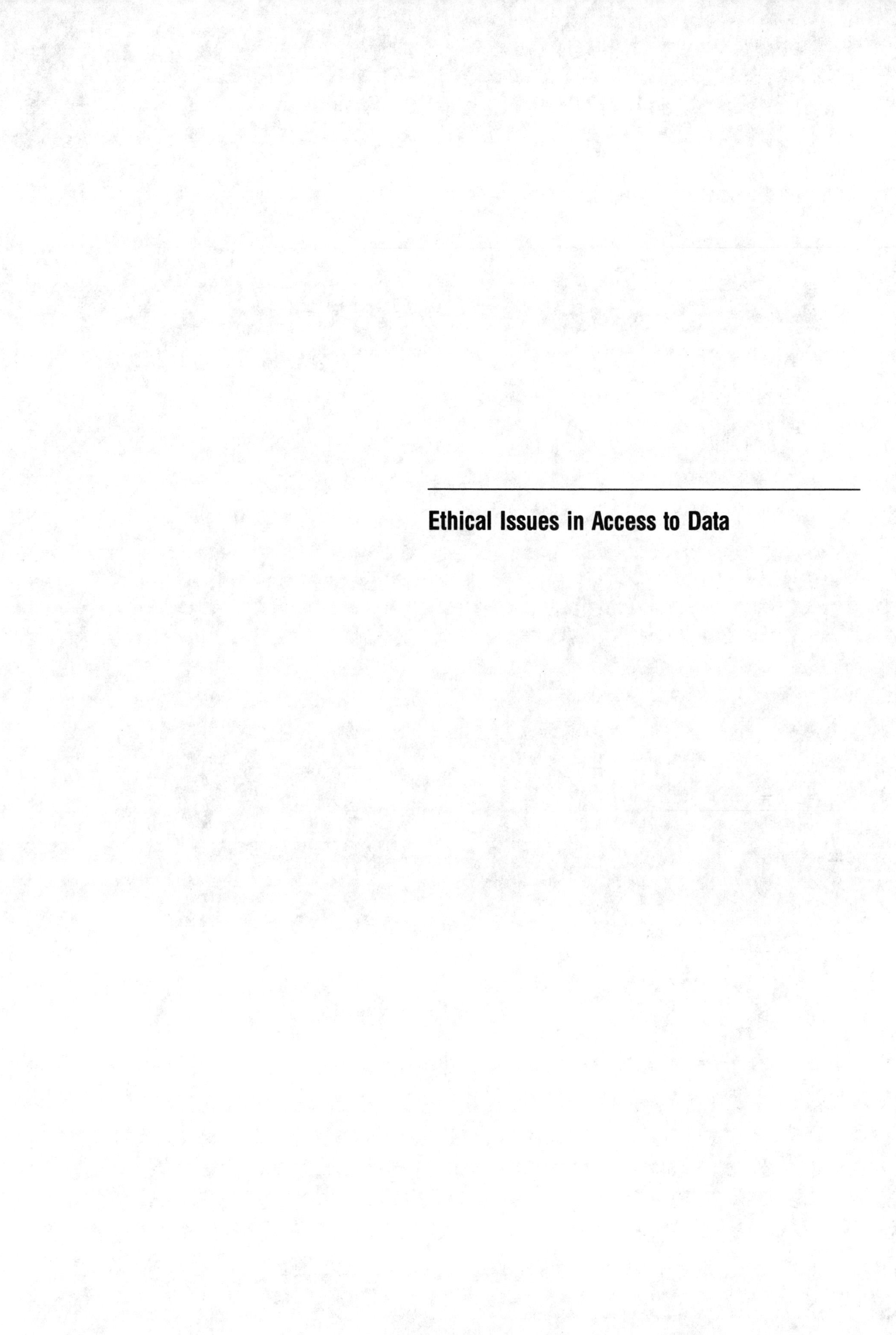

Ethical Issues in Access to Data

Analysis, Requirements and Development of a Collaborative Social and Medical Services Data Model

Risa B. Bobroff M.S., Cynthia A. Petermann M.S.,
J. Robert Beck M.D., and Gregory J. Buffone Ph.D.

Medical Informatics and Computing Research Program
Baylor College of Medicine
Houston, Texas

ABSTRACT

In any medical and social service setting, patient data must be readily shared among multiple providers for delivery of expeditious, quality care. This paper describes the development and implementation of a generalized social and medical services data model for an ambulatory population. The model, part of the Collaborative Social and Medical Services System Project, is based on the data needs of the Baylor College of Medicine Teen Health Clinics and follows the guidelines of the ANSI HISPP/MSDS JWG for a Common Data Model. Design details were determined by informal staff interviews, operational observations, and examination of clinic guidelines and forms. The social and medical services data model is implemented using object-oriented data modeling techniques and will be implemented in C++ using an Object-Oriented Database Management System.

INTRODUCTION

Delivery of social and medical services should be community based, providing ready access to the segment of the population served. Attainment of this goal requires an organizational infrastructure and computing and communication system capable of supporting geographically distributed clinics. To support these needs and to anticipate future expansion of distributed ambulatory services, the data model developed for the Baylor College of Medicine Teen Health Clinics (THCs) must be easily extensible and as well as serve the immediate needs of the clinics.

The Teen Clinics are representative of a medical and social care clinic. Spanning five sites throughout the city of Houston, Texas, the clinics provide a variety of free services to teenagers in Harris County. The services include family planning, Sexually Transmitted Disease (STD) screening and treatment, Case Management, patient education and counseling, school physicals, and prenatal and postpartum care. The clinics exhibit many of the problems typically associated with medical and/or social service clinics: patients may visit any of the clinic sites, making continuity of care difficult; clinic specific and aggregate statistical data are time consuming to acquire; manual and electronic data interchange with external entities are complex and time consuming; redundant and loosely coordinated data entry requires manual reconciliation of inconsistencies and is prone to errors and omissions.

The data modelling and implementation described here are integral parts of the Collaborative Social and Medical Services System (CSMSS) Project. The CSMSS is intended to provide the computing and communications support to fully integrate the Baylor College of Medicine Teen Health Clinics and address the problems enumerated above. We selected the THCs as the initial development domain for this data model due to the established needs of the clinics and the feasibility of designing an appropriate model. The THC environment is large enough to be representative of clinical and social service delivery, yet small enough to be understood and addressed in a reasonable time frame.

This paper describes a bottom-up process for developing a generic outpatient medical and social services data model. We present an evaluation of the high level data model and a strategy for testing the model in the clinics.

BACKGROUND AND RELATED WORK

Database Systems

Earlier systems, including the Clinical Information System (CIS) at Columbia Presbyterian Medical Center and the Virtual Database System (VDB) at Harvard Medical School Children's Hospital, used a relational model for their database implementation [1, 2, 3]. However, these system developers encountered a number of problems related to the difficulty of using relational tables to represent clinical data, including: negative performance impact from the use of full normalization; the need to keep table definitions constant over time despite changing data needs; and the challenge of displaying a meaningful view of the data to the user. In particular, the CIS project developers devised a generic extension table for each standard table in the database in order to accommodate differences in clinical findings. The VDB project required developers to denormalize data and store more than one type of data in the same table to achieve performance goals. They also mapped their hierarchical data representation to a set of tables that could be joined together, of necessity hiding the intuitive hierarchical nature of the data.

Object-Oriented Database Management Systems (OODBMS) are inherently well suited for representing and manipulating complex data models since the database stores data as persistent objects using the programming language's object representation. This storage mechanism alleviates the need for the compromises discussed above. OODBMSs offer more flexible mechanisms for schema evolution, for class inheritance, and for the introduction of new, related data types. These features are important in a generalized medical and social model as they make it easier for institutions to add new information to the data model, such as new tests or procedures. Furthermore, OODBMSs have the advantage of embedding data relationships within the model using direct links, as opposed to progammatical or dynamic relationships via relational joins, hence improving performance and the ability to present a logical view of the data model [4]. This implementation detail expedites many database operations, such as reviewing a list of recent test results for a patient. Rather than searching through the entire table of test results for a particular patient, there is a direct link from a patient to the corresponding test results.

JWG

The American National Standards Institute (ANSI) Health Informatics Standards Planning Panel (HISPP) / Message Standards Developers Subcommittee (MSDS) Joint Working Group (JWG) for a Common Data Model (CDM) is working to define and maintain a common data model for the health care industry. The JWG has published a Framework document that describes the notation and representation of the CDM and has generated a High-Level Data Model (HLDM). The HLDM consists of two diagrams: Subject Areas, showing the grouping of high level objects by subject; and Major Relationships, illustrating the relationships between the high level objects. This high level model was developed abstractly, i.e. top-down, by the JWG and is intended to serve as a guideline for model developers. A major goal of the JWG is to build a repository of the combined data models of each of the Standards Developing Organizations (SDOs), such as HL-7 and ACR-NEMA, in an effort to unify the data models of the independent SDOs and ease inter-standard communication [5].

METHODOLOGY

We used a number of sources to determine the elements in the data model. These included observations of operations and informal interviews with clinic staff members; the clinic Medical Protocols documents; the set of forms filled out by the staff; the reports generated by the clinics; discussion groups with representative clinic staff members; and the JWG HLDM subject definitions [5].

The informal interviews, observations of staff members, and examination of forms focused on data needs, storage (in the patient chart, in a notebook, etc.), and access. This input was used to define the classes, attributes, and relationships between classes in the model. For example, a number of objects were defined from the contents of the Patient Registration form including *PersonalData*, *EducationHistory*, *EmploymentHistory*, and *EmergencyContact*. The Medical Protocols helped enumerate the services provided by the clinics, define the attributes of each service class, determine default values and data ranges for those attributes, and describe typical services performed based on purpose of visit. A typical case is a six month visit during which the health care provider screens the patient for oral contraceptive side-effects, collects vital signs, collects specimens for gonorrhea, chlamydia and syphilis tests, discusses safe sex with the patient and reviews the proper use of the contraceptive method being used.

We used the JWG HLDM subject definitions as an initial guideline for our model development. We did not use the objects or the relationships between objects specified in the HLDM Major Relationships diagram in our development process, as we wanted to derive our own representation based on the Teen Clinics. Consequently, our model does not include all of the subject areas and high level classes specified in the JWG HLDM, as we, like the SDOs, are only developing the parts of the model that are within our application domain. We used the JWG recommended notation, a modified version of Coad and Yourdon [6], for representing our data model.

Several design goals strongly influenced the model's development. First, access control to the system is based on user role, with exceptions. To keep the access granularity high, classes are designed so that every attribute within a class may be viewed by all members of designated roles. For example, the *PersonalData* class contains a person's name, social security number, address(es) and phone number(s). A researcher gathering statistical data would not have access to this data. The write-once semantics of the database also influenced the design. In practice, the clinics amend data by crossing out the old data and replacing it with new data. Correspondingly, each database object instance is written once, and, aside from dynamically adding links to other instances, will never be updated. The data model will support amending data. Another design goal is utilizing semantic meaning in the data. For example, different test results appear in different formats. Rather than store all of the results as a generic string, each test is represented as a separate class, all of which are subclasses of the class *TestService*. Since the model is being implemented in C++, each test subclass can provide a method that translates its results to a common format for generalized handling. By keeping each result type separate, the user will be able to perform result specific comparisons on the data. Finally, the application data model contains attribute data types, while a separate data structure stores default value and range specifications for data in the application data model [5]. Separating these two types of data allows for greater domain independence, as each user may specify the dictionary(ies) to be used at any time. In addition, one clinic may easily maintain values and defaults different from the other clinics. This feature is important to the Teen Clinics, as the default populations the clinics serve differ by clinic location.

IMPLEMENTATION

The data model is being implemented in C++ using an OODBMS. We believe C++ and the OODBMS will ultimately facilitate extension of the model within the current domain or to other domains, provided the new domains follow the generalized structure defined for JWG HLDM and the THC. For example, during the model development process, the clinics added a number of new questions to their patient history form regarding sexual, physical, and mental abuse. To support this new function, an *AbuseHistory* class was added to the data model. When adding a new domain, the corresponding new tests and patient history classes may be added as subclasses or components of existing classes. Each new class inherits or implements a default data access interface from its superclass. In particular, if a predefined query listed all pending test results for a patient, adding a new test subclass would automatically add these tests to the search context, without requiring any changes to system code.

Another feature provided by the OODBMS is simplified data migration. In the case of the Teen Clinics, patients are not seen for general care after their 20th birthday. The OODBMS provides a mechanism by which we can migrate data on older patients to a different database. Longitudinal studies of clinic data may still access the relocated data by explicitly connecting to the archive database.

One significant drawback to OODBMSs is that object-oriented query languages are not well developed. Although some vendors provide an SQL interface, it is usually quite limited and data model navigation and queries must be implemented in the development language. This limitation makes user ad-hoc queries difficult to handle. However, a common object database standard has been proposed and published, and is supported by the major OODBMS vendors [7]. In the future, this standard may provide a common query language for OODBMSs. Despite this potential, a drawback to both types of systems remains -- the user must understand the entire data model to be able to query it. However, unlike relational systems, in which the attributes used to join tables would have to be explicitly stated externally to the database system, OODBMSs embed the relationships between classes in the model itself. This characteristic can also be a drawback to OODBMSs as the embedded relationships impose a structure on the data elements that is not present in relational systems.

EVALUATION

Comparison with the JWG HLDM

We generated a high level view of our data model and compared it to the data model presented by the JWG. Figure 1 shows how the two models compare. Since we divided our classes into subject areas based on the JWG HLDM, we expected our model to be a subset of the JWG model. However, until this figure was examined, we could not fully anticipate how the relationships we defined would compare with the JWG. We generated our high level model for comparison by extracting all of the classes contained in our model that are included on the JWG HLDM. We then compared the relationships between those classes contained in each model. We made one abstraction: since the Teen Clinics work minimally with finances and claims, we abstracted all of our financial classes into

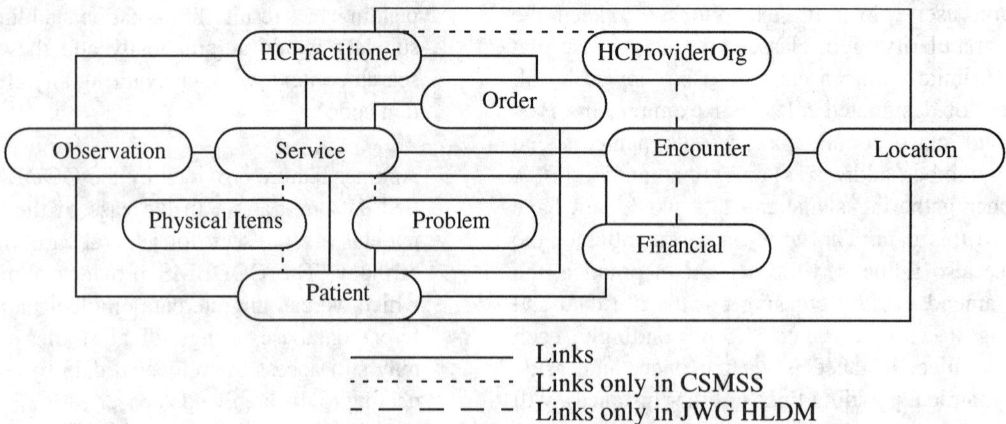

Figure 1. High level data model.

one representative *Financial* class, and did the same for the JWG HLDM.

The models are quite similar, as one would expect, given the thoughtful preparation of both models. This finding is also reassuring as it confirms that generalized models will be useful for system design and implementation. With a few exceptions, all of the connections between high level classes matched. One exception is the JWG HLDM relationship between *Encounter* and *Financial.* This relationship did not exist in our model because the claim forms used by the Teen Clinics are based on services, not encounters. Since encounter information can be accessed by traversing the relationship from service back to encounter, any necessary encounter information is still accessible using our model. Similarly, the JWG HLDM contains this same relationship, between *Service* and *Encounter*, and *can* therefore also derive encounter information from services.

The other major difference between the models is our relationship between *Problem* and *Service.* One might interpret this relationship as implicit in the JWG HLDM for the following reason. In the JWG HLDM subject definitions, *Problem* is contained in the *Observations* subject, and an *Observation* is reported to be the result of one or more *Services*. However, this relationship is not explicit in the JWG HLDM. Our research implied that an assessment service resulted in a problem definition, resulting in our adding a direct relationship between the two classes.

Our model contains one relationship not present in the JWG HLDM, that is, the relationship between *Health Care Practitioners* and *Health Care Provider Organization.* In our model, a health care practitioner belongs to one or more health care provider organizations. Also, our model includes some *relationships* not yet specified in the JWG HLDM: *Physical Items* to *Service* and *Physical Items* to *Patient.*

Comparison with Data Collected

Before review with clinic staff members, we inspected every form and report used by the clinics to ensure that every data item is represented in or can be derived from the data model. We also verified that every data item in the data model was used by a form or report. These checks were performed by generating a list of data items, sorted by source. The contents of this list was then compared to the data model, ensuring complete coverage. Then, each attribute of the data model was checked for use in the textual list.

Comparison with THC Operations

The model was reviewed with the clinic staff by walking through each form for each type of clinic visit, ensuring that we knew about all the patient data collected on a form (in the margins, etc.). We also distributed to each staff member a list of tasks performed, forms used, and report contents based on job description. Staff members returned the lists with their feedback.

Our intention is to deploy CSMSS initially at two sites, evaluate its performance, and then install the system at the remaining sites. During the phased deployment the clinics will maintain the small database system currently in use. At the end of each month, the monthly report will be generated using both systems and compared.

Before installing CSMSS in the clinics paper based versions of the forms will be used to collect clinic data. After clinic hours, staff members will enter the data from these forms into CSMSS. After data entry is completed, the standard clinic practices will be performed on this data: a nurse will audit the charts; a staff member will enter lab data; the billing clerk will generate claim forms from the new data; and a clerk will produce a monthly report. This investigation will be conducted to ensure that the format and content of the data stored by CSMSS fulfills the Clinics needs.

CSMSS is intended to be an active test environment with subsequent development of end user tools and multimedia facilities. Furthermore, feedback from the staff on the entire system and the data being stored by the system will be used to continuously improve the system.

Comparison with Other Domains

Other clinics affiliated with Baylor College of Medicine have expressed interest in the data model. After the Teen Clinic implementation is completed, we plan to evaluate the generality of the model by extending it to the domains of these additional clinics.

CONCLUSION

A number of data modelling questions arose during the design. These included: determining when to use an attribute to differentiate similar objects versus when to subtype the class; deciding when to create a direct relationship between two classes and when to use transitivity; deciding when to use an attribute to explicitly state a value, and when to use a link to an existing class (e.g. specify the name of the staff member who performed a service, or link to that staff member object); specifying mutual exclusivity in the data model using links (e.g. a patient may have a genitourinary exam or a pelvic exam, but not both). Comparison to analogous models which have been tested by implementation and use would be helpful in resolving these issues.

It is beyond the scope of this model to fully incorporate laboratory or other ancillary support models. Nevertheless, it would be advantageous to have generalized models for these areas that could be referenced or linked for purposes of completeness and implementation. The development of such data models and the means for referencing them for design and implementation purposes are needed. For example, a detailed model of the laboratory process and data could be combined with this model, thereby eliminating redundant terminology and conflicts in representation that arise from independent representations of the data relationships. We expect that our model will evolve concurrently with the CDM.

We are exploring methods of presenting the data model to the user to allow for ad-hoc queries and to eventually provide the user the means to extend the data model, as necessary.

In this paper we present the process followed for bottom-up development and implementation of an extensible data model for an outpatient medical and social service environment. We compared our model with the HLDM from the JWG. We are in the process of implementing the model and expect the use of an OODMS to accelerate implementation and improve maintenance efficiency and extensibility as we apply our system architecture and data model to other clinical domains.

Acknowledgments

The work reported here was supported in part by grant LM04905 from the National Library of Medicine. We thank the staff of the Baylor College of Medicine Teen Health Clinics for their help in this project.

References

[1]. C. Friedman, G. Hripcsak, S. B. Johnson, J. J. Cimino P. D. Clayton. A Generalized Relational Schema for an Integrated Clinical Patient Database. Proc. of the 14th Annual SCAMC, Wash., D.C., 1990.

[2]. S. Johnson, C. Friedman, J. J. Cimino, T. Clark, G. Hripcsak, P. Clayton. Conceptual Data Model for a Central Patient Database. Proc. of the 15th Annual SCAMC, Wash., D.C. 1991.

[3]. R. W. Stahlhut, D. P. McCallie, Jr., D. M. Waterman, D. M. Margulies. A Relational Model for Clinical Objective Results. Proc. of the 15th Annual SCAMC, Wash., D. C., 1990.

[4]. R. G. G. Cattell, Object Data Management: Object-Oriented and Extended Relational Database Systems. Addison-Wesley Publishing Company, Reading, MA, 1991.

[5]. ANSI/HISPP MSDS JWG for a Common Data Model IEEE P1157 Medical Data Interchange Working Group. Trial-Use Standard for Healthcare Data Interchange -- Information Model Methods. June, 1994.

[6]. P. Coad, E. Yourdon. Object Oriented Analysis, 2nd Edition. Yourdon Press, Englewood Cliffs, NJ, 1991.

[7]. R. G. G. Cattell Editor, The Object Database Standard: ODMG-93. Morgan Kaufmann Publishers, San Mateo, CA, 1993.

Evolving A Legacy System: Restructuring The Mendelian Inheritance in Man Database

Peter Li, Ph.D., Laurie Kramer, Stuart Pineo, and David Kulp
Genome Database, Johns Hopkins University, Baltimore, MD

Mendelian Inheritance in Man (MIM) is an encyclopedia of medical genetics that has been in electronic form for over 30 years. In its lifetime, MIM has undergone many organizational and software changes. In 1994, a major transition was made based on three basic principles: industry standards, open systems architecture, and extensibility. The resulting MIM database allows users to navigate to other genomic databases, permits the delivery of multimedia information, and improves the quality of data. The new MIM database also improved its administration because of 1) an internal format that enforces consistency; 2) a lower maintenance cost of software; and 3) a better ability to migrate MIM content. In addition, the new architecture will allow MIM easily to adopt emergent technologies as they mature.

INTRODUCTION

MIM is a comprehensive collection of literature reviews for the field of medical genetics [1]. It is authored by Dr. Victor A. McKusick at the Johns Hopkins University, School of Medicine and has been maintained in electronic format since 1963. Initially, entries recorded in the MIM database were mendelizing traits (phenotypes) reported in the literature. However, as the science of genetics evolved, entries about genes were also added to the database. Consequently, MIM began to evolve as a "gene catalog." Currently, there are 6,600 entries. Each entry is assigned a 6-digit number for identification. The total text size is 27 megabytes, 40 percent of which are 52,000 references.

The MIM editorial system, i.e., the repository that supports the editing and distribution of MIM entries, had not been updated for the last 10 years. It only supported three specific UNIX accounts for editing and the data were made available to users through only two media. The first medium is the printed book form, published once every 2 years since 1963. The second medium is the terminal-based online version of MIM (OMIM), using the "Information Retrieval eXperimental Workbench" (IRX) programs developed in collaboration with the National Library of Medicine in 1985 [2].

When compared to other genomic databases [3], many of which are less than 10 years old, the MIM repository was based on outdated principles and technologies. It was a classic example of a legacy system developed without applicable standards, constrained to a centralized machine, and based on proprietary code that could not be migrated easily [4]. Consequently, it was increasingly difficult to connect MIM information with other genomic databases and to provide MIM information through user-friendly means.

In order to maintain MIM's usefulness, it had to evolve to new standards and to meet new expectations. For example, the technology for accessing information through CDROM and Internet have matured and users want to be able to navigate to and from other genomic databases. However, the characteristics of the legacy system makes this evolution very difficult. Different strategies were considered, ranging from encapsulating the MIM system with a shell to migrating the data and software onto new architectures. We chose the latter approach because the encapsulation approach would not sufficiently resolve the limitations of the system.

MIM required a different approach for migration than the traditional databases of the business world because it is a text-oriented database. Text databases are under intense research from the information retrieval community [5][6], in part because of the difficulty of prescribing a single structure for the many unrelated flat files, e.g., as found in news and print archives. However, a subset of these wide-spectrum text databases is characterized by files that come from a single source or relate to a single topic, e.g., bibliographic databases. For these databases, it is easier to determine a single structure (schema) to which all contents can be converted. Once in this structured format, one can maintain consistency and integrity of the entries through database techniques.

MIM is an ideal candidate to evolve to a structured form because it is a collection of text files that comes from a single source and relates to a single topic. There are many approaches to defining structure for documents. One approach is based on the presentation format, such as titles, headers, and paragraphs. Another approach is based on large-scale semantic constructs, such as sections of text and the reference list. The restructuring of MIM took a third approach based on small-scale constructs. For example, instead of one structure for a whole reference list or a single reference, we broke down the references into components: authors, titles, journals, etc..

This paper describes the challenges and solutions encountered while making this evolutionary transition for the MIM database.

PROBLEMS AND GOALS

The previous major revision of MIM software resulted in the UNIX file system as the file repository and UNIX text editing as the main method for updating the entries. The problems of this system can be described from three perspectives: structure, maintenance, and access.

The structural problem relates to the fact that MIM entries were essentially flat text files and the software did not perform automatic structural validation. All errors (typographical and semantic) were only detected by proofreading. However, many errors were not found and accumulated until book publication. At this time, errors were discovered and corrected as the book production programs broke down while processing files with errors or when the pre-book comprehensive proofreading was done. While the flat files gave the most freedom to the writers in layout and presentation, they created a context where the information is organized only for textual editing and presentation. To provide automated validation, our solution was to use fine grain structure, so that structured contents could be verified against each other without natural language parsing. A goal for the new MIM system was to define the structure and then to enforce it. Furthermore, as the structure of MIM evolves with time, the enforcing mechanism must be simple to adapt and the conversion of existing entries to new schema must be simple to perform.

The MIM database maintenance problem is a result of its legacy nature. The software is dependent on specific UNIX directories, files, and accounts. For example, the checkin and checkout programs that transferred the files in and out of the repository were processing files in the home directories of specific UNIX users. As changes were made in the operating system and in staff personnel, increasingly complicated modifications to the software were required. In addition, all programs that access MIM information were developed in an adhoc fashion, with very little reuse of existing software, nor was the code written in a format that facilitated reuse. For example, the programs for the book typesetter cannot be used for generating the files for the IRX system. The previous MIM software was based on 4,000 lines of UNIX sh code, 2,000 lines of UNIX lex code, and 4,000 lines of C code. A second goal for the new system was to improve reuse, capacity, and capability without sacrificing adaptability. In addition, a framework of extensibility should be at the core of the system so that the MIM database can migrate to other architectures with ease.

Last, the delivery of MIM information to users was limited to the book form, the IRX-based OMIM, and the IRX-derived flat files for Internet access. It lacked the navigational features needed to interoperate with the many new genomic databases that have been recently deployed. In the recent years, the technologies for novel methods of accessing information over the Internet have matured: Wide Area Information Servers (WAIS), gopher, and World-Wide-Web (WWW) [7]. In addition, CDROM (multimedia) environments have also gained wide acceptance. MIM users were expecting to receive MIM information through these new methods. Therefore, our third and final goal was to ensure that the new MIM structure and software were designed to simplify the transporting of MIM information to new environments and to facilitate new ways of accessing MIM information.

A major underlying concern for all these goals was that the new MIM repository had to be of production quality and not a research system. Therefore, it had to be robust enough for heavy concurrent usage and provide sufficient throughput for on-demand access and editing sessions. In addition, three overriding principles were used when developing this new system: industry standards, open system architecture, and extensibility.

APPROACHES

We addressed the structural problem of MIM by tagging the elements in a MIM entry and then ensuring that the content of each tag was appropriate for the tag and the tags were in the correct order. The ISO 8879 standard, Standard Generalized Markup Language (SGML) [8], was used for such tagging or mark up of MIM documents. SGML provided a method of specification (Document Type Definition, DTD) that defines the structure of the document in terms of the tags and defines whether documents that have been tagged conform to a particular DTD. Because SGML is an international standard, many commercial and public domain software support the processing of SGML DTD's and tagged documents.

The software problem of MIM was best solved by using an open architecture, i.e., nonproprietary systems with standard application interfaces. This type of architecture allows vendor independence and future evolution. Unlike SQL, there are no standards widely accepted for text retrieval. In addition, we could not find a SGML-based textual database management system (DBMS) that was within our budget constraints. Consequently, we opted for in-house development, but made sure that it would be easy to migrate when an appropriate candidate DBMS is found. The software engineering tools and environment used for the Genome DataBase (GDB) [9] were adopted for MIM. These tools provided automatic set up, versioning, and common access for groups of users.

The solution for accessing MIM information in different distribution media was based on a set of filtering programs that convert the SGML-based MIM files to the appropriate format required for that particular medium. For example, if the typesetter can directly process SGML, then no conversion is needed. In fact, the eleventh edition of the MIM book was directly printed from SGML. The other formats (IRX, word-processing, and WWW) were given their own independent programs. This approach ensured the extensibility of the system for future methods of access.

Although the database implementation was done in-house, the problem of editing MIM files remained. SGML has a set of rich, i.e., "complex," features to minimize the intrusion of "tags" in the flow of the document, thereby allowing rapid keying of SGML tagged content using text editors and minimizing storage space. Plain text editors are not acceptable as editing tools because MIM staff writers are not experts in SGML rules. Therefore, we needed a tool with automatic enforcement of tags and their order. As a result, for the staff writers, we used a commercial SGML editing package that actively enforces the DTD-driven structure and provides a graphical user interface similar to the popular word processors used in the PC domain.

RESULTS

SGML Encoding for MIM

SGML does not convey any semantic information associated with the tags. It is up to the application domain or program to determine the meaning of the tags, i.e., whether it encodes semantic or formatting information. Since we chose to specify the MIM structure in terms of the semantic content, the tags relate to the meaning of the enclosed content. For example, a reference in MIM: "Fitzsimmons, J. S.: Familial recurrence of achondroplasia. Am. J. Med. Genet. 22: 609-613, 1985." can be tagged as:

```
<REF REFNO="13">
<AUTHOR>Fitzsimmons, J. S.</AUTHOR>
<TITLE>Familial recurrence of achondroplasia
  </TITLE>
<JOURNAL>Am. J. Med. Genet.</JOURNAL>
<VOLUME>22</VOLUME>
<PAGE>609-613<PAGE>
<DATE>1985</DATE>
</REF>
```

The start and end tags are "<label>" and "</label>", respectively, and they enclose a specific construct denoted by "label." This approach for defining the DTD for MIM ensures independence from distribution media because all formatting, including rearrangement, is performed as an independent step. It also offers the best approach for migration to traditional databases. Since direct editing is through a commercial SGML-based editor, writers never have to manually enter the tags as text string, so the minimization features of the SGML tags were not used. This, in turn, simplified the code for the parse engine because the start and end tags of all SGML constructs were always matched.

The choice of using SGML to specify structure also facilitated the evolution of MIM entries. Since the conversion in January 1994, the schema for the references has been changed three times to reflect more accurately the actual information content. Each time, the DTD modifications were carried out with minimal effort and the supporting software was updated with similar ease.

Validation of MIM Entries

Although SGML encodes the parts of MIM entries, it is unable to validate the semantic correctness of the contents. On the other hand, semantic validation is an open-ended problem that requires natural language processing in a narrative text file. A compromise was made: citations in the text that point to references in the reference list are checked for correct matching. For example, "...reported by Fitzsimmons (1985)..." can be tagged as: "...reported by <CIT REFNO="13"> Fitzsimmons (1985)</CIT>...," but only if there exists exactly one reference whose sole author is "Fitzsimmons" and the date of publication was 1985. When an exact match is found, the REFNO attribute of CIT will be assigned the REFNO attribute of the corresponding REF. This feature provided a bonus for the WWW users, because the citations are then presented as hypertext links to the references.

Most citations in MIM text follow a uniform convention, thus they can be automatically detected and matched against the references. However, after further analysis, the convention has four possible outcomes: (1) valid citation that uniquely points to a reference, (2) ambiguous citation that points to more than one reference, (3) problem citation that points to a missing reference, and (4) possible citation that may point to a reference. The semantic validation program will find all cases and properly tag them for correction.

Repairing Errors

The conversion to SGML was performed for the MIM database on January 1, 1994. Afterward, all editing activity occurred under the SGML-based editor. Therefore, all potential problems in the text files had to be identified and marked for later correction. The heuristic used was very sensitive and, to our knowledge, did not miss any problems, but the trade-off was a high false-positive rate. Out of 6,500 MIM entries and 50,000 references prior to conversion, only 3,500 entries and 35,000 references were converted without any identifiable problems. Excluding semantic problems, e.g., uncited and ambiguous citations, approximately 1,500 entries with 3,000 references were tagged as having potential structural problems. Out of these, only 500 entries with 1,000 references had real syntactic problems that required editing, e.g., a missing separator between author list and title in the original flat file which resulted in a "error" tag. The other 1,000 entries with 2,000 references were false-positives due to the sensitivity of our heuristics, e.g., the presence of a title delimiter inside the title because the original title contains it. Despite the high false-positive rate, the correction phase took an acceptable three person-months to perform. Overall, MIM had problems in 10 percent of the entries, but in terms of references, only 2 percent. This reflects the excellent proofreading skills of the MIM staff.

After the conversion to SGML and the correction of structural problems, we looked for semantic problems by examining the component fields of MIM. This was very useful for identifying inconsistent usage of a particular field. For example, all text tagged with JOURNAL was extracted, sorted, and printed for review. Initially, there were 1,800 distinct journal spellings, of which 120 were obvious variants, such as abbreviated vs. nonabbreviated names. However, about 100 variant spellings cannot be easily resolved and these will require a library literature search to correct.

These syntactic and semantic variants did not pose a problem in the flat-file version of MIM because the user, through natural language, can almost always determine the actual name of the journal or separate the authors from the title. However, these variants have to be corrected prior to cross-linking these references to references in the Medline database.

UNIX File System Repository

Since a suitable SGML-based DBMS couldn't be found, we had to develop a robust, in-house text database. The existing repository was based on the UNIX file system and the only problems were related to the software that managed this repository, as described above. Therefore, we adopted this architecture and merged it with the software engineering environment, but completely rewrote the software.

The previous system only dealt with three writers and, therefore, did not need robust concurrency control. In contrast, the number of active writers could now reach ten or more and robustness became critical. We used the UNIX atomic command "mkdir" [10] as a concurrency control semaphore to enter critical code sections that directly manipulate database files. For example, to lock a MIM entry for update or retrieval, the command "mkdir $LOCK/$sig" is executed, where "$LOCK" is a global lock directory, and "$sig" is a signature for a database resource, in this case, the MIM number. Only the first "mkdir" command will succeed in creating the signature directory. All other "mkdir" with the same signature will fail and have to wait (or abort) until the first user has completed the transaction and released the lock by executing "rmdir $LOCK/$sig". This had the additional benefit of creating a directory for temporary files and simplifying rollback of modifications.

Revision Control System (RCS) [11] was used as the method for maintaining file history, but its locking method was not used as write locks for the writers. The reason was that 6,500+ entries cannot be effectively maintained in one UNIX RCS directory. Thus, three levels of directories, each covering two digits in the 6-digit MIM number, were used. For example, the file for MIM entry 214355 is located in the directory $MIM/db/210000/214300/214355, along with all the status files relating to 214355. The variable "$MIM" specifies the root directory of the MIM database. All editing is performed in a separate directory, $MIM/edit, and the software manage the transfer of files between the two.

Instead of the traditional database transaction control mechanism, we retained the RCS approach of checkout/checkin. This was managed by UNIX shell scripts. Since its inception, the system has handled peak loads of 350 updates per work day, with 50 entries checked out at any one time, without problems. This peak activity is about 10 times higher than normal, based on statistics gathered over the last 2 years; it occurred during the time immediately post-conversion, when a major effort was made to correct errors.

The validation and processing of MIM files were performed by PERL scripts [12]. A total of 3,000 lines of UNIX sh code and 7,000 lines of PERL code comprise the new system software. Although the code size did not decrease from the previous system, the functionality had increased dramatically. Instead of spreading the code across sh, lex, and C, the new code relies only on sh and PERL. The objective is to simplify long-term software maintenance because expertise in fewer and higher-level languages is needed.

Converting SGML to Different Media

In order to ensure that the contents of an entry are tagged according to their semantic nature, we eliminated any text alignment formatting by removing all line breaks and extra spaces in the file prior to processing. Consequently, in order to distribute the MIM files to a particular medium, a filter program had to be built according to the requirements of the medium and generated the necessary formatting codes. The benefit from this strategy is that MIM files can be generated for any media without additional editing because it only has semantic SGML constructs. Another benefit is that formatting can be adjusted by the software and all media-specific MIM files can be made to reflect the new format almost immediately.

As it turns out, the increase in code required by the individual filter programs is minimal. For example, the filter programs for IRX, WWW, and word processing share large portions of code. The resulting design used a 400-line PERL core engine to parse the SGML-encoded text and another 500 lines specific to each filter program. Out of the 500 lines, however, only 200 have to be written de novo with the remainder copied from a basic template with minor modifications. Using the core facility, the filter program for WWW was completed within one week after the initial request.

DISCUSSION

This newly evolved MIM database was planned, developed, and executed based on the principles of industry standards, open systems, and extensibility. It took two person-years of software development time for the conversion to SGML-based structured text and the completely rewritten system software. Afterward, it took three person-months of corrections to resolve the remaining structural problems. The end result of this transition provided new features for navigating to external databases, allowed multimedia information, and improved the consistency of data. The advances for the support staff maintaining the MIM database include structured editing, simplified code maintenance, and better migration capability. We believe our approach of fine grain structuring with SGML and conversion to an open, extensible system has application for other flat-file, text-oriented databases. The principles used for MIM can also be used for porting other legacy systems.

The work reported here, the conversion to structured documents and the consolidation of software, is only one step among many that the MIM system will undertake. There are several projects under development. The first is the migration toward a relational administrative database, which will provide open architecture and standard. The second project is the compilation and cross-linking of references into a citation database to provide access to Medline abstracts. A third project is the search for an appropriate SGML-based text DBMS and retrieval engine that can make full use of the SGML structure.

Mendelian Inheritance in Man is one of the oldest active databases in the medical field. Its users range from researchers to clinicians and, now through the Internet, the general public. Part of its longevity is the result of providing the expected services to its users. As long as it continues to evolve and meet these challenges, MIM will remain valuable to scientists and the public. We hope that this most recent evolution of MIM will take it to the 21st century as a flagship database in the field of medicine and genetics.

REFERENCES

1. McKusick, V. A.: Mendelian Inheritance in Man. 10th Edition. Johns Hopkins Press: Baltimore. 1992.
2. Harman, D., Benson, D., Fitzpatrick, L., Huntzinger, R., Goldstein, C.: IRX: An Information Retrieval System for Experimentation and User Applications. Proc. RIAO 88 Conf., 840-848, 1988.
3. Lawton, J., Burks, C., Martinez, F.: Overview of the LiMB database. Nucleic Acids Research. 17:5885-5899, 1989.
4. Nassif, R., Mitchusson, D.:Issues and approaches for migration/cohabitation between legacy and new systems. Proc. ACM 93 SIGMOD. 471-474, 1993.
5. Leoffen, A.: Text Databases: A Survey of Text Models and Systems. ACM Sigmod Record 23(1): 97-106, 1994.
6. Salton, G., Allan, J., Buckley, C.: Automatic Structuring and Retrieval of Large Text Files. Communications of ACM. 37(2): 97-108, 1994.
7. Obraczka, K., Danzig, P. B., Li, S.-H.: Internet Resource Discovery Services. IEEE Computer. 26(9): 8-22, 1993.
8. Goldfarb, C. F.: The SGML Handbook. Oxford University Press: New York. 1992.
9. Li, P., Emmel, T. C., Campbell, J.: Virtual Development Environment-A database software engineering system based on UNIX tools. (in preparation).
10. Leffler, S. J., McKusick, M. K., Karels, M. J., Quarterman, J. S.: The Design and Implementation of the 4.3BSD UNIX Operating System. Addison-Wesley: Reading. 1989.
11. Tichy, W. F.: RCS-A system for Version Control. IEEE Software Practice and Experience. 15(7): 637-654, 1985.
12. Wall, L., Schwartz, R. L.: Programming perl. O'Reilly & Assoc.: Sebastopol. 1991.

ACKNOWLEDGEMENTS

The authors wish to thank Drs. V. A. McKusick, P. L. Pearson, K. Fasman, and Mr. C. Brunn for their support on this project. In addition, the system was refined with the advice and help of the MIM staff of C. Bocchini, P. Foster, and T. Hentges. Finally, many thanks to P. Foster for her editorial assistance. The work was funded by NIH 5P141HG00586-03 and DOE DE-FC02-91ER61230.

The Development of a Data Security Model for The Collaborative Social and Medical Services System

Ross Dargahi, Dave W. Classen, Risa B. Bobroff, M.S., Cynthia A. Petermann, M.S., Dennis R. Moreau, Ph.D., J. Robert Beck, M.D., and Gregory J. Buffone, Ph.D.

Medical Informatics and Computing Research Program
Baylor College of Medicine
Houston, Texas

ABSTRACT

This paper presents the development of the Collaborative Social and Medical Services System's (CSMSS) data security mechanism. This mechanism was synthesized from an analysis of the CSMSS problem domain, and from a study of the methods used by modern operating systems and database management systems.The resulting mechanism is more flexible and expressive than traditional access control methods and is generally applicable to the management of privacy and multi-provider access.

INTRODUCTION

According to The World Health Organization, "the road leading to health for all by the year 2000 passes through information" [1]. The truth of this statement is evident in the growing requirement for electronic access to medical record systems, and the explosion of research in the area of computerized patient record systems (CPRS) [2][3][4][5].

For CPRSs to be successfully deployed and used, it is imperative that the needs and expectations of both health care providers and patients be addressed. Generally these expectations mandate that a CPRS be able to manage the rich domain of information required for clinical medicine as well as maintain maximum protection of patient information in both storage and use. That is, the information's confidentiality, reliability, and integrity must not be susceptible to compromise. The importance of privacy with respect to medical information cannot be overstated. According to the American Health Information Management Association, "...Without such assurance (of privacy), the patient may withhold critical information which could affect the quality of care provided, the relationship with the provider, and the reliability of the information maintained" [6].

Protection of patient information, within a given system, is largely provided by system and data security. System security addresses the issue of protection from unauthorized access. This includes provision for hardware, software, communications, and users security [7]. Data security is concerned with the protection of data from accidental or intentional disclosure to unauthorized persons or from unauthorized modification or destruction [8].

Current system security mechanisms provide an acceptable level of system security; for example, Project Athena's Kerberos authentication system [9] provides network based client-server authentication, as well as encryption based on secure keys. Such a system can be incorporated into a CPRS to provide appropriate system security. Unfortunately, there is presently no satisfactory mechanism for providing a complete or even adequate solution to the data security problem faced by CPRSs. In fact, a literature review of confidentiality issues indicates that data security remains a key issue when discussing the comprehensive automation of medical records [3].

In this paper, a methodology for analysing the data security requirements of a CPRS along with its application to the CSMSS problem domain is described. The results of this analysis are the basis for developing a data security model for the CSMSS upon which a spectrum of policy based access control strategies may be built.

0195-4210/94/$5.00

AN ANALYSIS OF THE DATA SECURITY NEEDS OF AN OUTPATIENT CPRS

CPRSs pose an interesting data security problem. On the one hand is the desire to provide an open system for maximizing information sharing among health care practitioners and limited but sufficient access to researchers; on the other is the very real need to protect patient privacy. Furthermore, since the data is used in the day to day delivery of health care, it must ideally be: rapidly deliverable (there cannot be delays which impair the function of the health care practitioners); available on request (the system must be fault tolerant, that is not subject to the failure of software, hardware or communications); and distributed (information should be available to authorized personnel in different locales). These conflicting goals must be effectively managed by the data security model.

To realize the data security needs of a CPRS, one must understand the methods in which data will be accessed. There are four general use categories: patient care, social services, administration, and research [4]. These use categories exert different requirements upon the CPRS. The four use categories are normally further subdivided on the basis of specific roles. For example, patient care may be partitioned into the organizational roles important for the delivery of health care. Typical roles would be: physician, nurse, and nurse practitioner. Each role performs a defined set of tasks. Each task has a required set of inputs and produces a set of outputs. These relationships play an important part in the analysis model and its application to the CSMSS as described next.

The Analysis model and its Application to the CSMSS

The problem domain covered by the CSMSS design is the Baylor College of Medicine Teen Health Clinics (THC). The THCs are comprised of five geographically distributed clinics providing teenagers in the Harris County Hospital District with such services as: family planning, screening for and treatment of sexually transmitted diseases, prenatal and postnatal care, and patient education and counseling. A six step process is employed in determining clinic data security needs [10]. Each step will be detailed along with its application to the THCs.

The first task involves discovering and classifying the roles to be considered for the CPRS. This process examines the clinic's current organizational structure and extracts any roles that will require use of the CPRS. These roles are then broadly classified under the four use categories previously described. Interviews are conducted with staff members for each role in order to further understand its function and appropriateness as a part of the CPRS. The interviews may also result in the definition of new roles suitable only in the context of a CPRS; for example, a need for a data entry or transcriber role might be revealed. These emergent roles are defined by classification and further interviews. This iterative process continues until all the potential roles have been discovered. At the THCs, the roles identified are typical of many outpatient facilities and are illustrated in Table 1.

TABLE 1. Baylor College of Medicine Teen Health Clinic Roles

Clinic Roles	**Patient Care**	**Social Services**	**Administrative**	**Research**
Administrative Secretary			■	
Billing Clerk			■	
Clerk			■	
Community Services Aid		■	■	
Director			■	■
Health Educator		■	■	
Medical Assistant	■	■	■	
Nurse	■		■	
Nurse Manager	■		■	
Physician/Nurse Practitioner	■		■	
Project Coordinator			■	
Research Assistant				■
Social Services Coordinator		■	■	
Social Worker		■	■	

As previously discussed, each role in a clinic has a set of tasks which the person engaged in that role is responsible for performing. The goal of the second step in the analysis process is to define the tasks associated with each role. Observations of how the clinic staff work together to perform a single patient centered function, as well as interviews with staff members are used to define and refine the role specific tasks. The goal of the interviews is to derive, for each role, a set of tasks with crisp boundaries and minimal functional overlap (except in cases where it is appropriate for the performance of the task). In addition, the interviews should identify any role overlap by exposing those tasks which are performed by more than one role. It should be noted that it is often permissible for there to be role overlap and task redundancy; in many cases this is required for maintaining patient safety, meeting legal requirements, or ensuring the efficiency of clinic operations. In the case of the THCs, it was frequently found that one role performed the tasks of another due to the limited availability of staff to perform the required task.

With both the clinic roles and tasks defined, the input and output for each task must be analyzed. Questionnaires serve an important capacity in this step. Questions are centered around the data requirements of a task (task input), and the data produced by the execution of a task (task output), and they are framed in terms of a metaphor familiar to the clinic staff. Questionnaires for the THCs used forms, logs, and reports as the entities for uncovering task data and access requirements. Task input was specified in terms of the forms accessed to provide the input for a task, and task output was specified in terms of the forms, logs and reports generated or updated by the execution of a task.

With a knowledge of the roles, the tasks associated with those roles, and the input, output, and data access requirements for those tasks, it is possible to define the aggregate data requirements of a given role within the clinic. For the THCs the data requirements for a given role were determined by gathering all forms, logs, and reports required by the set of tasks associated with that role.

The next step is to discover any exceptions which may be applicable in the given health care environment. This process involves identifying the scenarios that would require the normal data security mechanism to be overridden, and defining any consequent processing, such as audit trails, which would be necessary in such instances. No exceptions were discovered at the THCs

Finally, the findings and conclusions are compiled into a matrix and are then verified with the clinic staff. Rows in the matrix represent the roles defined for the clinic, and columns represent the data requirements of each role. In the case of the THCs, this would be the forms, logs, and reports used by a task. The intersection of each row and column indicates the access permissions for the respective role/data element combination. The matrix is iteratively refined with the clinic staff until an acceptable policy is agreed upon.

The authors believe that the process presented above represents a generic six step process for analyzing the data security requirements in any health care setting. The next section examines the advantages and disadvantages of existing data security mechanisms for use in the CSMSS.

Existing Data Security Mechanisms

Data security is of importance to the designers of both operating systems (OS) and database management systems (DBMS). Clearly, such systems must provide an acceptable level of security for the resources they manage. CPRSs must address these same concerns as well as additional issues, as they provide similar services in the context of health care information management. The fundamental requirements of a data security model for a CPRS should also include:

- Flexibility. The model must be able to support a broad range of security policies. In particular it must provide both a generalized means of control that can be based on user role and required access, as well as provide for exception handling at the data element level.
- Speed. The model must not hinder the timely delivery of health care information. In addition, both emergency and multi-location access should be feasible.
- Ease of administration. The model must be easy to use and administer. Given the requirements for clinical consultation, practice coverage, and resident and fellow education, the system must be able to maintain an appropriate level of access and privacy.

The feasibility of using existing security models to address these issues is described below.

Operating Systems

The prevailing strategies for operating system data security are: access control lists, capability lists, multi-level security, and access matrices. The strengths and weaknesses of each will briefly be discussed.

Access Control Lists (ACL) have the advantage of providing fine grained access. However, with ACLs searching for a user's access privileges can be computationally expensive; furthermore ACLs are not easy to administer, as it is difficult to determine system-wide access rights for a given user since the rights data is localized by data element[12].

Capability Lists (C-Lists) also have the advantage providing fine grained access. C-Lists also localize permissions by user [12]; this makes data security administering on a per user basis a lot simpler. However this localization has the disadvantage of making it particularly difficult to revoke access to a given data element. [11].

Multilevel Security has the advantage that it ensures only upward information flow through the model.

This makes administering this model very easy. However, this method is also quite inflexible, since it is not possible to make exceptions when using this model. Due to its rigidity multilevel security can only express limited types of policy [13].

Access Matrices have the advantage of providing a very flexible approach to security by permitting a localized view of access either by data element, or user. The disadvantage of access matrices is that they tend to be sparse, and can become quite large and wasteful of system resources [11][12].

Database Management Systems (DBMS)
Although operating systems generally provide data security for the information stored in their file systems, DBMSs usually need much finer grained access control than provided at the granularity of a file. For this reason many commercial DBMSs provide their own data security mechanism.

Relational DBMS (RDBMS) provide security through the Grant/Revoke and view mechanisms. Grant/Revoke has the advantage that it can restrict access to a table or view (discussed next) by restricting the query language[14]. It's disadvantages are that it is not able to limit access to the individual rows in a table, and it does not scale well to a language with more than a small set of terms. Views can confine the user's view of the rows of any given set of tables [15]. Unfortunately, the restriction that views place on table rows tend to be too static and too coarse grained for the level of flexibility required by a CPRS. Views are also sensitive to changes in their constraining clauses and to changes in the underlying data model, thus they can be quite difficult to administer.

Object Oriented DBMS (OODBMS) are a relatively new entry into the commercial DBMS market. Consequently, OODBMS vendors are not offering particularly innovative solutions to security issues. However, there is ongoing research in the area, including extending the relational security model to OODBMSs [16] and using security constraints to enforce mandatory and discretionary security [17].

From the foregoing discussion it is clear that none of the traditional data security mechanisms, in and of itself, is sufficient for meeting the requirements of the CSMSS, as established in the analysis of the THC project. Furthermore, they do not support a level of flexibility consistent with the intention of constructing a domain independent CPRS infrastructure. Consequently, in order to meet the needs of the CSMSS, a hybrid data security strategy has been synthesized. This strategy is presented in the next section.

CSMSS DATA SECURITY STRATEGY

The CSMSS strategy is based on an extended access matrix model hybridized with parameterized role assertion and segmentation to facilitate access to dynamically allocated data elements. Specifically, the rows of the access matrix represent roles and the columns represent data segments.

Segmentation of data resources permits the logical collection of data element types into related groups, thus allowing them to be managed as a single entity. Since there are likely to be far fewer segments than data element types, this adaptation pre-empts one of the chief disadvantages of access matrices, large matrix size.

In order to represent finer grained data security without generating additional segments and roles, parameterized roles have been introduced. Parameterized roles allow the specification of a constrained relationship between roles and data resources. For example, consider restricting access to a certain patients medical records to only her physician; this is possible by parameterizing the physician role by the patient identifier.

Thus far the CSMSS data security model permits security restrictions to be placed upon data element types by role and even permits finer grained restrictions via parameterized roles. However the system must provide, for special cases, still finer grained access by permitting restrictions to be placed upon individual data elements. This is imperative for protecting such information as HIV test results or social worker notes. However, defining access constraints to specific data elements within the access matrix would imply creating a new column for each restricted data element. This results in an unconstrained, and therefore unacceptable, growth in the matrix. A solution is to introduce an auxiliary security mechanism for managing exceptional access control to dynamically created data elements. The mechanism selected is based on the access control list paradigm. Since it is being used for exceptional cases, there should be little overhead placed on the system, as a rapid table lookup will determine whether a ACL entry exists for a given data element.

Finally, it should be noted that the CSMSS data security paradigm can support domains which require either a open/closed (information is generally unrestricted) or a closed/open (information is generally restricted) security model. In the former, the access matrix and ACL entries register restrictions; in the latter, they register permissions.

CONCLUSION

Data security policy is generally quite dynamic. Roles and tasks may evolve over time; new roles and tasks may be created, and old ones may be retired. For example, new medical procedures can redefine the process involved in completing a task as well as the inputs and outputs associated with a task. Organizational constraints can also change the tasks associated with a particular role. Furthermore, legal constraints can place mandatory requirements on specific types of data[5]. For these reasons, a coherent process for evolving the data security policy as well as a flexible architecture that can support change must be in place.

This paper has presented a six step data security analysis methodology that was applied to the THCs to derive the specific needs for this component of the CSMSS. This analysis and a study of the current security models used by OSs and DBMSs resulted in the development of a generalized hybrid data security paradigm synthesized in part from existing security models. It is felt that the flexibility of this model will realize the broad spectrum of policy based access strategies demanded by CPRS including the CSMSS.

Acknowledgments

This work has been supported, in part, by grant LM04905 from the National Library of Medicine.

The authors wish to thank the staff of the Baylor College of Medicine Teen Health Clinics for their help on this project.

References

[1] Weiss, W.V., *Health Care: conflicting opinions tough decisions*, NC Press Limited, Toronto, 1992.

[2] Chueh, H.C., Barnett, G.O., "Client-server, Distributed Database Strategies in a Health-care Record System for a Homeless Population", *Journal of the American Medical Informatics Association*, Vol. 1, No. 2, March/April 1994.

[3] Benjamin, C.D., and Baum B., "The automated medical record: A practical realization?", *Topics in Health Record Management*, Vol. 9, No. 1, 1988.

[4] Henkind, S.J., Orlowski, J.M., Skarulis, P.C., "Application of a Multilevel Access Model in the Development of a Security Infrastructure for a Clinical Information System", *Proceedings of the Seventeenth Annual Symposium on Computer Applications in Medical Care*, Washington, MD, October/November 1993.

[5] Dick, R.S, Steen, E.B., Eds., *The Computer Based Patient Record: An Essential Technology for Health Care*, National Academy Press, Washington, DC, 1991.

[6] American Medical Record Association. "Confidentiality of patient health information", position statement of the American Medical Record Association, Chicago, 1985.

[7] Martin, J., *Managing the database environment*, Prentice-Hall, Englewood Cliffs, NJ, 1983.

[8] Martin, J., *Computer Data-Base Organization*, Prentice-Hall, Englewood Cliffs, NJ, 1977.

[9] Miller, S.P., Neuman, B.C., Schiller, J.I., and Saltzer, J.H., *Section E.2.1: Kerberos Authentication and Authorization System*, M.I.T. Project Athena, Cambridge, MA, December 21, 1987.

[10]Orr, G.A., Brantley, B.A., "Development of a Model of Information Security Requirements for Enterprise-Wide Medical Information Systems", *Proceedings of the Sixteenth Annual Symposium on Computer Applications in Medical Care*, Baltimore, MD, November 1992.

[11]Peterson, J.L., Silberschatz, A., *Operating System Concepts*, Addison Wesley, Reading, MA, 1986.

[12]Tanenbaum, A.S., *Modern Operating Systems*, Prentice-Hall, Englewood Cliffs, NJ, 1992.

[13]Bell, D., Grimson, J., *Distributed Database Systems*, Addison-Wesley, Reading, MA, 1992.

[14]Date, C.J., An Introduction to Database Systems, Volume 1, Addison-Wesley, Reading, MA, 1986.

[15]Pratt, P.J., *Database Systems Management and Design*, Boyd and Fraser, Boston, MA, 1987.

[16]Kim, W., "Architectural Issues in Object-Oriented Databases", *Journal of Object-Oriented Programming*, Vol.2, No. 6, March/April 1990.

[17]Thuraisingham, M.B., "Security in Object-Oriented Database Systems", *Journal of Object-Oriented Programming*, Vol. 2, No. 6, March/April 1990.

The Bioethics Online Service - An Implementation of a Bioethics Database and Information Resource

Arthur R. Derse, M.D., J.D., and Steven R. Krogull, M.S.
Medical College of Wisconsin, Milwaukee Wisconsin

ABSTRACT

Ethical analysis is crucial to decision making in biomedicine and health care, necessitating rapid access to diffusely disseminated sources of information pertinent to bioethics. We developed the Bioethics Online Service to provide this access and to provide a forum for discussion of bioethical issues. The service, originally designed as a local resource, was expanded to allow Internet access and now enjoys widespread extramural use. We have logged over 8,000 users from our campus, around the state, the nation, and 42 other countries. This model has shown promise in utility and ease of access, and is being used as the template for other informatics developments on our campus and beyond.

PURPOSE

The next several years will bring significant changes in American health care and the way it is provided to persons of different ages, gender, socioeconomic status, and geographic locations. Ethical analysis is crucial to the evolution of these changes; and access to scientific, economic, legal, philosophical, and health policy information is crucial to ethical analysis.

Institutional ethics committees, ethics consultants, primary care physicians, health care institutional administrators, health care legal counsel, and students in the health care field need to obtain information about bioethical issues quickly and accurately. Additionally, there is an increasing interest on the part of the public to learn about and participate in the discussion of issues in bioethics. At present this is not an easy task.

Part of the problem is that information about bioethics is disseminated diffusely. Court decisions, state statutes, journal articles, newspaper accounts, professional society and association position statements, federal and state government agency decisions, and published hospital ethics committee decisions add to the information base in bioethics each day. No one source can be relied upon for up-to-date, pertinent bioethics information — be it the medical library of a medical school, law school, or philosophy department, or through a legal case update service, administrative journals, or news service.

Another part of the problem is that the need for information is often time-critical. Ethics committees, ethics consultants, physicians, nurses, attorneys, and ethicists need accurate, recent information urgently. In fact, the Wisconsin Ethics Committee Network (WECN), a statewide consortium of over 180 hospital and long-term care facility ethics committees, sponsored by the Medical College of Wisconsin (MCW), found itself in need a time-efficient and appropriate means for its members to communicate about its activities and resources.

For busy individuals seeking ethics information, the task of synthesizing these disparate materials is formidable. One needs the expertise of the clinician, the ethicist, and the lawyer to pull together the pertinent information, to explain how the information applies to specific cases, and to show where the information fits into the larger picture. It was exactly this type of synthesis delivered through a centralized resource that WECN members and other bioethics experts wanted.

METHODS

In response to these needs, we developed the **Bioethics Online Service**, which was inaugurated in June, 1993 at MCW. This service consists of these features:

- The **Bioethics Database** is an update service which provides MCW-produced abstracts of pertinent bioethics journal articles, legislative actions and court decisions. It also provides an intermittent commentary about current bioethics issues. Online information is updated every week and the database is searchable by key words. Over 550 abstracts are available at this time.

- The **Bioethics Bulletin Online** publishes articles of interest from the Medical College of Wisconsin's Bioethics Bulletin.

0195-4210/94/$5.00

- The **Bioethics Resources** section serves as an archive and clearinghouse for ethics and ethics committee policies and other resources.

- The **Bioethics Reference Texts Online** area electronically publishes (with publishers' and authors' permission) helpful reference texts and position statements on bioethics topics. This section currently contains over 50 entires from about ten texts.

- The **Bioethics Discussion Forum** facilitates discussion of current bioethics cases and topics.

- The **Bioethics Center News and Announcements** section posts current bioethics news and announcements from the Medical College of Wisconsin and other academic and professional sources.

- The **Wisconsin Ethics Committee Network (WECN) News and Announcements** section posts current bioethics news and announcements from the Wisconsin Ethics Committee Network, a consortium of ethics committees from acute and long term care facilities in Wisconsin. The Bioethics Online Service acts as a core communications vehicle for WECN members.

- The **Directory of U.S. and Canadian Bioethics Networks and Centers** directs users to other resources in bioethics.

- Through **Electronic Mail**, users can communicate personally with other users of the service, Bioethics Center faculty, and other individuals worldwide through Internet.

Technical Implementation

The Medical College's Office of Research, Technology, and Information has successfully partnered with the Bioethics Center to implement the Bioethics Online Service through MCW's Medical Information Network (MIN). This internal network is tied to Wiscnet for state-wide communications, Internet for national and international access, and services such as America Online for convenient connection to the Internet. This configuration offers points of access for faculty, staff, students, other professionals and lay public. Thus, the Bioethics Online Service can be accessed by anyone with a computer, a communications program, and a modem from almost any location.

In the course of developing this service, several internal and external database and information management programs were evaluated. Gopher emerged as the system of choice to facilitate access from multiple routes, provide a highly structured (menu-based) method for information organization and retrieval, and implementation costs were minimal using existing computer and staff resources. This standard Internet tool is a text-based data system, searchable, easy to implement and maintain. Gopher will allow search and retrieval of text, files, telnet resources, sounds and graphics. Gopher runs under UNIX on a VAX at MCW which is connected to the Internet through the Wiscnet network. Usually, Gopher requires that the user have "client" software. However, MCW's telnet and dial-in connection system provides a Gopher client as part of a menu choice to connect to the Bioethics Online Service.

In analyzing the content to be housed in the Bioethics Online Service, the subject matter was discovered to be very diverse. The most common resources consist of tables of contents from pertinent journals, journal articles, advance sheets from court decisions, garnering newspaper stories, and other resources, (e.g. books sent for review). Our own set of key words (N=1450) were identified and developed by our abstracter with input from MCW Bioethics faculty based upon trends in the literature. These key words facilitate the Gopher search as the current implementation of Gopher does not support multiple-word phrase searches nor boolean logic in a search strategy. Also, a structured keyword system will help us to prepare for the possibility of eventually evolving toward a true database program supporting all of the searching and reporting functions this type of service requires.

The selection of Internet for our service was based upon the increasing ease of connectivity and access to the Internet among academic, business, and individual users. Internet is the Transmission Control Protocol/Internet Protocol (TCP/IP) based world wide network system connecting more than 2,000 other networks including wide-area networks, midlevel and regional networks, and campus and organization local networks in the U.S., Canada, Mexico, Japan, Europe, New Zealand, and Australia, with estimates of more than 1 million computers connected, and 15 million users. Wiscnet, our link to the Internet, is a state-wide high-speed logical network that connects academic institutions in Wisconsin.

Because of the demand for an interactive case discussion service through which subscribers from the bioethics, legal, medical, and philosophical communities could exchange ideas and information about specific or hypothetical cases, we sought to provide online interactive functions including public posting and archiving of information. At present, the technical implementation of the Gopher interface does not support these functions without linking traditional bulletin board software (BBS) to the Bioethics Online Service.

The few available UNIX versions of bulletin board software that were reviewed were felt not to have an appropriate interface for the Bioethics Online Service. Other (PC and Macintosh) BBS software packages were considered, but these required additional separate systems. All of these systems require significant input and organization from system operators (sysops) or discussion group moderators, which would add significant burdens to our limited human and financial resources.

Therefore, we turned to an automatic mailing list processor, Listproc, to address these needs. This list processor supports automatic enrollment of users, distribution of cases and subsequent commentary, and links to existing Gopher-based services. This link allows the list processor to be mirrored to a local campus bioethics news group and the main Gopher-based Bioethics Online Service. Thus, Gopher serves as a permanent, read only archive sorted in reverse chronological order, while the mirrored list processor and news group allow for on-going discussion among participants using either service.

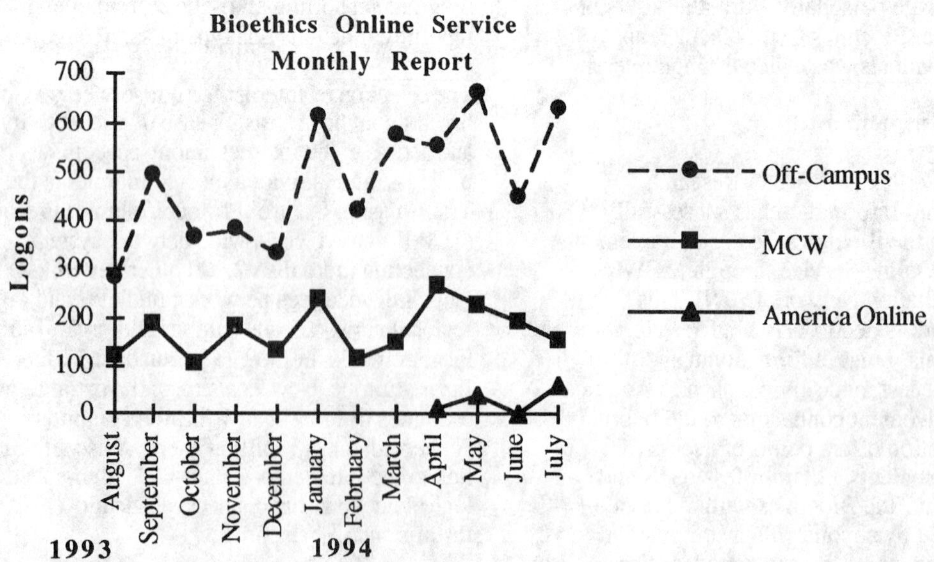

RESULTS

Initially, the Bioethics Online Service was meant to be a communication and information resource for WECN members (N= est. 500). The Bioethics Online Service was demonstrated at regional WECN conferences and ethics committee meetings. However, though initial interest was enthusiastic, few WECN members participated. We found that the majority of WECN members were not computer literate and did not know the fundamentals of telecommunication. Secondly, those who knew about telecommunication had a difficult time learning to navigate their local route of access to connect to MCW through the Internet. Different access sites had different procedures and variable costs for gaining connection. To address these problems we initiated a series of outreach and training seminars. Unfortunately, the staff time was a significant factor. To address these limits on staff resources, we attempted to enlist librarians and information specialists located within or proximate to a user to demonstrate the service.

Interestingly, when we analyzed the numbers of users by where the connection originated, we found that our extramural use far exceeded our intramural use, i.e. the Internet was our most common route of access, and the vast majority of connections were not from WECN members. Nonetheless, on our campus use has fluctuated around a mean of approximately 175 log-ons per month and our off-campus average is 476 per month.

Additionally, the Bioethics Online Service has been used in education at MCW. Our Masters students in Bioethics have used the Service in conjunction with course work for research and professional development, and medical students have used it as an introduction to various topics in bioethics. A clear advantage of the Service format identified by these users is its 24 hours per-day accessibility from any location.

The Bioethics Online service has attracted national attention. America Online (AOL), the nationwide information service with over 700,000 subscribers, has chosen the Bioethics Online Service as a "featured" database for their Internet users because of exemplary presentation of material with value and interest to their users and because it is, in their words, a reliable and well-maintained resource.

Future Plans

The Bioethics Online Service plans to enhance its role in the dissemination of bioethics information. In coming months, we plan to establish these new features:

1) an ethics committee fact file to allow rapid access to information specifically designed to aid ethics committees, including an ethics committee case directory, which will collect information about and analyze ethics committees' case consultations;

2) a bioethics educational programming clearinghouse, for the dissemination of information and ideas about bioethics teaching and research;

3) comprehensive retrospective searches of Medline and other sources such as legal databases to make sure that no significant information items have been neglected.

4) a biweekly current headline bioethics news update service.

We also plan to establish these new links:

1) an affiliation with a national bioethics organization as its official bulletin board,

2) a link to the national freenet system with access for Omnifest, the local freenet.

CONCLUSION

Through the Bioethics Online Service, the Bioethics Center at the Medical College of Wisconsin will help local, national, and international audiences of health care professionals, students, institutions, and the lay public confront the ethical challenges posed by continued scientific advances.

As a result of our endeavors, other educational institutions have expressed plans to create online services based on the Bioethics Online Service. We applaud these efforts and look forward to the development of similar services worldwide.

Acknowledgment

The authors wish to acknowledge the contributions of these individuals in the development and implementation of the Bioethics Online Service (BOS): Michele DeYoe, M.L.S., BOS Abstracts Format Editor and Program Coordinator of the Office of Research, Technology and Information, Mary Olson, B.A., BOS Abstracts Content Editor and Senior Research Associate, Center for the Study of Bioethics, Rob Gatter, J.D., BOS Abstracter, and Perry Brunelli, B.S., BOS Technical Director and Acting Director of Information Technology Systems.

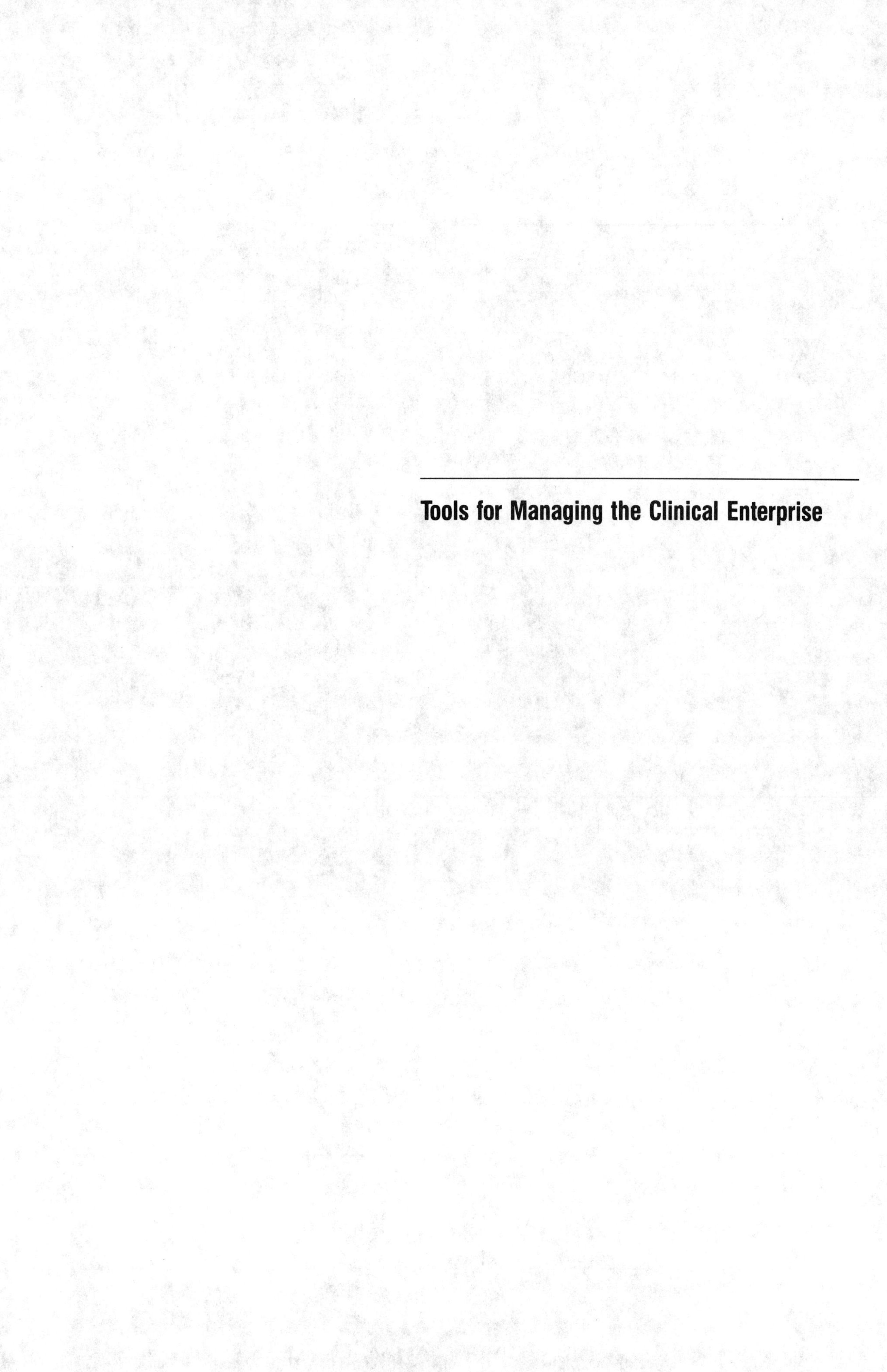

Tools for Managing the Clinical Enterprise

Modelling and Eliciting Organisational and Information System Requirements for Medical Information Systems

Andrew Blyth
Centre for Software Reliability, The University of Newcastle Upon Tyne,
Newcastle Upon Tyne, NE8 7RU. England.

Abstract

In this paper an outline of a modelling technique will be presented that allows for the encapsulation and analysis of the social and technical aspects of an organisational information system. This notation is used to construct and analyse both the static and dynamic models of organisations and organisational behaviour. The construction and analysis is achieved through the use of concepts such as role and responsibility. The conceptual modelling framework is then applied to a case study. This case study is based upon an accident and emergency department of an inner city hospital situated within the centre of Dublin, Ireland.

INTRODUCTION

In [3] the assertion is made that computers are not just instrumental means of production, they also condition and mediate social relationships. This mediation can take the form of decisions being made by the computer that have a direct impact on a person's life. For example, a medical information system is just a pure information system but also a safety critical system and an agent of change. The issues associated with the adoption and application of a medical information system are not just availability of service and integrity of information, but also how the information system will change the work patterns of the organisation. Conventional systems analysis has largely concentrated on information processing rather than taking a wider view of the problem which would consider the The framework presented within this paper views an information system as a socio-technical system. That is to say that it attempts to model the wider issues that surround and information system both at the social, behavioural, technical and moral level. This is achieved through the merger of the concepts of role and responsibility, and a linguistical model of interactions, within a modelling framework.

One of functions of this modelling framework is for it to act as a medium of communication. This is so that both the problem owners and problem solvers can build up a consensus that they are specifying and reasoning about the same problem. Another purpose of the modelling framework is to facilitate in the representation and validation of the problem.

By modelling an organisation and how it manipulates its resources and value system we are empowering it with the ability to model itself and its role within a society. This ability provides an organisation with the capability to embrace change and view it in a positive manner [5]. As a result organisations can at last begin to explore the consequences of adopting an information system and plan for the futhure.

THE BASIC CONCEPTS

The modelling concepts are perhaps the key aspect that makes this framework different from more conventional approaches to design. Enterprise modelling [1] provides a framework for representing and reasoning about the IT system as a component of a wider environment that is the organisation whose needs it is designed to serve. We have found that this form of modelling ensures an adequate representation of the structural and organisational aspects of the problem. It makes explicit policy issues and assumptions that cannot easily be stated. A major characteristic of the modelling framework presented in this paper is that responsibilities and relationships are modelled rather than activities. This enables us to elicit, capture, and represent information in the context of those who use it.

The enterprise modelling language has been designed to represent the structure of organisations. It has two related but distinct purposes: 1) to identify the requirements owners and their positions and roles within the organisation in order to demonstrate completeness of the requirements elicitation process, and 2) to identify the user community (and others affected by the proposed IT system) and their roles and responsibilities within the organisation in order to demonstrate completeness of the requirements modelling process.

0195-4210/94/$5.00

The Concept of Role

The our concept of role [1] allows us to distinguish: a) agents, and the relationships between them; and b) the network ofactivities that interact through information flows and are structured into tasks and operations. Our modelling framework enables us to represent and analyse the relations between these ('a' and 'b') and to represent the way in which they operate in real organisations.

The Concept of Agency

Our aim is to describe and reason about organisations that embody both a social and a technical system. These however comprise one single system, a socio-technical system, and as such cannot be described or modelled only in terms of state and behaviour as a purely technical system might be, since there is a fundamental difference between social and technical systems. It is to be able to differentiate between social and technical objects (i.e. between people and computers) that we introduce the idea of agency [1]. A machine may perform the same tasks as a person, but the person will hold responsibilities for those tasks in contrast to the machine which cannot hold responsibility. The person is said to be an agent and hold the agency.

Responsibility Modelling

We will define responsibility as a relationship between two agents regarding a specific state of affairs [4], such that the holder of the responsibility is responsible to the giver of the responsibility, the responsibility principal. We will define responsibility consists of: a) who is responsible to whom; b) the state of affairs for which the responsibility is held; c) the nature of realtionship(these include peer, power and service) d) the type of responsibility (these include accountability, blameworthiness, legal liability). A computer can not be held responsible for any things as responsibility implies issues such as culpability and restitution. Clearly a computer can not be punished for its actions, so we need to examine where that responsibility might lie. Thus if an information system is making a decision, or even helping in the making of a decision, then it needs to be clear when, where and to whom the responsibilities lie.

Service Modelling

The life cycle that we go through for a service from negotiation, delivery to restitution are depicted in Figure 1. This diagram forms a framework from within which the problem solver can begin to examine how the current system functions and how an information system may assist the organisation in the meeting of its objectives.

Each stage defines its own set of issues and concerns. For example, in the stage restitution we can examine the nature of that restitution by answer questions such as, to whom do we make restitution and who makes its, as well as does this restitution involve any litigation. For each stage we can examine the conditions under which we can engage in this stage and the conditions under which we exit this stage, as well as the organisational objects manipulated in that stage.

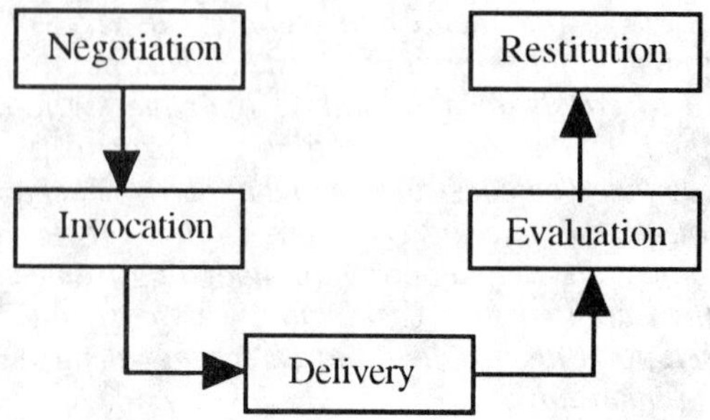

Figure 1 The Service Life Cycle Model

Within the negotation stage we would want to examine the conversation which leads to the definition of a service, the agents and the relationships associated with its invocation, delivery, evaluation. For example, within this section we could want to specify how and by whom a service will be evaluated. Issues such as when can some one engage in this conversation, with whom should the conversation be engaged and under what conditions can the conversation be engaged are just a few of the questions that we would seek to answer in this section. In addition, within this stages we would also want to examine what responsibilities and resources where created and manipulated as signs of the services invocation and evaluation.

For the invocation phase of the service life cycle we would want to examine issues such as under what conditions can the service be invoked. We would also want to examine the conversation concerned the services invocation and look at things such as what happens in the invocation fails, and what access rights on resources and responsibilities are required. Within the delivery phase of the service life cycle we can examine how a service is delivered, what organisational objects are manipulated by that delivery and whom is to delivery the service and to whom is the service to be delivered. Again we can examine the roles that these agents or agencies play within the whole of the life cycle.

For the evaluation phase we would want to examine issues associated with how the service was to be evaluated and by whom. In addition, we would want to make clear by examination the conditions under which the evaluation phase of the service life cycle model is started and terminated. Questions such as what metrics will be used, are their any legal methods to evaluate this service and how is this service to be payed for, all fall within the scope of this phase of the service life cycle model. For example we could now examine the question, is the evaluation of the service the same agent or agency who delivers it?

The restitution phase of the service life cycle model is concerned with issues such as how is payment to be made for this service, or how does the consumer of the service get legal compensation for anything that has gone wrong.

THE CASE STUDY - THE CITY HOSPITAL

Introduction

This case study is taken from an accident and emergency (A&E) department located in an inner city hospital of Dublin. Various social, economic and political factors conspire to make this case study interesting. For the purposes of this paper however, a condensed problem domain will be presented without generalisation and analysed from only one perspective. It should be remembered though that this problem forms part of a bigger problem, which in turn fits into the social, economic, and political environment of the country.

Characterisation of an A&E Dept

The primary function performed by the A&E department is to provide accident and emergency services to the public. This has evolved into a second function, which constitutes provision of low-grade medical services to the local populace, where patients use the A&E department as an alternative to general practice.

The A&E department is functionally related to a number of other departments within the hospital upon which it relies for services, e.g., pathology, radiology, pharmacy, and central administration. The A&E department internally consists of a small set of separate and distinct entities, e.g., senior nurse, consultant, junior doctors, junior nurses, and receptionists.

For the purposes of this case study we will concentrate on one aspects of the nurse's role within the A&E department. By modelling this role we will attempt to derive requirements. The role of the junior nurse upon which we will focus is that of administering drugs to the patient.

The Role of the Junior Nurse

Under Irish law, the person who administers a drug is responsible for the effect that the drug has on the patient,. Thus, if the wrong drug is prescribed and administered, the person is held responsible under the law. This gives rise to the nurses having to perform, and being taught to perform, some of the functions normally associated with a doctor. When administering drugs to a patient, one nurse administers the drug while another nurse observes to makes sure that the correct procedures are followed and that the recommended dosage of a particular drug is administered. Both nurses then sign for the drugs in the patient's records. Drug usage is monitored by the chief nurse as the unit contains little stocks of drugs, particularly controlled drugs such as morphine. The junior nurse is responsible for ensuring that the use of such drugs is recorded.

If the nurse is unhappy with the diagnosis, she can refuse to administer the drug. Within the health service it is impossible for anyone to be forced to administer a drug. Should the nurse decide upon this course of action, she is required to report it to the chief nurse. The resolution of this conflict then becomes the responsibility of the chief nurse. Should the chief nurse be unable to resolve this situation, she may also invoke a higher authority (the hospital's central administration) to deal with the situation. It then becomes their responsibility. Within the A&E department, there are therefore two management structures: one for the doctors with the consultant at their head; and one for the nurses with the chief nurse at their head. These two management structures only come together in the central administration of the hospital.

Modelling the System

The purpose in modelling the organisational system from the perspective of the junior nurse is to elicit, represent, and validate requirements that have either a direct, or an indirect, impact on the Organisational Information Technology system. In Figure 2, the rectangles represent the agencies or agents that contain the structural and functional roles. The structural roles are connected together with lines of double thickness, while the functional relationships are connected together with lines of a single thickness. The functional roles (*problem owner, problem repair*) are shorthand for the kind of behaviours (conversations) that the the various agencies or agents may engage in (e.g., the problem owner can report the existence of a problem, and the problem repairer can mend it). The structural roles (*consumer, supplier*) are shorthand for the framework of responsibilities that permit and give meaning to these behaviours i.e. it describes the nature of the 'social' relationship between the two agents.

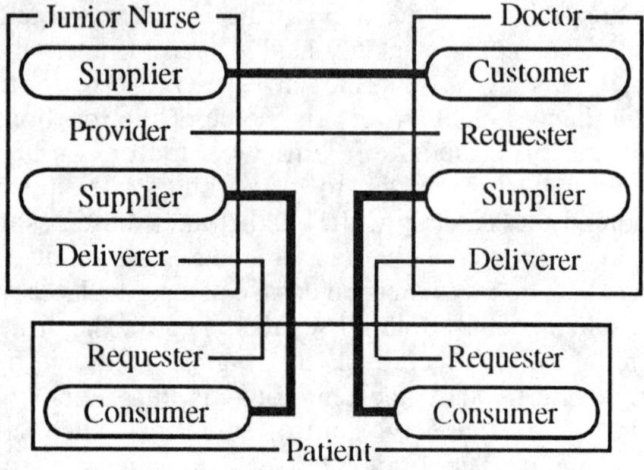

Figure 2 An Overview of the Structural System

The lines that join the functional and the structural roles represent the fact that a relation between two agents may be one of interaction or one of responsibility. Responsibility and interactions are related to each other through activities such that responsibilities only arise and are fulfilled through interactions. In short, the links between them are functional and structural relationships.In the role relation diagram depicted in Figure 5, the doctor and nurse have to negotiate for the delivery of a specified service to the patient. Due to the nature of the relationship, the structural relationship that exists between them is that of supplier - customer. The requester - provider functional relationship that is associated with the doctor - nurse structural relationship denotes the negotiation process by which the doctor attempts to persuade the nurse to perform a service. The service that the nurse performs is the delivery of health care to a third agent, i.e., the patient. As a result of the delivery of this service, both the doctor and the nurse fulfill their responsibilities.The structural relationship between the nurse and the doctor is one of customer - supplier. The nature of the conversation between them is one of negotiation, as the doctor is attempting to convince the nurse to treat the patient in a prescribed manner. As the nurse is legally responsible for any treatment he/she administers, he/she has to decide if she believes that the prescribed treatment for the patient by the doctor is appropriate and adequate. In order for her to make a decision she has to perform a brief diagnosis based on the information that she has access to.

The conversations that a nurse would engage in to administer some drugs to a patient at the request of a doctor will now be modelled. In the following diagrams, a rectangle is used to denote a speech act, and a triangle is used to signify those points in a conversation where different courses of action may arise (mental acts). In addition an oval is used to denote an instrumental act, and a rounded rectangle is used to express the starting or terminating points of the functional unit. The notation is described and explained in detail in [2].

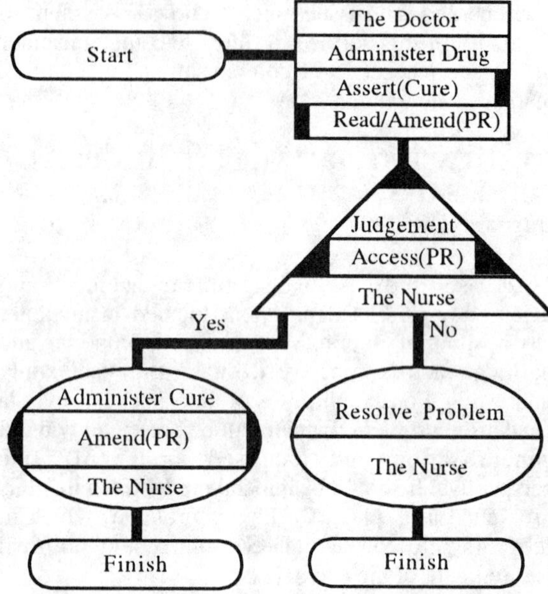

Figure 3 A Conversation Diagram of the Nurse's Decision

In Figure 3, the conversation begins with the doctor requesting the nurse to administer a drug to the patient. In so doing he/she needs to have read and write (read/amend) access to all the patient's records (PR) so that they can be augmented by adding what drug he/she thinks is required. In requesting the nurse to administer a drug to the patient, the doctor is asserting an informational attribute and mirroring this assertion in the patient's records by recording it there. This informational attribute is the proposition that a particular drug is what the patient requires as part of their cure at this point in time.

The nurse now has to make a decision as to whether he/she is going to administer the drug. The law consequently generates several direct and indirect requirements on the organisational information technology system. From the nurse's perspective, if the correct decision is to be made, then access to all the informational objects and attributes related to the patient is required. The nurse must be able to review them and form an opinion of what ails the patient so that a cure may be formulated and administered. In the above diagram, the term *Access(PR)* is used to express the accessing of all the informational objects and informational attributes related to the patient. Having identified that accessing of records is required, the nature of the accessing itself can be explored. We find that the nurse may only read and that under these conditions is not allowed write access. Thus a nurse may read the result of a test that has been performed on the patient, but may not request that a particular test be performed. We may also look at the mental act and ask the question, "what type of decision is it?" For example, is it a decision for which a set of rules governing the outcome may be given? Or is it a decision that calls upon the individual to make some kind of value judgement? The latter kind is a mental act that one may want a computer to assist in the making of, but not one that one would want the computer to make. The decision that the nurse is required to make is a value judgement due to legal aspects of the resulting action. For this reason, the nurses have special educational needs. Consequently, they are not just to be taught to apply a dressing or administer a drug; they are required to make informal diagnoses upon which they act. Thus they need to be taught how to make them and what information they need to make them.

The decision has two possible outcomes: either the nurse can choose to administer the drug, or he/she can refuse. Because of the legal aspects of the system, under no conditions can the nurse be forced to administer the drug Thus, should he/she decide to refuse the doctor's request then he/she must invoke steps to resolve the conflict. We may point to the oval which represents the conversation that the nurse would engage in to resolve the conflict and ask "what informational objects and attributes are required by this conversation?" From the perspective of the hospital, these steps are formally defined and clearly stated for all to see. Assume, however, that the nurse decides to comply with the doctors request.

SUMMARY

The most common problem of requirements engineering in the design and implementation of complex IT systems is combining differing representations of the system and its environments. The operational, organisational, and social environments of a system all possess different characteristics. Hence the core of this approaches philosophy is its advocation of involving policy makers/problem owners throughout the design of the system. It is a process of shifting the balance of responsibility between system owner and system designer away from the 'owner states, designer solves' model towards a relationship in which the problem solver helps the problem owner understand the problem and the problem owner helps the problem solver understand the implications of possible solutions.

Furthermore, used in the context of enterprise modelling, interaction analysis and role relations diagramming have shown, through the use of various case studies, their usefulness in dealing with an organisation's requirements and policies. A major advantage is the degree of flexibility it places within the analyst's control.

ACKNOWLEDGEMENTS

I gratefully acknowledge the contributions made by our colleagues in the ORDIT project to the ideas presented here. In particular we would like to thank Jarnail Chudge, John Dobson, Ros Strens and Alan Underwood for their input on this paper. We also gratefully acknowledge the support of the University of Newcastle upon Tyne and HUSAT Research and Consultancy and financial support afforded by the ESPRIT programme of the CEC (ORDIT Project) and by SERC (Bainbridge Project).

REFERENCES

[1] A.J.C.Blyth, J.Chudge, J.E.Dobson and M.R.Strens, The ORDIT Approach to Requirements Identification, in COMPSAC '92, pp. 356-361, 1992.

[2] A.J.C.Blyth and J.Chudge. The Role of Interaction Analysis in Requirements Engineering, IFIP WG 8.1, Como, Italy, 1993

[3] P. Ehn, Work-Oriented Design of Computer Artifacts, Arbetslivscentrum, Stockholm, 1988, (ISBN 91-86158-45-7).

[4] R.Strens and J.Dobson, Responsibility Modelling as a Technique for Organisational Requirements Definition, Intelligent Systems Engineering, Spring 1994.

[5] T.Winograd and F.Flores, Understanding Computers and Cognition, Addison Wesley, 1987.

A Decision-Support System for the Analysis of Clinical Practice Patterns

E. Andrew Balas, M.D., Ph.D., Zong Rong Li, Ph.D., Joyce A. Mitchell, Ph.D.
Donald C. Spencer, M.D., Edward Brent, Ph.D., Bernard G. Ewigman, M.D., M.S.P.H.

Health Services Management Program, Medical Informatics Group, and
Department of Family and Community Medicine
University of Missouri-Columbia

Several studies documented substantial variation in medical practice patterns, but physicians often do not have adequate information on the cumulative clinical and financial effects of their decisions. The purpose of developing an expert system for the analysis of clinical practice patterns was to assist providers in analyzing and improving the process and outcome of patient care.

The developed QFES (Quality Feedback Expert System) helps users in the definition and evaluation of measurable quality improvement objectives. Based on objectives and actual clinical data, several measures can be calculated (utilization of procedures, annualized cost effect of using a particular procedure, and expected utilization based on peer-comparison and case-mix adjustment).The quality management rules help to detect important discrepancies among members of the selected provider group and compare performance with objectives. The system incorporates a variety of data and knowledge bases: (i) clinical data on actual practice patterns, (ii) frames of quality parameters derived from clinical practice guidelines, and (iii) rules of quality management for data analysis. An analysis of practice patterns of 12 family physicians in the management of urinary tract infections illustrates the use of the system.

INTRODUCTION

There continues to be a widespread concern that medical practice variation, outcome variation, and the limited impact of new scientific information on practice patterns indicate an urgent need to improve the quality of health services in many areas [1]. Studies documented that physicians often agree with medical practice guidelines but actual practice patterns remain unchanged [2].

Continuous quality improvement, a major goal of physicians and health care organizations, requires the ability to alter medical practice patterns [3]. Compliance with accepted practice guidelines is an important issue but the use of guidelines to develop and implement quality improvement programs is still difficult. The individual differences in information needs and appropriate actions are often not recognized. In recent years, various interventions have been recommended but information methods seem to play the critical central role (e.g., education, reminders, feedback).

Several studies have indicated that health care providers are capable of changing their practice styles when confronted with credible information on how they compare to the practice styles of their colleagues [4]. Therefore, comparison to the performance of colleagues is often part of the analyses of clinical practice patterns. Unfortunately, the amount of information on practice styles is often overwhelming and important differences remain undetected.

The aims of this project were to assist groups of health care providers in translating accepted clinical practice guidelines into measurable quality improvement objectives, to compare actual practice patterns with objectives, and measure differences among providers in practice style.

CYCLE OF ANALYSIS

Continuous quality improvement focuses on processes instead of individuals, evaluates through measurement and data, and interprets detected defects as opportunities for improvement. The data processing functions, knowledge bases, and inference engine of QFES were designed to support the critical steps of clinical quality improvement (Fig. 1):

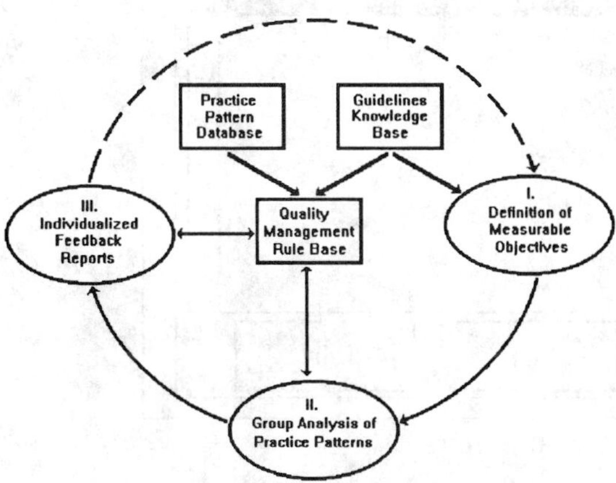

Figure 1 System Structure

I. Definition of a quality improvement plan requires identification of measurable objectives. The system supports the use of a variety of performance-based measures for the purpose of comparing individual data with those of some comparison group. This process is supported by providing a structure for the definition of quality objectives and also a library (knowledge base) of quality parameters (see knowledge representation). The user of QFES can select, edit, and also supplement the practice parameters readily available in the knowledge base (Fig. 2). The quality improvement plan is not only a list of specific objectives but also an important point of reference for subsequent analyses of practice patterns.

II. Evaluation of group performance and variation is based on actual practice data and the quality improvement plan. Analyses of practice variation can generate a large number of data and detection of clinically significant or costly differences can be difficult. The production rules of QFES assist interpretation by detecting significant discrepancies between recommendations and practice patterns and by identifying clinical practice variation among providers. The system combines the following methods in the analysis of practice patterns:

- Four measures are calculated: (i) crude utilization describes the provider-specific frequency of using a selected procedure without adjusting for case-mix differences; (ii) standardized utilization is the crude utilization divided by the utilization expected on the basis of the case-mix of the analyzed provider and practice pattern of his or her peers, (iii) relevant utilization which measures the use of the procedure in the group of eligible patients, and (iv) deviant utilization which measures the use in the group of ineligible patients, as defined by an established clinical practice guideline. Expected utilization is the average utilization rate of the physician group weighted with the number of patients of the analyzed provider in each severity categories.

- The system can express all above listed measures of utilization in three different ways: (i) number of procedures (clinical activities) ordered or performed, (ii) utilization rate (frequency of using a selected procedure), and (iii) cumulative cost effect (annual number of procedures multiplied by the unit costs). For example, the standardized utilization can be expressed as an excess or shortage in the number of procedures performed or ordered by a particular provider.

- The knowledge base of quality management rules and corresponding inference engine assist the interpretation of practice data in the analyses of group performance. The calculation of data leads to a data-driven search which generates messages about significant discrepancies and makes recommendations for possible interventions. The group analyses of data can overview the use of several procedures by all participating providers or, alternatively, can focus on a selected procedure.

III. Based on the results of group

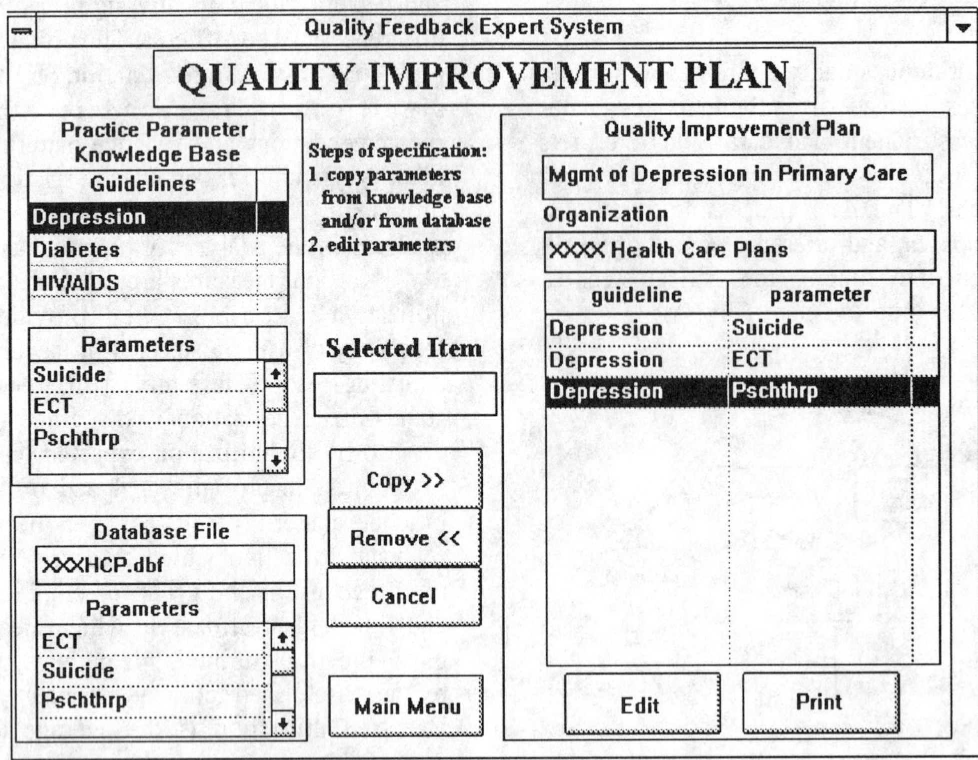

Figure 2 Selection of Quality Parameters

analysis, <u>individualized feedback information</u> will be available for the participating providers. Feedback and corrective action are considered the last steps of quality improvement projects and the QFES is designed to support these steps. Providers will be informed only about those aspects of their practice patterns which indicate achievements or need for improvement.

KNOWLEDGE REPRESENTATION

The unique approach of QFES is the separation of guideline specific and quality management knowledge. Through this separation, the QFES system can effectively handle the recommendations of various and evolving clinical practice guidelines. The user of the system gets full support for modification and supplementation of the structured knowledge which was made available by abstracting clinical practice guidelines. Guidelines can be edited in the knowledge base to make a permanent change or during the process of quality improvement plan development. In the latter case, the knowledge base (library of clinical guidelines) remains unchanged. The current version of the QFES system was built on a Level-5 platform [5] and uses one practice database and two knowledge bases:

<u>Guidelines Knowledge Base</u> This knowledge base is a frame-based representation of clinical quality parameters. Definition of the quality improvement plan requires the identification of measurable objectives and widely accepted clinical practice guidelines are available for this purpose in many areas. However, clinical practice guidelines are usually developed for one-on-one patient care and measures of practice patterns are rarely mentioned. Identification of measurable quality improvement objectives in published clinical practice guidelines requires considerable effort. To support the users of QFES, a library of quality parameters is available for the definition of quality improvement objectives. In the Guidelines Knowledge Base, each quality parameter is described by a name, numerator (procedure), denominator (clinical condition), target range, and a few quotations justifying the

target range with references. The definition of a parameter also includes supportive evidence beyond the quotation from the guidelines (e.g., results of meta-analyses, randomized clinical trials, or other types of original research). The user can copy selected parameters or entire guidelines (sets of parameters) to the quality improvement plan (Fig. 2).

Practice Database The analysis of practice patterns requires cumulative data about the patient care decisions from each participating provider within the specified time period. The input dBASE file consists of seven fields: name of the provider group, beginning and ending dates of the data collection period, provider name or identifier, name of the severity group, number of cases seen by the particular provider in the specified severity group, name of procedure, and number of procedures ordered for the patients of the particular severity group. In comparison to other clinical systems, the size of the practice database is small. Based on six severity groups and 10 parameters, an analysis of the practice patterns of 50 providers would require about 6000 data items (50X6X10 multiplied by two for the numerator and denominator). The size of practice database does not depend on the length of analyzed period or number of procedures performed. This simple and concise structure of cumulated practice data allows calculation of all major utilization measures, including crude utilization, case-mix adjusted utilization, and relevant/deviant utilization.

The Practice Database of the system is a collector of information for the analysis of variation and deviation. The necessary data are defined by the selected clinical practice parameters (measurable objectives). Most commonly used administrative databases do not have sufficient data for the comparison of practice patterns with the specific recommendations of clinical guidelines. However, matching data from different sources can often provide the necessary information. For example, in the analysis of management of diabetes the provider-specific number of patients with diabetes can be identified in the diagnosis-procedure database and the corresponding number of glycosylated hemoglobin determinations can be retrieved from the laboratory database. In developing the QFES system, it was anticipated that the information has to be obtained from variety of sources (e.g., computer file of patient-physician encounters, referral database, or manual chart reviews). It is an obvious advantage to have a comprehensive electronic patient records in place but the lack of such system is not prohibitive.

Management Rule Base This knowledge base is a production rule-based representation of the logic of quality management. In the analyses of clinical practice patterns, many different utilization rates need to be evaluated. In addition, variation and deviation are frequent observations but, often, reflect only random variation or practically insignificant differences. The management rule base contains specific production rules to detect substantial variation in the use of observed procedures or deviation from the recommendations of clinical guidelines. The IF part of the rules specifies the deviation or variation in practice patterns which needs attention and the THEN part specifies a corresponding message of recommendation. One group of rules defines criteria for sending the messages specified in the evidence section of the clinical practice parameters (e.g., if the difference between the recommended rate and the utilization rate of the analyzed provider exceeds 20% then present the listed evidence). The other group of rules interprets practice variation and generates additional messages (e.g., if the utilization rate of the analyzed provider is below the average of the physician group by more than two standard deviations then send a statement on that difference). Through the evaluation of a series of production rules, the QFES system can analyze practice data, compare them to quality improvement objectives, and make recommendation for further actions.

QFES is based on the integration of object oriented techniques, expert system technology, and traditional procedural programming. Objects in the knowledge base were created via class declarations. To facilitate future knowledge sharing, the Management Rule Base and Guidelines Knowledge Base were structured similarly to the logical modules of the Arden Syntax. QFES operates in a Windows environment and has a graphical user interface. Most interactions are menu- and mouse-driven.

CONCLUSIONS

The QFES was first used to analyze practice pattern data in the management of urinary tract infections. The source of data was Callaway Physicians, a non-profit family practice center providing fee-for-service care in Fulton, Missouri. The medical office uses the COSTAR system to support the documentation of patient care. The sample of the study consisted of patients who were diagnosed with cystitis, pyelonephritis, or urinary tract infection during a six month period. A retrospective chart review used a form designed for the analysis of urinary tract infection episodes. The case-mix analysis was based on the recently published clinical practice guidelines for the management of urinary tract infections in adults [6]. The analysis documented that several questions and procedures were used with significantly varying frequencies by different providers. Practice parameters for other applications of the QFES are currently under development (diabetes, depression, and HIV infection/AIDS in primary care).

According to a survey by the American Medical Association, more than half of physicians are subjected to either clinical or economic profiling [7]. It is anticipated that the prevalence of physician profiling will continue to rise. However, most available physician profiling systems produce reports which have no relationship with established clinical practice guidelines. Furthermore, analyses of clinical practice patterns focus on a single selected procedure and not on the process of care. Expensive or hazardous procedures are often subjected to analysis of practice variation. However, it can be very difficult to interpret variation when other clinical actions surrounding the arbitrarily selected procedure are not analyzed. Continuous quality improvement requires reengineering of clinical processes and, therefore, utilization data are needed on the entire sequence of actions. The QFES supports the full spectrum of process analysis and the evaluation can be based on a series of parameters derived from established clinical practice guidelines. The system provides a new structure for knowledge elicited from the medical literature and takes advantage of the common principles and implementation aspects behind the major content differences of various guidelines.

ACKNOWLEDGEMENT

This project was supported in part by grant number HS07715 from the Agency for Health Care Policy and Research.

REFERENCES

1. Soumerai SB, McLaughlin TJ, Avorn J. Improving drug prescribing in primary care: A critical analysis of the experimental literature. Milbank Quarterly 1989;67:268-317.

2. Lomas J, Anderson GM, Domnick-Pierre K, Vayda E, Enkin MW, Hannah WJ. Do practice guidelines guide practice? The effect of a consensus statement on the practice of physicians. N Engl J Med 1989;321:1306-11.

3. Berwick DM. Continuous improvement as an ideal in health care. N Engl J Med 1989;320:53-6.

4. Buck CR, White KL. Peer review: Impact of a system based on billing claims. N Engl J Med 1974;291:877-83.

5. Information Builders. Level 5 Object for Microsoft Windows: Reference Guide, 1994

6. Stamm WE, Hooton TM. Management of urinary tract infection in adults. N Engl J Med 1993;329:1328-33.

7. Emmons DW, Wozniak GD. Profiles and feedback: Who measures physician performance? In Gonzalez ML (Ed) Socioeconomic Characteristics of Medical Practice, AMA,1994.

Caregiver Involvement in a Large Clinical Systems Project

Stephanie Sales, RNNP; Peter Mathews, MD; Doug Gamblin, MS, RRT; Steve Gee, BS
CareGiver Workstation Project
Kaiser Permanente, Northern California Region, Oakland California

ABSTRACT

The Kaiser Permanente Northern California Region (KPNCR) CareGiver Workstation (CGW) Project's mission is to develop and implement a clinical workstation system that will enhance each caregiver-member interaction and aid in the decision-making processes of direct patient care in the inpatient and outpatient settings.

The requirements analysis approach for CareGiver Workstation (CGW) is based on the belief that extensive caregiver involvement will provide a better understanding of the diverse needs of Kaiser Permanente Northern California Region (KPNCR). In order to involve as many caregivers as reasonably possible, CGW included a 16 member caregiver core team and 6 different Medical Centers in the requirements definition process. The Medical Centers are referred to as "focus facilities". A "focus group" (caregiver team) at each selected focus facility consisted of a site coordinator and a 24-30 person multidisciplinary team involving physicians, nurses, therapists and other caregivers. The Medical Center selection process identified facilities that provided the best cross-sectional representation of KPNCR.

The Lead Focus Facility participated in the initial round of requirements definition activities. These sessions assisted in the design of a simulation that was used at five additional Medical Centers to validate requirements. The five additional Focus Facilities participated in simulation review sessions. Feedback from these sessions was used to revise the simulation and update the requirements document. Caregivers from all six focus facilities and other identified groups participated in a requirements survey to assist CGW with identification of high priority features.

Caregiver commitment and continuing involvement are essential for the success of CGW. The development of an initial system that can benefit the largest group of caregivers requires extensive user input and evaluation.

INTRODUCTION

The Kaiser Permanente Northern California Region (KPNCR) CareGiver Workstation (CGW) Project's mission is to develop and implement a clinical workstation system that will enhance each caregiver-member interaction and aid in the decision-making processes of direct patient care in the inpatient and outpatient settings. The system is expected to meet the information system needs of a 2.5 million member Health Maintenance Organization (HMO) and the Region's 30,000 caregivers located at 15 hospitals and 32 clinic offices throughout northern California . CGW has defined a caregiver as any person who provides care directly to a patient. Caregivers include physicians, nurses, therapists, etc. CGW is a large-scale development project which embraces the traditional medical informatics concepts of the Electronic Medical Record, Order Entry & Communications, Decision Support, Clinician Data Capture and Data Presentation. This system will have a significant impact on the delivery of patient care throughout KPNCR.

Caregiver and Information Services (IS) expertise are essential for successful system development and implementation. Therefore, the responsibility for the project is shared by caregivers and IS. The project is jointly managed and staffed with caregivers and IS both accountable for the planning, budgeting and caregiver involvement activities.

CAREGIVER INVOLVEMENT

Management Structure

To obtain adequate caregiver involvement a multilayered strategy was implemented. Different caregiver roles and responsibilities were identified and included in the project plan.

The first layer involves the project's management structure. A full-time Caregiver Manager co-

0195–4210/94/$5.00 © 1994 AMIA, Inc.

manages the project with an IS Manager and a Chief Clinician that represents the physician community. The co-management structure provides for the needs of all users to be represented in decisions affecting the project plan. In addition, a caregiver works on the leadership team with specific responsibility to direct the project communication efforts. This individual, the Communication Administrator, coordinates and helps to manage the caregiver involvement strategy.

Caregiver Core Team

The second layer of caregiver involvement is comprised of the Caregiver Core Team. The Caregiver Core Team includes 16 caregivers (5 nurses, 7 physicians, a respiratory therapist, a unit assistant, a medical assistant and a management engineer) from medical centers throughout KPNCR. The Core Team meets once a week to provide input, direction and critique to the clinical systems development process. Issues are often debated by the Core Team and recommendations are forwarded to Project Management. The Core Team serves as the primary source of system requirements and estimates of cost and benefits. In addition, the Core Team provides a caregiver perspective to the vendor evaluation process.

Focus Facility Involvement

The third layer of caregiver involvement includes caregivers from the Medical Centers. Invitations were extended to all Medical Centers in KPNCR to participate as a CGW "focus facility". Each facility administrative team viewed a presentation describing the CGW Project and the focus facility process. The goal of the focus facility selection process was to identify a combination of six facilities that would provide a cross-sectional representation of KPNCR. Although nearly all facilities indicated a desire to be a focus facility, six facilities were selected based on criteria that included geographic location, facility size, specialty services, clinical information systems experience and administrative support. These six medical centers were selected to participate in identification, validation and prioritization of caregiver requirements.

One of the selected medical centers was chosen as the "lead focus facility". The facility identified an administrative nursing sponsor and a physician sponsor to provide administrative support for focus facility activities. In addition to local sponsorship, the facility also selected a caregiver to function as the facility coordinator. The coordinator works closely with the CGW project team to plan and organize focus facility activities. The facility sponsors and coordinator recruited twenty five caregivers (8 physicians, 8 nurses, 9 others) from the facility to view the early development of requirements simulation software and provide insight for the system analysts. The caregivers included a mix of novice and computer-literate individuals. The caregivers at the facility are responsible for assisting with validation of initial functional requirements, enhancing the system design and providing a "frontline" perspective to the project.

The five additional focus facilities were organized in the same manner as the lead focus facility. Twenty five to thirty caregivers from each facility attended a four hour education session and 4 four-hour sessions to review, validate and prioritize the system's functional requirements. Each of the focus facilities also participated in a 109-question requirements survey to assist in prioritizing system features. The requirements survey was also distributed to selected KPNCR committees and caregiver peer groups.

General Caregiver Involvement

To provide opportunities for involvement of caregivers not associated with the focus facilities, additional activities were organized. Caregivers were interviewed by project analysts to identify issues regarding workflow and data needs. Other caregivers volunteered to be shadowed by an analyst while performing their daily tasks to determine workflow in the "real-life" setting. Presentations were delivered to all interested departments or groups. Individuals interested in the project were added to a contact list for future follow-up. Newsletters, video conferences and a "hot line" were all established to provide contact avenues for the caregiver community.

REQUIREMENTS AND SIMULATION

The primary objectives for Phase II of CGW are to identify the functional requirements of a clinical information system, evaluate the healthcare information systems vendor market, and evaluate the resource requirements associated with custom system development. The caregivers were very involved with identification of the functional requirements. The initial requirements for CGW were developed between June 1993 and January 1994, using the Caregiver Core Team as the primary contributors. The IS systems analysts, all with clinical experience, also conducted interviews and workflow observations which contributed to the requirements. The analysts compiled this information to create the final requirements draft.

The requirements are a detailed description of the caregiver needs of an information system. After completion of the requirements document it was necessary for it to be reviewed by a larger group of caregivers to validate and add to the requirements. Since it was unreasonable to have a large caregiver audience unfamiliar with information systems terminology review the written requirements, a computerized simulation was built to visually communicate the requirements for evaluation and validation. This simulation system was developed using Visual Basic on PC clones. The platform chosen to develop the simulated system allows for quick creation and modification of computer screens. Initial screens were developed by the user team, analysts and programmers from the requirements document.

Simulated requirements viewed by the lead focus facility: 9/93-12/93

1) Access to clinical data
2) Order Entry & Communications
3) Charting in response to an Order (Vital signs, I/O, etc.)
4) Physical exams and structured forms entry
5) Progress notes and free text entry

Simulated requirements viewed by all focus facilities after initial input and prioritization: 2/94-5/94

1) Access, orders, charting
2) Caregiver specific review of all features

The simulation was reviewed by the user team prior to the presenting it to the focus facility. At the focus facility, the caregivers were organized into two groups of approximately 12 caregivers. One group met in the morning and the other in the afternoon. The simulation session began with a short introduction of the requirements in the simulation that day. The group was then separated into subgroups of six caregivers at a computer terminal. Each caregiver was given the opportunity to be the "mouse driver" and actually operate the simulation. One of the systems analysts facilitated the session by guiding the caregivers through a clinical script from which the simulation was developed.

The caregivers viewing the simulation were encouraged to provide uninhibited criticism. All comments and suggestions were considered valid. The systems analysts were specifically instructed not to tell the caregivers what the system would do for them, but to ask the caregivers what they want the system to do for them. The analyst asked questions such as "Would this function work for you? Why or why not? What else would you need? What other functions would you need?". The caregiver responses were recorded by scribes and the requirements and simulation were updated based on the information collected.

The simulation represents the caregivers' conceptual view of the assistance a computer system can provide them in accomplishing their complex tasks. The simulation was also used as a communication tool to show other caregivers the eventual uses of a clinical information system.

Table 1. Caregiver numbers and hours

Caregiver Group	Number	Hours
Core Team	17	5848
Focus Facilities	185	3940
Interviews	76	152
Observations	15	60
Presentations	1083	1083
Totals	1376	11083

The Kaiser Permanente Northern California Region (KPNCR) CareGiver Workstation (CGW) Project's mission is to develop and implement a clinical workstation system that will enhance each caregiver-member interaction and aid in the decision-making processes of direct patient care in the inpatient and outpatient settings.

SURVEYS

The simulation itself could not provide all the information needed to proceed with developing and prioritizing system features. The development team and the caregivers completed the requirements identification process, but additional input was needed to prioritize system features. A survey was developed to query the caregiver population on the urgency of system features.

A 109-question survey was developed from the requirements document. Questions were divided into 5 categories:

I. Care Support
Questions 1-15
II. Viewing Clinical Information
Questions 16-34
III. Order Entry and Communications
Questions 35-65
IV. Care Documentation
Questions 66-109
V. Demographic information

The survey was designed to determine the importance of certain system features. Each question was rated by the caregiver on a scale from 1 to 5, with 1 "not at all important" and 5 "extremely important". The survey was initially administered to the focus groups and selected committees. Two hundred and one surveys were returned. It was also distributed at presentations to clinical groups and to specific individuals on the project contact list.

Example of high priority survey results: (numbers indicate the mean result for that item)

I. Care Support
•Obvious indication for abnormal results not viewed (4.55)
•Simple management of job related tasks (4.53)

II. Viewing Clinical Information
•Patient medication lists with dates and dosages (4.53)
•Viewing patient lab results (4.48), physician notes (4.47), summary problem list (4.46), allergies and adverse reactions to medications (4.37).

III. Order Entry and Communications
(types of orders desired)
•Laboratory (4.64)
•Pharmacy (4.60)
•Consults (4.25)
•Nursing and Diagnostic Imaging (4.12)

IV. Care Documentation (types of documentation)
•Patient problems and diagnosis (4.63)
•Document findings from the patient interview & examination (4.62)
•Document medication administration (4.38)
•Documentation devices should be located on the nursing station (4.86), in the physician office (4.77) and in the exam room (4.29)

In addition, the survey validated that having a partial order entry system (e.g. inpatient only), was not desirable and that caregivers would like to have some level functionality immediately, rather than wait for new technology to mature. (Such as voice recognition, pen computing, handwriting recognition, etc.) The survey results also indicated that there were very few differences between physicians, nurses and other caregivers in the placement of the top 3 or 4 items in each section.

The surveys were instrumental in planning the development strategy of the CGW. The results of the surveys were used to divide the features into three "levels". Level I contained the critical features for a useful system and will be pursued first. Level II includes features that will be added after the initial system features are available to all KPNCR. Level III includes all additional features necessary to allow the paper chart to be replaced with an electronic medical record.

Next Steps

The next phases of the project will continue to involve caregivers in all activities. After the completion of the analysis phase and selection of a development approach an initial test Medical Center or "beta site" will be selected. The beta site will focus on reengineering care as well as the technical implementation of CGW. All caregivers at the beta site will be involved in the reengineering efforts and system implementation activities. Analysis of the effect of automation on the beta site will assist the project determine the implementation processes for all of KPNCR.

References

1. E. M. Rogers, Diffusion of Innovations Third Edition. The Free Press, New York, 1983

2. R. Grayson, Kaiser Permanente, "MOCIS Phase I Evaluation Report". Kaiser Permanente, Oakland, June 1993

3. J Dewey, MD, P. Manning, BA, S. Brandt, MD, "Acceptance of Direct Physician Access to a Computer-Based Patine Record in a Managed Care Setting" Proceedings from SCAMC, November 1993

Tools & Approaches for Contemporary Problems in Health Administration

Building a Database of Data Sets for Health Services Research

Sandra J. Frawley, Ph.D.
Center for Medical Informatics and Department of Epidemiology and Public Health
Yale University School of Medicine, New Haven, CT

The Database of Data Sets (DB/DS) for Health Services Research will be an online searchable directory of data sets which are available, often with restrictions and confidentiality safeguards, for use by health care researchers. The DB/DS project is aimed at a wide audience, and intends to include a very broad range of health care data sets, ranging from state hospital discharge data bases, to national registries and health survey data sets, to institutional clinical databases. The intended users are the same community of researchers, policy-makers, administrators and practitioners who are served by the National Library of Medicine's current bibliographic databases. This paper describes a pilot phase of the DB/DS project in which the issues involved in creating such a database were explored with an initial set of 20 representative data sets.

INTRODUCTION

A Database of Data Sets (DB/DS) for Health Services Research is under development by the National Library of Medicine through its recently created National Information Center on Health Services Research and Health Care Technology. Growing out of work on the Unified Medical Language System Information Sources Map, the DB/DS will be an online searchable directory of data sets which are available, often with restrictions and confidentiality safeguards, for use by health services researchers.

With the establishment of the Agency for Health Care Policy and Research (AHCPR) in 1989, Congress set out as national priorities 1) the conduct of medical effectiveness research, and 2) the creation of clinical practice guidelines based on the results of past, present, and future research. The importance of bringing such information to clinical practice is an important theme of the health care reform proposals being considered in 1994.

Recognizing that time, resources, and sometimes ethical considerations will frequently not permit the use of prospective clinical studies to explore the efficacy of clinical treatment and patterns of care, various organizations, including the Institute of Medicine, have urged that researchers be given better information about and access to previously collected data (1). It is likely that research funding will be increasingly available for secondary analysis of data rather than for primary data collection and analysis. As a result, there is a major need to store information about such data sets in an organized fashion so that it can be searched easily by diverse researchers.

Health services researchers, broadly defined, span the spectrum from social scientists who study the organization and financing of medical care to clinicians who evaluate the relative effectiveness of alternative medical treatments. Among the social scientists, there is historically a greater tendency to utilize national or state data sets that have been collected by organizations other than the researchers themselves. With research questions focusing more on community patterns of disease and the outcomes of individual diseases and procedures, epidemiologists and clinical researchers have been less interested in the use of previously collected data. Rather, the emphasis has been on prospective, primary data collection efforts and using randomized clinical trials to evaluate treatments. Recently, however, there has been extensive discussion and debate about the feasibility and desirability of using existing administrative and clinical data sets for researching medical effectiveness issues (2-5).

The DB/DS project is aimed at a wide audience, and intends to include a very broad range of health care data sets, ranging from state hospital discharge data bases, to national registries and health survey data sets, to institutional clinical databases. Data sets sponsored or created by government agencies, private foundations, private corporations, and health care institutions will be included. The intended users are the same community of researchers, policy-makers, administrators and practitioners who are served by the National Library of Medicine's bibliographic databases such as MEDLINE, Health Planning and Administration, and Health Services/Technology Assessment Research (HSTAR).

A central issue in building the DB/DS is determining how best to code (catalog) the various data sets to serve the needs of health services researchers.

Researchers looking for secondary sources of data often start by asking where they can find information about a particular population they want to study, e.g., elderly Hispanics with congestive heart failure. As a result, the coding of a data set has to provide an accurate description of its content: the unit of analysis (the entities about which data has been collected) and the variables (the data items collected). The researcher also needs to understand the methodology of data collection and the quality of the data produced, both of which will affect the suitability of the data set for the researcher's purposes. In many instances, the researcher may want to combine data from several sources, so issues of linkability among data sets become important. Technical issues such as the formatting of data files and the electronic media in which the data set is available may determine whether the researcher will be able to analyze the data at his/her institution. Finally, he or she needs to understand the data access procedures, e.g., any restrictions that apply, from whom the data set can be acquired, and the likely cost.

This paper describes a pilot phase of the DB/DS project in which these issues were explored with an initial set of 20 representative data sets.

RELATED WORK

The need for flexible access to data sets is widely acknowledged. Two examples of systems which have approached this problem are described below.

The Centers for Disease Control and Prevention (CDC) recently made 24 public health databases available for on-line searching and data analysis through CDC WONDER (6). This system contains various data sets from national health and hospital discharge surveys as well as textual and bibliographic databases such as the Morbidity and Mortality Weekly Report. CDC WONDER users can search with keywords and be directed to the relevant databases. Because the data are stored online, users have immediate access to the information and can download selected data into personal computers.

On a much larger scale, though with less user search and analysis capability, are the data set archives developed by the Inter-university Consortium for Social and Political Research (ICPSR) at the University of Michigan (7). Started over thirty years ago, the archives now contain about 600 gigabytes in more than 30,000 machine readable data files, including a substantial number of health-related data sets. Users may search an online directory of ICPSR data sets using a SPIRES interface or a gopher server. A small number of frequently requested files are stored on a Sun workstation and made available to users by network file transfer protocol. Most data sets must be purchased in magnetic tape, CD-ROM, or diskette format.

Several differences between these programs and the NLM's new database are important to recognize. The NLM does not plan to archive coded data sets, nor put them online. Instead, detailed information about the contents, format, purpose, source, restrictions on use, and availability will be maintained online in a searchable database. Many data sets that will be coded are proprietary. Others exist as institutional information systems, from which data would have to be extracted for research purposes.

SELECTING DATA SETS FOR THE DB/DS PILOT PROJECT

During the pilot phase of the DB/DS project described in this paper, the goal was to develop an efficient yet robust coding scheme that would capture the information researchers will want to know about a data set, using a pilot group of 20 data sets. We wanted the 20 data sets chosen for initial coding to be representative of the great variety that will eventually be contained in the database. As a result, the main emphasis was on selecting data sets with different contents in terms of the units of analysis and types of information collected. Not surprisingly, the pilot group also showed wide variety in size, sponsorship, methodology, and accessibility.

Although the DB/DS project is not designed to be an archive of data sets, it became clear that accurate coding requires that a hard copy, or machine-readable copy, of the data set documentation be available to the coder. As a result, it is necessary to assemble this material as a reference tool during the coding process even though the actual data files themselves will not be acquired. Data sets that are created by federal government agencies and sold through HCFA, the NTIS or CDC tend to have extensive documentation available for users, including data dictionaries, data instruments, codebooks and tape layout descriptions. This material frequently includes the instructions originally given to the data collection team. Other data sets were established for institutional use and without the expectation that external researchers might utilize the data. These data sets often do not have documentation that can be made readily available to external users, even when there exists internal documentation appropriate for the needs of institutional users.

The listing below shows the group of 20 data sets coded for the pilot study.

Clinical Records

1. Duke DataBank for Cardiovascular Disease (Duke University Medical Center, Durham, NC)
2. HELP System Data Base (LDS Hospital, Salt Lake City, UT)

Discharge Summaries

3. Healthcare Cost and Utilization Project, 1988-1994 (AHCPR)
4. National Hospital Discharge Survey, 1988 (NCHS)
5. NY State Hospital Discharge Data Files, 1991 (NY State Department of Health)

Claims Records

6. MEDSTAT Market Scan Data Base (MEDSTAT Systems)
7. Quality Care MEDPAR File, 1988 (HCFA)
8. Standard Analytical Inpatient Public Use File, 1992 (HCFA)
9. Standard Analytical Physician/Supplier Public Use File, 1991 (HCFA)

Epidemiological Surveys

10. Tecumseh Community Health Study, 1959-1969 (Victor Hawthorne, et al.)

Health/Behavioral/Social Surveys

11. National Medical Expenditure Survey, 1987 (AHCPR)
12. National Health Interview Survey, 1988 (NCHS)
13. National Long Term Care Survey, 1982-1984 (DHHS)
14. National Survey of Access to Medical Care, 1982 (Ronald M. Andersen and Lu Ann Aday)

Disease Registries

15. ARAMIS - Arthritis, Rheumatism, and Aging Medical Information System (American Rheumatism Association)
16. Cancer Surveillance and Epidemiology in the United States and Puerto Rico, 1973-1977 (National Cancer Institute)

Birth Registries

17. Natality Detailed Data File, 1988 (CDC)

Data About Practitioners

18. AMA Physician Master File, 1992 (American Medical Association)

Data About Programs and Facilities

19. National Evaluation of Rural Primary Health Care programs, 1979-1982 (Cecil G. Sheps and Edward H. Wagner)
20. National Nursing Home Survey, 1985 (NCHS)

CODING THE DATA SETS

The main purpose of the pilot project was to explore the issues that arise in coding a representative group of data sets, and to develop an initial coding strategy which will be refined over time as the project evolves. In the coding scheme developed during the pilot project, 42 fields are available to describe the data sets, although not all fields are used for each entry. Some are free text, while others require that selections be made from pre-defined choices. The basic data provided for each data set include its name and any alternative names, the source (creator), a general description of the data set and the purpose for its creation, the person who prepared the entry, and the date of the entry.

Content of the Data Set: Roughly half of the fields deal with the content of the data set. After this content is summarized in a free text general description field, a series of fixed choice fields provide more precise information: whether the data set uses a standard vocabulary or coding scheme, such as DRG or CPT; whether it contains a standard or minimum set of variables, e.g., UB-82; the unit(s) of analysis; the setting(s) of data collection; the timeframe; geographic locations and level of detail; age groups included; ethnic groups included; and a listing either of individual variables (if fewer than 25) or of categories of variables.

Methodology: Methodology fields provide information on the universe, the sample size, sampling procedures, and mechanisms of data collection. A free text field allows for brief comments on methodology issues.

Published References: Two fields are intended to assist researchers in using the published literature to learn about a particular data set. The REFerences field gives citations to publications describing the data set, while STUdies contains citations to publications which have analyzed the data set. In addition, an eventual goal is for the DB/DS to contain a unique identifier for each data set that can be published in research reports and included in NLM database citations.

Accessibility: Accessibility fields describe the restrictions which may be placed on data use and access and also list address and cost information about the providers (vendors) of the data set.

Linking Data Sets: Many data sets are produced as part of annual or periodic surveys and other data collection efforts, e.g. the National Hospital Discharge Survey, the National Health Interview Survey, and the Natality Detailed Data File. Common data elements appearing over time facilitate longitudinal investigations. Other data sets can be linked together because the same personal identifier, e.g., patient number or physician license number, is used, as in various Medicare files. Probabilistic matching algorithms are being developed to permit data file linking even when common identifier numbers are not used (8). When links to other data sets are known, they can be described in the Related Entries field.

Technical Information: Information about technical documentation, the editing of data, the quality of data, the size, format, and structure of electronic data are provided in technical information fields. As described previously, the availability of technical information in the written documentation is quite variable.

CODING ISSUES THAT AROSE

In this section we discuss certain problematical issues that arose in developing a coding strategy for the pilot group of data sets.

Quality of the Data

After questions of content, perhaps the most critical issue for researchers is the quality of the data. This has proved to be the most difficult to capture within the coding scheme because there is usually not very much discussion of data quality in written documentation. In addition, quality may be highly variable from item to item within a data set. Researchers will be able to draw some inferences about quality from coded information about sampling and data collection methods.

An excellent source of information is likely to be the principal investigator or research director in the organization which created the data set. Over time however, this information becomes more difficult to retrieve. Personal memories fade and data producing organizations rarely invest many resources in documenting the decisions associated with data collection and production (9). Similarly, other researchers who have used the data set could have useful insights into data problems and limitations. It would be an interesting challenge to create a vehicle within this proposed database for researchers to communicate their discoveries about a data set.

Coding Tried and Discarded, and Why

An early version of the DB/DS coding included a field to indicate the likelihood that a data set could be used for each of 17 types of health services research. The different types of health services research, ranging from treatment effectiveness and outcomes studies to cost and utilization assessments, were based on discussions in recent publications of the Institute of Medicine, the NLM, and the AHCPR. We soon recognized, however, that it would be difficult for a data set coder to make a definitive judgment about the suitability of a data set for a particular purpose, and that researchers themselves have the responsibility of making such determinations. Furthermore, we were aware that in the dynamic field of health services research, 17 brief phrases were not likely to be a satisfactory statement of the breadth and depth of research concerns.

We also did not attempt to rate data sets according to the AHCPR's medical effectiveness criteria for database content (10). Two of these criteria are that treatment information and outcome information be included. There is a vast difference in the amount and usefulness of treatment or outcome data which appear in a discharge abstract, for example, and that which might appear in a computer-based patient record or observational study record. Rather than make judgments about the adequacy of treatment and outcome information, it appeared more reasonable to use the Variables or Variable Categories field to describe what treatment- and outcome-related data items actually appear in the records.

DISCUSSION

In performing this pilot analysis, we have attempted to look at a range of different data sets that illustrate a variety of issues that need to be confronted both in coding and in using the DB/DS. A number of interesting issues arose, as discussed below.

Great Variation in Number of Data Items
There were extreme differences in the number of variables included in different data sets. A few, e.g., Cancer Surveillance, contained only a handful of variables which may be handled by explicitly listing those variables. Other data sets, e.g., National Long-Term Care Survey, contained thousands of variables which therefore had to be summarized. Since even exact variable names can obscure the meaning of a data item, e.g., "Claim Non-Covered Day Count," coders will not always be accurate in describing the content of data items when summarizing large numbers of variables. As a result, facilitating user access to documentation, such as data dictionaries, codebooks and instruments, would be very helpful. We are exploring the possibility of making documentation available on the Internet via FTP so that researchers could immediately learn data definitions and see the actual wording of questions.

Differences in Scope and Accessibility
Many data sets, e.g., National Hospital Discharge Survey, exist as a public use file, readily available for purchase. Other data sets, e.g., the AMA Physician Masterfile, are very large files, from which researchers typically request a subset dealing with a particular specialty or region. Still other data sets, e.g., HELP, are large dynamic clinical information systems, from which a customized subset of data would be extracted with appropriate safeguards for patient confidentiality and with institutional approval.

Through the data set coding, users of the DB/DS should be informed about special procedures they must follow in order to gain access to institutional data. For example, external researchers have entered into collaborative efforts with Duke researchers to utilize the DataBank for Cardiovascular Disease.

Single vs. Multiple File Structures
While many data sets exist as a single file, others have multiple data files, each with a different unit of analysis and format, but all linked together because the information was gathered as part of a single research effort. To accommodate complex data sets such as the National Health Interview Survey, the coding scheme has the flexibility to allow differentiation of the content and technical descriptions of the various parts.

SUMMARY

Our experiences in the pilot phase of database development have suggested that coders will find great variation in the information they will have to work with in coding data sets. The coding scheme is evolving to be highly, even redundantly, descriptive, but not to require evaluative judgments by coders. We cannot anticipate all the inquiries and methods that health services researchers will bring to this database, and we are content to let users make their own judgments after following the leads we can offer.

Acknowledgements: This work was supported in part by NIH contract N01 LM13537 from the National Library of Medicine. The author would like to acknowledge the participation of Betsy L. Humphreys and Marjorie A. Cahn of the National Information Center on Health Services Research and Health Care Technology at the National Library of Medicine, for whom this work was performed.

References

[1]. Harris-Wehling J, Morris LC, Eds.: Improving Information Services for Health Services Researchers: A Report to the National Library of Medicine. (Washington, D.C.: Institute of Medicine), 1991.
[2]. Kane RL, Lurie N: Appropriate effectiveness: A tale of carts and horses. QRB 18(10):322-6, 1992.
[3]. Grady ML, Schwartz HA, Eds: Medical Effectiveness Research Data Methods. USDHHS, Public Health Service, AHCPR Pub. No. 92-0056, July, 1992.
[4]. Statistics in Medicine 10(4), 1991, entire issue.
[5]. International Journal of Technology Assessment in Health Care 6(2), 1990, entire issue.
[6]. Freide A, Reid JA, Ory HW: CDC WONDER: A comprehensive on-line public health information system of the Centers for Disease Control and Prevention. American Journal of Public Health 83:1289-94, 1993.
[7]. Inter-university Consortium for Political and Social Research: Guide to Resources and Services, 1993-1994, (Ann Arbor, MI: ICPSR), 1993.
[8]. Roos LL, Wajda A: Record linkage strategies. Part I: Estimating information and evaluating approaches. Methods of Information in Medicine. 30(2):117-23, 1991.
[9]. David MH: Systems for Metadata: Documenting Scientific Databases. SSRI Workshop Series, 9221, (Madison, WI: University of Wisconsin), 1992.
[10]. AHCPR: Feasibility of Linking Research-Related Data Bases to Federal and Non-Federal Medical Administrative Data Bases. USDHHS, Public Health Service, AHCPR Pub. No. 1991-0003, April, 1991.

Providing Easy Access to Distributed Medical Data

Bill Lord, Mark Tucker, Aninda DasGupta, and Mike Shneier
Philips Laboratories, Briarcliff Manor, New York

Many hospitals are fragmented along departmental boundaries, leading to islands of information about patients. This makes data integration difficult, and therefore can increase hospital costs and reduce patient care. This paper presents an architecture to provide uniform and transparent access to computerized data and functions available in this kind of heterogeneous computer environment.

INTRODUCTION

This paper presents an architecture to assist in accessing data and executing functions in a heterogeneous and fragmented information-gathering environment such as a hospital. The work is a component of a project undertaken to address problems that arise when medical practitioners need to access information from diverse sources[5]. A number of potential applications are envisaged, for example, reviewing a patient's record before a visit, preparation for interventions or surgery, producing diagnostic reports following a visit or procedure, and tele-consultations. Our project provides the information and tools needed to generate reports and review current patient records. A prototype application has been developed in the domain of cardiology.

Many of our goals are shared by other groups [7, 8, 12]. For example, the Hermes workstation project at Erasmus University in the Netherlands tries to integrate existing hardware and software into a physician's workstation [8, 9] without requiring substantial reprogramming. Our Data Server is a more general version of the Data Translator, Command Generator, and Network Facilitator modules that they have implemented, but the goals of hiding the details of communications protocols, the location of data, and the command language needed to retrieve the data are the same. Marrs et. al. at Washington University School of Medicine in St. Louis have implemented a system that integrates data from distributed heterogenous systems overnight, providing a global, unified view of this data by duplicating it on a central server[7]. Our Data Server provides the same global, unified view of the data, but without creating a new database.

The Current Dilemma in Medical Informatics

A typical hospital is made up of islands of information. Figure 1 shows a representative subset of a hospital's collection of computer systems. These systems are usually built around departments in a hospital, with each department storing the information it collects in its own computer system. Without a network between these systems, data from one department's computer system is often printed to paper, carried or faxed to another department, and then either scanned, re-entered manually or kept as paper. In fact, most patient records are still paper based even though almost 40 percent of their records were originally computer-generated [2].

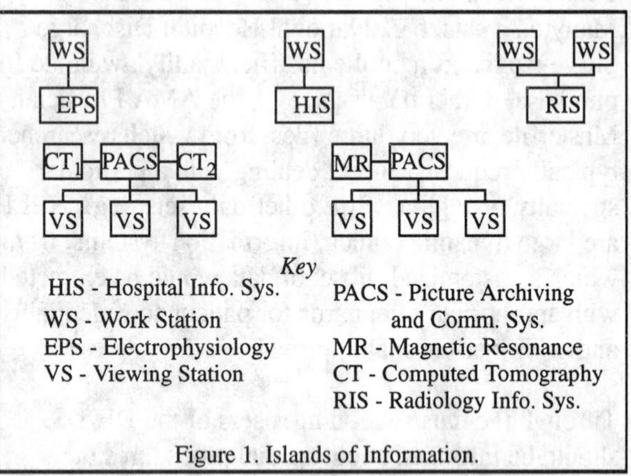

Figure 1. Islands of Information.

Simply networking different departments together is not sufficient to provide access between departments. There is still the potential problem of each system having a different operating system and/or database query language since each department typically chooses the computer system that best suits its needs. To obtain information from the islands requires knowledge specific to each system that will be accessed. The premise behind our work is that end users and application programmers want to be insulated from the details of data access. They want to think only in terms of available functionality and data models. They do not want to have to think in terms of protocols, data and function location, and data formats. Thus, we have developed methods to hide these system-specific details. Our solution focuses on information access techniques that enable site-independence. It is designed to allow the system to be introduced at a new location without requiring additional programming.

Possible Solutions

A common approach to integrating information from a large number of sources is to use a hub concept, in which a central location serves to integrate and often to store the information. In most of these systems (e.g., [3, 6, 7]), the information sources are expected to transmit information to the hub at scheduled times or as it becomes available. The hub integrates the information and responds to queries from users or other systems. It can also redistribute information. An advantage of the hub concept is that it is relatively easy to implement and may simplify the problem of maintaining consistency in the data. Disadvantages are that the hub has to store copies of all information, that network traffic is increased, and that the hub can potentially become a bottleneck.

The approach that we have taken is based on what we call a Data Server. The Data Server presents a single data model for the collection of a hospital's data. It functions by having knowledge of where and how requested data are stored, not by storing all data in a central repository. The data server accepts requests and forwards them to the appropriate system in the proper format for that system.

What the hub systems and the Data Server have in common is that they both hide from the user the idiosyncrasies of the information sources. While a hub system stores data, the Data Server stores information on how and from where to retrieve and manipulate data. In both cases, a connection to the equipment must be built. If there is no well-defined query language (such as SQL) and the system does not support HL7 [4], then a custom data interface must be written and installed on the system.

Our initial goal for the Data Server was to provide database access to all hospital data without needing knowledge of where the data actually reside. In the same way that we want to provide uniform access to data, we also want to be able to access the collection of available functions (such as image processing, for example) from all the hospital's systems in a uniform way.

The purpose of this paper is to discuss the architecture and various configurations for our Data Server. To set the stage for this, we give a brief overview of what a simple Data Server configuration does and how it works.

OVERVIEW OF THE DATA SERVER

The Data Server provides uniform and transparent access to electronically available information in a hospital. The Data Server unifies all communication needs and provides common entry and exit points for exchanges between different systems. The Data Server is the only system that needs to know all the communication protocols and database query languages used in hospitals, clinics, or satellite offices. When it receives a request, the Data Server must determine where to find the necessary information and must also know how to ask the owner of the information to retrieve it. It often has to break a request into a number of simpler requests, each of which is sent to a different information source using the language expected by that source. Information may be returned in any order and at any time, so the Data Server has to reconstruct the answer to the request, remembering which pieces belong to which requester, and send the answer using the proper protocol back to the user. Because many systems that supply information are dedicated to information-gathering, they may not be able to accept or respond to requests except at specified times. Thus, the Data Server must handle queues both for requests and for responses. The architecture allows for more than one Data Server to operate at the same time, so bottlenecks can be avoided.

Data Dictionaries

Data Dictionaries are a key resource of the Data Server. Data Dictionaries give the appearance, and are accessed as if they were simple tables of a relational database. However, instead of containing the actual data sought, they contain the precise descriptions needed to retrieve the data requested from its source. Entries include information about the device on which the requested information is stored, how to format a query for that device, how to interpret a response from the device, and if needed, how to expand the single query into a collection of multiple queries. This latter information allows for both simple and complex queries to appear to the requesting application program as simple requests. For example, a request from an admissions workstation for the description of a patient's last hospital visit will be expanded in the Data Server into requests to one or more devices for a date, location, and problem for that visit. These results will be collected on the Data Server, formatted into a single response and sent back to the requesting workstation. Specifying how to interpret results from various systems allows for the data server to run functions on collected data to adjust for mismatched schemas before sending the results back to the requesting application. An example of this would be an entry in the Data Dictionary that specifies that a function to convert pounds to kilograms be run whenever a patient's weight is obtained from the hospital's Hospital Information System (HIS).

We have developed a graphical user interface for specifying the layout and contents of the data dictionaries. This specification will typically be done by a system administrator who is knowledgable about the data schemas of each of the individual systems that is to be integrated into the virtual database of the Data Server. The Data Dictionary can be set up as a single global view of the union of all the data from all the systems in the hospital, or it can be set up to have a collection of multiple views of either all the data or various subsets of it.

Data Server Functions. We model how the Data Server works at the function level after work in the object oriented systems community [11]. This model requires all systems on a network to support a standard way of registering their addresses and what they can offer to others, as well as an authentication and access control mechanism. The Data Server becomes a distributed services broker, acting as an intermediary between clients (processes needing services) and service providers (processes controlling access to services). Services may include much more than information retrieval or storage. The client does not need to know where on the network the services are provided, or how the desired results are generated. Similarly, the server does not need to know for which clients it is providing the information (assuming that the authentication and security aspects are properly dealt with). Two evolving standards activities that address this architecture are the ISO/CCITT Open Distributed Processing (ODP) effort and the Object Management Group's Common Object Request Broker (CORBA) [10, 11].

Data Server Components

The Data Server consists of three kinds of components: client adapters, a request processor, and server adapters.

Client Adapter. The client adapter accepts incoming requests in a particular protocol from a client and calls an interface to the request processor. The role of the adapter is to convert system-specific protocols to and from a standard format. A client, in our terminology, is any process that requests information from a Data Server. Client adapters can be built for any known protocol. Currently we have client adapters for ACR-NEMA 2.0, HL7, and an internal protocol [1, 4]. These adapters can all run within a single process, or run as separate processes. More than one of each kind of adapter can run simultaneously. It is possible to have one adapter per client. A client adapter can run on the same system as the request processor portion of the Data Server, or separately.

Request Processor. The request processor supports different kinds of requests. Our discussion focuses on one class of request, data queries. The request processor for data queries consists of a request parser that creates request objects, and a request engine that executes them. In the request parser, queries are parsed (broken down) into atomic database calls. The collection of atomic calls forms the main content of a request object. These atomic database calls consist only of requests that are simple enough to be handled even by the least sophisticated of databases. For example, a query to find all of the reports written for all catheterization procedures performed on patient Jane Doe, would be broken in to three simple requests: 1. Find *Patient ID* given *Patient Name* of Jane Doe, 2. Find all the *Procedure IDs* for catheterization procedures performed with the *Patient ID* returned from the first simple request, and 3. Find all the *Reports* associated with all the *Procedure IDs* found in the second simple request. When sent to the request engine the atomic calls consist of three parameters: a relation name, an attribute name to search in, and the attribute's name from which to obtain the result. When the request is ready to be processed, a fourth parameter is added: the value to search for. If the original query to the request processor ends up as more than one atomic call, then each atomic call may have to go to a different system.

The request engine sequentially takes each atomic call and determines which process on the network can answer it. We refer to these processes as "servers," which usually, but not necessarily, run on a system other than the Data Server. Examples of typical servers are HIS and RIS systems. The atomic call is passed on to the server adapter for the server that holds the desired information. After passing on the atomic call, the request engine is free to service another request object. Further processing of a request object can be resumed after the server replies. After an atomic call is completed and the request engine is re-entered, the results of the atomic call will be used as the search values for the next atomic call

Server Adapter. A server adapter fulfils two purposes. First, it determines if the system to which the request is destined can handle multiple requests or not. Second, when the request is ready to send, the server adapter translates the parameters given by the atomic call into a system-specific request needed to obtain the desired information. If the information server can handle multiple requests, the request is sent out. If not, the request is put on a queue for that system. Because the server adapter may be required to maintain a queue for the server, only one server adapter can exist for each server. Server adapters can run one per process, or grouped into one or more processes.

DATA SERVER ARCHITECTURES

There is a lot of flexibility in the architecture for putting together the components of the Data Server. The simplest architecture has all three Data Server components running in the same process. This configuration is shown in Figure 2 and is based on the representative systems of a hospital presented in Figure 1.

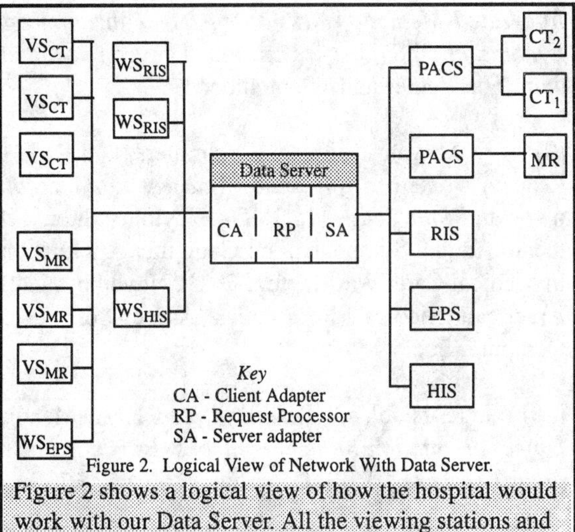

Figure 2. Logical View of Network With Data Server.

Figure 2 shows a logical view of how the hospital would work with our Data Server. All the viewing stations and the workstations would get information they needed from the data sources via the data server. Thus allowing for location hiding.

However, this configuration can lead to a bottleneck. We address this potential problem in two ways. First, most requests made to the Data Server are of low bandwidth while the answers may require high bandwidth. For example, a request for a patient's cine loop from a recent catheterization could be less than 100 bytes long. The data set requested could be on the order of tens of megabytes. Sending this from the archives system to the requester via the Data Server could take twice as long as sending it directly, and would tie up valuable resources. Instead the archives can either send the data set directly to the requestor, or send the requestor enough information about accessing the data that the requestor can then access it directly.

The second approach we have taken to alleviate the problem of a Data Server becoming a bottleneck is to have parts of the Data Server duplicated, and running in a distributed environment. One logical configuration is to use a client adapter and request processor for each cluster, and a server adapter for each information source. Each client adapter/request processor pair can run separately in its own address space, or they can co-exist in a process with the client. Similarly, a server adapter and server can run separately or within the same process. Figure 3 shows different configurations of the Data Server.

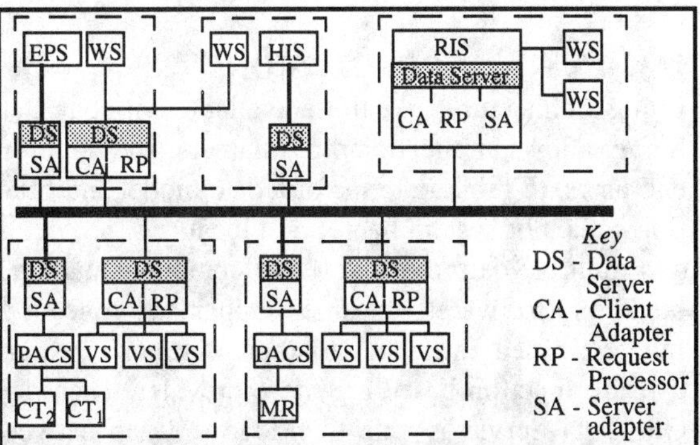

Figure 3. View of Network With Distributed and Redundant Components of the Data Server.

In this figure we see that the client adapter / request processor pair in the Electrophysiology Department runs as a separate process and is shared by the workstation associated with the hospital information system. The Radiology Information System has all three components of a Data Server compiled in with its code and all running as one process. The Magnetic Resonance cluster and the Computed Tomography cluster show typical configurations for cluster based topologies.

FUNCTION BASED INTERFACES

In the preceding sections we examined the use of the Data Server to provide uniform access to data. By expanding on the idea, the Data Server can become a means to uniformly access many of the other functions offered by the systems in a hospital, such as image processing, text processing, and drug interaction checking. In a manner similar to how it keeps knowledge of where data reside and the protocols required to retrieve them, the Data Server can also keep track of where available functions reside and how they can be executed.

In an ideal setup, each system on a network would advertise its capabilities and provide a standard method of accessing them. In this case the Data Server, if necessary at all, would only have to act as the "yellow pages." Because this ideal world does not exist yet, the Data Server is designed to give the appearance that it does.

Functions do not have to be a one-to-one mapping to the actual functions of the various systems on the hospital's network. For example a function on the request processor may advertise that it can supply annotated images, when in fact no system in the hospital supplies this capability directly. Instead the request processor has to retrieve the image in question from a PACS system, and then retrieve the dictation from another system and combine the two files together in the appropriate multimedia format for return to the requesting system.

CONCLUSION

Using architectures like those available with our Data Server allows application programmers, and therefore end users, to think in terms of a data model and function calls, not system names and locations, protocols, and multiple data models. Many computer manufacturers and software companies support the concept of function-based interfaces to their systems. Systems that are function based are more prevalent each day. Our Data Server is able to bridge the gap between older and current day systems, providing the benefits of seamless data integration and function specification.

References

[1] *ACR-NEMA Dig. Imaging and Comm. Stds. Ctee.,* ACR-NEMA 300-1985:Digital Imaging and Communications. 1985

[2] M. L. Cannavo. *Fitting radiology into the hospital of tomorrow.* Diagnostic Imaging, pages 131-133. April 1990.

[3] A. C. Curtis. *Multi-facility integration: An approach to synchronized electronic medical records in a decentralized health care system.* In Lun et al., editors, Proceedings of the Seventh World Congress on Medical Informatics (MEDINFO 92), Geneva, Switzerland, September 1992, pages 138-143. IFIP and IMIA, North-Holland.

[4] Health Level Seven, 900 Victor's Way Suite 122, Ann Arbor, MI 48108. *Health Level Seven: An Application Protocol For Electronic Data Exchange In Healthcare Environments.* Version 2.1.

[5] H. K. Huang, R. L. Areson. *Multimedia demands integrated databases.* Diagnostic Imaging. Vol. 15, #11. November 1993.

[6] S. B. Johnson, P. D. Clayton, D. Fink, et al. *Achievements in phase III of an integrated academic information management system.* In Lun et al., editors, Proceedings of the Seventh World Congress on Medical Informatics (MEDINFO 92), Geneva, Switzerland, September 1992, pages 117-123. IFIP and IMIA, North-Holland.

[7] K. A. Marrs, S. A. Steib, C. A. Abrams, and M. G. Kahn. *Unifying Heterogeneous Distributed Clinical Data in a Relational Database.* In Safran, editor, Seventeenth Annual Symposium on Computer Applications in Medical Care, Washington, D. C., November 1993. American Medical Informatics Association, McGraw-Hill. 1994. Pages 644-648.

[8] E. M. van Mulligen. *An Architecture for an Integrated Medical Workstation, Its Realization and Evaluation.* Ph.D. thesis, Erasmus University, Rotterdam, The Netherlands, September 1993.

[9] E. M. van Mulligen, T. Timmers, and D. F. F. Leao. *A framework for uniform access to data, software and knowledge.* In P. D. Clayton, editor, Fifteenth Annual Symposium on Computer Applications in Medical Care, Washington, D. C., November 1991. American Medical Informatics Association, IEEE Computer Society Press.

[10] J. R. Nicol, C. T. Wilkes, and F. A. Manola. *Object orientation in heterogeneous distributed computing systems.* IEEE Computer, 26(6):57-67, June 1993.

[11] Object Management Group, Framingham Corporate Center, 492 Old Connecticut Path, Framingham, MA 01701-4568. *The Common Object Request Broker: Architecture and Specification.* OMG Document Number 92.12.1, 1991.

[12] J. R. Scherrer, R. Baud, D. Hochstrasser, and O. Ratib. *An integrated hospital information system in Geneva.* M. D. Computing, 7(2):81-89, 1990.

Computer Tools to Support Collaborative Organization Design: Definition and Analysis of the Work at The Vanderbilt University Hospital and Clinic

Dean F. Sittig, Ph.D.

The Informatics Center, Vanderbilt University, Nashville, TN

In November, 1993 The Vanderbilt University Hospital and Clinic (VUH/TVC) convened a 10-member Collaborative Organization Design (COD) team that represented a diagonal slice through the organization. This team, lead by Gelinas & James, an outside consulting firm, was charged to develop, recommend, and implement a new organizational design which would promote a stronger patient focus, increased efficiency, and lower costs. The COD process is structured to inspire and enable employees to rebuild their organization so that it can respond to the challenges and opportunities that exist within their environment, to customer needs, and their own aspirations. This manuscript describes several of the computer tools which were utilized in the definition and analysis of the work of patient care at VUH/TVC. Specific examples of the findings from this phase of the work are utilized to illustrate their use and value.

INTRODUCTION

At no time in recent history have all the financial resources of academic medical centers been under direct attack simultaneously as they are today. To compete successfully in this new health care environment, academic institutions must reduce their costs dramatically while maintaining or even improving the quality of health care that they deliver (UHC, 1993). In response to these imparitives many organizations are in the midst of some sort of corporate reorganization (Boyce, 1992), be it restructuring (Bostrom, 1993), reengineering (Hammer, 1993) redesigning their organizational charts (Penchansky, 1993), empowering their employees (Dveirin, 1993), implementing total quality management (TQM) (Hamilton, 1993), or continuous quality improvement (CQI) programs, cross-training their employees (Lyons, 1992), implementing team management (Kerfoot, 1992; Meyer, 1994), or trying to change their organization's culture to name but a few of the current topics in organizational change. Most of these change efforts result in only temporary improvements in quality or reductions in cost in a limited area of the organization. The depth and scope of the change that is required and the resources that must be brought to bear are often sorely underestimated (Gelinas, 1992).

In an attempt to overcome these shortcomings, the Vanderbilt University Hospital (VUH) and Clinic (TVC) convened a 10-member collaborative organization design (COD) team, representing a diagonal slice through the organization, to review all aspects of the current organization and then suggest several major new directions.

What is Collaborative Organizational Design?

Collaborative organizational design (COD) is an organizational redesign process structured to inspire and enable members of the organization to rebuild their organization so that it can respond to the challenges and opportunities that exist within their environment, to customer needs, and their own aspirations (Gelinas, 1992). One of the most important tenets of the COD process is that before profound change can occur, everyone within the organization must agree on the problems. Therefore, the COD process is designed so that those expected to do the rebuilding will understand, be involved in, and support the entire process.

Simply stated, the COD process utilizes the best techniques from organizational systems theory, organization redesign, work reengineering, visioning, collaborative problem solving, and quality improvement programs to create a clear and easily understood process which will have a major impact on the organization (Gelinas, 1992).

The COD process is divided into six phases: Education and Planning, Definition and Analysis, Mission and Vision, Design, Implementation Planning, and Implementation and Evaluation. The specific goals for analyzing the work of VUH/TVC within the Definition and Analysis phase were:

1. To define, analyze, and document the current state of work surrounding patient care at VUH/TVC.
2. To identify strengths and problems of current work processes and their root causes.
3. To obtain agreement on definition and analysis of the work at VUH/TVC among all organization members.

0195-4210/94/$5.00

This manuscript describes several of the computer tools that have proved useful during the definition and analysis phase of this work. Specific examples taken from the work done are used to illustrate computer tool usage.

BACKGROUND

Vanderbilt University Hospital (VUH) is a 661-bed tertiary care academic medical facility located on the campus of Vanderbilt University in Nashville, TN. In Fiscal Year 1993 (FY'93) there were 28,126 inpatient admissions. The Vanderbilt Clinic (TVC) is an outpatient clinic physically connected to VUH. In FY'93 there were 408,000 outpatient visits. VUH/TVC currently employs over 5000 people of which over 1400 are nurses and 530 are housestaff. In addition, there are over 630 attending physicians on staff.

Why computer tools?

The collaborative organization design process is, by its very nature, highly interactive involving a large percentage of Vanderbilt's 6,000 members. Computer tools can help support this process in several different ways. First, they provide a rapid method for documenting in a neat and orderly fashion all the work that the various groups do. For example, flow charting tools can be used to diagram the current work processes (see figure 2). Second, they provide an on-line method for helping groups focus on the central problems during brainstorming sessions. For example, a computer-based Affinity Diagramming tool allows group members to identify different aspects of a particular problem that are responsible for a portion of the problem (see figure 3). Third, use of the OptionFinder (Option Technologies, Inc.) electronic balloting software enabled groups of over 80 individuals to express their level of agreement (or disagreement) with specific questions and then to see the overall group response instantaneously. Finally, computer-aided instruction has the potential to change the way students of all kinds learn by providing the new information at the time that it is needed (just-in-time) rather than just-in-case it is needed as we often do now. Specifically, the Continuous Improvement Toolkit provides on-line instructions and examples for use, as well as, the theory of the continuous quality improvement methodology behind the Toolkit (Bourne, 1993).

The Continuous Improvement Toolkit (CI Toolkit)

The CI Toolkit was developed by John R. Bourne, Ph.D. Director of the Center for Intelligent Systems at Vanderbilt University in conjunction with Northern Telecom's Quality Department. The CI Toolkit leads one through the various phases of a complete continuous quality improvement project. Specifically, the CI Toolkit allows one to identify and document the customers, the products and services the organization delivers to those customers, the suppliers of the input materials, flowchart the work processes, assign performance measures to the steps in the work process (i.e., time, cost, number of defects, and customer satisfaction), determine present performance, identify benchmarks against which the present performance should be compared, identify/prioritize opportunities for improvement, and develop an improvement plan. The CI Toolkit also includes a suite of quality tools such as a fishbone, or cause and effect diagram, control charts, Pareto Diagram, scatter plots, and histogram. We utilized the CI Toolkit's flow charting capability to document current work processes at VUH/TVC (fig 2).

Analysis of Work Processes at VUH/TVC

Work Processes are sets of interconnected activities, organized in time, through which the inputs obtained from the suppliers are transformed into deliverables which we provide to our customers (see figure 1). Some work processes may be contained solely within a single department, although most work processes cut across traditional departmental boundaries. Work processes are vital to the very existence of the organization. Clear organizational strategies, logical reporting relationships, and a skilled, committed work force are all necessary, but can not overcome flawed work processes.

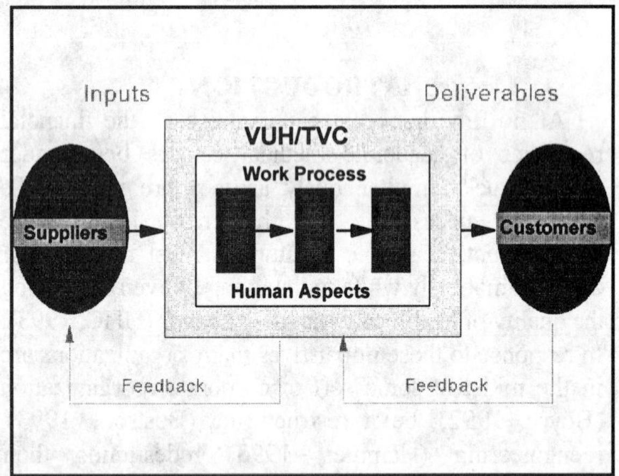

Figure 1. A Diagram showing how the work processes transform the inputs, received from the suppliers, into deliverables which we give to our customers. The human aspects of the organization reflect on the willingness and committment of the workers to actually do the work. Customer feedback is used to help us make improvements in our work processes. In addition, we provide feedback to the suppliers to help them deliver supplies which better meet our needs (from Gelinas, 1992).

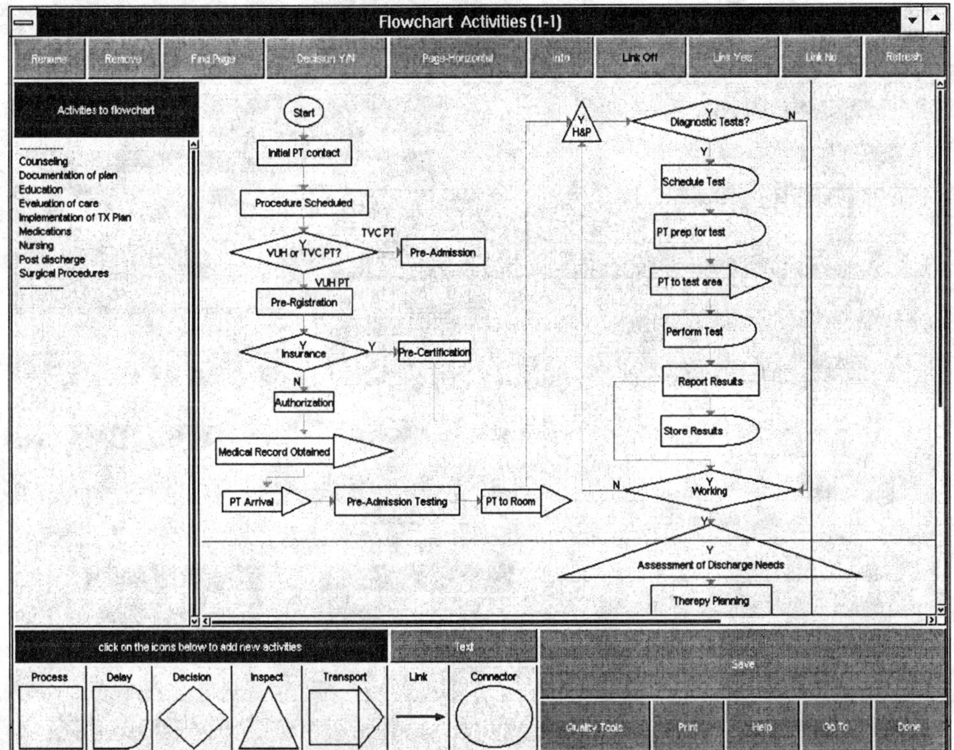

Figure 2. A sample screen from the CI Toolkit showing a partial flowchart of the patient care work process .

Following identification of the core work processes of VUH/TVC, we began a series of meetings with small groups of employees in an attempt to identify the root causes of some of the most serious problems faced by the institution. At several of these meetings, participants engaged in brainstorming activities. In response to these meetings, we developed a computer-based version of the Affinity Diagramming tool.

The Affinity Diagram Tool

The Affinity Diagram method is derived from the KJ Method developed by Dr. Kawakita Jiro. Briefly, the Affinity diagram uses the affinity between partial, piecemeal items of verbal data to help one understand the structure of the overall problem in a systematic fashion. To construct an Affinity Diagram using the new tool one:

1. Decides on the theme or topic to be discussed.
2. Begins collecting verbal data (i.e., facts, inferences, ideas, or opinions). This process is typically unstructured and is referred to as brainstorming.
3. These ideas are then iteratively arranged and rearranged on the computer screen as related ideas begin to coalesce.
4. Once the ideas, concepts, or opinions are arranged in a neat and organized fashion, the group begins to state their "belief" in the correctness or importance of each item.

The Affinity Diagram tool we have created then utilizes the Dempster-Shafer theory of evidence to combine and propagate these beliefs throughout the diagram (Gordon, 1984). Currently our tool only allows one person's beliefs to be input into the system, but it would only require a small change in the code (but a large change in the physical hardware, i.e., multiple machines connected by a network) to allow the entire group to "vote" on importance or relevance of each item.

Findings from the Work Process Analysis

During the myriad meetings with employee and customer focus groups, we identified several strengths of VUH/TVC. The following list provides an overview of these findings.

Strengths Identified:
We take care of patients who need our help.
Most staff want to do a good job.
We can obtain most (test, consultation, information, etc.) that is needed.
VUH/TVC is a "fine teaching laboratory".
There is an administrative commitment to improve and develop a better organization.
VUH/TVC has the potential to be great.
There are "pockets" of staff trying to help.

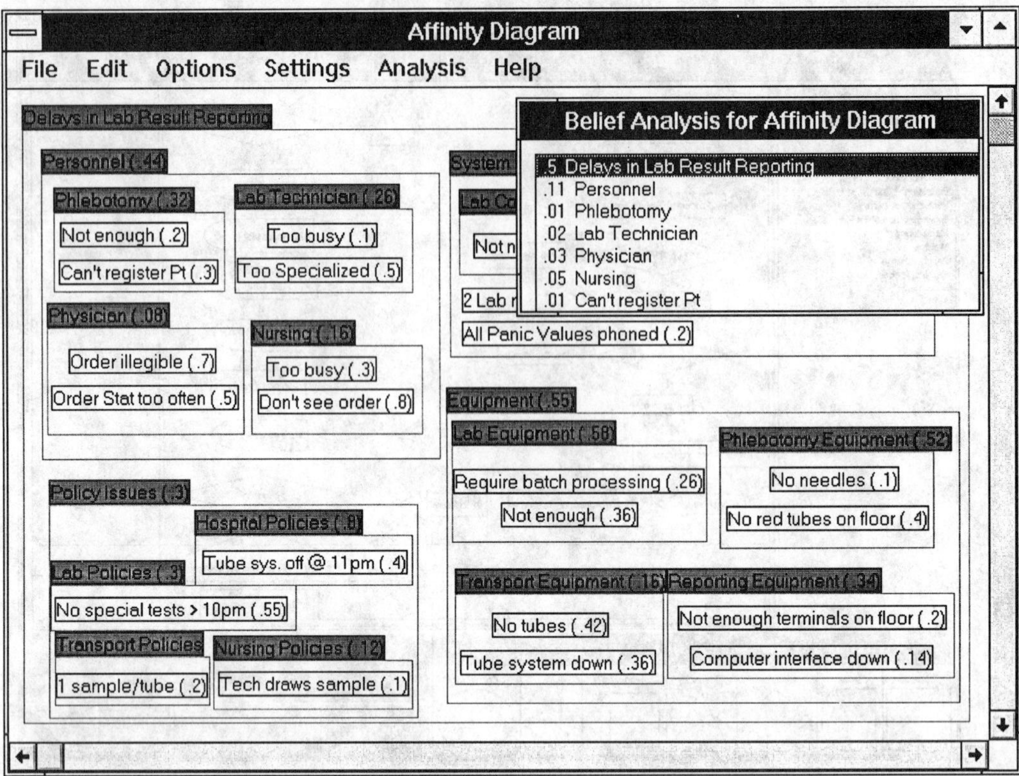

Figure 3. Sample screen from the Affinity Diagram tool. The small window in the upper righthand corner shows a portion of the belief calculations based on the Dempster-Shafer theory of evidence.

In addition, a myriad of problems surrounding the patient care work process were identified. The following list was an attempt to identify the root causes of the many problems.

Problems/Causes Identified:

1. Accessing the services provided is difficult.
2. Patients/families needs and expectations are not always a priority.
3. Data are initially entered incorrectly or not available.
4. There is inappropriate/inefficient use of services and resources.
5. Information/data is non-existent or difficult to access and no systematic feedback mechanism exists.
6. Faculty and staff do not understand how their decisions/actions affect other departments or the institution as a whole.
7. Communication throughout the organization is difficult.

Finally, these focus groups identified several of the major impacts of the problems which result from the root causes identified above.

Impacts Identified:
Patient treatment is delayed.
Patients get mad and do not come back.
There is increased patient cost.
There is decreased patient, staff, & faculty satisfaction.
There is increased length of stay.
Physicians send patients elsewhere.
There is reduced reimbursements from payors.

OptionFinder: Interactive Meeting Software

The OptionFinder (Option Technologies, Inc.) hardware and software set-up enables a large group of people to vote and have the groups' responses displayed immediately following the vote. Briefly, OptionFinder utilizes individual, wireless, portable keypads (3"x 6" x 1") which communicate with a central receiving station via radio waves. The central receiving station is connected to an IBM-compatible 386 with 4 Mb of RAM (min. config.) and approx. 20Mb of disk space .

OptionFinder not only helps teams work together more effectively during a meeting, but can also help teams learn to work together to organize, plan, and facilitate meetings. We utilized the OptionFinder in two large meetings (approximately 80 participants each) at which the findings from the work process analysis were presented (see Figure 4).

To what extent do the findings from the work process analysis match your view of VUH/TVC?
1. Off Target.
2. Needs Work.
3. I can Live with it.
4. Close.
5. Bull's eye.

Figure 4. A replica of one question the audience was asked to answer.Participants chose answer from menu.

Immediately following this question, we were able to show the following bar chart of their responses.

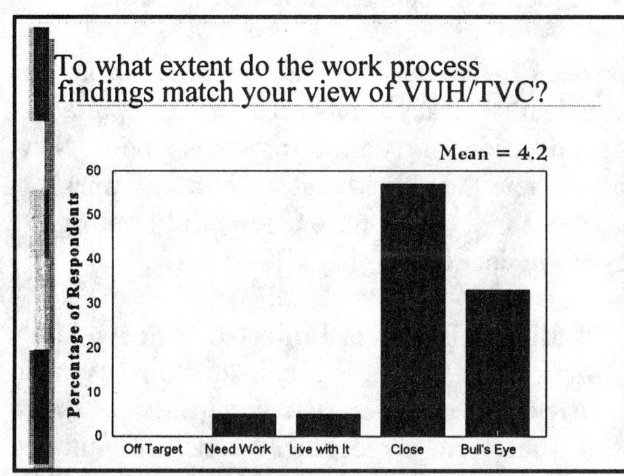

Figure 5. Graph of audience response.

DISCUSSION & SUMMARY

Use of the computer tools described in this manuscript has enabled the COD team to accomplish a great amount of work in a short time. We originally planned to use the CI Toolkit during meetings (via projection equipment) to record the work processes as they were identified. Even though the flow charting tool is easy to use, we found that using large Post-it notes was even faster and easier. The CI Toolkit found its major use following the meetings to document the work that had gone on.

The Affinity diagramming tool was likewise found to be most useful as a documentation tool. When we have the hardware necessary to allow us to use the Affinity diagramming tool's ability to combine the votes from a large group, then it may become useful as a realtime meeting facilitation tool.

Finally, the OptionFinder software has been instrumental in our success. As we have repeated in nearly every meeting, the main tenet of the COD process is that we cannot hope to to agree on the solutions if we cannot agree on the problems. The OptionFinder, in conjunction with the CI Toolkit and Affinity Diagramming tool, have allowed the COD team to move on into the Mission and Vision phase with good agreement by all the major stakeholders within VUH/TVC on the problems, root causes, and impacts identified.

REFERENCES

[1] Bostrom J. Zimmerman J. Restructuring nursing for a competitive health care environment. Nursing Economics. 11(1):35-41, 54, 1993.

[2] Bourne JR. The Continuous Improvement ToolKit Users' Manual. CIS, Press. 1993.

[3] Boyce RA. The organizational design of hospitals A critical review. Australian College of Health Service Executives, Monograph Series No. 1. North Ryde, Australia, 1992.

[4] Dveirin GF. Adams KL. Empowering health care improvement: an operational model. Joint Comm. Jour. Quality Improvement. 19(7):222-32, 1993.

[5] Gelinas MV & James RB. Creating profound change through collaborative organization design. Vision/Action: The Journal of Bay Area Organization Consultants. pgs. 1-8; 1992.

[6] Gordon J & Shortliffe EH. The Dempster-Shafer theory of evidence. n Rule-based Expert Systems: The MYCIN experiments of the Stanford Heuristic Programming Project (eds. Buchanan B & Shortliffe EH), Addison-Wesley, Inc., 1984.

[7] Hamilton J. Toppling the power of the pyramid. Team-based restructuring for TQM, patient-centered care. Hospitals. 67(1):38, 40-1, 1993.

[8] Hammer M. & Champy J. Reengineering the corporation: A manifesto for business revolution. HarperCollins, Inc., 1993.

[9] Kerfoot KM. Uecker S. The techniques of developing self-managed teams: the nurse manager's role. Nurs. Econ.. 10(1):70-1, 78, 1992.

[10] Lyons RF. Cross-training: a richer staff for leaner budgets. Nursing Management.23(1):43-4, 1992.

[11] Meyer C. How the right measures help teams excel. Harvard Bus. Rev. May-Jun:95-103; 1994.

[12] Penchansky R. Macnee CL. Ensuring excellence: reconceptualizing quality assurance, risk management, and utilization review. Qual. Rev. Bull. 19(6):182-9, 1993.

[13] University Hospital Consortium (UHC). Competing in the maturing healthcare marketplace: Strategies for academic medical centers. 1993.

[14] Wheatley K. OptionFinder Users' Manual. 1994.

Acknowledgements

This work was supported in part by grants R29 LM05284 and G08 LM05443 from the National Library of Medicine. A special thanks to the members of the VUH/TVC Design team for their tireless efforts.

A FRAMEWORK FOR "NEED TO KNOW" AUTHORIZATIONS IN MEDICAL COMPUTER SYSTEMS: RESPONDING TO THE CONSTITUTIONAL REQUIREMENTS

Vincent M. Brannigan, J.D.
Professor, Law and Technology
University of Maryland at College Park
College Park, MD 20742
(301) 405-6667 vb15@umail.umd.edu

"Need to Know" systems which restrict access to computerized data to those with a specified need for the data have been described as part of the solution to the problem of privacy in health care information systems. However, no operational "need to know" system is described in the medical literature. Recent legal developments in constitutional privacy protection make a "need to know" system mandatory, not optional. In sophisticated information systems users can utilize the unique characteristics of the system itself to implement a high level"need to know" system, based on the institution's own patient treatment pattern. This article provides an analytical tool for helping to define a "need to know" system with reference to the specific problems of health care institutions.

INTRODUCTION

There is widespread agreement among health care policymakers that computerized medical data should be restricted on a "need to know" basis.[9,14] Such a system would be required by the Fair Health Information Practices Act now before Congress.[10] Limiting access to those with a "need to know" has been adopted as a policy by the British Medical Association. [13] Ethics scholars have indicated that any use of patient data without consent must be based on some substantial need for the information,[11] and clinicians have recognized "need to know" as the proper automated implementation of the Hippocratic oath. [7]

Despite these pronouncements, some organizations persist in avoiding the process of effectively determining who should have access to medical data.[12] Some institutions claim to have a "need to know" system but simply assume that everyone on the staff needs to know everything about every patient, or assume that audit trails will identify privacy invaders so they can be held "responsible". However these approaches do not comply with the current developments in the law of privacy.

A series of legal decisions have defined protection for patient's privacy rights. The most important recent decision on medical privacy is Doe v. New York, where the United States Court of Appeals found that individuals have a **constitutional** right of privacy in data concerning HIV status.

> **"Individuals who are infected with the HIV virus clearly possess a constitutional right to privacy regarding their condition.... There is, therefore, a recognized constitutional right to privacy in personal information.[6]**

While the Court of Appeals cited the well known Supreme Court case of Whalen v. Roe it clearly went beyond Whalen in defining the constitutional right of privacy.

Restriction of data access to the smallest number of persons possible has ben one of the major concepts of constitutional privacy analysis. In Whalen the Supreme Court specifically noted that the data was available only to those officers who clearly needed access to the data for accepted official purposes. Under **Doe** it would appear that a carefully structured "need to know" system is a constitutional imperative.

Obviously agreement on the desirability or inevitability of a "need to know" system does not answer the question who truly "needs to know" which pieces of data. This article also will not answer that question. The purpose of this article is to develop a logical characterization of medical functions so that a "need to Know" system can be created.

PRIVACY IN CONSTITUTIONAL LAW

Finding privacy to be a constitutional right does not automatically protect individuals from injury. In the United States, Constitutional rights are essentially "negative" in that they only protect individuals against "governmental" actions. Such rights have no formal effect on non governmental actors. The constitutional right to privacy is therefore necessarily limited to governmental infringement on rights. As with many constitutional rights, balancing of the right of privacy against other legitimate social concerns may be needed.[3] In particular society may demand some compromise to protect public health. Further, a reasonable court might find that few patients would run substantial health risks to protect medical privacy. On the other hand, governments often find it inevitable that they incorporate public constitutional rights into laws regulating private conduct, and state courts might be encouraged to expand the common law right of privacy.

NEED TO KNOW: DEFINITIONS

Developing a "need to know" system requires a sophisticated understanding of medical, social, legal and technological requirements for both privacy and the provision of health care.[1]

Some medical users believe that if data would be useful to a medical professional then that user has a "need to know". Under this thinking a medical researcher has a "need" for any data that might help in research. But in constitutional analysis even a socially desirable activity can only be carried out in a manner which minimizes the intrusion on the protected right. For example, researchers would rarely if ever "need" the patient's identity. As a result privacy protection often requires changes in otherwise convenient methods of administration. It is critical to understand that cost and administrative convenience have rarely been allowed to be balanced against constitutional rights:

"administrative convenience does not justify a policy that otherwise runs afoul of the Constitution"[8]

For example, patient identifiers are often used to simplify administrative tasks. Human names are easily remembered, and may contribute to preventing mistakes in the administration of health care. However, use of names is simply a custom, not a necessity. Distinguishing between those privacy risks which are necessary and those which simply represent administrative convenience is one of the most important tasks in privacy analysis.[2]

For this paper the legal criteria for a "Need to Know" is defined as the **smallest intrusion on the patient's privacy which will permit completion of a well defined socially accepted task.**

NEED TO KNOW: PRIVACY PROTECTION

In the field of computer science, there is a rich literature of methods of implementing privacy protection systems, however it is normally assumed that the job of deciding who should have access to the data has already been done. Few if any medical models of "need to know" have been published, and there is no literature examining the special hazards and opportunities of information systems to create a functional "need to know" system.

A substantial gap exists between the information specialists and the medical community over privacy protection. Information specialists often do not know who needs the information and for what purpose, and the medical community has no idea what privacy protection system might be available. As a result, privacy protection tends to be sacrificed to administrative convenience in the turf battles among the various medical specialties and the administrative and information communities.[2] As networked systems and telemedicine develop and hospitals forge computer links with other health care providers the problems will get worse. Who decides which provider gets access to what data? [5]

The special privacy disclosure hazards of information systems have been widely documented, but information systems also have special privacy protection advantages. Access to data can be controlled dynamically, the data can be easily subdivided and segregated, and real time alerts of security violations can be provided. Basing access to computerized information systems on the historical system of access to paper records both ignores the increased risk of computer systems and the possibility of introducing novel privacy protections. [4]

NEED TO KNOW: DIMENSIONS

Normally data access rights have been structured as

"layers", where privileges are greatest on the inside and lowest on the outside. Developments in health care and information systems have rendered such a model obsolete. A consultant, for example, might have a high "need to know", but only for a limited time. Others might have a longer durational "need to know", but only of limited information. Some medical information might be needed by some, but not all clinicians. A pharmacist, for example, rarely needs to know the name of the patient for whom a prescription is being filled. The pharmacist only needs to know that the prescription is authorized, will be delivered to the correct patient and that it does not conflict with other medications for the patient. None of this requires the patient's identity.

"Need to know" should therefore be classified along a series of **DIMENSIONS**. Dimensions are used to categorize the relationship between the data and the person making the request. Dimensions describe the type of patient data, the type of health care provider, the type of data action and so forth. These dimensions can be articulated and classified independently, but interact dynamically. Each dimension affects data access authorization. The core assumption is that each health care worker stands in a definable relationship with each portion of a patient data file.

Using these dimensions computer systems can provide customized "need to know" functionality. Such systems are a product of the examination of the individual institutional health care environment. However a proper dimensional framework assures that key decisions about access are made by policy makers in a deliberate manner. A series of dimensions can be created:

Patient File Dimension

Each patient file is composed of least 5 dimensions:

Identifier information: information which can be used to discover the patient's identity but is not needed for treatment, such as name, birth date, Social security number or universal identifier.

Identifiable information: any information which might be used to generate an identifier, but is otherwise relevant to treatment, such as the date of injury.

Coded identifier: alphanumeric linking tool used to ensure that all data on a patient is linked together. It can be generated for each admission.

Standard medical data: clinically significant medical data which is not "restricted data" as defined below.

Restricted data: data is "restricted" because of its unusual sensitivity and lack of broad medical significance. The classification of restricted data is a social determination and might include categories such as elective abortions, some mental health data, and some pharmaceutical data.

Under either standard or restricted data there might be further subdivisions such as free text or patient codes. Since free text is inherently more capable of creating a security violation, greater access limitations might be justified.

Health Care Worker Dimension

Health care workers are divided by their status in relation to the patient:

Treating team: Health care practitioners directly engaged in regular care of the patient. These would be the people who are routinely allowed to write or execute orders on a patient, and normally have a legitimate knowledge of the patient's identity. The treating team includes several subcategories.

Category 1 members can add members of the treating team and set access. This might be the responsible health care provider.

Category 2 members need general access to patient files. This would include anyone with direct patient responsibility.

Category 3 members need limited access. These are support staff who perform limited functions

Consultants: Health care practitioners who need contact with the patient's data but are not part of the treating team. Consultants usually do not routinely need identifier information or permanent access. Second opinions are treated as a consultation. Usually consultations are addressed to specific individuals, but may be addressed to departments, who then designate the individuals.

Clinical supervision: This category defines the medical authority to review care on specific patients and initiate changes (e.g. clinical quality assurance)

Referral: Authority to transfer a patient to a new treating team, at the same or another institution.

Medical support services (e.g. tests, procedures, pharmacy,transcription): These can be distinguished from consultations when they do not require transmission of the patient file, and are addressed to departments. Support services can use coded identifiers. If identified information is needed, the service is normally a consultation.

File Access Duration Dimension

Duration of access to the patient file is an independent dimension. Even a treating physician may not need access when a patient has left the hospital. Support staff rarely need access when they are not on duty. Some only need access when a specific procedure is being performed. Possible limited dimensions include:

1) access during specific hospitalization, treatment, consultation or referral.

2) timed access (e.g. night coverage)

3) access to archive data only, prevents access to live data on patients currently being treated.

Data File Transaction Dimension

This dimension specifies what transactions are permitted in the file. Some examples include:

Read authority: Authority to read the file

Write authority: Authority to write entries to a file

Copy authority: the right to make copies of a file, for example by down loading to a remote system.

Change authority: authority to determine that an earlier entry should be overruled, either to correct an error or change the record. This is not an edit authority, in medical records all entries must be preserved.

Data Base Authority Dimension

This dimension defines the ability of the user to scan or browse the data base, rather than get information on specific identified patients. Because patient identity can be generated data base authority represents one of the most significant threats to privacy. Users with data base authority can be classified into several groups:

Quality assurance, Cost Control, Long Term Planning and Research: These categories of users review the data base for purposes other than clinical care for a given patient. As just one example these persons might be given access to archived data without identifiers.

Administration, bed control and staff scheduling These and similar tasks require access to current treatment and prognosis data, but not identifiers. An expert system or trusted intermediary might be used to stratify non archived data for immediate administration purposes. Insurance reimbursement can normally use coded identifiers, after an authorization is obtained from the insurer.

System staff: The question of data base access to confidential data by the system staff raises special security problems. However they normally should have no need to know identified data.

Emergency Access Dimension

The system must be arranged to allow temporary emergency access by any health care worker, for example in a typical "code" situation. However the use of emergency access would trigger an immediate quality review, to determine why no authorized user was present and a security review to assure that no security breach was involved.

IMPLEMENTATION

Each institution has to implement the system by examining its own operations and assigning access dimensions. A recent ACM article describes the typical corporate privacy policy as "drift ... until the organization perceived some sort of external threat" and that organizational policies often did not match organizational practice. [12]

Certain principles should govern Need to know systems:

No one should have access based simply on a speculative need under rare circumstances

The emergency override provides an adequate response to any genuine need, and system authorizations can be altered through experience with the system.

Routine access to identifier data should be based solely on the patient's clinical needs.

The key evaluation is whether the patient needs the health care worker to have the identifier data.

Outside access to identified patient data should be strictly limited

Special security precautions are needed before passing data outside the secure system. This means that telemedicine and other extended access to records demands special analysis.[7]

CONCLUSION

The consequences for violating individual's constitutional rights are substantial in both financial and operational terms. System operators can expect detailed scrutiny of their decisions on who gets access to medical data. A "need to know" system appears to be a constitutional requirement. Administrative convenience will not be accepted as a substitute.

Determining who "needs to know" patient information is a special task totally apart from technical "security" analysis. The introduction of information systems initially replicates existing information access environments. However privacy protection often requires confronting traditional methods of operation.

The structure for "need to know" systems proposed here does not attempt to define who "needs to know", rather it defines the appropriate questions which will allow a prototype "need to know" systemto be created. By examining the information flow in a variety of specific environments it is possible to create a wide variety of "need to know" systems suited to the special needs of divergent communities and institutions.

REFERENCES

[1] Brannigan V. **"Computerized Patient Information under the Privacy Act: a Regulatory Effectiveness Analysis"** Pro. 16th Sym. on Com. App. in Med. Care, McGraw Hill 1992: 741-4

[2] Brannigan, V., and R. Dayhoff. **Medical Informatics: The Revolution in Law, Technology and Medicine**, J. of Legal Medicine, Vol 7:1-53.

[3] Brannigan, V., **Patient Privacy, A Consumer Protection Approach**, J. of Med. Sys, 1984, 7:501-505.

[4] Brannigan V. and Beier B. **"Standards for Privacy in Medical information systems: A Technico Legal Revolution"** Proceedings 14th Symp. on Comp. App. in Med. Care, IEEE 1990:266-270

[5] Brannigan V. **Protection of Patient Data in Multi-institutional Medical Computer Networks: Regulatory Effectiveness Analysis** Proc. of the 17th Symp. on Comp. App. in Med. Care, IEEE, Washington D.C. 1993: 59-63

[6] Doe v. New York 15 F.3d 264 (2nd Cir)1/28/94

[7] France FHR Gaunt PN **The need for security- a Clinical View** Int J. Bio Med Comput 35 (Suppl 1) (1994) 189-194

[8] Flores v. Meese 942 F.2d 1352 1991, (US CCA 9th) citing Reed v. Reed, 404 U.S. 71, 76-77, 30 L. Ed. 2d 225, 92 S. Ct. 251 (1971)

[9] Gostin LO, Turek-Brezina J, Powers M, Kozloff R, Faden R Steinauer ED **Privacy and Security of Personal Information in a New Health Care System** JAMA 1993; 270: 2487-2493

[10] H.R. 4077 March 21 1994

[11] Kluge EHW, **Health Information, Privacy Confidentiality and Ethics** Int J. Bio Med Comput35 (Suppl 1) (1994) 23-27

[12] Smith J, **Privacy policies and Practices: Inside the Organizational Maze**, Communications of the ACM Dec. 1993 36: 105-122

[13] Tonks, A **Information Management and Patient Privacy in the NHS**: Brit. Med. J. 307: 6914 P 1227;Nov. 13, 1993

[14] U.S. Congress Office of Technology Assessment: **Protecting Privacy in Computerized Medical Information** Government Printing Office 1993

Section IV

Networks and Standards

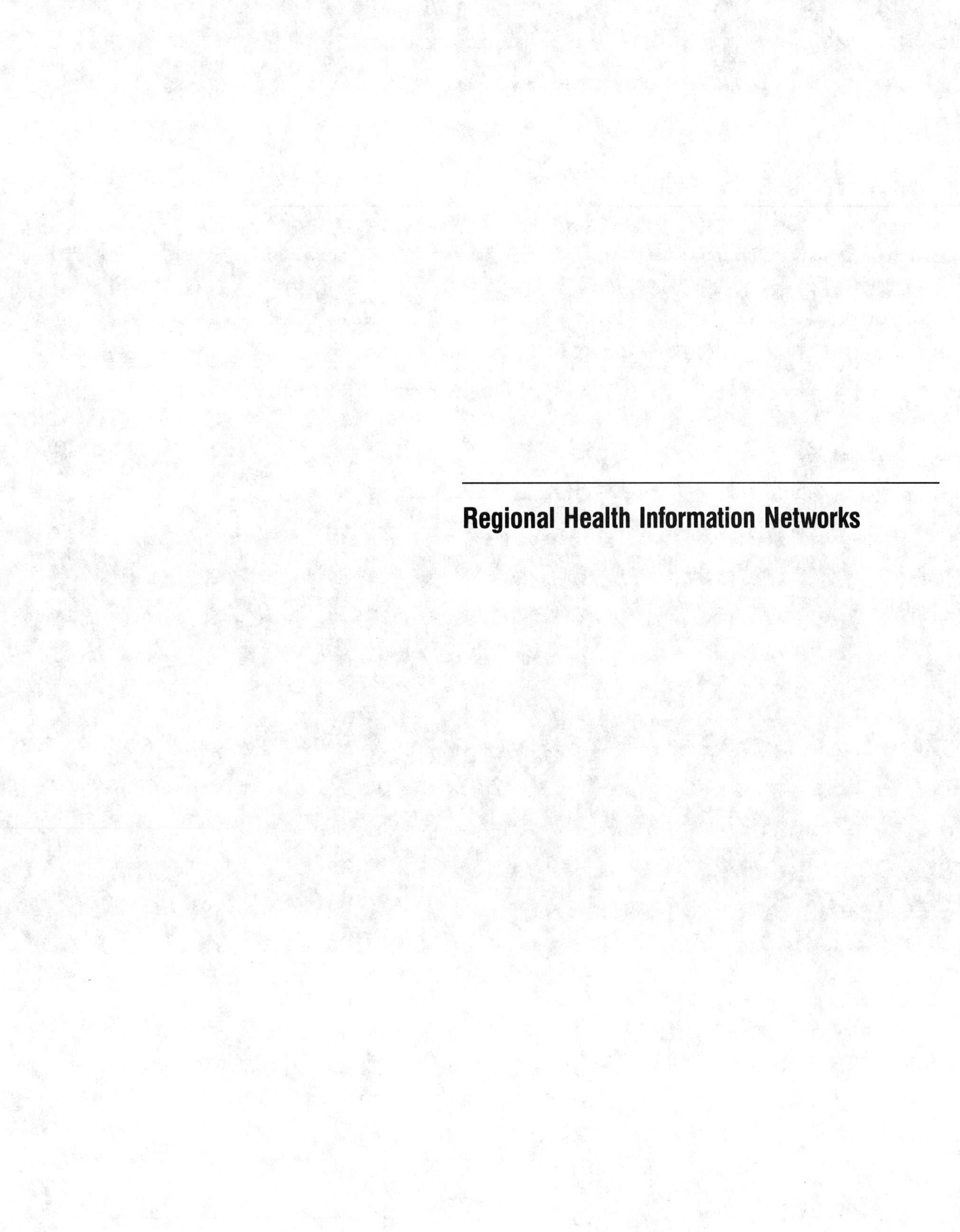

Regional Health Information Networks

Regional Health Information Networks: The Wisconsin Health Information Network, A Case Study

Kim R. Pemble, M.S.
Wisconsin Health Information Network

ABSTRACT

It is projected that by the turn of the century, ninety percent of diagnostic procedures and seventy percent of therapeutic procedures will occur outside a hospital setting [2,3]. Additionally, according to a 1992 study by Arthur D. Little, during any given physician office visit, as much as 30 percent of the required diagnostic data and information required by the physician is unavailable [4]. Driven by ever increasing demands for convenience and accessibility, health care continues to evolve into an environment where the importance of data and its relative availability to the requester are diverging. This paper will present the concept of a regional or community health information network (RHIN or CHIN). Specifically, the Wisconsin Health Information Network (WHIN) will be used as a case study.

PROBLEM/CHALLENGE

During the life of a patient, his or her movement through the "continuum of care" exacerbates the relative inaccessibility of information to the wide base of providers and other legitimate authorized viewers. This "continuum" includes primary care physicians, specialists, clinics, hospitals, reference laboratories and diagnostic centers. During a visit with any given provider, there is a need for current, complete and accurate information regarding the patient. Yet, according to an Arthur D. Little study, 30% of the diagnostic data (e.g. lab results, consults, patient history) are unavailable to the care provider during that office visit.[4]

Recent advances in implementation of integrated systems and computer based patient records is improving the data availability within a given institution, however the "continuum" of care is not constrained to a given hospital or integrated delivery system (Figure 1). There remains a growing need for access to patient clinical and demographic data for care providers and other authorized medical information users (e.g. payors, employers, laboratories, health care consortiums) within a community or region.

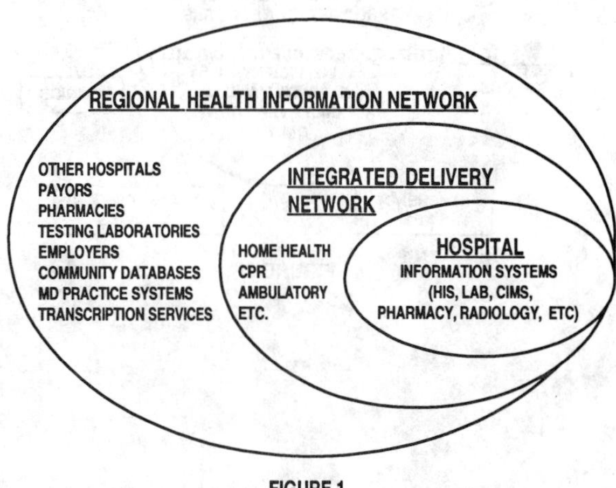

FIGURE 1

Examples of the data involved in this communications quagmire include:

- Patient Identification
- Patient Demographics
- Referral Requests
- Laboratory Results
- Transcribed Documents (e.g. Laboratory, Radiology,
  Surgical, History and Physical)
- Medical Records Abstracts
- Graphic Images (e.g. ECG, Pulmonary Function Tests)
- Radiographic Images
- Claims
- Eligibility Verifications
- State Required Testing Results and Other Community Databases

In the current paradigm (Figure 2), access to this data is gained through countless phone calls, proprietary networks to selected components of the community structure, the U.S. Postal Service and couriers. The advent of a Regional Health Information Network provides access through a means that incorporates a common "look and feel" to a broad spectrum of applications, regardless of originating host system(s) or application software. This access is through dial connections to a system serving as a switch (routing transactions) which is integrated with various medical information providers' systems (Figure 3).

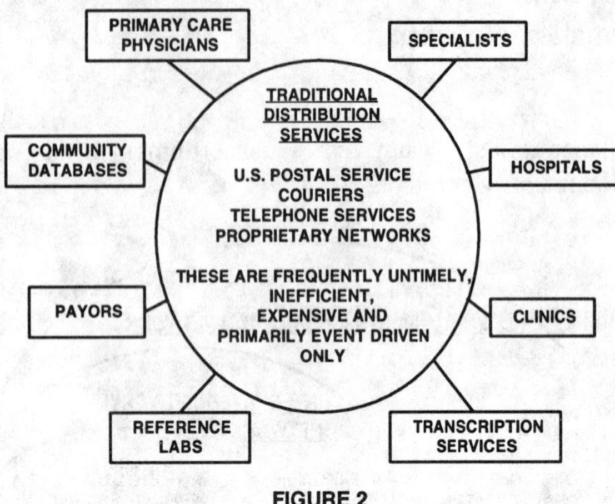

FIGURE 2

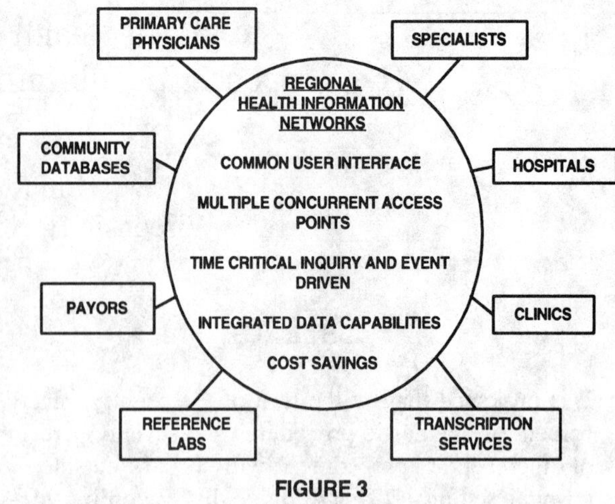

FIGURE 3

REGIONAL HEALTH INFORMATION NETWORKS

There are three components to the Wisconsin Health Information Network (WHIN): Information User Interface (e.g. physicians, physician office staff, hospital departments, clinics, pharmacies, laboratories), The Network Switch and the Information Provider Interface (e.g. hospitals, clinics, laboratories, pharmaceutical services, library services, transcription services, HIS, Laboratory Systems, Transcription Systems etc.). (Figure 4)

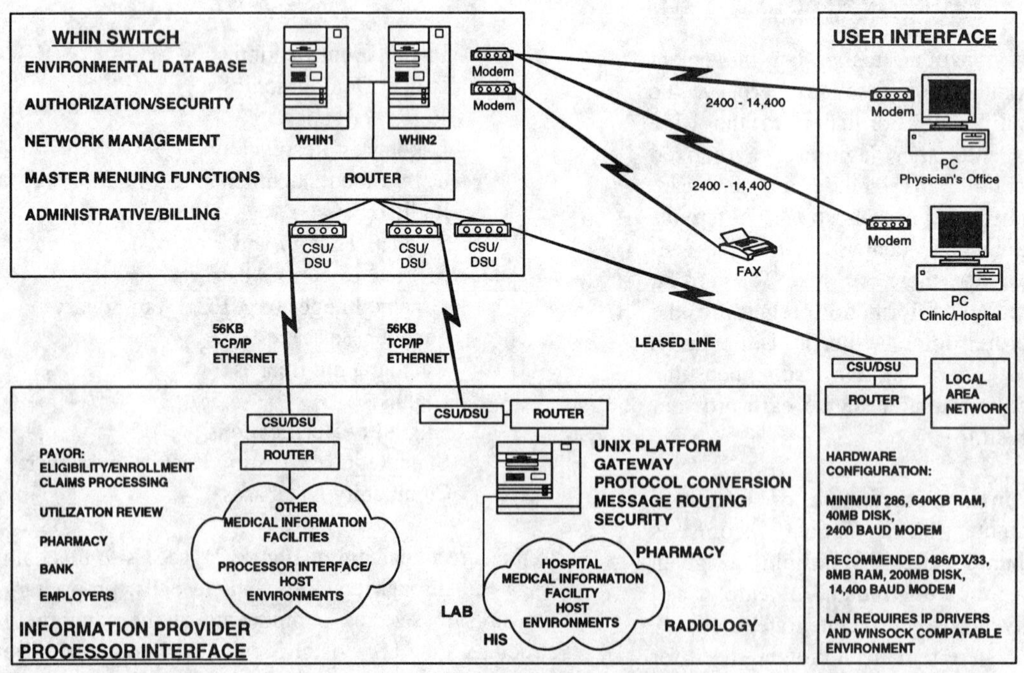

FIGURE 4

Information Provider Interface

Integrating the systems environment of a medical information provider, while maintaining the provider's investment in application hardware and software, is the role of the Processor Interface (PI). Functioning as an interface engine, the PI establishes the bridge between any system/protocol that is to provide information to the network and the network protocol. Interfaces may be established in a peer-to-peer manner, by direct SQL access to databases, or by "scraping" data from application screens. To date, interfaces have been developed to IBM mainframes, DEC/VAX and Hewlett Packard platforms. Network protocols that have been interfaced include SNA/3270, LU6.2, DECNET, and TCP/IP.

Location of the PI may be either at the WHIN site, executing on the WHIN hardware or, depending on the environment, at the medical information provider site executing on client provided, WHIN specified hardware. Connections from the medical information providers to the network are typically 56KB leased lines (point to point) or through frame relay services. As band width requirements rise, ISDN, T1 or greater connections can be implemented.

The interfaces are designed to support request/response communications, initiated by an information user, as well as "event-driven" processing, which are transactions initiated by a host system.

Network Switch

Providing the server side of a client/server relationship, the switch runs on a redundant SUN SPARC UNIX platform, utilizing TCP/IP and HL/7 protocols. The switch maintains all network user authorization and authentication information as well as managing all routing functions for the network. In addition to request/response and event-driven processing, the switch also provides electronic mail services, outbound fax service and deferred request processing. During the period January 1, 1994 through July 31, 1994, a total of 19,724 calls were received by the network, processing clinical and claims transactions. 73.3% of transactions were clinical and 26.7% financial.

Information User Interface

Utilizing a common user interface, information users may access data from medical information providers that have authorized this access. The common user interface (UI) is currently based on a DOS, Microsoft Windows or Novell platform. This interface provides the client element of the relationship with the network switch.

With the common user interface, patient demographics from Hospital A and Hospital B are accessed through the same means and displayed in the same manner. Data components that may not be supported in one environment may be indicated as 'not provided'. Similarly, laboratory results are accessed in one consistent manner, although results display may vary, depending on such parameters as normal ranges and test code groupings.

By providing a common access point to a wide range of medical information providers, this UI and the network to which it connects replaces the proprietary network connections and printers typically found in a physician office setting. Connection to the network is the only physical login the user is required to supply. All other host logins are managed at the software level.

Access to WHIN from the user interface is accomplished through a dial connection. Speeds from 2400 baud to 14.4 baud are currently supported. Again, as requirements dictate, additional bandwidth through V. Fast and ISDN connections is available. There are also UNIX and Network versions of the User Interface.

Information Flow

There are two models for the flow of data/information on the network, the primary method is a request/response structure and the second is 'event driven'. Using request response, users connect to the network and send requests for information regarding patients to medical information providers. Security surrounding the ability to make these requests is outlined in the following section.

In the 'event-driven' model, the medical information provider systems are the initiators of the data flow. Messages are routed through the network to the indicated recipient(s) and filed in an electronic mailbox until they are read by the user. These messages may also be delivered via network outbound fax capabilities. Confirmation of delivery is returned to the indicated initiator through the e-mail service which is a part of the network. These event-driven messages are viewed in the same manner as the on-line request response messages.

SECURITY

Although a detailed discussion of the security implemented at WHIN would require a separate paper, the following is presented as a high level overview of some security points.

Access to the network switch is gained through a user ID and password. The phone number dialed is managed by the software and hidden from the user. All traffic on the dial connection is encrypted and requires a copy of the User Interface to break. Additionally, access to the network requires the UI software and authenticating serial number assigned to each copy during installation.

Authorization from a medical information provider is required for any user to submit requests to, or receive messages from, that host environment. Access and viewing capabilities may be granted on a medical information provider, system or data element level. In addition to the security of the network, all security developed at the medical information provider system is supported and maintained through the processor interface.

No data is stored on the WHIN switch, other than as an element of an electronic mail message, an event driven message or deferred response waiting to be read. Once deferred or event driven messages are read, or reach an age of 30 days, they are purged.

WISCONSIN HEALTH INFORMATION NETWORK: STATUS REPORT

As of August 1, 1994, there are eleven (11) hospitals or medical centers (Children's Hospital of Wisconsin, Community Memorial Hospital, Froedtert Memorial Lutheran Hospital, Sheboygan Memorial Medical Center, St. Luke's Medical Center, Sinai Samaritan Medical Center, St. Mary's Hospital, St. Mary's Ozaukee, Trinity Memorial Hospital, Valley View Medical Center and Wausau Hospital) signed on the network (six of these are live with the remainder in various stages of PI development), three (3) payors (one in pilot testing), one nursing home and two ambulance companies. Over 1000 physicians, authorized physician office staff members and hospital departmental staff are subscribers to the network. It should be noted that several of the mentioned medical centers and hospitals are competitive entities participating on the same network.

Monthly transaction volumes average in excess of 40,000 from more than 3,100 calls to the network. Response time, although very dependent on the performance of host systems providing responses to requests, averages 3-7 seconds. Current functions available include patient demographics, transcribed documents, laboratory results, pharmacy orders, medical records abstracting, electronic mail, outbound fax, electronic claims submission, patient search and patient census by physician. Distribution of data requests by type, most frequent first, is:

Clinical:

- Patient Search
- Patient Visit and Insurance Information
- Transcription Data
- Patient Census
- Medical Procedures/Episodes
- Laboratory Results
- Physician List

One of the WHIN medical information provider participants had previously implemented a proprietary network for physicians to access their host based systems. WHIN was implemented as a replacement for this proprietary network. During a three month period in 1993, a study group of 24 physicians was monitored to compare their usage of WHIN to the same group's previous use of the proprietary network during the same three month period in 1992. Data services that were monitored for the study were available from both networks.

First quarter 1992 total requests to proprietary network 3,189

First quarter 1993 total requests to WHIN network 11,274

The study showed WHIN usage had a two hundred fifty four percent (254%) increase over the proprietary network. Even allowing for fluctuations in patient volumes, this appears to demonstrate the added value that WHIN brings to this physician population.

Additionally, WHIN offers other services than those included in this study (e.g. E-mail, electronic claims submission, claims status and eligibility inquiry).

In addition to community participation, ownership in the Wisconsin Health Information Network is open to health care related entities in the State. WHIN currently employs 16 full time staff, including installation/training/Solution Center (Help Desk), technical development/network management and sales/marketing.

BENEFITS

According to a 1992 study [4], there is potential for an annual savings of more than 30 Billion dollars by providing physicians and other authorized users telecommunications access to patient information.

Areas where benefits are projected:

Hospital:

- reduction in calls to medical information providers requesting information
- savings from developing proprietary networks including hardware, software, support staff, help desk, training
- reduction in repeated tests
- improved public image due to anticipation and preparation for preadmitted patient arrivals
- reduction in postage, courier costs and staff time to distribute results
- electronic eligibility verification

Physician:

- improved access to critical patient clinical data
- electronic eligibility verification
- electronic claims submission and tracking
- electronic explanation of benefits
- reduced pre-authorization time
- reduced telephone tag with pharmacies for filling and refilling prescriptions
- reduced staff time in obtaining results and other patient information
- improved communications with hospitals and colleagues

A detailed cost benefit study of WHIN is projected in the near future. Until that time, we can only relay the subjective feedback regarding benefits realized from WHIN's clients:

> "The biggest benefit is the cost savings", said Dr. Richard J. Battiola, saying that the network has cut down immensely on ordering multiple tests for patients. [6]

> "Networks like this are very important in reducing our medical costs," says the supervisor of the administrative office for Dr. Joseph Shaker. [7]

The author wishes to thank his colleagues at WHIN and all the clients of the Wisconsin Health Information Network for their assistance in making WHIN a success, allowing the writing of this paper.

REFERENCES

1) Steinman, Jack, "An Extended Enterprise Computing Solution: Wisconsin Health Information Network", Proceedings of the Thirteenth Annual Conference on the Use of Clinical Information Systems, March 14, 1993, pages 35-36.

2) Gabler, James M., "Shared Information Boosts Competition in Healthcare Networks", Computers in Healthcare, March 1993, pages 20-26.

3) Zinn, "Enabling Technologies Build Bridge to 21st Century", Computers in Healthcare, December 1992, pages 28-33.

4) Little, Arthur D., "Telecommunications: Can It Help Solve America's Health Care Problems?", July 1992, reference 91810-98.

5) Singer, Charles F., "The Singer Report on Managed Care Systems and Technology", report number 21, April 4, 1994.

6) Stewart, Janet Kidd, "Doctor Likes Medical Info Network", Chicago Sun-Times, November 18, 1993 page 56.

7) Sharma-Jensen, Geeta, "On line: Ameritech looks into the future", The Journal (Milwaukee), February 1, 1994 pages 1 and 7.

HUBNET: Wide Area Network Utilization of Local Area Network Medical Reference and Communication Resources

John W. Loonsk, M.D.*, John E. Schweigel, M.S.*, David Carr, B.S.**
*Office of Medical Computing
School of Medicine and Biomedical Sciences
**Computing and Information Technology
State University of New York at Buffalo

The State University of New York at Buffalo School of Medicine and Biomedical Sciences and its associated teaching sites have developed and partially implemented a regional Wide Area Network (WAN) in Buffalo and Western New York. The school wishes to use this WAN to deliver reference and communication resources to students, residents and faculty. The richest pool of easy to use reference and communication resources are PC software programs that are intended for individual workstations or at best, client - server, Local Area Network (LAN) implementation. HUBNET (Hospitals and University at Buffalo Library Resource Network), a project of the School of Medicine and the Library Consortium of Health Institutions in Buffalo offers integrated presentation of many such LAN resources over this regional WAN. The system crosses many institutional boundaries and reaches physically remote sites in a complex mix of information systems environments with few issues related to performance. The system design provides a level of ease of use that has brought many new users into active computer use while addressing integration into diverse information systems settings and networking environments.

INTRODUCTION

The School of Medicine and Biomedical Sciences of the State University of New York at Buffalo has eight teaching hospitals that are distributed throughout the city of Buffalo and Western New York. This geographic distribution and an increasing emphasis on primary care put significant demands on the school's ability to communicate with and support its students, residents and faculty at the clinical sites in which they work. Electronic resources, especially those that can be offered through a consistent and easy to use interface, can potentially enhance communication across this wide area and allow remote access to many of the support resources of the medical school and university. The geographic distribution of the medical school is complicated by a wide variety of information systems and network environments making the task of consistent and distributed presentation of materials difficult. These different systems complicate the school's ability to offer more than simply the lowest common denominator of electronic resources. Through the Western New York Health Sciences Consortium, an alliance of the teaching hospitals and the School of Medicine, a city-wide FDDI ring has been established. The medical school and four of the eight teaching hospitals have contracted for FDDI service with the provider NYNEX for multi-year connectivity to a city wide FDDI ring. Two other teaching hospitals have ethernet level connections with the medical school via microwave and fiber optic media, and several other associated hospitals and primary care sites have developed T1 level connection to this FDDI ring.

HUBNET is a reference and communication system which resides at the School of Medicine and Biomedical Sciences and is offered as a subscription service across the FDDI / T1 WAN. The impetus for the HUBNET system arose from discontent with the existing environment which included a university MiniMedline system, single-workstation CD-Plus Medline systems installed in several hospitals and hospitals and individuals using on-line fee based Medline access. Many of the hospitals in the consortium were facing increased Medline costs as they moved from single Medline workstations in their libraries to many networked access points. The hospitals and the university were also facing increasing costs and the need for greater technical expertise to mount and support the increasing number of on-line resources becoming available. In addition, there was also a desire to make the resources at the

0195–4210/94/$5.00

different clinical sites consistent, so that students, faculty and staff would not have to learn new systems as they moved from site to site. This is especially important because of the shared undergraduate and graduate training programs that exist in this consortium environment.

PLATFORM CHOICES

While investigating the different possibilities for presenting the Medline database, it became clear to the HUBNET committee that the most attractive interface, based on ease of use and search capabilities, was the Microsoft Windows CD-Plus search engine. While some users may find fault with specifics of the search engine and some may desire wholly different access software, few can argue that the software domain defined by Microsoft Windows and the DOS applications that can be run within Windows offer the largest pool of easy to use electronic reference resources. Additional resources were important as the HUBNET committee also wanted to create as rich a support environment as possible. The HUBNET committee noted that a Windows or Windows compatible workstation was the defacto standard for workstations in the associated hospital libraries and at hospital clinical sites and therefore decided to offer Microsoft Windows CD-Plus Medline. However, the committee did not want to exclude existing Macintosh and Unix workstations completely. Also, quality dial-in access and easy installation of the networked offering in the diverse environments of the networked sites were desirable. Finally all of this needed to be delivered in an environment with constrained resources, limited technical support and many political and technical hurdles.

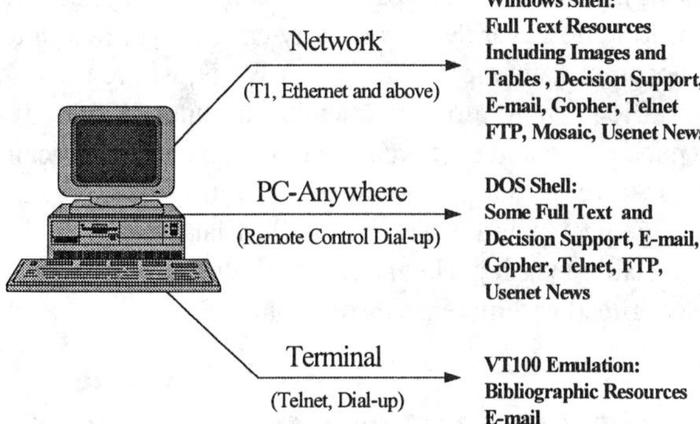

Figure 1: HUBNET Access Methods and Available Resources

In order to meet the diverse needs of this environment three methods of HUBNET access were developed, with differing amounts of resources available via each of the access methods. The resources available in each method are constrained by the technical possibilities of that method. Generally, the number of resources available is inversely proportional to the variety of computer platforms that can access the system using that method.

"NETWORKED" HUBNET ACCESS

The full range of HUBNET resources is available via direct access to a series of four Novell file servers that comprise "Networked" HUBNET.

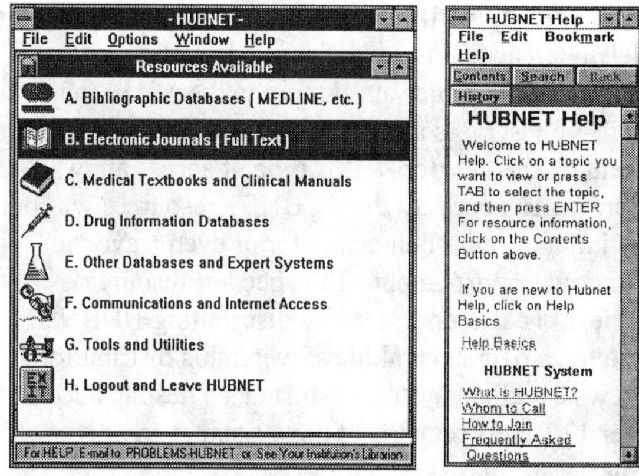

Figure 2: "Networked" HUBNET Interface

This HUBNET presentation is available to any Microsoft Windows capable computer that has a direct network connection to the WAN, allowing access to the following resources:

- full Medline database (1966 to present)
- Cinahl
- CancerLit
- Health
- Current Contents
- 19 full text electronic journals (NEJM, JAMA, Annals of Internal Medicine, etc.)
- six textbooks of medicine (Scientific American Consult, Merck manual, etc.)
- two drug information databases
- two expert systems,
- electronic mail and scheduling software
- Gopher, Mosaic and a Usenet News reader
- menued telnet and ftp

There is also an on-line account application program which allows guest users to request a full HUBNET account. These resources are offered in a graphical menu system which has on-line HUBNET help describing where information is available and how to get started with a specific program in addition to the help systems of the individual applications.

"Networked" HUBNET access is achieved by IPX Ethernet II connection to one HUBNET Novell server. This connection is made by running a Novell workstation shell, enabling Novell support in Windows and a single drive mapping, which enables a Windows (or OS/2) computer on the WAN to put a HUBNET Icon on their local desktop. When the user clicks on the HUBNET icon, username and password dialog boxes are presented and user input is automatically verified on another Novell server where HUBNET accounts are maintained. Valid user information initiates attachment to the rest of the HUBNET servers and presentation of the HUBNET menu on the desktop. This type of access allows users quick access to the HUBNET resources without having to reboot their computer or even leave the Windows environment. The speed of resource retrieval is also optimized by distributing HUBNET resources over several file servers; this distribution allows excellent system performance despite a load of over 120 users on parts of the system at any given time.

IPX on the WAN

"Networked" HUBNET access uses the IPX Ethernet II networking protocol native to Novell file services. Offering IPX file services out to a complex WAN environment was a major issue in the development of HUBNET. The initial commitment of the WAN networking committee was to support only TCP/IP communications as in the Internet and other complex networking environments. Unlike TCP/IP networking schemes where "firewalls" can be readily constructed, incorrectly configured IPX network servers can cause considerable problems for other IPX network servers. In addition Novell servers learn about and advertise information about other network resources. Network managers at the university and at the clinical sites were wary of these institutional resources being advertised across institutional boundaries.

The solution to the firewall issue was to set up a dedicated ethernet network on the university's Wellfleet router on which the HUBNET servers would be located. This network was configured so that it did not receive advertisements of file services from other networks (Server Advertisement Protocol - "SAP" is turned off to this network). Accordingly, the servers on this special network do not "know" about other file services and therefore cannot advertise these services to others. There are several additional filters in place where the university router is attached to the FDDI ring. The university router drops all outgoing IPX SAP traffic except for the file services from the HUBNET Novell servers (this is basically a static SAP table). This filter stops any additional university servers from being advertised to the hospitals. The university router drops all incoming packets destined for socket 0x0452. This filter prevents any incoming SAP from the hospitals. The University also drops incoming traffic destined for socket 0x0456 (the diagnostic socket) which was implemented to cure a stalling problem that developed university-wide do to an interaction of Arcserve's client software NLM (at a hospital) with the Clarkson packet driver version of Novell access shell. The clients would experience what looked like a stall in server access which was actually an endless string of Routing Information Protocol (RIP) requests. The software was trying to seek out clients to back-up.

The diagnostic socket issue is avoided if clients are running ODI instead of "packet driver" Novell shells. ODI is very desirable on clients because it also enables much better IPX WAN performance through the use of Novell's large packet and packet burst protocols. IPX in WAN environments has been inhibited in the past because each packet sent requires an acknowledgment and each packet could only be 512 bytes large (1/3rd of ethernet and 1/9th of token ring). On a LAN this can cause considerable network traffic, however there is usually enough bandwidth to accommodate the need, but in a WAN, where the IPX traffic must go through at least one router, the fixed packet size and its concomitant acknowledgment can cause very poor performance. Novell version 3.12's large packet and packet burst allow larger and variable length packet sizes which decrease network overhead and increase throughput.

INTEGRATING WINDOWS ON THE WAN

One of the design goals of the HUBNET system was to position it on a "clinical desktop" along with terminal access windows to hospital information systems applications and other programs. Work done by ourselves [1,2] and others [3] describes methods for directing the user through coordinated Windows on a desktop and associating reference materials with the content and context of other work on a clinical desktop. To achieve this type of parallel positioning, the HUBNET system needed to be a Microsoft Windows application itself with the ability to check user authenticity, attach to Novell file services and map network drives from within Windows. We did not want users to have multiple login procedures or are required to exit and restart Windows (with its associated time delay) in order to gain network access. Additionally, we needed a system that could easily accept software updates and the changes that they frequently involve, and which would allow the addition of new software with minimal restructuring. We achieved these goals by using a combination of Winbatch software for Windows (Wilson Windoware) and a Windows menu program (Saber menu for Windows - Saber Software Corporation).

We first use Winbach to authenticate the user against the bindery of one Novell server, then to connect to other file servers and map network drives within the Windows environment. We also use Winbatch to check local tag files which are copied into the Windows and system directories of local PC's or networked Windows installations. These tag files list the current versions of executable files and .dll files that are copied to local or locally networked Windows directories. These files are moved to a local installation because some poorly designed software demands that certain files must be in specific places and to improve WAN performance in some circumstances by accessing local vs. remote files.

The final result step in the compiled Winbatch program is the execution of the Windows menu. The menuing program allows easy configuration of the individual software programs that make up the HUBNET system. Through the menu, software can also be offered selectively to users on the basis of membership in groups on the authentication server.

REMOTE DIAL-IN ACCESS

Even with the development of a regional WAN, good dial-in access is important for users at home and for users at sites which do not have enough computers to justify a T1 link. Dial-in is possible through the university dial string; users are attached to a terminal server and can attach to HUBNET via the VT100 emulation that is described below. Better dial-in access, however, is offered through PC-Anywhere remote software and a series of PC's on HUBNET's own dial string. Incoming calls are automatically forwarded to the next open line by the phone system. An available phone line connects the user to a PC running PC-Anywhere host for DOS software. This dial-in access was first offered to hospital libraries that did not have network connections, but proved to be very popular among PC users who could get mouse control and bounce bar, menued access to DOS applications on the HUBNET system. Many of the HUBNET Windows resources (Citation databases, full text journals, some textbooks, e-mail, Gopher, Telnet, FTP, Usenet News, etc.) have DOS analogs that access the same data or Internet resources. Many Macintosh users have found that they too can access these resources, despite the lack of a Macintosh shell and the poor WAN capabilities of Appletalk, by running SoftPC and PC-Anywhere in combination. This solution certainly does not maintain the Macintosh interface and some Macintosh users find it to be unacceptable on older, slower machines.

TCP/IP ACCESS FOR DOS APPLICATIONS

Retaining access for other operating systems in the university and hospital environments was an important consideration. Limited resources and technical staff made it desirable to offer TCP/IP telnet access to networked, non-Windows computers and to computers that could not run PC-Anywhere. VT100 terminal access to DOS applications was realized by using a Xyplex terminal server placed on the ethernet network with 10 serially attached personal computers connected to the HUBNET Novell file servers via IPX. The terminal server has a rotary configured on it which allows clients connecting by telnet to find the next available PC. Once connected to a PC through the terminal server the user controls the PC via VT100 keystrokes and can run the citation databases and e-mail programs. Users can download search sets via ftp or kermit directly to their PC in this configuration.

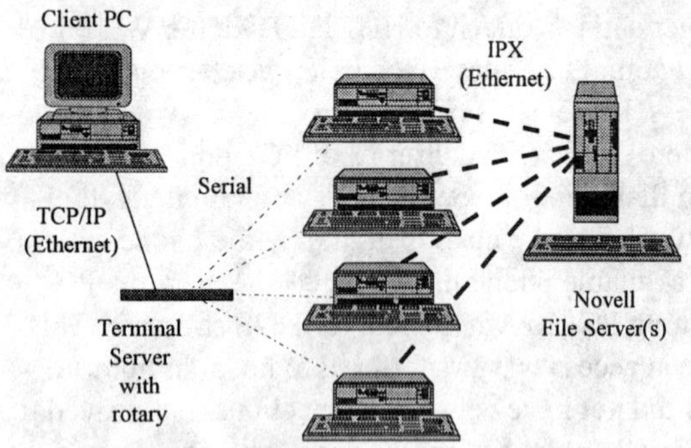

Figure 3: DOS Applications via VT100

SYSTEM USAGE

HUBNET has met the needs of its participating institutions by providing easy to use, networked access to citation databases across a WAN. The system has exceeded many expectations by offering more full text and Internet resources than had been anticipated by virtue of the savings generated through shared access and by virtue of the ease with which LAN resources can be installed and updated. In the eight months that HUBNET has been fully functional 3,800 user accounts have been established on the system. Anecdotally, many of these users are new to electronic reference and communications and many others are using resources in new ways (printing out articles for rounds, calling up information on the spot to answer patient care questions, signing out via e-mail). While full usage statistics will be available for presentation with this paper in November, it is already clear that the communications and full text resources of the system are being used much more heavily than was first expected and that the consistent interface implementation and help systems have expanded the number of programs users are comfortable using frequently.

REFERENCES

1) Loonsk, John W., Designing Educational Application Workgroups, *Proceedings of American Medical Informatics Association (AMIA), Annual Education and Research Conference*, June, 1990.

2) Loonsk, John W., Lively, Rick E., TinHan, Erik, Litt, Harold., Implementing the Medical Desktop: Tools for the Integration of Independent Information Resources. *Symposium on Computer Applications in Medical Care (SCAMC)*, November, 1991.

3) Cimino, James J., et al. The Medline Button, Symposium on Computer Applications in Medical Care (SCAMC), November, 1992.

4) Shifman MA. Clyman JI., et. al. NetMenu: Experience in the Implementation of an Institutional Menu of Information Sources, Symposium on Computer Applications in Medical Care (SCAMC), pgs. 554-8, 1993.

5) Ketchell DS. Fuller SS., et. al. Collaborative Development of a Uniform Graphical Interface. Symposium on Computer Applications in Medical Care. (SCAMC), pgs. 251-5, 1992.

Expanding M NET: Lessons from the Development of a Referring Physician Computer Network

Jocelyn G. DeWitt, Ph. D.*, Kurt A. Riegel, ** Michael P. Miotto,**
*University of Michigan Medical Center
**International Business Machines, Inc.

ABSTRACT

M NET, the University of Michigan Medical Center's statewide referring physician computer network, was implemented as a pilot project in 1990. After three years of design, development and implementation, M NET has progressed from its pilot project status to a production system within the institution's strategic plan for hospital networking.

This paper describes the evolution of M NET from a small pilot project to its current production status encompassing all clinical departments and hundreds of physicians across the state. The lessons learned from the pilot, the requirements of both the referring physicians and the Medical Center, and the development of a flexible and robust network architecture to allow network expansion are addressed.

INTRODUCTION

The need for efficient, reliable and easy access to hospital and clinical information by referring physicians has been well documented in the literature.[1,2,3,4] Numerous implementation strategies for various computer and telephone based information systems have been described.[5,6] Many hospitals view this provision of information access as key to maintaining a referral base, establishing new referral source relationships, and, now with health care reform issues at the forefront, providing a service that differentiates them from competitor hospitals hoping to establish referral relationships with the same audience. Concurrently, these information services must be cost effective in their approach and in the rationale for their implementation.

Similarly, referring physicians view information access as being crucial to providing high quality follow-up care to patients referred to tertiary institutions. They often find that this information access allows them to provide ongoing quality care in remote locations through literature search capabilities, consultant resources using electronic mail and other means, and bulletin board functions alerting them to health care news of particular interest to them. Referring physicians are looking for ways to provide high quality, yet cost-effective health care and see easily accessible information as critical to that endeavor.

The University of Michigan Medical Center (UMMC) launched its own referring physician computer network in 1990 after several years of requirements gathering and institutional preparation.[7] This pilot project, developed in conjunction with IBM, spanned three years until the fall of 1993, when the full production implementation of M NET began. This paper describes the transformation of M NET from a pilot project to its current production status. The lessons learned from the pilot, the requirements of the referring physicians and the UMMC, and the implementation of an architecture to allow for network expansion are addressed.

PILOT IMPLEMENTATION

As a referring physician computer network, M NET's primary purpose was to facilitate the dissemination of information from the University of Michigan Medical Center to its referring physicians across the state. The information disseminated included clinical records, such as discharge summaries and procedural reports; CME course information; general information on Medical Center departments and services; a restaurant, shopping and lodging guide; maps and directions to the Medical Center; and functional capabilities such as electronic mail and Medline access. A graphical user interface was designed for easy retrieval of the available information. Computer workstations consisting of an IBM PS/2 Model 70, an IBM 4019 LaserPrinter, a U.S. Robotic Courier V.32 bis modem, and an IBM 8515 XGA high resolution monitor were loaned to the participating referring physicians during the pilot project. Twenty sites across the state encompassing 45 physicians comprised the external pilot network participants. Adult and pediatric cardiology were the two internal hospital pilot departments.

In order to accommodate the complexity of the UMMC hospital-wide information system and plans for substantial network growth, the initial M NET network architecture was designed for change and expansion. Rather than building M NET-specific function into existing departmental systems or the hospital mainframe, a three-level approach was used. This approach called for a dedicated server to be placed between the hospital data sources and the external referring physician machines, allowing for improved flexibility and control of network function. The pilot network architecture that resulted from these considerations is shown in Figure 1.

The hospital mainframe electronic mail system served as the initial collection point for reports sent to referring physicians from clinical departments. The M NET server was an IBM PS/2 model 80 running OS/2. This machine would transfer reports from the mainframe and distribute them to local mailboxes for each referring physician. M NET client machines running a custom-built user interface would then dial into the M NET server and retrieve patient reports, electronic mail, and other data.

Subsequently, the M NET project has been elevated to a production system within the Medical Center's information system initiatives. All clinical departments are now able to participate in M NET by providing the clinical information pertinent to the patients sent by their referring physicians. Additionally, all referring physicians across the state may now become M NET participants, resulting in an ever increasing number of network users.

The following sections discuss the lessons learned from the pilot project and the strategies that were implemented as a result of those lessons.

LESSONS LEARNED

At the end of three years of pilot implementation, data collection and requirements gathering, it was learned that, in general:

1. A large percentage of referring physician offices do not have computer systems to run their practices. Most common is the use of a personal computer or terminal used solely to access a contract billing service.

2. Most referring physicians are not yet comfortable using computers to manage their patient data and do not have online practice management systems in their offices. Therefore, they still prefer paper copies of information to include in their patient files.

3. Physicians are not the primary users of the computer. Office staff and nurses are more likely to be the daily computer operators. Physicians use the computer for specific functions such as electronic mail and literature searches.

4. Providing a computer to a referring physician is not sufficient impetus for a physician to use the computer, especially if the computer is able to receive information from only one institution. Similarly, a referring physician will not

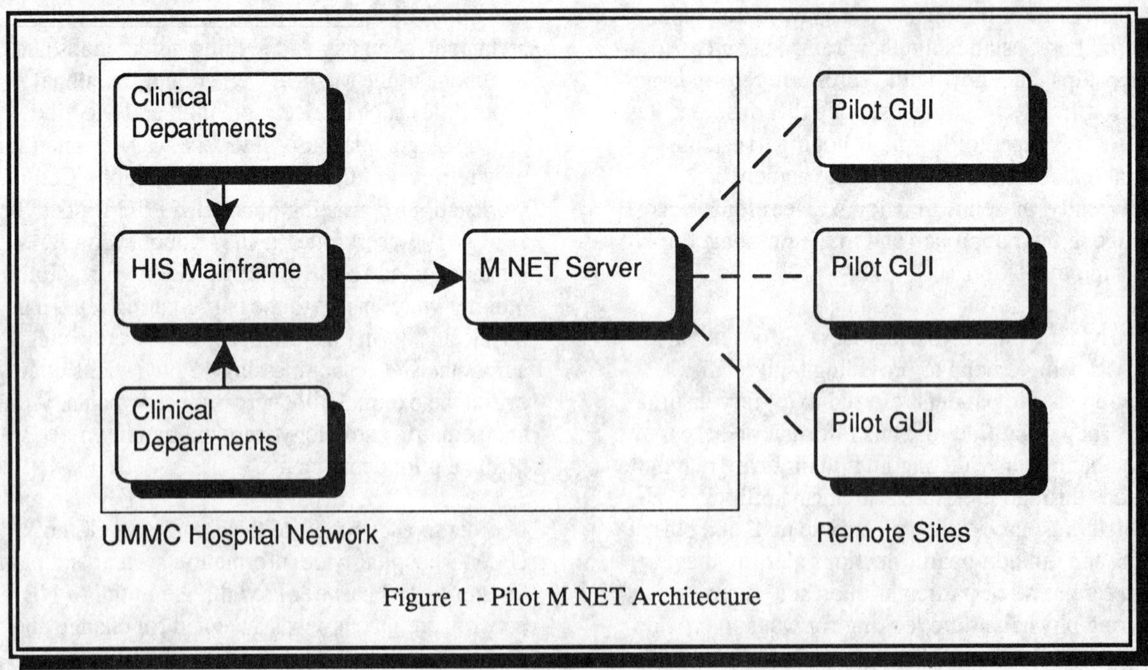

Figure 1 - Pilot M NET Architecture

purchase a computer to access a single institution's information.

5. Referring physicians are most interested in receiving clinical information regarding their patients as quickly as possible. Complementary data, such as CME course information, restaurant and lodging information, and Medical Center services are of less use and interest to them.

6. A referring physician computer network must provide adaptability to a variety of back end networks and data sources to allow the incorporation of all clinical data sources.

7. A referring physician computer network must also provide for the integration of a variety of front end interfaces to support the creation of a variety of delivery platforms to meet user requirements.

PROJECT STRATEGIES

Given the knowledge gained from the referring physicians who participated in the pilot project, the conceptual framework for production implementation of M NET was revised and expanded. This section describes the strategies implemented as a result of pilot project experience. These strategies will be discussed in terms of delivery options, program functions and system architecture.

Delivery Options

Originally it was determined that information would be delivered to the referring physician office via a single computer interface. While valid as a long-term strategic goal for referring physician networking, that decision became an obstacle to many of the referring physicians receiving the information they required. Without computers in their offices, and without working knowledge of and comfort with computers, it was premature to expect the physicians and office staff to embrace a single technology. Therefore, several additional options for delivering the information to the referring physicians were developed. Physicians would then be able to choose which option best met their environment and information needs. The M NET delivery options now available are: 1) M NET with the custom designed user interface designed for and used during the pilot phase of M NET; 2) M NET on Lotus Notes (a commercially available groupware software package), that runs on the Windows or Macintosh operating systems; 3) M NET integrated into a commercially available office practice management system; 4) M NET by fax, which allows information to go automatically to a referring physician fax machine; and 5) M NET on DOS, a query-based program for referrers with minimal equipment availability, but who require the ability to conduct ad hoc searches for patient information.

This range of options allows the Medical Center to tailor the information system solution to the unique environment of each referring physician office. These options also allow for a dynamic office environment; as the office infrastructure becomes more sophisticated the M NET implementation scheme will change to meet that growth.

M NET on Lotus Notes has received the most development effort of the new options. Its flexibility in terms of platform, data integration, image management capability and expansion provide for significant development opportunities. Using Notes, each physician office can define and develop unique functions for its own use. Because the user interface is standard across all the functions within Notes, there is no additional training required when new functions are added. Additionally, a commercially available, standardized delivery vehicle allows the M NET staff to concentrate on information content rather than support of the application itself. Simplifying the network support requirements is of particular interest given the size of the state of Michigan and its rural geography. Once a Lotus Notes M NET site is installed and the users trained, all program updates and enhancements can be completed on line.

Purchasers of a practice management software package (Genius Solutions) are able to run M NET through a module on that package. Data sent to these offices from the UMMC flow directly into the patient database within the practice management software. M NET is available through the purchase and installation of this software package, eliminating the need for offices to run two separate systems to manage their offices and to access the UMMC.

M NET by fax has allowed offices with no computer to receive information on their patients as readily as offices with computers. Similar to most of the other M NET options, physicians in these offices do not have to request the information, as it is sent to them automatically from the M NET server.

The M NET on DOS option is specifically designed for physicians with less powerful computer systems.

However, it provides flexible capabilities that allow ad hoc queries to the Medical Center on any patient referred by that physician.

Program Function

The functions provided within each of these M NET options have also been reconsidered. Referring physicians are concerned primarily with obtaining timely and valid clinical information about their patients. In addition to this clinical information, M NET provided complementary data for patient, office staff and physician use. Much of this peripheral information was transferred to the new platforms because of high utilization during the pilot project. This information included electronic mail; library and Medline access; CME course brochures and registration functions; a catalog describing hospital departments, clinics, services and procedures; and maps and directions to the Medical Center. Information that was not accessed frequently and deemed unimportant to the referring physician was eliminated. These discontinued functions included directories of restaurants, hotels, and shopping areas; a journal club listing abstracts of selected articles by discipline; research protocols; and a list of the computer assisted instructional materials available at the Medical Center. As the referring physician requirements change these functions will be reassessed to determine their usefulness and may be reintegrated into the M NET program in similar or revised form.

Network Architecture

Since the development of the pilot architecture, there have been numerous changes in the data sources, data access mechanisms and presentation vehicles that comprise M NET. Moreover, it has become apparent that this type of change can be expected to continue as the project continues to evolve and expand. Fortunately, the basic architectural approach of placing a middleware layer between the data sources and the delivery platforms has allowed for this kind of change. The current architecture of the M NET network is shown in Figure 2.

The M NET server, running OS/2 on an IBM PS/2 model 95, continues to act as the intermediary between the data sources and the delivery platforms. This level of software control has made it possible to accommodate relatively major changes to the network with relatively minor effort and with little or no disruption to participating departments and users.

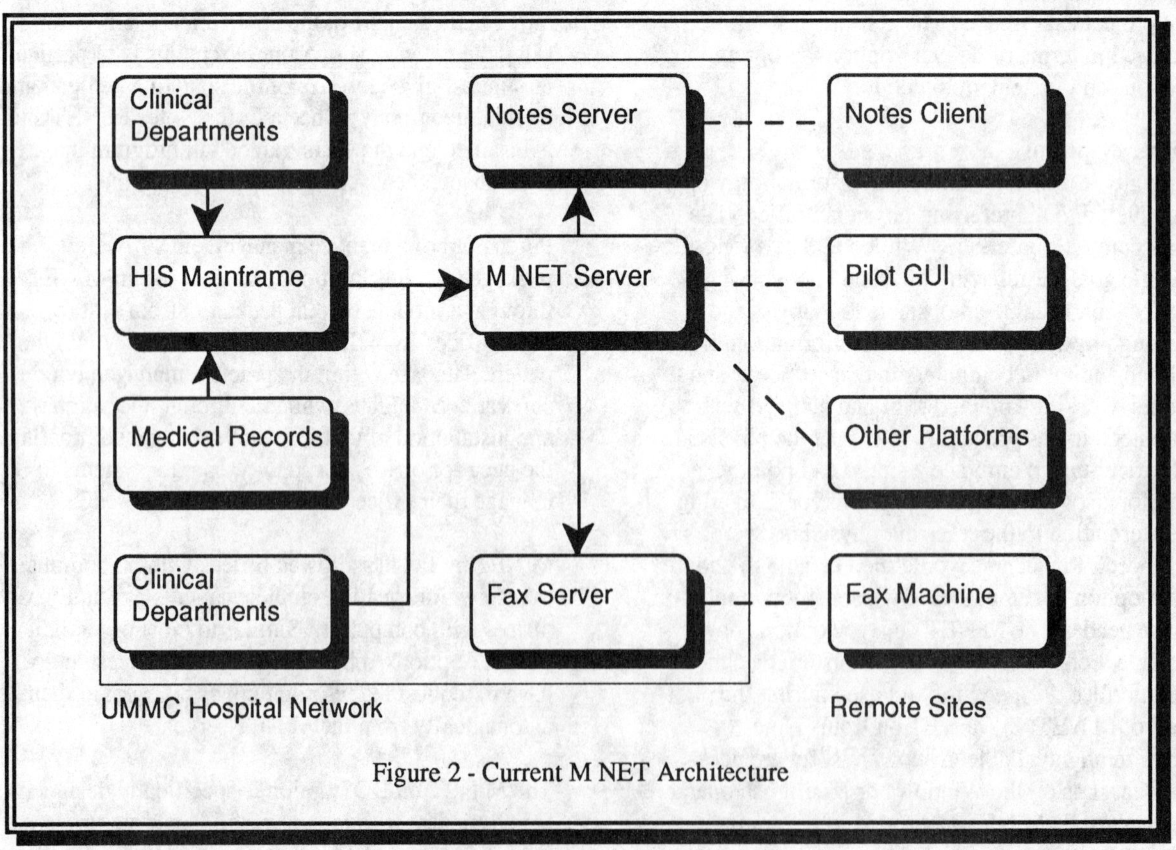

Figure 2 - Current M NET Architecture

Use of the mainframe electronic mail system has ended and been replaced with access to a VSAM database of clinical results. This database acts as a common collection point for results from clinical departments publishing their data internally. By accessing this database, M NET is able to make a substantial portion of UMMC clinical data available to outside physicians.

In addition to this central data source, several departments make their data directly available to M NET through a variety of mechanisms. Pathology and radiology data are to be published through open relational databases. Other departments send their data from extracts of proprietary databases running on a variety of platforms. Several additional types of data sources, in particular message routing systems supporting HL7, are expected to be integrated into the network within the next several months.

The variety of data delivery platforms that are now part of M NET (e.g. M NET on Lotus Notes and fax) were straightforward to incorporate into the basic three-level architecture. Additional servers were added to manage the unique characteristics of the Lotus Notes and fax platforms. These servers receive data from the M NET server through existing program interface tools, and then pass the data along to their respective client machines.

This three-level approach, incorporating data sources, delivery mechanisms, and an intermediate or middleware layer for data formatting, routing and control, has proven to be a robust, flexible, and maintainable structure for this type of physician network. In spite of the changes that have occurred in data access and end user functionality requirements as the project has moved from pilot into production stages, the network architecture has remained essentially unchanged.

CONCLUSION

The flexibility inherent within the basic network architecture as well as the functions provided by the program allow M NET to meet the continuously changing needs of the UMMC and the physicians who refer patients to the Medical Center.

Four system characteristics will help support the continued expansion of the M NET network. First, referring physicians are able to receive information through the vehicle that best meets their needs, whether that is an IBM compatible or Macintosh computer, or a fax machine. Second, the type of information the referring physician is able to receive can be tailored to meet his or her needs. Some physicians prefer to receive only clinical data, while others elect to receive a full complement of Medical Center information in addition to clinical reports. Third, as new data sources within the hospital are identified (such as new departments, new clinical procedures, or revised clinical reports), they can be integrated into the M NET network with minimal effort. And finally, the network structure will allow expansion of M NET to other referral sources, such as additional hospitals, clinics, and managed care organizations.

This paper has discussed the development of the M NET referring physician computer network and its evolution from a pilot project to a fully implemented production system. The lessons learned from this evolutionary process should assist others in the implementation of similar information networks. Clearly, a growing number of medical centers will include this type of physician network in their overall information system strategy as a means of expanding their relationships with outside referral sources and other health care providers.

References

[1]. Beck J, Krages K, Ash J, Gorman P. Outreach to Oregon Physicians and Hospitals: 5000 by 2000. Annuals New York Academy of Sciences 1992; 670:91-97.

[2]. Jacknowitz L. West Virginia CONSULT: Enhanced Information Access for Health Care Practitioners in a Rural Environment. Annuals New York Academy of Sciences 1992; 670:163-70.

[3]. McElroy T. Hospital-Physician Bonding: The Ultimate Strategy. Michigan Hospitals 1988; 9:27-9.

[4]. Parsons D. Progress and Problems of Interhospital Consulting by Computer. Annuals New York Academy of Sciences 1992; 670:1-11.

[5]. Holt N, Crawford M. Medial Information Service via Telephone: The Pioneer of Physician Consultation Services. Annuals New York Academy of Sciences 1992; 670:1-11.

[6]. Reis H, Brenner D, Robinson J. Multimedia Communications in Health Care. Annuals New York Academy of Sciences1992; 670:155-62.

[7]. Ten Haken J, Calhoun J, Ellison J, Miotto M. Proceedings of the Sixteenth Annual Symposium on Computer Applications in Medical Care. M NET: A Statewide Referring Physician Computer Network. McGraw-Hill, Inc. 1992; 814-5.

A Frame-Relay Approach for a State-Wide Health Information Network

Reed-Fourquet LL, Beaudin S, Courtway P, Pappanikou J, Trask J,
Durand D, Bonacci J, Rhodes K, Pendleton R, Vogler E, Lynch JT,MPH

ABSTRACT

An approach for a frame-relay implementation is described which is intended to establish connectivity between the health care providers in the state of Connecticut with a gateway to the internet. While other health care networking efforts have based the interconnectivity efforts on direct connections to the internet for each institution, our design takes a more cost effective approach by establishing a private health care network with a single entry point to the internet. This will not only provide the advantages of internet connections to all participating providers, but it will also isolate intrastate patient care traffic from the internet, reserving internet traffic for those information needs not available within the statewide network. In addition to the network solution, an extensive user support infrastructure is also presented.

INTRODUCTION

As is well documented in the literature, the need for health care providers to begin an information sharing effort is essential not only to maintain and minimize health care costs, but to improve the quality of patient care. The network described will answer this need by providing a communications infrastructure upon which powerful information sharing applications can be built.

As a central membership organization, the Connecticut Hospital Research and Education Foundation (CHREF) can provide a point of coordination to manage a cooperative effort among multiple health care facilities. We will provide centralized services in order to implement and maintain the network. These services will include, but not be limited to, education, administration, help desk, and network management. Details for these services will be addressed in the sections to follow.

EXPECTED USAGE AND BENEFITS

There are a number of benefits to health care providers which will be realized from this networking effort. The resources available on the health information network will directly benefit physicians, nurses, administrators, radiologists and researchers. These professionals will have access to a growing set of resources which will assist in patient management and care, consultations, and information sharing. This in turn will benefit all those patients seeking health care from these providers.

SHARING OF PATIENT DATA

CHREF currently maintains a statewide patient database for all of the acute care facility discharges in the state. This data is used by our "Toward Excellence in Care" program to perform comparative patient outcome studies for our member institutions. It is also used for resource utilization studies to assist members in monitoring and reducing health care costs. Currently, data is collected via tape on a monthly basis and is processed in batch mode. Study results are printed and mailed to participating institutions. The data highway which would result from this networking proposal would serve to allow this process to migrate to an on-line service, allowing for more timely dissemination of quality indicator and utilization results.

Access to the statewide patient database would be a tremendous service to both the health care provider and the researcher. By making the patient medical history available to the provider, administrative time to gather patient history would be minimized, and the patient would have more immediate access to a better informed provider. The ability to electronically transfer patient information while the patient is enroute has a wealth of potential for savings in both administrative costs and expensive duplication of testing. In terms of improved patient care, the health care provider would be better served if such data could be examined before the patient arrival. As demonstrated by our "Toward Excellence in Care" program, this database is a valuable resource for epidemiological studies. By making this database available on-line to the researcher over the network, many outstanding epidemiological questions will begin to be answered.

WORLD-WIDE INFORMATION SHARING

Access to the internet will allow providers to gather and exchange information with literally a world of other health care providers and researchers. Medline is one of the most valuable resources available to the medical community today. Desk-top access to the most current medical literature would be a valuable asset to any health care facility. New databases are available every day on the internet, which will allow providers access to the most current treatment techniques and genetic testing methods. European efforts have made available bone marrow donor databases. Similar efforts in this country would be invaluable to both the provider and the patient, and once they are available, our health care facilities will be in a position to query the data. Nutrition database efforts are underway in this country which would assist healthcare nutritionists in assessing the dietary needs of their patients. Nurses will have at their disposal a vast amount of nursing practice and educational resources as well as professional conferences and bulletin boards. Access to any available on-line federal health care regulation information would also be a valuable resource to health care administrators.

COMMUNICATIONS INFRASTRUCTURE

The network will not only address the specific areas mentioned, but will provide a basic electronic communications infrastructure for our healthcare professionals. Electronic mail and file transfer capabilities will bring our health care facilities up to speed in the electronic age reducing large volumes of paper communications, and otherwise providing for a more efficient means of communication. This basic infrastructure would make available to health care professionals access to world-wide collaborators and specialists. Medical treatment centers are notably absent from most of the hazard and disaster information computer networks. In establishing a communications infrastructure, this lack of inclusion can be addressed. Efficient communication and participation in early warning systems can minimize casualties in times of disaster.

MULTIMEDIA

This network infrastructure will also play an important role in the establishment of multimedia applications for healthcare, consultation, and administration. There are a multitude of advanced testing techniques which produce images and films for analysis. The ability to send these images over a network would allow for consultations in a timely manner, without moving the patient. This is not only a cost effective method of information sharing, it also minimizes risk to the patient. Although the development of information sharing standards are in the early stages, success in this area is imminent. Our network structure is designed to insure that this technology can be implemented with minimal effort as well as minimal additional cost with respect to the network infrastructure.

NETWORK DESIGN

Connecting each of the above facilities on an individual basis to the internet through a standard mid-level network provider would be rather expensive. Each connection requires a connection from the local site to the internet provider in addition to the provider fees. Instead, what we propose is to create a state-wide network of health care providers using a standard value added network carrier, and provide a single gateway to the internet from a central site, thus allowing the institutions to share a larger bandwidth. A T1 connection is capable of transporting 23 times as much traffic for only 2-4 times the price, and only a single installation fee is incurred. By dealing with the local carrier, additional savings are realized since the distance to the local connection is generally less. This approach is not only much more cost effective, but it also isolates from the internet intra-state health care network traffic.

Due to the voluminous nature of health care information, high band-width capacity will be necessary. It is important that the tariffs for the wide area network be offered at a fixed monthly rate rather than on a per usage basis. This will be imperative as multi-gigabyte database queries and multimedia applications become more prevalent. A poorly designed database search could itself cost on a per packet basis more than the fixed monthly fee. Based upon the status of the current technology, the best option for the wide area network will be frame relay. This will provide significant bandwidth for the participants at very reasonable monthly rates.

Frame relay technology is based upon the establishment of permanent virtual connections (PVC's) between network members. Because there has been no connectivity among independent health care institutions, the inter-institution bandwidth requirements can only be estimated. However, by providing a single 56.7 kbps connection between each participant and CHREF, all inter-institution traffic can be maintained. Subsequent analysis of traffic patterns may warrant further dedicated interconnectivity between some institutions. Based upon this approach, the central site will require high bandwidth capacity as well as a high performance router. It is anticipated that 56.7 kbps will be an underestimate based upon potential uses of the network, however, since many applications are still in the developmental stage, the higher bandwidth is not yet warranted as the cost to upgrade would roughly equivalent to three months of underutilization waste. .

In order to maximize the ability to maintain

service to each site, the wide area network provider will be contracted to service the network hardware. This contract stipulates that there will be a single point of contact for wide area network problems up to and including the router. This will minimize any potential problems of wide area network components falling out of the jurisdiction of a given vendor. Staff at CHREF will be the primary contact for the provider, but service can be initiated from the remote sites.

Some of the larger facilities have plans to extend networking services to their affiliated laboratories, clinics, and other healthcare institutions not represented in this proposal. These sites will obtain additional bandwidth in order to further facilitate the statewide healthcare networking effort.

These larger sites will be equipped with T1 access to the network. The remaining institutions will begin with a 56.7 kbps access to the network with a single PVC to the central site. Because the current maximum bandwidth for frame relay is T1, the central site, CHREF, will need to support multiple high band width T1 access lines to the frame relay network. Because traffic which needs to access the internet is anticipated to be less than the intra-state traffic, and due to bandwidth limitations of the internet provider, a single T1 access line to the internet will be provided from the central site.

IMPLEMENTATION

The network implementation is a 4-phase process. Phase I of the implementation will involve networking those sites with representation on the network advisory committee. We will refer to this phase as a prototype. Phase II will involve adding those sites that have a skilled network team. The experience gathered in networking these institutions will be documented, and will be used for Phase III, which will involve networking those institutions that are network ready, but do not have an internal network management team. Phase IV will involve networking those institutions that are not yet network ready.

In order to work through the technical details of the network design, installation, and maintenance, a Network Advisory Committee has been established. This committee is a two tier group. The upper tier is composed of information system directors. This group will assist in upper level management decisions, and will serve as primary consultants for policies and procedures which may be required for network management. The lower tier of this committee is composed of network specialists. This tier will serve as technical consultants for both the design and implementation of the network. This group will be responsible for implementing and testing the prototype.

In order to coordinate the installation and maintenance of each network site, and to maximize communication, a Network Communications Conference will be established. The conference is intended to establish a formal communication forum for network issues including implementation schedules, education, troubleshooting, and general information dissemination.

The prototype will involve connecting those sites represented on the network advisory committee. These sites are not only well supported in network communications, but they have been involved in the network design. This prototype will be used in order to work out any unanticipated connectivity problems, and as a benchmark for network utilization studies. This effort will be used as a learning process in order to gather additional experience with the set-up. The prototype experience will be documented and used as a baseline for subsequent implementation phases. Based upon the background obtained from this implementation experience, a formal implementation approach will be tabulated in order to minimize implementation problems as subsequent sites. The prototype phase will be coordinated through the Network Advisory Committee. This group will, as part of the prototype, implement an electronic conferencing method in order to maximize communication potential and to minimize travel.

Once the prototype is sufficiently tested, phase II is initiated. This will involve bringing on-line those sites with strong network support capabilities. This effort will test the deployment techniques developed during the prototype. Based upon feedback from these sites, the implementation methods will be refined so as to minimize difficulties in subsequent installations. Because the target sites for this installation phase are well supported, additional experience with the network will be obtained with minimal interruption and time expenditure. This phase will involve coordination between the central network support specialist and the network representative from the health care site. While the implementation details for each site may be somewhat different, the central network support specialist will be encouraged to visit these sites in order to maximize the experience level of this individual for subsequent installations.

Before embarking on phase III of the installation, an educational program will be sponsored at CHREF in order to provide the information system personnel with sufficient information to prepare for both the installation and maintenance of the networking equipment. Any additional information learned during either the prototype or during phase II will be disseminated at this time as well. Should there be a need for additional educational programs for installation and maintenance, multiple programs will be provided.

Those sites that do not currently have a network in place will need additional assistance in order to establish a link to the internet. Minimally, a personal computer with a network card, TCP/IP, a hub, cables, and installation. Because these sites may wish to implement a more extensive solution, a list of systems integrators will be provided. The central network support specialist will work closely with these sites to assist in finding resources for the sites' internal network structure, however, the responsibilities of the central network support specialist will end at the router.

Because the current network design is based upon anticipated usage, a tuning effort will be necessary. The first tuning analysis will be performed on the pilot sites. Any changes in Permanent Virtual Connection designation will be applied to phase II sites. Similarly, a performance analysis will be performed prior to phase III and phase IV implementation.

LOCAL SUPPORT

User support for each local site will primarily be the responsibility of the information systems staff of each participant. Support at this level will therefore be in an indirect manner. Each site will be asked to designate an information systems representative to the Network Communications Conference. This will provide a formal vehicle for information transfer as well as a primary point of contact for maintenance and enhancement purposes. Educational programs will be offered to members of this group such that they will be better prepared to provide local network support. As appropriate, members of this conference and members of the Information Systems Conference will sponsor educational programs to end-users in conjunction with the many other conference groups of the Connecticut Hospital Association (CHA).

CENTRAL HELP DESK SUPPORT

In addition to the user support for each local site, there will be central support services provided. These services will include a help desk coordinator. This individual will be available for telephone support and basic troubleshooting. This individual will assist in identifying the source of a given problem, and will be apprised of the appropriate measures to be taken to address the problems. The central network specialist will provide technical support to the help desk, but the help desk coordinator will serve as the primary liaison. In addition to troubleshooting support, the help desk coordinator will be responsible for identifying and researching value added services on the internet which might benefit health care institutions. Those functions which require systems integration will be referred to the network specialist and the project coordinator for further investigation. For those services which require no further integration, the help desk coordinator will investigate the features and user procedures, document instructions for use, and disseminate the instructions to the remote site contact. Those services with sufficient merit will be referred to the Information Systems Conference for an educational seminar. A newsletter targeting the end-user will be established and disseminated to the user community.

ELECTRONIC HELP DESK

In order to better service the network user community, an electronic help desk will also be established. This electronic help desk will be based upon an e-mail function. While central network support personnel will primarily be responsible for responding to items listed in the electronic help desk, this forum will be supplemented by the technical members of the Network Advisory Committee.

EDUCATIONAL SERVICES

As mentioned above, educational services will be provided to both user groups and user support personnel. These services will include investigation into value added services and databases on the internet relevant to health care and health care administration. Newsletters, instructions and bulletins will be used as a conveyance vehicle to inform the user community of available features. Seminars and training sessions will be offered centrally.

COOPERATION AND COMMUNICATION

Because of the nature of the membership organization, CHREF as and affiliate of CHA, has at its disposal a means of establishing and maintaining communication and cooperation among member health care organizations. This is an essential component of any effort which intends to collect and distribute information from among multiple independent parties. CHA has in place several conferences of health care professionals which generally meet on a monthly basis. This is a natural vehicle to establish consensus, standards, and information exchange. It also provides a means of educating members in the midst of change. By tapping into these conferences, members of the Information Systems Conference hope to identify the information system needs of each group, and use the conference structure to provide appropriate educational services to each group.

Information systems professionals from acute care hospitals have also begun to take on a role in establishing and providing information services to affiliated physician offices, laboratories and pharmacies. By establishing consensus and cooperative design efforts within this group, CHREF can be assured that changes and migration are uniform within the state, and thereby minimize the duplication of effort.

REFERENCES

Bergman, R. A doctor in the network. Physician links improve access to critical data. Hospitals. 1993 May 5;67(9):24-6.

Butler, D. L., and Anderson, P. S. The use of wide area computer networks in disaster management and the implications for hospital/medical networks. *Ann N Y Acad Sci*. 1992 Dec 17;670:202-10.

Dayhoff, R. E., and Maloney, D. L. Exchange of Veterans Affairs medical data using national and local networks. *Ann NY Acad Sci*. 1992 Dec 17;670:50-66.

Flaherty, G. The health information network. *Aust Fam Physician*. 1993 Apr;22(4):563-5.

Fry, P. A., Using integration technology as a strategic advantage. *Top Health Inf Manage*. 1993 Aug;14(1):25-39.

Gardner, E. Milwaukee network would be a first. *Mod Healthc*. 1992 May 4;22(18):30.

Haigh, P. J. Healthcare reengineering via network technologies: a critical combination. *Computer Healthcare*. 1993 Nov;14(12):36, 38,40.

Holliday, C. R., and Pfiffner, E. B. Fiber optics: health care needs a public network. *Hospitals*. 1991 Nov. 20;65(22):64.

Konsynski, B. R., and McFarlan, F. W. Information partnerships--shared data, shared scale. *Harv Bus Rev*. 1990 Sep-Oct;68(5):114-20.

Lafrance, S. Building strong networks eight ways. *Healthc Inform*. Jan;10(1):42-4.

Lemke, H. U. Communication networks for medical image transmission. *Strahlenther Onkol*. 1993 Sep;169(9):512-20.

Lemkin, P. F. Xconf: a network-based image conferencing system. *Comput Biomed Res*. 1993 Feb;26(1):1-27.

Lim, P. MediNet: Singapore's nationwide network. *Ann Acad Med Singapore*. 1990 Sep;19(5):656-61.

Ostbye, T. et al. Establishing an international computer network for research and teaching in public health and epidemiology. *Eur J Epidemiol*. 1991 Jan;7(1):34-8.

Regan, B. G. Computerized information exchange in health care. *Med J Aust*. 1991 Jan 21;154(2):140-4.

Rosenthal, L. E. Information networks and their impact upon medicine. *Ann Acad Med Singapore*. 1990 Sep;19(5):621-6.

Soergel, D. et al. A network model for improving access to food and nutrition data. *J am DietAssoc*. 1992 Jan;92(1):78-82.

Sparks, S. M. Electronic networking for nurses. *Image J Nurs Sch*. 1993 Fall;25(3):245-8.

Streety, M. A. Connecting healthcare providers. An effective computer network can create durable relationships. *Health Prog*. 1991 May;72(4):60-4.

Wagner, G. Test driving Iowa's FDDI superhighway. *Healthc Inform*. 1993 Jul;10(7):90- 2,94.

Wagner, G. The Iowa Medical Information Network: a concept. *J Med Syst*. 1992 Jun;162(2-3):73-86.

Wear, L. L., and Pinkert, J.R. Computer Networks. *J. AHIMA*. 1993 Oct;64(10):28-30, 32, 34-7.

Weser, A. J. Hors, J., and Persijn, G. Transplant-euro-computer-network--European initiative to support communications between transplant facilities. *Transplant Proc*. 1993 Dec;25(6):3067-8.7.

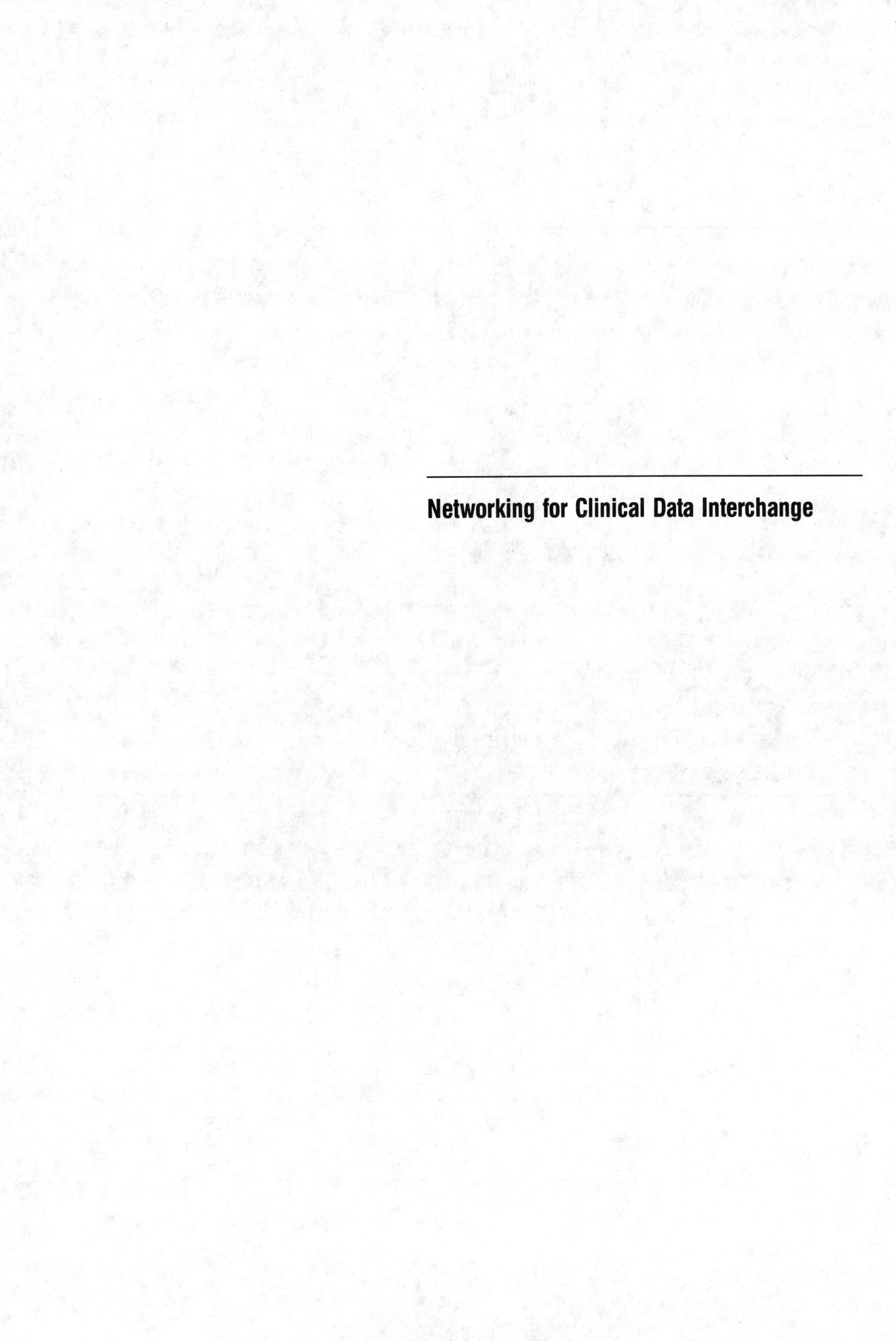

Networking for Clinical Data Interchange

An X-Protocol Based Medical Teleconsultation System Using Low or High Speed Networks. A Specific-Design Approach.

Antonio Dueñas, Miguel A. González, Adolfo Muñoz, Carlos H. Salvador.
Lab. Bioingeniería, Clínica Puerta de Hierro, Madrid, Spain.

The objective of this proposal is to provide solutions for the necessities of teleconsultation or telediagnosis among medical professionals, using work stations within the X-Windows environment and applicable in communication lines with an extensive range of bandwidths and operating system independence. Among the advantages sought are savings in transportation, improvement in the quality of the medical attention provided and continued training for the medical professional.

INTRODUCTION

The present state of the technologies dealing with information sciences and telecommunications favors the emergence of proposals aimed at bridging the geographical distances between groups of professionals. In particular, in the case of medical professionals, a typical scenario arises when a doctor reviewing a patient's folder has some doubt about the interpretation of a given document and prefers to consult a colleague with greater expertise in that area. If the specialist is nearby, the doctor can take the document to him. Frequently, however, this is not the case and the only solution is to discuss the problem over the telephone, which does not always clarify the doubt and is often awkward since the document must be described verbally. On these occasions, this model of teleconsultation would be extremely useful. The system described here is part of a larger application, evolution of the one presented in [1], and includes tools for acquisition of documents by scanner, database managing, electronic transfer of patient folders and a user interface designed for medical professionals.

Document

A document will be considered to be any bidimensional image produced by medical equipment. It is digitized by scanning a transparent or opaque original of any size, in color, grays or monochrome. The TIFF file format is employed.

Approach

Systems that deal with the problem of collaboration among professionals that are separated by a physical distance can be classified on the basis of one of two approaches:

1.- Shared windows system: extends existing single user applications by augmenting a window system so that it supports the sharing of the application interface by multiple dispersed users [5].

2.- Collaboration aware application: a specific application designed to directly support multiple cooperating users [3].

The former is more useful for taking advantage of an existing application base for cooperative use. The specific design of the application is considered to be more appropriate for our situation since it allows greater freedom of exact adaptation to the needs of the physicians. These needs are not precisely defined as yet, but will be established throughout the period of evaluation.

On the other hand, from the programming point of view, frequently the development of a communications module focuses too much on the hardware level being too dependent on this or on the operating system, in the attempt to enhance efficacy by taking advantage of the available bandwidth [4]. The solution offered here potentially can be used on any machine with X-Windows, regardless of the operating system, factors which do not imply a significant reduction in performance. The development and evaluation were carried out using a SUN SPARCstation IPX with SunOS 4.1.3.

It is also important to point out that no restrictions or controls have been established with respect to contending user actions, for example, when two users attempt simultaneously to move the document within the window (scroll), one moving it upward and the other downward. These actions are dealt with asynchronously, that is, they are all carried out, but the one that remains is the last one performed by any of the users involved. The proper use of this freedom is left up to the users themselves, who are provided with a voice channel.

DESCRIPTION

To define teleconsultation, it is assumed that it

involves a general physician and a specialist or two specialists. The teleconsultation session will develop according to the following steps:

0.- Depending on the speed of the communication line the document(s):
   a) They will have been transmitted previously (if <64 Kb/s).
   b) They will be transmitted immediately before step 1.- (if >64 Kb/s but <2 Mb/s) by means of the utility designed for that purpose.
   c) Each one is sent automatically in step 3 (if >2 Mb/s) (approximate speeds).

1.- Voice contact with the specialist is established by normal telephone, preferably with "free hands" feature to facilitate the use of the mouse. If both agree that to hold the session at that time, then...

2.- The consulting user selects the location corresponding to the specialist from a menu that appears in the document window. The specialist receives notification in the center of his screen, identifying the consulting user and the document. Having confirmed, by means of a button provided in the notification, his acceptance to discuss the document,...

3.- A window, identical to that on the screen of the consulting user, that is, containing the same document in the same position and with the same dimensions, appears on the specialist's screen. From that moment on, any movement of the mouse made over the document by either of the two users will be faithfully reflected in the other screen with a second, larger, colored cursor. The same occurs if the mouse is moved by pressing button 1 (scroll) or 2 (magnifying glass), if the window is moved or iconized, if the brightness of the image is changed, etc. If the cursor goes beyond the edge of the window or if other windows are moved or changed, no modification will appear in the remote screen; thus, the rest of the windows are "private".

The handling by the user of a document or events, which are capable of being reflected in a remote terminal, can be classified according to one of three categories:

1.- Window configuration. This encompasses the events that affect the arrangement of the window on the screen, that is, those that alter the placement or dimension, iconization or visibility.

2.- Directly related to movement of the mouse. The particular features are that:
   a) Temporal peaks with large amounts of information can be produced (when the mouse is moved).
   b) The maximum permitted latency (from the moment the action of the user occurs at one end until it is reflected at the opposite end) must necessarily be short. If it were too long (>0.7 s), it would affect the subjective feeling of agility perceived by the users since there is practically no delay in the voice line. In addition to making it possible to follow the remote cursor by drawing a second cursor in the local window, this category includes the options for scroll, magnifying glass and marking.

3.- Editing of the contents of the window or document as such. This includes those actions that modify the image to improve viewing, for example, a change in brightness or angle. The latency can be somewhat longer than in the preceding category since it is considered together with the time employed in editing, which is greater than in the above cases.

In all three cases, and of special importance in the third, the transmission to the remote station of an order for a change to be made takes place prior to its execution in the local station; thus, the processing time overlaps. For example, the time elapsed between the moment a gamma correction is requested at one end and is carried out at the remote end is only the latency of the communication, not the sum of the latency and the time needed to calculate the gamma correction.

IMPLEMENTATION

The practical use of the above features will be done through the facilities for communications between clients provided by X-Windows. This is possible since, with the client-server philosophy on which X-Windows is based, it makes no difference whether the client and the server are using the same machine or different machines linked by a TCP/IP network since it is the X-Protocol that isolates the system from these differences. The ultimate objective is to take advantage of the suitability of the communications capacities inherent to X11.

There are three possibilities:

1.- **cut-buffers** is a simple but limited form of communication between clients.

2.- **selections** is the most potent and standardized method since release 4 of X [2].

3.- **properties**, used in most cases in communications between the window manager and other clients. Both the cut-buffers and the selections make use of properties.

The direct property system was chosen because it

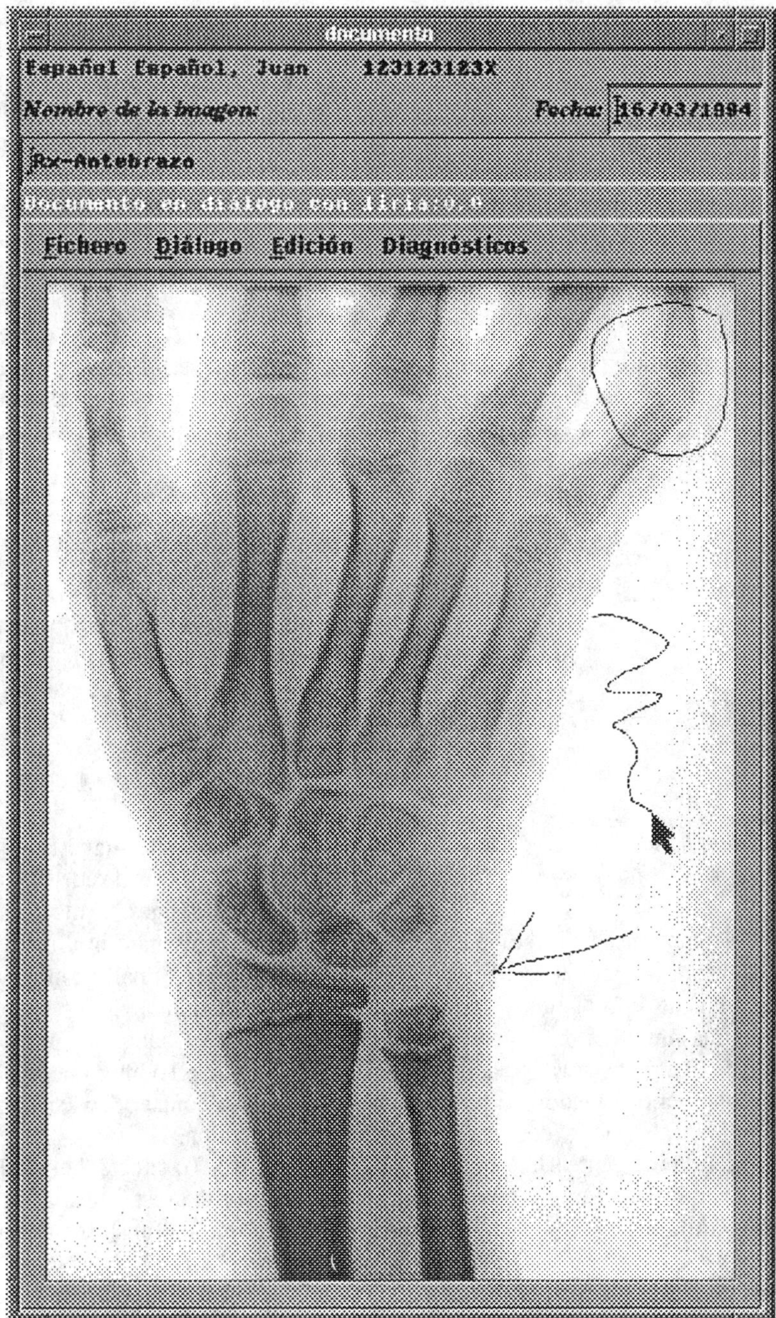

Fig 1: Document window during a teleconsultation session

satisfied our needs since the properties allow the association of arbitrary information with a window, placing it at the disposal of other clients or applications storing it in the server. The properties are referenced by atoms as a means of nickname. A given atom and a given window identify a single property. For properties that are not predefined, in the first call to function **XInternAtom**(), with the name of the property (in the form of a string) as argument, a new atom is assigned to it. This same atom will be assigned to each and every client who calls XInternAtom() with the same name and will remain in the memory of the server while it is active. The properties can contain structures or raw data. They remain set until the window is destroyed, which takes place when the client exits, except in the particular case of a root window which is never destroyed.

Briefly, the procedure would be is follows:

Initially,

myatom = XInternAtom(mydisplay, "TELECONS",

```
False);
```

and whenever an incident is to be communicated to a remote client,

```
XChangeProperty(mydisplay, mywindow, myatom,
mydeed->type, 8, PropModeReplace, (Deed
*)mydeed, sizeof(Deed));
XFlush(mydisplay);
```

mywindow will always be the toplevel window of the application, which does not have to be visible. The toplevel window of the application is located in the remote display by searching for the name among all the applications by using **XQueryTree()** and **XFetchName().**

The **Deed** structure contains the information necessary in each case to properly reproduce the local action in the homologous remote window. It can take the form of a union since it can be different in each case:

```
typedef union _Deed {
    int type;
    AnyDeed myanydeed;
    ConfigDeed myconfigdeed;
    EditDeed myediteed;
    . . .
} Deed;
```

for example:

```
typedef union {
    int type;
    Window w;
    Position x, y;
    Dimension width, height;
    . . .
} ConfigDeed;
```

When the incident being communicated is the creation of a new document window, after creating the homologous window with the information gathered from the data structure transmitted in the property, a table with the two is updated at both ends to establish, from that moment on, the remote window to which the events detected in the local window correspond. To gather the information being sent in the remote display, it is sufficient to inform the **MainLoop** of the XtToolkit of the attention routine:

```
XtAddEventHandler(myapptoplevel,
PropertyChangeMask, False, deedrcvEH, NULL);
```

This Event Handler will read the information and proceed to:

```
XGetWindowProperty(mydisplay, myapptoplevel,
myatom, 0, sizeof(Deed)/4, False,
AnyPropertyType, &actual_type, &actual_format,
&nitems, &bytes_after, (Deed *)mydeed);
```

If this method is applied to the transmission of mouse events, the result is not sufficiently valid for low speed (9600 b/s). As was mentioned above, the events generated by moving the mouse are critical due to their large volume during peak times and the limited tolerance to increasing transmission latency. This is due to the fact that the transmission of properties is of lower priority for the server. Thus, it is necessary to adopt a particular solution for mouse movement which consists in only accepting events occurring within a certain time span for transmission. A value of 100 ms (10 events/s) was empirically selected for this interval, rate which provides more than acceptable subjective quality without exhausting the 9600 b/s limit. To perform all this, a periodical interrupt is installed:

```
PRDTO = 100;
XtAppAddTimeOut(XtWidgetToApplicationConte
xt(toplevel), PRDTO, perioTO, NULL);
```

perioTO which, every 100 ms, picks up the last event involving a movement, disregarding those occurring before:

```
while(XCheckMaskEvent(yourdisplay,
PointerMotionMask | ButtonMotionMask,
&myxevent));
draw_remote_cursor(): /* in local display */
```

Thus, regardless of the speed with which the mouse is moved, there will always be a maximum controllable number of events per second, in this case 10.

EDITING

As a result of the suggestions of actual users in the initial trials, it was decided to increase the options for editing the images themselves during the dialogue. These are presented in a menu bar in each window. The utilities finally included for use during teleconsultation are:

1.1.- Move. Change the position of the window.

1.2.- Resize. To alter the height or width.

1.3.- (De)Iconize. To substitute for a symbolic representation.

1.4.- Raise. To situate the window in the foreground, in front of the rest.

1.5.- Close. To finish the consultation regarding this window.

2.0.- Remote cursor. Larger than the local cursor and brightly colored. Always activated.

2.1.- Scroll. If the dimensions of the document surpass those of the window, the window can be moved around over the document by moving the mouse while pressing the left button.

2.2.- Marking. By pressing the middle button, a line is drawn by the cursor as it moves, in both the remote and the local window.

2.3.- Magnifying glass. Pressing the right button augments the area surrounding the cursor to a 2:1

scale.

3.1.- Mirrors. Horizontal and vertical symmetry.
3.2.- Turn. ±90°.
3.3.- Brightness. Changes in intensity.
3.4.- Contrast. Changes in percent or threshold.
3.5.- Gamma correction. y = x**n; n≤≥∈ [0,1]
3.6.- Restore. Return to the original image.

EVALUATION

The demonstrations and laboratory tests have awakened a great deal of interest among the end users. Several of their suggestions for improving the system have been taken into consideration. However, demonstrating its true validity will require its continuous use within a program of evaluation in circumstances resembling a real situation. At present, the possibilities of the system are being studied in depth in a a pilot demonstrator set up between a health care center and a referral hospital approximately 40 kilometers away. It is tested mainly for transmitting radiologic images (at a rate of 20 a day), problem which is presently being solved by a specialist at the health care center who goes to the hospital twice a week.

CONCLUSIONS

The result is a relatively simple, but robust, application that constitutes the basis for applying teleconsultation in many cases that are currently being handled by less efficient means. Aside from the possibilities of the system itself, there are additional factors, such as:

1.- It is practically independent of the operating system to be used, which means that it can be installed in existing stations. The only requirement is the availability of an X11R4 or higher.
2.- It is also quite independent of the type of communications and its bandwidth. Only TCP/IP or DecNET protocol support is needed, whether it is installed in the same machine or via router in its local network. It has been exhaustively and satisfactorily tested in these cases:
    a) Modem at 9600 or 14400 b/s (V.32 and V.32bis) with error correction (V.42) and via PPP (Point-to-Point Protocol). In this case, the percentage of bandwidth occupancy when the mouses of both users are fully active is nearly 100% (the limit being 10 positions/s and at 9600 b/s), but never reaches saturation.
    b) ISDN at 64 and 128 Kb/s. Equally valid. Connection and disconnection are much more rapid. The surplus bandwidth is serviceable for data and the second B-channel for voice.
    c) Ethernet. In this case, real time transmission of documents is permitted, as well (during the session), avoiding the need to prepare it beforehand. Logically, in other broad band networks (ATM, FDDI), its performance can be expected to be equally satisfactory.

ACKNOWLEDGEMENTS

This work has been supported by the Fondo de Investigaciones Sanitarias de la Seguridad Social, Spain (FIS 92/0412 and FIS 94/0142).

Reference

[1]. C. Blanco, A. Muñoz, A. Dueñas, M.A. Gonzalez, C.H. Salvador. Medical workstation for the management of the transplantation unit of a hospital. proc. Fifth IEEE Symposium on Computer-Based Medical Systems. Durham, 1992.

[2]. D. Rosenthal. Inter-Client Communications Conventions Manual. MIT X Consortium. 1991

[3] J.M. Ng, E. Chang, Horace H.S. lp, K.Y. Kwok, Y.K. Lee, H.H. Tsang. A Multimedia Conferencing System for Co-operative Medical Diagnosis. Proc. Sixth Annual IEEE Symposium on Computer-Based Medical Systems. 1993.

[4]. S.J. Dwyer. Teleradiology using switched dialup networks. IEEE Journal Selected Areas in Communication (vol. 10, #7). 1992.

[5]. H. Abdel-Wahab, M.A. Feit. XTV: A Framework for Sharing X Window Clients in Remote Synchronous Collaboration. Proc. IEEE Communications for Distributed Applications and Systems. Piscataway, N.J. 1991.

A High-Speed Network for Cardiac Image Review

Jonathan L. Elion MD FACC and Robert R. Petrocelli
Brown University and The Miriam Hospital, Providence, RI

A high-speed fiber-based network for the transmission and display of digitized full-motion cardiac images has been developed. Based on Asynchronous Transfer Mode (ATM), the network is scaleable, meaning that the same software and hardware is used for a small local area network or for a large multi-institutional network. The system can handle uncompressed digital angiographic images, considered to be at the "high-end" of the bandwidth requirements. Along with the networking, a general-purpose multi-modality review station has been implemented without specialized hardware. This station can store a full injection sequence in "loop RAM" in a 512 x 512 format, then interpolate to 1024 x 1024 while displaying at 30 frames per second. The network and review stations connect to a central file server that uses a virtual file system to make a large high-speed RAID storage disk and associated off-line storage tapes and cartridges all appear as a single large file system to the software. In addition to supporting archival storage and review, the system can also digitize live video using high-speed Direct Memory Access (DMA) from the frame grabber to present uncompressed data to the network. Fully functional prototypes have provided the proof of concept, with full deployment in the institution planned as the next stage.

INTRODUCTION

This paper describes the implementation of a prototype of the **Cardiac Image Network**, a high-speed network for multi-institutional sharing and viewing of full-motion cardiac images. Using Asynchronous Transfer Mode (ATM) networking, a scaleable approach to real-time image review over local- and wide-area networks is now possible. The design of the full network is presented, and the results of the initial laboratory prototypes described. This technology permits diagnostic-quality full-motion cardiac studies to be accessed and reviewed at distributed sites, as easily as current lab reporting systems.

DESIGN GOALS

The specific goals of the project are to:

- Deploy a comprehensive, fully scaleable ATM network for high-speed transmission and interactive review of full-motion image sequences
- Implement a file server with a virtual file system to handle on-line (high-speed disk), near-line (mounted tapes), and off-line (on the shelf) storage
- Develop a multi-modality cardiac image review station capable of receiving and displaying uncompressed image data at 30 frames per second (bandwidth requirement of 7.5 megabytes per second using 8-bit pixels and 512 x 512 images)

Several aspects of the Cardiac Image Network are particularly noteworthy, in contrast to other approaches:

- The public utilities can be used to extend the network, smoothly integrating local (LAN) and wide-area networking (WAN) functions.
- High bandwidths can be achieved, supporting real-time image display without compression. The same network design can be scaled down for lower bandwidth applications (such as traditional image archiving systems).
- It is designed to improve the allocation of medical resources and accelerate appropriate cardiac care. It should have an immediate and direct effect on health care delivery and costs.
- The design is fully scaleable, suitable for both large and medium-sized institutions. While designed for images initially, the database can be easily extended for handling non-image data.

ASYNCHRONOUS TRANSFER MODE

Asynchronous Transfer Mode (ATM) networking is an emerging standard for simultaneous handling of video, voice, and data [1]. It is central to the design of the Cardiac Image Network, and has several distinct advantages over previous networking approaches:

- ATM network is based on a network of switches and dedicated host links, so aggregate bandwidth increases as hosts are added. Shared media LANs, on the other hand, can saturate with just a small number of hosts, and have a greater cost since statistical aggregation of trunks is lacking.
- ATM offers an open-ended growth path, not locking into a single physical medium. Different systems can use the same format, interconnecting LANs, switches, and public networks. This permits a network design strategy that makes use of

0195-4210/94/$5.00

existing facilities while providing a smooth growth path as components are upgraded.

- Previously, the protocols to implement a Local Area Network (LAN) were different from those used for a Wide Area Network (WAN). ATM, on the other hand, uses the identical protocols (same cell format) for both LANs and WANs, thereby eliminating the artificial barriers between them.

ATM offers the following desirable design characteristics:

- The protocols for interfacing with user applications are based on published industry standards [2].
- Commercial products use ATM to connect workstations, and to do the necessary switching. Fully functional networks can be implemented now, without waiting for full deployment of large ATM switches by the public utilities.
- The technology is fully scaleable. Small prototype systems developed to provide ATM services within a single location can be extended to provide services between locations.

Final details of nation-wide ATM deployment have not been finalized (carrier-to-carrier interconnection, fully switched circuits, etc.). Current systems still permit full use of ATM advantages in a metropolitan area, using "switched virtual circuits" tunneled within dedicated fiber lines.

PREVIOUS WORK

NYNEX Media Broadband Services

NYNEX has developed a network-based multimedia communications to support collaborative work between users at geographically remote locations [3], and trial of the NYNEX Media Broadband Services (MBS) was recently completed at several hospitals in Boston [4]. MBS and its MEDOS operating system are proprietary, rather than being built on industry standards, and the software is currently only available on a limited number of hardware platforms. High-speed applications and video services have not yet been demonstrated. The collaborative review of coronary angiograms developed as part of these trials uses a synchronized control scheme (local and remote viewers synchronized over the network), rather than achieving real-time data transmission.

Project Zeus

Washington University has completed a technical feasibility project creating an ATM network for their campus, referred to as Project Zeus [5]. This project confirms the technical feasibility of ATM networking concepts, and has provided an important platform on which to build applications. Unfortunately, much of the hardware development for Project Zeus was based on a computer company that is no longer selling workstations. The video that was demonstrated was based on a JPEG coder-decoder, and is not appropriate for the diagnostic imaging project we are proposing.

Sony CineNet

This is primarily a digital video distribution system, based on the RP-125 digital video standard. This is at the center of Duke's digital angiography archiving program [6]. While the video is transmitted digitally, the result is not a general-purpose computer network, and no "out of band" communications are possible over the network. An additional computer network would need to be added to implement the virtual file system and other control functions. Wide Area Network strategies may be possible, but only by sacrificing the many advantages of ATM listed previously.

Review Stations

Several workstation-based systems have been described for the presentation of image or multimedia information [7,8]. These systems were not intended to be used for real-time display of high-resolution motion sequences, or for high-speed network interfacing. We have previously reported on the development of a personal review station for digital angiography. The system was designed to expand to handle full-motion uncompressed studies, but currently uses JPEG compression to compensate for the relatively slow speed of existing devices [9]. The review station has been demonstrated for the viewing of images from optical and magnetic disk, and high-speed tapes.

High-Speed Medical Image Networks

Several high-speed networks have been reported for Picture Archiving and Communications Systems (PACS) functions [10,11] and image review, but the reported bandwidths are still well below those required for cardiac imaging [12]. A parallel operating image buffer system has been used to increase the effective speed [13], but still could not break through the speed requirements. The implications of Wide Area Networks for image transmission has been examined [14], but with the exception of Project Zeus, none have looked at the ATM technology.

Network-Based Image Archives

The PACS system currently running at UCLA is considered to be large-scale [15], generating an average of 2 gigabytes a day of image data. By comparison, the digital output of a medium-sized cardiac catheterization laboratory is 4 to 8 gigabytes per day (assuming 8 patients per workday, and 0.5 to 1.0 gigabytes per patient). The archival requirements for the Cardiac Image Network are clearly at the "high end" of what is currently implemented.

NETWORK DESIGN

Fully Scaleable ATM Network

The Cardiac Image Network is designed to provide integrated access to real-time and archived multi-modality image data. To fully achieve this objective, it must be possible to convey digital image data in real-time among several target hospitals. The nature of ATM technology allows network development to be based at a single site, with the same hardware and software capable of connecting several sites as the public utilities ATM switches are installed.

The basic elements of the approach for a single site are presented in Figure 1. The File Server uses a Unix workstation running a commercially-available Virtual File System (VFS) and a large-capacity RAID disk. The VFS makes a series of disks, tapes, cartridges, and other on-line and off-line storage media all appear as a single contiguous file system to the software. The details of migrating files on and off of the high-speed RAID disk are all handled by the VFS.

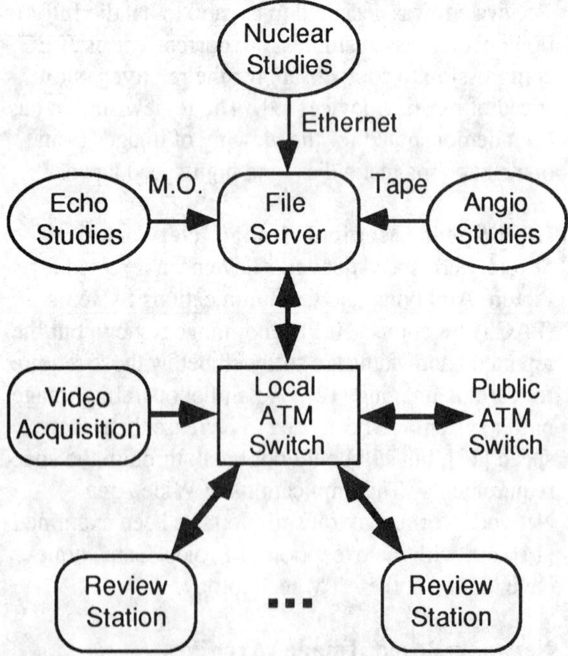

Figure 1: Cardiac Image Network at a single site (bold arrows are ATM connections).

Only the pathways for image data are shown; other non-image data (lab values, reports, etc.) could be handled in the future, but are not part of the initial system implementation. Nuclear cardiology studies are available by a direct Ethernet connection. The echocardiographic studies are read from a magneto-optical disk, and angiographic studies are imported from computer tapes.

More sophisticated electronic interfaces to external imaging systems are anticipated, and can be implemented using a workstation with an ATM adapter added to the network. The video acquisition module acts in this manner, digitizing video and making it available on the ATM network.

Network Design

Each node in a fiber-based ATM network is interconnected by a high performance "contentionless" switching array. This switching fabric permits the addition of connections without any degradation in network performance. The ATM network requires a central switch, station adapters for the workstations and the fiber optic connections from computer systems back to the switch. Our prototypes were implemented with commercially-available components. A standard ATM switch cluster provides a 2.5 gigabit per second switching array, can accommodate up to 16 network connections, and features support for standard network routing and data transmission (TCP/IP). Workstations are connected to the network using interface adapters that connect to the EISA bus.

Multi-Modality Review Workstations

The prototype software for angiographic review has been implemented using X-windows and Motif on a Hewlett Packard 735 workstation. Customized display software permits grayscale images to be stored in the workstation RAM at their native 512 x 512 resolution, then be interpolated up to 1024 x 1024 and displayed at 30 frames per second. Additional display controls allow setting of brightness, contrast, gamma settings, and edge enhancement. Similar software has been developed for the display of echocardiographic images (originating on a magneto-optical disk storage system that is part of the Hewlett Packard Sonos 1500 system used for clinical studies).

The review station is a client on the network, and communicates with a server managing the image files. Control messages between client and server uses the UDP layer (thereby permitting "many-to-one" connectionless service), while file transfers use the TCP/IP layer (connection-oriented). Virtual file system software on the server manages the migration of image files between on-line storage (RAID disk), near-line storage (tape or optical drives), and off-line storage (unmounted cartridges on the shelf).

Real-time Image Acquisition
A commercially available frame-grabber with programmable phase-lock loop capabilities has been integrated into the network (no additional time-base corrector is needed). The system can acquire video signals and transfer them to the host computer using high-speed Direct Memory Access (DMA).

Industry Standards and Portability
Whenever possible we have sought to eliminate hardware dependencies and make the software portable to a variety of platforms. The following industry standards have been used in the design of the system:

- Unix Sys/V Operating System, X11 windowing system, Motif Graphic User Interface, and ANSI C programming language
- Asynchronous Transfer Mode ATM network transmission layer
- Transmission Control and User Datagram Protocols (TCP/IP and UDP/IP) networking protocols. TCP/IP provides a connection-oriented reliable delivery service on top of ATM to provide data to review stations. UDP/IP provides service for low-priority loss-tolerant traffic for low-bandwidth administrative functions.

Initial Prototype
As proof of concept, we have developed a prototype client-server application based on these designs This prototype initially ran with a dedicated ATM link between two workstations, and has now been extended to allow several review stations to connect to the server through an ATM switch (refer to Figure 1, above). The prototype has been used to evaluate the performance of several of the critical system components. We have confirmed the following performance using uncompressed image data:

- **Screen Rendering:** 512 x 512 8-bit images can be interpolated to 1024 x 1024 and displayed at 33 fps. Faster performance has been achieved on a newer workstation, but only 30 fps is required (traditional viewing rate for digital angiography).
- **Video Acquisition:** This has also achieved 30 fps using Direct Memory Access (DMA) to transfer from frame grabber to host memory.
- **ATM Transfer Rate:** The TCP/IP protocol used has approximately 40% overhead, but still sustained 64 megabits/second rates between the server and the client (60 megabits/second need to transmit a 512 x 512 8-bit image at 30 fps).

FULL NETWORK DEPLOYMENT

A full client-server based implementation of the network system has been completed, as described above. The Virtual File System (VFS) allows the client to access the entire patient library as if it was a large on-line file system (the VFS handles the migration of large data files between disks, tapes, and shelves). Plans for full deployment within one institution are now being completed. Planning with the local telecommunications company has also begun, with plans being finalized for an ATM switch to be installed in the central office shortly.

The extension of the Cardiac Image Network to connect multiple institutions is shown in Figure 2. Each hospital's local ATM switch and network remain intact, with the local ATM connected to the public ATM. Network addressing is resolved using the standard IP addressing scheme, so that no change in the local software or hardware is needed.

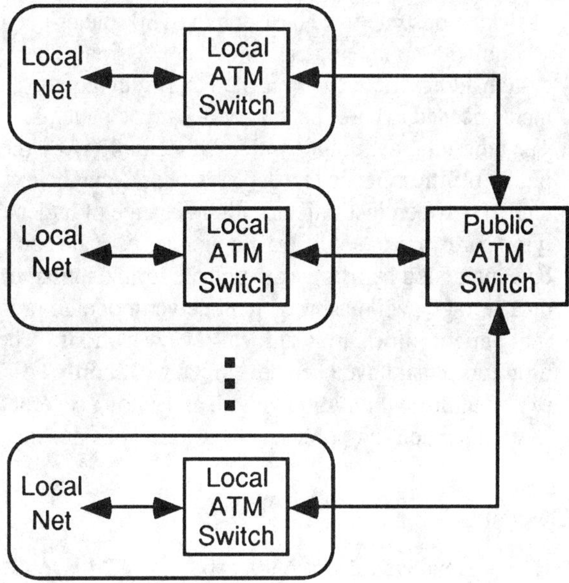

Figure 2: Multiple hospitals interconnected with public utility ATM switches

Studies are planned to look at the impact of the network on patient care within a single facility (using a multi-modality review station on the Coronary Care Unit to review echocardiograms, thallium studies, and coronary angiograms). Once the service is extended to affiliated hospitals, a study will examine the impact of the network on resource utilization. This is especially timely as new cardiac catheterization laboratories at several of the affiliated hospitals perform diagnostic studies only; patients are transferred for angioplasty or coronary artery bypass surgery. The ability to review images "live" (with the patient still in the cath lab of the referring hospital) should help with scheduling of limited resources at the receiving hospitals. Finally, it is planned to use the video acquisition capabilities of the network to allow review of echocardiographic video tapes and coronary catheterization films between hospitals. Patients often have diagnostic studies at one hospital and are then subsequently admitted emergently to another hospital (the ambulance stopping at the closest hospital), providing a need to transmit diagnostic studies between hospitals on an urgent basis. The Cardiac Image Network provides the technology to do this.

SUMMARY

A high-speed network for the storage, transmission, and review of full-motion cardiac image studies has been developed. This represents a significant advance in speed and image quality over what has been previously demonstrated; we have achieved 30 frames per second with no image-degrading compression. The system addresses the highest end bandwidth requirements needed to care for acutely ill cardiac patients. The emerging availability of ATM technology by the public utilities means that ATM networks can be extended between institutions with no change of underlying hardware or software. Economies of scale can be appreciated by using a central site for the massive data storage, while using a client-server model to present patient information at local review stations. The prototypes that have been developed will shortly be extended throughout the hospital, and among several hospitals when the public ATM switch goes on-line.

References

[1] Broadband ISDN ATM aspects - ATM layer functionality and specification. ANSI Draft Standard T1S1.5/92-002R3, March 1992.

[2] ATM user-network interface specification, version 2.0. ATM Forum, June 1992.

[3] Reis H, Brenner D, and Robinson J. Multimedia communications in health care. Ann NY Acad Sci, pages 257-268, 1992.

[4] Robinson J. Final Intercompany Priority Council status report on the MBS trials. NYNEX Technical Report, 1993.

[5] Cox Jr JR, Gaddis ME, and Turner JS. Project Zeus. IEEE Network, pp 20-30, March 1993.

[6] Cusma J. Which media are most likely to solve the archival problem. In 5th Internat Symp Cor Arteriography, Rotterdam, Netherlands, June 1993.

[7] Kitanosono T, Kurashita Y, Honda M, Hishida T, Konishi H, Mizuno M, and Anzai M. The use of multimedia in patient care. Comp Meth Prog Biomed, 37(4):259-63, 1992.

[8] Dayhoff RE, Maloney DL, Kuzmak PM, Sadan A, and Majurski W. Integrated imaging workstations using MS-DOS and UNIX/X Windows. Proceedings - The Ann Symp on Comp Applic Med Care, pages 965-7, 1991.

[9] Elion JL. A personal digital cine review station. In 5th Internat Symp Cor Arteriography, Rotterdam, Netherlands, June 1993.

[10] Stewart BK, Honeyman JC, and Dwyer III SJ. Picture archiving and communication system (PACS) networking: Three implementation strategies. Comp Med Imaging & Graphics, 15(3):161-9, 1991.

[11] Stewart BK, Dwyer III SJ, and Kangarloo H. Design of a high-speed, high-resolution teleradiology network. Journal of Digital Imaging, 5(3):144-55, 1992.

[12] Stewart BK, Lou SL, Wong WK, and Huang HK. An ultrafast network for communication of radiologic images. Am J Roent, 156(4):835-9, 1991.

[13] Reijns GL and Kayser A. Communications for a picture archiving communications system with a parallel operating image data base. Journal of Digital Imaging, 6(1):55-64, 1993.

[14] Baxter KG, Wetzel LH, Murphey MD, Rosenthal SJ, Haines JE, S, Caresio JF, Templeton AW, and Dwyer SJ. Wide area networks for teleradiology. Journal of Digital Imaging, 4(1):51-9, 1991.

[15] Wong AW, Taira RK, and Huang HK. Digital archive center: Implementation for a radiology department. Am J Roent 159(5):1101-5, 1992.

A TELEMEDICINE DISTRIBUTED SYSTEM FOR COOPERATIVE MEDICAL DIAGNOSIS

Enrique J. Gómez PhD, Francisco del Pozo PhD, Jose A. Quiles MS,
Marcos Sanz MS, Hellmer Rahms, Juan J. Vaquero MS,
Pilar Cano MS, M. Elena Hernando MS, M. Teresa Arredondo PhD.
Grupo de Bioingeniería y Telemedicina - GBT
E.T.S.I. Telecomunicación - Universidad Politécnica de Madrid

ABSTRACT

Telemedicine is changing the classical form of health care delivery, dramatically increasing the number of new applications in which some type of distributed synchronous cooperation between health care professionals is required. This paper presents the design and development of a telemedicine distributed system for cooperative medical diagnosis based on two new approaches: 1) a distributed layered architecture specially designed to add synchronous computer supported cooperative work features either to new or existing medical applications; 2) the definition of a methodological procedure to design graphical user interfaces for telemedicine cooperative working scenarios. The cooperative work is supported by a collaborative toolkit that provides telepointing, window sharing, coordination and synchronization.

Finally, we have implemented and installed the telemedicine system in clinical practice between two hospitals, providing teleconferencing facilities for cooperative decision support in haemodynamics studies. This specific implementation and a preliminary evaluation were accomplished under the Research Project FEST "Framework for European Services in Telemedicine" funded by the EU AIM Programme.

INTRODUCTION

Over the last decade, a series of social, political and economic changes in western societies have been influencing the evolution of the traditional health and social care models. Several aspects make it necessary to revise current concepts of the means to provide health care, making extensive use of the present state of information and telecommunications technologies; namely: demographic changes, increased health costs, need to improve the quality of medical care, fulfillment of social equity, and opening of new markets.

Telemedicine, a fundamental pillar of that IT&T supported health care, can be defined as the flexible, easy and rapid access to shared and remote medical expertise and resources by means of telecommunications and information technologies, no matter where the patient, the relevant information or the resources are located [1].

The need for computer-supported cooperative work (CSCW) [2][3][4], and particularly for synchronous cooperation, become a fundamental generic service common to many Telemedicine applications whenever a group of professionals wishes to collaborate simultaneously to achieve a common final goal.

Distributed medical communication systems have been developed to provide medical care and education services between remote hospitals. Some of them allow specific cooperative medical applications [5][6][7]. Very few experiences involving general multimedia CSCW architectures for medical consultations are reported [8]. All these research experiences are usually envisaged to make extensive use of broadband network facilities.

This paper presents a general distributed architecture for computer-supported cooperative working tools, designed to support synchronous cooperation tasks, especially suitable for Telemedicine applications. The other critical component which conforms this type of application, the graphical user interface (GUI), is also presented, mostly addressing the definition of a methodological procedure to design GUIs for Telemedicine cooperative working scenarios.

Figure 1 shows the general scenario: the medical teleconference for cooperative diagnosis. The communication service that supports the CSCW is based on any existing metropolitan or wide area network (MAN/WAN).

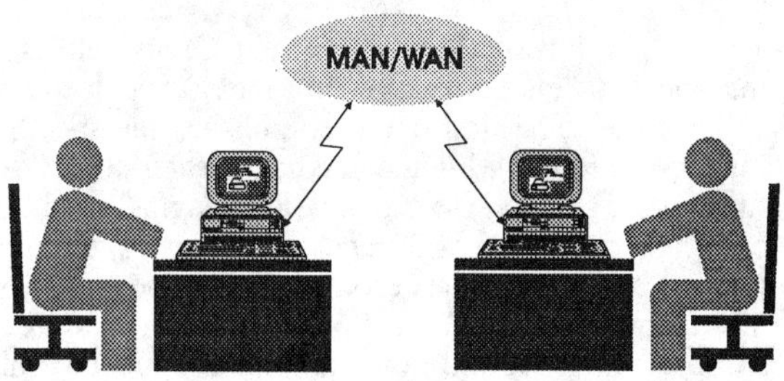

Figure 1. Synchronous Medical Teleconference

The proposed architecture has been implemented in a real pilot to allow both validation of the technology and assessment the usability of the system. A cooperative work scenario for haemodynamic studies was selected.

THE CSCW LAYERED DISTRIBUTED ARCHITECTURE

The architecture for synchronous groupware can be centralized or distributed [10]. In the case of centralized solutions, the application and its data are located at a single site. The application maintains links with several displays so that all the participants have the same view of the system. The main problem with a centralized architecture is the communication and processing bottleneck produced when the application has to attend to the different displays. It also involves additional inconveniences such as its low tolerance to errors.

Our distributed architecture replicates the application code and data at both user sites: two application instances are thus created. The internal structure of these instances is shown in figure 2, where we can see the layered software structure and common data (those needed by both user professionals in order to work in a cooperative manner). This architecture is thus arranged to isolate functions within layers and to achieve a high degree of independence between the functions supported by the collaboration tools and those specific to the application. This approach permits any medical application, based on a window system, to operate directly in multi-user mode without substantially altering the existing code. Below, we describe the layers in terms of their functionality and the protocols of information exchange among them.

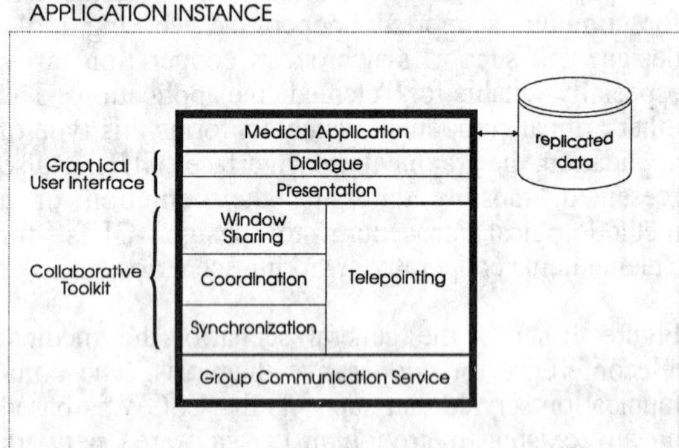

Figure 2. Layered Structure in Application Instances

Two upper layers, Application and Graphical User Interface, normally exist in all interactive medical applications. The first one accomplishes the specific functions required by the medical professionals to fulfill their goals, for example, managing medical case histories, processing and animation of medical images, and so on. The second one is responsible for the support of the communication between system and user: information presentation and dialogue with the medical user.

The Collaborative Toolkit provides synchronous cooperative functions in a transparent manner to upper layers. These functions are telepointing, window sharing, coordination and synchronization. The synchronization function allows the tasks of the application to start and finish at the same time at both sites, preventing problems derived from differences in the processing performance of a specific workstation. The coordination function enables the control of the medical professionals' interactions with the computer system; thereby, at a given moment, only one of them can interact with the cooperative application. This application control is activated by the system, rather than by the user, in a manner referred to as a coordination technological protocol. The window sharing function automatically allows WYSIWIS implementation. Finally, the telepointing function forwards each user pointer to the remaining screens [9].

The Collaborative Toolkit provides utilities that enable the applications to select the windows to be shared. Other functions allow the application to signal the beginning and end of user actions, thus ensuring coordination and synchronization. Internally, this Toolkit picks up all the events produced in the shared windows, subsequently transmitting them to both local and remote applications. Communication between the Collaborative Toolkits is achieved by means of an internal protocol based on token-passing that determines which user has permission to actively participate at a given moment. This technological protocol, unlike sociological protocols, conceals the activity of the moderator from the user during the cooperative work session.

The Group Communication Service allows communication among different application instances [10]. This layer has to support the session joining and exiting operations and both group and single message sending, as well as message consistency and sequence supporting. In our case, it is based on Sun ToolTalk [11], a communication service that links different applications. Although this service assumes a very limited number of message exchanges between application instances and, thus, is not appropriate for hard real-time systems, it is entirely suitable for our cooperative system because our layered distributed architecture minimizes the message exchange between application instances.

USER INTERFACE DESIGN METHODOLOGY

The design procedure of GUI's with high *usability* [12], suitable for systems that support cooperative work between health care professionals, was developed taking into account the results and recommendations of certain research projects [13][14], the state of the art in the area of tools for the development of *GUI's [15]*, and the experience of our research team [16].

The main steps of this methodology, repeated in an iterative cycle, are as follows:

1. Product description. The Telemedicine Service capabilities and features and the information architecture must be described in a structured way (by filling out a questionnaire).

2. *Context of use description.* To produce user requirements, also in a structured way, a *Context of Use Questionnaire* must be completed including: descriptions of the system users, the user tasks to be performed with the system, and the physical,

technical, and organizational environment in which the system is going to be used [16].

3. *Task analysis.* A hierarchical task analysis is performed to assist the functional specification. It consists of the decomposition of user tasks (also referred to as *objective tasks*) into simpler sub-tasks identifying the hierarchical structure.

4. *Enabling task analysis.* In order to allow a complete functional specification, the *objective tasks* must be decomposed into smaller fractions, which are called *enabling tasks* because they allow the user to access the specific system capabilities [17].

5. *Functional specification of the user interface.* A *State Transition Network* is produced taking into account the decomposed tasks (objective and enabling) and preserving the possible parallelism between them. *State* defines the group of tasks that can be performed by the user at each moment.

6. *Specification of the user interface metaphor.* A system metaphor must be selected to show a coherent view of the system to the users, taking into account their previous knowledge, to simplify the cognitive complexity of the system.

7. *Specification of man-machine dialogue.* In this stage, we select the interaction procedures and the dialogue style according to the selected system metaphor.

8. *Specification of graphical scenarios.* Keeping in mind the system metaphor, a graphic representation must be assigned to each of the simplest tasks after decomposition. Each system state (group of tasks) is then converted into a graphical scenario (group of graphical representations of tasks). The transitions in the *State Transition Network* define the transitions between graphical scenarios.

9. *User interface development.* The graphical scenarios should be implemented with a *User Interface Management System* (*UIMS*), observing general design guidelines with respect to dialogue, general screen layout, colors, etc., and specific guidelines concerning system functionality.

IMPLEMENTATION EXAMPLE: COOPERATIVE DECISION MAKING IN HAEMODYNAMIC STUDIES

Medical problem

To implement and validate the proposed general architecture, we have integrated it into an existing application developed within the European Research Project FEST- "Framework for European Services in Telemedicine" (EU funded, AIM Programme). The final goal of this application is to provide a cooperative decision-making telemedicine service to be shared among several regional hospitals and a specialized haemodynamics center. Haemodynamic studies were selected since they require medical personnel and equipment that is affordable only to major hospitals. Smaller clinical sites send their patients to the corresponding referral hospital for an angiographic study. In routine clinical therapy, patients requiring therapy (e.g. angioplasty, atherectomy, valvuloplasty,...) visit the referral hospital twice, where they undergo two catheterization sessions, with all the associated risks, plus additional inconveniences: extended hospital stay, twice the personnel and material costs and reduced catheterization service yield.

Telemedicine CSCW services are intended to contribute as follows: after viewing the just acquired images of the patient, the referring cardiologist could discuss the case with the haemodynamist, consultation that would help in arriving at a diagnosis and deciding the most convenient therapy in "real time"; that is, while the patient is still in the catheterization laboratory and surgical treatment is still possible. The timing constraints for this operation (less than 30 minutes) are very strict.

Additional tools and services complete the CSCW service in the Telemedicine scenario described above: image import from the digital angiography equipment, image transmission, case study handling tools: static and dynamic image viewing and voice communication.

User interface design

Here we deal only with the most relevant decisions taken during application of the user interface design methodology to the medical problem depicted above.

- In order to adapt the system to the *Context of Use* of the cooperative diagnosis, it was decided to implement a telepointing device with no type of dialogue control, assuming both users are at the same level within the organizational hierarchy (as was also described in the *Context of Use*).
- The main objective tasks established at the first level of hierarchical decomposition consisted of: a. identifying images of interest; b. viewing and animating images; c. showing images and animation to another physician; d. speaking with the other physician; and e. cooperating in the diagnostic decision.
- The main *enabling task* is the *image transfer task* which must be performed before cooperative viewing because the system does not support it in real-time.
- A real world metaphor was selected, designed on the basis of the physicians' routine work and the real objects they used; this selection also took into account the users' description in the *Context of Use*: the users had no experience with workstations or with any kind of window environment, and very limited experience with information systems.
- The most appropriate dialogue style for a real world metaphor is direct manipulation of graphical objects, which are, in this case: *box file* (patient information), *wastebasket*, *film tapes* (medical images), *telephone, phone list*, *television*, *postbox*, and *box to be sent by post*; the latter two objects are used to perform the enabling task mentioned above, in such a way as to be compatible with the metaphor selected.

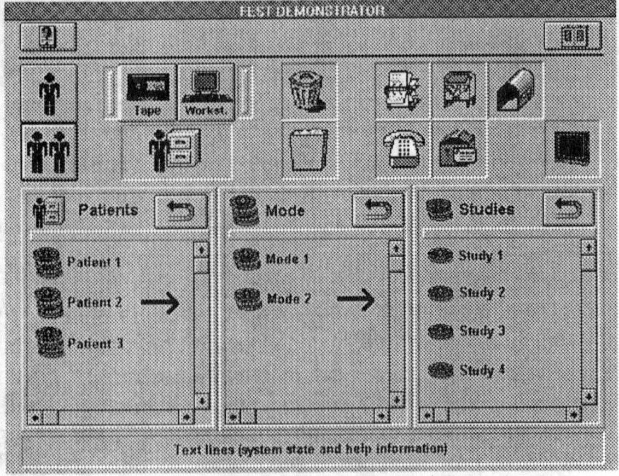

Figure 3. User Interface Main Screen of the FEST Application

Figure 3 shows an example of the user interface for the main screen of the FEST application which was developed with a User Interface Management System (UIMS) for Motif Toolkit. The upper section of the screen displays the real world objects that the physician will use to perform the diagnostic task. This section is equipped with buttons to select actions, such as retrieving data from the digital imaging system, storing data in the backup tape and switching between local and cooperative work. The middle section of the screen consists of *handlers* with the content of the *patient's box file* (*image tapes*), finally showing the *study tapes*, which can be moved within the *television* object to display the medical images. The user interface is completed with a *help* button, an *exit* button in the upper corners and a text line in the bottom section to show the system state and some permanent help information.

System Implementation

The CSCW distributed system was developed in two stages. First, a local medical workstation, based on the X-Windows system and the OSF/Motif toolkit, for decision making in angiography was fully implemented in the specialized center. It was designed with no additional specification for coping with its further integration into our distributed architecture. Second, this local system was integrated on the basis of the Collaborative Toolkit and the Group Communications Service.

A communication network was set up to support all components of the FEST application installed between two clinical sites (30 km apart): Hospital General Vall d'Hebrón in Barcelona (HVH) as the referral site and the Hospital de Manresa (HM) as the referring site.

As illustrated in Figure 4, the network infrastructure consists of:

- A Local Area Network at the HVH site, used to import image series from a Philips digital imaging system (DCI) to the demonstrator workstation (DWS) where the medical application is running. It also allows the DWS to access the remote bridge, as will be described in the following paragraph.
- The link between HVH and HM demonstrator workstations was initially a leased line at 64Kbps using synchronous V35 modems and high speed remote Ethernet bridges with real-time hardware compression; in addition, an ISDN 2B+D link for 128Kbps operation is currently being installed.

Remote bridges are used to allow an Ethernet extension, transparent to all application nodes. Moreover, the use of TCP/IP provides a virtual and safe local area network between the two clinical sites.

RESULTS

The FEST cooperative medical diagnosis system is currently installed and used in clinical practice to link the two Spanish hospitals mentioned above. The results of a preliminary system evaluation [19][20] in real clinical sessions have shown:

- The appropriateness of a technological coordination protocol in this type of cooperative diagnosis applications where time is critical, and users have to focus only on the main tasks supported by the diagnosis application, remaining unaware of the coordination issues.
- Users did not perceive any significant delay in telepointing and in the other synchronous collaborative functions. When compared with other existing centralized architectures, our CSCW distributed architecture optimizes the message exchange between application sites, allowing its implementation on low bandwidth communication lines.

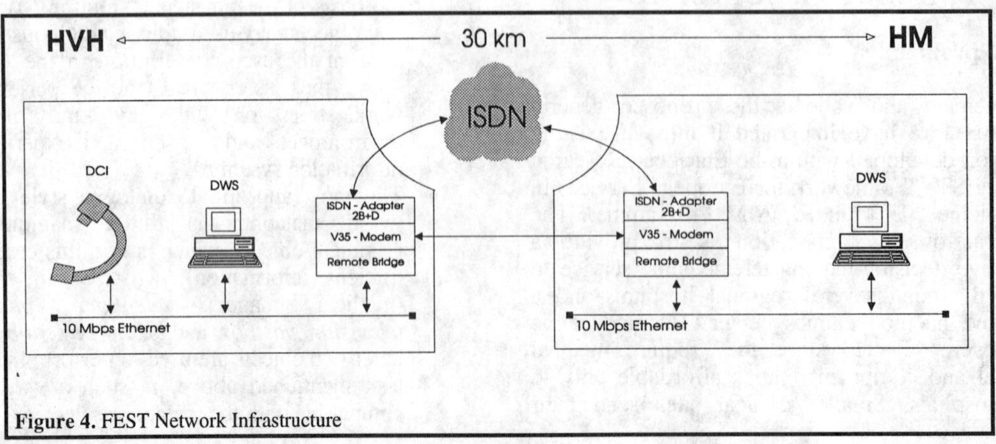

Figure 4. FEST Network Infrastructure

- The feasibility of our design and development approach to cope with the addition of synchronous cooperative working features to an existing local medical application. First, the system was developed in two separated stages with no relevant integration problems, as described above. Second, due to the user interface consistency for both local and telemedicine cooperative applications, the adaptation of regular users to the synchronous CSCW service was very efficient.
- The capability of the user interface design methodology to minimize the number of user interactions necessary to reach a cooperative diagnosis, and to drastically reduce the system learning time.

CONCLUSIONS

The need for synchronous cooperation is essential in many information technology applications where groups of professionals collaborate simultaneously to achieve a common final goal. This situation is especially relevant in Telemedicine services and applications.

This paper has presented a layered Telemedicine distributed architecture to define and implement the main functions of a cooperative distributed and synchronous application. These functions are clearly separated from the application and network infrastructure and provide mechanisms for their implementation in the different existing window systems.

The other critical component which conforms this type of applications, the graphical user interface, was also addressed, with the definition of a methodological procedure to assure the usability of the system.

Finally, we have carried out a real clinical implementation to demonstrate and validate the advantages of new architectural and methodological approaches to the design and development of telemedicine distributed systems for cooperative medical diagnosis.

ACKNOWLEDGMENTS

This work is supported in part by EU - AIM FEST project no. A-2011, and by grants CICYT TEMA TIC 92-1288-PB and TELEMEDICINA TIC 93-1279-E. Special thanks to Dr. I. Anivarro, Dr. J. Soler and Dr. E. Domingo, at Hospital Vall d'Hebrón and to Dr. J. Reig at Hospital Manresa, Barcelona, Spain.

Reference

[1] AIM-1993, 'Research and technology development on telematic systems in health care', DG XIII- Adv. Infor. Med., Commision of the European Union, 1993.

[2] Ellis C.A., Gibbs S.J., Rein G.L. 'Groupware. Some Issues and Experiences' Communications of the ACM. 34(1):38-58, 1991.

[3] Rodden T., Blair G.S. 'Distributed Systems Support for Computer Supported Cooperative Work' Computer Communications. 15(8):527-538, 1992.

[4] T. Hoshi, F. Nakamura, S. Nakamura. 'Broadband ISDN Multimedia Workstations and Tele-Working Systems', Hitachi Review, 40(3):217-222, 1991.

[5] F. Del Pozo, C.H. Salvador, M.A. González, A. Dueñas. 'Relevant Issues in Multimedia Dialogue Sessions of Medical Professionals', Proc. 13th Ann. Int. Conf. IEEE EMBS, 13(3):1349-1350, 1991.

[6] S.T. Treves, E.S. Hashem, B.A. Majmudar, K. Mitchell, D.J. Michaud. 'Multimedia Communications in Medical Imaging', IEEE Journal on Selected Areas in Comm. 10(7):1121-1131, 1992.

[7] M.E. Goldberg, E.R. Ritenour. "A Teleconferencing System", SCAMC 1993; 17:803-807.

[8] L. Orozco-Barbosa, A. Karmouch, N.D. Georganas, M. Goldberg. 'A Multimedia Interhospital Communications System for Medical Consultations', IEEE Journal on Selected Areas in Comm. 10(7):1145-1156, 1992.

[9] Nakajima A. 'Telepointing Issues in Desktop Conferencing Systems' Computer Communications. 16(9):603-610, 1993.

[10] Kirsche T., et al 'Communication Support for Cooperative Work' Computer Communications. 16(9):594-602, 1993.

[11] SunSoft, Mountain View California. 'ToolTalk 1.0 Programmers Guide', 1991 .

[12] Booth, P. 'An Introduction to Human-Computer Interaction'. Lawrence Earlbaum Associates.

[13] ETSI, 'Guide for Usability Evaluations of Telecommunications Systems and Services' ETSI DTR/HF 3001, 1993.

[14] Maissel, J., Dillon, A., Maguire, M., Rengger, R., Sweeney, M. 'Context Guidelines Handbook'. MUSIC, Esprit Project 5429, 1991.

[15] Myers, B.A., Rosson, M.B. 'Survey on User Interface Programming'. Human Factors in Computing Systems: Proceedings SIGCHI'92, ACM, New York, pp. 195-202, 1992.

[16] Sanz, M.F., Gómez, E.J, Trueba, I., Cano, P., Arredondo, M.T., del Pozo, F. 'A pen based system to support pre-operative data collection within an anaesthesia department'. SCAMC 1993;17:321-325.

[17] Byerley, P., May, J., Whitefield, A., Denley, I. 'The Enabling States Approach: Designing Usable Telecommunications Services'. IEEE Journal on Selected Areas in Communications, 9(4):524-530, 1991.

[18] FEST AIM Project A-2011. 'Report on Operational and Functional Requirements of the Demonstrator' Deliverable 1. EEC Brussels. 1992.

[19] Sanz M.F., Gómez E.J., del Pozo F., Arredondo, M.T., Cano P., Rahms H. 'User Interface of a Cooperative Diagnosis System for Health Care Professionals' V Int. Symp. on Biomedical Engineering. Sep. 1994.

[20] FEST AIM Project A-2011. Deliverable 27: 'First Report on the Usage and Application Functionalities', 1993.

Simulation Studies of a Wide Area Health Care Network

James G. McDaniel, Ph.D., School of Health Information Science, University of Victoria, Victoria, British Columbia, Canada

There is an increasing number of efforts to install wide area health care networks. Some of these networks are being built to support several applications over a wide user base consisting primarily of medical practices, hospitals, pharmacies, medical laboratories, payors, and suppliers. Although on-line, multi-media telecommunication is desirable for some purposes such as cardiac monitoring, store-and-forward messaging is adequate for many common, high-volume applications. Laboratory test results and payment claims, for example, can be distributed using electronic messaging networks.

Several network prototypes have been constructed to determine the technical problems and to assess the effectiveness of electronic messaging in wide area health care networks. Our project, Health Link, developed prototype software that was able to use the public switched telephone network to exchange messages automatically, reliably and securely. The network could be configured to accommodate the many different traffic patterns and cost constraints of its users.

Discrete event simulations were performed on several network models. Canonical star and mesh networks, that were composed of nodes operating at steady state under equal loads, were modeled. Both topologies were found to support the throughput of a generic wide area health care network. The mean message delivery time of the mesh network was found to be less than that of the star network.

Further simulations were conducted for a realistic large-scale health care network consisting of 1,553 doctors, 26 hospitals, four medical labs, one provincial lab and one insurer. Two network topologies were investigated: one using predominantly peer-to-peer communication, the other using client-server communication. The client-server model was less expensive to operate but also less responsive to message priorities.

INTRODUCTION

Several large projects have implemented and evaluated generic wide area health care networks. These projects are the Inter-Institutional Information Exchange (3I) project [1], the Advanced Informatics in Medicine (AIM) Strategic Health Informatics Network for Europe (SHINE) [2], and others [3, 4]. As well, there are smaller prototype networks initiated by university hospitals (see for example [5, 6]). Networks are also being developed by telephone and insurance companies, for example, Ameritech [7] and Blue Cross and Blue Shield [6]. The intent of these networks, that are usually targeted at physicians, medical labs, hospitals and payors, is to support telecommunication for several diverse types of complementary health care applications.

In all but a few projects, there has been no documented effort to determine the behaviour of the proposed network and its operating cost. Although telephone companies have performed extensive analyses on the queueing behaviour of switches and telephone networks [8], little of this work has been extended to health care networks. In most cases, application network designers assume that the underlying third-party telecommunication services are adequate to support the application. This assumption can be justified as the telecommunication carriers expand their networks to meet increased demand. However, by omitting these analyses, researchers are unable to determine the dependency of network performance and cost on topology and traffic congestion.

Traffic patterns are sensitive to time of day and type of health care facility. Some institutions like hospitals and medical labs are mainly information sources. Others, like payors, are information sinks. As well, the volume of transactions varies by size and type of facility. For example, the communication traffic of a physician's office is a fraction of that of a hospital. The content of some transactions is time-sensitive. For example, the rapid delivery of lab test results is likely to be more critical than billing claims. The design criteria for a cost effective network should optimize the network configuration to meet the information exchange requirements.

This research investigated the behaviour and operating cost of a wide area health care network. It was based on actual prototype software that has been developed for the public switched telephone system. First the behaviour of mesh and star networks with symmetric loading was simulated and analyzed. Then a simulation study was performed on two models of a realistic large scale network. The results of the study were used to estimate the operating cost of the network.

BACKGROUND

One common method to estimate network performance and cost is to perform a static analysis of the network based on message characteristics, network demand and resources [9]. This type of analysis can be used to calculate an estimated response time and operating cost but the designer must make a number of assumptions about the network loading and the characteristics of network components.

A static analysis for a health care network has been described by van Lierop *et al* of the Dutch GEIN project [10]. They estimated the cost of implementing and operating an Electronic Data Interchange (EDI) network in the region of Breda, The Netherlands, consisting of three hospitals, 180 specialists and 165 GP's. They determined that one million messages would be exchanged annually. Costs were calculated based on the communication cost of a limited set of EDI transactions and the support organization needed to administer the network. The study concluded that Breda was too small to support the EDI infrastructure.

This author was unable to find other detailed analyses of wide area health care networks. It is probable that similar techniques have been used to estimate the cost of nearly all prospective networks. It is unlikely that an analysis has been conducted to determine the dynamical behaviour of a network and the cost of operating a network designed to accommodate the time-varying demands of its applications.

METHODS

Health Link [11] was a research project in which communication software was designed, developed and tested, surveys were conducted at two medical clinics, network simulations were performed and a field test was conducted for a prototype network. The simulation studies described in this paper were based on the properties of the communication software, the expected telecommunication requirements of GP's that were extracted from the surveys, and performance benchmarks that were measured in the field test.

Network Description

The *Health Link* software was designed to automatically store and forward messages using a connection-oriented protocol. It is capable of scheduling messages for pickup and delivery. Nodes can be configured to originate calls only or to both originate and accept calls. The network can be configured to support peer-to-peer communication, client-server communication and other variants. The software can use any underlying communication network that can be accessed by a serial connection but it has been designed specifically for the public switched telephone network.

A *Health Link* network is composed of one or more subnets. Depending on its routing table, a node can communicate directly with a peer in the local subnet or it can communicate with a gateway server that stores and forwards messages to the destination in the local subnet or to another gateway in a remote subnet. No message is ever transmitted more than three times from its source to its destination. The routing table for each node can be configured independently.

Every message is processed before it is sent. A Message Authentication Code (MAC) is calculated and the message is compressed and encrypted. A digital signature is generated and encrypted using the RSA public-key cryptosystem [12]. The reverse procedure is followed once a message is received. Message processing is interrupted when messages are exchanged because the MS-DOS operating system, under which the software executes, does not support preemptive multi-tasking.

Network Demand

Two clinics that participated in the field test were surveyed to determine their procedures, patient load, and the nature and volume of external communications. A messaging network would need to support the communication traffic shown in Table 1. Applications, such as making referral appointments, that are better suited for on-line communication are not shown. Messaging requirements for specialists, hospitals, medical labs, the provincial lab and the government payor were extrapolated from the messaging requirements of the GP's.

Table 1: Estimated Message Traffic for Principal Network Users

Type of Message	Source	Destination	Messages Per Day	Message Size (characters)
Medical lab test report	medical lab	GP	20/GP	175
Provincial lab test report	provincial lab	GP	3/GP	175
Emergency report	hospital	GP	2/GP	200
X-ray report	hospital	GP	2/GP	300
Lab test report	hospital	GP	2/GP	250
Operating room (OR) report	hospital	GP	2/GP	1000
OR booking	GP	hospital	2/GP	175
OR booking confirmation	hospital	GP	2/GP	175
Outpatient clinics	GP	hospital	2/GP	175
Specialist referral	GP	specialist	3/GP	1000
Specialist referral	specialist	specialist	3/source	1000
Specialist report	specialist	GP	5/specialist	200
Health insurance claim	GP	government	1/GP	2000
Insurance claim confirmation	government	GP	1/GP	100
Medical record transfer	GP	GP	3/GP	1000
Medical record transfer	hospital	hospital	10/destination	500

Discrete Event Simulation Modeling
Discrete event simulation models [13] were constructed for the nodes and gateway servers. Simulation transactions, that were computational analogs of messages, were subjected to equivalent processing and queueing delays.

Canonical Steady State Models: Symmetric mesh and star node clusters were simulated using a program that exploited cluster symmetry through a multi-nodal driver. Each node in a cluster was assumed to have a single communication port. For star clusters, network performance was analyzed for a varying number of gateway ports. The number of messages exchanged during the simulations were nominally 3,000 messages and 1,000 messages for the mesh and star clusters, respectively. The results of the discrete event simulations were validated by performing analytic studies [14] on the same models.

Large-Scale Dynamical Models: Simulations were based on a realistic asymmetric model describing the health care system in the Province of Saskatchewan, Canada. In this analysis, a program was written that used a rule-based object-oriented approach to construct the network topology. Events such as message creation and connection initiation were determined by random events constrained by time schedules and node configurations. Eight subnets were defined for a network of 1,585 nodes (see Table 2). In the course of a simulated day, approximately 80,000 data messages were exchanged. Except for those data messages from the provincial lab, all messages were acknowledged by the destination node upon receipt.

Analyses of two models were performed. One was based on peer-to-peer communication among the physicians, hospitals and gateway servers within a given subnet. This model configured those physicians who were in the same subnet as one or more labs, to poll those labs six times daily. In cases where a lab delivered data messages outside its subnet, it forwarded the messages at medium priority to the gateway server without delay.

The second model was based on client-server communication within each subnet. Each node within a subnet delivered messages to its gateway server and polled the gateway server for messages. Polls were scheduled hourly. Gateway servers exchanged messages among subnets without delay.

Model Parameters: Table 3 shows some of the timing parameters used by the simulation models. All communication links were 2,400 bits per second serial connections. The base processor at each node was assumed to be an Intel 80386SX25. The number of serial ports at a node determined the CPU factor that was used in calculating the message processing times. For example, a computer with two ports was assumed to have twice the CPU power of the 80386SX25.

Table 2: Composition of the The Saskatchewan Model

Region	GP's	Specialists	Hospitals Municipal	Regional	Medical Labs Private	Provincial	Insurer
Moose Jaw	46	8	0	2	0		
North Battleford	92	16	0	4	0		
Prince Albert	92	16	0	4	0		
Regina	245	185	4	0	2	1	1
Saskatoon	338	299	4	0	2		
Swift Current	46	8	0	2	0		
Weyburn	46	8	0	2	0		
Yorkton	92	16	0	4	0		
Total Nodes	997	556	8	18	4	1	1

Message priority was implemented by using priority holding delays. Messages were collected in a mailbag that was held for the least priority delay of any one of the enclosed messages. A connection was initiated when the priority delay expired or when the receiver initiated a connection. For the steady state simulations, high, medium and low priority delays were zero, three and five minutes, respectively. For the dynamical simulations, these parameters were zero minutes, three minutes and four hours, respectively. Data messages were exchanged at either high or medium priority. Acknowledgment messages were exchanged at low priority.

The payload of data messages was fixed at 1,000 characters for the steady state simulations. The mean payload of messages sent in the dynamical simulations matched the message sizes shown in Table 1. Acknowledgment messages carried no payload.

Calibration: The timing parameters shown in Table 3 were measured in benchmark tests. The effective data exchange rates were taken from a stress test conducted over a period of three months at four different sites. The stress test was run using an automatic driver at each node that sent messages timed according to a Poisson distribution. The stress test analysis produced a performance curve for an actual four node cluster. For each simulation program, the performance of a modeled four node cluster was matched to the actual cluster.

Model Initialization: Two methods were used to compensate for the bias caused by starting the simulations from an empty and idle state in which there were no messages. For the steady state simulations, swamping [15] reduced the initialization bias to less than two percent on the mean message delivery time. For the dynamical simulations, a warm-up period of one simulated day removed the bias.

Table 3: Simulation Parameters

Timing Parameter	Value
Dial time (sec)	15
Ring and connect time (sec)	12
Relisten time (sec)	14
Modem reset time (sec)	10
Line idle detection time (sec)	60
Effective full-duplex data rate (bps)	362
Effective half-duplex data rate (bps)	770
Minimum wait between retries (sec)	180
Fixed protocol overhead (sec/msg)	2
Message processing time (sec/msg)	21

Calculating Standard Error: Simulations were conducted in a series of independent replications with random starting points to estimate the standard error of various performance measurements [13].

RESULTS

The results of the two series of simulation studies are given in turn. The simulations of the steady-state models provided insight into the behaviour of a network where all nodes were similar. The simulations of the dynamical models explored the behaviour of similar topologies in a realistic environment where the nodes experienced stochastically cyclical, asymmetric loads that characterize the health care system.

Canonical Steady State Models: The studies performed on the mesh and star node clusters indicated that both topologies are capable of supporting the anticipated mean load of 50 messages per day per node. Mesh clusters with up to 1,000 nodes would have an operating region from zero to 12 messages per hour per node. The cluster exhibits uniform performance in this region, achieving end-to-end delivery of medium priority messages, each having a data payload of 1,000 characters, in under 8 minutes.

Changes to the priority delay can affect the throughput as well as the performance of the mesh cluster. For small clusters, the number of messages exchanged during a single connection increases with the priority delay thus increasing port efficiency. The impact of the priority delay on throughput decreases as the number of nodes in the cluster increases.

The performance and throughput of star clusters depend on the capacity of the gateway server. The cluster exhibits long end-to-end message delivery time for both light and heavy network loads. When the cluster is lightly loaded, nodes rarely connect with the gateway server to send and receive their messages. When the cluster is heavily loaded, the gateway server is under contention. A star cluster is able to exceed the throughput of a mesh cluster if the server is configured with a sufficient number of ports. For example, a throughput of 15 messages per hour per node can be achieved in a 1,000-node cluster with 250 server ports. This configuration results in a mean end-to-end message delivery time of one hour.

Priority holding delays have little beneficial effect in star clusters. Increasing the delay has the effect of improving the throughput of the sender but there is no benefit to the receiver. Messages are held by the gateway server for pickup regardless of their priority. Priority delays have a negative impact on performance since they increase the message holding time at their source.

Two general observations were also made:
1) message processing requires as much time as does communication and 2) if an acknowledgment message is sent to confirm the delivery of each data message, the cluster throughput is reduced by nearly 40 percent.

Large-Scale Dynamical Models: Ideally, the models chosen to represent a network in the Province of Saskatchewan, Canada would optimize performance and operating cost. Moreover, we were interested in exploring the differences between peer-to-peer and client-server communication. However, optimization of these two models is difficult because of the many configuration and scheduling parameters. Examining the results is equally problematic as there are many interesting outcome measurements. A few of the more prominent observations follow.

The analyses of the peer-to-peer and client-server models indicate that both topologies can be used for a wide area health care network. The two models differ with respect to performance and operating cost. In order to make the mean end-to-end message delivery times comparable between the two models, each node in the client-server model was scheduled to poll its gateway server at a mean rate of once per hour. This resulted in mean end-to-end data message delivery times of one hour, 23 minutes for the peer-to-peer model and one hour, 24 minutes for the client-server model.

The peer-to-peer model exhibited the same sensitivity to priority delays as did the mesh model. Figure 1 shows two cumulative density functions for medium priority messages sent among physicians, one for messages exchanged among subnets and one for messages exchanged within the same subnet. Figure 2 shows the same functions for the client-server model. Table 4 gives a comparison between the two figures. The delivery time of messages exchanged in the client-server model was almost ten times that of messages in the peer-to-peer model; a consequence of the hourly polling frequency by the destination nodes in the client-server model.

The telecommunication cost of the peer-to-peer and client-server models was evaluated. The telephone and Datapac (a public packet switched network) tariffs were applied to the traffic patterns and volumes derived from the simulation models. The more economical service, voice telephone or packet switched communication, was chosen for each node. Table 5 shows a comparison of telecommunication monthly basic access and usage charges before applying several cost-optimizing strategies.

Figure 1: Mean End-To-End Delivery Time for Medium Priority Messages Sent Among Physicians in the Peer-To-Peer Model

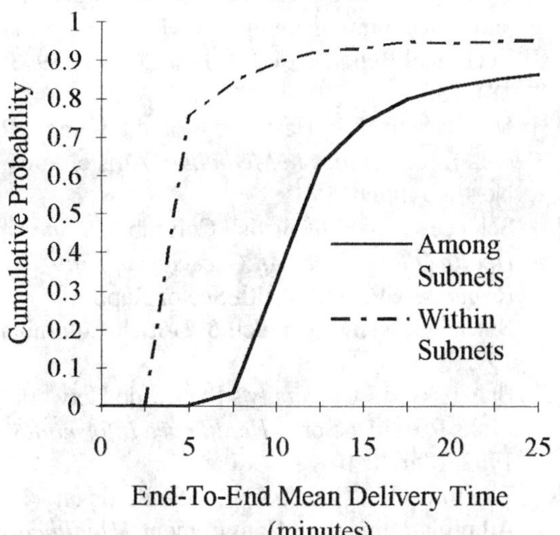

Figure 2: Mean End-To-End Delivery Time for Medium Priority Messages Sent Among Physicians in the Client-Server Model

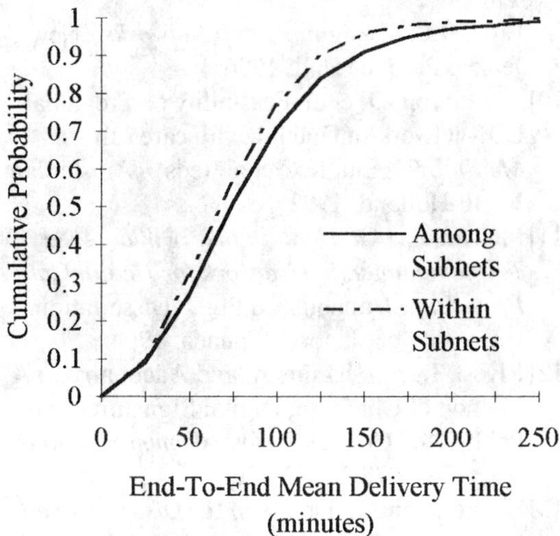

The peer-to-peer model relied heavily on telephone communication. Each node was supplied with at least one dedicated communication line, because every node in this model was configured to accept calls. This is not a prerequisite as there are devices available that sense the communication mode of incoming calls. The peer-to-peer model incurred long distance telephone charges within each subnet. Although ideally a subnet would be defined within single local dialing area, Saskatchewan has a widely dispersed population that is 37 percent rural.

Table 4: A Comparison of Medium Priority Messages Sent Among Physicians

Simulation Model	Among Subnets	Within Subnets
Peer-To-Peer		
Sample size	5,361	8,845
Median delivery time	11:40	4:10
Mean delivery time	22:59	9:03
Client-Server		
Sample size	5,537	9,064
Median delivery time	1:17:30	1:11:40
Mean delivery time	1:26:44	1:16:59

Table 5: A Comparison of Monthly Telecommunication Charges ($Cdn)

Telecommunication charges	Peer-To-Peer	Client-Server
Telephone access	57,722	6,653
Datapac access	2,420	3,563
Long distance telephone	77,293	0
Datapac usage	7,849	52,050
Datapac volume discount	-706	-4,029
Total charges	144,578	58,237
Charge per node	91.22	36.74

For the client-server model, because all call connections terminated at the gateway server, it was possible to use public Datapac ports. Universal Datapac Access (UDA) was used which included long distance telephone charges in the total Datapac usage charges.

The telecommunication cost of both models can be reduced by tuning call connection schedules. A saving of approximately five dollars per month can be made without significantly changing the behaviour of either model. Other gains may be realized by configuring hybrid networks that are better suited to the traffic patterns and the tariff schedules.

CONCLUSION

Two series of simulation studies were conducted for a telephone-based wide area network. Canonical mesh and star model networks were examined. The mesh network was more sensitive to message priority than the star network. The mesh network also was able to deliver messages in a shorter time than the star network. The star network could be configured to have a greater throughput than the mesh network. Both networks are easily capable of meeting the projected demands of a wide area health care network.

Simulation models with two topologies for a large-scale wide area health care network were constructed. These studies indicated that both peer-to-peer and client-server topologies are practical. The simulation of the peer-to-peer topology predicted that message delivery can be expedited by setting message priority but at a telecommunication cost that is greater than that of the client-server topology. The telecommunication cost in Canadian dollars of a network delivering 1,100 messages per month per node was predicted to range from $32 to $87 per month per node. This is a per-message cost of between $0.03 and $0.08.

The communication networks that were modeled by these studies rely on low speed telephone and packet switched technologies that are accessible to nearly all users. Although these technologies do not allow for high speed broadband communication that is needed for transmitting large messages such as digital radiographic images, it does support the transmission of smaller messages that are more commonly exchanged by health care providers.

The simulation techniques used in this research can be extended to other geographic regions, other applications and other telecommunication technologies. Simulations such as these could predict the behaviour and operating cost of a network before undertaking its costly installation.

ACKNOWLEDGMENTS

Support for this research was given in part by the Science Council of British Columbia under HDF #43-89, MART #90/91-11, HDF #7-91, and Technology B.C. #179 (T-3) Grants. Much of the financial support for my studies has been given by the University of Victoria and the Medical Research Council of Canada.

Reference

[1] Hasman, A., Arnout, P.C. and Boon, P. The 3I Project. In: *Telematics in Medicine*, Duisterhout, J.S., Hasman, A. and Salamon, R. (eds.). Amsterdam: North-Holland, 1991: 163-173.

[2] Commission of the European Communities DG XIII Information Technologies and Industries, and Telecommunications. AIM 1993. Annual Technical Report on RTD: Health Care. 1993: 181-186.

[3] Duisterhout, J.S., Hasman, A. and Salamon, R. (eds.). *Telematics in Medicine*. Amsterdam: North-Holland, 1991.

[4] Science Council of British Columbia. *Sharing Health Information: An Overview of Fifty Projects*. SPARK Health Sector Report. Burnaby: Science Council of British Columbia, 1992.

[5] Bahensky, J. University's Statewide Network Links Rural Doctors. *Healthcare Informatics* 1992, March: 10-12.

[6] The Impact of EDI & ANSI Standards on Administrative Cost Containment. *Healthcare Informatics* 1992, November 9(11): 90-96.

[7] Ameritech advertising brochure, Chicago, circa 1993.

[8] Briley, B.E. *Introduction to Telephone Switching*. Reading: Addison-Wesley Pub. Co., 1983.

[9] Ellis, R.L. *Designing Data Networks*. New Jersey: Prentice Hall, 1986.

[10] van Lierop, D. et al Feasibility of a regional EDI-network in Dutch health care. In: *MedInfo 92*, Lun K C et al. (eds). Amsterdam: North-Holland, 1992: 89-93.

[11] McDaniel, J.G. *Health Link: A Wide Area Telecommunication Network for Health Care Providers*. Unpublished Ph.D. Dissertation. University of Victoria, Canada, 1994.

[12] Rivest, R. L., Shamir, A. and Adelman, L. A Method of Obtaining Digital Signatures and Public-Key Cryptosystems. *Communications of the ACM* 1978,2: 120-126.

[13] Banks, J. and Carson, J.S. II. *Discrete-Event System Simulation*. Englewood Cliffs: Prentice-Hall, 1984.

[14] Kleinrock, L. *Queueing Systems, Volume I: Theory*. New York: John Wiley & Sons, 1975.

[15] Banks, J., Carson, J. S. II and Sy, J. N. *Getting Started with GPSS/H*. Annandale: Wolverine Software Corp., 1989.

Computer-Based Patient Records: Capturing the Data

PEN-Ivory: The Design and Evaluation of a Pen-Based Computer System for Structured Data Entry

Alex D. Poon and Lawrence M. Fagan

Section on Medical Informatics
Stanford University School of Medicine
Medical School Office Building (MSOB X215)
Stanford, CA 94305-5479
poon@camis.stanford.edu

ABSTRACT

PEN-Ivory is a pen-based computer system that uses structured data entry for creating patient progress notes. Users make simple gestures such as circles, lines, and scratch-outs to enter medical findings from a controlled vocabulary. The result of an interaction with PEN-Ivory is a computer-generated patient progress note in English prose.

We designed PEN-Ivory's user interface in a principled way. We first created multiple working prototypes, each differing in one of three user-interface characteristics. Then we empirically evaluated the prototypes in a controlled, experimental setting for their efficiencies in enabling users to create patient progress notes. The prototype that allowed the fastest data entry had the following three user-interface characteristics: it used a paging form, used a fixed palette of modifiers, and made available all findings from the controlled vocabulary at once.

INTRODUCTION

Traditionally, physicians have recorded clinical findings in the form of handwritten progress notes. This enduring use of handwriting and paper-based medical records is not surprising. Paper is easy to use, portable, and facilitates the jotting of quick notes and simple sketches. But the use of pen and paper is not without problems. Handwritten patient charts are often illegible, missing, and poorly formatted [1, 2].

Many physicians now use recording devices to dictate their notes, which are later transcribed by specialized staff members into typewriters or word processors. While this method of documentation saves time for the physician, the transcription process introduces not only the potential for transcription errors, but also a delay between the time a physician generates a note and the time the note becomes accessible [2].

But perhaps the most important drawback of handwritten and dictated information is that it is unstructured and not coded, and therefore difficult to process with computers. The advantages of coded data entry are well documented [2]. For example, coded medical data can be used as input for medical expert systems, systems for outcomes analysis, billing systems, and research databases.

Because of the problems of illegibility, chart accessibility, and non-coded data, many researchers have created computer systems that can be used to record medical findings in a structured way. However, computer systems for clinical data entry are not widely used in practice. They are generally more difficult to use [2-4], less time-efficient [5, 6], and less flexible than using paper and pen [1, 2, 7]. Furthermore, large computer terminals have been shown to interfere with the physician-patient encounter [3, 7].

The need for systems that allow and encourage direct data entry by physicians is well known. The Institute of Medicine's Committee on Improving the Patient Record calls the development of such systems "the single greatest challenge in implementing the computerized patient record" [2]. Shortliffe and Barnett have blamed awkward human-computer interfaces for being the biggest factor in inhibiting the clinical use of computers [1].

The goal of the PEN-Ivory project is to develop a computer system that realizes the benefits of coded data entry, but takes advantage of the conveniences of paper and pen. This idea is not a new one. There are at least five other pen-based computer systems for medical charting [6, 8-11]. PureMD, developed by Développement Purkinje Inc., is the most comprehensive, allowing physicians and dentists to enter information from a database of over 50,000 possible clinical observations [10]. However, none of these projects have empirically evaluated the merits of alternative user-interface characteristics for such pen-based systems.

In this paper, we describe the design and evaluation of PEN-Ivory, a pen-based system for writing patient progress notes using structured data entry. First, we give a general description of the system and its user interface. Then, we describe how we designed the system in a principled way by creating multiple working prototypes that differ in just one user-interface characteristic. Finally, we present the results of a preliminary experiment in which we evaluated the different prototypes in a controlled, laboratory setting.

SYSTEM DESCRIPTION

PEN-Ivory is derived from another system, Ivory, that uses a mouse and keyboard interface for data entry [12]. Like Ivory, PEN-Ivory uses a SOAP (subjective, objective, assessment, and plan) format for its progress notes. Currently, PEN-Ivory employs structured data entry for only the subjective and objective sections of the note. We are presently extending the vocabulary to include the assessment and plan portions.

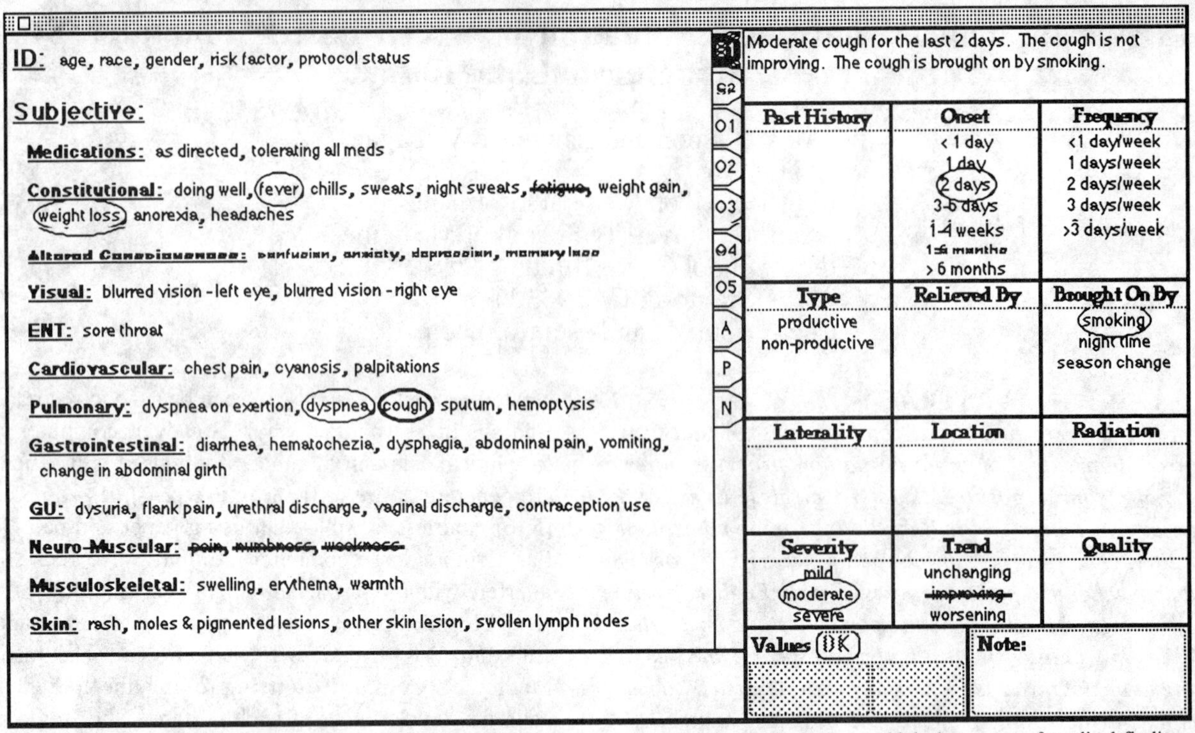

ID: age, race, gender, risk factor, protocol status

Subjective:

Medications: as directed, tolerating all meds

Constitutional: doing well, fever, chills, sweats, night sweats, ~~fatigue~~, weight gain, weight loss, anorexia, headaches

Altered Consciousness: confusion, anxiety, depression, memory loss

Visual: blurred vision - left eye, blurred vision - right eye

ENT: sore throat

Cardiovascular: chest pain, cyanosis, palpitations

Pulmonary: dyspnea on exertion, dyspnea, cough, sputum, hemoptysis

Gastrointestinal: diarrhea, hematochezia, dysphagia, abdominal pain, vomiting, change in abdominal girth

GU: dysuria, flank pain, urethral discharge, vaginal discharge, contraception use

Neuro-Muscular: ~~pain, numbness, weakness~~

Musculoskeletal: swelling, erythema, warmth

Skin: rash, moles & pigmented lesions, other skin lesion, swollen lymph nodes

S1 S2 O1 O2 O3 O4 O5 A P N

Moderate cough for the last 2 days. The cough is not improving. The cough is brought on by smoking.

Past History	Onset	Frequency
	< 1 day 1 day 2 days 3-6 days 1-4 weeks 1-6 months > 6 months	<1 day/week 1 days/week 2 days/week 3 days/week >3 days/week
Type	**Relieved By**	**Brought On By**
productive non-productive		smoking night time season change
Laterality	**Location**	**Radiation**
Severity	**Trend**	**Quality**
mild moderate severe	unchanging ~~improving~~ worsening	

Values OK

Note:

Figure 1. PEN-Ivory's user-interface. The left side of the screen represents the encounter form on which the names of medical findings are listed. The right side represents the attribute palette, used to augment findings with specific modifiers. Users draw circles, lines, and scratch-out gestures to interact with the system. Currently, the selected finding is cough, shown with a bold circle on the left.

PEN-Ivory currently runs on an Apple Macintosh™ computer connected to a Wacom handwriting tablet. The Wacom handwriting tablet consists of a digitizing tablet integrated with a backlit LCD display. Figure 1 shows a screen shot of PEN-Ivory's user interface. The screen is divided into two main areas. The left side represents the encounter form on which the names of medical findings are listed, while the right side represents the attribute palette, used to embellish findings with specific modifiers.

Users interact with the encounter form and attribute palette with a set of three simple gestures: circle, line-out, and scratch-out.

Circle

Circling a finding in the encounter form signifies that the patient exhibits that particular finding. Multiple findings may be circled with a single stroke of the pen.

Once a finding is circled, the user may enter more information about that particular finding by circling items out of pre-defined lists of modifiers in the attribute palette. The contents of the palette change depending on the finding that was circled.

Line-Out

Drawing a horizontal line through a finding or modifier signifies that the patient does not exhibit that particular finding or modifier. As with circling, multiple findings may be lined-out with a single stroke.

Scratch-Out

Leaving a finding untouched signifies that a finding's status is either non-assessed or unknown. Scratching-out a finding or modifier that has previously been assessed returns its status to the non-assessed or unknown state. Multiple findings or modifiers may be scratched-out with a single stroke.

Handwritten Notes

Users may also take handwritten, free-form notes that are stored as electronic ink. This allows the user not only to draw sketches and diagrams that are printed out along with the note, but also to record information that cannot be easily expressed in PEN-Ivory's controlled vocabulary. PEN-Ivory does not attempt to translate the handwritten notes into text.

Progress Note Text Generation

As the user interacts with the encounter form and the attribute palette, PEN-Ivory generates English text based on the information that the user has entered. The user may toggle between viewing the encounter form and the generated progress note. Figure 2 shows an example of a generated progress note. The user may directly interact with the finding and modifier terms in the progress note by using the same set of gestures as in the encounter form.

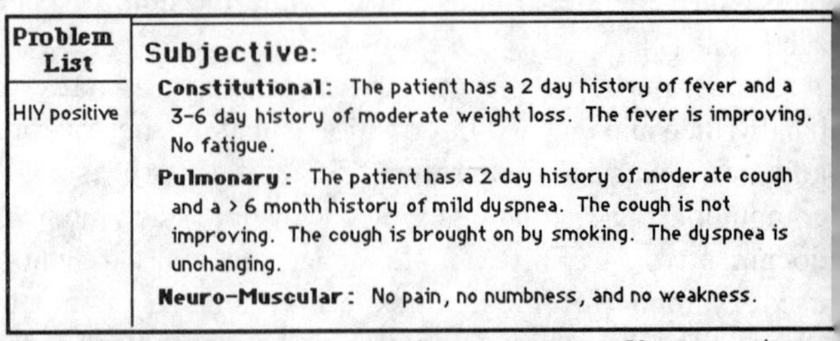

Problem List	Subjective:
HIV positive	**Constitutional:** The patient has a 2 day history of fever and a 3-6 day history of moderate weight loss. The fever is improving. No fatigue. **Pulmonary:** The patient has a 2 day history of moderate cough and a > 6 month history of mild dyspnea. The cough is not improving. The cough is brought on by smoking. The dyspnea is unchanging. **Neuro-Muscular:** No pain, no numbness, and no weakness.

Figure 2. A PEN-Ivory generated progress note. Users may interact with the note using the same gestures they use in the encounter form.

USER INTERFACE CHARACTERISTICS

In designing PEN-Ivory's user interface, we created multiple prototypes that differ in one of three *user-interface characteristics*. The three user-interface characteristics are scrolling vs. paging, dynamic vs. fixed palette, and all findings vs. subset of findings.

Scrolling vs. Paging

The encounter form in which the findings are displayed can be listed either as one long *scrolling* list of findings, or as a series of *pages* of finding. The advantage of a scrolling form is that it allows for greater flexibility with regard to which findings can be displayed on the screen at once. The advantage of a paging form is that it enables the user to remember the location of particular findings by both their page numbers and their positions on the pages. For instance, a user might remember that subjective gastrointestinal problems are always listed on the bottom of page S2.

We hypothesize that the paging encounter form is faster and easier to use because of the paging form's greater ability to allow users to remember findings by screen location. This hypothesis relies on the premise that users can become sufficiently familiar with the forms that they can take advantage of such positional memory [13].

Dynamic vs. Fixed Palette

Users can elaborate upon a particular finding by selecting items from the attribute palette. For instance, "headache" is a basic finding, while the attributes "every day," "worsening," and "no past history" are attributes that can embellish "headache."

A *fixed attribute palette* is one that is always visible and whose location and size on the screen are fixed. Another characteristic is that the categories of attributes have fixed absolute positions within the palette. Figure 1 shows an example of a fixed palette showing the attributes for the finding cough. Notice that empty attribute categories are still shown in the palette. Because all of the 14 attribute categories are always shown, the positions of the categories remain fixed regardless of the finding being modified. For instance, the categories "Severity," "Trend," and "Quality" are always shown at the bottom.

A *dynamic attribute palette* is one that pops-up on demand and whose location and size on the screen are not necessarily fixed. In addition, the absolute positions of the attribute categories within the palette may change, depending on which categories are relevant for the finding being modified. Figure 3 shows an example of a dynamic palette for the finding cough. Notice that because only those attribute categories that are relevant for cough are shown, the positions of the categories may change depending on the finding being modified.

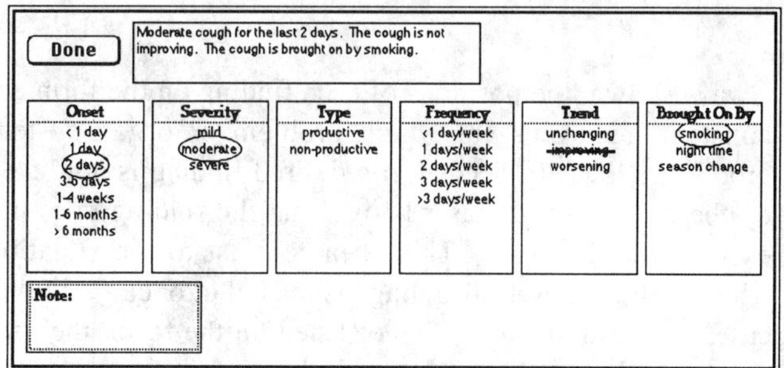

Figure 3. A dynamic, pop-up attribute palette for the finding cough. Notice that empty attribute categories are not displayed, and that the user must explicitly dismiss the palette by touching the "Done" button.

Our hypothesis is that the fixed palette will be faster to use than the dynamic one, because it permits the user to memorize the absolute location on screen of the attribute categories. Like the first hypothesis, this hypothesis relies on the assumption that users are able to take advantage of positional memory [13]. We also believe that users will like the fixed palette over the dynamic one because the fixed palette does not require an explicit dismissal step.

All Findings vs. Subset of Findings

The Ivory vocabulary consists of over 1000 basic findings. Findings can be grouped logically by either problem or organ system. A problem group consists of only those findings that are relevant for patients with that particular problem. For instance, "AZT Intolerance" is a problem group that consists of 83 findings which are appropriate for patients who are AZT-intolerant. An organ system group consists of findings that belong to a particular organ system, such as all findings related to the heart. We refer to problem groups and organ system groups more generally as finding groups.

We developed two different methods for using finding groups. The first displays only a *subset of findings* based on a particular finding group. The second displays *all findings* all the time, while highlighting those for a loaded finding group.

In the prototypes that display only a subset of findings at once, users must first specify the problem or organ system groups whose findings they want displayed. This allows users to work with a more manageable subset of the over 1000 findings. Users can load in additional finding groups if the currently loaded groups do not contain all the findings they wish to enter.

In the prototypes that display all findings at all times, finding names from loaded finding groups are highlighted on the screen for emphasis. Thus, although all 1000 findings are made available at once, only a small subset are highlighted, allowing users to ignore the findings that are less relevant.

The advantage of displaying only a subset of findings is that only those findings that are relevant for a particular problem or organ system group are shown, resulting in a much shorter list of findings.

We recognize two advantages of displaying all findings. First, because all findings in the database are always shown, the positions of each finding on the form are constant, regardless of which problem or organ system groups are loaded. Second, if a desired finding is not listed on the form, then the user knows that the finding does not exist in the database. This is in contrast to the situation where only a subset of findings is loaded at once — in that case, if a desired finding is not listed on the form, the user cannot easily know whether the finding is simply not part of the loaded finding groups, or if it does not exist in the vocabulary at all.

We hypothesize that displaying all findings is superior to displaying only a subset, because of its ability to allow users to remember findings by position regardless of the finding groups loaded. As do our other hypotheses, this hypothesis relies on the abilities of users to memorize, over repeated use, screen locations of user-interface elements. Our hypothesis also relies on the premise that users can easily ignore extraneous information presented on a display, an ability that Nygren has observed of computer users [13].

EXPERIMENTAL RESULTS

The goal of the experiment was to discover empirically the better design for each of the three interface characteristics. We conducted a preliminary experiment in which we timed users entering progress notes with one of the PEN-Ivory prototypes. Our user group consisted of fifteen students from our division, five of which were medical doctors. Table 1 shows the average times for entering a finding using each of the five PEN-Ivory prototypes we tested.

Table 1. Average times and standard deviations for entering a finding using each of the five PEN-Ivory prototypes tested.

Prototype	Average Time Per Finding (sec)	Standard Deviation (sec)
PFA (paging, fixed, all)	16.13	09.18
SFA (scrolling, fixed, all)	19.64	13.97
PFS (paging, fixed, subset)	26.00	27.26
SFS (scrolling, fixed, subset)	26.33	32.48
PDA (paging, dynamic, all)	18.19	11.44

Scrolling vs. Paging

For evaluating the scrolling encounter form against a paging encounter form, we compared prototypes PFA to SFA and PFS to SFS. PFA was faster than SFA by an average of 3.51 seconds per finding, with $p < .025$ using a paired sample, two-tailed t test with 63 d.f. However, there was not a significant difference in speed between PFS and SFS. This suggests that a paged form is significantly faster than a scrolling form when showing all findings, but are virtually equal when showing only a subset.

Dynamic vs. Fixed Palette

For comparing the dynamic palette to the fixed palette design, we compared prototype PFA to PDA. We found that the fixed palette was faster than the dynamic one by an average of 2.06 seconds per finding, with $p < .05$. Upon close examination of the timing data points, we found that much of the extra 2.06 seconds of the dynamic palette was due to the extra time that the system needs to create the dynamic pop-up views on the fly.

All vs. Subset of Findings

For evaluating the design of displaying all findings against the design of displaying only a subset of findings we compared prototypes PFA to PFS and SFA to SFS. PFA was faster than PFS by an average of 9.87 seconds per finding, with $p < .005$. Furthermore, SFA was faster than SFS by an average of 6.69 seconds per finding, with $p < .20$. This suggests that showing all findings is significantly faster than showing just a subset, especially when using a paging form.

We noticed that the main reason for the slowness of PFS and SFS was that users were often unsure if a particular finding was already loaded in as part of the current finding group. They spent much of their time loading in finding groups even when the desired finding was already displayed on the encounter form. These instances also account for the high standard deviations seen in designs PFS and SFS — in some cases, users spent well over a minute trying to load in finding groups. In contrast, those using PFA and SFA never had to waste time loading in additional findings.

FUTURE RESEARCH DIRECTIONS

We identify at least three potential research directions for our work with PEN-Ivory: continuing the interface characteristic study, generalizing our study results to other domains, and comparing PEN-Ivory to writing and dictation.

Interface Characteristic Study

In this paper we have described the results of a preliminary experiment in which we compared five PEN-Ivory prototypes using fifteen users. This preliminary experiment has shown that we can detect measurable significant results with the current study design. However the user group for our study was composed of fifteen students from our department, all who are frequent computer users. A pragmatic next step is to repeat the study with a larger set of computer-naive physicians.

Generalizing Results

The results from the experiment show, for instance that a paging form works better for users than does a scrolling form. One potential research goal is to find what application domains these results apply to best. For example, for what applications and tasks does a paging form outperform a scrolling form? Is this finding a PEN-Ivory specific finding, or can we generalize it to other applications? Another way in which we could attempt to generalize the study results is to determine empirically the boundaries for which the results hold. For example, does a paging form work well if there are over 100 pages? Is a fixed attribute palette feasible if there are 40 attribute categories instead of 14?

PEN-Ivory vs. Writing and Dictation

Our experiment indicates that the PEN-Ivory interface that performed the best was the one that used a paging form, used a fixed attribute palette, and displayed all the findings all the time (PFA). An important question still remains however: are physicians willing to use PEN-Ivory? We suspect that the answer to this question depends greatly on how efficiently physicians can use PEN-Ivory as compared to writing and dictating, the traditional ways of creating progress notes.

Users who tested the fastest prototype, PFA, averaged 16.13 seconds per finding to enter. Instinctively, this seems much slower than writing and dictation. However, all of the users in our study group had never used PEN-Ivory before, and therefore were unaccustomed to the interface and the layout of the findings. Furthermore, we noticed that their times improved with each patient case. For the first case, the users averaged 20 seconds per finding, while for the third case, users averaged 13.78 seconds per finding. We speculate that over continued use, the times would drop even lower.

To approximate how fast expert users might reasonably become, we ran the study using one of the authors as the user. Because the author was intimately familiar with both the interface and the layout of the findings, he was able to complete the three cases with an average of 6.05 seconds per finding. For comparison, the same author also recorded the three patient cases using paper and pen. On average, he was able to write each finding in 8.0 seconds. This informal experiment suggests that as users become more familiar with the interface, they may be able to generate patient progress notes with PEN-Ivory as fast as they do with pencil and paper. We plan to study this hypothesis formally.

ACKNOWLEDGMENTS

We thank Keith Campbell for creating the Ivory system from which this work was derived. This work would not have been possible without his contribution. We also thank Dr. Jeanette Sison for helping to create the patient cases for the PEN-Ivory experiments, and Tom Moran, Ted Shortliffe, and Terry Winograd for their enlightening advice and continued support. And finally, we thank those who graciously lent their time and effort by participating in the PEN-Ivory experiments.

Primary support for this research is provided by the Department of Defense. Additional support was provided by the CAMIS project (LM-05305) and Apple Computer.

References

1. Shortliffe, E., Barnett, G. Medical Data: Their Acquisition, Storage, and Use, in *Medical Informatics: Computer Applications in Health Care,* E. Shortliffe et. al., editors. 1990, Addison-Wesley: Reading, Massachusetts. p. 37-69.
2. Institute of Medicine. *The Computer-Based Patient Record: An Essential Technology for Health Care.* 1991, Washington D.C.: National Academy Press.
3. O'Dell, D.V. Increasing Physician Acceptance and Use of the Computerized Ambulatory Medical Record in *Symposium on Computer Applications in Medical Care.* 1991. Washington D.C.: McGraw-Hill, Inc.: p. 848-852.
4. Hammond, W.E., and Stead, W.W. Adopting TMR for Physician/Nurse Use in *Symposium on Computer Applications in Medical Care.* 1991. Washington D.C.: McGraw-Hill, Inc.: p. 833-837.
5. Urkin, J., et. al. A Computerized Medical Record with Direct Data Entry for Community Clinics in Israel in *Symposium on Computer Applications in Medical Care.* 1991. Washington D.C.: McGraw-Hill, Inc.: p. 838-842.
6. Gelman, M.A. The Right System for the Write Reason in *American Medical Informatics Association Spring Congress.* 1994. San Francisco, CA: p. 83.
7. Luff, P., et. al. Tasks-In-Interaction: Paper and Screen Based Documentation in Collaborative Activity in *CSCW.* 1992.
8. Swearingen, R., Brown,. T. Requirements and Benefits of a Successful Pen-Based Data Entry System in *American Medical Informatics Association Spring Congress.* 1994. San Francisco, CA: : p. 101.
9. Essin, D., Lincoln, T. Design Criteria for Event-Driven Pen-Based User Interfaces in *American Medical Informatics Association Spring Congress.* 1994. San Francisco, CA: p. 100.
10. Lussier, Y., et. al. PureMD: A Computerized Patient Record Software for Direct Data Entry by Physicians Using a Keyboard-free Pen-Based Portable Computer in *Symposium on Computer Applications in Medical Care.* 1992. Baltimore, MD: McGraw-Hill, Inc.: p. 261-264.
11. Rich, C., Jr. Pen Computer Clincial Encounter Recorder in *American Medical Informatics Association Spring Congress.* 1994. San Francisco, CA: p. 62.
12. Campbell, K., et. al. A Computer-Based Tool for Generation of Progress Notes in *Symposium on Computer Applications in Medical Care.* 1993. Washington D.C.: McGraw-Hill, Inc.: p. 284-288.
13. Nygren, E. Reading Documents in Intensive Care I: Pattern Recognition and Encoding of Characteristics of the Information Media. 1991, University of Uppsala: CMD-21/91.

Using the PEN&PAD Information Model to Support Hospital-Based Clinical Care

Heather A. Heathfield[1], Nicholas R. Hardiker[2] and John Kirby[2]
[1]Computing Department, Manchester Metropolitan University, Manchester, UK
[2] Medical Informatics Group, University of Manchester, Manchester, UK

ABSTRACT

The PEN&PAD model for clinical record systems has been successfully used for medical records in both General Practice and hospital-based care. This paper describes experiences of using the model for developing computer-based nursing records. Results from this work show that there are some problems with directly applying the model to the nursing domain. Whilst the main purpose of the nursing record is to document and communicate a patient's care, it has several other, possibly incompatible, roles. Furthermore, the structure and content of the information contained within the nursing record is heavily influenced by the need for the nursing profession to visibly demonstrate the philosophical frameworks underlying their work. By providing new insights into the professional background of nursing records, this work has highlighted the need for nurses to clarify and make explicit, their uses of information, and also provided them with some tools to assist in this task.

INTRODUCTION

In 1988 the Medical Informatics Group at the University of Manchester began looking at the specific problem of computerising General Practice records, with the aim of producing systems that were both useful and usable by doctors [1]. A prototype clinical workstation for General Practitioners was developed and underwent extensive field trials. Users were highly enthusiastic about the prototype system, which proved to be sufficiently flexible and expressive to capture detailed clinical information in an intuitive and efficient manner. This work resulted in the identification of several requirements of an electronic medical record [2] and progressed to the definition of an information model capable of meeting these requirements [3]. The group also developed several tools and techniques to support the project including a User Centred Design Methodology, a novel technique of data entry called Predictive Data Entry [4] and the GRAIL formalism. GRAIL (Galen Representation and Inference Language) is a semantic network language with subsumption and multiple inheritance which can be used to express both the terminological model necessary to guide data entry and also the semantics of clinical observations. GRAIL was developed specifically to support the clinical requirements of computer-based clinical records and is currently being used in the specification of a medical terminology base as part of the GALEN Project (Generalised Architecture for Languages, Encyclopaedias and Nomenclatures), under the auspices of Advanced Informatics in Medicine Initiative [5].

The second and current phase of the PEN&PAD project began in 1992 and is sited in an elderly care ward of a small NHS hospital in the UK. One aspect of the work has addressed issues of collaborative care, while another aims to evaluate the approach developed in phase one for use in hospital-based care. The initial presupposition was that these tools and techniques would be easily transferable from the the domain of General Practitioners to clinical care in hospitals. While this assumption proved to be true for doctors' clinical records, our attempts to apply the approach to nursing records have been less successful and have uncovered several philosophical, professional and cultural barriers to the introduction of information systems to nursing practice.

This paper discusses our attempts to use the PEN&PAD approach in the nursing domain. We begin by discussing the general requirements for nursing record systems and briefly describe a prototype system for the display and manipulation of nursing data. More importantly, we look at requirements for data entry in nursing care planning. We describe the technique of Predictive Data Entry developed in phase one of the project and show how it is used in a prototype care planning system. The results of our evaluations using Predictive Data Entry in nursing are described. Finally we discuss the wider implications of using the PEN&PAD information model in light of the of our evaluation results.

HOSPITAL-BASED NURSING CARE

The prime requirements of computer-based clinical record systems are the need for flexible and intuitive data viewing and manipulation facilities and use of recognisable clinical concepts such as a patient record, problem, daily record entry or laboratory result. Storing patient data as natural language or in a "semi-structured" manner (i.e. as composite strings) does not provide sufficient semantics to support these requirements.

Using GRAIL to represent the underlying patient data, we have developed a nursing system which enables users to view and manipulate data in a flexible and intuitive manner. The system is based on a folder (similar to an A4 ring binder) metaphor in which there are several pages or sections, including a summary page, basic patient information page, medication page, results page, progress and evaluation notes page and care plan page. This prototype has been evaluated in several user workshops and was enthusiastically received [6].

Data Entry in Care Planning

The major role of the Nursing Care Plan is to provide a unique protocol of care which can be consulted by the patient. This accounts for the highly discursive and personalised manner in which the record is written. This style of writing is seen by the nurses as central to their professional identity and differentiates their perspective on patient care from that of the other practitioner groups. Furthermore, nurses do not deal exclusively with clinical terms, and often base their observations on the immediate environment of the patient. For example, a nurse may record that the patient "cannot walk further than the end of their garden" or that "their neighbour Anne pops in to do the cleaning every Friday".

Most existing computer-based care planning systems provide the nurse with a list of single terms or pre-defined composite phrases as the only available options for describing observations of the patient. These are seen as unacceptable by nurses as they are inflexible and not sufficiently expressive to capture data for individual patients.

The PEN&PAD philosophy is that users should be provided with data entry forms that contain all basic terms and phases that are sensible to apply in a given situation. The user is then free to combine these terms, in as much or as little detail as they wish, to form accurate and precise statements about the patient. The key idea is compositionality of observations using atomic concepts or qualifiers. This form of data entry is named "Predictive Data Entry" in that it predicts all sensible terms and phrases that can be applied in a given situation [4] and has been used in several other studies (eg. [7] and [8]) Given the vast possible numbers of situations or contexts in which patient observations may be made, it is not possible to enumerate the contents of every data entry form. Instead, the GRAIL model of terminology is used predict the contents of a data entry form.

Methods

The contents of the actual data entry forms are dynamically generated from a GRAIL model of nursing terms. In order to determine which terms should appear on a given data entry form, we carried out several discussions with one or more nurses, until we had an agreed set of terms for each nursing topic and context in the study (topics mobility and elimination in the contexts of prior needs, goals, and actions).

We then produced a GRAIL model which represented the semantics of these terms, using inheritance links and user-defined links. A semantic link might be "with-support-at" which can relate the term "sitting balance" to the term "head", (which in natural language translates to "sitting balance with head support"). An inheritance link might be "bed sitting balance is-a-kind-of sitting balance", thus if we have a link that asserts "sitting balance with-support-at the back " is a sensible statement, then through the notion of inheritance, we can also say that "bed sitting balance with-support-at the back" is sensible.

GRAIL models are produced as text files, using specific keywords to indicate the relationships between terms, and then compiled into a GRAIL network, each concept being classified and positioned in the network as appropriate. The GRAIL software is written in Smalltalk-80 and runs on Hewlett Packard Workstations (apollo series 700).

Figure 1 shows a Predictive Data entry form for nurses to record problems/needs concerning mobility in stroke patients (based on the Activities of Living Model). It is generated from a GRAIL network which contains terms relevant to the nursing assessment of stroke patients.

Care planning data (as shown on the data entry form in figure 1) is entered in the context of a care plan page. The care plan page consists of several panes, each of which corresponds to a different stage in the care planning process (eg. Prior Ability, Problems and Needs, Goals and Actions).

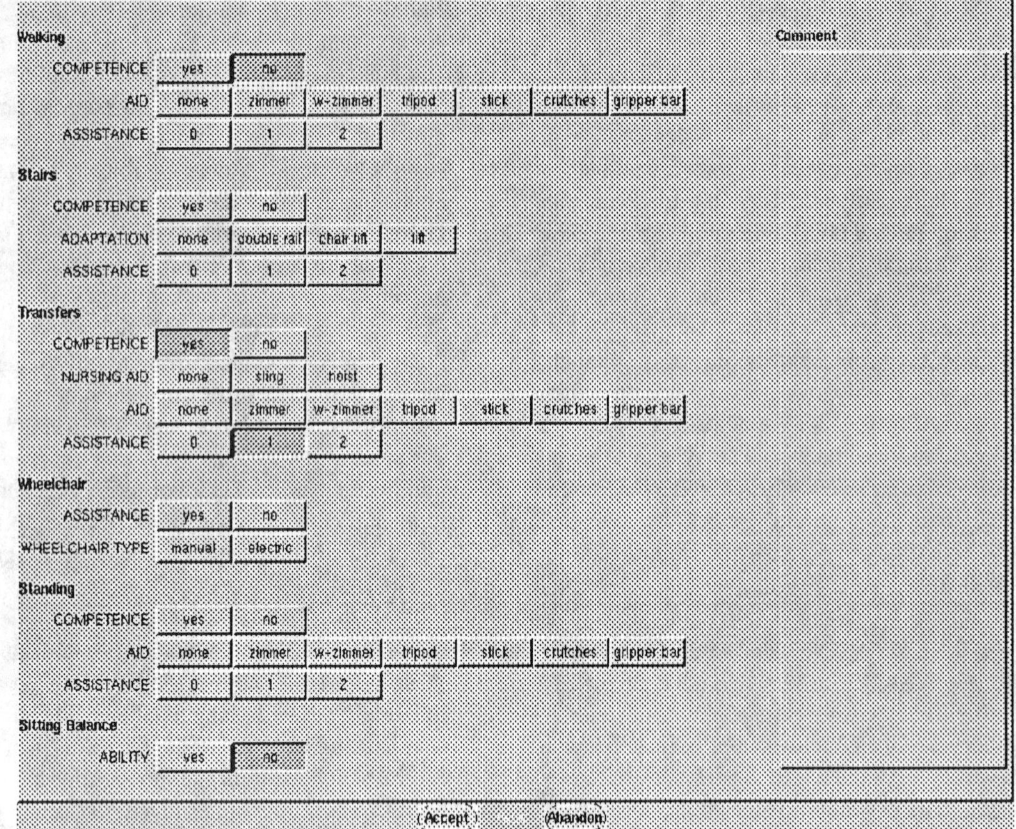

Figure 1. A Predictive Data Entry form for recording mobility problems/needs for stroke patients

Individual sections of the care plan are filled-in as required using Predictive Data Entry forms. As each Predictive Data Entry form is completed and accepted by the nurse, the information recorded is displayed in the relevant pane on the care plan page.

The Predictive Data Entry technique for entering care plan data was evaluated by nurses in user workshop:

• User Training. The first part of training involves the evaluator giving a demonstration of the system to the user, complemented by commentary and explanations. The user then carries out several training tasks and assistance is provided as necessary.

• Evaluation Scenarios. The user is asked to carry out a set of tasks, reading them from a paper script, without the aid of the evaluator if possible. These tasks are based around real situations that may arise on the ward.

• Observations. We observed the users carrying out the evaluation scenarios and made notes of any problems encountered or items of interest that occurred.

• Questionnaires and discussion. The users were asked to complete two sections of a questionnaire. The first section (completed before training) asked about general computer experience and attitudes to computerised patient records. The second section, (completed after the evaluation scenarios) asked about specific aspects of the system. After the evaluation exercises had been completed, users were engaged in a general discussion which gave then a chance to offer their opinions in a less structured manner.

EVALUATION RESULTS

A total of 10 Registered Nurses, including 2 ward managers, performed evaluations on the system. The evaluation questionnaires were put as questions with multiple choice pre-set answers (with space for comments), and also open-ended questions. An example of the former might be "How easy to understand are the care plans?" with possible replies "very/quite/average/ not easy/difficult", whilst an example of the latter might be "What is your impression of the care plans?". The results were collated by counting the number of replies in each category for the multiple choice questions, and classifying comments into obvious themes for the open-ended questions. Some of the replies are presented below.

In response to the question "Do the forms contain the right level of detail?", three nurses replied "too little" and seven "about right". When asked "Are there other things that ought to be added to the form?" the responses were "none" or cited administration data such as review dates, rather than additional descriptive terms concerning the patient. In response to the question "How well do the forms enable you to say what you would want to say about a patient?", four nurses replied "well", four replied "average", and two replied "poor". When asked "What is your overall impression of the forms?" two nurses replied "very good" and eight replied "good". On a general level, four users thought that it was "very" easy to use the computer to create a care plan, two thought it "quite" easy, and three thought it "average". When asked to compare the computer-based approach to the current paper-based one, the majority of users replied that it was easier and the same speed or faster using the computer system. Responses to the question "Can you imagine using this approach to care planning on a regular day to day basis?" were reserved, with five nurses replying "possibly" and four "definitely".

In the discussions held after the evaluation and questionnaires had been completed, nurses were more forthcoming about their reservations and critical of the plans produced. Many nurses were particularly concerned about their plans becoming standardised and not reflecting the individual nature of care.

We also performed limited experiments transforming the data displayed in the care plans into a more English-like form, yet the output was still seen as unacceptable to the majority of nurses. However, when asked to point out specific areas where the care plan was inadequate the nurses found it difficult to articulate their concerns.

DISCUSSION

These results appear to be contradictory and somewhat inconclusive given that although Predictive Data Entry forms were generally perceived by nurses as sufficiently expressive and flexible to capture most of the information necessary to formulate care plans, the resulting care plans themselves were perceived as lacking sufficient information to carry out patient care. These are preliminary results based upon only ten evaluations. Furthermore, none of the nurses involved had any previous experience of computer-based care planning systems. Whilst this latter fact is necessary to ensure that the requirements work we carry out with users is not influenced by their prior experience with other systems, it does not enable us to compare our system with others which is also important. However, our future plans do include such comparative evaluations with users from another site who do have experience with other systems.

Our work has raised a number of complex issues concerning the computerisation of nursing records:

- The contradictory nature of our results led us to the observation that nursing care plans fulfill several, possibly incompatible, roles. While the primary purpose of a care plan is to document and communicate a patient's care, several other roles were identified. These included: a legal document; a notebook; a things-to-do list; a record of alibi in the event of misadventure; a prompter for the hand-over of care from one nurse to another or simply a record of the presence of a nurse [9].
- As argued in [10], nurses have traditionally found it very difficult to define and describe patient care without devaluing the skill required. A variety of frameworks have been introduced to assist in this task, including the nursing process and models for nursing practice (e.g. [11]). These frameworks however have little regard for the structure or content of the information needed for patient care.
- The purpose of the nursing record is still not fully understood and much of the valuable information contained within nursing records is "swamped by mandatory obligations or culturally driven information" [9]. Therefore, attempts to develop and evaluate nursing information systems are problematic.

The recording practices of doctors and other clinical staff differ significantly as illustrated by our work in the nursing domain, and it is not obvious whether the PEN&PAD model is directly transferable from medicine to nursing care, given the strong philosophical, professional and cultural barriers that exist. While we believe that the model can capture the actual information content of the nursing record, this are other issues that must be addressed. The nursing profession must first clarify the disparity between what the nursing record is supposed to do and what it represents before we can consider introducing information systems. However, our work has been useful in that it does highlight the need to do this and provides some tools to assist in the task.

The situation is further complicated by the introduction of various abstracting mechanisms in nursing. For example, controlled vocabularies, such as Nursing Diagnoses, define a subset of terms and phrases that can be used to describe patient care and so restrict the information model (which should consist of all of those things that can be sensibly said about what nurses have heard, seen, thought or done). Minimum data sets, which have been devised to serve specific purposes and often conflict with the recording needs of daily nursing care, are process models of what ought to be done. Basing computer record systems on such abstractions renders the information they record distorted and useless for all except a single pre-defined purpose. As we have argued in [2] clinical information, as it is generated and used during patient care, is the only sound basis for a model of the clinical record. Our work in care planning has not made this argument any less valid and is valuable in that it has made explicit the multiple and often conflicting roles of nursing care plans. We can use this insight to contribute to the current debate over the structure and content of care plans [9], and can assist nurses in finding solutions.

This work has illustrated that the development of clinical information systems is not reliant simply on the strength of the technical solutions employed. Rather there are other, potentially more powerful, factors which affect the usefulness and acceptance of an information system. In particular there are social and cultural issues that need to be addressed before we can consider computer-based clinical records.

One method of influencing these factors is through education, moving from the current situation where learning by example is the norm, to more theoretically based learning. Another method is to conduct evaluations of the system on the ward, rather than an isolated laboratory evaluation, with the hope that routine use of the system will reveal to nurses that much of the information written in care plans is not necessary to daily care. We are currently setting up field trials on the ward with our system with the hope of exploring these issues further.

These observations reflect the general awareness of the medical informatics community, that is beginning to widen its considerations away from purely technical matters, to address human, cultural and organisational issues [12].

References

[1] Howkins TJ, Kay S, Rector AL, Goble CA, Horan B, Nowlan A, Wilson A. An overview of the PEN&PAD project. MIE 90; Lecture Notes in Medical Informatics NO. 40. Berlin. Springer-Verlag 1990: 73-8.

[2] Rector AL, Nowlan WA, Kay S. Foundations of an electronic medical record. Methods Inf Med (1991) 30: 179-86.

[3] Rector AL, Nowlan WA, Kay S, Goble CA, Howkins TJ. A framework for modelling the electronic medical record. Methods Inf Med (1993) 32: 109-119.

[4] Nowlan A and Rector A. Medical knowledge representation and predictive data entry. In: Lecture Notes in Medical Informatics 1991; 44 (Springer Verlag, M Stefanelli, A Hasman, M Fieschi, J Talmon (Eds) 1991).

[5] GALEN, General Architecture for Language, Encyclopaedias and Nomenclatures in Medicine. Project 2012, AIM Initiative, EC. Technical Annex.

[6] Heathfield HA, Hardiker N, Kirby J, Tallis R, Gonsalkarale M. The PEN&PAD Medical Record Model: A Report of its Use in the Development of a Clinical Record System for Hospital-based Care of the Elderly. Submitted to: Methods Inf Med April 1994.

[7] Kuhn K, Zemmler M, Reichert C, Heinlein D, Rosser D. Structured data collection and knowledge-based user guidance for abdominal ultrasound reporting. In: Safron C (ed) Proc 17th SCAMC}, McGraw-Hill, New York, 1993, 311-315.

[8] Benoit RG, Canfield K, Teilelbaum S, Cushing B, Stamp N, Durham A, Ondrish A, Woodman M, Bame W. Frame-based clinical data entry: design issues for physician acceptance. In: Lun KC, Degoulet P, Piemme TE, Rienhoff O (eds) MEDINFO 92, North-Holland, Amsterdam, 1992, 1280-1285.

[9] Hardiker NR. Towards an information infrastructure for nursing: a critique of the nursing record. Information Technology in Nursing (1994) 6.1: 7-9.

[10] Dukes S, Copp G. Hidden nursing. Nursing Times 1992; 88, 17: 40-2.

[11] Pearson A, Vaughan B. Nursing models for practice. Butterworth-Heinemann Ltd 1991.

[12] Heathfield HA, Wyatt J. Philosophies for the design and development of clinical decision-support systems. Methods Inf Med 1993; 32: 1-8.

Getting the Data In: Three Year Experience With A Pediatric Electronic Medical Record System

Isaac S. Kohane, Division of Endocrinology, Children's Hospital and Harvard Medical School, Boston, MA

The Clinician's Workstation (CWS) has provided the full-functionality of an on-line electronic patient record for outpatient pediatric clinics over the past 3 years. The implementation of the CWS built upon a substantial effort in integration of data from various sources. This paper addresses the subsequent design issues which had to be resolved in order to enable both physician and transcriptionist-driven data entry and retrieval, notably selecting a feasible mixture of controlled vocabulary and free text. Some of the consequences of these design decisions on clinical care, clinical education, clinical and basic research are reviewed with examples from the last three years.

INTRODUCTION

Over the past 5 years, the trend towards implementing a fully-electronic medical record has accelerated considerably. Comprehensive electronic medical record systems (EMRS) have been discussed for decades [1], but comprehensively implemented in relatively few sites (e.g. Regenstrief [2]. HELP,[3], TMR [4]). There have also been several efforts to develop workstation-based, graphics-intensive on-line patient charts (e.g. PWS at Hewlett Packard/Stanford, [5]). These efforts only addressed the specific requirements of pediatric EMRS tangentially. I describe here the design and performance of a pediatric EMRS—the Clinician's Workstation (CWS)—built upon a "client-server" architecture. The CWS has been in operation for three years, first in the Division of Endocrinology and more recently in the Divisions of Nephrology and Nuclear Medicine.

The data-integration efforts that led to the development of the CWS will only be briefly touched upon as these have been published elsewhere[6,7]. Rather this paper focuses on the task that McDonald et al. [8] have termed "the difficult side of medical record systems," namely data acquisition and in particular acquisition of data from clinicians. This focus includes the tradeoffs that have made between clinician acceptance, and the requirements for controlled, coded vocabularies. It also describes the technological solutions and organizational solutions required to implement these tradeoffs. The consequences of our* design choices are illustrated by providing a few illustrative examples of how the CWS can be used to 1) improve clinical efficiency, 2) enable clinical and basic science research and 3) quantify some aspects of clinician performance. Those aspects of the CWS that are specific to the practice of pediatrics will be emphasized.

*Several members of the Division of Endocrinology, particularly Drs. Majzoub and Crigler, were influential in the design process. This work was supported, in part, by the Charles Hood Foundation.

Summary of Current CWS Functionality.

The current version of the CWS is implemented on Macintosh computers networked to the Integrated Hospital Information System (IHIS). The IHIS has as its centralized data repository, an Oracle database stored on several Digital Equipment Corporation VAX computers (the "VAX Cluster"). The CWS retrieves and displays all pertinent administrative, financial and clinical data residing on the VAX Cluster. These data include: demographics, visit history with associated procedure and diagnostic codes, inpatient pharmacy orders, inpatient laboratory studies which are entered into the IHIS through other departmental applications (e.g. the Cerner laboratory system). Users of the CWS enter additional clinical documentation into the IHIS through the CWS interface. These data include: problem lists, patient-provider relationships, bedside measurements, history, past medical history, family history, review of systems and other components of clinic notes or letters to referring physicians. Access to this information is controlled by assigning data access/modification privileges to various provider roles. The CWS serves to maintain *all* clinical data/documentation of patients seen by *all* clinicians in each participating clinic. Data displays are designed to follow the metaphor of the paper chart as possible but employ other metaphors where appropriate.

The client program on the Macintosh computers was written in Hypercard. Transactions with the Oracle data-base are communicated through SQLNet protocols (Oracle Corporation) running over a hospital-wide ethernet network.

DESIGN CONSIDERATIONS

Goals

At the outset we set the bounds on the technological solutions we envisaged by insisting that we meet, within a 1.5 year implementation project plan, the following goals.

1. The CWS would be universally used within each clinic in which it was deployed.

2. Clinicians should be able to rapidly enter free text and coded data items as part of the routine workflow in the care of their patients.

3. Clinicians who did not wish to perform data entry should be able to dictate the clinic visit into a tape recorder and have transcriptionists enter data. This alternate route should not provide less coded and objective information than the direct entry method.

4. Provide entry and display screens that are useful and familiar to pediatricians.

5. Provide sufficient accurately coded and quantified data to support automated clinical event monitors, clinical research, and outcomes research.

6. Avoid redundant data entry: From a single entry of data from a clinic visit, all other documentation (e.g. clinic notes, letters to referring physicians) should be generated.

7. Training requirements would have to be minimal in order to accommodate the large number of transient clinicians rotating through our clinics.

Constraints

Further we were constrained by the following limitations:

1. Voice-recognition and handwriting recognition technology was not mature to reliably and accurately encode terms for the relatively unconstrained domain of pediatric histories.

2. We could not guarantee that each clinician could always have immediate access to a workstation for data entry. Each clinic was provided with between 5 to 7 Macintosh computers networked to the IHIS. This limitation has since been made moot by the collapse of hardware costs but was a significant consideration in our original design.

3. In the late 1980's, off-the-shelf client authoring tools for SQL-compliant data-bases were scarce and had limited capabilities.

4. Post-hoc parsing of free text (e.g. [9]) is not sufficiently accurate to achieve goal 5 (above).

IMPLEMENTATION

The approach we took for the task of clinician-driven data entry was three-fold: 1) an electronic form was created in the CWS for data-entry 2) clinicians were given a variety of paper-based equivalents to the electronic form and 3) an ongoing program of clinician feedback and software modification was implemented. These three components are described below.

Electronic Form

The purpose of the electronic form is to enable data entry to be performed at very close to the speed of unrestricted typing. The user of the form tabs from field to field within the form and is only prompted upon detection of potential data entry errors.

If a patient has already been seen once, then the CWS automatically retrieves the following items which therefore do not have to be entered by the clinician: patient/parent's address, the address of referring clinician(s) and laboratory studies at the time of the visit. Each clinic using the CWS can define those data elements that they wish to be encoded for later systematic analysis. In the Endocrine clinic these include standard anthropometry (e.g. height, weight, arm span) and sexual development information (e.g. testicular size, Tanner staging). Within the form, a field is created for each such data element in the order that the clinic providers are accustomed to. As the provider enters the values of these data, a clinical data extraction program associated with each field is triggered. The default program, which can be customized, stores the content of the field in a clinical data table on the server. Bookkeeping details such as the date the clinical finding was observed, the time of data entry and the code of the data type are automatically determined by the data extraction program. For some data elements, the default data extraction program has to be modified for specialized data validation. For example when one of the testicular short axis measurements are entered, the data extraction program checks whether this measurement is less than the long axis. If not, it offers to switch the two measurements. We have summarized below the three most important classes of coded data elements: physical exam bedside measurements, patient:provider relationships and problem lists. The non-coded fields in the electronic form merely tag the sections of the unrestricted or "free" text of the clinical note (e.g. family history) so that the program which generates the letters to referring physicians or the clinical note for the chart can manipulate and position the text fragments appropriately.

Physical Exam. The tempo and pattern of growth and development of children is among the most sensitive measures of health. Many disorders can be first detected through careful inspection of the growth and development data routinely acquired during the course of regular pediatric visits [10]. We have consequently encoded several standards for the progression of growth and development parameters (e.g. blood pressure, height, sexual staging) with age. Where possible we have encoded longitudinal standards obtained for the many distinct populations that pediatricians will follow (e.g. Turner's Syndrome, Down's Syndrome, late and early puberty).

These encoded standards serve to improve data validation (e.g. through automated identification of implausible changes in standard deviation score for height) by the default data extraction program of the electronic form. They also have enabled us to generate data displays that are familiar to pediatricians such as the growth chart in Figure 1. This chart was generated using one [11] of several standards for growth and another standard for predicting adult height from bone age [12].

Patient:Provider Relationships. Particularly in tertiary-care centers, many providers participate in the health-care of each patient. Furthermore, a large fraction of these same providers (fellows and residents) will only follow these patients for a few years. To prevent unintended gaps in patients care, we chose to explicitly enter patient:provider relationships as part of the data entry process. Every clinic visit document has a primary signatory and a large subset of them also have a secondary signatory (if the attending physician sees the patient with a fellow or resident). Clinicians "sign" the documents generated from the electronic form by entering their unique provider identification number. This populates a patient:provider relationship table on the server data-base in the IHIS. The table also stores the time that the relationship was established and the role that the provider serves for the patient (e.g. supervisory, primary or research).

Problem Lists. Problem lists serve to quickly summarize a patient's course. They can also serve to identify subpopulations of clinic patients of relevance to clinical or basic science research or outcomes studies. As part of the data entry process, each patient is assigned one or more problems (e.g. autoimmune thyroiditis) from a vocabulary that is specific to each clinic. Each vocabulary term is classified in a nosology to permit aggregation of these subpopulations (e.g. to find all patients with thyroid disease). Unfortunately most standard controlled vocabularies do not provide sufficiently fine-grained descriptors for all the pathophysiological disorders we would like to capture. Therefore, for each clinic using

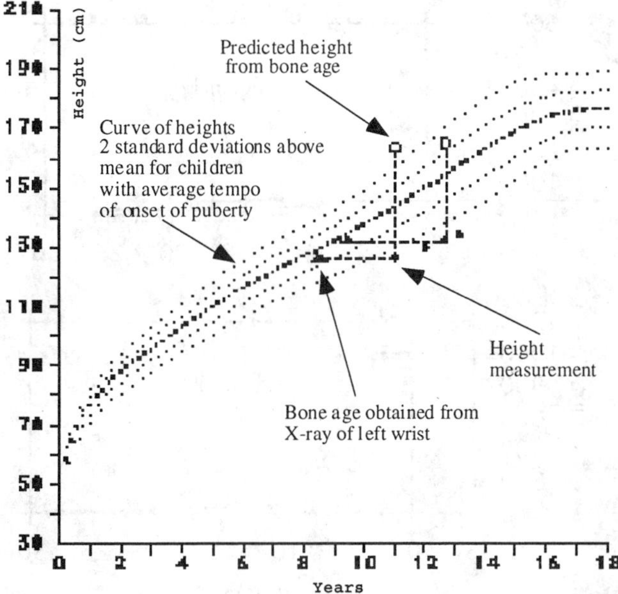

Figure 1: Growth Chart

the CWS, the clinicians must arrive at a consensus vocabulary for problems. These vocabularies are periodically updated. We are now considering requiring for each such consensus vocabulary, a set of mappings to the ULMS vocabulary[13], which even though not as fine-grained is standardized.

Paper Forms

As noted in the design considerations section, we did not want participation in the CWS data entry to be limited by access to workstations or clinician resistance to use of computers. Therefore, we created paper equivalents of the electronic form that clinicians use for taking notes during the course of the patient visit. For each field in the electronic form there is an equivalent labeled area on the paper form in identical order.

Many clinics at Children's Hospital still use the traditional paper chart, therefore the paper form is backed with "carbonless" pressure-sensitive paper so that a duplicate copy of the notes can be left in the paper chart before the electronic version is generated. If the clinician does not directly enter the documentation of the clinic visit into the CWS, a transcriptionist will enter the documentation either using the paper form or a taped, dictated summary. Any clinician dictating the documentation for a clinic visit follows the same order that the data appears on the electronic and paper forms. Index cards listing the data elements in order have been provided for this purpose.

Clinician Participation

Clinician acceptance of the CWS was recognized as the principal hurdle from the outset. Consequently, physician and nursing staff in the target clinics were appraised of major design decisions at regular intervals during the design process. The appearance and function of the electronic and paper forms have undergone several revisions since the onset of the design process.

We found that the transcriptionists and administrative staff were among the more frequent users of the CWS and that the success of the entire project depended critically on their ability to use the client program efficiently. Bottlenecks became rapidly apparent both in the automated auditing of the transcription process performed by the CWS and in the comments coming from the administrative staff. These comments led to repeated streamlining and simplification of the data entry process as well as automation of mundane but onerous ancillary tasks (e.g. addressing envelopes, creating address lists of patients followed by a particular physician).

Our approach to user participation in the design process has dictated an incremental, clinic-by-clinic adoption of the CWS rather than attempting a hospital-wide implementation. Given the lessons learned during the course of its deployment and the varying requirements of each clinic, this seems to have been a prudent course.

RESULTS

Since its first deployment in July of 1991, the CWS data-base has accumulated the records of 3100 patients (i.e. 100% of patients seen in the clinic). Excluding reports generated by other departmental applications (e.g. radiology, pathology which are accessible through the same CWS interface) 6500 visit forms were completed. In the process, 38,000 individually coded clinic measurements were automatically entered into the data-base as well 3400 problems (using the clinics' controlled problem list vocabulary). As the first 2.5 years of its deployment were restricted to a single clinic, we anticipate rapid growth in these numbers in the near future.

In this section we describe the impact of the CWS deployment with a few selected examples that we have organized into four rubrics that we have found to represent important uses of the CWS.

Clinical Care

The most obvious consequence of implementing the CWS is the availability of the patient record. Whereas previously, at best records were missing or misplaced for approximately 5% of patient visits, we now have immediate access to documentation on all visits to clinics where the CWS has been deployed. With the hospital-wide ethernet network, these records can be viewed, with proper authorization, throughout the institution.

In the Division of Endocrinology, there are 19 physicians who use the CWS and approximately 20 visiting physicians (fellows from other institutions and housestaff from Children's Hospital) per year. Electronic data entry is performed by only 15% of clinicians whereas 20% submit the paper forms with handwritten entries and 65% submit taped dictations.

By selecting 100 clinic visits from immediately prior to the deployment of the CWS and 100 one year after its deployment, the time from a patient visit to the sending of a letter to the referring physician declined from approximately 3 weeks to 2.1 weeks (the null hypothesis of the mean follow-up time in the two periods being equal was rejected with $p < 0.05$). Many factors may have contributed to this trend other than the CWS client-server application. These include the effect that the paper forms may have had in standardizing the data acquisition behavior of clinicians. It could also be explained in part by other factors such as changes in administrative staff.

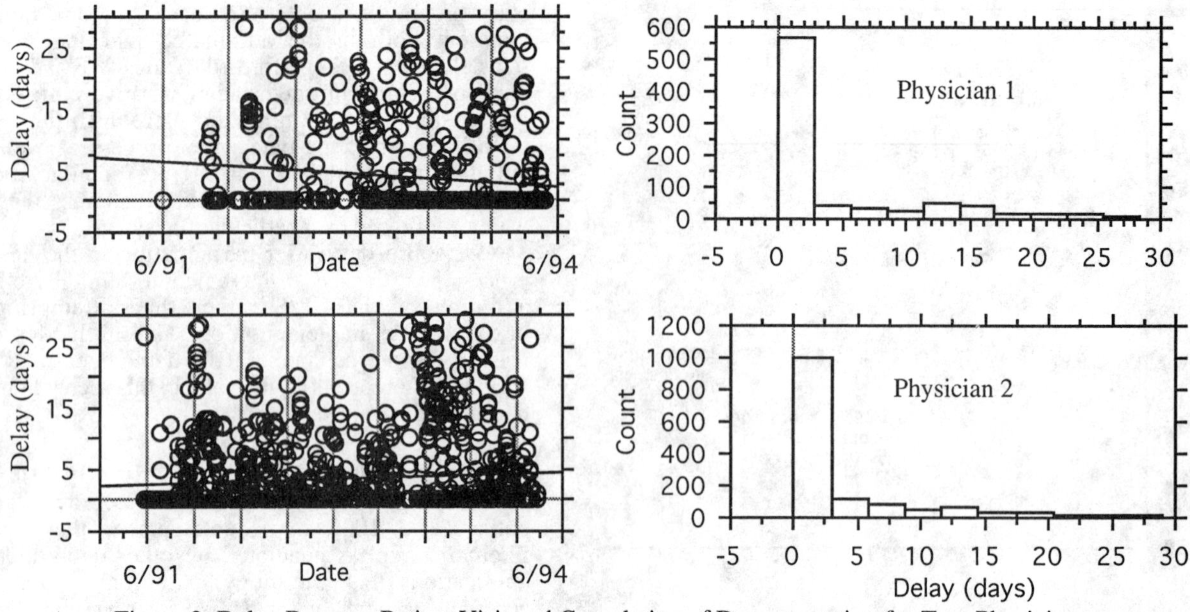

Figure 2: Delay Between Patient Visit and Completion of Documentation for Two Physicians.

Nonetheless, in the absence of controlled trials, these results are encouraging. We note however, that the model of the CWS use is designed for tertiary care clinics. In other settings, such as high-volume primary-care clinics, it may present a suboptimal model for entry of clinician-derived data.

Quality Assurance

During the process of generating a clinical document such as a clinic note or a letter to a referring physician, the CWS enters a large amount of bookkeeping detail which has enabled us to implement several quality assurance programs. This includes the identity of the clinicians involved, the transcriptionists, the date of the clinic visit, the date the document was first created, the date it was last modified and the date "published" (at which point it can no longer be edited). Although we are still in the process of picking those monitors or filters that will be the most useful, we illustrate here (Figure 2) one potentially interesting application. In these graphs we illustrate the delay between the date the patient was seen and the date the letter to the referring physician was completed. One of the two physicians clearly has a lighter clinical load (spends a greater percentage of time in basic research) and is less prompt in completing the documentation although the plotted regression line shows some steady improvement over the past three years. These plots do not control for patient case mix.

Clinical Research

The CWS has already enabled several clinical research projects that would otherwise have been prohibitively labor intensive, to get underway. This includes a study of the dose-response relationship for growth hormone in growth hormone-deficient patients [14], and a review of outcome predictors in patients

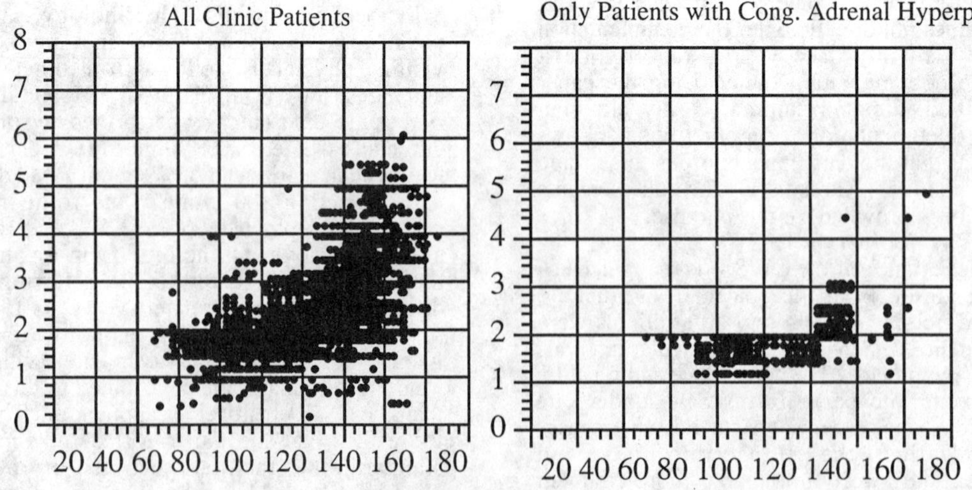

Plots of Long Axis of Testicle (cm) vs. Height (cm)

Figure 3: Graphs for Clinical Research from the CWS

with non-classical adrenal hyperplasia (in progress). As clinical data continues to accumulate as a side-effect of routine health-care documentation, we anticipate that not only will we be able to quickly generate cost-effective clinical studies but we will be able to generate new, comprehensively documented, standards for a variety of pediatric parameters (e.g. problem-specific growth curves). Again, only to illustrate the capabilities of the CWS, we show (in Figure 3) a graph of testicular dimension (long axis) plotted against total standing height. These parameters are plotted for both for the entire clinic population and for also for those patients with congenital adrenal hyperplasia. Although somewhat whimsical in their specifics, these graphs demonstrate how the various kinds of coded data (in this case bedside measurements and problem lists) stored by the CWS can be used to aid clinical research.

The emergence of reasonably robust interapplication protocols on personal computers (as the CWS is implemented on the Apple Macintosh we have used the AppleEvents protocol) has enabled us to display, in real-time, within commercial graphical applications (e.g. Deltagraph from Deltapoint or Excel from Microsoft) the results of queries initiated in the CWS client application. Figure 3 was generated in this way. The interapplication protocols have also enabled us to automatically route clinical alerts from the CWS to the electronic mail system.

Basic Research

We have found that the CWS can serve to generate a low-cost bridge between basic research and clinical practice. For example, for a collaborator interested in the specific gene defects leading to obesity, we were able to generate a list of all patients with a very high weight for height (using pediatric standards encoded in the CWS) and who did not have known CNS malignancies (obtained from the coded problem list). The CWS enabled another researcher to find a group of patients with combinations of neuroendocrine insufficiencies from which she identified a novel mutation of the Pit-1 gene [15].

CONCLUSION

The Clinician's Workstation's implementation has have largely met the goals that we set for ourselves in the design stage. Initial results over the first three years of deployment suggest that the specific combination of free text and controlled vocabularies we have chosen is effective in meeting these goals. Further, as the users of the CWS become more familiar in its use and as its data-base has become more substantial, we have begun to see it used for clinical productivity and research in ways we had not anticipated.

Nonetheless, five years after we implemented the first prototypes, some limitations have become apparent. The tools we chose to implement the client application have relatively poor performance and versatility as compared to the client-building tools available today. Also, the cost of high-performance hardware and the capabilities of system software have reached levels that make technologies such as pen or voice recognition potentially viable. If these technologies result in a much higher clinician acceptance of direct data entry, then a much larger portion of the visit documentation could be encoded in controlled vocabularies. The current CWS information infrastructure will permit us to explore the added value of these tools in the near future.

REFERENCES

1. Greenes, R. A.; Pappalardo, A. N.; Marble, C. W.; Barnett, G. O. Design and implementation of a clinical data management system. *Comput. Biomed. Res.* 1969, *2*, 469-485.

2. McDonald, C. J.; Blevins, L.; Tierney, W. M.; Martin, D. K. The Regenstrief Medical Records. *MD Computing* 1988, *5*, 34-47.

3. Pyror, T. A.; Gardner, R. M.; Clayton, P. D.; Warner, H. R. The HELP system. *Journal of Medical Systems* 1983, *7*, 87.

4. Stead, W. W.; Hammond, W. E. Computer-based medical records: The Centerpiece of TMS. *MD Computing* 1988, *5*, 48-62.

5. Tang, P. C.; Annevelink, J.; Fafchamps, D.; Stanton, W.; Young, C. Y. Physician's workstations: Integrated information management for clinicians. In: *Proceedings Symposium on Computer Applications in Medical Care.* P. D. Clayton, Eds., Washington, DC: McGraw-Hill, 1992:569-573.

6. Margulies, D.; McCallie, D. P.; Elkowitz, A.; Ribitsky, R. An integrated hospital information system at Children's Hospital. In: *Proceedings SCAMC.* Washington, DC: 1990:699-703.

7. Kohane, I. S.; David P. McCallie, J. A dynamically reconfigurable clinician's workstation with transparent access to remote and local databases. In: *First Annual American Medical Informatics Conference.* Snowbird, Utah: 1990:

8. McDonald, C. J.; Tierney, W. M.; Overhage, J. M.; Martin, D. K.; Wilson, G. A. The Regenstrief Medical Record System: 20 years of experience in hospitals, clinics and neighborhood health centers. *MD Computing* 1992, *9*, 206-217.

9. Salton, G. Development in automatic text retrieval. *Science* 1991, *253*, 974-980.

10. In *Nelson Textbook of Pediatrics*; 12 ed.; R. E. Behrman and V. C. Vaughan, Ed.; 1983; pp. 186-194.

11. Hamill, P. V. V.; Drizd, T. A.; Johnson, C. L.; Reed, R. R.; Roche, A. F. In *Vital Statistics Report*Rockville, MD, 1976; Vol. 25.

12. Greulich, W.; Pyle, S. *Radiographic Atlas of Skeletal Development of Hand and Wrist*; Stanford Press: 1959.

13. Sheretz, D.; Tuttle, M.; Blois, M.; Erlbaum, M. Intervocabulary mapping within the UMLS: the role of lexical matching. In: *Proceedings SCAMC.* R. Greenes, Eds., Washington, DC: IEEE Computer Society Press, 1988:201-206.

14. Kohane, I. S.; K.Faizan; Adjanee, N.; Najjar, S. S. Can cost effectiveness of growth hormone be improved? *Pediatric Research (Suppl.)* 1993, *33*, S51.

15. Cohen, L. E.; Wondisford, F. E.; Radovick, S. A novel mutation in the phosphorylation consensus sequence of the Pit-1 gene in a patient with dysregulation of prolactin and thyrotropin secretion. In: *76th Annual Meeting of the Endocrine Society.* Anaheim, CA: 1994:Abstract #6.

Computer-Based Patient Record: The Essential Data Set Approach

K. Moidu, M.D., Ph.D., J.J. Falsone, M.D., S. Nair, M.D.
Beulah Hinds Center for Health Informatics, Section for Pulmonary and Critical Care Medicine,
Norwalk Hospital, Norwalk CT 06856

Abstract

The clamor for data to study the impact of care, to evaluate clinical performance and justify resource utilization is increasing. The data in demand normally should exist in the record of a clinical encounter. Advances in information technology and software techniques have provided us with tools to develop and implement computer-based patient record systems. The issues that constrain development are integral issues of clinical medicine, such as the variability in medical data, specialized practice of medicine, and differing demands of the numerous end-users of a medical record. This paper describes an approach to develop a computer-based patient record. The focus is on identification of the essential data set by infological data modeling and its implementation in a commercially available package for a physician's office.

INTRODUCTION

The paradigm shift in health care management from monitoring the "process of care" to evaluating the "outcome of care" is driven by economic forces[1]. The foundation of all scientific decisions is information. Inadequate information places a decision maker, who may be: a physician, a nurse, an administrator or a clinical epidemiologist, in a dilemma. In the normal course of events much of the desired information would be in a clinical encounter record.

Paper based patient records have natural limitations, such as legibility, access and availability round the clock.

In a medical record due to lack of structure there is either excessive detail or a paucity of clinically relevant data. Computer adds value of automation to information and a computer-based medical record would provide care providers timely access to accurate data [2]. The panel on Computer based Patient Record (CPR) called by the Institute of Medicine has reviewed the need along with the current information technological advances. In conclusion explicitly state that technology is no longer a barrier [3].

At Norwalk, a practice based outcomes research study in chronic obstructive pulmonary disease has been initiated with application of Informatics tools and methods [4]. The emphasis was on developing a CPR to serve as a common tool for data collection from multiple sites. Later apply the structured approach perfected in Medical Informatics research to make explicit the knowledge that lies in our patient records from past clinical experience [5,6]. This feed-back to the care providers would result in clinical practice of high quality and introduce cost effectiveness in care.

The key challenges addressed in the Informatics approach were the issue of data taxonomy, coding, nomenclature, clinical classification using clinimateric indexes and developing a CPR to serve as a uniform data collection tool. In a recent review article Feinstein recommends such an approach to clinical research [7].

In this paper the approach to definition of data is outlined Then describe electronic implementation of the data set in a commercial application, the Medical Electronic Desktop [MED].

BACKGROUND

In computerization of patient records the earlier direction was to replicate the paper based patient record and techniques employed were to manage free text. In information systems that permit free text entry, either there is not adequate data to reconstruct the reason of clinical encounter [8]. Else, there is so much data that we drown in information as in the case at an academic center that led to abandonment of a CPR experiment [9].

Developers to make a CPR must address the three major problems:

- Structure, as in layout
- Semantics, as in issues of interpretation and coding
- Content, as the level of detail in data collected.

Weed, presented a revolutionary orientation for recording a clinical encounter in what he described as the "problem oriented medical record" [10]. As an

0195-4210/94/$5.00

organizational format it was most appropriate for a quick review of the clinical encounter record. It provided the design stimulus for many patient record computerization projects. The issue of structure has more recently found attention from many quarters. The Sub-Committee ASTM E31.12 of the American Society for testing and materials circulated a draft report that outlines a generic structure and describes the architectural design of a CPR [11].

Medical data, as Prof. Blois emphasized, is the central issue for medical Informatics research [12], since that is the subject of medical computing [13]. The issue of semantics and management of the large terminology base has led to the development of coding schemes. The UMLS Meta-thesaurus project is designed to tackle the problem of the numerous coding schemes utilizing computer power [14]. The appropriateness of the various coding systems is under evaluation by a working group of the Computer-based Patient Record Institute.

The matter of content remains a neglected issue. Insufficient detail or lack of uniformity patient data makes it difficult to compare performance of different hospitals and there is an information gap [15]. Uniformity in content is desirable, specially to compare and evaluate effects of interventions [1, 16]. One needs to insure the content is adequate to reconstruct the clinical encounter [17]. In a multi-center research study, the *essential data set* approach was identified as one approach to develop health application software that could be used at multiple sites. The uniform data collection tool made it possible for experiences from the sites to be compared [18].

Figure 1 Decision Making Role Analysis of the Essential Data Set

	@ First encounter	during History	during Physical	during Follow-up	for summary	for research	Action Initiated
Nocturnal Cough Starts immediately							
after an hour							
>3 hours							
Stops when patient sits-up							
Does the patient complain of wheezing							

THE ESSENTIAL DATA SET APPROACH

An *Essential Data Set* (EDS) is the core data set that is essential to support decision making in a clinical setting. Elements in an EDS should be adequate to enable a clinician to describe the health status at the time of the encounter. In a retrospective mode enable evaluation of prior provider actions and resource utilization at the clinical encounter. An *Essential Data Set* for a clinical domain must include the data elements required to support clinical decision making, by all levels of care providers. Indirectly the same data elements should support administrators to monitor the resource utilization and researchers to evaluate the impact of the care provided. All data elements may not be required by all the care providers, at all sites or by the administration must be kept in mind. Duplicate elements may be eliminated, and some qualifications need to be made so that the set is definable.

A data element in an *Essential Data Set* for a clinical domain must fulfill some of the following criteria:

- easy to collect, preferably at the least cost
- provide information related to health status
- assist in risk and clinical assessment during encounters
- reflect the actions or interventions undertaken
- should assist in assessment of an outcome or have a predictive value for an outcome
- should reflect the actual outcomes.

Defining the EDS

Data modeling, a recognized technique used in systems development process was applied in identifying the EDS. In data modeling the objective is to identify information requirements of application users. A group of pulmonary physicians was led by a trained medical Informatics specialist with prior experience in defining a data set.

The infological modeling approach as described by Sundgren [19] was adopted, first performing information analysis and then *normalization*. In an infological data model, data specification is in purely logical terms. An object can exist independent of any property or relationship pertaining to it. The first step was enumerating the data list from the soft situational perspective. The list was normalized and reduced from a functional perspective and finally a second normalization after an analysis of the data for its traditional decision making use. See form used in Figure 1. An EDS was thus defined to record an encounter with a chronic obstructive pulmonary disease patient.

The essential data set was organized in a paper format of a standard medical record. This was used for data extraction during review of charts. Many data elements were added as the records required to support research need greater detail. To support outcomes research elements to assess functional capacity were included.

Electronic Implementation

The next step was to implement the pulmonary EDS in a software to provide the project with common data collection tool. The first option was to develop the entire software application package using commercially available application programs, as in a previous experience [20]. The other option was to use an available package for a physician's office and modify it to incorporate the pulmonary EDS.

After an evaluation of available packages, Medical Electronic Desktop© a commercially available package developed by JAM Software of Australia, was selected. The package runs on Apple Macintosh computers with the simplest available configuration. The 'click and run' user *interface* of a Macintosh computer is easier with a shorter learning curve appropriate for clinicians who are busy.

The package is stable and designed for use in the physician's office. It has four components:

MED Patient - the patient record management component.

MED Maker - a utility tool-box to modify the MED Patient to modify the record system and the knowledge base.

MED Extract - a tool to support extraction of data from the patient record to any statistical package for analysis of data.

MED Billing - To include practicing clinicians into the study the financial management aspect has to be kept in mind. The availability of such a component was considered important to gain acceptance for a common data collection tool.

The access to the system requires an electronic key, (See Figure 2) a log is maintained by a time date stamp for all interactions (See Figure 3). Data driven support functions can be easily implemented using the tool box. The pulmonary EDS was incorporated along with the knowledge base in to the Medical Electronic Desktop using MEDmaker. The effort to incorporate was approximately 4 man-weeks of effort. It allowed the project group to maintain a clinical focus while developing of the CPR - MED-Pulmonary.

Figure 2 Log-in using electronic security key

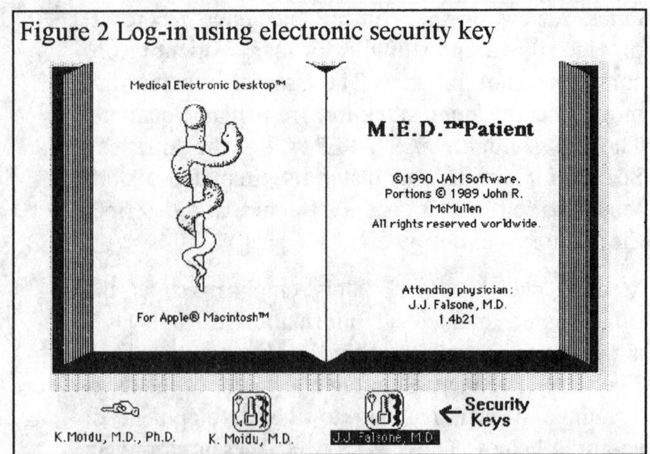

Figure 3 Date and time stamp and log record

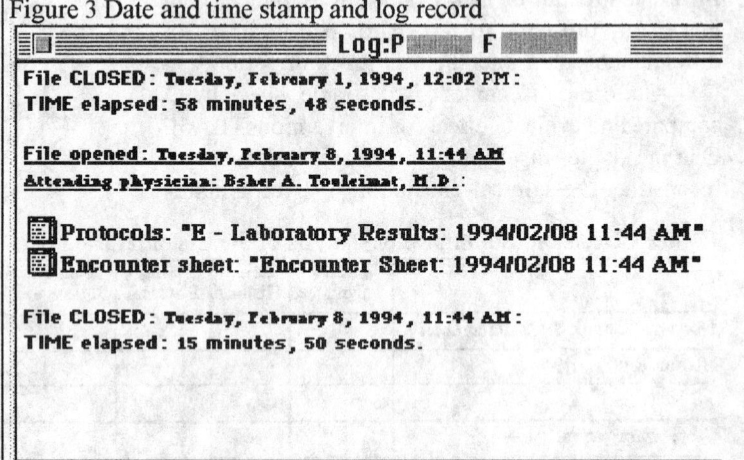

DISCUSSION

In traditional research with a statistical design manual data collection and management, a small set of variables are collected. On the assumption that all change is reflected in that small set and all other data elements can be excluded. The use of computers has often been limited to data analyses.

In an I*nformatics* approach the power and potential of the computer must be fully utilized. If there is to be a significant shift in the research paradigm towards an Informatics approach then the computer

Figure 4: Data entry and retrieval of salient features of same encounter

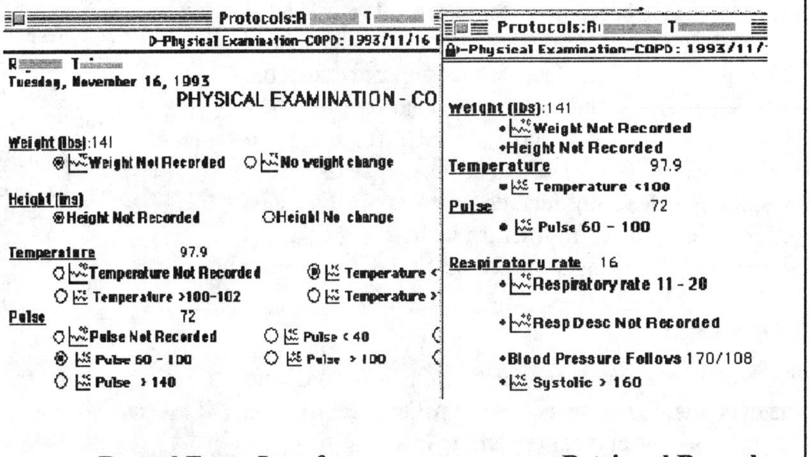

Record Entry Interface **Retrieved Record**

must be introduced in data collection and management. This would enable us to collect greater detail, in essence collect all data variables that may influence a clinical situation under study. It would also permit us to collect data prospectively and analyze it retrospectively applying the natural criteria to stratify the cohort. The data collection tool designed as an instrument to support the clinical care provider would improve the data quality, as the collector of data is also the first user of the data.

A critical step in the project was defining of the pulmonary EDS. It was with an objective to collect detailed History and Physical examination findings in a clinical setting. It was extended, at this stage to assure thorough data collection. The pulmonary-EDS will be reduced in the future as the redundant data elements are removed, just as a clinician through years of practice adopts short cuts. The principle objective of the CPR in this case is to support in data collection in a physician's office for the outcomes research study.

The expansive data set comes with an overhead of time, it took almost an hour (See in Figure 3) and was a major hurdle to initiate the pulmonary fellows to use the system in the busy clinical settings. However, subsequent encounters required around 4 - 11 minutes for up-dating a record. The value of the detailed first history was later appreciated by the clinical staff in the follow-up encounter, led one of them to state "I now really know more about the patient in a shorter time." The relevant details collected can be retrieved on review, making data reduction an automated process (See Figure 4).

The ease with which one could set data driven reminders made the system acceptable to the clinical staff. The reminders list provided them with a powerful tool to provide team care, sharing plans for clinical work-up and follow-up. It also provided them with a list of reminders for communication with the patient, such as advice on smoking cessation, vaccination, or a therapy. See figure 5. The pulmonary-MED system was used in the pulmonary clinics for recording all cases. The implementation strategy was the "agent of change" approach, where a member of the clinical team was trained with the intention he will provide a role model and train the fellows as they rotated through the clinic.

The pulmonary-MED system has security in terms of access limited by a digital key. There is also security in the detailed log maintained, that identifies the end-user and a summary of actions of the end-user. The system manager is able to define the access levels, but not make alterations in a record.

Availability of tools such as MED makes it possible to focus on the clinical issues in the development of a computer-based patient record. Under the guidance

Figure 5. Opening a patient file leads to a pop-up reminder appearing

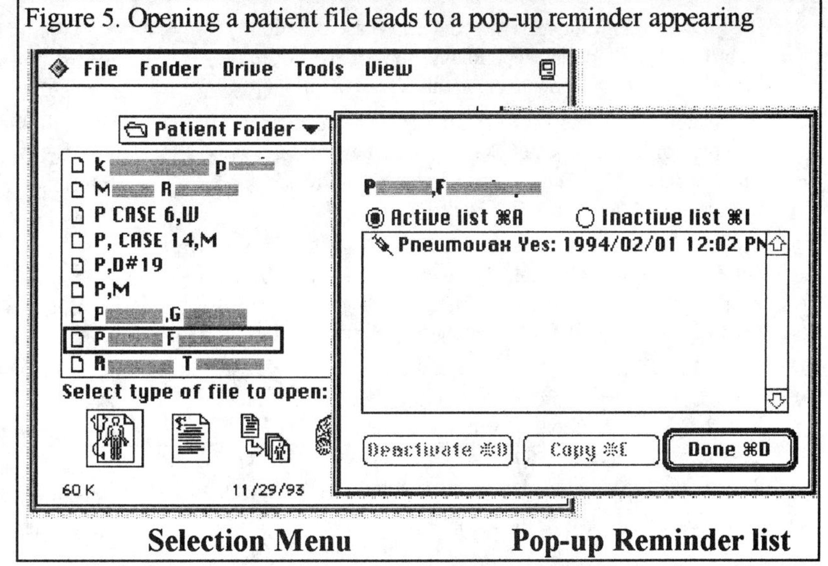

of a Medical Informatics expert and some assistance it would be possible to get a system up and running in a short time. Data content is the critical element of a computer-based patient record, it must have clinical relevance. The EDS approach is currently gaining acceptance. The data set provides the knowledge base and design foundation for IMR [Intelligent Medical Record] a CPR system used in clinical training of medical students at Norwalk Hospital. Medical Informatics, as an applied science to strengthen the infrastructure in its research must address problems 'inside medicine' [21].

CONCLUSION

The Essential data set approach is a method to define the contents of a computer-based patient record. The participation of clinical experts is essential to make the system responsive to clinical decision making needs. In the new systems architecture, with a client-server database; with the EDS defined for each clinical domain a hospital wide patient record system could be developed. The shared data elements would provide the foundation for horizontal logical integration.

***Acknowledgment**: The authors wish to thank JAM Software for providing the Medical Electronic Desktop for the project and the Pulmonary Fellows for being patient and cooperative.*

Reference

1. AR. Tarlov, JE. Ware, S. Greenfield, et.al.. The Medical outcomes study. JAMA. 1989. 262; 925 - 930.
2. K. Moidu, O. Wigertz. Computer based information systems in primary health care— Why? J Med Systems 1989; 13; 2: 59-65.
3. R.S. Dick, EB. Steen. The computer-based patient record - An essential technology for Health Care. Washington, D.C. National Academy Press, 1991.
4. K. Moidu, J. Falsone, S. Nair, et.al.. Informatics support for primary care COPD outcomes research. Proceedings of Third Primary Care Research Conference, Atlanta, GA. 1993. pp:79.
5. MG. Walker, RL. Blum. Towards Automated Discovery from Clinical Databases: The RADIX Project; In Eds. Salmon, R., Blum, B., Jorgensen, M. Proc. of MEDINFO 86, Washington. North-Holland, 1986, 32 -36.
6. SI. Chowdhury. Computer-based support for knowledge extraction from clinical databases. Linköping studies in science & tech, Dissertation No 240. Sweden, Linköping University. 1990.
7. AR. Feinstein . Clinical Judgment Revisited: The Distraction of Quantitative Models. Ann Intern Med. 1994; 120: 799-805.
8. WM. Boon. Data-entry support for better registration of the computer-based medical record. In eds. Barber B, Cao D, Qin D, Wagner G. Proc. of MEDINFO 89. 1989, 2: 737 - 740.
9. MR. Dambro, BD. Weiss, CL. McClure, AF. Vuturo. An unsuccessful experience with computerized medical records in an academic medical center. J Med. Edu. 1988; 63: 617-623.
10. LL. Weed. Medical Records, medical education, and patient: The problem oriented record as a basic tool. Cleveland. Case Western Reserve Press. 1971.
11. G. Murphy. Task Chair for ASTM standard 1384-91. Standard guide for description for content and structure of an automated primary record of care. Draft Circulated. 1993
12. MS. Blois. What is it that computers compute? MD Comput 1987; 4(3):30-33.
13. OB. Wigertz. Medical Data the subject matter of medical computing. Methods of Information in Medicine (Special Issue) 1988: 3-10.
14. BL. Humphreys, DAB. Lindberg The Unified Medical Language System Project: A distributed experiment in improving access to biomedical information. In: Lun KC, Degoulet P, Piemme T, Rienhoff O (eds). Proc. of MEDINFO 92. North-Holland. 1992; 2: 1496-1500.
15. National Association of Health Data Organizations. Fostering Uniformity for Health Care Assessment Data Gathering. (Final Report) Washington DC., National Association of Health Data Organizations. 1989.
16. World Health Organization. Priority research for health for all. European Health for All Series No 3. Copenhagen, European Regional Office, World Health Organization, 1988.
17. K. Moidu, AK. Singh, K. Boström, et.al. Towards an essential data set: applicability in the domain of maternal health services. Methods Inf Med 1992; 31(3):182-92.
18. K. Moidu. Application of an essential data set based computer system in support of maternal health services. International Journal of Bio-medical Computing 1992 (31) 3,4 : 159 -175.
19. Sundgren B. Conceptual Design of Data Bases and Information Systems. Lecture Notes. Sweden, Linköping, Dep. Computer and Information Science. 1984.
20. K. Moidu, AK. Singh, K. Boström, et.al. MCHS: An Application software for family welfare programmes. Medical Informatics. 1992. 17; 4: 279-291.
21. Nayemi-Rad F, Trace D, Moidu K, Carmony L, Booden, T. Applied Medical Informatics: Informatics in Medical Education. TIHM. 1994. 14 (4): 40-50.
22. PL. Reichertz. Preparing For Change: Concepts And Education In Medical Informatics. Comput Methods Programs Biomed 1987;25(2):89-101.

Making Standards Work for Sharing Patient Data

A Proposal for a National Health Care Identifier

Barry R. Hieb, M.D., Digital Equipment Corporation
representing ASTM E31.12

ABSTRACT

This paper describes a proposed standard for the creation of a national health care identifier being developed under the auspices of the ASTM. The standard includes the desired properties of such an identifier and a description of existing identifier schemes. It includes a proposed identifier scheme, descriptions of how the proposed scheme would function, and an evaluation of how well the proposed scheme meets the properties outlined in the standards document. This paper provides a partial summary of the material contained in the proposed standard.

INTRODUCTION

The establishment of a robust national identifier to meet the needs of health care has been a longstanding goal of the United States medical establishment. Earlier studies have explored the possibilities and limitations of record linkage without the use of a unique identifier (1). The identifier issue has been brought into sharper focus as the implications of the Computer-Based Patient Record are considered (2). Much of the debate on the identifier topic has focused on the merits and deficiencies of using the Social Security Number (3) as the identifier since it is frequently viewed as the only viable candidate for such a function. This article will describe an alternative candidate - the Universal Healthcare IDentifier (UHID.) The UHID is the result of a 2 year standards development process by ASTM committee E31.12 on medical informatics chaired by Dr. Elmer Gabrieli. During the summer of 1994 the standard is undergoing balloting for acceptance as a formal standard (4).

PURPOSE

The purpose of this article is to describe the proposed standard and identify some of its features and benefits. For purposes of accuracy and clarity much of this article will consist of ***selective quotes in italics*** of portions of the proposed standard. The UHID standard consists of three parts. The initial part defines the properties which a candidate national health care identifier must possess in order to meet the needs of health care in the United States. The second part contains descriptions of some of the existing identifier schemes. The third part defines a recommended implementation of a UHID and provides an evaluation of how adequately it meets the criteria defined in the inital part of the document.

FUNCTIONS

The proposed standard establishes four basic functions which a candidate national health identifier should meet:

This guide sets forth the fundamental considerations for an UHID that can effectively support at least four basic functions:

(1) positive identification of patients when clinical care is rendered;

(2) automated linkage of various computer-based records on the same patient for the creation of lifelong electronic healthcare files;

(3) providing a mechanism to support data security for the protection of privileged clinical information;

(4) enable the use of technology for patient records handling to keep health care operating costs at a minimum.

The proposed standard then goes on to define thirty criteria that describe more detailed requirements for any candidate identifier. Each criterion is given as a titled entry which describes that requirement. Included below are selected entries from the list of criteria contained in the proposed standard.

6-3 Atomic

A UHID should be a single data item. It should not contain subelements which have meaning outside of the context of the entire UHID. Nor should the UHID consist of multiple items which must be taken together to constitute an identifier.

This criterion implies that a collection of data items (e.g. name, date of birth, mother's maiden name) does not qualify as an identifier.

6-5 Content-free

The UHID should not depend on possibly changing or possibly unknown information pertaining to the person.[1]

6-7 Cost-effective

The UHID system chosen should achieve maximum functionality while minimizing the investment required to create and maintain it.

6-9 Disidentifiable

It should be possible to create an arbitrary number of UHIDs which can be used to link medical information concerning specific individuals but which cannot be used to identify the associated individual. These are Encrypted Universal Health Care Identifiers (EUHIDs). EUHIDs should, with the exception of disidentification, have all of the properties attributable to UHIDs including verification (cf. section 6-30, page 12). It should be clear to all users whether a specific identifier represents a UHID or an EUHID. The EUHID scheme should be capable of generating a large number (at least hundreds) of EUHIDs for a single individual.

An EUHID creates an alias which can be used to link information without identifying the corresponding individual[2]. The need for multiple EUHIDs arises from the wide variety of anticipated uses for disidentification and the inability to reconcile conflicting operational requirements between these various uses.

6-10 Focused

The UHID should be created and maintained solely for the purpose of supporting health care. Its form, usage, and policies should not be influenced by the needs or requirements of other activities.

6-12 Identifiable

It must be possible to identify the person associated with a valid UHID. Identifying information may include such standard items as name, birthdate, sex, address, mother's maiden name, etc. This information is not incorporated in the UHID but is associated with it by linkages.

6-19 Permanent

A UHID, once assigned, remains with that individual. It is never reassigned to another person even after the individual's death.

6-27 Unique

A valid UHID or EUHID identifies one and only one person. A person should have only one UHID. (Note that for purposes of disidentification a person may have an arbitrary number EUHIDs as defined in section 3-11, cf. page 4.)

6-30 Verifiable

A user should be able to determine that a candidate identifier is or is not a valid UHID without requiring additional information. This should support the ability to detect accidental misinformation such as typographical errors. It is not meant to be able to preclude intentional misinformation.

A UHID should have a mechanism - such as check digits - to enable the user to perform a consistency check to ensure that the identifier is valid.

After listing the criteria for an identifier as partially outlined above the standard goes on to discuss several topics that are related to the identifier. The first of these sections discusses the need for Temporary Patient Identifiers to be used when a UHID is not available. This is followed by a discussion on encrypted identifiers (EUHIDs.) EUHIDs are the method whereby the identification scheme supports the disidentification requirement listed in 6-9.

. . . . Essentially an EUHID creates an alias which can be used to link various information items without knowing whose information is being linked. It is generally assumed that such an alias would be used for ordering a single patient care episode, e.g. a sin-

[1]*Including content in the UHID makes it impossible to assign the "correct" identifier if that information is not known. It also leads to invalid situations if the information changes: e.g., what happens to an identifier based on gender if the person has a sex-change procedure?*

[2]Note that the standard spells out the requirements for disidentification but does not attempt to determine the policies and procedures under which such disidentification capability will be used.

gle hospitalization, or a single procedure such as a sensitive laboratory test. As a result, the system must be capable of creating multiple (hundreds or more) EUHIDs to cover potentially large numbers of care episodes for a given individual. . . .

Since EUHIDs are used to provide disidentified patient information linkage it is important that they not contain content relating to the individual. Items such as sex, birthdate, names, etc. must be excluded from EUHIDs to prevent compromising their disidentification function.

An EUHID must be revealable in order to serve its linkage function. Thus, it should be possible to print it on reports, store it in databases, etc. in a manner analogous to a person's UHID without compromising its disidentification function.

[Two examples of possible EUHID use may be helpful. A hospital wishes to order a sensitive test (e.g. HIV) on a patient. The institution obtains an EUHID for the patient and uses it to label the sample. When the results are obtained the institution can then take appropriate action to link the result to the patient depending on the results of the test and the applicable rules and regulations.

In the second example a researcher wishes to obtain a blinded patient population for research. She provides the number of patients needed and the type of information needed on each patient to an authorized health care information agency. The agency gathers the needed information on each patient and links it using an EUHID. The disidentified information is then provided to the researcher for use. If at some later date the information needs to be unblinded this can be done by provinding a link between each EUHID and the corresponding UHID.]

The proposed standard concludes by listing some of the policy decisions which will be required in order to implement a national identification scheme. It is noted that these policy decisions - while essential to the implementation of any national identificaion system - are beyond the scope of the ASTM standards effort.

Two appendices are attached to the proposed standard. The first appendix describes some of the existing identifier systems in use in the United States and Europe. Identifiers reviewed in this section include the Social Security Number, the Swedish "Personal Identity Number", the Danish personal identifier, and the identifier used in Finland. A novel scheme based on geographic information is also included (5).

PROPOSED IDENTIFIER SCHEME

The second appendix to the proposed national identifier standard outlines a candidate implementation scheme. It begins by describing the nature and structure of the proposed identifier. Figure 1 provides an overview of the structure of this proposed identifier. It consists of a 16 digit Sequential Identifier (SI), a single character delimiter, 6 check digits, and 6 encryption digits. The SI provides a unique number for each individual. The delimiter marks the boundary between the SI and the check digits. The check digits implement an error detection scheme which is able to ensure the validity of the UHID to a certainty level of one part in one million. The encryption digits provide the ability to create up to one million EUHIDs for each person. As shown in Figure 1, a full identifier constitutes 29 digits but leading and trailing zeroes may be truncated to provide a compact identifier which would typically be on the order of 16 or 17 digits.

Appendix 2 of the proposed standard goes on to briefly describe each of the subcomponents of the UHID and provide usage examples showing how the proposed identifier would be used to support three typical activities: assigning a UHID to a person, generating an EUHID, and decrypting an EUHID,

The proposed UHID uses check digits to support the verification requirement stated above in section 6-30. The next section of the appendix discusses how these check digits are computed for both UHIDs and EUHIDs. Tables needed for this computation are included. The final section of appendix 2 contains a preliminary evaluation (by one of the authors) of the candidate identifier against the 30 criteria listed in section 1 of the document. Each criterion is evaluated on the following scale:

1 - not supported
2 - minimally supported
3 - inadequately supported
4 - adequately supported
5 - fully supported
X - cannot be rated

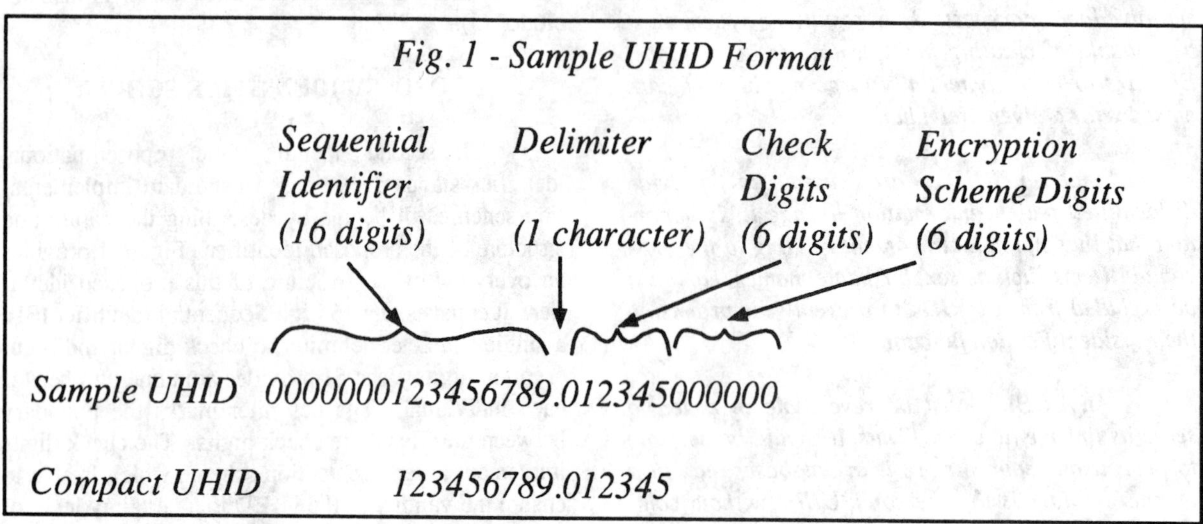

Fig. 1 - Sample UHID Format

The summary of this evaluation is provided in the following table.

UHID EVALUATION SUMMARY

Evaluation Category	*Number of Criteria*
1	*0*
2	*0*
3	*2*
4	*5*
5	*18*
X	*5*

From this evaluation it can be seen that the proposed scheme appears to adequately meet all but two of the criteria listed in the standard. The two criteria which were deemed to be inadequately supported were cost (because creation of a new UHID system would likely require a significant financial investment) and the limited ability to "split" an identifier which has inadvertently been assigned to two individuals.

CONCLUSION

The debate concerning the future of health care in the United States makes the present time particularly appropriate for an evaluation of the need for a national health care identifier. Most discussion on this topic to date has been focused on the merits and demerits of the use of the Social Security Number, largely because of the lack of any viable alternative.

Many disadvantages of the SSN have been identified. However, it has the perceived advantages of cost-effectiveness and rapid implementation. The UHID scheme discussed in this proposed standard provides the opportunity to open a debate on the question of whether it is feasible to create a more functional identifier in a timely and cost-effective manner.

REFERENCES

1. Newcombe, Howard B.: Handbook of Record Linkage; Oxford University Press, Oxford, England, 1988.

2. Health Data in the Information Age Use, Disclosure, & Privacy. Molla S. Donaldson & Kathleen N. Lohr, editors, Committee on Regional Health Data Networks, Division of Health Care Services, Institute of Medicine, Washington, D.C., National Academy Press, 1994.

3. Federal Register, November, 1922, The Social Security Number, policy and general procedures.

4. ASTM: Guide for the Properties of A Universal Healthcare Identifier. (Proposed standard in balloting process. To obtain a copy contact Dr. Elmer Gabrieli, CBML, 4 Cambridge Center, Cambridge, Mass. 02139)

5. Carpenter, Paul and Chute, Christopher: The Universal Patient identifier: A Discussion and Proposal, Proceeding of the 17th Annual Symposium on Computer Applications in Medical Care, p. 49-53, 1994.

A standardized message for supporting Shared Care

Peter J. Branger[1,2], Aleksander van 't Hooft[1], Joop S. Duisterhout[1], Johan van der Lei[1]

1. Department of Medical Informatics
2. Department of General Practice
Erasmus University,
P.O. Box 1738, 3000 DR Rotterdam
The Netherlands

ABSTRACT

As health care becomes more complex, interest in the benefits of coordination of care has increased. Especially patients that are being treated jointly by more than one physician (shared care), are vulnerable to adverse effects resulting from inadequate coordination and communication. We describe a study in which care providers support shared care by using computer-based patient records for data storage, and structured electronic data interchange as a means of communication. In this study, we are aiming at the development and implementation of protocols for shared care.

1. INTRODUCTION

Shared care is a situation in which physicians jointly treat the same patient. Patients requiring shared care are, for example, patients suffering from chronic disorders, such as diabetes mellitus, obstructive pulmonary diseases, and cardiological disorders. To be effective, shared care requires coordination of activities. Fletcher states that: "*When many different providers are involved in a patient's care, it is possible that the process will not be integrated into a meaningful whole; such care is subject to failures of communication*" [1].

For a number of health problems, shared care protocols have been developed, involving allocation of tasks between health care providers from different disciplines [2]. Optimal communication is considered to be a vital aspect of shared care, both from medical and cost effectiveness points of view [3]. Previous studies, however, have indicated that paper-based information exchange between care providers needs to be improved, both in terms of content of information exchange [4] and in timely deliverance of this information [5,6].

Nowadays, new technologies are emerging that have considerable potential for supporting physicians in delivering shared care. Computer-based patient records, which in recent years have penetrated Dutch health care, are gradually replacing paper records: physicians themselves use these systems to store textual data during consultations. In addition to recording medical data, computer-based patient records also assist the physician in monitoring risk profiles, screening of patients, and conducting follow-up [7]. These systems are able to exchange information using computer-to-computer communication. This communication is known as Electronic Data Interchange (EDI), and is defined as "*the replacement of paper documents by standard electronic messages conveyed from one computer to another without manual intervention*" [8]. In the Netherlands general practitioners judged the use of EDI favorably for medical care [9].

Current EDI implementations, however, focus on small segments of the medical record. An example of such an implementation is the laboratory test report, with which laboratories can transfer test results electronically to general practitioners. To support shared care, not only limited subsets of the medical record may have to be transferred, but the whole medical record, including the structure of it.

In this paper we describe the implementation of a procedure for EDI-based communication between physicians jointly treating diabetes mellitus patients. We also describe the evaluation study that we are presently performing.

2. DESIGN CONSIDERATIONS

In this section we describe the present state of computer-based patient records in the Netherlands, message syntax standards used, and the user interface requirements of the EDI message handler.

2.1 Patient Records

In the Netherlands, several computer-based patient record systems, designed using specifications formulated by professional organisations of general practitioners, are available [7]. These systems allow the general practitioner to replace the paper patient record with a computer-based patient record. The overall structure of such a computer-based patient record supports problem-oriented and episode-oriented recording of information, and SOAP coding [10,11]. Using SOAP-coding, the physician divides the information in Subjective information (the complaint of the patient), Objective information (findings like blood pressure), Assessment by the physician, and Plan (e.g. medication or referral). Using that overall structure, the physician may code detailed content of the patient record, such as reasons for encounter, diagnoses, medication, referrals, laboratory tests, and risk factors. The physician uses the system during patient consultations to inspect and record clinical data.

2.2 Message Standards

Several message standards are available for electronic communication. The HL7 standard, used for example in the United States, provides common data segment and message definitions, for communication across various systems within hospitals [12]. In Europe, the ISO syntax standard EDIFACT has been adopted as the standard for defining messages [13]; each message consists of a number of segments. Each segment starts with a segment tag (e.g. UNH), contains a number of data-elements, and ends with an apostrophe. Segments that logically belong together may be grouped and thus form a segment group. Data elements, segments, and segment groups may be conditional or mandatory.

In The Netherlands, coordination of the standardization of health care messages is performed by a national organization. At present, several standardized messages are available for a variety of purposes. One is a message for data exchange between physicians [14]; in this message, however, only physician-, patient- and hospital identifying data are structured, and all medical data is transferred as free text. Consequently, using this message, the receiving system is unable to integrate the data into the computer-based patient record. In order to support shared care, a message is needed that can also transfer the structure of the data in a computer-based record in order to allow integration of records from multiple sources.

2.3 User Interface Requirements

With EDI, messages can, in principle, be sent and received without human intervention. For patient-related communication, however, the physician has to match incoming messages with the patients in his practice, because in the Netherlands there does not exist a unique patient-identifying number. The computer-based patient record assists the physician by matching patient-identifying data (e.g. name, date of birth, gender) in an incoming message with known patient records; verification of the proposed match is subsequently performed by the physician.

In addition, fully automated data exchange is not desirable for several other reasons. First, in order to prevent an excessive growth of the amount of data in the computer-based patient record, the receiving physician needs to be able to select data from the message that can be discarded. Second, when composing a message, the sending physician may want to exclude from a message information that he considers to be irrelevant for the receiving physician, or a threat to the privacy of the patient involved.

3. IMPLEMENTATION

As discussed in section 2.2, currently available messages do not allow transferral of structured data. Therefore, we developed a new message, called MEDEUR, using the EDIFACT standard and already existing segment definitions. In this section we describe the structure of MEDEUR and the implementation of this message in the computer-based patient record system Elias.

3.1 MEDEUR message standard

MEDEUR, is designed for integrated patient data exchange between computer-based patient records. The message can contain both administrative and medical data. It can be used for transmission of a complete medical record, or sections of it. Table 1 shows the sequence number of the different segment groups (first column), whether it is mandatory or conditional (second column) and a short description of contents (third column). In total, 12 segment groups can be distinguished:

Segment group 1 contains identification (such as name, address, i.d. number) of sending physician (first occurrence) and receiving physician (second occurrence).

Segment group 2 contains identification (such as name, address, i.d. number, insurance data) of the patient involved (first occurrence). If required,

Table 1 - Contents of MEDEUR message

Segment group	Mandatory / Conditional	Description
1	M	Physician identification
2	M	Patient identification
3	C	General medical characteristics: sequence number
.. 4	C	.. Description
.. 5	C	.. Procedures planned
6	C	Patient encounter information - Type (e.g. consultation) - Date and time
.. 7	C	.. Free text lines
.. 8	C	.. Measurements (coded)
.. 9	C	.. Diagnoses (coded)
.. 10	C	.. Medication (coded)
.. 11	C	.. referrals (coded)
12	M	Authentication data

identification of persons related to the patient can be included in the next occurrence(s) of segment group 2.

Segment groups 3, 4, and 5 contain general medical characteristics of the patient, such as risk factors (e.g. smoking), and medical problems (e.g. diabetes mellitus). It also specifies the procedures planned by the physician in relation to the risk factors or medical problems (e.g. kidney function checkup in case of a diabetic patient). Every medical characteristic has a sequence number, described in segment group 3: segment groups 4 and 5 are nested within group 3 and describe the medical characteristic. The description may be coded, in which case also the identification of the code list used (e.g. ICPC or ICD-9) is included.

Segment group 6 contains the patient-encounter-oriented medical data. It specifies type of encounter (consultation, home visit, medical procedure), date and time of the encounter, and identifies (if needed) the physician involved in the encounter. The message contains one occurrence of segment group 6 for every patient encounter: each message may contain descriptions of up to 99 encounters. Segment groups 7 to 11 are nested within segment group 6: The data in these segment groups can be linked to a specific problem, already specified in segment group 3.

Segment group 7 contains that part of the data from the consultation that is in free text format.

Segment group 8 contains measurements that were performed (e.g. blood pressure, cholesterol etc.). Measurements may be specified with a code and the name of the code list used. Other data items include the date that the test was performed or the date that the test result became available, the result of the test, the unit, and the normal value range.

Segment group 9 contains diagnoses: these diagnoses may be coded, and the code list used (e.g. ICPC or ICD-9) can be specified.

Segment group 10 contains details about the medication prescribed by the physician during the consultation. It specifies identification of the medication (if desired coded according to e.g. brand name or chemical components), amount, dosage, for which diagnosis it was prescribed, and the specialism of the prescriber.

Segment group 11 contains details about other specialisms that the patient has been referred to, and data about outcomes of these referrals.

Segment group 12 contains information that can be used for authentication procedures.

```
<1>   UNB+UNOA:1+500011774+500003170+940731:2127+1
      08E'UNH+2100+MEDEUR:1:1:IT'BGM+UPD'DTM+13
      7+1994:07:24'NAD+EMP+123456+Dr. Sending'
      NAD+EMP+654321+Dr. Receiving'PNA+PAT+999999+
      Patient name'
<2>   SEQ+P+1'DTM+194+1989:10:22'CIN+DI+T90.1+ICP++
      Insulin dependent Diabetes Mellitus'
      SEQ+P+2'DTM+194+1991:03:27'CIN+DI+K86.0+ICP++
      Primary hypertension'
<3>   GIS+C'DTM+007+1994:08:08'INV+LM+102:LOC:Gluco
      se'RFF+G3:1'RSL+N+17.2+mmol/l'RNG+NRM+:3.5:4.5
      'DLI+O+0'CLI+MED+13617893:KMP::Ins mixt 10/90
      novolet 3M'RFF+G3:1'DLI+P+0'CLI+MED+13180789:
      KMP::Capoten 25MG Tablet'RFF+G3:2'DLI+P+0'
<4>   AUT+1234+4321'UNT+2100+27'
```

Figure 1 - Simplified example of a MEDEUR message, describing a patient consultation. The message can be divided into four parts: **part <1>** contains E-mail numbers (UNB), name and i.d. number of sender (NAD, first occurrence) and receiver (NAD, second occurrence), and patient and i.d. number (PNA); **part <2>** Contains problems the patient is suffering from, with a sequence number (SEQ), starting date (DTM), ICPC code, and a description (CIN); **part <3>** contains the data gathered during the consultation, such as lab tests (INV), the problem the test relates to (RFF, in this case to diabetes mellitus), the test result (RSL), and the normal value range (RNG); prescribed medication (CLI), the problem the medication relates to (insulin for the diabetes, and capoten for the high blood pressure); **part <4>** contains the authentication data and the message trailer.

Where possible, the use of code lists is supported: diagnoses, referrals, measurements, reason for encounter, and medication can be coded. In addition to this coded data, there is ample space to include free text. This free text can be used for data that cannot be placed in dedicated segments, or for additional data that is collected for research purposes. Figure 1 gives an example of a MEDEUR message.

3.2 MEDEUR Message handler

The computer-based patient record system Elias already contains a communication module that allows it to exchange EDIFACT messages with other information systems, via telephone lines and e-mail services [9]. We designed a user interface that enables the physician to send and receive MEDEUR messages.

To send a MEDEUR message, the physician first specifies the patient and the period about which he wants to report. Elias then creates a MEDEUR message, based on the information stored in the computer-based patient record. The physician can, before the message is actually sent, edit the message by specifying what data to discard, and add text to the message.

The patient data in received MEDEUR messages can be stored directly into the computer-based patient record, with exactly the same structure as that of the patient record the data came from. Prior to storing the data, the physician can select and subsequently discard the data from the received message he considers to be irrelevant.

4. PRESENT STATE

To evaluate the benefits of EDI for the support of shared care, we are conducting studies in which general practitioners and internal medicine consultants share data about patients with diabetes mellitus.

In the Netherlands the general practitioner functions as a gatekeeper between primary and secondary care. Typically, patients first consult their general practitioner. If considered necessary, the general practitioner refers the patient to a specialist. The specialist will report the results of the treatment back to the general practitioner. Therefore, the general practitioner is the central physician and the ideal person to coordinate shared care.

In a number of Dutch cities, we are introducing electronic communication between physicians. In the city of Apeldoorn, 64 general practitioners provide care for approximately 120,000 persons. Of these 64 general practitioners, 40 use the computer-based patient record system Elias. Apeldoorn has one hospital, with 10 internal medicine consultants. Two of these consultants provide medical care for 80% of all diabetics referred to the outpatient clinic. An electronic communication network is available, and is already used by physicians to transmit data, such as laboratory reports and admission/discharge reports [9].

We installed the MEDEUR message handler at the practices of 25 general practitioners. At the outpatient clinic of one of the two diabetes mellitus treating consultants, we installed an Elias system, tailored to the information needs of that consultant, and the MEDEUR message handler. Starting January 1994, this consultant and the 25 general practitioners exchange data about consultation outcomes, using MEDEUR messages. Code lists are used for coding reasons for encounter, measurements, diagnoses, referrals, and medication.

Using the implemented inter-physician communication, we are conducting studies to evaluate the benefits of EDI for shared care; these studies consist of two phases.

Phase 1: Prior to the intervention, we study 260 (randomly selected) medical records of diabetes mellitus patients that both treated by general practitioner and internal medicine consultant. We evaluated (1) the type of information routinely collected; and (2) communication frequency with the co-treating physician. Furthermore, we investigated patterns in laboratory test ordering and medication prescribing of general practitioner and consultant.

Phase 2: Starting after the introduction of the MEDEUR message handler, we receive a copy of each transmitted MEDEUR message. This copy does not contain patient or physician identifying data. From these message flow measurements we can deduct (1) which information is routinely collected by the physician; (2) which information is considered relevant for the receiving physician; (3) which information from a received message is considered relevant by the physician.

The results of these studies may lead to the definition of a communication protocol between primary and secondary care providers, specifying frequency and content of communication.

5. DISCUSSION

Computer-based patient records, installed in general practices and used during consultations, have become a widely accepted component in the Dutch health care process [9]. These systems are able to assist the physician with recording medical data in a structured manner.

Using computer-based patient records and EDI, we have created an environment which enables the efficient exchange of information [9]. Moreover, using the standard message MEDEUR, it is possible to exchange patient information between computer-based patient records in such a manner, that the semantic structure of the information can be rebuilt in the receiving system. By doing this, physicians can share the information about patients that are jointly treated.

Previous studies have shown that existing paper-based communication is insufficient [4-6]. With the introduction of computer-based patient records and EDI, the opportunity to exchange <u>all</u> patient data is available. This could, however, lead to an information overload, especially when different care providers fail to agree on their role in the delivery of care and the information requirements of that role.

In the Netherlands, at present, no protocols exist that explicitly specify the role of co-treating physicians. Ideally, such a protocol should include a description of (1) the division of tasks; (2) guidelines for record-keeping; (3) guidelines for communication, both in terms of frequency, content, and a definition of consultation outcomes that should trigger communication activities. The use of these protocols should not only prevent medication conflicts and duplication of diagnostic tests, but should also guarantee that necessary procedures (like yearly checkup of the kidney function in diabetic patients) are being performed. We expect that EDI will facilitate the development of shared care protocols. Future studies will have to evaluate the impact of EDI and shared care protocols on the delivery of care.

6. References

1. Fletcher RH, O'Malley MS, Fletcher SW, Earp JAL, Alexander JP. Measuring the continuity and coordination of medical care in a system involving multiple providers. *Medical Care* 1984;**22**:403-1
2. Powell J. Shared-care. *Practitioner* 1991;**235**:761-2
3. Constantino M, Hoskins PL, Fowler PM, Pech C, McFarlane R, Flack JR, Forrest J, Yue DK, Turtle JR. Interaction between diabetic patients, their general practitioners and a hospital diabetic clinic. *Med J Aus* 1991;**155**:515-8
4. Hull FM, Westerman RF. Referral to medical outpatients departments at teaching hospitals in Birmingham and Amsterdam. *BMJ* 1986;**293**:311-4
5. Williams EI, Fitton F. General practitioner response to elderly patients discharged from hospital. *BMJ* 1990;**300**:159-61
6. Mageean RJ. Study of "discharge communications" from hospital. *BMJ* 1986;**293**:1283-5
7. Van der Lei J, Duisterhout JS, Westerhof HP, Van der Does E, Cromme PV, Boon WM, Van Bemmel JH. The introduction of computer-based patient records in the Netherlands. *Ann Intern Med* 1993;**119**:1036-41
8. Walker RJ. *First steps in EDI: Proceedings of COMPAT '89.* Munich: Blenheim Online, 1989.
9. Branger PJ, Van der Wouden JC, Schudel BR, Verboog E, Duisterhout JS, Van der Lei J, Van Bemmel JH. Electronic communication between providers of primary and secondary care. *BMJ* 1992;**305**:1068-70

10 Weed LL. Representation of medical knowledge in PROMIS. In: Blum BI, editor. *Computers and medicine: Information systems for patient care.* New York: Springer Verlag 1984:83-108

11. Weed LL. *Medical records, medical education, and patient care: The problem-oriented record as a basic tool.* Cleveland, Ohio: Press of Case Western Reserve 1971
12. Cahill BP, Holmen JR, Bartleson PL. Mayo foundation electronic results inquiry, the HL7 connection. In: Clayton PD, editor. *Fifteenth Annual Symposium on Computer Applications in Medical Care.*New York: McGraw-Hill 1993:516-520
13. ISO 9735. *Electronic Data Interchange for Administration, Commerce and Transport (EDIFACT) - Application Level Syntax Rules.* Geneva: United Nations Economic Commission for Europe - Trade Division, 1988.
14. Hasman A, Ament A, Arnou PC, Van Kesteren ACA. Inter-institutional information exchange in healthcare. *Int J Biomed Comput* 1992;**31**:5-16

This work is supported by the Dutch Ministry of Health (Grant I92061, Ministerie van WVC), ANOZ health-insurance corporation, the Dutch Association of General Practitioners (LHV), the Netherlands Asthma Foundation (Nederlands Astmafonds) and IMS Nederland bv.

The standard data model approach to patient record transfer

Kip Canfield, PhD, Marcelo Silva, BS
Laboratory for Healthcare Informatics
University of Maryland, UMBC

Kerry Petrucci, PhD CRNP
Department of Physiological Nursing
University of Washington, Seattle

ABSTRACT

This paper develops an approach to electronic data exchange of patient records from Ambulatory Encounter Systems (AESs). This approach assumes that the AES is based upon a standard data model. The data modeling standard used here is IDEF1X for Entity/Relationship (E/R) modeling. Each site that uses a relational database implementation of this standard data model (or a subset of it) can exchange very detailed patient data with other such sites using industry standard tools and without excessive programming efforts. This design is detailed below for a demonstration project between the research-oriented geriatric clinic at the Baltimore Veterans Affairs Medical Center (BVAMC) and the Laboratory for Healthcare Informatics (LHI) at the University of Maryland.

INTRODUCTION

Patient records exist to improve patient care, ease administrative and financial reporting, and allow research access to healthcare data. Computer-based patient records (CPR) have advantages in each of these areas. Electronic patient records are more accessible to providers and therefore can improve continuity of care [1]. Henrion [2] estimates that the cost savings from information technology would be 4 percent of the total health care costs by the year 2000. Cross-patient research access to patient records is prohibitively expensive except with database records. An important theoretical advantage and practical problem for CPR is transfer of patient record information over networks. This is needed for creation of research repositories, quality control for patient care and billing, and consultation by remote providers. Evaluation of this CPR transfer demonstration project supports the following propositions concerning the standard data model approach to patient record transfer and replication.

Proposition 1 - Information Density

The information density required in a well designed AES is only possible with some type of data model. This implies that transfer of a patient record should contain the data model information. A data model contains much implicit information about the enterprise. For example, in an E/R model that is meant to be implemented on a relational database management system (RDBMS), all of the relationship data is implicit in the foreign keys of the ultimate relational tables. This information would be difficult to code for transfer of a patient record without reference to the data model. An example of this relationship-oriented information would be a link between each physician order and the patient problem that it addresses. Such a link would allow audits of all resources expended for a specific problem.

Proposition 2 - Efficiency and Reliability

Industry standard tools already exist for certain data modeling techniques and relational database architectures and they offer an efficient way of enabling the implementation of the standard data model patient record transfer. The industry standards for IDEF1X data modeling [3] and RDBMSs have sufficient penetration that a rich set of interoperable, multivendor tools for CASE (Computer-Aided Software Engineering), scripting methods, and querying with a standard language such as Structured Query Language (SQL) are available. Examples of these tools are used in the demonstration project and evaluated.

Proposition 3 - Communications

Existing methods of communications on the Internet, such as e-mail and FTP are sufficient to implement the standard data model patient record transfer approach for complex text data. The use of industry standard database tools produce text script files that are easily compressed, encrypted, and transferred on the Internet. This allows developers to largely automate the routine tasks associated with patient record transfer without regard to vendor or platform.

Each of these propositions is argued to be supported by this patient record transfer demonstration project. The data model used documents an AES that is used for real patient data and is in regular use at the Baltimore site. The patient record transfers are real patient data that have been made anonymous for the purposes of this project. Each procedure described in the project methodology is tested in a realistic simulation and discussed below.

AES DATA MODEL DESIGN

This data model was developed for a CPR system named GERI at the BVAMC. The clinic has a defined workflow for placing volunteer research candidates into one of four research demonstration projects involving smoking cessation, exercise programs, nutrition, and stroke rehabilitation. The volunteer research candidates (hereafter referred to as patients) consist of veterans who have one or more cardiac risk factors and meet the criteria for one or more research protocols.

We chose a database development system from Gupta Technologies Inc. (the SQLWindows development system for the MSWindows client and the SQLBase Netware database server). This product is an RDBMS with client/server network connections.

The core of the GERI CPR is the care planning module, which is the clinical interface to the system. Figure 1 shows this interface. It allows clinicians and researchers from various disciplines to see all patient information. Dynamic views, order entry, and reporting are supported. The remainder of this section describes relevant portions of this interface in order to show the level of complexity in the transferred patient data.

Fig. 1. The Main GERI Window.

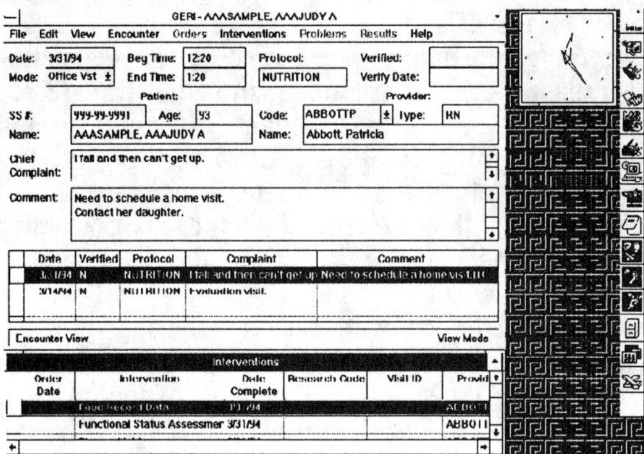

The CPR is encounter-based in that all displayed information is specific to the selected encounter. The separate table window *Interventions* at the bottom of the GERI window in Figure 1 lists all patient events for the selected encounter. Intervention is a broad term that is here used to describe any direct or indirect care or other documented event for a patient in an encounter. It includes the carrying out of typical orders, surveys, examinations, procedures, etc. For example, the patient had a functional status assessment on 3/31/94. The user can control the content of the bottom window in Figure 1. For example, the user can view current problems, or pending orders in that window instead of interventions.

An important feature of this care plan is the fact that all orders (or non-orders) are linked to problems (or a protocol) in the record [4]. This allows more detailed information for quality assurance, billing, and clinical research. "Accurate measures of resource consumption also constitute the bridge between the use of an AES [ambulatory encounter system] for traditional quality or payment purposes (or both) and the current push toward continuous quality improvement (CQI)." [5]

This interface is based on the simplified data model in Figure 2 (the actual data model has more than 20 entities and the data dictionary is a more complex multi-entity object). The data model that produced this interface revolves around the concept of a patient *encounter*. This is an encounter between a patient and a provider of some type.

The complex information contained in this data model is captured with the graphical user interface (described above) that allows linking of data elements and simultaneous data element browsing. This data complexity is captured economically in the data model. The argument for Proposition 1 is that the information density of this kind of patient information is possible to transfer with a standard model.

Fig. 2. The Simplified Data Model

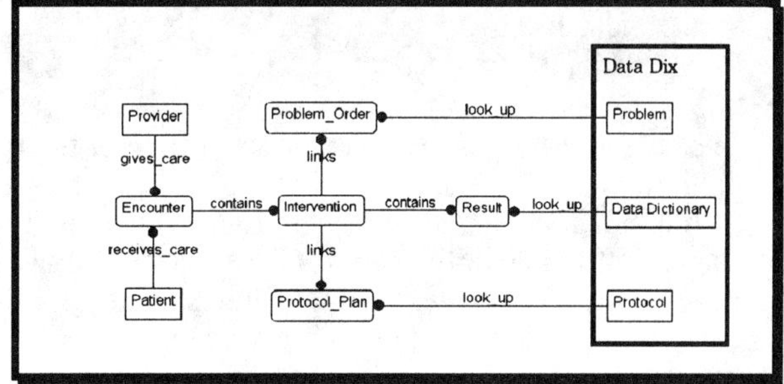

This case study shows the complex interrelated data elements required for AESs. Without a model, all assumptions about the relationships in the data would have to be contained in the transfer document and there may be an impedance mismatch with the target database. This section has shown that certain aspects of complex patient information such as the time-oriented, protocol-driven, and linked data of this case can be represented economically using the data model. The issue of economy of representation leads to Proposition 2 and is discussed below.

PROJECT METHODOLOGY

The methodology used in this project to transfer patient records between sites is dependent upon semi-standard SQL-based RDBMSs and a common portion of the data model described above. Simple programs unload patient data from the relational tables into text script files that can be run at the receiving site to update their database. This methodology requires a minimum of program development and user expertise, but relatively extensive standardization. It is our position that this standardization is worth the effort in order to reap the demonstrated benefits of information density, efficiency, and ease of communications. Whether such standardization is politically or logistically possible in the current healthcare information systems context is not in the scope of this paper, although it is now a key theme of healthcare informatics [6]. The transfer methodology has the following steps.

Sending Database Task Steps:

1. Extract patient information from each table of the sending database.
2. Create a text script file to update the receiving database.
3. Compress and encrypt the script file with a password.
4. Log the transaction.

Receiving Database Task Steps:

5. Uncompress and unencrypt the script file.
6. Run the script against the receiving database.
7. Log the transaction.

The database at each site must have a portion of their data model in common. Each site may have additional (non-shared) tables and additional (non-shared) attributes in the shared tables, but they must have a core of tables and attributes exactly in common. Because of this flexibility, the only real tool restriction with this shared model is the requirement of a RDBMS from any major vendor. The extraction program (Step 1) is very simple. Every table in the model is queried for any rows linked to a particular patient ID (and possibly in a particular date range). This requires a simple SQL query for each table in the model. All of this data is written to a single text file that becomes a SQL script for updating the receiving database. The script file (Step 2) is a sequence of SQL queries that are automatically run one after another. For example, the following 'insert' statement would be one of many in the script (one for each table in the shared model).

```
INSERT INTO SYSADM.PROBLEM
VALUES(:1,:2,:3,:4,:5,:6,:7,:8,:9,:10,:11)
\
5,"DIAM","",44,10002,1993-06-10,,"O",,,$long,
6,"ATH","",40,10002,1993-06-10,,"O",,,$long,
7,"ATH","",81,10022,1993-06-23,,"O",,,$long,
8,"STOC","",79,10002,1993-06-23,,"O",,,$long,
10,"STOC","",81,10022,1993-06-23,,"O",,,$long,
/
```

Note that this implementation of the 'insert' command supports bind variables. Each bind variable (such as ':1') corresponds by position with the comma separated block of text delimited with the forward and backward slashes. Every line of this text block is inserted as a record into the receiving table with this one SQL statement. This is a very non-standard feature across RDBMSs and would require the most development and coordination efforts. Imports, exports, and the SQL Data Definition Language (DDL) are the most non-standard elements of RDBMSs and SQL. Both sites in this demonstration project used Gupta's SQLBase database server and therefore did not deal with this standardization problem. This required development for multivendor interoperability is minor compared to methods that do not share a data model, common SQL Data Control Language (DCL), and relational database implementation.

The script resulting from these two steps is a (human-readable) text file that is sent by the sending site. The receiving site simply runs this script file against the database that is updated with the transferred patient(s') data. All linked information and referential integrity are preserved because the data model is replicated at each site. Compression and encryption of the script file (Step 3) can be performed with any applicable utility. The only requirement is that both the sending and receiving sites have the same program. Password access to the encrypted file secures the patient data to the limits of the encryption scheme and the security procedures of the provider sites. We used the shareware utilities PKZIP and PKUNZIP for this step. This utility may not be very secure and therefore not adequate for real operations, but it precisely demonstrates the concept. The sender's log file (Step 4) records any standard information that each site requires such as the identification of the sender and any notes relating to the transfer. This log may update a table on the senders database and a copy of this log is sent with the data to the receiver.

The receiving site must uncompress and unencrypt the script file (Step 5) and run the script against their database (Step 6). In the case of Gupta's RDBMS, Step 6 is accomplished simply by using a 'Run Script' option that sequentially executes any SQL statements in a script file. This utility is offered by many vendors and would be a relatively simple utility to add to any RDBMS. The sender's log file can automatically update the receiver's log table (Step 7), documenting the transaction.

A crucial factor in sharing patient data is a common data dictionary for healthcare terminology. This is a difficult problem and this methodology allows a relatively simple way to share a standard data dictionary between sites. Once a truly standard terminology is available, it could be substituted. Script files can be created with the same methodology as above to transfer the data dictionary information between sites. In this demonstration project, both sites use the same data dictionary.

Relational database schemas to create patient databases are also easily transferred as scripts in this same way. There are many data modeling CASE tools on the market that allow a developer to graphically define a data model and then automatically generate a SQL script that will create the tables and indexes for that model in a target RDBMS. Because of the non-standard nature of current DDLs, these tools typically generate a custom script for the RDBMSs of most major vendors.

DEMONSTRATION PROJECT RESULTS

This demonstration project was performed to test support for the last two of the three initial propositions. It is not a controlled experiment, but a proof of concept exercise. In order to test the methodology for efficiency, reliability, and ease of communication, we developed an application that implements the seven steps in the patient record transfer methodology. This application works within the GERI patient record application as a menu item. It performs the steps in the methodology in a way that requires minimal training of personnel already using GERI. The user initiates a patient record transfer in the context of a displayed patient record by choosing a menu item 'Transfer' under the 'File' menu and sees a dialog box where all transfer actions are performed.

The user specifies a script filename and emails a log note for the transfer. For this demonstration project, there was only one destination site and therefore that did not need to be specified. The transfer application creates and compresses the script file with a password, and the initiator sends this file (by FTP) to the receiving site. At the receiving site, the receiver uses a batch file to uncompresses the script and run it against the database. An email message from the sending site notifies responsible users of the transfer and sends the log information. An email message from the receiving site acknowledges the transfer.

The demonstration project tested this application of the transfer methodology with a one week trial. Real patient data (stripped of identifying information such as name and SSN) was sent from the BVAMC (sending site) to LHI (receiving site) over the Internet. A person (at each site) was responsible for sending the information from Baltimore and updating the database at LHI. These tasks required no knowledge of the database or the methodology other than that necessary to perform the duties. The person at the sending site received an email message asking to send a record for a particular patient. This person then enters GERI, opens that patient's record and uses the transfer application. The person at the receiving site opens the transfer application (outside of GERI in a SQL tool) and updates the database. This trial transferred only entire patient records (all records corresponding to one patient) and did not support specific date ranges.

The trial had 3 phases. The first phase transferred a script from the BVAMC to LHI that created the database. This step simulates setting up a database at a repository site, a consultant site, or remote site for a clinic. This was accomplished in one step with a script that created the tables, the indexes, and the stored commands. This task requires no database experience other than the knowledge of how to run the script. The second phase transferred a script that contained the data dictionary tables. This step simulates providing updates of the data dictionary for remote sites to keep all sites in synch. The third phase transferred 10 patient records between the BVAMC and LHI. This process was conducted over a week-long period. Email was used for notification and logging of each transaction. The first two transfers required phone support to complete the training. All of the remaining eight transfers were successful and required no additional support. This trial demonstrates that this methodology is logistically simple to implement and does not require large support resources.

DISCUSSION AND EVALUATION

Each of the propositions discussed in this paper assume that the patient record transfer methodology is driven by computer-based clinical automation techniques that integrate well into current database, communications, and CASE tool technologies. Techniques that do not integrate well with current technologies will not be adopted due to cost and scarcity of expertise. As database architectures and their tools change, the specific methodology, such as that given here, would also change, but the three propositions would stand. The following conclusions about the three initial propositions are supported by the demonstration project.

The demonstration project shows that complex patient data (data with relationships) can be transferred easily between environments with a common subset of a standard data model. This standard data model is a higher level standard than HL7 in the sense that HL7 is a standard for exchanging transaction-oriented messages between (possibly) heterogeneous systems, while the standard data model approach to patient record transfer is a systems-oriented standard that assumes more than a common terminology for transactions. It assumes standard relationships. The Joint Working Group for a Common Data Model has begun working on just these kinds of standards [7]. Their work can form a basis for this type of inter-site communications.

This study has assumed that this data model is implemented in an RDBMS but this is not a requirement. Other more general (than SQL) representation systems can and will be developed. For example, the SQL scripts can be wrapped in a language/protocol such as Knowledge Query and Manipulation Language (KQML) [8] to supply the transport and performatives for use on an internetwork using intelligent agents. The content language may change from SQL to KIF (Knowledge Interchange Format) for greater flexibility and generality, but the basic concepts of this study would remain.

The methodology described here is efficient because it offers integration with the user interface, uses existing standards, co-opts the work of vendors, and offers ease of development. These methods requires network resources that are available over the Internet or other private networks such as Community Health Information Networks (CHINs). Currently, stable technology and network infrastructure exist to support extensive patient care repositories for research, DSS, and education. They also have relevance to clinical care. For example, the methods described here are easily modified to produce executable single patient versions of the CPR that could be sent over the network as a self-contained CPRs to providers doing consults. The methodology is not, however, currently reliable because of known problems with TCP/IP transport and lack of a principled procedure for tracking the log files and other inter-site communications. The reliability of the Internet transport is now being aggressively addressed in research and commercial areas. The log file procedure to ensure database integrity is an area for future work.

The barriers to the benefits of these methods are also due to organizational issues and communications problems. It is a complex management challenge to deploy information systems in an organization. It is even more difficult for inter-organization standards to be agreed to and implemented. This paper has developed and tested a method for CPR transfer that is designed to soften these very difficult problems. We are planning a more extensive and realistic test of this methodology between the VAMCs at both Baltimore and Seattle.

Reference

[1]. McDonald, C.J. & Barnett, G.O. in Medical Informatics: Computer Applications in Health Care, eds. Shortliffe, E., et al., Addison-Wesley:Reading MA, 1990, pp. 181-218.

[2]. Henrion, M., Silva J., Cost Savings from Information Technology in the US Health Care Reform: Insights from Modeling, *Healthcare Information Management*, 8(1), 1994 pp. 23-28.

[3]. Bruce, T.A. Designing Quality Databases with IDEF1X Information Models, Dorset House:New York, NY, 1992.

[4]. Beeler, G., Gibbons, P., & Chute, C. Development of a Clinical Data Architecture. In M. Frisse (Ed.), 16th SCAMC, McGraw-Hill:Baltimore, 1992, pp. 244-248.

[5]. Goldfield, N. Ambulatory encounter systems: Implications for payment and quality. *J. Ambulatory Care Manage,* 16(2), 1993, pp. 33-49.

[6]. Hammond, W., McDonald, C., Beeler, G., Carlson, D., Barnett, L., Bidgood, D., & McDougall, M. Computer Standards: Their Future within Health Care Reform. In Proceedings of the 1994 Annual HIMSS Conference, Phoenix AZ, 1994.

[7]. Beeler, G. HISPP/MSDS Joint Working Group for a Common Data Model Report of Meeting Sept. 20-21, 1993.

[8]. Finin, T., et al. Specification of the KQML Agent-Communication Language. Technical Report EIT TR 92-04, Enterprise Integration Technologies, Palo Alto, CA, 1992.

Using a meta-model to build a Connection Service in an object oriented medical application development environment

François-Christophe Jean[1], Jean-Jacques Mascart[2], Alain Codaccioni[2], Marion Lavril[1], Dominique Sauquet[1] and Patrice Degoulet[1]

[1] Medical Informatics Department, Broussais University Hospital, Paris
[2] Centre de Traitement de l'Information Médicale des Armées, Paris

Interoperability is a key issue in distributed health information systems. This paper presents the design and implementation of the Connection Service (CS) component of the HELIOS medical software engineering environment. An exchange message meta-model based on CEN TC251 recommendations and a message description language are proposed. Using this meta-model, the CS is able either to interpret messages expressed in a given syntax (e.g., EDIFACT, ASTM) and map them to the application objects or to automate the translation of the messages in another syntax. It is concluded that this meta-model approach contributes to the management of semantic heterogeneity.

INTRODUCTION

Defining a hospital as a set of resources dedicated to the improvement of patients' health is generally widely accepted. These multiple resources, hosted by different entities (e.g., administrative units, clinical wards, laboratories, radiology departments) that may be scattered within the hospital buildings, need to communicate to serve the hospital role. In addition, the recent and rapid development of *telemedicine* imposes the easy connection of the hospital wards to various external medical information producers or consumers, which may dispose of dedicated and efficient computerized data management systems. In that context, the "classical" Hospital Information System (HIS) concept may be progressively replaced by the notion of Health Information Networks seen as logical aggregations of different entities that will cooperate in the processing of medical information. The underlying architecture of such systems needs to be open to provide the end-users with the ability to access the required information transparently whatever its nature or localization. Transparency may be provided by a virtual environment (e.g., a medical workstation [7]) that gives the user the illusion of working with a single application on a single machine (i.e., his station) whatever the complexity of the underlying hidden system. To be really transparent for the end-user, an open system must be based on a strong integration of its parts. Four integration axes are generally distinguished. *Presentation integration* ensures a common look and feel among the system components, *data integration* allows to share information elements, *control integration* coordinates the components interactions while *communication integration* allows distributed components to interact, generally through message passing. Obviously, communication among specialized information processing components is a prerequisite to any distributed information system. Unfortunately there exists, even in the single field of health care, an increasing range of "standards" dedicated to the transfer of medically relevant information [9][11]. These standards cover raw data exchanges (e.g., ADT messages or lab results coded using *ASTM, HL-7* or *EDIFACT* syntaxes) as well as "complex" information interchanges (e.g., image or medical instrumentation data transferred using *ACR-Nema/DICOM* or *MIB* protocols) [5]. The problem facing the distributed health information systems developers is then twofold: 1- how to integrate easily a component based on a given (new) standard (i.e., *syntax*) in a running framework to comply with the "plug and play" paradigm, 2- how to deal with *semantics* integration since heterogeneous systems will necessarily lead to heterogeneous semantics when seen from the communication integration point of view.

In this paper, the strategy developed within the HELIOS European project will be presented. A multi-syntax prototype will be described and a semantic integration perspective, related to applications development requirements, will be introduced.

MEDICAL EXCHANGES MODELING

In the described context, we were only concerned by a small subdomain of distributed systems interoperability: interaction between a medical application and several medical data servers (e.g., patient identity or lab results servers). In that restricted area, modeling the domain of exchanges reveals a high level that allows to define a meta-model to specify explicitly the semantic correspondences between different "worlds" as shown in figure 1.

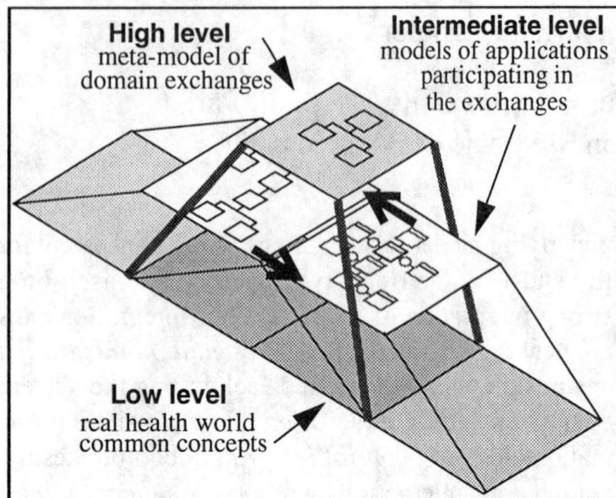

Figure 1 The meta-model of message exchange

Such an approach has been followed by the European normalization committee devoted to medical informatics (*CEN TC 251*). This authority proposes a methodology (described in [3]) that isolates a *"meta-syntax" level* allowing the separation of the structural and semantic definitions of the messages from their implementations (which are directed to particular syntaxes). The methodology is organized around three key points:

- The *Domain Information Models (*DIM*)* are object oriented conceptual models that specify the *subjects*, *classes* and *objects* (together with their *relations*) participating in information exchange and which represent common concepts in health care.
- The *General Message Descriptions (*GMD*)* are subsets of the DIMs identified by considering the objects (representing a selected amount of information) involved in an exchange *scenario*.
- The *scenarios* describe the interactions between the different communication parties for a given purpose (e.g., request for a service or report from a performed service).

The final step of the CEN methodology is the implementation of the different GMDs in one or several syntactic formats (e.g., ASTM E-1238, HL-7, EDIFACT, ASN.1). In the following paragraphs, we shall describe how, in the HELIOS project, the GMDs are used as foundations for a generic automaton dealing with the syntactic part of exchanges.

A META-SYNTAX IMPLEMENTATION IN THE HELIOS FRAMEWORK

HELIOS *Connection Services* design

HELIOS is an object oriented software engineering environment, dedicated to the realization of distributed multimedia medical applications [2]. The framework is constituted from several independent and cooperative software components, organized along the object-oriented paradigm, federated by a communication channel: the *HELIOS Unification Bus* (HUB) as shown in figure 2. Each component is specialized in the management of a particular aspect of medical applications, both at development and run times. Among the components plugged on the HUB, the *Connection Services* (CS) is responsible for the easy integration of applications, developed with the HELIOS framework in broader clinical information systems.

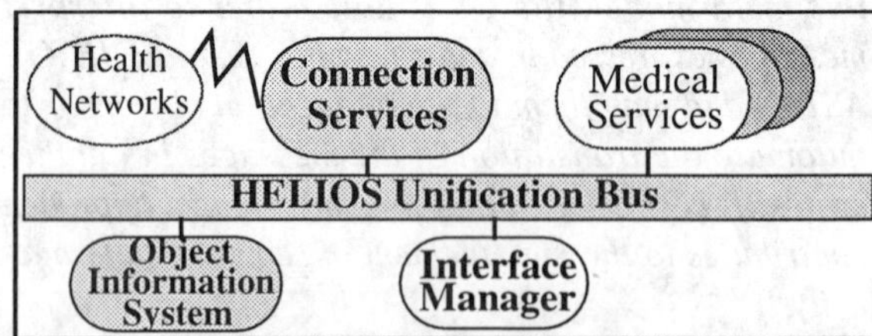

Figure 2 The HELIOS framework

As any HELIOS component, the CS must be seen from two points of view:

- At application development time it has to provide the developers with a ready-to-use (but flexible) set of communication tools. This set comprises the "connectors" to different message transportation protocols and the different syntax interpreters that a developer may use to connect his application with the desired "remote" service. However, as considered before, these tools are of no use without the ability to map the remote application semantics (conveyed by the received messages) to the one used in the application under development. To reach this goal, the CS works in close collaboration with the *Object Information System* (OIS) development database [6], which is the data and knowledge repository that manages the model of exchanges, records the required normalized nomenclatures and directs the scheme of application under development.
- At run time, the CS has to behave as a transparent gateway between the operational application and the remote service, interpreting the exchanged messages and affecting the relevant slots of the application objects with the message field values.

Functional description of the Connection Services

Figure 3 presents the logical organization of the CS component. It can be seen that it brings together functional modules that cover the different topics presented before.

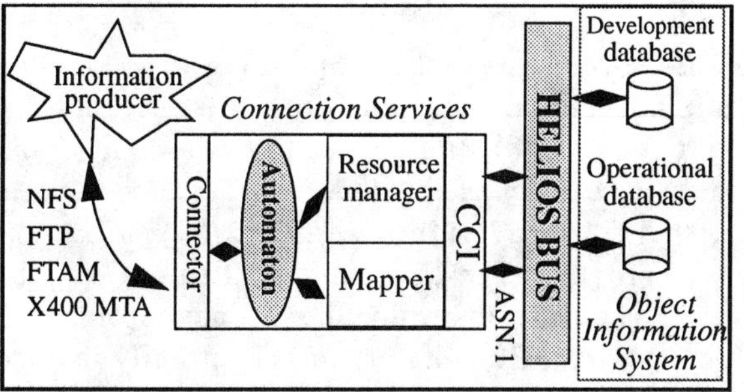

Figure 3 Functional architecture of the CS

1. A set of "*connectors*" allows the transfer of information between a HELIOS application and the foreign producer/consumer.
2. An *automaton* interprets/codes the messages expressed in a normalized medical exchange syntax.
3. A *resource manager* allows the automaton to know the "legal" construction of messages in a given syntax. The manager is supplied either with flat resource files that describe the messages, segments and fields or with imports of those descriptions coming from the OIS development database.
4. A *mapper* is responsible for the assignment of the internal representation slots with the message field values.
5. The *Component Communication Interface* (CCI) is the standard HELIOS feature that allows the connection of any component on the HUB and to code/decode data in ASN.1, which is the internal HELIOS coding scheme.

The next section will present the implementation solutions that deal with multi-syntax and multi-semantics message passing. Through the example of an incoming message (but the process is of course bi-directional), we will show how the different components of the CS collaborate, at run time, for processing a message.

PROTOTYPE IMPLEMENTATION

From a meta-syntax perspective, it can be seen that most of medical information exchange messages share a common *logical* structure. Actually, at an *abstract* level, a message consists of the information elements identifiers (e.g., headers, segment names), of the composition of the relations between these elements (e.g., repetition factor, presence status) and of a content allowing the generation of valid message instances. It is therefore possible to define a generic way of *describing* a message whatever its target translation into the specifications of a given coding system.

The resource manager

To provide the developers with a relative independence towards a given "interpretation" (or evolution) of a normalized syntax, two levels of message descriptions have been considered and implemented as "*resources*".

- The first resource describes the legal *segments sequence* for a given normalized message. Each segment is characterized by its name, a maximum number of repetitions and a status (i.e., `Mandatory`, `Required`, `Optional` or `Conditional`). It can be combined with others to form a segment group (written between `[]`). As illustration*, the message `MEDPID` (patient identification) begins as follow:

  `UNH1M BGM1M DTM2M [SG1 NAD1M]1M ...`

- The second resource describes the legal *fields sequence* for a given normalized segment. In addition to the field status, information for mapping the field to a slot (i.e., instance variable) of the internal representation may be present as in the following excerpt that describes the EDIFACT coded address of a patient.

  `MEDPID:ADR1 3901M{I01} [C053 3769M"I01" 3906M(99) 3906O(31) ...`

  Between {} is expressed the fact that the field value is the occurrence discriminator of a repetition, "" denotes a control constant, while () and <> refer to entry index numbers in the mapper array. At development time, the developers dispose of resource editors to maintain these descriptions. At run time, the automaton will use the loaded descriptions to accept (or reject) incoming messages and to pass relevant field values to the mapper. For outbound connections, the resources guarantee the correctness of the generated messages.

The automaton

The automaton is a three-step process: 1- to receive the data flow (i.e., message) from the connector 2- to load and parse the relevant resource for processing the flow 3- to produce an intermediate representation of the message to be passed to the mapper. To know which resource it has to use, the automaton may negotiate it with the communication party or determine it from the decoding of the first received message ele-

* The examples are given using the EDIFACT target syntax (currently promoted in Europe) but the same scheme had been applied without modifications for ASTM and HL-7.

ments. The intermediate representation core consists of the association of a data element, read from the message, with a reference (index number), coming from the resource. In the given example, when the automaton comes across a message field, identified from the processing of the resource to be the second 3906 field of the MEDPID:ADR1 segment, it passes to the mapper the value of the field (e.g., "4915 St. Elmo Avenue") read from the message, together with the reference affected to 31 (value read from the formal description). In that message, *31* will correspond to the position of the "patient address" mutator in the mapper array. As a side effect, the combined use of the automaton and the resources manager permits to translate a message expressed in one syntax (e.g., *ASTM*) to the same one expressed in another dialect (e.g., *EDIFACT*).

The mapper and the internal representation

The mapper establishes the transition between the syntactic (i.e., intermediate representation) and semantic (i.e., internal model currently limited to GMD representations) "worlds". The major goal of this implementation is to enable both the automaton and the mapper to remain invariant even if new messages or new GMDs come out. In fact, the only parts allowed to be changed are the resources and the GMDs manipulated through structured editors. To reach the required generic level, an *abstract* class is implemented as the root from which all real classes must be derived. Thanks to the inheritance principle of object orientation, together with the dynamic binding facilities attached to C++ virtual functions, the abstract class is able to manage an array of pointers to the instance variables *accessors* and *mutators* of its children. An indirection is then made possible from the intermediate slot reference passed (i.e., index in the virtual array) to the corresponding attribute mutator. In the given example, dereferencing the 31st mutator (*SetAddress*) will affect the "patient address" instance variable with "4915 St. Elmo Avenue". The automaton and the mapper are generic since they manipulate only the abstract root class virtual functions that will be dynamically bound, at run time, to real GMD instances accessor/mutators. If a new class, derived from the existing GMD hierarchy, needs to be linked with the application under development, the resource editor places the address of all the class accessors/mutators in the root array and the corresponding indexes in the associated resource.

When all the relevant fields of a message have been processed this way, the last (HELIOS specific) step begins: sending an *ASN.1* encoded message to the HUB connected application. This is devoted to particular methods of the GMD classes that translate their structure into a tagged ASN.1 SEQUENCE type. Then a normalized "HELIOS message" can be sent to the application through the CCI.

RESULTS

The CS connectors set currently supports the following normalized transport protocols: file sharing through *NFS*, file transfer using *FTP* or *FTAM* and message transfer using *X400*. The automaton can deal with *ASTM*, *HL7* and *EDIFACT*. *ACR-Nema* support is in progress. The CS is fully written in *C++*, the corresponding parts within the OIS are implemented in *Smalltalk*. Running platforms currently include Digital (MIPS based under Ultrix and AXP under OSF/1), Sun and HP workstations, PC under Windows and Macintosh. The Connection Service prototype will be used as a component of a Ward Information System to link a hypertension application both with patient identity and lab results servers.

DISCUSSION AND CONCLUSION

The described approach separates clearly the low level generic "machinery" of message coding/decoding from the higher level of semantic mapping. The realized prototype demonstrates that it is realistic to combine heterogeneous distributed open systems with exchange normalization, since the considered level is a meta-syntax (e.g., CEN GMDs). Standardization allows indeed programs to be written independently from the applications that may use them if they comply to the implicit data model of the syntax. However, it is known that total interoperability will not be reached without *semantics* sharing [10]. In the open distributed medical applications development context, semantic integration is required since developers have to deal with multiple application models. Semantic mismatches are in fact among the more difficult problems to solve when building distributed information systems. In the literature [8][12][13], four levels of such mismatches are generally considered. *Data model* and *structural conflicts* are revealed when the different components of a system were not implemented using the same formalism or when different representations are used to model the same data structure. *Descriptive conflicts* occur when a single concept is characterized by different sets of attributes depending on the considered component. More complex are the *semantic conflicts*, where the different applications do not share exactly the same domain model or the same concepts inside a common domain. Several authors, such as [1] and [4], have proposed different approaches based on meta-models to deal with divergent semantics thanks to the use of well-defined mapping procedures allowing to convert one model to another. A comparable approach is followed by [14] where *mediators* play the role of surrogates or "intelligent interfaces" between several distributed information systems. Similarly, in the distributed information systems field, it seems necessary to refer to a common meta-model to be sure that a message can be understood by the communication parties. However, a universal and unique meta-model is neither realistic nor desirable. In that respect, we propose to extend the presented architecture in a way that allows to consider different meta-models within the connection component.

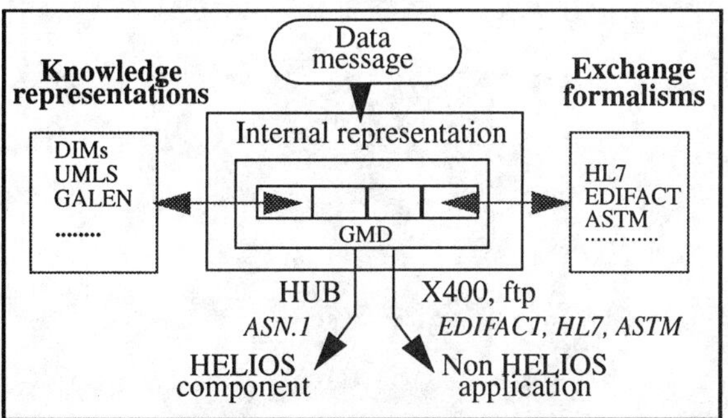

Figure 4 An extended functional model for the CS

In such an architecture, the semantic part described in the CEN methodology (i.e., the DIMs) could be used together with other "meta-model approaches" like UMLS or GALEN's Grail. Implementation of multi meta-models will open the way to a component allowing to transpose the semantics of messages as it transcodes their syntax. Integration of remote objects will thus become possible from the very beginning of new applications development, since the developers can reuse already modeled and implemented objects. Health care professionals' workstations could then be opened to various services, available as soon as they comply with the architectural standards of distributed computing. It is then possible to consider for the near future the next step represented by total interoperability between health applications.

Acknowledgments

This work has benefited from the financial support of the Commission of European Union (AIM contracts A1004 and A2015) and Digital Equipment Corporation (ERP FR018).

References

[1] Barsalou T, Gangopadhyay D: M(DM): An open framework for interoperation of multimodel multidatabase systems. *Proceedings of the 8th International Conference on Data Engineering*, Phoenix IEEE, February 1992.

[2] Degoulet P, Jean FC, Meinzer HP, Engelmann U, Baud R, Rassinoux AM, Jagermann C, Sandblad B, Cordelle D, Wigertz O: The HELIOS Medical Software Engineering Environment. *Comp. Meth. Prog. Biomed.* (in press).

[3] De Moor G, Segers D, Schilders L: Towards a meta-syntax for medical EDI. *Int J Biomed Comp.* 1994; 34(1-4):319-330.

[4] Gangopadhyay D, Barsalou T: On the Semantic Equivalence of Heterogeneous Representations in Multimodel Multidatabase Systems. *SIGMOD RECORD*; 1991; 20(4):35-39.

[5] Hammond WE. The role of standards in creating a health information infrastructure. *Int J Biomed Comp.* 1994; 34(1-4): 29-44.

[6] Jean FC, Thelliez T, Mascart JJ, Degoulet P: Object-oriented information system in the HELIOS medical software engineering environment. *Proc. 16th SCAMC.* 1992; pp. 595–599.

[7] Jean FC, Lavril M, Degoulet P: A Software Engineering Approach For Medical Workstation Development. *Int J Biomed Comp.* 1994; 34(1-4):249-260.

[8] Kim W, Seo J: Classifying Schematic and Data Heterogeneity in Multidatabase Systems. *Computer.* 1991; 24(12):12-18.

[9] McDonald CJ: Standards re-revisited. *M.D. Computing.* 1991; 8(2):74-76.

[10] Nicol JR, Wilkes TC, Manola F: Object orientation in Heterogeneous Distributed Computing Systems. *Computer.* 1993; 26(6):58-67.

[11] Schilders L, Segers D: Medical EDI Message Specification and Interchange Formats. *Progress in Standardization in Health Care Informatics.* De Moor et al. (Eds), IOS Press, 1993; pp. 149 - 155.

[12] Spaccapietra S, Parent C: Conflicts and correspondence assertions in interoperable databases. *SIGMOD RECORD.* 1991; 20(4):49-54.

[13] Urban SD, Wiu J: Resolving semantic heterogeneity through the explicit representation of data semantics. *SIGMOD RECORD.* 1991; 20(4):55-58.

[14] Wiederhold G: Mediators in the Architecture of Future Information Systems. *Computer.* 1992; 25(30): 38-48.

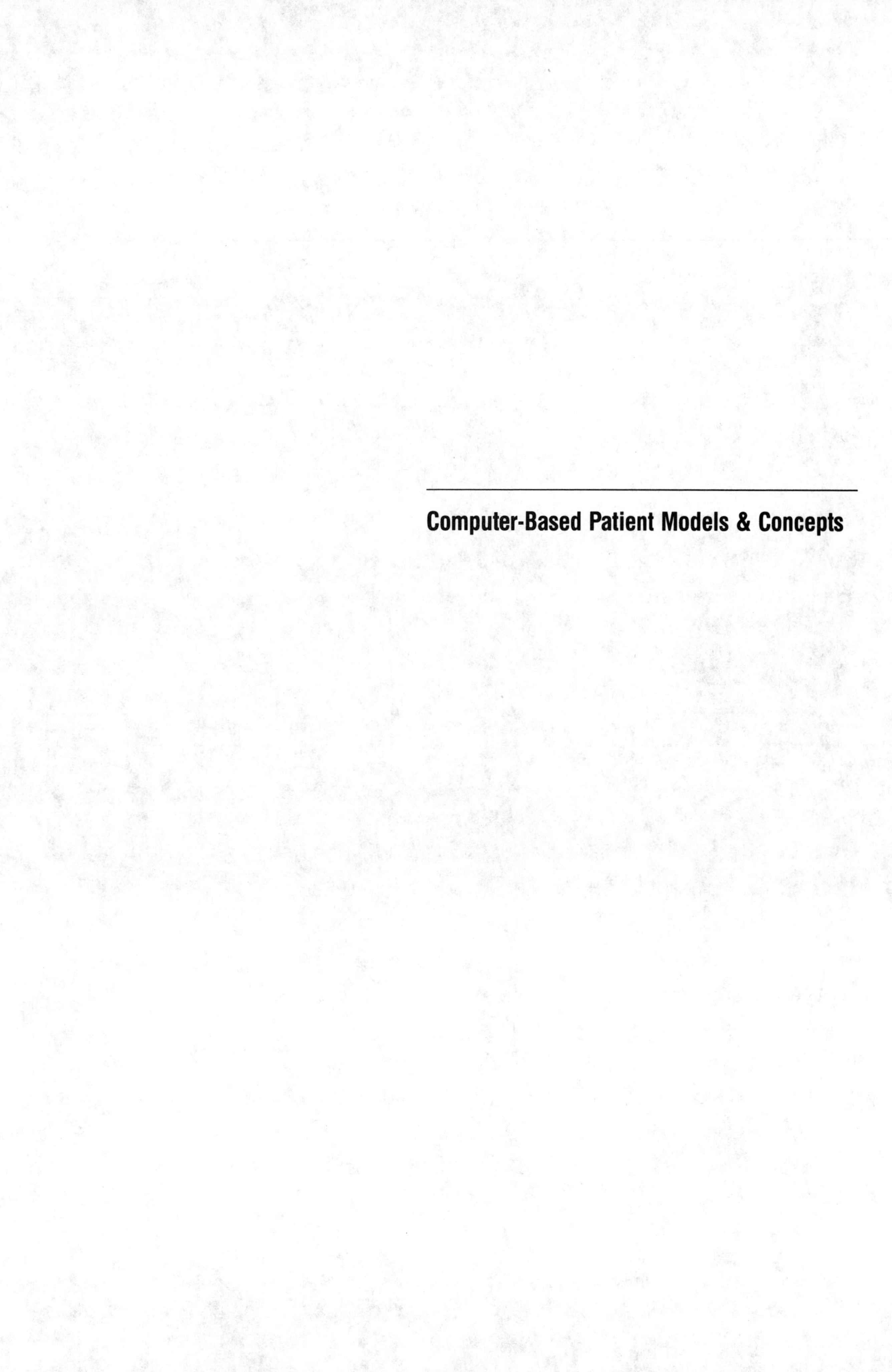

Computer-Based Patient Models & Concepts

A Business Case for Health Informatics Standards

Margret Amatayakul; Edward E. Heller, MD; and Gary Johnson
Computer-based Patient Record Institute

ABSTRACT

The acceleration of health informatics standards development has both value to health care delivery as well as economic value to the nation's economy. This paper describes the business case for standards development to enable development and implementation of computer-based patient record systems.

INTRODUCTION

Economic benefit is derived from both reduction in cost as well as improved product. A healthier populace is the product of an effective health care delivery system. Reduced health care costs is the result of a more efficient health care delivery system.

A healthier populace is a more productive populace, leading to greater economic gains through lower insurance costs, fewer sick days, decreased accidents, greater attention to detail, etc. Health accrues from many factors, but some include emphasis on wellness, patient education, patient responsibility for lifestyle factors, patient participation in the care process, improved care delivery by providers, etc.

Many of the benefits of improved health care and cost reduction can be derived from effective and efficient use of information. The health care delivery system today suffers from a wealth of data but limited means to put the data to good use. Information technology has not been fully developed and thus not widely adopted in health care delivery.

Again, many factors contribute to the fact that systems to manage health information are not widespread. Significant among these factors are the nature of health data itself (significantly text-based and multi-media), the manner in which it is captured, the speed with which it must be accessed in many cases, and the heuristic way in which it is processed by caregivers.

STANDARDS

A lack of standards which would enable better capture, processing, storage, retrieval, communication, and presentation of data is a significant factor which has contributed to the lack of information technology utilization in health care.[1]

Significant progress in standards development would help to achieve many of the economic benefits.

A dictionary definition of "standard" provides that a standard is something established by authority as a rule for the measure of quantity, weight, extent, value, or quality.[2] Standards development organizations describe six principal types of standards: test method, specification, practice, terminology, guide, and classification.[3]

Standards in health informatics may be any of the six types of standards, though most commonly specifications (e.g., content for a computer-based patient record), practices (e.g., health data interchange), terminology (e.g., medical vocabulary), guides (e.g., properties of a universal healthcare identifier), and classifications (e.g., code system).

Standards may be established in one of five ways: through rules, policies, and practices exclusively defined by and uniquely used by a company; through industry groups or professional associations; by the government in regulation, and by independent standards development organizations.[4] While any of the groups my use a consensus process, true consensus standards are developed by neutral organizations which have brought together people with a diversity of backgrounds, expertise, and knowledge. Consensus standards usually have the greatest acceptance because they have had the widest input and review.[5]

In health informatics, the primary source of standards has been groups other than neutral organizations. Most vendors and providers have had to develop their own specifications. The health care industry has borrowed from other industries in some cases (such as for bar codes). Professional specialty groups have been the primary source of vocabularies and code systems. Government, or quasi-governmental accreditation groups have regulated much of the content of health data to be retained. Consensus-based, voluntary standards development organizations have initiated work in the health informatics standards arena only fairly recently.

BUSINESS CASE FOR STANDARDS

It may be because the standards development organizations for health informatics are the "new kids on the block," that they have not drawn as much attention, are not as productive, and their products have not met with as wide acceptance as standards generated from such types of organizations in other fields. Another contributing factor to the lack of standards in health informatics is that the professionals needed to populate standards groups have tended to focus more on their own professional specialties. Certainly, the health care industry with its "charitable" history has not been one to have funds to support voluntary standards development organizations without seeing direct and immediate benefit, and have not viewed the standards activity from a business case perspective. Finally, informatics, itself, has not received the attention it deserved in a field so overwhelmingly, and rightfully, devoted to the care of people's ailments and injuries.

Standards, however, can provide real economic benefit by lowering the cost to produce product, integrate product throughout a system, and maintain product. In recent years, the value of health information has come to be much more widely understood. There follows, then, that standards applied to health information systems will enable more economically viable product development and more widespread dissemination of such products.

A standard description of the concept of the computer-based patient record would enable vendors to plan and design products. It would assure that known features existed and that specified information could be generated.

Completion of work that has already been initiated on health data interchange standards would provide the capabilities of information transfer among internal and across external systems. The notion of a lifetime health record for a patient can only truly be obtained through a complete and comprehensive set of health data interchange standards.

Standards to ensure confidentiality and security provide the assurance that the data captured and maintained in computer-based patient record systems and moved across a health information network is safeguarded, complete, and accurate.

Lifetime health records also depend on standards for linkage of patient data across the continuum of care. There must be a standard way, either to identify patients or link records of patients. There must also be identifiers for providers and site of care to facilitate information interchange.

Finally, computer-based patient records systems in a health information infrastructure depend on the ability to process data they contain. Such ability to process data depends on either the ability to process text into structured form or the input of structured data. While this is primarily a function of provider preference and technological advances, either (and both may well be the norm for the future) require standards for vocabularies and code sets. To enhance communication a common structure by which vocabulary and code systems can be developed is essential.

SYSTEMS

The Institute of Medicine patient record study committee defined a computer-based patient record as "an electronic record (i.e., a repository of health care information about a single patient) that resides in a system specifically designed to support users through availability of complete and accurate data, alerts, reminders, clinical decision support systems, links to medical knowledge, and other aids."[6] The committee identified 12 attributes such computer-based patient records and record systems should possess:

1. Patient's clinical problems/current status.
2. Measurement of the patient's health status.
3. Logical basis for all diagnoses or conclusions.
4. Linked with other clinical records of a patient.
5. Accessible only to authorized individuals.
6. Accessible in a timely way at all times.
7. Allows selective retrieval and formatting.
8. Linked to local and remote knowledge, literature, bibliographic databases.
9. Assist clinical problem solving with decision analysis tools, clinical reminders, etc.
10. Defined vocabulary.
11. Manage and evaluate the quality and costs of care.
12. Flexible and expandable.

The committee also noted, however, that the computer-based patient record does not exist in such a form, although significant progress has been made at certain sites.[7]

Standards would enable these attributes to be designed into products and used effectively by caregivers.

A patient's clinical problems/current status should be available instantaneously to a caregiver, yet today requires either an historical account by the patient or person accompanying the patient, or access to very limited information such as might be available on an arm band or other such limited set of data. Unless the provider is very familiar with the patient, care must often depend on observation alone.

The collection of the patient's health status depends on a longitudinal record and a standard vocabulary scheme. Such information must be provided over time by both the caregiver and patient directly.

Logical basis for diagnoses or conclusions follows from all information keyed accessible and generally keyed to the diagnosis. While not specifically recommending a problem-oriented structure, the Institute of Medicine committee's vision included the ability to make logical inferences from data.

Obviously linkages of patient's records requires a standard means of identification, or other system of linkage.

Limited accessibility requires confidentiality and security standards. Timely accessibility requires standards for information retrievability within the technology.

Selective retrieval and formatting requires that the technology depends on standard structures that can be presented as desired by the caregiver or others legitimately using the information.

While linkages to local and remote knowledge, literature, and bibliographic databases have been available for some time, they have not been available in the manner which is easy to use directly with patient data. Coupled with clinical problem solving and decision analysis tools, clinical reminders, etc., the technology becomes a powerful tool to deliver care.

The attribute of defined vocabulary reflects the frustrations of communication problems when describing patient conditions, treatment methodologies, and other factors relating to health care.

The first ten attributes contribute to better management and evaluation of the quality and cost of health care.

Finally, the attributes of flexibility and expandability reflect the need for advancing technologies.

INFORMATION BENEFITS

Since the computer-based patient record is still in the conceptual stages, it is impossible to quantify with precision the benefits that can accrue from such a system. Qualitatively, the benefits can be enumerated based on extrapolation of benefits from components which have already been implemented and on comparison with benefits from information technology implementation in other industries. The Computer-based Patient Record Institute has enumerated the following major categories of benefits in its Standards Acceleration Project proposal:[8]

- Improved patient care is the primary benefit. Better information systems in providers offices, and at the patient's bedside or in their homes will help health care professionals improve care by accessing lifetime patient data, knowledge databases, online expert systems, and other professionals for help with diagnosis and therapy. The patients will be able to make better choices about their health care and to participate more fully in their care.

- Reduced waste from repetitive tests and potentially even therapies not only reduces cost directly, but reduces actual danger to the patient. A significant waste also is the burdensome paperwork.

- More efficient care can result from systems which provide for electronic monitoring done at alternate sites, more quickly, and with better data. Better information systems will also enable the shift from the medical model of patient care, centered on episodes of sickness, to one centered on prevention and wellness.

- Improved financial management has been the primary target of information technology to date, but would be much more fully enhanced with complete clinical information as a resource; while ensuring greater confidentiality through focused, rather than shotgun, access to health data.

- Improved research results from aggregated health data, which is not only collected online, but organized and structured using standard vocabulary and code structures so as to make aggregate data meaningful.

- Improved learning occurs by both the health professional and the patient with greater access to health care data.

- Wider health care coverage can be provided through telemedicine and other technologies which expand the usefulness of information.

- Support for health policy formulation is achieved through adequate data to make judgements about the quality and cost of health care and the health of the nation.

ECONOMICS

Quantitatively, several estimates of savings or cost reductions directly attributable to the health care delivery system are available. Arthur D. Little suggests that "electronic management and transport of patient information" can reduce health care costs by more than $30 billion per year.[9] Examples of where these savings accrue include: reductions in repetitive diagnostic studies due to inaccessible information; reductions in medication errors from illegible entries, lack of access to alerts concerning contraindications and other protocols; reductions in misdiagnosis from incomplete and/or inaccessible information; improved selection of both more effective and efficient diagnostic studies and medications due to accessible knowledge bases; reductions in administrative overhead resulting from more rapid and direct transmission of patient data for claims processing and clinical utilization; and reductions in the paperwork burden of caregivers.

Several studies confirm such savings.[10, 11] For example, through computerized drug order entry and more effective reporting, one health care system has significantly reduced the number of adverse drug reactions and post-operative infections, and determined that such reductions save $1,939 for each episode of an adverse drug reaction and $14,000 for each post-operative infection.[12]

These benefits will be realized over a period of time and in stages. Some benefits will accrue immediately in systems which exist today. A hospital or physician office which has more than one information system application will benefit from completion of health data interchange standards permitting greater connectivity at reduced cost for customization. Confidentiality and security standards can both simplify and thus reduce cost of system implementation as well as alleviate concerns of both patients and providers. Resolution of identifiers for patients, providers, and sites of care will significantly reduce administrative costs of linking patient data.

Benefits which will have an impact in the near-term include those which describe the concept of the computer-based patient record, and its content and processes. This will have a two-fold impact: First, it will enable vendors to develop products which can be implemented in multiple sites. Today, a lack of standards precludes vending products across institutions and makes research and development of products very costly. Second, a standard description of content will greatly enhance the ability to access and utilize data for health care planning, policy setting, public health, research, and other information purposes. Vendors will know what content requirements exist and government, researchers, accrediting agencies, planners, and others will know what data is available. It will be accessible at much lower cost and much more rapidly, permitting much more timely implementation and utilization of policies and practices that impact health care.

Longer term benefits from standard vocabularies and code systems will further enhance utilization of patient data for improving the health of the nation.

Benefits also accrue to the economy as a whole. Cost reductions in the health care delivery system directly benefit government and employers. A healthier populace makes a more productive populace, also benefiting employers.

Standards, specifically, benefit vendors of information technology, permitting them to invest in research and development of systems which they are assured will meet user needs, be legally acceptable in all states, and operate with other systems. Standard systems drive down unit costs and make them more accessible to purchasers.

It is estimated that the current (1993) health information technology market is $7.5 billion and will grow to $11 billion by 1996.[13] Considering that an average size hospital may spend between $2 and $6 million on a computer-based patient record system,[14] growth in this market could easily double by 2000. In a study conducted by the Health Information and Management Systems Society, respondents indicated that they expected health care reform to accelerate greatly (39 percent of respondents) or somewhat (40 percent of respondents) the advancement of information technology in health care.[15] This same survey conducted over the period of 1992 through 1994 revealed that information technologists see increasing importance on implementation, specifically of computer-based patient records, and integrating existing systems to share information across department and increasing the use of computers by physicians and nurses (prerequisites to implementing computer-based patient records) as extremely important. The speed with which computer-based patient records are seen as needed to be adopted is seen in the increase in importance placed on this by the technologist respondents from third place in 1993 to second place in 1994 given a list of top 10 information systems priorities in health care across the US.[16]

Widespread product development and implementation, such that would double growth, however, depends on standards. Without standards to ensure that products meet the needs of the user community, are legal in all states, and inter-operate with other systems, vendors cannot make the investment necessary to develop and broadly market computer-based patient record systems.

Developing products which meet standards lowers unit costs making them more accessible to providers. Accelerating the standards development effort not only makes the economic benefit accrue more rapidly, but reduces redundant standards development which complicates development of interoperable systems and keeps prices higher.

SUMMARY

Standards acceleration is the key to ensuring that complete and accurate health information is available to care for patients and to manage the health care delivery system. Standards enable product development, which in turn puts the tools into the hands of the users. There are economic benefits for patients, providers, government, and industry.

ENDNOTES

1. Koop, C. Everett and Edward H. Shortliffe. "The Roles of Information Infrastructure in Health and Health Care." White Paper, National Research Council, October 5-6, 1993.
2. Amatayakul, Margret. "Healthcare Computing Standards: Making Sense out of the Alphabet Soup," *Journal of the American Health Information Management Association.* November 1991, Vol 62, No. 11, pp. 74-78.
3. ASTM, "Guide to Standards." Public Relations Brochure, 1990.
4. Ibid.
5. ANSI, "75th Anniversary Booklet." Public Relations Brochure, 1993.
6. Dick, Richard S. and Elaine B. Steen, Editors. *The Computer-based Patient Record: An Essential Technology for Health Care.* Committee on Improving the Patient Record, Division of Health Care Services, Institute of Medicine, National Academy Press, Washington, DC 1991.
7. Ibid.
8. Computer-based Patient Record Institute, "Proposal to Accelerate Standards Development for Computer-based Patient Record Systems," Version 3.0, April 29, 1994.
9. Arthur D. Little. "Can Telecommunications Help Solve America's Health Care?" September 1993.
10. Board of Directors, AMIA. "Standards for Medical Identifiers, Codes, and Messages Needed to Create an Efficient Computer-stored Medical Record," *J. of the American Medical Informatics Association*, Vol. 1, No. 1, Jan/Feb 1994, Position Paper.
11. CPRI Work Group on CPR Systems Evaluation , *CPRI Compendium*, Version 1.0, 1993.
12. Grandia, Larry, Presentation at SCAMC, 1993.
13. Dorenfest, Sheldon. "Creating a 'Top 100' Firm: The Lessons of History," *Healthcare Informatics*, June 1994, p. 49.
14. Dick, Op Cit.
15. Healthcare Information and Management Systems Society, Annual Leadership Survey, 1992-1994.
16. Ibid.

A Powerful Macro-model for the Computer Patient Record

van Ginneken AM, Stam H, Duisterhout JS
Department of Medical Informatics, Erasmus University
PO Box 1738, 3000 DR Rotterdam, The Netherlands

ABSTRACT

Especially in the Netherlands, the introduction of computer patient records (CPRs) in primary care has been relatively successful. Specialists usually maintain more extensive records than general practitioners and it has proven to be a great challenge to design a CPR that is useful and practical for specialized care. In this paper, we present the design of a CPR for use by specialists in an out-patient clinic. The philosophy underlying the design is that specialists may keep record in a relatively conventional way, while, at the same time, the system motivates them to add structure to their data. Data can be presented in various views, each suitable for one or more specific tasks. The potential to benefit from these views depends on the degree of structure in the recorded data. Since a CPR has to be faithful and permanent, explicit representation of observations, insights, and evolution of insight is also supported. The CPR system is in a final stage of implementation and will be evaluated in a clinical setting in summer 1994.

INTRODUCTION

Although the paper medical record (PMR) is still the most widely used medium for storage of patient data, advances in computer technology and an increase in complexity of health care have made the shortcomings of PMRs more apparent [1-4]. Depending on the viewpoint, different shortcomings are recognized. From a pragmatic point of view, the PMR can only be consulted in one place at a time, the legibility of hand-written sections may be poor, and information may be missing or difficult to find if the document is not well organized. Paper records often contain redundant information as a partial compensation for the fact that multiple views on the contents cannot be created dynamically. Where forms provide structure in the presentation of data, they introduce inefficiency at the same time, because they lead to sparse data storage: a form has to accommodate a large variety of possibilities while only few of those will apply to a certain patient. From the viewpoint of research, retrieval from PMRs involves a labor intensive search. Additionally, interpretation of the contents may be hindered by lack of standard terminology and completeness of data. While collecting data for analysis, transcription errors may occur. Furthermore, the PMR is passive: it cannot check the validity or plausibility of data and it cannot produce warnings for abnormal data or prompt for information in the context of a research protocol.

Electronic storage of patient data already provides a solution for part of these shortcomings: data can be accessed from several locations at the same time and legibility is no longer an issue. However, reduction of the other shortcomings requires more than storing free text. When information is identifiable in the record data can be presented in several views, thereby eliminating the need for redundancy. These potential advantages have lead to a great interest in CPRs, and the Medical Records Institute has encouraged their use. However, the benefit of such records highly depends on the amount, type, and reliability of the information they hold.

Although it is recognized that the degree of structure in a CPR determines much of its potential benefits [2,5], there is a tension between these benefits and the effort of structured data entry [6]. Physicians may prefer a few selections of predefined items over typing free text, but as soon as structured data entry involves a battery of menus and forms, they will refrain from data entry by computer. As a result, the most widely used CPR systems have clerical personal enter data that physicians record on system print-outs [2,7-9]. The physicians may use the system for consultation of information but they still make notes on structured forms. It is obvious that data entry by others than the physician himself is prone to transcription errors [10].

In the Netherlands, about 26% of the general practitioners (GPs) have completely replaced their PMRs by CPRs [11]. The efforts by professional organizations and support by the government have played an important role in this success. Yet, the records kept by GPs are far less extensive than those usually maintained by specialists. Therefore, because of the quantity of information involved, the step to computerized recording is more difficult to take for specialists. In our research, we focused on the development of a CPR for the out-patient clinic of a

0195-4210/94/$5.00

medical specialist, the internist in particular. In the following sections, we will present the philosophy behind our work, our CPR model, and discuss how the philosophy comes to expression in that model.

PHILOSOPHY

Even when physicians cannot directly be motivated to enter data by computer, there is still the challenge to expose the physician to the (potential) benefits of a structured CPR. Nygren has conducted important research on the use of PMRs by physicians [12]. He found that the clinical question greatly influences how the PMR is searched for relevant data. The ordering and structure of documents is vital to the efficiency of this search. Where Nygren provided insight in the type of information that physicians need in several clinical situations, Rector formulated foundations for CPRs [13]. These foundations constitute important criteria that CPRs should meet, with emphasis on the faithfulness and permanence of these records. The studies mentioned, have been the basis for the philosophy of our model. The following requirements have been the starting point of our research:

1) In order to be faithful and permanent, the record should allow for recording of observations, insight, and evolution of insight.
2) Allow for record keeping that offers options for structuring, but lets the physician free to choose for free text, at least for history and physical exam.
3) Offer views on patient data, each suitable for one or more specific tasks. The interface should motivate the physician for more structured data entry by making apparent how he can benefit from it.
4) Support structured data entry by intelligent and flexible anticipation of what the physician may want to describe.

THE MODEL

In our CPR, we distinguish 1) the macro-structure and 2) the micro-structure. The macro-structure comprises the components of the medical record, such as history, physical exam, lab data, diagnoses, problems, and the relationships between these. The micro-structure involves a detailed formal representation of the findings that otherwise constitute the free text portions history and physical exam [14,15]. Within this paper, we restrict ourselves to the model of the macro-structure.

Record keeping involves recording of information over time. Fig. 1 shows the three basic components of the macrostructure and how these are related to time and to each other.

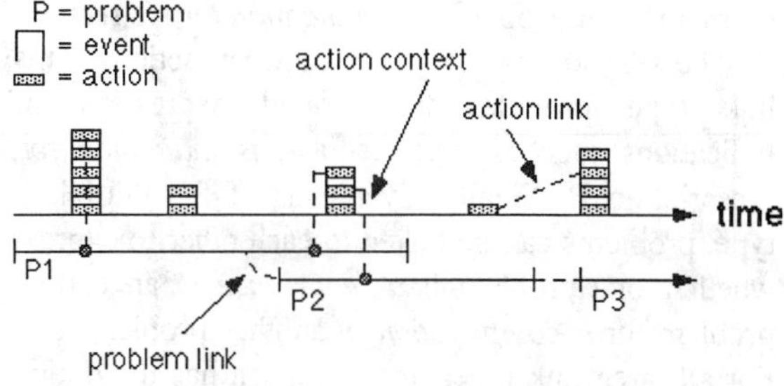

Fig 1 The three basic components of the CPR model with their relations to time and to each other.

Actions are the smallest units of information in the macro-model. Examples are a history, a physical exam, a lab result, and a prescription. Some of these actions, such as history and physical exam, have no further structure in the macro-model and are represented by one text field. Others consist of a number of specific fields: testname, value, and units in case of a lab result, and drug name, dose, frequency, and total amount in a case of a prescription. The *event* embodies a set of one or more actions that belong together in the sense that they can be considered to have been entered at one moment, have been discovered at one moment, are valid from one moment, and originate from the same source. The most typical example is the patient visit, but one lab report with several test results is also an event. Which actions may be described within a certain event type is defined in the model. The event-action model leaves room for several degrees of structure: a physician may choose to use only the action "summary" for all his text, whereas another physician may decide to partition his information over different actions, such that history, physical exam, diagnosis, etc., can be distinguished. The events and their actions represent what the physician has observed or done (decided).

The third component in the macro-structure is the *problem*, which was introduced by Weed [16]. Problems constitute conditions for which the patient is being evaluated and/or under treatment.

Besides structuring direct observations and decisions, the physician can add structure on a higher level by defining links between the basic components of the model. The first type of link, between an action and a problem, is called the action context and provides for the possibility of problem-oriented record keeping: observations, test orders, and treatments can be put in the context of a problem. There are several predefined descriptions to express the meaning of the link. Examples are: the physical exam *is related to* problem A, or problem A *is indication for* lab request B. The second type of link is between actions. This link type provides for refined expression of indications such as: test result A *is indication for* prescription B. Finally, by means of the third link type, problems can be linked to each other to express whether one problem is *a recurrence of* an earlier problem, or *a complication of* another problem, etc. For all three link types, the physician has the option to also express the meaning of the link in his own words. Action context, action-action links, and problem-problem links reflect the physician's insights.

The requirement that the patient record is permanent, i.e. not editable afterwards, calls for the need to record evolution of insight. The physician must be able to record that he realizes **now** that some condition has been present **since** some moment in the **past**. A series of such entries would document evolution of insight. This will be illustrated with a diagnosis. A diagnosis is an action in the sense that it reflects the physician's decision about the medical label for the patient's condition. When a diagnosis is entered, it is mandatory to define its status: certain, under consideration, certainly not, or cured. Since the insight with respect to the status of a diagnosis can change, recording the status of a diagnosis is also an action. When recording the status of a diagnosis, three dates are recorded: 1) the moment of data entry, 2) the date since the physician has his current insight about the status, and 3) the date since when the status should be regarded applicable. With these three dates a physician can record **now** that he knows **since a week**, that the patient has condition A since **2 years**. An example is illustrated in Fig. 2.

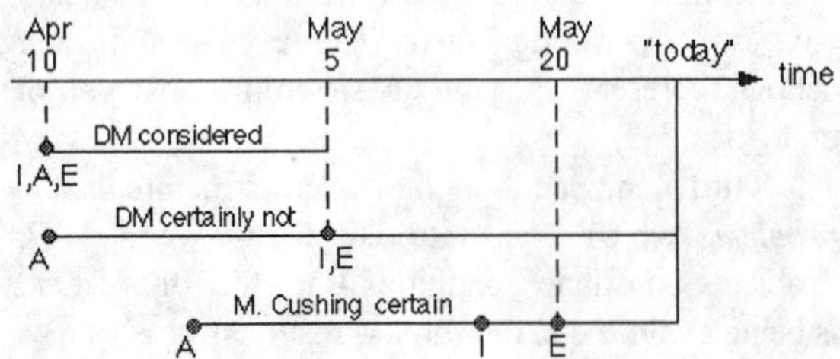

Fig 2. A schematic representation of recording insight and evolution of insight regarding the status of a diagnosis.

The example in Fig 2 shows that Diabetes Mellitus (DM) was entered on April 10 as being *under consideration* since April 10. On May 5th, the physician realized that the patient did not have DM and changed the status of that diagnosis to *certainly not* since April 10. A few days before May 20, the results of a test in late April leads to the conclusion that the patient suffers from Cushing's disease. On May 20, the physician enters that he knows since a few days, that the patient had Cushing's disease for *certain* since at least the date of the test.

When re-evaluating test orders and treatment in the past, it is important to realize that insights **then** may differ from insights **now**. Although it is presently known that the patient suffers from Cushings' disease, all actions on May 2nd were still based on the suspicion of diabetes.

Assessing the insights on a date in the past has its equivalent in a PMR in looking through the pages on or prior to that date. For the current insights one would start this search from the present backwards. The explicit representation of evolving insight is important for medical audit and decision support that involves temporal reasoning [17].

Besides the temporal aspects of recording, each observation and insight is always recorded with its author and its authorizer. The authorizer is the person, who is responsible for data entry into the CPR. The author represents the source of the information. In most cases, the authorizer is also the author, but it may happen that a neurologist conveys his insights to the treating physician. When the treating physician enters these insights into the CPR, he may record the neurologist as the author while he himself is the authorizer. Knowledge about the author, will facilitate consultation of the original information when the data is too concise or suspect for potential errors in transcription or interpretation.

PRESENTATION OF PATIENT DATA

As Nygren made explicit, it is important to present data in various views, each suitable for performing one or more specific tasks. Since the CPR can never "know" in advance which clinical question the physician wants to answer, the default view on the data should be based on anticipation of what the physician most likely wants to see. From there, the physician should be able to call for other views in an efficient manner, depending on his needs. In an out-patient clinic, the most frequent reason for consultation of a patient record is to obtain or recall the clinical picture of the patient. Our default view is based on that goal and is called the "patient profile" (PPF). Since the profile constitutes a view, it does not simply compare to a page in the PMR. The profile represents which information on the patient is currently valid and involves a set of data from different parts of the CPR. The data presented are: problems, past history and sensitivities, medication and test results since last visit, dates of all previous visits, and those diagnoses, that are currently certain or under consideration. In a PMR, gathering this set of data may involve browsing through many pages. Drugs may have been prescribed on several dates in the past: the physician has to judge whether or not one or more of these have to be prolonged. Sensitivities may be visible on the cover of a paper chart, but they can also be hidden somewhere in the volume. Test results require browsing through several lab or X-ray sheets to see what the latest results are. In the PPF, all this information is retrieved by the system and presented to the physician in one view. Although the default date of the PPF is today, the physician can enter any date since the CPR was started, and the PPF will present the information and insight that was applicable on the specified date.

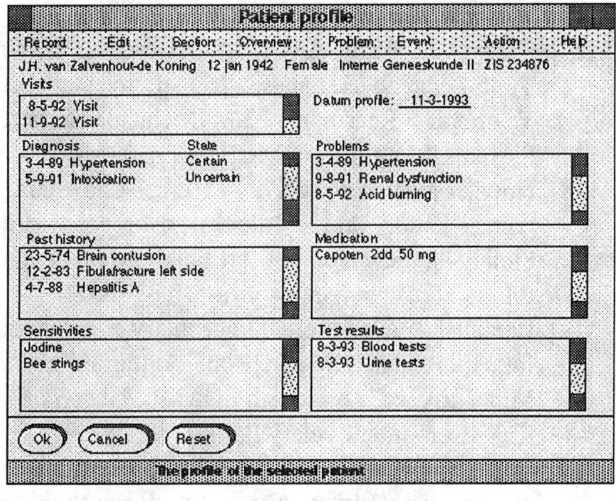

Fig 3. This patient profile window is derived from its Dutch equivalent. The PPF gives an overview of the patient data as they were valid on the specified date in the upper right part of the screen.

Besides serving as a view on the data, the PPF is also designed to provide immediate access to other information in the record, either by the option to call for another view or by zooming in on the data presented. The chronological overview presents a chronologically ordered list of all events that are stored in the CPR. Within this list, the physician has the option to limit his scope to events of a certain type such as "visit", or "blood test results". He can further refine his scope to a certain problem. Hence it is possible to ask for all visits linked to the problem "renal dysfunction". Whether or not a view has been defined, selection of one of the events in the list gives direct access to the "page" involved. From there, the physician can step back or forward in time, within his scope.

The zoom-option corresponds to looking up a certain page in a PMR, such as the notes of a visit and the contents of test results.

DISCUSSION

The CPR model fulfils the objective of being faithful and permanent by its explicit representation of observations and insights in relation to time and source. The model also supports temporal queries for research or decision support. Drawing from the experience with Dutch GPs and other systems in ambulatory care [2,7-9], it seems that structured data entry via a controlled vocabulary is a relatively large step for medical specialists, especially for data conventionally recorded in free text [18-21]. Therefore, we have chosen to give the physician the option to keep a CPR that is fairly conventional in its degree of free text and structure. We believe that physicians will ultimately be motivated to add more structure to their records when the possible views on the data enhance their awareness of the potential benefits. When the patient profile only shows the dates of recent visits and nothing else, the physician may regret that he simply wrote all his information and decisions as free text in the summary fields of the patient visit screen. Even when he decides to record diagnoses as separate actions, it may happen that the PPF shows a cystitis as a diagnosis, that has been certain since a year. Such an experience may motivate the physician to also record when a diagnosis is no longer valid. Similar motivations can be given for separate recording of problems, prescriptions, and other actions. Likewise, the option to specify scopes in the chronological overview may stimulate the user to specify links between actions and problems. Finally, intelligent and flexible support of structured data entry on micro-structure level is the subject of a parallel research project that is beyond the scope of this paper [14,15]. However, the CPR model does already have the slots for this encoded descriptive information.

PRESENT STATUS

The macro-structure model of the CPR will be evaluated in a clinical setting in summer 1994, tailored to the domain of cardiac failure. The CPR will be running as a service on the Hermes workstation, which supports access to and analysis of a variety of data from different databases [22].

CONCLUSION

Although we have ample experience with CPRs in primary care, developing a CPR, suitable for specialists, remains a great challenge. It is our philosophy that a CPR for specialists should allow its user to start record keeping in a way he can relate to, and from there encourage him to evolve into a record keeper that can enjoy the benefits of a structured CPR. Evaluation of our CPR in a clinical setting will reveal to which extent our philosophy applies and provide us with further insight in the use of patient data by specialists.

REFERENCES

[1] Institute of Medicine. Dick RS, Steen EB. The Computer-Based Patient Record: An Essential Technology for Health Care. Washington DC: National Academy Press, 1991.

[2] McDonald CJ, Barnett GO. Medical-record systems. In: Shortliffe EH, Perreault LE, eds. Medical Informatics: Computer Applications in Health Care. Reading MA: Addison-Wesley, 1990: 181-218.

[3] Komaroff AL, The variability and inaccuracy of medical data. Proc. of the IEEE, 1979;67:1196.

[4] Koran LM. The Reliability of Clinical Methods, Data and Judgments. N Engl J Med 1975;293:642-46 and 695-701.

[5] Whiting-O'Keefe Q, Simborg DW, Epstein WV, Warger A. A Computerized Summary Medical Record System Can Provide More Information Than the Standard Medical Record. JAMA 1985;254:1185-92.

[6] Reiser J. The Clinical Record in Medicine. Part 2: Reforming Content and Purpose. Ann Intern Med 1991;114:980-85.

[7] Blum BI, ed. Information Systems for Patient Care. New York: Springer-Verlag, 1984.

[8] Mc Donald CJ, ed. Computer-stored medical record systems. MD Computing, 1988;5:1-62.

[9] Barnett GO. The application of computer-based medical-record systems in ambulatory practice. N Eng J Med, 1984;310:1643.

[10] Safran C, Porter D, Lightfoot J, et al. ClinQuery: A system for the online searching of data in a teaching hospital. Ann Intern Med 1989:751-6.

[11] Van der Lei J, Duisterhout JS, Westerhof HP, et al. The Introduction of Computer-Based Patient Records in the Netherlands. Ann Intern Med, 1993;119:1036-41.

[12] Nygren A, Henriksson P. Reading the medical record. I. Analysis of physicians' ways of reading the medical record. Comput Methods Progr Biomed, 1992;39:1-12.

[13] Rector AL, Nowlan WA, Kay S, et al. Foundations for an electronic medical record. Meth Inform Med, 1991;30:179-86.

[14] Moorman PW, van Ginneken AM, Wilson JHP. Investigating and modelling the structure and contents of endoscopy reports. In: Lun KC, Degoulet P, Piemme TE, Rienhoff O, eds. Proceedings of MEDINFO '92. Amsterdam: North Holland, 1992:944-8.

[15] Moorman PW, van Ginneken AM, van der Lei J, et al. A Model for Structured Data Entry Based on Explicit Descriptional Knowledge. Accepted for Meth Inform Med.

[16] Weed LL. Medical Records, Medical Education, and Patient: The Problem-Oriented Record as a Basic Tool. Cleveland OH: Case Western Reserve Press, 1971.

[17] Kahn MG. Fagan LM, Tu S. Extensions to the Time-Oriented Database Model to Support Temporal Reasoning in Medical Expert Systems. Meth Inform Med , 1991;30:4-14.

[18] Nowlan WA, Rector AL. Medical knowledge representation and predicitive data entry. In: Stefanelli, ed. Proc. of artificial in medicine Europe. Springe-Verlag, 1991:105-116.

[19] Bernauer J. A controlled vocabulary framework for report generation in Bone-scintigraphy. In: Miller RA, ed. Fourteenth SCAMC. New York: IEEE Computer Society Press, 1990:195-9.

[20] Bell DS, Greenes RA, Doubilet P. Form-based clinical input from a structured vocabulary: Initial application in ultrasound reporting. In: Frisse ME, ed. Sixteenth SCAMC. McGraw-Hill, 1992:789-90.

[21] Campbell KE, Musen MA. Creation of a systematic domain for medical care: the need for a comprehensive patient-description vocabulary. In: Lun KC, ed. MEDINFO 92. Amsterdam: Elsevier Science Publishers, 1992:1437-42.

[22] Timmers T, van Mulligen EM, van den Heuvel F. Integrating clinical databases in a medical workstation using knowledge-based modelling. In: Lun KC, Degoulet P, Piemme TE, Rienhoff O, eds. Proceedings of MEDINFO '92. Amsterdam: North Holland, 1992:478-82.

Ethical Implications of Standardization of ICU Care with Computerized Protocols

Alan H. Morris, M.D., Thomas D. East, Ph.D., C Jane Wallace, BSN, James Orme, Jr. M.D., Terry Clemmer, M.D., Lindell Weaver, M.D., Frank Thomas, M.D., Nathan Dean , M.D., James Pearl, M.D., Brad Rasmusson, M.,D.
Pulmonary Division, LDS Hospital, 8th Avenue and C Street, Salt Lake City, Utah 84143

ABSTRACT

Ethical issues related to the use of computerized protocols to control mechanical ventilation of patients with Acute Respiratory Distress Syndrome (ARDS) are identical to the ethical issues surrounding the use of any therapy or intervention. Four ethical principles must be considered: nonmaleficence, beneficence, autonomy, and distributed justice. The major ethical challenges to computerized protocol use as a specific application of clinical decision support tools are found within the principles of nonmaleficence and of beneficence. The absence of credible outcome data on which ARDS patient survival probabilities with different therapeutic options could be based is a constraint common to most ICU clinical decision making. Clinicians are thus deprived of the knowledge necessary to define benefit and are limited to beneficent intention in clinical decisions. Computerized protocol controlled decision making for the clinical management of mechanical ventilation for ARDS patients is ethically defensible . It is as well supported as most ICU therapy options.

INTRODUCTION

A systematic overview of ethical implications of a new therapy requires consideration of four basic principles in biomedical ethics: nonmaleficence (do no harm), beneficence (do good), autonomy (respect for patient self direction), and distributive justice (be fair) [1, 2]. When the decision to treat has been made, and the only choice remaining relates to the technique or process of delivering the treatment, issues usually considered under the purvue of the principles of autonomy and distributive justice become less important. The importance of the principles of nonmaleficance and of beneficence remain undeminished. While nonmaleficence is frequently the overriding principle, the committment of the health care professions to provide benefit to patients is virtually universal [1]. Striking a reasonable balance between the principles of nonmaleficence and beneficence is a frequent challenge in serving the patient's best interest [3]. In effect, a risk-benefit assessment must be made, and is best made with sound data on which to base probability estimates of outcome for the treatment options under consideration. For patients with life-threatening hypoxic respiratory failure, the acute respiratory distress syndrome (ARDS), the outcome of interest is patient survival [4]. Unfortunately, credible outcome data are generally unavailable for many medical problems, including ARDS [5]. Only about 15% of medical interventions are supported with any scientific data [6, 7], and only 0.7% of interventions were reported to be supported by at least moderately strong scientific evidence [6]. Care must be exercised when choosing treatments without credible scientific outcome data, since potent modern interventions can induce harm as well as good. Mechanical ventilation for life-support of ARDS patients has both the potential for good (benefit) [8-10] and the potential for harm [11-16]. This paper addresses the ethical implications of using executable computerized protocols to control mechanical ventilation of patients with ARDS.

PROTOCOL CONTROL OF CARE

Virtually all clinical trials employ protocols. These protocols include definitions, patient selection criteria, procedural rules, and guidelines for conduct of the trial. They generally provide some specific instructions, but not enough detail to adequately control the moment to moment process of care. Algorithms usually contain non-specific, judgment requiring suggstions like "optimize PEEP" or "maximize antibiotic therapy." While these are useful general statements and concepts, they are not executable instructions. Clinical algorithm texts and other published guidelines contain many such general instructions [17-21]. While general instructions are of value for their conceptual content, they fail to standardize therapy because they are conceptual in focus and require judgment by the clinician before steps in the algorithm can be carried out. The application of general guidelines is associated with variation of practice by different clinicians [22]. Finally, guidelines in general have so far failed to significantly impact the practice of medicine or its cost [5, 23, 24].

Computerized protocols eliminate unnecessary variation in clinical care [25], thus standardizing clinical care and imposing control on the clinical care process. This control can be expected to reduce noise introduced by the clinical caregiver and thereby increase the signal-to-noise ratio for ultimate clinical outcomes [26-29]. Unaided humans are not capable of providing the persistent commitment to detail and to decision making logic (rules) necessary to effect standardization of care comparable to that achieved by an executable computerized protocol. The hectic ICU environment makes it even more difficult. Since treatments must be applied in a uniform manner to comparable patients before one can evaluate the

0195-4210/94/$5.00

outcome of a particular medical intervention, this standardization of care is of importance [30].

DEVELOPMENT & IMPLEMENTATION

Computerized protocols [26, 27, 31] were developed to control the intensity of care of patients enrolled in a randomized clinical trial in which ARDS patient outcome after extracorporeal support was compared with that after mechanical ventilation alone [9]. We reasoned that standardization of therapy would increase the interpretability and credibility of our clinical trial results. Our protocol-control goals were to ensure uniformity of care, equal intensity and frequency of monitoring, consistent decision making logic, and common therapeutic targets (e.g., PaO_2).

Published protocols for respiratory management of ARDS did not provide the detail and specific instructions we were seeking[17-19, 21, 32-34]. We developed protocols for controlling continuous positive pressure ventilation, pressure controlled inverse ratio ventilation [35], low frequency positive pressure ventilation-extracorporeal CO_2 removal, and continuous positive airway pressure.

The protocols were initially developed and used at the bedside in paper-based flow diagram form. After about 7,000 hours of around the clock use, the protocols were computerized using the LDS Hospital Health Evaluation through Logical Processing (HELP) information system [36, 37]. The HELP system provides bedside access, through computer terminals, to a fully integrated real time computerized patient data base for every patient. Computerized protocols automatically generated therapy instructions, 24 hours a day for the clinical care team, on each patient's bedside workstation [27, 38]. This bedside expert system controlled mechanical ventilation 95% of the time in routine around-the-clock clinical application. In 72 ARDS patients, 92% of 19,455 computerized protocol instructions were accepted and followed by the LDS Hospital clinical staff [27]. The protocols achieved the PaO_2, target of 59 mm Hg in patients supported extracorporeally as well as in patients supported only with traditional mechanical ventilation [9] in spite of the dramatic differences between the two therapies. Intensity of care, for which the number of changes of FIO_2 and PEEP per day were surrogates, was also almost identical in both groups of patients even though one group received prolonged extracorporeal support. Survival of ARDS patients supported with computerized protocol was four times the expected rate from historical controls [9]

These protocols are now used routinely for ARDS patients in the Shock Trauma/Intermountain Respiratory Intensive Care Unit at the LDS Hospital and have been used for over 50,000 hours in over 150 ARDS patients. The protocols have been exported to a personal computer platform and are currently being used in a clinical trial at one hospital in Los Angeles and one hospital in Houston. At these two hospitals 94% of 4,531 computerized protocol instructions in 12 ARDS patients have been accepted and followed by the clinical staffs of these two institutions (protocol performance is indistinguishable from that at the LDS Hospital).

AUTONOMY & DISTRIBUTED JUSTICE

The principle of autonomy requires patient participation and the acquisition of informed consent for application of new or non-standard treatments [1, 2]. Two opposing arguments can be mounted regarding the need for informed consent for the use of computerized protocol control of mechanical ventilation for ARDS patients. Firstly, computerized protocol control could be viewed as new and innovative non-standard therapy with undefined risks and benefits. One could argue that since much medical decision making requires frequent knowledge domain changes, protocol control of decision making will not likely be successful. Informed consent would then be mandatory. Secondly, computerized protocol control could be viewed as a decision support tool that merely formalizes and standardizes common practice. The forethought and concensus development required for protocol generation [25, 26] leads to a more precise and detailed articulation of the explicit and implicit rules applied in standard clinical practice (albeit with variability) [22]. Decisions under protocol control would, therefore, be made with more forethought and planning than would be decisions made individually by an independent practitioner [5]. Certain iterative therapies, such as mechanical ventilation, can be considered tasks within a single knowledge domain, and thus would be amenable to computerized protocol control. In this argument protocols are viewed as an extension of the common practice of generating guidelines [5] such as critical paths, routine sets of orders, etc., all of which are efforts to standardize care. Informed consent would then not be mandatory. At the LDS Hospital, the Institutional Review Board has accepted the latter argument and we do not require that informed consent be obtained for the use of computerized protocol control of mechanical ventilation.

The principle of distributive justice raises no obstacles to the use of computerized protocol control as long as it is applied to all appropriate patients without prejudice.

NONMALEFICENCE AND BENEFICENCE

The principles of nonmaleficence and beneficence are the source of major challenges to protocol control of care. These challenges are frequently couched in questions like "How can you be sure the protocol incorporates the right clinical care?" or "Physicians must be free to decide so the best therapy can be chosen for each individual patient." The use of computerized protocol control challenges the traditional authority of medical experts. Protocol control might thus be viewed as a threat, rather than as a complement, to the clinical *status quo*, in light of the common belief that medical experts maximize patient benefit by individualizing decisions.

Computerized protocols for mechanical ventilation of ARDS patients actually generate decisions that are no less individualized than decisions in many other clinical care domains. Firstly, other treatments such as drug therapy for hypotension or for infections are standardized with respect to drug dose, frequency and route of administration. Secondly, the mechanical ventilation support of ARDS patients is not standardized by computerized protocols. It is the computerized protocol logical elements and the decisions that result from error signals that are standardized. The actual treatment instructed by the protocol varies from patient to patient. The input data and the computerized protocol output instructions are both patient-specific. The standardized logic of the protocol generates individualized treatment instructions in response to the individual patient's unique physiologic expression of ARDS.

Beneficence can involve both the conferring of benefit on the patient and the intent to confer benefit without such achievement. The intention to do good is sometimes persuasive in itself [1]. For the critically ill ICU patient with ARDS, for whom the decision to provide mechanical ventilation has already been made, the overriding outcome variable is patient survival. Intentions to do good or to be benevolent pale in importance with actions that achieve increases in survival. Outcome data that can lead to credible estimations of survival probabilities for different treatment options become crucial to clinical decision making, whether protocol controlled or not. Unfortunately necessary data are unavailable and many complex clinical decisions must therefore be based on the clinician's intention to do good. The intention to do good is often insufficient [29, 39-42], although laudable [1].

Many ARDS clinical trial design flaws, and many clinical objections to performing clinical trials for patients with ARDS or other life-threatening problems, are based on "ethical concerns" originating in the expert or authoritarian paradigm that has been the foundation of the traditional patient-physician relationship. The physician is the expert and posesses the requisite training, knowledge, and experience to provide the advice necesary to guide the patient towards a favorable outome. In this process, the patients "best interest" is served by provision of the "best available" therapy [43]. The physician's "belief" in the superiority of a therapeutic choice is cited as a foundation of ethical decision making [43] and of the fiduciary nature of the physician-patient encounter [3, 43]. The absence of such a belief in the face of therapeutic options constitutes the state of "equipoise" within an individual physician (individual equipoise) or within the medical community (clinical equipoise) [43, 44]. When equipoise is present, randomized clinical trials comparing therapeutic possibilities seem justified. A number of concerns can be raised in response to this traditional view. Firstly, the implicit assumption that physician belief is a reliable reflection of the best information is not responsive to general human limitations with information processing [28, 29, 35, 45, 46]. Ignoring these limitations raises physician "belief" to a level of undeserved importance. Physician "belief" in the superiority of complex therapies may, in fact, undermine the fiduciary relationship that should exist between physician and patient [3, 43] by exposing the patient to undesirable therapy.

Secondly, the "belief" of the adherents of a particular policy, in itself, provides no justification for the policy. The belief is no more than an opinion. The policy can only rationally be justified by data or arguments. Belief can be based on credible outcome data or on unfounded conjecture. Belief is commonly based on considerations that fall on a continuum between credible outcome data and unfounded conjecture. Belief insufficiently grounded in credible outcome data, even when based on extensive personal and medical community experience, can mislead well intended clinicians to make decisions that fail to benefit and even bring harm to their patients. The results of the Vineberg procedure for angina pectoris, with its 75% positive placebo effect [47], and of the Cardiac Arrhythmia Suppression Trial (CAST) with its unexpectedly high mortality associated with effective suppression of premature ventricular beats following myocardial infarction [41] are graphic examples of this danger. Other important examples are easily found and include O2 therapy for neonatal respiratory distress [40], gastric freezing for upper gastrointentinal hemorrhage, laetrile for cancer, rapid I.V. infusion of 5-FU for colorectal cancer, intrarterial infusion of chemotherapeutic agents for colorectal liver metastases, hydrocortisone after myocardial infarction [30], splenectomy for Gaucher's disease, and frontal lobotomy. It is of interest, therefore, to find belief, in itself used as a justification for some of the most consequential and onerous decisions in critical care medicine [43, 48, 49]. To be fair, it must be acknowledged that some workers demand that physician opinion be based on reliable actuarial data [39, 49, 50], but this does not appear to be a universal expectation. It is rapidly appreciated that belief itself is neither sufficient nor even always necessary for the effectuation of correct therapy. The steadfast belief of the medical adherents of Laetrile therapy did not make the therapy correct, nor could it justify the conduct of a clinical trial [49]. Just as the individual practitioner cannot invoke idiosyncratic good intentions as a defense, so also should this avenue of defense be forbidden to the expert committee that may be charged with defining a standard of care for the medical community. Poorly supported opinion, no matter how well intended, does not gain accuracy by being offered by a dozen experts rather than by one practitioner.

The common clinical concerns raised about computerized protocol controlled care are reflections of the strength of the authoritarian paradigm and of the beliefs of the clinicians that practice within this paradigm. Open discussion of the limitations of such beliefs when bereft of supporting scientific data has been an effective means of overcoming these clinical concerns in the LDS Hospital and in the hospitals, in Los Angeles and Houston, to which the computerized mechanical ventilation protocols have been exported.

SUMMARY

The ethical implications and challenges raised by the use of computerized protocol control of clinical decision making appear to be identical to the issues raised by therapeutic interventions in general, both in clinical practice and in clinical trials. In the absence of credible data concerning outcome (survival) probabilities for different therapy options, clinicians are forced to use intent rather than patient benefit as the operational decision driver regarding the principle of beneficence. The use of computerized protocols raises ethical questions that are qualitatively indistinguishable from those encountered routinely in clinical care. Available reports indicate that further development and evaluation of protocol control of care is clinically and ethically desirable.

REFERENCE

1. Beauchamp T, Childress J. Principles of biomedical ethics. (3 ed.) New York: Oxford University Press, Inc, 1989:470.
2. Jonsen A, Siegler M, Winslade W. Clinical ethics. (3 ed.) New York, NY: McGraw-Hill, Inc., 1992
3. Moline J. Professionals and professions: A philosophical examination of an ideal. Soc Sci Med 1986;22(5):501-508.
4. Morris A. ARDS and new modes of mechanical ventilation: Reducing the complications of high volume and high pressure. New Horizons 1994;2(1):19-33.
5. James B, Eddy D. CPI and practice guidelines. In: Horn S, Hopkins D, ed. Clinical practice improvement: A new technology for developing cost-effective quality health care. New York: Faulker & Gray, Inc., 1994: 271. vol 1).
6. Williamson J, Goldschmidt P, Jillson I. Medical Practice Information Demonstration Project-Final Report (Contract #282-77-0068GS).Baltimore, MD: Office of the Asst. Secretary of Health, DHEW, 1979
7. White K. Foreward. In: Payer L, ed. Medicine and culture. New York, NY: Henry Holt, 1988: 9.
8. Hickling K. Low volume ventilation with permissive hypercapnia in the Adult Respiratory Distress Syndrome. Clin Intens Care 1992;3:67-78.
9. Morris A, Wallace C, Menlove R, Clemmer T, Orme JJ, Weaver L, Dean N, Thomas F, East T, Suchyta M, Beck E, Bombino M, Sittig D, Böhm S, Hoffmann B, Becks H, Pace N, Butler S, Pearl J, Rasmusson B. A randomized clinical trial of pressure-controlled inverse ratio ventilation and extracorporeal CO2 removal for ARDS. Am J Respir Crit Care Med 1994;149(2):295-305.
10. Tobin M., ed. Principles and practice of mechanical ventilation.New York, NY: McGraw-Hill, Inc., 1994.
11. Slavin G, Nunn JF, Crow J. Bronchiolectasis, A complication of artificial ventilation. Br Med J (Clin Res Ed) 1982;285(6346):931-934.
12. Albelda SM, Gefter WB, Kelley MA, Epstein DM, Miller WT. Ventilator-induced subpleural air cytsts clinical radiographic and pathologic significance. Am Rev Respir Dis 1983;127:360-365.
13. Churg A, Golden J, Fligiel S, Hogg JC. Bronchopulmonary displasia in the adult. Am Rev Respir Dis 1983;127:117-120.
14. Tsuno K, Prato P, Kolobow T. Acute lung injury from mechanical ventilation at moderately high airway pressures. J Appl Physiol 1990;69(3):956-961.
15. Dreyfuss D, Saumon G. Lung overinflation: Physiologic and anatomic alterations leading to pulmonary edema. In: Zapol WM, LeMaire F, ed. Adult respiratory distress syndrome. New York: Marcel Dekker, Inc., 1991: 433-449. (Lenfant C, ed. Lung biology in health and disease; vol 50).
16. Dreyfuss D, Saumon G. Role of tidal volume, FRC, and end-inspiratory volume in the development of pulmonary edema following mechanical ventilation. Am Rev Respir Dis 1993;148:1194-1203.
17. Boutros AR, Hoyt JL, Boyd WC, Harford CE. Algorithm for management of pulmonary complications in burn patients. Crit Care Med 1977;5(2):89.
18. Don H, ed. Decision making in critical care. Philadelphia, St Louis: BC Decker Inc., The CV Mosby Company, 1985:Clinical decision making Series
19. Karlinsky J, Lau J, Goldstein R. Decision making in pulmonary medicine.Philadelphia: BC Decker, 1991
20. Armstrong R, Bullen C, Cohen S, Singer M, Webb A. Critical care algorithms.New York, NY: Oxford University Press, 1991:100.

21. Guidelines-Committee-Society-of-Critical-Care-Medicine. Guidelines for the care of patients with hemodynamic instability associated with sepsis. Crit Care Med 1992;20(7):1057-1059.
22. James B, Horn S, Stephenson R. Management by fact: What is CPI and how is it used? In: Horn S, Hopkins D, ed. Clinical practice improvement: A new technology for developing cost-effective quality health care. New York: Faulker & Gray, Inc., 1994: 39-54. vol 1).
23. Anderson C. Measuring what works in health care. Science 1994;263:1080-1083.
24. Walker R, Howard M, Lambert M, R S. Medical practice guidelines. West J Med 1994;161(1):39-44.
25. Morris A, James B. CPI and computerized protocols. In: Horn S, Hopkins D, ed. Clinical practice improvement: A new technology for developing cost-effective quality health care. New York: Faulker & Gray, Inc., 1994: 271. vol 1).
26. East T, Morris A, Wallace C, Clemmer T, Orme JJ, Weaver L, Henderson S, Sittig D. A strategy for development of computerized critical care decision support systems. Int J Clin Monit Comput 1992;8:263-269.
27. Henderson S, Crapo R, Wallace C, East T, Morris A, Gardner R. Performance of computerized protocols for the management of arterial oxygenation in an intensive care unit. Int J Clin Monit Comput 1992;8:271-280.
28. Morris A, Gardner R. Computer applications. In: Hall J, Schmidt G, Wood L, ed. Principles of Critical Care. New York: McGraw-Hill, 1992: 500-514.
29. Morris A. Paradigms in management. In: Pinsky M, Dhainaut J, ed. Pathophysiologic foundations of critical care medicine. Baltimore: Williams and Wilkens, 1993: 193-206.
30. Pocock SJ. Clinical Trials: A Practical Approach.New York, NY: John Wiley & Sons, 1983:266.
31. East T, Morris A, Gardner R. Computerized management of mechanical ventilation. In: Grenvik A, Ayres S, ed. Textbook of critical care. 3 ed. Philadelphia, PA: W. B. Saunders Company, In Press:
32. NHLI. Protocol for extracorporeal support for respiratory insufficiency collaborative program.Bethesda: National Heart and Lung Institute, Division of Lung Diseases, 1974
33. Shoemaker WC. A patient care algorithm for cardiac arrest. Crit Care Med 1978;4:157.
34. Bryan-Brown C, Shapiro B, Miller C, Kathirithamby K. A less invasive approach to monitoring acute respiratory failure. Med Instrum 1979;13(6):327-329.
35. East TD, Böhm SH, Wallace CJ, Clemmer TP, Weaver LK, Orme JF Jr, Morris AH. A successsful computerized protocol for clinical management of pressure control inverse ratio ventilation in ARDS patients. Chest 1992;101:697-710.
36. Pryor TA, Warner HR, Gardner RM, Clayton PD, Haug PJ. The HELP system development tools. In: Orthner H, Blum B, ed. Implementing health care information systems. New York: Springer-Verlag, 1989: 365-383.
37. Kuperman GJ, Garder RM, Pryor TA. HELP: A Dynamic Hospital Information System.New York: Springer-Verlag, 1991(Orthner HF, ed. Computers and Medicine
38. Henderson S, Crapo RO, East TD, Morris AH, Gardner RM. Computerized clinical protocols in an intensive care unit; How well are they followed? In: Miller RA, ed. Fourteenth Annual Symposium on Computer Applications in Medical Care. Washington, DC: IEEE Computer Soc Press, 1990: 284-288.
39. Chalmers T. A belated randomized controlled trial. Pediatrics 1990;85(3):366-369.
40. Silverman W. Human experimentation: A guided step into the unknown.Oxford, England: Oxford University Press, 1985
41. The Cardiac Arrhythmia Suppression Trial II Investigators. Effect of the antiarrhythmic agent moricizine on survival after myocardial infarction. N Engl J Med 1992;327(4):227-233.
42. Silverman W. Doing more good than harm. Ann NY Acad Sci 1993;703:5-11.
43. Truog R. Randomized clinical trials: Lessons from ECMO. Clin Res 1992;40(3):519-527.
44. Meinert C. Extracorporeal membrane oxygenation trials. Pediatrics 1990;85(3):365-366.
45. Miller G. The magical number seven, plus or minus two: Some limits on our capacity for processing information. Psychol Rev 1956;63(2):81-97.
46. Miller J. Living systems.New York: McGraw-Hill Book Company, 1978
47. Hulley S, Cummings S. Designing Clinical Research.Baltimore: Williams and Wilkins, 1988
48. O'Rourke P, Crone R. Pediatric applications of extracorporeal membrane oxygenation (Editorial). J Pediatr 1990;116:393-394.
49. Levine R. Ethics and regulation of clinical research. (2 ed.) New Haven: Yale University Press, 1988
50. Chalmers I. Minimizing harm and maximizing benefit during innovation in health care: Controlled or uncontrolled experimentation? BIRTH 1986;13(3):155-164.

Acknowledgements: This work was supported by NHLBI grant #HL36787, AHCPR grant #HS06594, the Respiratory Distress Syndrome Foundation and the Deseret Foundation (LDS Hospital).

Issues in System Design Clinical Models and Objects

An Information Model for Medical Events

Daniel J. Essin, MD LAC+USC Medical Center
Thomas L. Lincoln, MD LAC+USC Medical Center and RAND Corporation

ABSTRACT

Information gathered during the healthcare process is lost when forced into rigidly structured record-oriented databases. By contrast, content can be difficult to manipulate if stored as unstructured text. Spurred by the requirements of electronic publishing, military procurement and the Internet, new robust standards for structuring documents have been developed and deployed. These standards can provide a foundation for a document-based Electronic Medical Record System. In order to fully exploit this added flexibility, an information model is necessary to define both the direct and contextual content of documents. Once context, as well as fact, are recorded in formal structures, inferential techniques can either selectively extract knowledge and data from documents or aggregate data to create summaries so that all interested and authorized parties have a better chance of meeting their information needs from a single, permanent data source.

BACKGROUND

Information gathering is a cognitive activity. Our environment is filled with objects and situations that have the potential to yield information. The information that comes to our attention does so either as the direct result of our experiences, or as the result of reflecting on those experiences [1]. The discovery or recognition of these occurrences, and the subsequent generation of information from them, takes place in a discrete and episodic fashion rather than continuously. An information model describes when this cognitive activity will be translated into a machine processable representation and what content will be included.

Individuals intuitively know when to vary the structure of their notes to effectively capture or represent relevant context. To represent this informational environment in an electronic format, structure and content need be modeled separately so that the relationship between them can be dynamically adjusted to meet the evolving needs and expectations of the human users.

Models are abstract representations of concepts, forgoing detail in order to isolate and clarify a set of core properties. The design and function of any complex system depends on the participation of many concepts which, when expressed along with their inter-relationships, constitute the system's architecture (or model.) The architecture of Electronic Medical Records Systems (EMRS) can be expected to include models of requirements, workflow, transactions, security, data structure, denotational semantics (the semantics that provide the symbols and names necessary to signify meaning), and information content.

Of these models, perhaps the most fundamental are 1) the requirements model that describes what the system is expected to do and 2) the information model that identifies the information content that must be captured to fulfill the requirements. The popular system development methodologies contain implicit models of structure and denotational semantics. Although these can interfere with the full realization of requirements or with the graceful evolution of an implementation the "best" structure or semantic model cannot compensate for the failure to capture relevant information. Many successful healthcare information systems have responded to these constraints by restricting themselves to the processing of highly structured documents whose content can be mapped onto formal database structures.

Loosely structured documents offer a unique alternative that can address a broader range of applications and information [2,3]. There is a growing body of standards that address the formal structure and processing of loosely structured documents. For example, HyTime* [4], built on SGML† [5] provides a notation that defines a generalized hierarchy of document

* Hypermedia/Time-based structuring language ISO/IEC 10744
† Standard Generalized Markup Language ISO/IEC 8879

types and provides a means of recording and processing them. Since loosely structured documents can be formally described and processed, they are a good candidate for the foundation upon which to build an EMRS.

THE INFORMATION MODEL

The objective of the information model presented here is to address six observations. 1) Facts originate in events. 2) Facts require context to be informative. 3) Context is always rich and highly variable. 4) The temporal association of facts and events is a significant component of context. 5) Context is difficult to reconstruct; if it is not captured "up-front" it is usually lost forever. 6) Although information can be modeled separately, in practice the underlying structure and semantic models have a strong influence on the ability to fulfill the demands of the information model.

The moments during which information is recognized or synthesized are called *Information Laden Events* (ILE). If an individual makes only a "mental note" of information, it will have no direct impact on the actions of others now or in the future. The act of recording an ILE instantiates the factual or informational content of the event as part of the universe of known data. The term *Information Bearing Object* (IBO) [6]. will be used to describe the records of those events which become part of the accessible information (knowledge) base by virtue of being recorded by people or by devices or processes set into motion by people. The model describes the components that must (or may) be present within an IBO to insure that the facts and the context of the event are captured in a machine processsable representation.

Facts require context in order to be considered information. The model therefore requires a statement of "WHAT" happened (including the EVENT TYPE) to provide the fact as well as statements of "WHO", "WHERE", "WHEN", "WHY" and "HOW" to provide the context. Different event types have different minimal requirement for context below which the IBO would not be informative. Beyond that minimum, there are a wide variety of additional context-defining items that could be supplied. The information content increases as more context is recorded. The importance or relevance of additional information depends on the nature of the primary event and what unique circumstances may have occurred.

The following is a non-exhaustive list of the informational components that may be necessary to fully describe the content and context of an ILE. Each component can be expected to have substructure depending upon the nature of the event to be documented and the type of document being used to record the event.

WHO (acting in what capacity or role)
 To whom did it happen?
  A person, a group or association of people
  A legal entity, an *ad hoc* association
 Who did it?
 Who recorded it, checked it, approved it?
 Who looked at it, changed it, etc.?

WHAT kind of event is it?
WHAT thing(s) were involved?
WHAT detailed information was collected?
  Data elements ("fields")
  Structured notes
  Narrative
WHAT special circumstances were/will be involved?
WHAT other events are linked/related to this event?
WHAT happens next?
WHAT version is this?
WHERE did it/will it happen?
WHEN
  When did it/will it happen?
  When did it/will it expire/be retired?
HOW did it/will it happen?
  Orders
    Simple, Complex
  Procedures
WHY did it/will it happen?
  Assessment, Commentary, Annotation

To continue this formulation it is necessary to establish the fundamental properties of each component of the model and to explore the denotational semantics that may be required to represent them. They are:

1) persons
2) objects
  a) with a unique physical presence other than persons e.g. items of capital equipment with serial numbers, etc.,

b) objects that have a non-unique physical presence such as pi-mesons, Band-Aids, individual fresh carrots, etc.

3) points on a timeline

4) points in space

5) Assertions or retractions of fact or opinion along with supporting context. There may be many types of events including:

a) informational (descriptive) events

b) identity-defining events

c) complex entity, organization and association describing events

d) role-defining events

e) knowledge-defining events

f) rule-defining events

g) opinion-defining events

Persons

"Person" references literally represent people, not an abstract class. There are no subtypes of people. With the exception of the genetically determined links (if known) to mother and father, relationships between people are determined by applying inference to a collection of identity-defining and relationship-defining IBO's using a collection of rules that define relatedness. Several examples will illustrate the intended interactions.

The determination of siblings and family groupings requires inferential queries. To find an individual's brothers requires retrieving a rule (that defines a brother as any male offspring of an individual's mother), then searching for birth events involving the UID of the mother that produced male children followed by the retrieval of the necessary IBO's.

Age is another datum that must be inferred since it is not constant and can have a variety of context-dependent values. Even with birthdate information available, the age cannot be computed until the age context is defined. Is it the age today or the age at the time of some event?

Something as apparently simple as a person's name is subject to similar ambiguity. Just as with age, the question must be asked - Name as of "When" and for "What" reason? In many settings the name recorded as part of the birth event is not the legal name since there are a number of circumstances in which names change such as adoption, marriage, etc.

Inanimate Objects

Inanimate objects fall into two categories. Some objects are significant because they are expensive, dangerous or must have an individual identity for some reason. Such objects have some properties in common with persons and other complex entities. Other inanimate objects, especially consumable supplies, are treated differently in purchasing, receiving, inventory, distribution, and usage accounting.

Certain IBO's, such as documentation of surgical procedures, will need to indicate that various equipment and supplies were brought into the operating room, which were used, opened, applied to the patient, disposed of, etc. A semantic network describing the similarity between various objects would facilitate fuzzy searches such as "Find everyone who had intravenous therapy on March 12".

Spatial and Temporal Location

Every IBO should contain at least the date, time and location when it was created. In order for IBO's to be meaningful in the future or if transmitted to distant locations, the data that place an event in time and space must be global in nature so that the meaning is not lost. Most existing systems satisfy this requirement for dates but nor for time values. Times should be stored as Greenwich Mean Time (GMT) and all locations should be stored as a latitude, longitude, and elevation allowing for the indirect determination of the GMT offset.

The practice of describing locations in relative or colloquial terms is a great source of ambiguity as functions are moved from place to place while retaining familiar names. The GPS (Global Positioning System) Coordinates of any location can now be readily determined and make it possible to describe locations in absolute terms. Geographic Information Systems can translate the coordinate data into more familiar terms as needed. In addition, date and location data make it possible to properly interpret time both relative to Daylight Savings Time and changes in time zone.

Roles

Persons may assume, or be assigned, a large and unpredictable number of roles. The set of allowable roles changes as the organization evolves. Using IBO's to create and assign roles eliminates the need to identify the universe of allowable roles before a system is actually built. Many development methodologies, make role information a structural component of system design that is difficult to augment or eliminate at a later date.

Complex entities, represent a special case of role-definition. They originate in events that assert their creation. Subsequent events can then assign persons or other complex entities to roles within the new organization or association. Examples of complex entities are corporations, committees, ward-teams, group practice associations, etc. While in existence, complex entities can assume many, but not all, of the roles that can be assumed by persons.

Information and Knowledge

Several other types of knowledge are required to integrate a complete system:

1) Domain-specific knowledge, e.g. medical terminology and medical diagnoses;
2) Application structure and control information;
3) Ordered or unordered links between events;
4) Aapplication defined functions and rules;
5) Features that will support activity-tracking;
6) Rules defining security and user permissions and capabilities;
7) and, the ability to include multimedia data as part of "What", "How", and "Why" notations.

Denotational semantics are the subject of much active research. Organizations will have different needs in this area if they are centers of excellence in highly specialized domains or have evolved a unique institutional culture. The purpose of the information model is to explicitly accommodate a variety of denotational semantics, not to impose particular choices. When organizations using different semantics need to exchange information, pragmatic translations between semantics can be negotiated providing that a consistent information model is in use.

Knowledge can be represented using the same structures that represent "data." This will allow knowledge and data to be managed by the same tools. Likewise, the rules that define what data mean and the various ways that data should be validated, displayed and interpreted should reside in the database as computable entities.

Simple vs. Compound IBO's

Some events that occur take a long time to complete. The need to keep contemporaneous documentation will mean that some events may be composed of multiple IBO's. These can be termed Compound Events. The posting of correcting entries and other types of audit information may convert an event from simple to compound. Thus it will be necessary to provide retrieval functions that will aggregate the components of a compound event and merge them into a single record for display purposes.

Formal Elements of the Model

IBO's are composed of a series of statements about context and information. Both the IBO's and the statements within them are produced by generating functions.

Abstractly we have:

$\mathcal{D} = \{D_1, D_2, \ldots\ldots, D_n\}$ The set of domains of denotational semantics.

Every system uses a variety of denotational semantics. Some may adopted from external sources such as English, SNOMED [7], the MIB Semantic Model [8] or Univ. of Utah's Event Definitions [9] while others may be developed locally such as a hospital formulary or a list of approved abbreviations.

ε = { person, unique inanimate object, nonunique inanimate object, association} The set of entity types.

$E = \{ (\varepsilon, \text{role}) \}$ The set of entity references as entity-role tuples.

Entities are an important part of most statements since they are either involved as the subjects or objects of actions. References to entities usually include a role qualifier such as "a person acting in a capacity" or "a thing used for a purpose."

$\mathcal{C}$ = {event_type, location, time, etc.} $\forall \mathcal{C}, \mathcal{C} \in \mathcal{D}$. The set of context-describing elements mapped to various domains of denotational semantics.

κ = {data, knowledge, opinion, rules, etc.} $\forall \kappa, \kappa \in \mathcal{D}$ The set of knowledge-describing elements.

$\mathcal{A} = \{ A_1, A_2, \ldots\ldots, A_n \}\ \forall \mathcal{A}, \mathcal{A} \in \mathcal{B}$. The set of actions and processes.

$\mathcal{P} = \{\text{permissions, capabilities}\}\ \forall \mathcal{P}, \mathcal{P} \in \mathcal{B}$. The set of security-describing elements.

Each of the elements used to describe context, information/knowledge, actions and permissions is described using a specific denotational method.

$\mathcal{S} = \{ S_1, S_2, \ldots\ldots, S_n \}$ The set of statement constructor functions.

$\mathcal{O} = \{ O_1, O_2, \ldots\ldots, O_n \}$ The set of IBO constructor functions.

$X = \mathcal{S}(E, \mathcal{C}, \mathcal{A}, \mathcal{P})$ A contextual statement generated by statement construction function

$I = \mathcal{S}(E, \mathcal{C}, \mathcal{A}, \mathcal{P}, \kappa)$ An informational statement generated by statement construction function.

$IBO = \mathcal{O}(\{ X_1, X_2, \ldots, X_n\},\{I_1, I_2, \ldots, I_n \})$ an IBO is composed of a group of context statements followed by a group of informational statements.

Statements and IBO's are the output of a set of functions that take entity references, context, knowledge, actions and permissions as inputs. The functions can take many forms depending on the tactics and the strategy of a particular implementation. The components of these functions represent a convenient of checklist to be satisfied by any implementation.

SUMMARY

Regardless of the techniques used to structure documents, an Information Model is necessary in order to organize and describe the content. The information model delineates the content that must be present to insure that a description of an event is fully meaningful. The elements of this model can be applied to object-oriented structures or relational constructs as well as to loosely structure documents. Up to now, the hierarchical properties of objects and the notational complexities of relational databases introduced scale-up problems. These difficulties are markedly accentuated by the need to complete the design before releasing a product. The most common response of developers has been to avoided the added complexity that would be needed to fully qualify the context of an event. Requiring adoption of and adherence to an explicit Information Model is one way to insure that the next generation of systems are capable of capturing the context necessary to make the data informative over a long period of time.

REFERENCES

1. Norman D: "Things That Make Us Smart: Defending human attributes in the age of the machine," Addison-Wesley, 1993.
2. Lincoln TL, Essin DJ and Ware WH: The Electronic Medical Record: A Challenge for Computer Science to Develop Clinically and Socially Relevant Computer Systems to Coordinate Information for Patient Care and Analysis. The Information Society Journal, Vol. 9, No. 2 (Apr-Jun 1993).
3. Essin DJ: Intelligent Processing of Loosely Structured Documents as a Strategy for Organizing Electronic Health Care Records. Methods of Information in Medicine, 32:265-68, 1993.
4. Newcomb S, Kipp N, and Newcomb V: The 'HyTime' Hypermedia/Time-based Document Structuring Language, Commun. ACM, 24:11, (November 1991), 67-83.
5. Goldfarb C: "The SGML Handbook," Oxford University Press, 1990.
6. Guha RV and Lenat DB: Enabling Agents to Work Together, Commun. ACM, 37:7, (July 1994), 127-142.
7. SNOMED International: the systematized nomenclature of human and veterinary medicine [3rd ed.], Editors: Roger A. Cote, et al., College of American Pathologists & American Veterinary Medical Association, Schaumburg, IL, 1993..
8. Gottschalk HW and Wittenber J: "MIB Software - Semantic Model: ASN.1 Messaging for a pulse Oximeter," 14th Annual Symposium on Computer Applications in Medical Care, IEEE Computer Society Press, (November 1990), 220-225.
9. Fu LS, Bouhaddou O, Huff, SM, Sorenson DK and Warner HR: "Toward a Public Domain UMLS Patient Database," 14th Annual Symposium on Computer Applications in Medical Care, IEEE Computer Society Press, (November 1990), 170-174.

A High-Level Object-Oriented Model for Representing Relationships in an Electronic Medical Record

Robert H. Dolin, MD
Southern California Kaiser-Permanente
3111 W. Orange Av, Anaheim, CA 92804

ABSTRACT

The importance of electronic medical records to improve the quality and cost-effectiveness of medical care continues to be realized. This growing importance has spawned efforts at defining the structure and content of medical data, which is heterogeneous, highly inter-related, and complex. Computer-assisted data modeling tools have greatly facilitated the process of representing medical data, however the complex inter-relationships of medical information can result in data models that are large and cumbersome to manipulate and view. This report presents a high-level object-oriented model for representing the relationships between objects or entities that might exist in an electronic medical record. By defining the relationship between objects at a high level and providing for inheritance, this model enables relating any medical entity to any other medical entity, even though the relationships were not directly specified or known during data model design.

INTRODUCTION

There is a growing need to define, standardize, and model the complex informational needs of medicine. In 1991, the Institute of Medicine emphasized the need for computer-based patient records to improve the quality and cost-effectiveness of patient care [1]. In 1993, the American Hospital Association noted the importance of computerized data to evaluate the likely outcomes of alternative treatment options [2]. President William J. Clinton's American Health Security Act stresses the need for information on health outcomes and calls for national standards for information systems, clinical data, and minimal health data sets [3].

Computer-assisted data modeling tools and techniques are being used to help define the structure and content of medical data. Entity-Relationship (E-R) modeling [4] and Object-Oriented Analysis (OOA) [5] are two techniques in common use [6-9]. In E-R modeling, entities (such as ENCOUNTERS or PATIENTS) have attributes (such as SEX or ADDRESS) and relationships to one another (such as PATIENTS having MANY ENCOUNTERS). E-R models map directly into relational databases. In OOA, the E-R model is extended such that entities are referred to as objects, and inheritance is supported. Using inheritance, an object can inherit the attributes of another object. For example, if the object PERSON has attributes SEX and ADDRESS, and if the object PATIENT is a specialization of PERSON, then PATIENT inherits the attributes SEX and ADDRESS from PERSON. Object-oriented data models can map to object-oriented databases or to relational databases. The concept of the E-R relational 'primary key' remains valid in OOA, meaning that both E-R and OOA require a mechanism of identifying unique instances of entities or objects.

E-R and OOA tools graphically depict the relationship between any two entities or objects as a line connecting them. These graphical data model depictions become complex as the number of objects increases, particularly when there is a large number of relationship lines. An average data model contains 35 objects, a large model contains 110, and for domains with several sub-domains there may be 200 to 500 objects [5]. If all objects related to all other objects, the number of relationships would be calculable using the formula $n(n-1)/2$, where n equals the number of objects. The Message Standards Developers Subcommittee of the American National Standards Institute Healthcare Informatics Standards Planning Panel (ANSI-HISPP) has developed a rough-cut high-level data model of the healthcare domain wherein approximately fifty medical objects are discussed [7]. If each of these objects related to each other, the number of relationships would equal $n(n-1)/2 = 50(49)/2 = 1225$. In addition, objects of a single class may relate to one another, there may be more than one relationship between two objects, and normalization of each many-to-many relationship potentially results in a new object and relationship.

One approach to managing all these inter-relationships is to find an attribute that is common to all objects or entities. A consideration for this common attribute is TIME, meaning that two objects occurring at the same TIME for the same patient are assumed to relate to one another. For example, a patient having an ENCOUNTER at one TIME also has a PROCEDURE performed at the same TIME. One can infer that the PROCEDURE occurred during the ENCOUNTER. This solution will work in many situations, but in others, a precise relationship must be made and documented. A lab test result that was available during the time a patient was being seen does not necessarily indicate that the provider saw the result.

Obviously, every object will not need to relate to every other object. However there are a great number of required and potentially important relationships. The relationship of SYMPTOMS to PROBLEMS is necessary to support Weed's Problem-Oriented Medical Record [10]. Outcome analysis requires knowing the SERVICES that were provided for each PROBLEM [11,12]. Healthcare reform requires knowing the relationship between ORDERS and their INDICATIONS. When automated decision support is used, a provider may document the ALGORITHM used to arrive at a DIAGNOSIS or TREATMENT PLAN. Other relationships of potential interest include SYMPTOMS or RESULTS that support a DIAGNOSIS; ENCOUNTERS that address a certain PROBLEM; ORDERS generated during an ENCOUNTER; MEDICATIONS administered during a SERVICE or prescribed during an ENCOUNTER; and more.

Rather then attempting to exhaustively identify and define every potential relationship that might exist in an electronic medical record, the model described in this report provides a high-level mechanism for relating any two objects, whether they be instances of the same object, or two different objects.

DESCRIPTION OF MODEL

Figure 1 gives a brief review of the modeling techniques used in this report. The graphical representation of objects, entities and relationships are not fully standardized. The Medical Informatics Technical Committee of the European Committee for Standardization (CEN / TC251) represents object relationships slightly different in two of its preliminary standards documents [6,8]. United States medical informatics standards are commonly modeled using the representation described in [5]. This nomenclature is used by the ANSI-HISPP in describing its high-level data model of the healthcare domain [7] and by the Institute of Electrical and Electronic Engineers (IEEE) medical device communications standards [9]. The model described here will follow the representation described in [5].

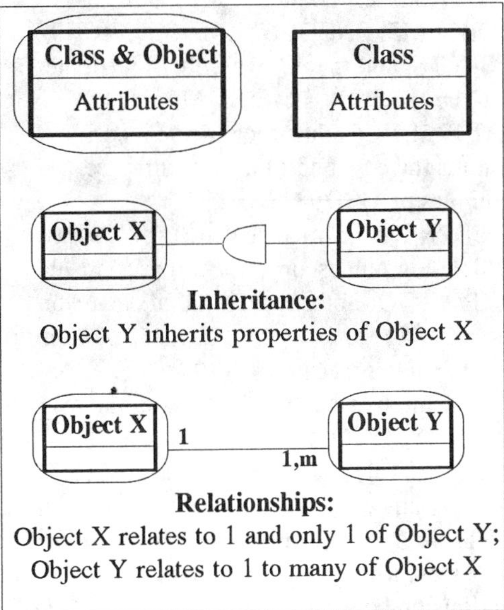

Figure 1. Object-Oriented Modeling Representation.

The high-level object-oriented data model for representing relationships among the objects or entities in an electronic medical record is shown in Figure 2. The object MEDICAL ENTITY OCCURRENCE represents the occurrence of a

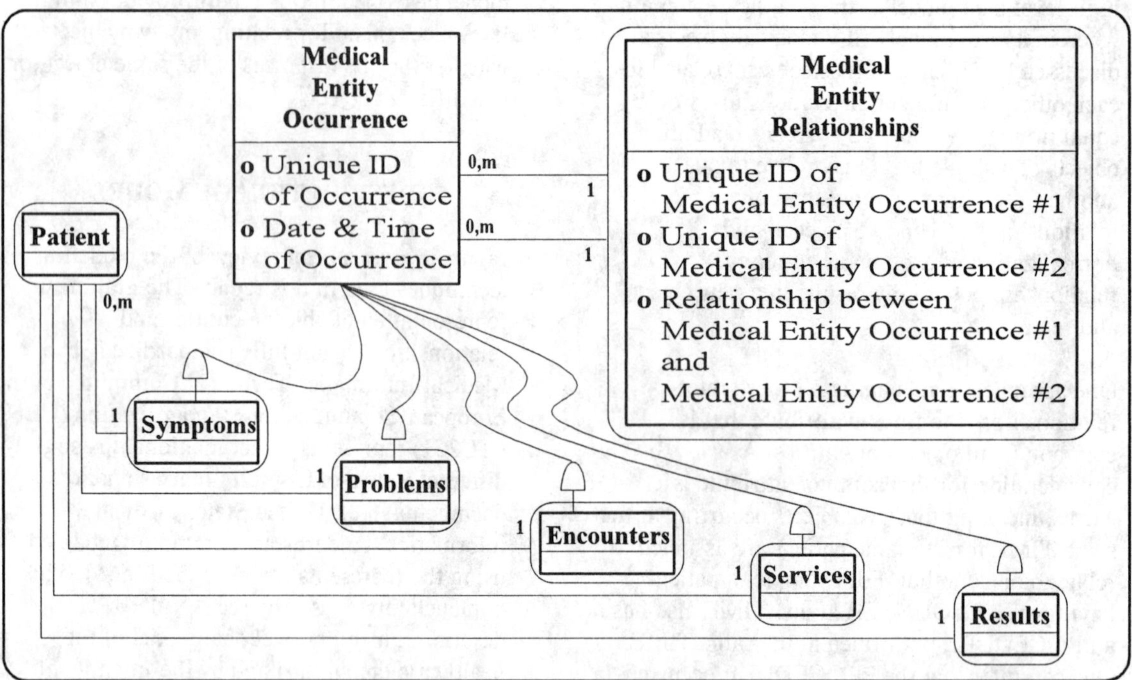

Figure 2. A high-level object-oriented data model for specifying relationships among objects in an electronic medical record.

medical entity at a specific date and time. Medical entities include SYMPTOMS, PROBLEMS, ENCOUNTERS, SERVICES, RESULTS, and more. They inherit attributes from the object class MEDICAL ENTITY OCCURRENCE, thus each medical entity contains the date and time of occurrence. Examples of MEDICAL ENTITY OCCURRENCES include the SERVICE of a Flexible Sigmoidoscopy on February 3, 1994; the SYMPTOM of Chest Pain that occurs on December 11, 1993; or the RESULT of a serum sodium value on March 24, 1994. The relationship between PATIENT and the medical entities SYMPTOMS, PROBLEMS, ENCOUNTERS, SERVICES, and RESULTS is zero-to-many on the PATIENT side, meaning a PATIENT can have at least zero and at most many instances of the entity occurrence. The relationship between each medical entity and PATIENT is one, meaning that each occurrence is specific to one and only one PATIENT.

MEDICAL ENTITY OCCURRENCES are associated with one another in a many-to-many relationship, since any entity occurrence may need to be related to one or more other entity occurrences. Because attributes are necessary to fully describe the relationship between two MEDICAL ENTITY OCCURRENCES, the many-to-many relationship is normalized resulting in the creation of the object MEDICAL ENTITY RELATIONSHIPS. This object has an attribute 'Relationship Between Medical Entity Occurrence #1 and Medical Entity Occurrence #2' which is used to describe the nature of the relationship between two MEDICAL ENTITY OCCURRENCES, such as SYMPTOMS that SUPPORT THE DIAGNOSIS OF a particular DIAGNOSIS, or ORDERS that ARE ORDERED BECAUSE OF particular PROBLEMS.

Note further in Figure 2, the attribute 'Unique ID of Occurrence' of object MEDICAL ENTITY OCCURRENCE. Several authors note the potential pitfalls of trying to determine a unique object identifier during data model design, and feel it is preferable to defer its consideration to the implementation phase [5,7]. While the model in Figure 2 does show a unique identifier for medical entities, it does not attempt to fully define what that identifier should be. But the model does include the unique identifier as an inheritable attribute. In this way, all specializations of MEDICAL ENTITY OCCURRENCE, such as SYMPTOMS and PROBLEMS, will have their own unique identifier structured in the same way. If each object structured its unique identifier in a different way, it would be difficult or impossible for a single table to store relationships between any two objects. But by providing for the inheritance of a common unique identifier, this model guarantees that all unique identifiers will have a common structure, thus enabling all specializations of MEDICAL ENTITY OCCURRENCE to be related to one another in MEDICAL ENTITY RELATIONSHIPS.

The unique identifier of an object is generally system dependent and implementation specific, therefore only general strategies can be described here. One approach is to use a standardized medical coding scheme, such as SNOMED International [13], to codify all medical entities. Then, a unique identifier might equal: Patient ID + SNOMED Code + Date & Time of occurrence. However, in a fully implemented electronic medical record, multiple providers may describe the same entity as it occurred at the same date and time. In fact, a single provider may describe the same entity herself again at a later date. Thus, the unique identifier may need to include Provider ID and Date & Time entered. Another approach is to allow the system to assign a unique sequence number to each entity occurrence, in which case the unique identifier of Patient ID + SNOMED Code + Sequence Number may suffice. However, if a given SNOMED code can be recorded in more then one table, the unique identifier may need to include the table name. In this case the unique identifier might simply be: Table Name + Sequence Number.

The following scenario illustrates how the proposed data model allows any object to relate to any other object. A patient seen in clinic today reports a symptom of chest pain that occurred three days ago. An electrocardiogram is performed and is normal. The provider orders a treadmill test. The clinic visit is an ENCOUNTER; chest pain is a SYMPTOM; the normal ECG is a RESULT; the treadmill test is an ORDER. Any of these MEDICAL ENTITY OCCURRENCES can be related to any other in MEDICAL ENTITY RELATIONSHIPS. This is shown in Table 1.

Table 1. Relating Medical Entity Occurrences.

ENTITY1 ID*	ENTITY2 ID*	RELATIONSHIP
Clinic Visit	Chest Pain	Elicited During
Clinic Visit	ECG	Ordered During
Clinic Visit	ECG	Reviewed During
Clinic Visit	Treadmill	Ordered During
ECG	Chest Pain	Reason for Order
Treadmill	Chest Pain	Reason for Order

* The actual values stored are the unique identifiers.

DISCUSSION

The preceding discussion has shown how any medical entity can be related to any other medical entity, with provisions to record the nature of the relationship. Other existing representations of medical information can be mapped directly into this model. Several authors have described the use of conceptual graph notation as a means of modeling descriptive findings, and the use of this notation is gaining popularity [14,15]. Conceptual graph notation maps onto relational data models and first-order predicate calculus, and is supported by the data model described in this report. Concepts or conceptual nodes in conceptual graph notation correspond to entity occurrences and conceptual relations map to attribute 'Relationship Between Medical Entity Occurrence #1 and Medical Entity Occurrence #2' of object MEDICAL ENTITY RELATIONSHIPS. The many-to-many relationship between MEDICAL ENTITY OCCURRENCES also supports the construction of polyhierarchies, and can therefore map to directed acyclic graphs [16] and semantic networks [17], which are other schemes used for representing information.

The process of defining, representing and managing all potential relationships in an electronic medical record using standard Entity-Relationship or Object-Oriented tools can result in a tremendous number of tables needing to maintained, and a pictorial view of the data model that is covered with hundreds to thousands of relationship lines and normalized relational tables. However, by defining a standard representation for the Unique_ID (or relational 'primary key') for each medical object or entity, relationships between all entities can be defined using the high-level object-oriented model defined in this report. Limitations to this model include the inability to show mandatory relationships, such as that between a SERVICE and its corresponding ORDER. However, this model does not preclude explicit representation of known mandatory relationships.

In summary then, standards in medical informatics continue to gain importance as the need for reliable electronic medical data grows. A standardized unique identifier allows an electronic medical record to record important relationships between any two medical entities even though the relationships were not directly specified or known during data model design.

Acknowledgments

Special thanks to the Southern California Kaiser-Permanente Patient Care Data Modeling Team.

REFERENCES

[1]. Institute of Medicine, Committee on Improving the Patient Record. The Computer-Based Patient Record: An Essential Technology for Health Care. Washington, DC: National Academy Press; 1991:190.

[2]. American Hospital Association. Toward a National Health Information Infrastructure. Report of the Work Group on Computerization of Patient Records to the Secretary of the U.S. Department of Health and Human Services, April 1993.

[3]. Clinton, WJ. American Health Security Act (Working Group Draft). The White House Domestic Policy Council, September 7, 1993.

[4]. Barker R. CASE Method - Entity Relationship Modeling. Reading, Mass: Addison-Wesley; 1990.

[5]. Coad P, Yourdon E. Object-oriented Analysis. 2nd Edition. Prentice Hall; 1991.

[6]. CEN (European Committee for Standardization)/ Technical Committee 251 - Medical Informatics. Project Team 009 - Data interchange methodology for administrative and clinical data using intermittently connected devices. Interim Draft. CEN/TC251/PT009. January 12, 1994.

[7]. HISPP/MSDS Joint Working Group for a Common Data Model, "Trial Use Standard for Medical Data Interchange--Information Model Methods" IEEE P1157.1, draft 1, 6/6/94.

[8]. CEN (European Committee for Standardization)/ Technical Committee 251 - Medical Informatics. Project Team 002 - Terminology and coding systems of medical procedures. Interim Draft. CEN/TC251/PT002. November 10, 1993.

[9]. Institute for Electrical and Electronic Engineers. Standard for medical device communications - Overview and framework. IEEE P1073. Andover, MA; IEEE; 1992.

[10]. Weed LL. Medical records that guide and teach. NEJM 1968; 278:593-600.

[11]. Rozewski CM, Yahnke DP, Gottlieb MS, Hoffmann RG. A process for obtaining patient clinical information in the ambulatory setting. Computers and Biomedical Research 1993; 26(5):482-495.

[12]. Ellwood PM. Shattuck lecture - Outcomes management: A technology of patient experience. NEJM 1988; 318(23):1549-1556.

[13]. Cote RA, Rothwell DJ, Beckett RS, Palotay JL (Eds). SNOMED International - The systematized nomenclature of human and veterinary medicine. Northfield, Il; College of American Pathologists; 1993.

[14]. Campbell KE, Das AK, Musen MA. A logical foundation for representation of clinical data. J Am Med Informatics Assoc 1994; 1(3): 218-232.

[15]. Bernauer J. Conceptual graphs as an operational model for descriptive findings. SCAMC 1992; 214-218.

[16]. De Vries W, Eidelman DH. Acyclic directed graphs for automatic image analysis of lung parenchymal geometry. Computers and Biomedical Research 1993; 26(4): 344-352.

[17]. Lindberg DAB, Humphreys BL, McCray AT. The Unified Medical Language System. In: van Bemmel JH, McCray AT (Eds). Yearbook of Medical Informatics. The Netherlands; IMIA Publications; 1993, pg 41-51.

An Infrastructure for Cooperation and Communication in an Advanced Clinical Information System

K. Kuhn[1], M. Reichert[2], M. Nathe[2], T. Beuter[2], P. Dadam[2]
[1]Medical University Hospital, University of Ulm, Germany
[2]Dept. Databases and Information Systems, University of Ulm, Germany

ABSTRACT

In a research project, organizational and technological requirements for an advanced clinical information system have been analysed, and a concept has been developed. From the application's perspective, medical personnel is more actively relieved from routine tasks by support of organizational tasks and by coordination of distributed activities. Program development is supported by a concept of simple and complex services with well-defined interfaces, and by the use of activity templates, i.e. pre-modeled activities describing possible sequences of services. The concept is based on an open systems approach, with a reliable and secure communication infrastructure. In addition, monitoring facilities are provided.

INTRODUCTION

In the development of hospital information systems, several trends of increasing importance are emerging. Today, physicians confronted with a massive load of data, that have to be intellectually processed and structured, tend to make mistakes, such as overlooking rare events [1].

An advanced computer-based system should therefore increase the availability of patient specific information and present it in a structured way. Moreover, it should relieve medical personnel from tracking the state of medical activities like processing of an order, and from caring about the timely collection of information about the outcomes.

In addition, medical and organizational tasks are highly interrelated, especially if scheduling is involved. In typical activities, several parties at different sites interact at various points of time. From modeling organizational aspects inherent in medical activities, and from an active support of cooperation, positive effects can be expected.

Furthermore, physicians have to select tests and interventions under aspects like invasiveness, efficiency and costs. Here, system support of medical guidelines [2] and consequently the representation of medical knowledge inherent in complex medical activities will become increasingly important.

The outlined need of systems playing a more active role has to be seen in the context of general tendencies in hardware and software development, that can also be observed in the medical environment. The number of heterogeneous and decentralized application modules is increasing, while centralized solutions, which tend to be too static, are going to play a less important role [3]. This development is combined with an increase in application-oriented programming skills and fewer personnel with system know-how in computing centres. Therefore, an appropriate software engineering environment *for developing secure and stable distributed applications* is mandatory. In addition, a reliable communication framework with *sufficient monitoring facilities* is needed.

This paper presents first results of a research project, which is aimed at the systematic analysis of organizational and technological requirements for an advanced hospital information system. The basic concepts developed and an exploratory prototype will be described.

0195-4210/94/$5.00

BASIC CONCEPTS

Distributed, heterogeneous systems are integrated by means of a *software bus* [4,5,6], which offers *services* to applications, and abstracts from heterogeneity and distribution (see Fig. 1). The concept of services with well-defined interfaces has been introduced to reduce the need of system know-how for application programmers.

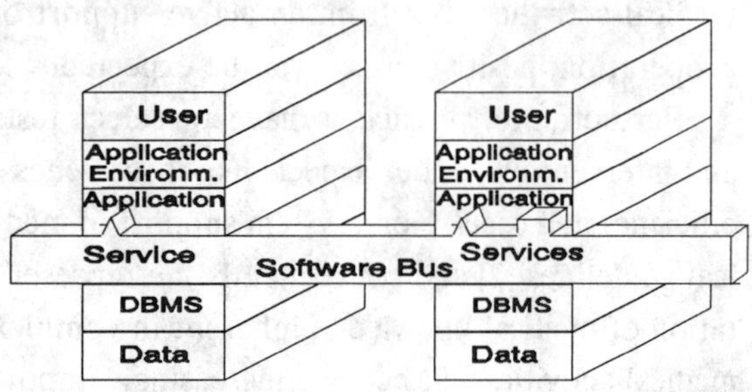

Figure 1. Simplified model illustrating the software bus [4].

Services are provided or utilized by application components called *agents* [7]. *Basic* services are executed by single agents. *Complex* services consist of several basic services executed in parallel or sequentially; they may be nested. Examples of complex services, which are typically handled by distributed agents, are the entry of an order into a local (e.g. ward) as well as into a remote (e.g. radiology) database, or the notification of a patient transmission to the local and to several remote (departmental, administrative) systems. To guarantee consistency, extended *transaction concepts* are used, if the two phase commit protocol is too restrictive [8,4]. For these cases, compensation methods necessary to undo each basic service have to be provided; these compensation methods are used for *semantic rollback* of complex services.

Organizational knowledge inherent in clinical tasks is being modeled under the *concept of medical processes or activities*, which are executed by several distributed agents over time. To *actively support and coordinate* the execution of typical activities like processing of an order (from order entry to transmission of the results, possibly including scheduling), or patient transmission, activity templates supporting the coordinated execution of services are used. Activities can be tracked by users, and, more important, by watchdog agents without need of user interaction. It is possible to react on problems and to issue reminders (e.g. in the case of unexpected delays or loss of a sample).

Descriptions of data, services, and agents are kept in a repository [9]. To support application programmers, medical data, especially the medical record, are managed under an object system which abstracts from distribution and from technical details like physical storage or replication. Services are built upon predefined (medical) object classes and upon methods for the access and management of objects and for graphical presentation.

The concept assumes the existence of a medical entities dictionary. As there are considerable research efforts in this area [e.g.10], this project intends to build upon their results.

Cooperation Infrastructure

As outlined, the system plays a more active role for users and for developers than a pure message handling approach. In addition and as a consequence, it has to maintain a consistent distributed state in the situation of concurrent, potentially interfering activities and in the case of system problems like node failures, network disruptions, or faulty service implementations. The components proposed for the necessary coordination of distributed services and their underlying communication infrastructure are shown in Fig. 2, which will be explained in the next sections.

Service Processing. Users interact with agents. Agents issue service requests, which are sent to the local task manager. The *task manager* stores the request. This persistent request handling is needed for requests that cannot be executed immediately (e.g. a service has to wait for remote

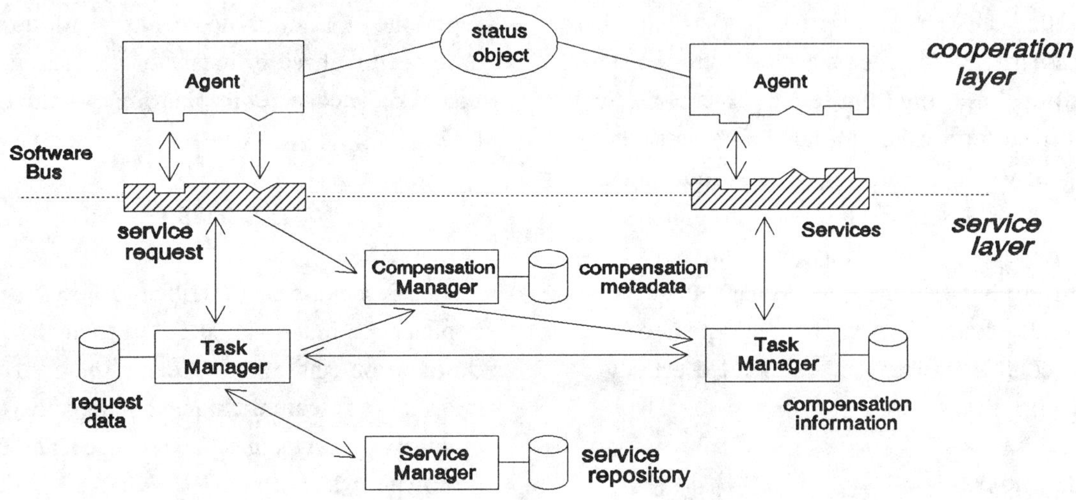

Figure 2: Cooperation Infrastructure (partial view)

user interaction) and for the case of system problems (e.g. a call has to be repeated if a remote system was not available). The task manager calls a *service manager* acting as a global request broker [11], which selects a task manager running on a node offering the requested service. The request is forwarded to the selected task manager, which activates the corresponding agent. This agent executes the service and results are passed back to the task manager on the client node. The client task manager removes the corresponding request entry from its logfile and forwards the results to the requesting agent. The information necessary to compensate a basic service is stored by the task manager at the host side.

In analogy to database transactions, services can be combined into blocks which represent complex services or activities, and which can be nested. A *compensation manager* receives the appropriate nesting information whenever basic services are executed; it also handles compensation requests.

Activity Modeling and Control. The *development* of distributed applications is difficult and error prone. Therefore, to the application programmer, a graphical tool [5] will be offered for *modeling* activities. Here, pre-modeled activities (activity templates) which are kept in the repository, can be used and modified. These activity templates describe

- the states an activity may go through
- the kinds of services that can be called in the context of the given type of activity (where services are classified as system-driven or as user-driven)
- possible state transitions (caused by service executions)
- data flow
- parameters holding auxiliary information like time constraints
- the call interface of the activity as a whole.

The *application programmer* is composing concrete activities using activity templates. The two main tasks are to assign (where still necessary) appropriate service implementations to the corresponding entries in the templates, and to connect the in/out interfaces of the activity to the application environment.

At *run-time*, an instantiated activity template is passed to the local agent which informs all other agents involved in the activity. Each activity in execution is represented by one global status object (logical view, see [12] for possible implementation details). This status object is modified by the participating agents according to the state transitions resulting from service executions. System-driven services are initiated automatically by an agent when a matching state is found in the status object. User-driven services are initiated by user interaction. Time constraints for state transitions are handled by watchdog agents querying the status objects. They enable the system to warn the user, if, for example, a scheduled activity is about to fail.

Further aspects

In this paper, the *basic* infrastructure has been presented in some detail. In addition, and to introduce "intelligent" system behavior, there a specialized agents like planning agents, scheduling agents, and knowledge agents [13]. These agents cooperate in order to support the planning, supervision and execution of complex medical activities according to medical guidelines. The planning agent takes into account dynamic inter-activity dependencies; as an example, an actual result of a laboratory examination may be needed before the next examination starts.

PROTOTYPE IMPLEMENTATION

Although some of the described manager components and the global data resemble a centralized approach, they have to be implemented in a distributed way. To better understand the interaction of modules, an exploratory prototype has been implemented based on UNIX, OSF/DCE, C++ and the relational DBMS INGRES. For presentation services, X11 and InterViews [14] are used. Example activities have been realized as distributed DCE applications. Task managers communicate by means of the DCE Remote Procedure Call mechanism. Authorization and authentification are based on the DCE security service. Service managers utilize the DCE cell directory service. Compensation data and task data have been made persistent by using INGRES. Object methods are implemented on top of the SQL level. Medical Logic Modules [13] have been realized by means of the classification-based knowledge representation system LOOM [15].

DISCUSSION

The basic idea of the described project was not to implement a functional HIS, but to analyse application problems and to relate them to recent informatics research. Under this objective, an exploratory prototype has been realized, and further prototypes will follow.

Related Work

In the HELIOS project [6], a software bus has been used in a comparable way. There are differences, however, in the scope and functionality of the services, as well as in mechanisms for error handling and guaranteeing consistency.

The Kernel $K/2_R$ [5] approach shows an increased functionality compared to HELIOS. S-transactions [8] and workflow management have been integrated.

For the medical environment, several approaches for integrating heterogeneous systems have been presented [e.g.3,16,17] which have resulted in functional systems.

An approach close to the one outlined has been described by Gangopadhyay and Wu [18]. The importance of modeling and automating medical processes is stressed by these authors in the same way as in our concept. Their approach is object-oriented as well, and they use a finite state machine similar to our description of state transitions.

Finally, there are parallels to the RICHE project [19], where knowledge servers and the idea of 'act management' have been introduced.

Conclusion

In actual systems of the medical environment, co-operation mechanisms of the proposed scope are not yet playing an important role. In our opinion, however, these concepts are definitely helpful. A positive effect on the coordination and support of (distributed) clinical processes as well as on application programming can be expected. The high level modeling approach is flexible, and it should help to reduce programming errors. Besides supporting program development at a higher level of semantics, the concept also provides a stable and reliable communication platform. In general, the acceptance of clinical systems will depend on their reliability and on the flexibility of both applications and application design.

Acknowledgement: The authors are grateful to Drs. G.Adler, K.Beckh, B.Böhm, H.Heimpel, M.Reinshagen, and A.Seibold for valuable discussions on application questions and to C.Heinlein for technical discussions. This work was supported by a research grant of the State of Baden-Württemberg, Germany.

References

1. McDonald CJ, Tierney WM. Computer-Stored Medical Records. JAMA 1988, 259:3433-3440.
2. Audet A-M, Greenfield S, Field M. Medical Practice Guidelines; Current Activities and Future Directions. Ann Intern Med 1990, 113: 703-714.
3. Clayton PD, Sideli RV, Sengupta S. Open Architecture and Integrated Information at Columbia-Presbyterian Medical Center. MD Computing 1992, 9: 297-303.
4. Kuhn K, Reichert M, Nathe M, Beuter T, Heinlein C, Dadam P. A Conceptual Approach to an Open Hospital Information System. In: Barahona P, Veloso M, Bryant J (eds) Proc 12th Intl Congr Europ Federation Med Informatics (MIE 94), Lisbon, 1994: 374-378.
5. Adomeit R, Deiters W, Holtkamp B, Schülke F, Weber F. $K/2_R$: A Kernel for the ESF Software Factory Support Environment. In: Systems Integration '92, Proc 2nd Intl Conf Sys Integration. Ng PA, Ramamoorthy CV, Seifert LC, Yeh RT (eds). Los Alamitos: IEEE Comp Soc Press, 1992: 325-336.
6. Jean FC, Jaulent MC, Coignard J, Degoulet P. Distribution and Communication in Software Engineering Environments. Application to the HELIOS Software Bus. In: Proc 15th SCAMC 1991, Clayton P (ed). New York: McGraw-Hill, 1992: 506-510.
7. Lee KC, Mansfield WH, Sheth AP. A Framework for Controlling Cooperative Agents. IEEE Computer 1993, 26(7): 8-16.
8. Elmargarmid AK (ed). Database Transaction Models for Advanced Applications. San Mateo CA: Morgan Kaufmann, 1992.
9. Hsu C, Bouziane M, Rattner L, Yee L. Information Resource Management in Heterogeneous, Distributed Environments. IEEE Trans SE 1991, 17: 604-25.
10. Cimino JJ, Clayton PD, Hripcsak G, Johnson SB. Knowledge-based Approaches to the Maintenance of a Large Controlled Medical Terminology. JAMIA 1994, 1: 35-50.
11. Nicol JR, Wilkes T, Manola FA. Object Orientation in Heterogeneous Distributed Computing Systems. IEEE Computer 1993, 26(6): 57-67.
12. Schill A, Malhotra A. Language and Distributed System Support for Complex Organizational Services. In: Conference on Organizational Computing Systems, 1991, SIGOIS Bulletin 12, 1991, no 2,3.
13. Heinlein C, Kuhn K, Dadam P. Representation of Medical Guidelines on Top of a Classification-based System. To appear in: Proc 3rd Intl Conf Information and Knowledge Management (CIKM), Gaithersburg, MD, 1994.
14. Linton M, Vlissides J, Calder P. Composing User Interfaces with InterViews. IEEE Computer 1989, 22(2): 8-22.
15. MacGregor R. The Evolving Technology of Classification-Based Knowledge Representation Systems. In: Sowa JF (ed) Principles of Semantic Networks. San Mateo: Morgan-Kaufmann, 1991, 385-400.
16. Van Mulligen EM, Timmers T, van Bemmel JH. A New Architecture for Integration of Heterogeneous Components. Meth Inf Med 1993, 32: 292-301.
17. Gierl L, Greiller R, Landersdorfer D, Müller H, Überla K. A User-oriented Protocol for Integrating Heterogeneous Communication Systems of Medical Facilities Using Ports. Meth Inf Med 1989, 28: 97-103.
18. Gangopadhyay D, Wu PYF. An Object-Oriented Approach to Medical Process Automation. In: Proc 17th SCAMC 1993. Safran C (ed). New York: McGraw-Hill, 1993: 507-511.
19. The RICHE Consortium: RICHE Final Report. Louveciennes, France, 1992.

An Object-Oriented Tool for the Generation and Management of Multimedia Patient Folders

Domenico M. Pisanelli[1], Fernando Ferri[2], Fabrizio L. Ricci[2]
Consiglio Nazionale delle Ricerche, 1-ITBM, 2-ISRDS, V. C. De Lollis 12, 00185 Roma, Italy
isrd1@vm.cnuce.cnr.it

ABSTRACT

Computer-based patient folders are evolving from the simple reproduction of traditional paper documents toward active tools, able to support the whole diagnostic and therapeutic process. The advent of multimediality has given emphasys to the idea of computerized folder, i.e. a collection of heterogeneous kinds of documents pertaining different media.

In this paper we present a tool implementing generation and management of multimedia patient folders showing its architecture and functionalities and the innovative interaction paradigms adopted. The tool realized allows medical users to choose the concepts desired in their target application and generates a customized patient folder management system by means of a friendly interface and without the need of a programming language. The system automatically created can be effectively employed for reporting and storing clinical cases.

1. INTRODUCTION

The patient folder is the essential support for documenting the process of care, but also for assisting ward management, filing and evaluation of health-care quality.

If we review the computer applications realized so far, it is clear that there is no model sharable by everyone. HL7 addresses the problem of structuring the electronic data exchange in healthcare environments [1], whereas in Europe standardization activity is carried on by the CEN with respect to the structure of the electronic patient record [2].

Each application implemented so far is optimized with respect to the peculiar function to be performed (e.g.: clinical support, data interchange, statistical analysis, legal documentation). Such heterogeneity reflects the different perspectives of the users and the quest for commonalities would be useless. Anyhow, an emerging trend during the years is the transition from passive documentation to active support. Among the most relevant achievements we may quote: the "Problem Oriented Medical Record", [3], the "Decision Directed Medical Record" [4] and more recently "PEN&PAD" [5].

This work was partially supported by the Commission of the European Union under the DG XIII - AIM programme, MILORD project.

Computer-based patient folders are less and less a mere reproduction of the traditional paper documents. The advent of multimediality has especially fostered their evolution toward an active tool, able to sustain the whole diagnostic and therapeutic process. From the concept of *medical record* as a structured set of information, emphasis has been given to the idea of *folder*, i.e. a collection of heterogeneous kinds of documents pertaining different media.

The question is no longer the definition of the model best fitting the physician's requirements, but the creation of a folder that from clinical requirements is able to adapt the information layout, namely which information has to be managed and in which way it must be shown.

In this paper we present a tool implementing generation and management of multimedia patient folders. In the next paragraph its architecture is sketched out, whereas the third one illustrates the innovative user-interaction paradigms adopted.

2. THE OBJECT-ORIENTED DESIGN AND THE ARCHITECTURE OF THE SYSTEM

Physicians usually do not share the same concepts in managing information about their patients. It is expected that every patient folder management system will include slots for personal data, main symptoms and diagnostic images. In addition, some physician might consider familiar anamnesis, others would like to see the staging of a disease and so on.

The tool described in this paragraph allows medical users to choose the concepts to be present in their target application starting from scratch or from a default configuration. It generates a customized patient folder management system by means of a friendly interface and without employing a programming language. The system automatically created can be effectively used for reporting and storing clinical cases. It will be always possible to modify its structure according to future requirements.

The tool supports multimediality, managing texts and images in an integrated way. The impact that such an

0195-4210/94/$5.00 © 1994 AMIA, Inc.

integration may achieve on the users is not to be stressed here. We plan to incorporate bio-signals and voice annotation in future releases.
The tool runs on Macintosh platform and has been developed using the Prograph® programming environment. A case-study has been carried out and resulted in the definition of a multimedia patient folder used experimentally by the 4th Surgical Clinic of the University Hospital of Rome. Since this project is carried on under a European Union funded initiative, English is the language adopted for the interface which must be shared and validated by the other partners. However, clinical data of the case-study are directly entered in Italian.

The overall architecture of the system is composed by the following five modules [6]:

a) patient folder designer
b) multimedia patient folder manager
c) presentation manager
d) user interface
e) user models manager

a) patient folder designer

Physicians use this module to define the structure of the folder. They choose the concepts relevant for their clinical purposes which will be included in the target application. This activity generates an object-oriented model of medical concepts, where the classic relationships hold: generalization (IS_A) and aggregation (PART_OF). Therefore different levels of abstractions may be defined and each concept may be broken down into more elementary concepts and vice-versa.
The taxonomy of concepts created by means of this model is isomorphic to the logical organization of data in the folder. Figure 1 reports a fragment of such an organization, as it might have been defined by a physician .

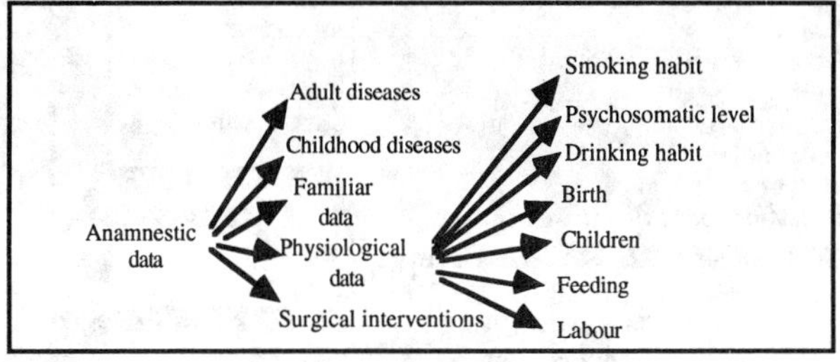

Figure 1
A fragment of a possible taxonomy of concepts

In this way it is possible to say that Adult diseases, Childhood diseases, Family data, Physiological data and Surgical interventions are not only Anamnestic data but also the concepts which in the patient folder constitute the anamnestic data. Likewise, Smoking habit, Psychosomatic level, Drinking habit, Birth, Children, Feeding and Labour are Physiological data.
Depending on his/her own particular specialization, a physician can organize the medical folder to suit himself/herself. Every physician is free to add or delete an exam and re-arrange the corresponding taxonomy of concepts in order to conform to his/her requirements.

Figure 2 shows the interface of the designer which manages these concepts. In the example shown "rectosigmoidoscopy" is being added and will be a slot in the patient folder that the tool is going to define. The picture shows also the features to be chosen for "rectosigmoidoscopy" In this case data type is "hypermedia", this means that the system will allow links between sentences and details of an image. The "Time dimension" window accounts for the temporal phases which are clinically relevant for the entities [6]. In this case all the phases make sense and the user enables them by clicking on the corresponding boxes.

b) multimedia patient folder manager

This module retrieves and stores the information that constitute the contents of the medical folders by means of a relational DBMS which is able to handle images and texts in an integrated way.

c) presentation manager

The presentation manager is the kernel of the system. It determines the access to the patient folder data by processing the users' queries (handled by the user interface module). According to the user profile, it also select which information the interface has to show and in which way.

d) user interface

The human-computer interaction is managed by this module. It follows the requirements reported in the user models manager which are processed by the presentation manager. The system is able to create run-time the windows needed to show the user's required information. Object-oriented design allows to encapsulate behavioral features into classes of objects and to propagate them by means of the inheritance mechanism (e.g.: from "endoscopic exam" to "duodenoscopy"). This capability is exploited in the interface management, with respect to data presentation and manipulation requirements (see §3).

e) user models manager

The acquisition and storage of user models is achieved by means of this module. The user model formalizes the knowledge needed to implement the interaction between the physician and the system. It stores assumptions on those user aspects relevant to the system's behavior in the interaction session.

3. THE INTERACTION PARADIGMS

The dynamic management of the interface is a peculiar feature of this tool. During the consultation phase of the patient folder the user may escape from the rigid structure given to the information in the designing phase. In this case the system sets up dynamically new clinical data views.

The patient folder management system is able to adopt three different interaction styles in presenting the information.

The *default presentation* provides a layout which replicates exactly the structure given to the patient folder in the designing phase. A traditional interaction is carried on, by means of an interface completely pre-defined which remains stable during the consultation.

The *selective presentation* leaves the user free to pick up the data to be shown on the monitor. Whereas in the previous interaction style, once a class of information is chosen (e.g. "anamnesis"), it must be fully visualized, here the user browses an index of information items (e.g. a list of laboratory exams) and selects among them the most relevant ones.

The *co-operative interaction* relies on the user model. Here the system has an active role and determines its behavior also without the explicit control of the user. In fact it can show not only the data selected, but also other related facts on the patient, if reported (e.g. data on the same apparatus) [7].

Figure 3 shows an example of a window dynamically defined by the system. It arranges semantically related information, allowing for hypermedia links between sentences and details of images. Multimedia features are exploited, by showing the "miniature" of a diagnostic image which, of course, can be fully visualized in a high resolution monitor (the concept of "miniature" in multimedia system has been introduced by Christodoulakis in 1986 [8]).

The system employs the following criteria to arrange the information to be shown to the user:

•*Consistency of visual organization with temporal organization.*

If a patient has been submitted to a certain exam more than once, the different instances of this exam must be shown according to their temporal order, left to right and top to bottom.

•*Information affinity*

If more than one anamnestic information is shown, they have to be grouped together and not mixed with heterogeneous information.

•*Consistency of visual organization with causal relationships.*

If there is a link of causality between two pieces of information, the visual organization must allow the user to read the cause first and then the effect.This criterium becomes particularly relevant whenever the user is pursuing a particular strategy.

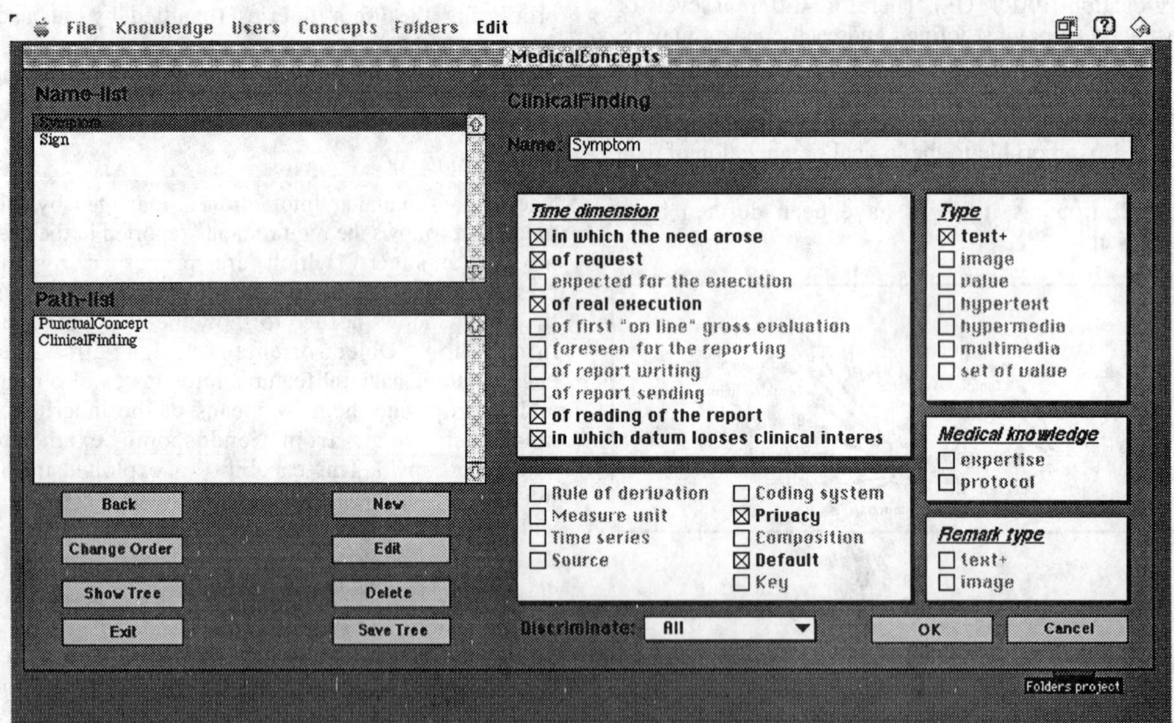

Figure 2
A sample video display output of the patient folder designer.

4. CONCLUSIONS

The ultimate aim of any computerized tool in medicine should be the improvement in the quality of care. This can be achieved also by means of a more effective information management. Its computerization, far from being trivial, is worthwhile only when aimed at improving efficiency in clinical data analysis and ward activity planning. Computerized medical folders can play a significant role by increasing the efficiency in handling clinical information and by supporting daily scheduling of ward activity.

The user must be able to handle images related to one or more patients, to make explicit semantic links with data of different nature, to navigate in a hypertextual support system, to visualize opportunely the data aggregation results, to query the system, possibly being supported by the system itself. The presentation of the patient folder as a hypermedia document is a convenient method to offer the clinical information to the user in an efficient way.

A patient folder management system should be also the active supporting tool for the creation of the physician's belief about the patient's state of health. It should be able to retrieve and to propose the most appropriate and useful information to the user. Our realization proposes a new philosophy for a patient folder management system, able to tailor the information to the user's belief, goal and knowledge about medical data.

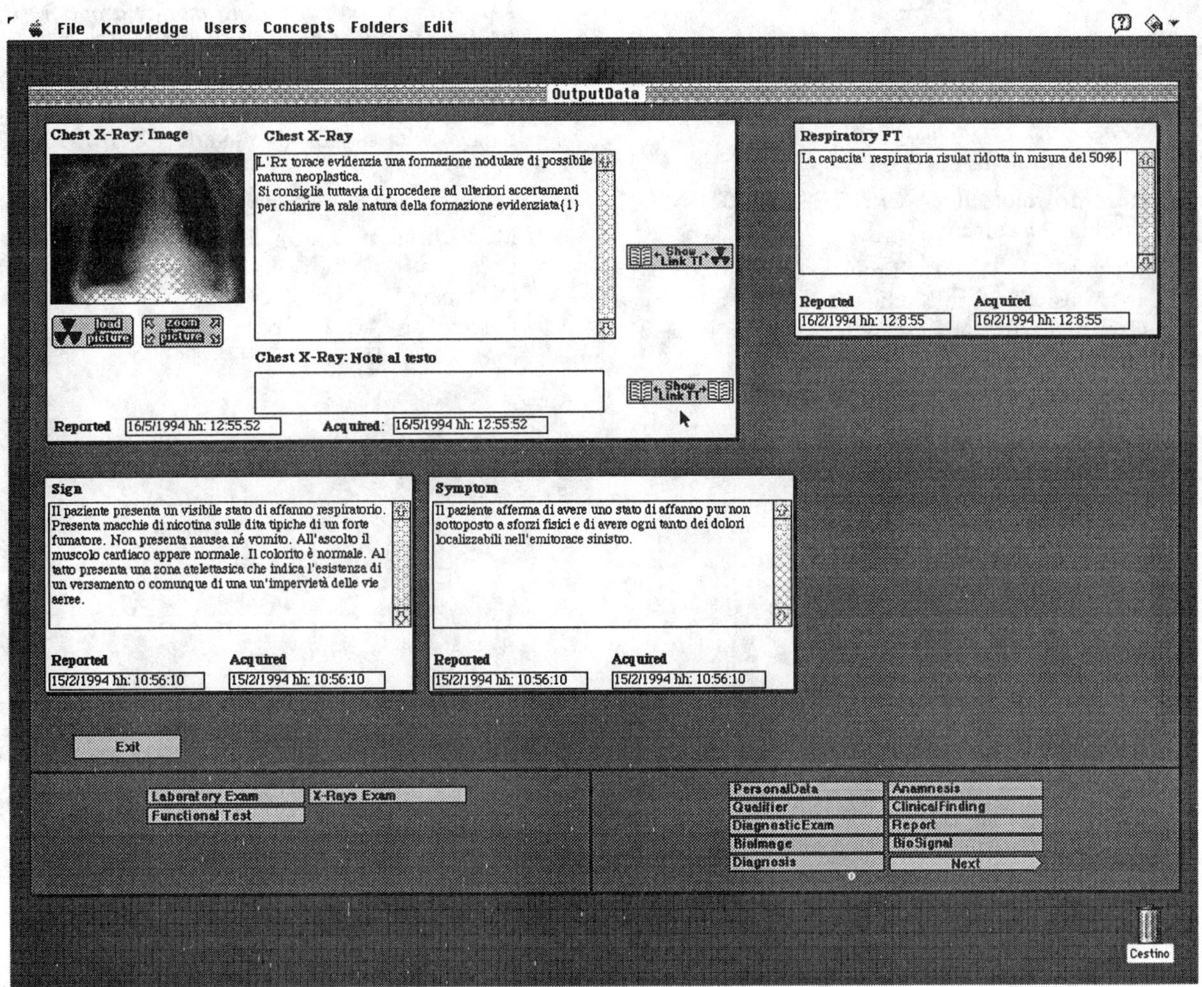

Figure 3
A set of windows semantically related of the multimedia patient folder.

ACKNOWLEDGEMENTS

Beside the authors the research group is composed by Fabrizio Consorti and other physicians of the 4th Surgical Clinic of the University Hospital of Rome. Special thanks should be given to Roberto Minarelli Della Valle and Fabrizio Tittarelli who actively participated in the design and development of the tool. We also would like to thank Luca Dan Serbanati for his precious suggestions on Object Oriented Analysis and Design and the anonymous referees for their interesting remarks. Last but not least, we thank Robert Thornton who revised the English.

REFERENCES

[1] Smith S, Dennis B (1991). "HL7: Facilitating Multiple Approaches to Systems Integration", *Computers in Healthcare,* pp.59-61.

[2] Hurlen P et al. (1994). "Electronic Health Care Record Architecture", CEN/TC251/PT011/N300 Working Document.

[3] Weed LL (1971). "The Problem Oriented Record as a Basic Tool in Medical Educations, Patient Care and Clinical Research", *Ann.Clin.Res.,* **3**, pp.131-134.

[4] Acheson HWK (1972). "The Clinical Record as an Aid to Continuing Education in General Practice", *British Journal of Medical Education,* **6**, pp.26-35.

[5] Nowlan WA, Rector AL, Kay S, Goble CA, Horan B, Howkins TJ, Wilson A (1990). "PEN&PAD: A Doctors' Workstation with Intelligent Data Entry and Summaries", in Miller R (ed.) *Proceedings SCAMC 90,* Los Alamitos (CA), IEEE-CS Press, pp. 941-942.

[6] Ricci FL, Pisanelli DM, Ferri F, Consorti F (1994). "Modeling the Structural and Behavioural Features of Medical Concepts: A Tool for Generating Multimedia Patient Folders", in: Barahona P, Veloso M, Bryant J (eds.) *Proceedings of Medical Informatic Europe (MIE) 94,* Participants' edition, pp.470-474.

[7] Ferri F, Minarelli Della Valle R, Pisanelli DM, Ricci FL (1993). "A Medical Folder Management System with an Adaptive Interface", *CNR-ISRDS Technical Report* 33-93.

[8] Christodoulakis S, Ho F, Theodoridou M, Papa M, Pathria A (1986). "Multimedia Document Presentation, Information Extraction and Document Formation in MINOS: A Model and a System", *ACM Transactions on Office Information Systems,* pp.345-383.

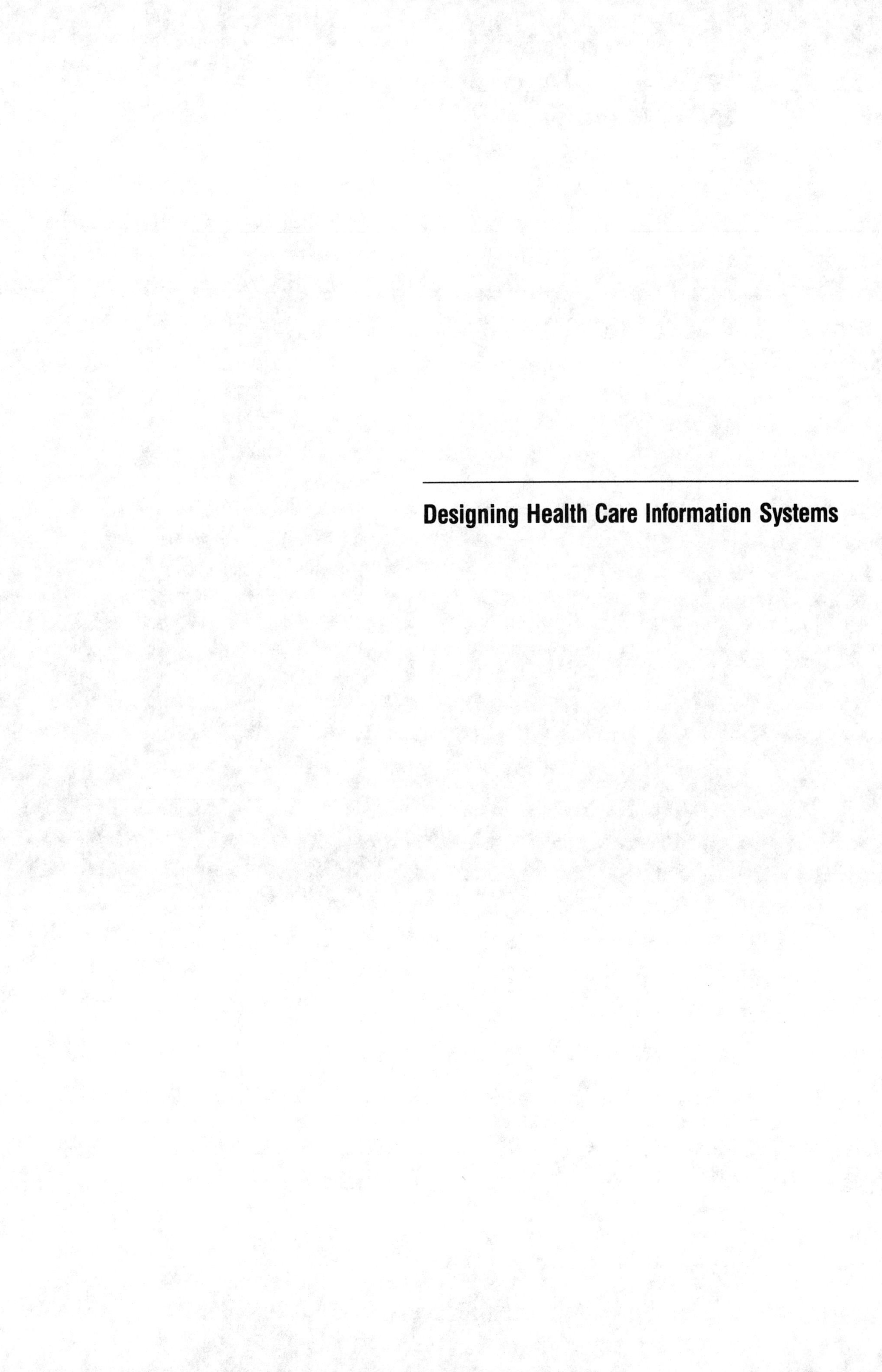

Designing Health Care Information Systems

New IEEE Standard Enables Data Collection for Medical Applications.

Robert J. Kennelly, ILC Data Device Corporation
Jan Wittenber, Hewlett-Packard Corporation

ABSTRACT

The IEEE has gone to ballot on a "Standard for Medical Device Communications", IEEE P1073. The lower layer, hardware portions of the standard are expected to be approved by the IEEE Standards Board at their December 11-13, 1994 meeting. Other portions of the standard are in the initial stages of the IEEE ballot process. The intent of the standard is to allow hospitals and other users to interface medical electronic devices to host computer systems in a standard, interchangeable manner. The standard is optimized for acute care environments such as ICU's, operating rooms, and emergency rooms. [1]

IEEE General Committee and Subcommittee work has been on-going since 1984. Significant amounts of work have been done to discover and meet the needs of the patient care setting. Surveys performed in 1989 identified the following four key user requirements for medical device communications:

1) Frequent reconfiguration of the network.
2) Allow "plug and play" operation by users.
3) Associate devices with a specific bed and patient.
4) Support a wide range of hospital computer system topologies.

Additionally, the most critical difference in the acute care setting is patient safety, which has an overall effect on the standard. The standard that went to ballot meets these requirements.

The standard is based on existing ISO standards. P1073 is compliant with the OSI seven layer model. P1073 specifies the entire communication stack, from object-oriented software to hospital unique connectors. The standard will be able to be put forward as a true international standard, much in the way that the IEEE 802.x family of standards (like Ethernet) were presented as draft ISO standards.

The standard will allow for data obtained from patient connected devices to be communicated to host computer systems for multiple purposes. Initial applications will be for data collection, enabling the development of systems for technologies such as computer based patient records. Longer term uses of the standard will include closed loop control of patient connected devices and rapid, robust reported of device status changes. The standard has been written to be accommodate these applications and is extensible for future applications. Prototype hardware has been demonstrated in conjunction with an anesthesia automatic record keeper at SUNY Stony Brook, at the AAMI show in May, 1994. Additional demonstrations have been performed at LDS Hospital and Hewlett Packard in January, 1994; at CEN TC251, Working Group 5 meeting in Madrid in March, 1994; IVAC and Imed in July, 1994; and the American Society of Anesthesiology in October, 1994.

HISTORY

The work of present AMIA members (R. Gardner, M. Shabot), starting in 1982, helped lead to the formation of an Institute of Electrical And Electronic Engineers (IEEE) standards committee in 1984. This committee was charged with writing the "Standard for Medical Device Communications", IEEE P1073. The work of this committee has been on-going since 1984 and been through several major revisions and iterations. The IEEE P1073 committee has also worked closely with several other standards developers to write a communications standard for the patient care setting. Several committees were consulted for expertise in the hospital environment. The work of the ASTM E-31.11 Technical Subcommittees, chaired by Clement McDonald (past President; AMIA), the HL-7 committees, and the X-12 committees helped to validate the requirement for the standard that the IEEE committee was working to solve. The latest revision of the IEEE standard was started in June, 1993, and was agreed to by the committee in January 1994 at a meeting at LDS Hospital. Portions of this standard have finally gone to ballot, and should be approved in December, 1994.

The P1073 Standard is written specifically for medical device communications. The primary focus is on critical care applications where multiple devices are used in a mix and match fashion. This critical care environment has safety, reliability, and ease of use requirements not met by standard computer hardware. The key user requirements identified by the committee in 1989 are: frequent network

0195-4210/94/$5.00 © 1994 AMIA, Inc.

reconfigurability; plug and play operation; the ability to associate a device with a specific bed, and thus a specific patient; accommodation of multiple topologies. These goals are all satisfied in the documents that went to ballot. The ability to meet these goals, interoperability of devices from different vendors, and patient safety are the major contributions of the P1073 standard.

INTENT OF THE STANDARD

A major obstacle to development and use of high level applications in hospitals has been the difficulty in getting patient data into the computer systems. The general lack of data communications available from patient connected devices has made data collection very difficult. Additionally, RS-232 connections are NOT standard, frequently giving different data types, on different pins, and changing from device model to device model. This problem exists even for devices produced by a single vendor. The P1073 standards solve the problem by allowing a local or remote Host Computer to collect data from all compliant devices. The standard also achieves interoperability amongst devices from multiple vendors. The standard is designed for the following example scenarios: (1) Automation of the recording and entry of information from medical instruments; (2) Providing clinical personnel better access to device status changes, such as alarms; (3) Automation of adjustments of device settings derived from computed parameters.[1] Use of complaint devices will enable medical informatics professionals to greatly expand their ability to implement systems level solutions.

APPLICATIONS

Medical applications of this technology will grow rapidly. LDS Hospital used previous prototype hardware to develop their HELP System. The improvements in outcomes based on the proper time to administer antibiotics has been previously documented.[2] SUNY Stony Brook has developed an anesthesia automatic record keeper that has been demonstrated using prototype P1073 hardware. This system is also used as a computer assisted instruction tool. The Mayo Clinic has a system in its coronary care units based on IEEE 1073 as of 1987. Cedar Sinai has a critical care system broadly based on IEEE 1073 concepts. Many applications previously presented at SCAMC and other symposia will now be clinically viable due to solution of the hardware problems.

Cantraine has done work in Belgium on computer controlled injection systems.[3] This work has been on going, yet frustrating, due to constantly changing hardware and software requirements. Each new pump, or new pump vendor requires a rewrite of software code, and possible rework of hardware connections. Cantraine is using computers and computer modeling to select appropriate drugs, evaluate the pharmokinetic, prepare infusion sheets, control of delivery, and synchronization of multiple pumps. This is representative of higher level applications, developed by practitioners, that the IEEE P1073 standard will enable.

Typical user developed applications, as produced today, require significant time, effort, and dollars be expended to get interfaces between the desired medical devices. Retrieval and formatting of this data is not routine. As much as one half of the total system design effort can be expended on the seemingly trivial detail of configuring the communications to run the application. This is compounded greatly by the constantly changing nature of data available from devices. Different firmware revisions of the same device may have greatly different data. The system or application designer has to account for the specific complement of devices, and design for the superset of possibilities. This effort has proven extremely challenging, and has stopped many applications from being developed. The solution of this dilemma will be one of the greatest contributions of the IEEE standard. It will allow creative practitioners to create new methods and applications, without needing to learn how every device communicates. Putting all of this creative energy into medical applications, rather than electronic manipulations will prove of tremendous benefit to the practice of medicine.

CLINICAL DEMONSTRATION

Using RS-232 to 1073 converter "matchboxes" and IBM plug-in Bedside Communication Controller (BCC) cards, hardware demonstrations have been performed during surgery at SUNY Stony Brook in New York. The matchboxes were Octagon Micro PC card cages with an XT computer card and a prototype 1073 card. The matchbox was programmed to accept data from a specific device. At Stony Brook, three matchboxes were used. These were programmed to convert data from three different devices to the IEEE 1073 format. The three devices were a Drager Narkomed 3, a Siemens 404 patient monitor, and an Imed Gemini infusion pump.

The matchboxes were controlled by prototype BCC cards plugged into a 80486 based personal computer. The PC was previously programmed to run an anesthesia automatic record keeper application developed at Stony Brook.

The matchboxes were connected to the RS-232 ports of the three devices and configured for the specific data stream of the device. All devices were polled by the matchbox for data to go into a 1,000 byte data table. This table will be replaced by future IEEE standards, 1073.1.x for a Medical Device Data Language, MDDL. The matchboxes then placed this table into their memory for transmission to the BCC. The BCC polled the matchboxes to receive the data table at 1 Megabit per second. The data was Manchester encoded for increased noise immunity. The cables between the matchboxes and BCC cards were then removed and replaced, as well as switched, to demonstrate plug and play, robust operation. The data was automatically collected whenever the cables were connected, with no further operator action.[4]

The prototype hardware used in this demonstration was approximately 80% compliant to the balloted physical layer standard and 60% compliant to the balloted transport profile, due to changes in the draft standard. Subsequent demonstrations were done on 100% compliant prototypes, after the available hardware caught up with the changes to the draft standard. These hardware demonstrations were shown at the AAMI conference, and the ASA Scientific exhibit.

The matchbox configuration used in these demonstrations is typical of what hospitals would need to use with legacy devices with RS-232 ports. These matchboxes convert the RS-232 to IEEE 1073, but need to be programmed for the specific devices they are connected to. Devices introduced after approval of the standard will likely contain the IEEE 1073 interface internally. Demand for such devices will be determined by hospitals. The manufacturers will only add 1073 when the users demand it. Standard products for both matchboxes and internal device communications controllers (DCC) will be available in early 1995.

HOSPITAL IMPLEMENTATION

The IEEE P1073 standard will alter data capture in critical care settings that implement the standard. Each bedside must have one or more BCC's. The BCC is the local communications controller, polling each device in a deterministic, negotiated manner. The BCC may be an intelligent device like a personal computer or simply a router to a remote host computer. The DCC's in devices cannot "speak" until they are polled. One of the major functions of the BCC is to get unambiguous association of devices with a specific bedside, and thus patient. The first version of the standard specifies a star topology so each device has its own cable to the BCC. This prevents a single wire failure (carts, people, scalpels can sever wires) from bringing the entire network down. Simple devices can use present microcontrollers to implement a 2400 Baud or 9600 Baud data rate in compliance with the standard. The use of ISO standard upper layers and object-oriented technology presents some extra communications overhead, but will prove well worthwhile at the first system change. More complex devices, or host systems, will use the 1 Megabit per second data rate. This will allow most clinical applications to function over the network. This data rate will support ECG waveforms, but is not intended for radiological use.

Higher level BCC functions can be developed to support many present user requirements. BCC's can be programmed to filter data so that only relevant data is sent on to the host computer. Filtering functions such as signal averaging, change data only, or low frequency data recording will be typical BCC filter applications. Many bedside applications can also be programmed into BCC's. Examples are anesthesia record keepers, computer patient records, or closed loop control systems. The likely initial BCC's will be one of three types: a PC with a BCC card; a patient monitor configured as a BCC; a simple, router BCC highly dependent on the host computer.

DCC's will also exist in several forms. New devices will integrate the DCC function with the device. Some vendors will put the DCC internal, while others will offer an external option similar to some present RS-232 options. These will be offered at all three data rates. Legacy devices will be brought into the network through "matchbox" RS-232 to IEEE 1073 converters. These will be programmed for a specific device and firmware revision, and mechanically connected to the device for their life together. Matchboxes will be re-programmable.

Upon physical connection to the network, an automatic connection sequence occurs between the DCC and BCC where device type and status are determined. The device and host negotiate a polling rate based on the request of the device and the available bandwidth of the BCC. If agreement is reached, the DCC is logically connected to the network and serviced by the BCC. The minimum polling rate is once per second to allow for robust capture of status changes, such as alarms.

There are several optional features for DCC's, while all features are mandatory for BCC's. This is sensible, since a BCC must accept any DCC, while a DCC doesn't need to support higher level features that are not appropriate for the function of the device. DCC's may issue interrupts to the BCC to request emergency service prior to the next scheduled poll. This feature is mandatory in high speed DCC's and is used in the connection establishment sequence. The interrupt function allows for any status changes to be communicated immediately. DCC's may also accept a time synchronization pulse from the BCC. This is used to align the time of day on different devices to within 1 millisecond.

BCC's and DCC's can both issue and receive indications of an intentional disconnect. This lets the device or BCC override alarms when network disconnection was intended. This was a major desire of practitioners.

The present star topology is extremely fault tolerant. The BCC deterministically knows the physical and logical status of all of its communications ports. The BCC will know if a device is still physically connected, even if the device is off or failed. Robust design of devices will allow DCC's to be "alive" even if their host is dead. This will allow for failure isolation in hospital systems, where DCC's can issue messages about the failure of their host to the rest of the system. This feature can be used to build very robust alarms at the system level, rather than the device level. Alarms can also be more robustly designed to allow for sharing of data between devices, or central analysis. Nuisance alarms can be greatly eliminated by comparing data from multiple devices. Even for simple devices, the BCC can use its polling mechanism to determine device operation. Since any working device that is plugged in must respond, and the BCC knows which ports have devices plugged in, it knows of device failures with no ambiguity.

SUMMARY OF THE STANDARD

The P1073 standards follow the Open System Interconnect (OSI) model for communications. The family of standards specifies all seven layers of the ISO communications stack. The documents that are being balloted are as follows:
IEEE P1073 - Framework and Overview of the Standard for Medical Device Communications;
IEEE P1073.1 - Framework and Overview of the Medical Device Data Language;
IEEE P1073.3.1 - Transport Profile;
IEEE P1073.4.1 - Physical Layer for Cable Connected Devices.
The standards are all written as applications or variants of existing ISO Standards, tailored to the bedside environment. It has always been the intention of the committee to use ISO Standards in the sub layers to enable P1073 to be adopted as an ISO Standard for international use. The standard specifies EIA485 transceivers and a defined subset of HDLC with additional capabilities for medical applications for the lower layers. The standard is compatible with IEEE 802.2 to allow alternate transport layers to be useable. The upper layers define a Medical Device Data Language (MDDL), the use of ASN.1, and Basic Encoding Rules (BER). The MDDL is based on object-oriented methodology and defines base classes that are used in other MDDL subsets. These subsets build on each other by means of object-oriented inheritance. MDDL also defines terminology based on SNOMED and the Universal Medical Device Nomenclature System (UMDNS). [5]

The balloted standard specifies a star topology, though others are possible and planned for. The future topologies anticipated are data bus, fiber, and wireless. Use of the ISO model allows for software written for one topology to be useable on the next.

The standard allows highly reliable, deterministic, automatic communications with devices though a Device Communications Controller (DCC). The DCC is internal to a device, or attached to legacy devices. These DCC's are slaves to a Bedside Communication Controller (BCC) which is the hub of the star. The star is connected using six wire, hospital unique cables and connectors. Devices may be plugged into any port of a BCC and communications will commence.

The standard offers two data rates, on the same wires. This accommodates simple devices with very low cost 2400 Baud data, and higher performance devices and systems with 1 Megabit. The standard also has several special function wires that allow devices to be time synchronized or to interrupt the polling routines with high priority messages. Finally, there are two wires that provide 12VDC power sufficient to power the DCC. [6]

CONCLUSION

The IEEE 1073 Standard for Medical Device Communications will begin to be available in early 1995. Standard, off the shelf, hardware will be available to device manufacturers and hospitals alike. The demonstrations performed to date show that the goals of the standard can be met. Plug and play operation of devices from multiple vendors will be achievable. Devices are able to be associated with a specific bedside. The network can be rapidly and frequently reconfigured. The hardware available in 1995 will allow practitioners, manufacturers, and system integrators to concentrate on true value added functions for hospital operations. The effort now being expended by nurses and doctors to write down data can be channeled into patient care. The effort being expended by information systems professionals on device interface can be expended on connecting hospital systems to get greater efficiencies in inventory management, billing, outcomes research, pharmacy operation, and litigation defense. The steps taken in 1994 and 1995 will be small ones, but they will lead to an explosion in hospital data usage in the second half of the decade.

REFERENCES

[1] IEEE P1073 Standard for Medical Device Communications, Draft 3.0, IEEE, New York, 1992

[2] R. Gardner, W. Hawley, T. East, T. Oniki, H. Young, "Real time data acquisition:recommendations for the Medical Information Bus (MIB), International journal of Clinical Monitoring and Computing, 1992

[3] F. Cantraine, "Computerdriven I.V. injection systems, State of the art, future developments", Acta Anaesthesiologica Belgica, 1988[2] IEEE P1073 Appendix B, Tutorial on System Operation, Rev. 0.01, IEEE, New York, 1994

[4] J. Gage, "Notes from Stony Brook", MD Computing, AMIA, 1994

[5] IEEE P1073 Appendix B, Tutorial on System Operation, Rev. 0.01, IEEE, New York, 1994

[6] IEEE P1073.4.1 Standard for Medical Device Communications, Physical Layer - Cable Connected Devices, Draft 4, IEEE, New York, 1994

Building a Children's Health Network: City-wide computer linkages among heterogeneous sites for pediatric primary care.

Larry Deutsch, MD, MPH, Michael Fisk, David Olson PhD, Joseph Bronzino PhD
Children's Health Network, Hartford Primary Care Consortium, Hartford, Connecticut

For many infants and children in our cities, quality of care and health status outcomes suffer due to poor continuity and coordination among ambulatory care sites. Despite proximity to technologically-advanced secondary and tertiary institutions, primary care services for children are fragmented, multiple-site use is common, and data flow among providers serving the same patients is primitive. Preventive and acute health care is often incomplete or redundant, and aggregate information for public health purposes is insufficient.

This paper focuses on the development of a city-wide computer-based pediatric health care network to improve provider decision-making and follow-through, parent role in their children's care, and community-wide data. A process of building consensus for a regional system is presented, addressing issues of establishing a uniform data base, coordination among heterogeneous institutions, system development, confidentiality, and integration with public health reporting and planning functions.

I. INTRODUCTION

In many urban areas infants and children are served by several medical institutions having advanced technical resources. Yet even with access to such facilities, rates of preventable morbidity and mortality remain high, particularly among impoverished, multi-cultural, and mobile populations; and quality of care is often poor, particularly in continuity and coordination, two critical information-dependent features listed by the Institute of Medicine (IOM) and scholars in primary care pediatrics [1]. In such settings in which fragmentation of services and multiple-site use are common, well organized medical records are often unavailable, thereby impairing the efficiency and success of clinical interventions and prevention efforts for children who visit community health centers, hospital emergency departments, and school-based clinics.

While increased access to children's services has been widely addressed, their quality and equality has received less attention. In a national survey, poor children were more likely than non-poor (15% vs 8%) to lack a regular source of ambulatory care (RSAC); and those with a regular source made 80% timely visits for routine care, versus only 48% for those without one. Furthermore, poor children more often (17% vs 6%) receive sick care at a site different from routine care, a discontinuity particularly for those who have access to a community clinic rather than a physician's office (40% vs 4%) [2].

The establishment of a computer-based system to share uniform information among institutions serving these families fulfills several patient record functions in clinical practice, as envisioned in IOM's recent volume [3]: storing data, guiding clinical problem solving, and supporting decision analysis, reminders and risk assessment. The presence of a uniform data base will permit longitudinal follow-up by clinicians and production of hand-held parent records in paper or magnetic copy for personal reference and presentation in new settings.

Such a system will also enhance the public health functions of community needs assessments and planning for efficient resource allocation among projects and agencies. A modern computerized city-wide system assuring individual confidentiality will permit small-area and aggregate data analysis and facilitate new wide-scale treatment outcome studies.

This paper presents the process undertaken to develop a computer-based health care records system for the pediatric community in greater Hartford, Connecticut and other cities.

II. PROCESS OF BUILDING A CITY-WIDE INFORMATION NETWORK AMONG URBAN PRIMARY CARE SITES

During the past year a Children's Health Network was formed in Hartford, supported by the Maternal and Child Health Bureau (Public Health Service). Three years earlier, a concept paper had been written and discussion begun by individuals from the city's three community health centers, three hospital outpatient departments (OPDs), and school-based health services. Initial submissions to two large foundations and requests for corporation hardware donations were unsuccessful. Subsequent work included formation of a multidisciplinary task force

0195-4210/94/$5.00

and data gathering, including a survey assessing multiple-site use of pediatric services. For off-hour visits at a major urban hospital OPD, indication of RSAC was 33% the same institution, 25% another public site, 22% none, and 20% private [4]. Prior records were frequently unavailable even with consistent site use.

Wider discussion and dissemination led to local foundation grants, multi-institutional and state health department support, and then federal funding. Multidisciplinary work groups and a steering committee have been formed to obtain input from community and provider sources, including hospitals, community health centers, school-based clinics, pediatric practices, visiting nurse organizations, technical firms, and city and state agencies. Groups address the following areas:

1. Consensus development and adoption of a uniform database for clinical encounters: we studied and expanded for pediatric use the Uniform Ambulatory Care Data Set proposed by the National Center for Health Statistics.
2. Implementation in the community as Network development proceeds: survey of existing hardware and software resources, compatibility, preferences for data entry method, format of parent-held native-language record, and technical and political obstacles to implementation among heterogeneous sites.
3. Technical features of system design and implementation (elaboration in following sections).
4. Creation of materials and techniques by consultant attorneys to assure security and confidentiality: concordance with individual patient/family preferences and institutional needs; specific informed consent documents and network liability provisions; and compliance with evolving transmission and security standards of federal agencies, professional organizations, and state and federal law.
5. Analysis of aggregate data: procedures for public health reporting and sharing information with outside agencies and researchers.
6. Evaluation: process; data validity and utility; and patient, community, and provider satisfaction.

Many issues remain to be resolved, with space limitations precluding discussion here: details of data base contents, coding methods, and unique identifiers remain tentative, as they should, pending national consensus in this time of intense activity. For current needs of consumers and providers, it appears necessary to proceed with system development and implementation, ensuring flexibility to modify and update upon critical review, comparison with experience elsewhere, and development of techniques and standards at local and national levels.

III. UNIQUE SYSTEM REQUIREMENTS

To support the needs of distributed health care for children as described above there are unique information requirements not present in traditional patient record systems [5]. These unique system requirements are:

- ensure access to patient records from any location,
- ensure that the data is available and on-line with acceptable speed during clinical encounters, at any time of day,
- support communication and information distribution throughout community while retaining security of information, and
- minimize cost of system introduction at each location.

To support these unique requirements we developed an information deployment strategy for heterogeneous systems. This information, to ensure it is current and always available, will be treated as mission critical data. This data criticality then needs to be applied to multiple users and multiple systems across a wide geographical area [6].

IV. ARCHITECTURE STRATEGY

A network supporting multiple users and multiple systems distributed across a wide geographical area requires a complex system architecture. This network architecture needs to be configured to address the needs of the users, overall system capabilities, health care organizations, and various federal and state regulations:

- Access to any child's records from any location,
- Security of access and data,
- Minimize or eliminate inability to access data,
- Interaction using inexpensive computers (e.g., PCs) and phone lines, and
- Ability to access services such as on-line health care databases (e.g., Medline searches).

To support these critical requirements two common architectures were considered: a) the Central Data Repository where the data is contained in one location and terminals access the information, and b) the Wide Area Network (WAN) approach with distributed databases. Both offer advantages as well as disadvantages.

Centrally Based Repository

The centrally based repository architecture involves a single data repository with terminals or computers accessing data on any child. When the child receives health care at any participating facility the information is accessed from the repository and new data transmitted back to it. Figure 1 shows the Centrally Based Repository architecture.

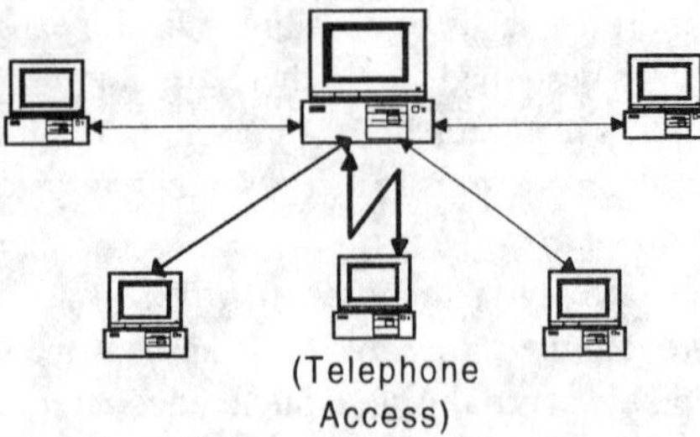

Figure 1. Centrally Based Repository

The advantages realized are:

- Data is in one location allowing consistent access, analysis and back up
- Services can be shared by all users (e.g., database accesses, peripherals)
- Records are available from any connected locations at any time

The disadvantages to this approach are:

- Repository based systems, unless through expensive redundancy efforts, present a single point of failure
- To support real time access from a large group the central computer of repository architectures require extensive and expensive resources, facilities, and equipment

Wide Area Network (WAN) Distributed Client Server Architectures (CSA)

WAN Distributed CSAs support multiple servers maintaining pediatric data for children assigned to a specific location. When a child arrives at a facility other than the one assigned, the appropriate provider computer will be accessed from the "foreign" provider. When health care is provided that server will update the required data back to the child's host server. Figure 2 shows the WAN distributed CSA.

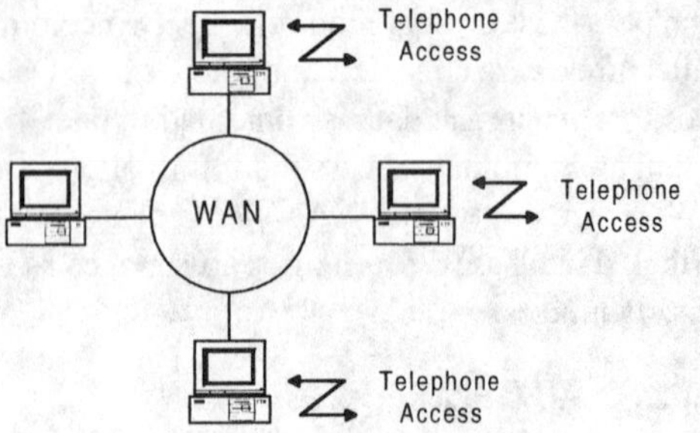

Figure 2. WAN Distributed CSA

Advantages for the Network are:

- Allows local control of data security
- Immediate access to data
- Optimum use of equipment
- Distribution of costs and decreased expenses

Disadvantages to this approach are:

- If server or line is off line, child data is unavailable to "Foreign" provider
- Accessing of remote data needs to be real time

V. DESIGN RECOMMENDATION

Since both architectures provide capabilities required for successful application of a database in support of the Children's Health Network, it was decided to implement a hybrid, hierarchical based Client Server Architecture with a major server providing the role of Central Data Repository. The distributed network will provide the real time, direct access support, with the repository receiving scheduled updates with access when distributed servers are off line. This hybrid architecture is shown in Figure 3.

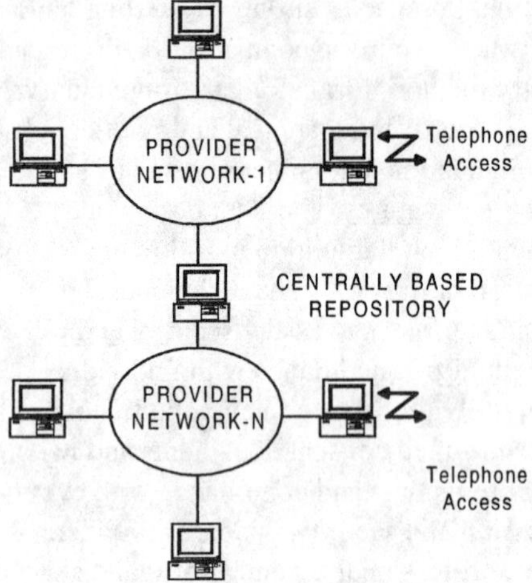

Figure 3. Hybrid Distributed CSA

Implementing a distributed CSA with a server providing the function of a central repository without the real time access (i.e., scheduled updates) provides advantages of both architectures. This approach also resolves data latency and retention needs [7]:

- Data is in one location allowing consistent access, analysis and back up
- Services can be shared by all users (e.g., database accesses, peripherals)
- Records are available from any connected locations at any time
- Allows ownership and control of data
- Immediate access to data

- Allows ownership and control of data
- Immediate access to data
- Optimum use of equipment
- Distribution of costs and decreased expenses

The disadvantage to this approach is:
- Cost is higher than a distributed CSA

Although it can be costly to implement a server as a central repository, this additional cost can be minimized by carefully selecting large servers as repositories.

To support this capability, the following network characteristics will be implemented:
- All computers will be Intel processor and Windows based
- Repository will retain all transactions and records shared by providers
- Overall architecture will be Client Server Architecture (CSA) and Structural Query Language (SQL) compliant.
- Support will be Integrated Services Digital Network (ISDN), 2400, etc.
- Providers (e.g. clients in CSA) with "foreign" patients, will automatically access identified provider (e.g. server in CSA)
- Upon a transaction, provider will update repository records
- If provider does not answer system, client and/or providers with "foreign" patients, will access the repository
- The provider will access the repository upon start-up and periodically to ensure data integrity

Building Block Approach

The overall goal of the project, if the prototype is successful, is to deploy the network in a broader geographical area. This will be done by applying a hierarchical posture to the repositories as the prototype network is expanded to the city, state, regional, and possibly national levels. Implementing in this method allows the development to proceed leveraging previous efforts including the prototype towards this final goal. This building block approach, will allow the network to expand throughout the city, region, state, and hopefully the country. The distributed CSA will minimize costs and retain ownership and privacy while the repositories provide data and access redundancy, information interchange between health care organizations, and a comprehensive overview (e.g., contagious outbreaks). In addition, the structure of the repositories position the network for easy integration into the National Information Infrastructure (NII) allowing an even broader interchange. This hierarchical based expanded hybrid design is shown in Figure 4.

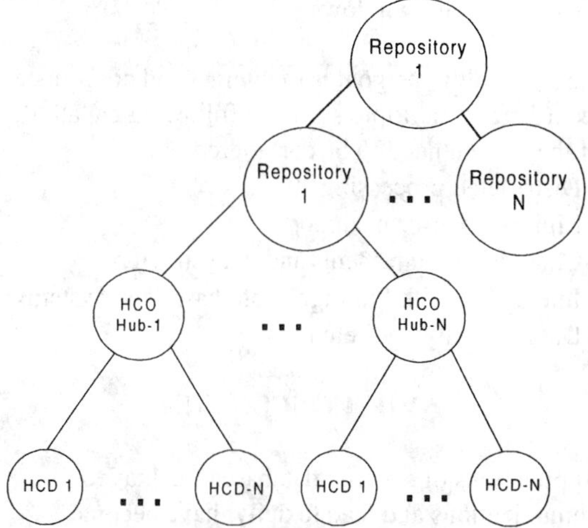

Figure 4. Hierarchical Expanded Design

The regionally (e.g., City, State) defined repositories are characterized as:
- Large organizations - hospitals, research institutes
- Community defined (e.g. City, County)

The Health Care Organizations (HCO) are:
- Hospitals (small/medium)
- Walk-in clinics
- Practitioner's organizations

The Health Care Deliverer (HCD) is characterized as:
- Small doctors offices
- Specialist
- Nurses - school, home care
- Facility or specialty defined (e.g. school)

VI. PROTOTYPE SYSTEM

The primary decision factor in the software to support the prototype system (i.e., one school, one hospital) is the means to retain and update all consented students records, and the ability to enter, track and report information associated with the students. This information includes:
- Students demographics
- Abstracted (coded) medical history and text
- Medical treatment and recommended follow-up.

Essentially the software required to support retaining, maintaining and updating this information is tasked to provide data management services.

As a result of overall implementations throughout the industry, the following system requirements for the school / hospital connection have been identified:

- Operates on a desktop 486 with modem support
- Supports client server architecture
- Operates with windows.

Since the ultimate goal is to interact and coordinate records from multiple sites, the following capabilities of the system need to be considered:

- Distributed processing
- Multiple platform support
- Changing requirements and data structures
- Interaction with "foreign" data bases and systems
- Data integrity and retention

VII. CONCLUSION

Applications of specific databases, such as for immunizations and lead toxicity, have become available, and a variety of comprehensive clinical systems for individual institutions are in place. But automated ambulatory record systems shared among distinct sites are not common; there are numerous obstacles to their design and implementation such as lack of standardization, incompleteness, inaccuracy, and security concerns [8]. Other problems include interface design for heterogeneous databases and political issues of data sharing among a variety of health institutions and agencies [9].

Even within a context of urban poverty and poor health, the technical capability to narrow the gap between reality and potential exists. Lack of systematic and patient-sensitive means to acquire and share data has impaired the consistency, continuity, and coordination needed for quality care and improved health outcomes for infants and children.

Development of this computer-based, client-server, distributed database system is underway. The design approaches mentioned above, (i.e., a transaction-based central database server with network/modem connectivity), will provide remote access while maintaining the integrity and security of the database. Although this system meets the needs of the pediatric community, similar strategies can be employed for developing a more complete patient-based record for the general population.

The implementation phase will enable us to test the data screens designed by our clinical work group and assess the utility of this effort. The key requirement for this system is to satisfy the clinical staff who need and use the information contained in the database. Only if the system is used by the clinical staff will it be successful.

Acknowledgment

This work is supported by Project # MCJ-097112, Maternal and Child Health Bureau (Title V, Social Security Act), Health Resources and Services Administration, DHHS. Thanks for technical assistance to Jennifer Poirier and Cass Frasher.

References

[1]. B. Starfield. Primary care: Concept, Evaluation, and Policy. Oxford University, New York, 1992.

[2]. Robert F. St. Peter, Paul W. Newacheck, Neal Halfon. Access to Care for Poor Children: Separate and Unequal? *JAMA* 267:20;2760-2764.

[3]. Richard S. Dick and Elaine B. Steen. The Computer-Based Patient Record. National Academy Press, Washington, D.C. 1991

[4]. Larry Deutsch, unpublished research.

[5]. David Trace, Frank Naeymi-Rad, David Haines, J.J. Shanthi Robert, Fabio DeSouza Almeida, Lowell Carmony, and Martha Evans, Intelligent Medical Record Entry (IMR-E) *Journal of Medical Systems,* Vol. 17, Nos. 314: 139-151 1993

[6]. Henry C. Chueh, M.D., M.S. and G. Octo Barnett, M.D., Client-Server, Distributed Database Strategies in a Healthcare Record Systems for a Homeless Population. Proceedings of 17th annual Symposium on Computer applications in Medical Care. McGraw Hill, Pg 119-124, 1994.

[7]. Bill Rosenblatt, UNIX RDBMS: The next generation, *February 1994, Advanced Systems:* 82-90

[8]. M.L. Grady, H. A. Schwartz. Automated Data Sources For Ambulatory Care Effectiveness Research. AHCPR, USDHHS, 1993.

[9]. K.A. Marrs, S.A. Steib, C.A. Abrams, M.G. Kahn. Unifying Heterogeneous Distributed Clinical Data In A Relational Database. Proceedings of 17th annual Symposium on Computer applications in Medical Care. McGraw Hill, Pg 644-648, 1994.

Medical Data Capture and Display: The Importance of Clinicians' Workstation Design

Ruth Dayhoff, Garrett Kirin, Steve Pollock+, Chylton Miller++, Seldon Todd+++
Washington Information Systems Center, +Kansas City V.A. Medical Center
++Leavenworth V.A. Medical Center, +++V.A. Medical Care Cost Recovery Office

Dept. of Veterans Affairs
8403 Colesville Rd, Suite 200
Silver Spring MD 20910
(301) 427-3700
E-mail: DAYHOFF@FORUM.VA.GOV

ABSTRACT

The Department of Veterans Affairs is developing, testing and evaluating the benefits of physicians' workstations as an aid to medical data capture in an outpatient clinic setting. The physician's workstation uses a graphical user interface to aid the clinician in recording encounter data. Various input devices including keyboard, mouse, pen, voice, barcode reader, and tablet are available on the workstations, and user preferences will be examined. Access to general services such as electronic mail and reference databases is also available. The workstation provides a wide variety of patient specific data from the hospital information system, including image data. The single data collection process by the clinician will also provide data for the cost recovery process.

INTRODUCTION

The Institute of Medicine's study of the computer-based patient record (CPR) identified the development of a technology that is sufficiently powerful and appropriate to the needs and preferences of health care professionals so that they can -- and will -- enter medical and other health care data directly into the computer as the single greatest challenge in implementing the CPR. It further noted that significant new technologies such as the graphical user interface can now support data entry by practitioners [1]. The VA is undertaking a project to evaluate the use of windows-based workstations with various input devices for clinician data capture. This study will be looking at user preferences for data entry technology and will compare workstations with other technology such as scannable encounter forms.

Others have reported work on clinical workstations. Some workstations were designed to present existing data, generally from networked hospital information component systems, to clinicians in an integrated manner, without allowing data entry [2,3]. Other workstations allow physician ordering for the Regenstrief system [4], clinical note entry for PEN&PAD [5], and problem list entry for the HELP system [6]. Recently several institutions have developed portable pen-based medical data entry systems for outpatient encounters and progress notes [7,8,9]. Results of this work is directly applicable to workstations performing the same functions. Various techniques have been tried in these studies to make the data entry process simpler and less time consuming. These include creating lists of input choices based on the context of the interaction [5, 10] and allowing multiple keyboard methods for choice selection [6]. These workstations generally use a keyboard and mouse or pen. Text data from the HIS may be displayed, but not images.

CLINICAL DATA CAPTURE WORKSTATIONS

Image capture and display workstations have been used by VA clinicians since 1990 [11]. They run the VA's hospital information system (HIS) with extensions that provide medical images as an integral part of patients' online medical records [12]. Over three years of experience has shown that physicians are willing and even eager to use the workstations in order to insert images into the patient record. The images included in the integrated online record seem to provide valuable information not adequately recorded in the traditional patient chart.

0195-4210/94/$5.00 © 1994 AMIA, Inc.

The entering of verbal descriptions is still a time consuming process, so more efficient methods of data capture are being examined. The automated data capture project described here has developed a graphical user interface to provide data entry capability in outpatient clinics and enhance existing imaging workstations in use at some V.A. Medical Centers.

There is ongoing discussion about appropriate metaphors for user interaction in a windows environment. Some prefer a user interface which imitates the paper chart, while others feel this is "not adequate for all aspects of clinical information processes" [13]. The user interface developed in this project is based on a main outpatient encounter window which summarizes all of the data to be collected for the visit (see Figure 1). Data entry occurs in dependent windows, and data then appears on the summary screen. This approach is similar to the Rooms metaphor [13] and was used by Nowlan et al [5].

The triage nurse enters the vital signs, chief complaint, and nursing note. The physician enters the type of visit, the procedures performed, the diagnoses or problems, and the narrative comments. Electronic signatures are used to verify all information.

A variety of input devices are available on the clinician workstations including: keyboard, mouse, pen, digitizing tablet, recorded voice, scannable forms automatically converted to ASCII data and

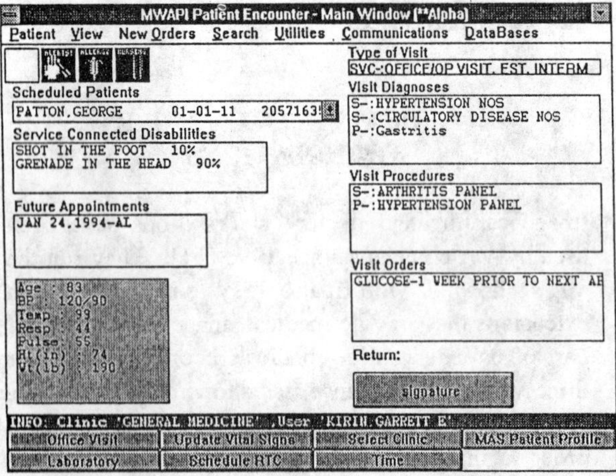

Figure 1: Outpatient encounter summary window

imported into the HIS database, and captured images. A clinician may use a single device for all interaction, or change devices during data entry, for example to make a diagram, handwrite a note or dictate.

INCENTIVES FOR CLINICIAN WORKSTATION USE

Clinician capture of data can be encouraged through the benefits obtained from the greater availability of data, the variety of patient data views, the range of data types available (structured and free text, images, electrocardiograms, anatomical drawings), and access to reference databases. Additional benefits are obtained by the institution due to availability of more accurate data for cost recovery and management.

The workstations access a variety of data from the hospital information system, including standard reports such as the patient's medication profile, health summary, progress notes, medical procedures reports, radiology reports, and laboratory results. These reports are often multiple pages and are therefore displayed in a window which can scroll or page for ease of review. Data presented at the workstation must be up-to-date and reflect the data in the main hospital system.

Images are available for review on the workstation using the "visual chart" option (see Figure 2) at some sites. Users may view all images pertaining to a particular patient, regardless of the hospital service that originated the images. For example, during a single hospital visit, a patient may have an endoscopy study, a biopsy read in pathology, an xray, an electrocardiogram and surgery. Image abstracts ("thumbnail" size images) will appear on an image menu, similar to that shown in Figure 2 and the user may select images to be viewed in full resolution. Images are displayed chronologically, and create a longitudinal record, including multiple hospital stays or outpatient visits.

Another benefit to workstation use is the availability of electronic multimedia mail from the graphical user interface workstation. Users may send and read mail conveniently. Mail messages may incorporate image, waveform, scanned document or voice data. This capability is being tested in a referral patient evaluation project between two test sites.

Finally, clinicians can access reference and other data sources from the workstation. Sources such as Medline, Micromedix, and CD-ROM data are being

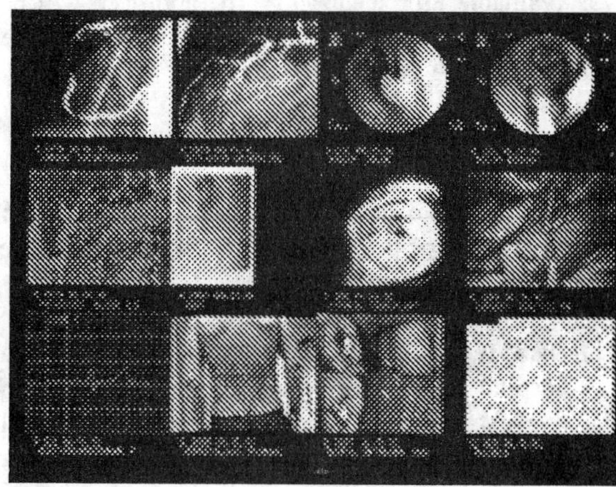

Figure 2: A true color Visual Chart summary of images for a patient is used to select images for full resolution viewing.

will be provided, depending on availability at the medical center.

REQUIREMENTS OF THE DATA CAPTURE PROCESS

The development process has followed the "VA structure model" where prototypes are developed and reviewed by a group of physicians and clinical users [18]. This has first been done by users at the initial test sites informally; it will be followed by more formal review. Suggestions are made for modifications. The resulting system is tested at alpha and beta test medical centers which provide feedback to the developers. Logging of system usage as well as user interviews will provide direct feedback and guide future development, as has been done for imaging workstation development [11]. There will be a formal evaluation of workstation use at the beta test sites, performed by an outside evaluation team.

Based on experience and the work of others, an automated data capture process must meet a number of requirements in order for physicians to willingly participate. These include:

- Data capture must be rapid. A typical outpatient visit may last only seven minutes. Data capture operations must be measured in seconds to avoid slowing physicians' work.
- Workstations must be simple to operate. Physicians cannot spend time figuring out how to do what they need to do. In many institutions, physicians rotate periodically, so training must be quick and easy.
- Input methods must be customized to the user. Different users prefer different input devices and screen layouts. Typing ability varies so different users will prefer keyboards, mice, and scannable forms.
- It must be possible to record various types of data. For example, some data is best recorded as structured text, others as captured images or annotated anatomical drawings.
- Finally, the record must be valuable to clinicians. Useful data must be collected and presented in a functional format; and data retrieval must be rapid.

IMPLEMENTATION OF SPECIFIC DATA CAPTURE METHODS

The use of a pointing device, such as a mouse or pen, for data entry requires that short to medium length lists of input choices be provided for user selection. These lists include the most commonly used terms for a specific clinic. We will examine whether the clinicians data capture task can be made easier if lists are created dynamically using patient specific information stored in the HIS. Users also have the ability to enter choices not on the lists. It is important to use the terms preferred by the clinician, but these must be mapped to standard terms for retrieval. The VA uses a standard clinical lexicon, which is updated as new terms are used. The clinician's own terms are recorded in addition to the standard terms so they can be displayed for the clinician reviewing the record.

Many clinicians prefer to dictate their narrative comments. The workstation allows voice dictation and records the audio data as a digital file. The digital voice file is stored on the network server and a transcription service directly accesses these audio files. These are transcribed to produce ASCII text files placed back on the network server and are linked to the patient's record automatically. They are then verified by the clinician before removal of the audio file.

Image data capture, including video capture of true color and black and white medium resolution images, is done using the workstations. Network interfaces have been developed to allow image acquisition directly from radiology PACS systems [14], image scanners, or electrocardiogram systems [15].

Another input mechanism to be tested at some sites and compared is the scannable form. There are commercial forms packages which allow automatic recognition of data entered on scannable forms [16]. These scannable forms allow entry of checkbox data, alphanumeric optical character recognition data, and scanned image areas. The same lists of commonly used diagnoses and procedures as described for the workstation may be used on these forms, and the same generic interface file may be used for input to the hospital information system. Check boxes are used as much as possible because of their greater reliability, however, alphanumeric recognition is used for entry of items not included in the most commonly used list. Scanned forms are printed individually for each patient scheduled for a clinic visit. This allows the inclusion of demographic and other data related to the patient and the customization of the lists to the clinic and even to the individual patient.

SYSTEM ARCHITECTURE

There are several alternative methods for creation of the graphical user interface. The VA has a policy of using standards that are hardware and software independent. The VA's hospital information system is written using the ANSI standard M language. M has developed a standard graphical user interface applications programmer interface (API) called the M Windowing API (MWAPI) [17]. Software for Microsoft Windows, Mac Windows and X Windows is identical from the programmer's perspective, and the software can be moved from one platform to another. The advantage of this approach is that the existing backend hospital information system software can be called directly in response to user actions. It is not necessary to write separate backend processor software.

An alternative choice is to use a non-M front end tool such as a platform independent windows code generation tool. The front end can be implemented using platform specific software such as Visual Basic for Microsoft Windows. User interface software must be written for each platform to be supported. This approach requires the writing of new backend and frontend software to incorporate the workstation functionality and enforce the VA's business rules.

The first phase of the VA's data capture workstation development uses the MWAPI approach. This approach was chosen because it could be implemented quickly and would allow the gathering very valuable user feedback. The approach will be evaluated after about a year, and decisions will be made for future versions.

DATA STORAGE MECHANISMS

Storage of the data that has been captured is an important part of the process. Data entered on the workstation falls into two access categories:

(1) Data requiring immediate storage within the hospital information system because changes to this data must be immediately available to all users. Examples of data which requires such a "live link" is vital signs, chief complaint, and nursing notes data. This is collected by the triage nurse, often within seconds of the time the physician sees the patient and needs to access the data. Problem list data is also shared by providers, the up-to-date problem list information must accessed for referral during the visit and changes must be rapidly updated following the visit. It is necessary to prevent multiple users from updating the problem list simultaneously through the use of locking mechanisms. It is difficult to meet these requirements with input mechanisms such as scannable forms.

(2) Data which may be processed in the background because only one user needs access at a time. This data is generally going to an HIS module which does not interact much with other modules or processes. Billing data can be processed in this manner.

We have implemented two mechanisms for transferring data to and from the data capture workstation. The first is the use of silent application programmer interfaces to the HIS modules. These are entry points in the software modules which may be called by the workstation to access or update data.

The second mechanism uses a generic interface file structure, which is a temporary file in which collected data is placed for processing by a background job. Any HIS module which needs data collected on the workstation will provide processing software to extract the data from the generic interface file and store it in package specific data structures. Therefore, the generic interface file is independent of the packages, and use of data can be extended to additional modules without modification to the user interface or interface file.

Data collected by the workstation is currently used by the following hospital information system modules: vital signs/nursing package, outpatient visit file (Patient Ccare Encounter module), billing package, radiology, pharmacy and laboratory packages (orders), and scheduling package (return visit).

CONCLUSIONS

We believe that technology now available will assist in clinical data capture by making the process easier. Proper design of a data capture workstation and its flexibility to satisfy clinician's individual preferences is critical to its clinical use. Other devices may be required to meet the needs of other clinicians. Clinician data capture will improve the quality of data for clinical care and billing because it is done by the person who knows the most about it. Use of the same data capture process for billing and statistical data assures more accurate accounting and management information.

REFERENCES

1. Dick RS, Steen EB eds. The Computer-Based Patient Record, National Academy Press, Institute of Medicine, 1991, p. 142.
2. Suermondt HJ, Tang PC, Strong PC, Young CY, Annevelink J. Automated Identification of Relevant Patient Information in a Physicians Workstation SCAMC 1993, pp. 229-232.
3. Hammond JE, Berger RG, carey TS, Fakhry SM, et al. Progress Report on the Clinical Workstation and Clinical Data Repository at UNC Hospitals, SCAMC 1993, pp. 243- 247.
4. Tierney WM, Miller ME, Overhage JM, McDonald CJ. Physician Inpatient Order Writing on Microcomputer Workstations, JAMA 269(3): pp. 379-383.
5. Nowlan WA, Rector AL, Kay S, Goble CA, Horan B, Howkins TJ, Wilson A. PEN&PAD: A Doctors' Workstation with Intelligent Data Entry and Summaries, Proc. SCAMC, 1990, pp 941-942.
6. Huff SM, Pryor TA, Tebbs RD. Pick from Thousands: A Collaborative Processing Model for Coded Data Entry. Proc. SCAMC, 1993, pp. 104-108.
7. Poon AD, Campbell KE, Fagan LM. PEN-Ivory: The Design of a Pen-Based System for Progress Note Creation, AMIA Spring Congress 1994, p. 99
8. Swearingen RL, Brown TA. Requirements and Benefits of a Successful Pen-Based Medical Data Entry System, AMIA Spring Congress 1994, p. 101.
9. Gelman MA. The Right System for the Write Reason, AMIA Spring Congress 1994, p. 83.
10. Lussier YA, Maksud M, Desruisseaux B, Yale P, St-Arneault R. PureMD: a computerized patient record software for direct data entry by physicians using a keyboard-free pen-based portable computer. Proc. SCAMC, pp. 261-264, 1993.
11. Dayhoff RE, Maloney DL. Exchange of VA Medical Data Using National and Local Networks, Annals of the New York Academy of Sciences - Extended Clinical Consulting, March 1993, 670: 50-66.
12. Dayhoff Ruth, Maloney Daniel, Kenney Thomas, Fletcher Ross. Imaging: A Multidisciplinary Application Spanning DHCP's Functionally Specific Medical Subsystems, Proc. MUG 1991.
13. Esterhay RJ. User metaphors for health care professional workstations. Intl Jl Bio-Medical Computing 34: 95-113, 1994.
14. Kuzmak PM, Dayhoff RE. A Bidirectional ACR-NEMA Interface between the VA's DHCP Integrated Imaging System and the Siemens-Loral PACS, SCAMC Proc. 1992.
15. Enison EJ, Dayhoff RE, Fletcher R. Graphical Electrocardiogram Waveforms as Part of an Integrated Hospital System's Patient Record, SCAMC Proc. 1993, pp. 373-375.
16. Teleform, Cardiff Inc.
17. MWAPI Standard, M Development Committee, c/o M Technology Association.
18. Brannigan V. Procurement of hospital information systems in the Federal Republic of Germany, MUG Quarterly XVII: 13-16, 1988.

ACKNOWLEDGEMENTS

The work of the Salt Lake City Information Systems Center on the Patient Care Encounter software, the Albany Information Systems Center on the billing software, and the other members of the DHCP Imaging staff is gratefully acknowledged. The Martinsburg and Kansas City V.A. Medical Centers have provided valuable user feedback.

Beyond Clients and Servers

Erik van Mulligen[1,2], Teun Timmers[1]
[1]Department of Medical Informatics, Erasmus University Rotterdam, The Netherlands
[2]University Hospital Dijkzigt Rotterdam, The Netherlands

Computer scientists working in medical informatics have to face the problem that software offered by industry is more and more adopted for clinical use by medical professionals. A new challenge arises of how to combine commercial solutions with typical medical software that already exists for some years and proved to be reliable with these off-the-shelf solutions [1]. With the HERMES project, this new challenge was accepted and possible solutions to integrate existing legacy systems with state-of-the-art commercial solutions have been investigated. After a period of prototyping to assess possible alternative solutions, a system based on an indirect client-server model was implemented with help of the industry. In this paper, its architecture is described together with the most important features currently covered. Based on the HERMES architecture, both systems for clinical data analysis and patient care (cardiology) are currently developed.

INTRODUCTION

After three decades of medical informatics and a large amount of local solutions available, the question arises whether a new approach might bring a solution to provide clinicians with the best possible computer support. This new approach could try to combine the current power of commercially available applications with the medical legacy systems into a medical workstation.

Exactly this was the main objective of the HERMES project when it was started about six years ago [2]. From a computer scientific point of view, the question arose whether it was technically possible to encapsulate existing software, both commercial and local developments without modification and make their functions accessible as a reusable component. An architecture that supports the integration of reusable components into medical workstations for various medical tasks and a user friendly interface through which the components can be addressed were the other two main objectives for the HERMES project.

The project started with the development of a prototype called MW2000, with which the technical feasibility of such an approach was tested [3]. The available computer power, network technology and ability of graphical user interfaces were assessed as being adequate, stable and mature enough for a medical workstation. From a user evaluation of the prototype MW2000, it was concluded that such an approach really can help clinical professionals with their task. With the help of industry, a HERMES consortium has formed that developed from experience with the prototype an open integration architecture, and based on that architecture medical workstations for clinical data analysis, for the outpatient clinic for patients suffering from heart failure and for occupational health care have been developed [4].

A project that addresses similar research questions is the HELIOS project [5]. Although their prime focus has not been the encapsulation of existing sofware in reusable components, but the creation of a software engineering environment that supports the structured development of new components, the technical mechanism is comparable. Through a software bus, components can activate functions resident in other components. Integration in this project is restricted to components that have been developed according within the HELIOS environment and integration of existing software did not receive much attention.

Integration architectures based on reusable components have been proposed by others. Greenes promoted this practice as a mechanism to build complex applications and reach a critical mass of functionality [6]. Outside medical informatics, the Object Management Group (OMG) proposed a Common Object Request Broker Architecture (CORBA), consisting of a common object repository [7]. In their view, each object has methods through which components can be accessed and data can be exchanged. Currently, a first implementation of CORBA is available. Other initiatives, such as Distributed Computing Environment (DCE) and Open Network Communication (ONC) Remote Procedure Calling (RPC) are less ambitious and mainly focus on transparent network-wide procedure calls (no brokering or encapsulation mechanism) [8].

CORBA, DCE, and RPC bind a call and the actual procedure at compile time. In HERMES, we use very late binding; at execution time, a generic call is delivered to a central broker, bound by this broker to a specific procedure call and finally this call is forwarded to a service and executed. With this feature, it is possible to very easily switch between alternative components that provide the requested functionality and (2) allows the broker to evaluate different break-downs of a generic call for particular criteria (such as speed, CPU-cost, reliability etc.).

In many research projects integration is limited to data. Projects such as IAIMS and Hewlett Packard's Physicians Workstation primarily aim at combining data from different (heterogeneous) sources [9,10]. Research topics in this direction are related to data semantics, modeling and communication. Earlier work in the field of integration investigated other communication mechanisms between the processes and sources involved in the integration [11,12].

In this paper, we will extend on the basic HERMES methodology that turns existing legacy systems into open reusable services and elaborate on those features that have proven to be esential for such an approach in the medical domain.

METHODOLOGY

Indirect client-server model

In the traditional client-server model, a client composes a request and forwards it to a server; the server on its turn will compose a reply and send it back to the client. In this model, the client selects the service (and host) that can solve the request. Furthermore, both client and server have to agree on the syntax and semantics of the message language in which the request and reply are expressed; any change must be implemented in both client and server. One solution to this is to reduce the mutual dependence between client and server by having a mediator that establishes indirect client-server communication. The task of this mediator is to do some interpretation and transformation of the requests that are exchanged between clients and servers.

HERMES utilizes as mediator a brokering mechanism that dynamically searches for a binding between a request of the client and the available procedures and data of the services. An overview of this mechanism is shown in Figure 1. This brokering mechanism is supported by a broker that reads an object-oriented database with all information about its environment: there are classes of requests with request instances, in the service classes instances identify the services that are available in the network, and a host class contains an instance for each host. Mandatory parameters for the various requests are specified as instances in parameter classes. Furthermore, a user is represented by an instance in one of the user classes. Relations between all these instances contain the operational knowledge of what service can handle what request, what mandatory parameters should be included in a request, on what host a service is resident and what preferred services are specified for each user.

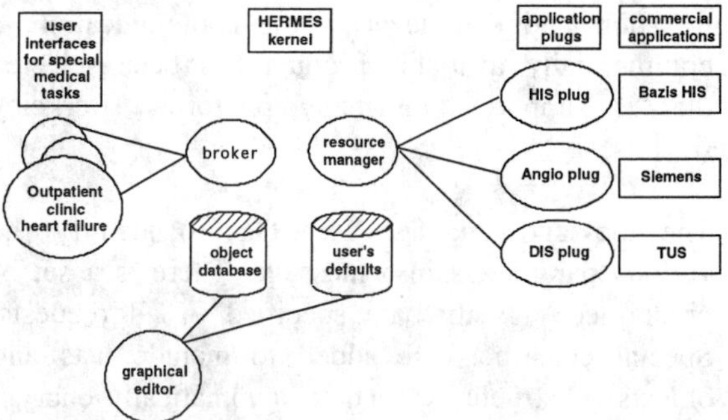

Figure 1. Overview of the HERMES indirect client-server architecture.

New requests, parameters, services, hosts, and users can be made operational by creating objects for them in an object database. Relations between objects specify the various bindings that have to be made; e.g. the relation 'can_be_handled_by' between a request and a service object defines that that service can handle that request. Through this broker, clients can directly benefit from newly installed services and hosts, without having to change the client. Furthermore, differences between the mandatory parameters for services that supply similar procedures are solved by the broker by adding these. The current brokering algorithm selects the first from a user-defined list of alternative services.

Resource manager

Although the client-server model offers an elegant mechanism to separate functionality into reusable services that can be shared by different clients, the disadvantage of all these separate processes is a significant increase of both computer load and memory use. From experience with the prototype integrated workstation, we learned that efficient resource management is essential to improve the throughput of systems that use a brokered client-server mechanism. Therefore, a resource manager has been inserted between the client and server communication that attempts to combine per user requests to already open service sessions. This strategy reduces the initial time to start a service and initialize a context. In addition, the resource manager will add user preferred parameters to requests and overrule the value of parameters set by the broker.

Message Language

Requests are composed by a client and follow the HERMES message language syntax. In this message language, all dependencies on the host's hardware and on the client process are avoided so that it can be passed between any host and process. For the transport and data level of the communication, a commercially available product has been selected that is supported on many platforms (Berkeley sockets).

The message language uses tags to identify the various parameters in a message. There is a set of predefined tags that are specified in all requests. Special constructs are added to include lists and objects (C-structures), and to automatically encrypt and decrypt data. One important feature of the HERMES kernel is that parameters do not necessarily have to be explicitly defined in the HERMES kernel. This allows dynamically construction of new parameters, thus freeing the kernel from having to know all possible parameters in advance. A special feature is the raw data type that can be used to pass data that does not follow the syntax; with this envelope feature 'foreign' messages (such as HL7) can be passed without having the broker and resource manager interpret this data for obedience to the syntax.

HERMES library

To free the developer from knowing how to express internal data structures and variables in the HERMES message language and to allow modifications or replacement of the message language by newly developed standard message languages (such as ASN-1), a special library has been provided. Both the client and the service use this library provided with HERMES as their stubs that translate between the internal data and request representation and the HERMES message language. The library consists of a set of high-level functions through which a client can, e.g., compose and send, and identify internal data that should be included in the request. Most importantly, we extended the stub's functionality so that it automatically includes parameters that are essential for the client's identification (hostname, username, process number, etc.). For the server, the library provides procedures that parse the message and construct an internal representation of its contents.

Callback mechanism

The HERMES library contains procedures that facilitate true asynchronous communication by installing a callback; this callback is automatically executed by the stub when an answer is received by the client. The server can use the same mechanism to install a callback for receiving requests. The stubs also handle several internal requests that are composed by the broker and resource manager to keep track of the status of clients and servers. Exception handling, connection termination, session management, and login handling are automatically provided by the stubs.

The HERMES library has been optimized for transmission of large data volumes (series of images or multi-record data for clinical research). In that case, data is automatically stored on a file to avoid internal memory problems.

Application Programming Interfaces

Developers can use the HERMES library to write macro procedures that allows them to define a procedure that composes a request for a service. The arguments of the procedure are passed as data for the request to the service. A set of these procedures forms the Application Programming Interface (API) for a service. These procedures are made available in libraries that can be linked with clients (see Figure 2).

Independence

One of the most important features of the HERMES integration architecture is its layered design that allows new commercial solutions that provide similar functionality to be easily put in. First of all, the broker mechanism allows a client to be truely independent from a service. Secondly, the HERMES library allows both client and server to use procedures without having to know the message syntax. The HERMES library procedures can be modified to generate messages according to a standard message language when available. Apart from this, client and servers can be developed separately, using different programming languages and operating systems.

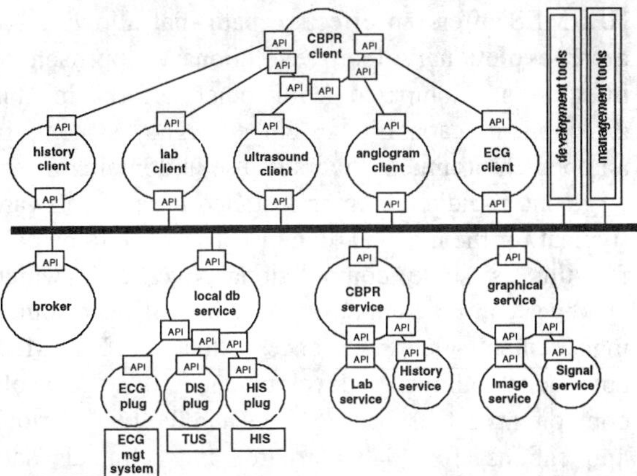

Figure 2. *Network of clients and services communicating through HERMES APIs which provide easy access to data and functions.*

Encapsulation

Another key feature of the HERMES integration architecture is its ability to embed legacy systems without modifications in a plug. This plug behaves to HERMES as a network-accessible true service, but translates incoming requests to the data format and instructions for the underlying system. These instructions can be either formulated as a batch for systems that accept batch processing or as a series of keystrokes for interactive applications. For integration of PC software, the plug can be enhanced with an additional layer between the plug and software that emulates a MS-DOS PC (commercially available).

Sessions

The notion of a session is important when integrating existing systems. Many of these systems are stateful, i.e. the meaning of an action is dependent on previous actions, and requires preservation of a context. Although a connectionless approach (with no notion of sessions) requires less resources and is much easier to realize in a network, it lacks this essential feature for encapsulation of existing systems. In addition, when clients share stateful services they can exchange information through the created context and avoid redundant interaction with the user to recreate the context. Of course, connectionless communication can be simulated in HERMES by shutting a session directly after creation. Note that the resource manager incorporates functionality to reduce the resource load of a session oriented communication mechanism by reusing open connections.

Data model server

All data available in the network is described in a data model. This description includes meta-data about the type, the range, the coding, the medical name, the size, keys, etc. and (medical) relationships with other data. This data model is supported by a data model server that offers other components (clients and services) the possibility to query for information. The data model contains per object a quadruple (dbms, database, relation, attribute) that exactly identifies where the data is located.

The data model server allows various conceptual views on the data. These views can be created by medical professionals and contain medical relationships between the data. The end nodes of this conceptual tree are links to attribute elements in the data model. These views can be modified independently of the underlying data model (and consequently database schema).

User-interface

All interaction with the user is window-oriented. In HERMES, the user-interface has been implemented with X11. Although most interaction with the user is handled by a client, it is not exclusively restricted to a client. Therefore, it is essential that the window systems, such as X11, enables remote services to interact with the user on the local host.

Secondly, in HERMES clients can be composed of subclients. To allow management of the windows of the subclients, their user-interfaces have to be integrated as part of the client's user-interface. This feature, called reparenting, is supported by X11 and included as a special option in the message syntax. The HERMES stubs contain code to automatically perform user-interface reparenting when this tag is included in the message.

ASSESSMENT

Flexibility and extensibility

The very late binding of a request to the actual call to a procedure in a service has proven to be a very powerful feature in the development of integrated medical workstations. Already during the development, similar functionality was offered by different applications. With one single client, we were able to switch between different services without having to rewrite a single line of code. Furthermore, it proved to be powerful for version control; depending on the user, different versions of a service can be accessed by the same client. New functionality could also be easily added by editing the broker's database with a graphical editor. However, no checks were included to preserve the correctness of the name space (i.e. duplicate requests can coexist). To improve the management of requests, a special editor has to be developed that ensures consistency.

Plugs

We created several plugs for batch-oriented systems and interactive systems with and without PC emulation. It appeared that writing a plug is not a trivial task and that only little of the code is generic. We divide a plug into three main modules: (1) translation of the data in the HERMES format to the application format, (2) generation of instructions for the application from the request, and (3) transformation of the application's output to the HERMES format. Code for step (1) can be generated more or less automatically. With a macro recorder interactive applications can be automated in step (2); for batch-oriented applications more programming is required. Step (3), transformation of the output is typically a manual programming job and little automated support can be given.

CONCLUSIONS

For introduction of open system technology and distributed processing in a medical environment, it is essential to provide an architecture that is able to cope with existing systems (both legacy information systems and systems from different vendors) without having to modify these systems. Furthermore, attention should be paid to develop a maximally flexible approach that allows systems to be replaced with new, preferably suited for operation in a client-server environment services without having to change all dependent applications/clients. A broker that binds requests to services and manipulates messages seems a suitable approach to this problem.

The price to be paid for a client-server approach is an increase in processor and memory load, which can be minimized by introducing a special server that monitors all running services and tries to combine requests to a single server process. The reusability of the server components in HERMES favours the development of medical applications for specific medical tasks rather than a generic application for various tasks. Our experience with building an environment for clinical data analysis and for the outpatient clinic for patients suffering from heart failure supports this.

HERMES offers an effective path that allows for a more evolutionary than revolutionary approach to integration. Compared with other efforts in this direction, its capability to embed legacy systems in an open environment favors its use in domains with a large and rapidly changing installed base of software (typical for the medical domain). The price to be paid for this is some computational overhead, which however can be compensated by intelligent resource management. Our experience is that the HERMES approach allows development of reusable components that can be shared by various applications for patient care and clinical data analysis.

Acknowledgement

Hewlett Packard Medical Products Group Geneva is greatly acknowledged for their financial support.

Reference

[1] Power LR. Post-facto integration technology: new discipline for an old practice. In: Hg PA, Ramamoorthy CV, Seifert LC, Yeh RT, eds. *Proceedings of the First Conference on Systems Integration.* IEEE Computer Society Press, 1990:4-13

[2] Van Mulligen EM, Timmers T, Van Bemmel JH. A new architecture for integration of heterogeneous software components. Methods of Information in Medicine 1993;32:292-301

[3] Van Mulligen EM, Timmers T, Van den Heuvel F, Van Bemmel JH. A prototype integrated medical workstation environment. Computers Methods and Programs in Biomedicine 1993:39:331-341

[4] Cornet R, Van Mulligen EM, Timmers T, A cooperative model for integration in a cradiology outpatient clinic. Accepted for SCAMC'94.

[5] Degoulet FJ, Coignard J, Scherrer JR et al.. The Helios European Project on Software Engineering. In: Timmers T, Blum BI (eds.) Software Engineering in Medical Informatics. Amsterdam: Elsevier Scientific Publishers. 1991:125-37

[6] Greenes RA. Promoting productivity by propagating the practice of "plug-compatible" programming. In: Miller RA, ed. *Proceedings of the 14th Annual Symposium on Computer Applications in Medical Care. Washington DC.* New York: IEEE Computer Society Press 1990:22-6

[7] OMG. The Common Object Request Broker: Architecture and Specification. OMG Document 91.12.1, X/Open publisher

[8] OSF. Introduction to OSF DCE. Englewood Cliffs, New Jersey: Prentice Hall, 1992.

[9] Young CY, Tang PC, Annevelink J. An Open Systems Architecture for Development of a Physician's Workstation. In: Clayton PD, ed. *Proceedings of the 15th Annual Symposium on Computer Applications in Medical Care.* Washington DC. New York: McGraw-Hill Inc. 1991:491-5

[10] Roderer NK, Clayton PD. IAIMS at Columbia-Presbyterian Medical Center: accomplishments and challenges. Bull Med Libr Assoc 1992;80:253-62.

[11] Sinha A. Client-server computing. Communications of the ACM 35, 7 (1992):77-97

[12] Wiederhold G. Views, objects and databases. IEEE Computer, 19;12:37-44

Evaluation of Computerized Health Care Strategies

Survey of Nurse Perceptions Regarding the Utilization of Bedside Computers

Diana Willson, R.N., B.S.N.
Medical Informatics Department, Intermountain Health Care

ABSTRACT

In December 1993, Intermountain Health Care (IHC) placed a moratorium on the installation of bedside computers in the acute care setting unless information could be obtained to justify resumption of these installations. A survey was developed and administered to nurses at two IHC hospitals. The survey results indicate that acute care nurses value bedside computers and believe that IHC should install them at other facilities. In addition, the acute care nurses estimate that they are using the bedside computers over 75% of the time during the day shift to document vital signs/measurements and intake/output quantities. Based on the results of this survey, IHC has decided to continue installing bedside computers in the acute care setting.

INTRODUCTION

Computerizing patient data not only allows for the production of financial and clinical reports, but can assist clinicians with automated decision support capabilities [1]. Patient data collected by nurses and other clinicians is playing an ever increasing role in the automation of real-time alerts and the generation of suggested interventions to improve patient care. Intermountain Health Care is committed to improving patient care and believes that automating the patient medical record is a crucial step in this process. Therefore, IHC is installing the HELP (Health Evaluation through Logical Processing) hospital information system at numerous IHC hospitals.

The question for IHC is where to install computers to optimize the collection of patient data. Bedside computers were installed on all units where the nursing information subsystem of HELP was implemented. The decision to install bedside computers rather than pod or centrally located computers was based on a 1989 study done on an acute care unit at LDS Hospital [2]. This study, designed to measure the impact of bedside computers, concluded that not only did nurses prefer bedside terminals but patient care and the incidence of real-time data entry increased.

In December of 1993, IHC placed a moratorium on the installation of bedside computers on acute care nursing units unless information could be obtained to support their continued installation. This decision was based primarily on the results of a study to measure the impact of the HELP nursing information system on an acute care nursing unit at McKay-Dee Hospital [3]. This study indicates that nurses spend 54% of documentation time at the nurses station and 21% in the patient room. This observed preference for documenting at the nurses station rather than at the bedside was unexpected and raises many important questions about what the computers at the bedside are being used for and when. Are the nurses using the bedside computers only during the day shift? What data are they documenting on the bedside computers? Why are they not using the computers at the bedside? IHC felt that more information about bedside computer use was needed in order to justify the continued installation of bedside computers in the acute care setting. A decision was made to conduct a survey of clinicians who use the bedside computers at LDS Hospital and McKay-Dee Hospital to determine nurse perceptions regarding the utilization of bedside computers.

METHODS

A survey tool was developed to answer the following four questions.

1. Given the cost of installing bedside computers, do the benefits justify their continued installation at IHC hospitals?

The survey question to answer this question is the following: "The initial cost of installing bedside computers is about $2000 per room. IHC would like your opinion as to whether the benefits of bedside computers justifies their continued installation and maintenance costs at IHC hospitals. Please circle your opinion. YES - the value of bedside computers justifies the cost of installation and maintenance. NO - As long as sufficient numbers of computers are available elsewhere, bedside computers are not necessary."

2. For specific applications/functions, what percentage of the time do users think they use the bedside computers?

The survey asks the users to indicate on a continuous scale (0=never, 100=always) the amount of time they use the bedside computer for various functions and to indicate if there is a difference between day (0700 - 1900) and night (1900 - 0700) shifts. Nine functions are listed on the survey.

3. How strongly do users feel about the reasons for and against using the bedside computers?

The survey asks the users to indicate on a continuous scale (0=never, 100=always) the degree each of the listed reasons influences where they use the computer. There are eight reasons listed for using the bedside computer and ten reasons for using computers not at the bedside.

4. What interventions do the users think would increase their use of bedside computers?

The survey asks, "What changes or interventions could IHC do to increase your use of bedside computers?"

The survey was administered anonymously to users of the bedside computers. At LDS Hospital these users are the nursing staff on the acute care and ICU units (RN's, LPN's, aides, critical care technicians) and respiratory therapists. At McKay-Dee Hospital, these users are the nursing staff on the acute care units and the float nurses. In order to reach the largest number of staff, the survey was administered primarily at the February 1994 staff meetings at LDS Hospital. Several different methodologies of survey administration were used at McKay-Dee Hospital. Out of a possible total sample size of 695 users, 327 were surveyed (47%).

SURVEY RESULTS

The results are presented in categories corresponding to the following four questions. While information was collected from ICU nurses and respiratory therapists, IHC's primary interest and the focus of this paper is the response of the acute care nursing staff (RN's, LPN's, aides).

1. Given the cost of installing bedside computers, do the benefits justify their continued installation at IHC hospitals?

Survey respondents indicate that they place value on bedside computers and are in favor of their continued installation at IHC hospitals. Figure 1 shows the percentage of users responding with a "NO" or "YES" to the question about whether the value of bedside computers justifies the cost of installation. 66% of the acute care nurses at LDS Hospital and 60% at McKay-Dee Hospital indicate that IHC should continue with the installation of bedside computers.

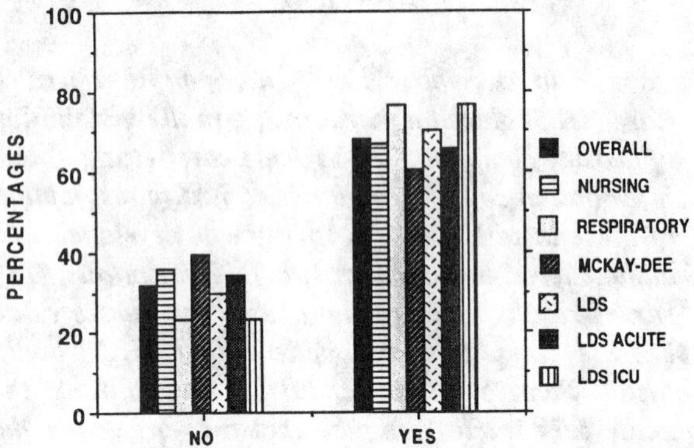

Figure 1. Does the value of bedside computers justify the cost?

2. For specific applications/functions, what percentage of the time do users think they use the bedside computers? The list of functions included in the survey are: chart vital signs/measurements, chart intake/output, chart physical assessment, chart therapy/treatments, edit data, care plans, review charting, review lab/xray results, order entry and other.

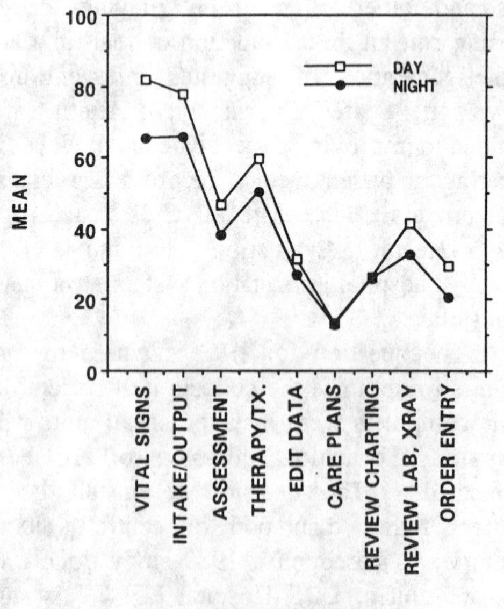

Figure 2. Acute care estimates of bedside computer use for various functions.

Figure 2 shows how acute care nurses at LDS and McKay-Dee Hospitals responded to the question asking them to estimate the percentage of the time they use the bedside computer for various functions and to indicate differences between day (0700 - 1900) and night (1900 - 0700) shifts. During the day, nurses estimate that 82% of vital signs/ measurements, 78% of intake/output quantities and 60% of therapies/treatments are documented on the bedside computer. At night, these estimates decrease somewhat to 65% of vital signs/measurements, 66% intake/output quantities and 50% of therapies/ treatments are documented on the bedside computer.

A comparison was made between those nurses who responded that the value of bedside computers justifies their costs (positive response) with those who responded that bedside computers are not necessary (negative response). Figure 3 shows that those nurses who respond positively to the value of bedside computers consistently indicate they use the bedside computers more than the nurses who feel bedside computers are not necessary.

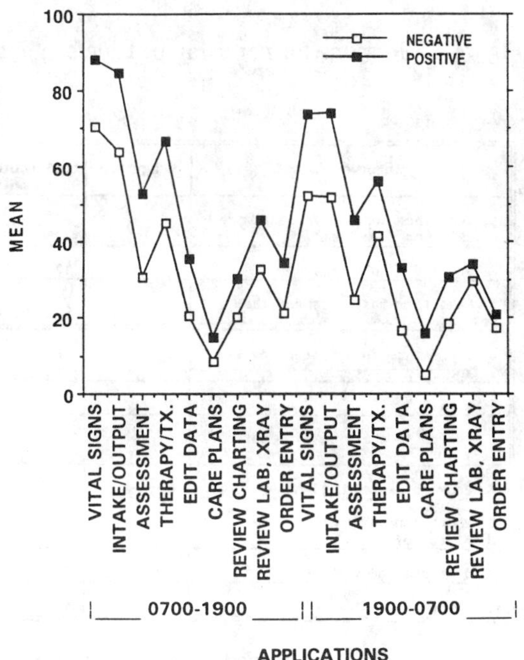

Figure 3. Comparison of acute care nurses who responded positively and negatively to the question about the value of bedside computers.

3. How strongly do users feel about the reasons for and against using the bedside computers?

The reasons listed in the survey for using the bedside computer and the mean scores for acute care nurses are:

1. At the bedside, I can enter patient data immediately as it is gathered. (mean 68)
2. I feel that patient data is more accurate if entered at the bedside. (mean 68)
3. The patient is already identified at the bedside so it saves me keystrokes. (mean 70)
4. It's easier for me to document at the bedside rather than try to remember it. (mean 67)
5. Entering directly into the computer saves me from writing it down first. (mean 63)
6. I like to complete nurse charting in a quiet environment. (mean 70)
7. I can involve the patient in the care giving process while in the room. (mean 59)
8. It saves me time to document at the bedside computer. (mean 64)

The acute care nurses indicate very little difference between these reasons. The mean scores are all grouped between 63 and 70 with the exception or the seventh reason (I can involve the patient in the care giving process while in the room.) with a mean of 59.

The reasons listed in the survey for using computers not at the bedside and the mean scores for acute care nurses are:

1. The computers in the rooms are more frequently "down" or broken. (mean 35)
2. I feel uncomfortable using the computer with family members in the room. (mean 54)
3. I prefer to sit down when I chart. (mean 64)
4. I prefer uninterrupted time to think when I chart. (mean 68)
5. It is too dark in the room to use the bedside computer at night. (mean 53)
6. It's easier to "batch" chart than chart individual items on one patient. (mean 46)
7. Using bedside computers doesn't fit into my work flow. (mean 41)
8. I'm just not in the "habit" of using the bedside computer. (mean 39)
9. I'm at the central station/pod for other reasons so I just chart there. (mean 50)
10. I prefer to be in the company of other nurses at the pod or nurse's station. (mean 36)

Acute care nurses indicate some differences between the reasons for not using the bedside computer. The range of means varies from 35 to 68. The top five reasons for not using the bedside computers are: (1) I prefer uninterrupted time to think when I chart, (2) I prefer to sit down when I chart, (3) I feel uncomfortable using the computer with family members in the room, (4) It is too dark in the room to use the bedside computer at night, and (5) I'm at the central station/pod for other reasons so I just chart there.

Those nurses who respond that the value of bedside computers justifies their cost (positive response) feel more strongly about the reasons for using the bedside computers and less strongly about the reasons for not using the bedside computers than the nurses who do not think that bedside computers are necessary (negative response) (see Figures 4 and 5).

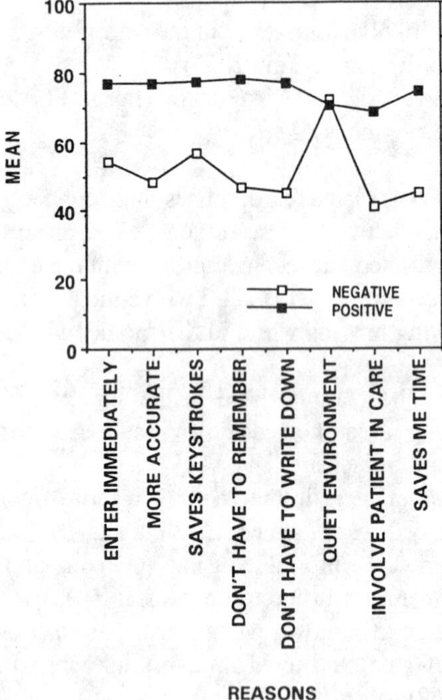

Figure 4. Reasons for using bedside computers.

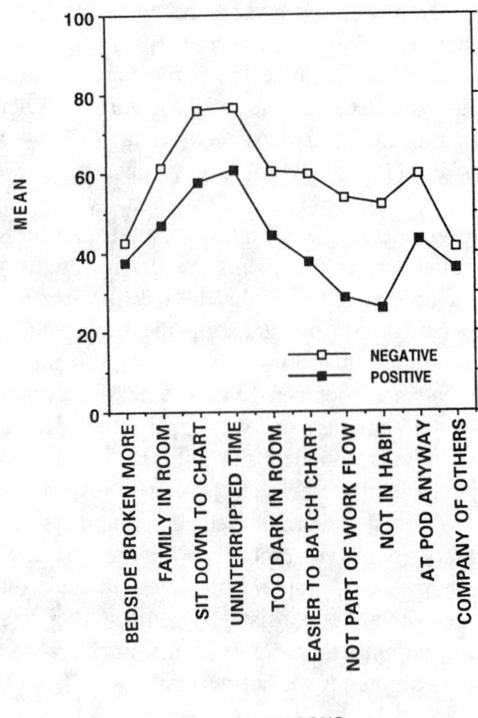

Figure 5. Reasons for not using bedside computers.

4. What interventions do the users think would increase their use of bedside computers?

The users' textual responses to this question were coded. Table 1 shows the coded comments that have more than 5 responses.

The nursing staff at LDS Hospital indicate that keeping the computers working and speeding them up are interventions that would increase their use of the bedside computers. While there is some question as to whether the computers at the bedside are really "down" more often and are slower than the computers at other locations, it is obvious that the nurses are concerned about these issues. LDS Hospital is committed to trying to improve these conditions.

Intervention	McKay-Dee only	LDS acute care only
1. Keep them working (repair more quickly, no down time)	1	22
2. Provide stools/chairs	7	10
3. Make them faster (speed them up)	1	9
4. Place them in a better location in room	0	12
5. Nothing	1	11
6. Prefer to chart outside patient room	2	6
7. Provide keyboard light	4	3
8. Shorten password (no sign-on, don't log off)	4	2
9. Decrease the work load	6	0
10. Other	12	9

Table 1. Suggested interventions to increase bedside computer use.

Placing the computers in a better location in the patient room is apparently another LDS Hospital specific issue. Most of the computers in the acute care patient rooms are located at the head of the bed, behind the bathroom door; the computers at McKay-Dee Hospital are located at the foot of the patient's bed. Providing stools/chairs and keyboard lights are suggestions from both hospitals.

DISCUSSION

Intermountain Health Care is committed to the computerization of the patient record for the purposes of providing comprehensive clinical and financial reports, supporting the clinician in decision making, automating alerts and providing other computerized decision support capabilities, and supporting clinical quality improvement and outcome studies. The question for IHC is not whether the data documented by acute care nurses should be computerized, but where should the computers be located. The survey results indicate that acute care nurses value bedside computers and are in favor of their continued installation at IHC hospitals. In addition, the nurses indicate very high use of bedside computers for the documenting of vital signs and measurements, intake and output quantities, and documentation of treatment and therapies. These are the same data elements, with the addition of medications and lab results, that have been identified by physicians at McKay-Dee Hospital as being the crucial ones for clinical decision making and are the most important to be documented "real time" (Mig Neiswanger, Nursing Information Systems Coordinator, McKay-Dee Hospital, personal communication, May 9, 1994). Based on the survey results, IHC decided to lift the moratorium on bedside computers in the acute care settings and to resume installing them at hospitals preparing to implement the HELP nursing information system.

Certainly, there is room for further research. Since the survey was completed, a new version of the nursing documentation software was installed at both LDS and McKay-Dee Hospitals. This software is, for the first time, able to capture with each data element, the user name/ID doing the documenting, which computer is being used, and the actual time that the data is being entered (not just the time the user charts that it is). Future studies should examine what is actually being documented at the bedside, not just the user's perception.

The survey indicates that there are nurses who value the bedside computer and those who do not. Those who are supportive indicate that they consistently use the bedside computers more and feel more strongly about the reasons for using the bedside computers than the nurses who do not feel bedside computers are necessary. What can explain the reasons for this dichotomy? Possibly, the differences can be attributed to nurse attitudes which could be measured with the Nurse Attitude Survey [4].

Based on the survey results, several avenues might be explored to enhance the use of bedside computers: keep the computers functioning and fast, provide stools/chairs for nurses, select optimal placement of computers in the patient room, provide keyboard lights for night-time documentation, and educate nurses as to the data elements that must be entered "real time" to not only assist clinicians in managing patients but to drive the automated decision support capabilities of the information system.

ACKNOWLEDGEMENTS

I want to thank the following individuals for their contribution to the development of the survey tool. from LDS Hospital: Reed Gardner, PhD, Co-Director of Medical Informatics, Brenda Rosebrock, RN, BSN, Clinical Information Systems Coordinator, Nancy Nelson, RN, BSN, Clinical Information Systems Coordinator and Karen Meyer, BS, Statistician; from the Salt Lake Valley Hospitals: Carol Ashton, PhD, Director of Nursing Research, and Diane Tracy, PhD, Research Analyst; from McKay-Dee Hospital: Mig Neiswanger, RN, BSN, Nursing Information Systems Coordinator; from the University of Utah: Linda Lange, RN, EdD, Assistant Professor and Director of Nursing Informatics

REFERENCES

[1] Kuperman, G.L. & Gardner, R.M. (1990). The impact of the HELP computer system on the LDS Hospital paper medical record. The Proceedings of the Fourteenth Annual Symposium on the Computer Applications in Medical Care, pp. 673-677. Computer Society Press.

[2] Halford, G., Burkes, M., & Pryor, T.A. (1989). Measuring the impact of bedside terminals. Nursing Management, 20(7), 41-45.

[3] Hinson, D.K., Huether, S.E., Blaufuss, J.A., Neiswanger, M., Tinker, A., Meyer, K.J. & Jensen, R. (1994). Measuring the impact of a clinical nursing information system on one nursing unit. The Proceedings of the Seventeenth Annual Symposium on Computer Applications in Medical Care, pp. 203-210. Computer Society Press.

[4] Burkes, M. (1987). Identifying and relating nurses' attitudes toward computer use. Computers in Nursing, 9(5), 190-199.

Academic Physicians' Assessment of the Effects of Computers on Health Care

William M. Detmer[1] and Charles P. Friedman[2]

[1]Section on Medical Informatics, Stanford University School of Medicine
[2]Laboratory for Computing and Cognition, University of North Carolina School of Medicine

We assessed the attitudes of academic physicians towards computers in health care at two academic medical centers that are in the early stages of clinical information-system deployment. We distributed a 4-page questionnaire to 470 subjects, and a total of 272 physicians (58%) responded. Our results show that respondents use computers frequently, primarily to perform academic-oriented tasks as opposed to clinical tasks. Overall, respondents viewed computers as being slightly beneficial to health care. They perceive self-education and access to up-to-date information as the most beneficial aspects of computers and are most concerned about privacy issues and the effect of computers on the doctor-patient relationship. Physicians with prior computer training and greater knowledge of informatics concepts had more favorable attitudes towards computers in health care. We suggest that negative attitudes towards computers can be addressed by careful system design as well as targeted educational activities.

In academic medical centers, substantial resources are now being directed towards development of clinical information systems. In many design schemes, the physician will be both entering data into the system and extracting information from it. For successful implementation of such systems, understanding physicians' attitudes towards computers will be important.

To understand how academic physicians view the effects of computers on patient care and job satisfaction, we distributed a questionnaire at two academic medical centers. We elicited physicians' perceptions of the effects of computers on health care and related those perceptions to demographic information, experience with computers, and knowledge of informatics concepts.

BACKGROUND

Eliciting and analyzing user attitudes can be an important component of good system design. Several methods are commonly used to study user attitudes. Detailed observation of users in the workplace can lead to a better understanding of attitudes and other important issues before or after a system is developed [1, 2]. However, this method may be time-consuming and may elicit attitudes from only a limited group of individuals. Cohort studies, where an investigator observes how attitudes change as the result of a new computer system, can often ascribe a change in attitudes to the effect of the new system [3]. However, this method requires that the computer system is operational. Survey studies, where an investigator studies a sample of a population with a questionnaire or similar instrument, can elicit subjects' attitudes before or after system development [4]. This method is time-efficient and inexpensive, but can suffer from problems with validity (i.e., questions may not accurately elicit the true attitude).

Many investigators have designed survey instruments to assess user attitudes towards information systems (for a review see [5]). In the medical domain, most instruments have been designed from the perspective of hospital-information-system managers [6, 7], nurses [8], or physicians [9-11].

We chose to modify and modernize a survey instrument developed by Teach and Shortliffe [9]. Their instrument, which focuses primarily on attitudes towards decision-support systems, assesses the acceptability of different computing applications, the expectations about the effects of computers on medicine, and the demands on system performance. Our instrument elicits attitudes about a more general set of applications while preserving portions of the original questionnaire to allow comparison with the original Teach and Shortliffe study.

METHODS

We distributed a 4-page, 106-item questionnaire to physicians at two medical centers—Stanford University and University of North Carolina at Chapel Hill (UNC). Eligibility criteria were that the subjects be full-time physician faculty members and be specialists or subspecialist in one of the following areas: internal medicine, surgery, radiology, or radiation oncology. We chose these specialty areas because they span a range of disciplines.

Eligible subjects received and returned the questionnaire through the campus mail. We sent out a second mailing four weeks after the first mailing to enhance response rate.

Computing Environment

The clinical computing environments at the two institutions were similar. Stanford provided electronic access to recent laboratory and radiology reports but had not yet deployed an integrated clinical information system. UNC was in the process of installing a clinical workstation that carries out transparent logon to multiple information servers, integrates information about a single patient from

0195-4210/94/$5.00

these disparate sources, and provides access to this information via a graphical user interface [12]. At the time of the survey, the workstation was becoming operational in outpatient clinics but had not appeared on inpatient services.

Questionnaire Content

Our questionnaire requested information in four areas: (1) demographic information, (2) experience with computers, (3) knowledge of informatics concepts, and (4) attitudes towards computers in health care. The attitudes section elicited from subjects their *demands* on future systems, their *priorities* for future system development, and their assessment of the *effects* of computers on health care. In this paper, we report on the "effects" section of the questionnaire and how responses in this section relate to demographic information, experience with computers, and knowledge of informatics concepts. We have reported on the "demands" and "priorities" sections elsewhere [13].

In the section eliciting demographic information, we asked subjects their age, gender, specialty, and the percent of time that they spent in the following activities: clinical care and clinical teaching, didactic teaching, research, and administration. We combined clinical care and clinical teaching into one category because we have observed that many physicians perform both tasks simultaneously.

In the section on experience with computers, we elicited how often subjects use computers, what types of computers they use, what tasks they perform with computers, and what types of training they have had in the use of computers. We asked subjects how they used computers by listing 10 tasks regularly performed by academic physicians and asking them to what extent they use computers for each task. Subjects rated how frequently they use computers to perform each task using the following scale: "never" (0), "sometimes" (+1), "often" (+2), or "always" (+3).

The section on knowledge of informatics concepts consisted of two parts: (1) a single-item self-assessment of overall sophistication and (2) a 18-item "test" of informatics knowledge. The test of informatics knowledge contained pairs of concepts (e.g., Free text <–> Coded data), and three statements to choose from: "I don't understand the distinction at all" (0), "I have a general appreciation of the distinction but couldn't define it" (+1), and "I can define the distinction precisely" (+2). We chose concepts that we believed were representative of important informatics concepts and concepts with a range of difficulty. We created a summary "knowledge score" by dividing the sum of the item scores by the number of items. Although self-perceptions of distinctions between concepts may be a less precise measure of knowledge than a test where subjects are asked to provide answers, we used this method because we were concerned that a true test of knowledge might discourage subjects from completing the questionnaire.

The section on the effects of computers on health care contained 17 questions each listing a potential effect of computers on patient care or job satisfaction. Subjects rated the effects of computers on health care as "highly detrimental" (–2), "detrimental on the whole" (–1), "neither detrimental nor beneficial" (0), "beneficial on the whole" (+1), or "highly beneficial" (+2). We created a summary "effects score," representing the overall effect of computers on health care, by dividing the sum of scores on individual questions by the total number of questions.

Statistical Methods

We used nonparametric statistics to test for significance between variables. We adopted this more conservative approach because many of our variables had ordinal values and because we did not want to assume that the distributions of answers to questions were normally distributed. To test for significance between two groups we used the Mann-Whitney rank-sum test, and to test for significance between three or more groups we used the Kruskal-Wallis test. For measuring the association between two variables, we used the Spearman rank-correlation test.

RESULTS

A total of 470 faculty members were eligible to participate. Table 1 shows the number of questionnaires returned and the response rate for each institution. The difference in response rate between institutions was highly significant ($\chi^2 = 42.8$, $p < .0001$).

Demographics

Subject characteristics are shown in Table 2. Subjects were predominantly male and spent the majority of their time performing clinical care and clinical teaching. We found no significant differences between the institutions on any demographic characteristics.

Experience with Computers

Respondents' experience with computers is shown in Table 3. More than 90% of subjects reported using a computer at least one hour per week ("regular computer users"). Subjects reported using computers

Table 1. Number of questionnaires returned and response rate for each institution

Institution	Questionnaires Returned	Response Rate
UNC	154/206	75%
Stanford	118/264	45%
TOTAL	272/470	58%

Table 2. Characteristics of questionnaire respondents

Age (mean ± SD)	46.3 ± 10.3
Male	82%
Specialty	
Internal Medicine	54%
Surgery	29%
Radiology	14%
Radiation oncology	3%
Primary Activity	
Clinical care and clinical teaching	63%
Research	30%
Administration	5%
Didactic teaching	2%

from 0 to 40 hours per week, with a mean of 9.7 hours and a median of 8 hours.

One third of subjects had some formal training in computing. Eighteen percent of subjects had taken computer science or related courses, 2% had formal training in medical school, 4% had formal training in residency, 2% had taken a CME course or participated in a CME-approved conference on computing, and 16% had participated in a computer workshop or conference that did not award CME credits. Age was not a significant determinant of whether a subject had any formal training. In addition, of the 26 subjects who received their medical education in the last decade (those under age 35), only one subject (4%) had a formal course in medical school and only five subjects (19%) had a formal course during residency.

Regular computer users rated how frequently they use computers to perform various professional tasks. Table 4 shows mean and median ratings of regular computer users for each task. A majority of respondents never used a computer to document patient information, obtain decision support, or schedule patient appointments. On the other hand, a majority of subjects always used computers to perform statistical analysis, prepare presentation slides, search the medical literature, and write documents (e.g., grants, research papers, and teaching material). We found no significant differences between institutions on experience with computers.

Table 3. Subjects' experience with computers

Regular computer users	91%
Hours per week (mean ± SD)	9.6 ± 8.83
Computer use	
Desktop computer at work	82%
Desktop computer at home	71%
Portable or notebook	35%
Computer training	
Formal courses	33%
Self-guided	50%
None	17%

Table 4. Frequency with which regular computer users use computers for various professional tasks*

Task	Mean	Median
Documenting patient information	0.36	0
Scheduling patient appointments	0.37	0
Obtaining advice on a specific patient's diagnosis or therapy	0.49	0
Teaching students and residents	0.80	1
Communicating with colleagues	0.98	1
Accessing clinical data	1.45	2
Performing statistical analysis	1.79	3
Preparing presentation slides	2.20	3
Searching the medical literature	2.30	3
Writing grants, research papers, etc.	2.41	3

*Scale: "never" (0), "sometimes" (1), "often" (2), "always" (3).

Knowledge of Computer Concepts

We asked subjects to rate their degree of sophistication with computers. Subjects reported themselves as "very unsophisticated" (16%), "unsophisticated" (16%), "neither sophisticated nor unsophisticated" (41%), "sophisticated" (19%), or "very sophisticated" (8%). Older subjects tended to rate their level of sophistication as lower than younger subjects (Spearman's $\rho = -.16$, $p = .009$). As a group, female subjects rated their level of sophistication lower than their male counterparts (Mann-Whitney, $p = .003$), this despite the fact that female subjects were significantly younger than male subjects (Mann-Whitney, $p < .0001$). The amount of time that subjects used a computer correlated significantly with self-reported degree of sophistication (Spearman's $\rho = .64$, $p < .0001$). In addition, subjects with formal training rated themselves as more sophisticated than those without formal training (Mann-Whitney, $p < .0001$). We found no significant correlation between self-reported sophistication and institution or specialty.

To obtain a more precise measure of knowledge, we also asked subjects to rate their knowledge of various informatics concepts. Table 5 shows the mean and median responses of subjects on each of 18 items. For the summary knowledge score, the mean (± standard deviation) was 1.08 (± 0.44), corresponding to an average response of "I have a general appreciation of the distinction but couldn't define it." The summary knowledge score correlated significantly with self-reported sophistication (Spearman's $\rho = .71$, $p < .0001$). As with the self-reported level of sophistication, the mean knowledge score was significantly higher for male subjects (Mann-Whitney, $p = .005$), younger individuals (Spearman's $\rho = -.22$, $p = .0005$), time spent using a computer (Spearman's $\rho = .54$, $p < .0001$), and formal training (Mann-Whitney, $p < .0001$).

Table 5. Subjects' assessment of their knowledge of various informatics concepts*

Informatics Concept	Mean	Median
Forward chaining ↔ Backward chaining	0.20	0
ICD9-CM ↔ SNOMED	0.40	0
Entities ↔ Relationships	0.46	0
Interpreter ↔ Compiler	0.57	0
Relational database ↔ Flat-file database	0.69	0
Free text ↔ Coded data	0.90	1
Client ↔ Server	0.95	1
Database ↔ Knowledge base	1.00	1
Field ↔ Record	1.01	1
Full-text database ↔ Bibliographic database	1.19	1
Images ↔ Graphics	1.21	1
Digital ↔ Analog	1.29	1.5
Electronic mail ↔ Electronic bulletin board	1.32	1
Sensitivity ↔ Positive predictive value	1.34	2
Data in memory ↔ Data on disk	1.57	2
Mainframe computer ↔ Personal computer	1.70	2
Floppy disk ↔ Hard disk	1.82	2
Hardware ↔ Software	1.85	2

* Scale from "I don't understand the distinction" (0), to "I can define the distinction precisely" (+2).

Table 6. Subjects' assessment of the effects of computers on various aspects of health care*

Effect of computers on:	Mean	Median
E1. Personal and professional privacy	- 0.31	0
E2. Humaneness of the practice of medicine	- 0.22	0
E3. The rapport between clinicians and patients	- 0.12	0
E4. Role of the government in health care	- 0.08	0
E5. Management of medical/ethical dilemmas	0.15	0
E6. The self-image of clinicians	0.18	0
E7. Clinician autonomy	0.22	0
E8. Status of medicine as a profession	0.25	0
E9. Patients' satisfaction with the quality of care they receive	0.34	0
E10. Enjoyment of the practice of medicine	0.57	1
E11. Interactions within the health care team	0.66	1
E12. Generalists' ability to manage more complex problems	0.68	1
E13. Costs of health care	0.84	1
E14. Quality of health care	0.94	1
E15. Access to health care in remote or rural areas	0.98	1
E16. Continuing medical education	1.15	1
E17. Clinicians' access to up-to-date-knowledge	1.49	2

* Scale from "highly detrimental" (–2) to "highly beneficial" (+2).

Attitudes Towards Computers in Health Care

Table 6 shows the mean and median responses of subjects on 17 questions relating to the effects of computers on health care. Of the questions asked, subjects rated most negatively the effects of computers on privacy (E1 and E4) and the doctor-patient relationship (E2 and E3). On the other hand, subjects rated most positively the effects of computers on physician education (E16 and E17). In between, subjects reported that use of computers would have a neutral or slightly beneficial effect on personal satisfaction (E6, E7, E8, and E10) and a more substantial effect on management of health care (E11–15).

For the summary effects score the mean (± standard deviation) was 0.44 (± 0.42), corresponding to a slightly favorable rating of the effects of computers on health care. We found that subjects with higher knowledge scores had a more favorable attitude towards the effects of computers (Spearman's $\rho = .27, p < .0001$). In addition, subjects with formal training had a more favorable attitude about the effects of computers than did subjects with no formal training (Mann-Whitney, $p = .03$). We found a significant difference between specialty groups in their assessment of the effect of computers (Kruskal-Wallis, $p = .004$): surgeons rated the effects of computers as more negative than other groups. We found no significant correlation between the summary effects score and gender, institution, or primary academic activity.

DISCUSSION

Our study describes the knowledge and attitudes of a sample of academic physicians at two institutions in the early stages of clinical information-system deployment. Because of limited response rate, particularly at Stanford University, we can not confidently generalize these results to all physicians at these institutions, nor to all such physicians at similar institutions. However, we believe these results do help sketch a picture of many academic physicians at such institutions.

On the positive side, respondents see the benefits of computers for their own education and as a source of information. The majority of subjects always used the computer to search the medical literature and rated questions regarding the self-education potential of computers as generally or highly beneficial. This may provide a point of leverage for system designers who are trying to persuade physicians to use computers to perform less desirable tasks such as order and data entry. Access to up-to-date information provided in the context of the display of clinical information may be one "carrot" that designers can offer physicians who otherwise may be reluctant to use new computer systems.

On the negative side, respondents appear somewhat concerned about computers because of the potential loss of personal and professional privacy. This fear has been confirmed in other studies, even in environments where information systems are more mature [14]. We believe these concerns should be addressed by both careful design of security features and clear communication with clinicians about how captured clinical information is going to be used.

Another concern of respondents is the effect of computers on the doctor-patient relationship; many believed that the computer will have a negative effect on the rapport between physicians and patients. As more computers are introduced into the patient-care environment, they will likely affect the process of care beyond just changing how clinical information is accessed. Although one study has shown no negative effect of physicians entering data into the electronic medical record during clinical encounters [15], concerns about computers intruding in the doctor-patient relationship will still exist. System designers will need to ponder how to introduce computers into clinical environments without harming the human aspects of patient care. Mobile, pen-based computers, which can be can carried to the bedside yet appear similar to a clipboard, may be one technology that will help in this regard.

We found that most respondents lacked formal training in computing or medical informatics. Even younger physicians had rarely had a formal course on computing during medical school or residency. Physicians with formal training, when compared to those without formal training, were more knowledgeable about informatics concepts and reported that computers would be more beneficial to health care. This result may reflect the effect of education on attitudes or just that those who see value in medical computing seek formal training. Future studies will need to ascertain whether educational programs for faculty would be of interest and benefit, and what topics these programs should address.

Acknowledgments

We would like to thank Jeremy Wyatt, Edward Shortliffe, and Robert Carlson for their help with both the study design and instrument design. We also thank Martha Faircloth for assistance with data entry. This work was conducted with the support of the National Library of Medicine under grant LM-07033. Computing facilities were provided by the CAMIS Resource, LM-05305.

Reference

[1] Kaplan B, Duchon D. Combining qualitative and quantitative methods in information systems research. *MIS Quarterly* 1988;12:871-586.

[2] Forsythe DE, Buchanan BG, Osheroff JA, Miller RA. Expanding the concept of medical information: an observational study of physicians' information needs. *Comput Biomed Res* 1992;25(2):181-200.

[3] Brown SH, Coney RD. Changes in computer anxiety and attitudes related to clinical information system use. *J Am Med Informatics Assoc* 1994;1(5):381-394.

[4] Kraemer KL, ed. *The information systems research challenge: Survey reserarch methods*. Boston: Harvard Business School, 1991.

[5] Zmud RW, Boynton AC. Survey measures and instruments in MIS: Inventory and appraisal. In: Kraemer KL, ed. *The information systems research challenge: Survey reserach methods.* Boston: Harvard Business School, 1991: 149-180.

[6] Zviran M. Evaluating user satisfaction in a hospital environment: an exploratory study. *Health Care Manage Rev* 1992;17(3):51-62.

[7] Bailey JE. Development of an instrument for the management of computer user attitudes in hospitals. *Methods Inf Med* 1990;29(1):51-6.

[8] Burkes M. Identifying and relating nurses' attitudes toward computer use. *Comput Nurs* 1991;9(5):190-201.

[9] Teach RL, Shortliffe EH. An analysis of physician attitudes regarding computer-based clinical consultation systems. *Comput Biomed Res* 1981;14(6):542-58.

[10] al-Hajjaj MS, Bamgboye EA. Attitudes and opinions of medical staff towards computers. *Comput Biol Med* 1992;22(4):221-6.

[11] Anderson RM, Donnelly MB, Hess GE. An assessment of computer use, knowledge, and attitudes of diabetes educators. *Diabetes Educ* 1992;18(1):40-6.

[12] Hammond JE, Berger RG, Carey TS, et al. The Physician's Workstation: an example of end user integration of information systems. *Proc Annu Symp Comput Appl Med Care* 1991:970-2.

[13] Detmer WM, Friedman CP. Demands of academic physicians on future medical information systems. *Proceedings of the 1994 AMIA Spring Congress* San Francisco, 1994: 55.

[14] Rind DM, Safran C. Real and imagined barriers to an electronic medical record. *Proc Annu Symp Comput Appl Med Care* 1993:74-8.

[15] Legler JD, Oates R. Patients' reactions to physician use of a computerized medical record system during clinical encounters. *J Fam Pract* 1993;37(3):241-4.

Transforming Information Use in Preventive Medicine: Learning to Balance Technology with the Art of Caring

Carolyn E. Aydin[1], Peter N. Rosen[2], and Vincent J. Felitti[2]
[1]Cedars-Sinai Medical Center, Los Angeles, CA
[2]Kaiser-Permanente Medical Care Program, San Diego, CA

CompuHx is an Interactive Health Appraisal System (IHAPS) used in the examining room to record patient information, assist in diagnosis, and provide a legible summary of findings. This paper describes Phase I of a longitudinal study in which 22 examiners (five system users and 17 non-users) responded to detailed surveys and interviews about the system. Findings indicated that both users and non-users had mixed feelings about the system's ease of use and impact on their jobs, but agreed that it would have value for their practice. Underlying their acceptance of the system was a common concern for maintaining a caring relationship with patients and not allowing computer technology to depersonalize the examining room. Examiners also expressed concerns about the implementation process.*

INTRODUCTION

The majority of work on computer use by clinicians has focused on informatics in hospitals and in specialty medicine [1]. Furthermore, the systems in use in outpatient settings seldom involve direct clinician data entry during the patient visit [2]. Most research on the use of computers in the consulting room comes from studies conducted in the United Kingdom where it is estimated that 75-90% of primary care physicians work in computerized practices and over 60% use computers during consultation [3,4,5,6,7].

This paper extends the literature on computers in the consulting room to the U.S. by reporting on Phase I of a longitudinal study designed to examine clinician, patient, and organizational outcomes of an interactive health appraisal system. The project is particularly important because it focuses on computerization of the health appraisal process in a large health maintenance organization, a setting likely to become increasingly important as health care reform unfolds.

The portion of the study described here was designed to: (1) describe clinician reactions to CompuHx in the examining room, (2) examine the individual and organizational variables influencing those reactions, and (3) determine whether clinicians who report more stress from uncertainty in patient care have more positive reactions toward a system designed to ensure thoroughness and assist in reaching a diagnosis [8].

HEALTH APPRAISAL

The Kaiser-Permanente Medical Care Program provides a detailed, complete history and physical examination to 50,000 members per year in the San Diego Department of Preventive Medicine. The majority of these patients are the "worried well," patients whose care does not require the traditional, costly, sickness-care portion of the organization [9]. Despite this fact, however, personal interactions with the clinician are an essential part of the health appraisal process for these patients. Recent interviews with 53 patients indicated that approximately 60% came with specific symptoms, concerns, or fears to discuss [10]. All examinations are performed by a nurse practitioner or physician assistant ("examiner"), with a physician always available for consultation. The minority needing further care are guided to the appropriate physician. Five of the 22 examiners are CompuHx system users.

COMPUHX IN THE EXAMINING ROOM

CompuHx is an Interactive Health Appraisal System (IHAPS) designed to utilize artificial intelligence, data base management, and computer graphics to create a fully detailed, legible medical record. CompuHx is designed to enforce thoroughness by (1) addressing all information contained in the original patient questionnaire, (2) ensuring that all information necessary for diagnosis has been obtained, and (3) recording/storing/reproducing the information in a legible, structured, and easily accessible medium. CompuHx is intended ensure the performance of the examiners and the quality of patient care.

Two categories of information are initially stored in the data base: patient history (based upon a questionnaire completed by the patient at home prior to the visit) and lab values. Stored in the examining room computer are almost 100 screens, each specific to a question in the medical history. When queried by the examiner, the program displays screens specific to questions answered affirmatively (or left unanswered) by the patient on the questionnaire. Each screen has color- and shape-coded icons covering the subsidiary questions necessary to fully detail a specific medical problem. Almost all entry is mouse-driven and screens are designed to aid the examiner in obtaining the necessary information, as well as recording that information and a diagnosis.

Following the patient history screens is a series of 20 screens to be used in similar fashion during the actual physical examination. Icons prompt the examiner to record all relevant information and diagnoses. At the end of the physical exam, the computer displays a list of all findings and diagnoses. The examiner eliminates findings that have been subsumed, prioritizes the diagnoses, relating a condition to a referral if necessary, and "ties" medications to a condition if prescribed. When complete, all information is sent back to the data base and a written summary of the patient history and medical examination is generated along with a "to do" list. A summary letter to the patient discussing the implications of findings is currently in alpha testing.

SYSTEM IMPLEMENTATION

Implementation of CompuHx began in 1991 with a computer installed in one examining room and was expanded to include one additional computer and examiner within the year. When the study began in Fall 1993, five of the 22 examiners had already volunteered to use CompuHx. Their experience with the system ranged from 1 month to two years. Four are currently using the system, with expansion to six planned shortly.

The implementation process has also included technical evaluation and ongoing development of the system itself. As part of this process, all histories completed using CompuHx are reviewed in detail by the Director of the Department of Preventive Medicine, who has sponsored and guided the development of the program. These reviews include the performance of the individual examiner on CompuHx as well as potential changes to the computer program itself and to the text of the report produced for a specific patient. This implementation process and its organizational context, along with other variables described below, may influence the attitudes of individual examiners toward the implementation of CompuHx.

PREDICTORS OF USER ATTITUDES

Characteristics of individual users such as age, job tenure, previous computer experience, prior attitudes towards computers in health care, and reactions to the stress of uncertainty in patient care can often help predict attitudes toward a new information system. Outcomes, however, are not always predictable. Age, job tenure, and previous computer experience, for example, have been shown to lead to both positive and negative attitudes in different settings. Measuring these background factors enables investigators to document their influence when considering their interaction with other factors in the organizational environment [11].

STUDY METHODOLOGY

Surveys

Phase I of the study began with a comprehensive survey completed by all 22 nurse practitioners and physician assistants (100% response) in the Department of Preventive Medicine. The survey was distributed with a letter explaining that all responses were confidential and would not be available to anyone in the organization. To ensure confidentiality, completed surveys were mailed directly to the investigator not affiliated with Kaiser-Permanente.

Because research has shown that prior expectations for a system are important in understanding later reactions to it (e.g., expectations confirmed, disillusionment, etc.), the survey gathered baseline information from all examiners, system users and non-users alike [12]. Respondents were instructed to answer either from their experience with the system (users) or their expectations about what using the system would be like (non-users). Statistical analyses (e.g., t-tests) examined differences between responses of users and non-users.

Independent variables included in the survey were basic demographic information, personal attitudes about the desirability of computer applications in medical care [13], and reactions to uncertainty in patient care [8]. Dependent variables included expectations or opinions about the accuracy, format, and ease of use of the system [14]; and the impact of CompuHx on numerous aspects of individual job performance and the performance of the department as a whole [15,16,17].

Interviews

Following completion of the surveys, moderately structured 10-20 minute interviews were conducted with 11 of the 22 examiners, including 3 of the 5 system users and 8 non-users. The interviewer was not affiliated with Kaiser-Permanente and respondents were assured that their responses were confidential. Examiners were asked what they knew about the system and how they had acquired the information, their opinions about CompuHx, learning to use the system, impacts on their job, the implementation process, interactions with patients and other clinicians, and other opinions they wished to share. Interview findings supplemented analyses of the survey data.

FINDINGS

Demographic Data

Survey responses indicated that the 22 examiners included 7 nurse practitioners, 14 physician assistants and one examiner who had both credentials. They had a mean of 8.7 years health care experience (range=1-18 years) and had worked in the department a mean of 4.4 years (range=4 months-14 years). Fourteen (64%) were female and 8 (36%) were male.

Thirteen examiners (59%) had no previous computer experience while 9 (41%) had experience with word processing or other computer applications. Three of the five CompuHx users (60%) had previous computer experience compared to six of the 17 (35%) non-users. Four of the five CompuHx users (80%) were male. Since CompuHx users had volunteered to use the system, demographic data indicate that male examiners and those with previous computer experience were more likely to volunteer. (In fact, the one woman who had used the system indicated that, while she was willing, she had initially been asked to use the system by the Director.)

Attitudes Toward CompuHx

Ratings of CompuHx System

Findings showed no significant differences in attitudes toward CompuHx between system users and non-users. Thus their data are combined in Tables 1-3 below.

Table 1
Ratings of CompuHx System
(N=22)

Scoring: 1=almost never, 3=almost half the time, 5=almost always

	Mean	SD
Content	3.75	0.64
Accuracy (alpha=.90)	3.82	0.58
Format (alpha=.89)	3.68	0.77
Ease of Use (alpha=.85)	3.18	0.82

Respondents' ratings (users and non-users combined) of the CompuHx system itself are shown in Table 1. The system received higher ratings for content, accuracy and format, but was rated as "easy to use" only "almost half the time." (Cronbach's coefficient alpha, a measure of internal consistency, is also given for scales composed of multiple questions.)

Impacts on Job Performance

Respondents (both users and non-users) rated different potential impacts on job performance. (See Table 2.) Findings showed respondents were uncertain about positive effects on their job performance, but agreed that (1) their performance will be monitored more, (2) top management sees the system as important, (3) training is sufficient, (4) external relationships with departments such as primary care will improve, and (5) the system is a good teaching tool for new grads.

Table 2
Impacts on Job Performance
(N=22)

	Mean	SD
1=strongly disagree, 3=uncertain, 5=strongly agree		
Positive effects on job performance (alpha=.89)	3.15	0.58
Performance monitored more	3.82	0.73
Top management sees system important	3.86	0.64
Training sufficient/adequate (alpha=.63)	3.68	0.72
Improves external communication/ relationships (alpha=.85)	3.57	0.74
Good teaching tool for new grads	3.64	1.18
1=strongly disagree, 4=neutral, 7=strongly agree		
Makes job easier/interesting/fun/ pleasant (alpha=.89)	3.73	1.43
Makes job more stressful	4.23	1.38
Increase overall ease/quality of department's work (alpha=.89)	4.52	1.16
System worth the time and effort required to use it	4.64	1.22

Overall, respondents also felt it would make their job slightly less easy, interesting, fun, and pleasant and slightly more stressful. Higher standard deviations, however, indicated wider diversity of opinion on these questions. Finally, examiners slightly agreed that the system would increase the ease and quality of their work and would be worth the time and effort to use it.

Predictors of Attitudes toward CompuHx

Individual characteristics such as gender, age, experience, or prior computer use did not predict attitudes toward CompuHx. Opinions about the impact of computers on the role of the clinician, however, significantly predicted attitudes toward CompuHx [13]. Respondents who felt that computers would diminish the clinician's role (i.e., be hard to learn, diminish clinician judgment, be a less efficient use of clinician time, depersonalize practice, and alienate clinicians from their patients, alpha=.89) had significantly more negative attitudes toward CompuHx. (See Table 3.)

Table 3
Correlation of Computer Impact on Clinician Role with Selected Impacts on Job Performance
(N=22)

	Diminish Clinician Role
Positive effects on job performance	r=-.63 p<.002
Makes job easier/interesting/fun/ pleasant	r=-.75 p<.0001
Increase overall ease/quality of department's work	r=-.61 p<.003
System worth the time and effort required to use it	r=-.73 p<.0001

Uncertainty in Patient Care and CompuHx

Respondents also answered 13 questions designed to measure reactions to uncertainty in patient care (alpha=.89) [8]. Higher scores indicate greater stress. While Stress from Uncertainty did not correlate with attitudes toward the system, CompuHx users (M=2.37) did show significantly less stress from uncertainty in clinical practice than did non-users (M=3.21), $t(18.5)=3.57$, $p<.003$. It is unclear, however, whether those with greater tolerance for uncertainty volunteered to be the first users or whether using the system contributed to their higher tolerance for uncertainty. In other research, males and physicians in practice longer have shown less stress from uncertainty. There were, however, no significant gender or time differences in the present study, although, understandably, examiners in this preventive medicine setting showed less stress than did physicians in other settings [8,18].

Interview Findings

Interview findings indicated that respondent attitudes toward the system clustered around four themes: (1) quality control, (2) depersonalization of patient care, (3) time concerns, and (4) the implementation process.

Thoroughness and Quality Control

Most respondents mentioned the thoroughness of the examination enforced by the prompts in the CompuHx system as a benefit for patient care. Some respondents (both users and non-users) were concerned, however, that the program might not allow enough space for open-ended responses or direct patient quotations.

Depersonalization of Patient Care

Ten of the eleven examiners interviewed brought up the potential for depersonalizing patient care when the examiner's attention is focused on a computer terminal or keyboard and not on the patient. As one respondent noted, this is a "psychological and social visit" for these patients. "They come for the time and attention." While most CompuHx users didn't feel that it was a problem, they mentioned making a concerted effort (especially while they were first learning the system) to maintain eye contact with patients. One user noted that it was too disruptive to use the computer while conducting the physical exam. Rather, he enters the data into the computer after the patient leaves. A non-user described mastering the computer system and continuing to meet patients' needs at the same time as an "art" that would have to be learned. Both users and non-users also noted that many patients may be pleased with the thoroughness of the computerized exam, feeling they get more time and attention from the examiner.

Time

Time was a third recurring theme. Both users and non-users noted that, because the program's thoroughness and enforced responses do not allow examiners to use their clinical judgment to skip certain areas of questioning, examinations using CompuHx take more time and have an impact on examiner productivity. Some non-users, however, hoped the computer system might help them speed up their history taking.

Implementation Process

The fourth area of concern was the implementation process. Because implementation has been intertwined with continuing system development and modification, considerable time is spent by both the Director of Preventive Medicine and the examiner in reviewing and correcting the final report for each patient. Furthermore, each examiner learning to use the system becomes something of an apprentice to the Director, altering their working relationship, at least for a time. Some examiners expressed unwillingness to use the system until all modifications were complete, not wanting to spend the time editing reports or, perhaps, subject themselves to the close scrutiny of the department Director.

DISCUSSION

This case study provides baseline data on provider reactions to CompuHx in a one organization. While the sample is small, 100 percent of the department's 22 examiners responded to the survey. This high response rate, combined with interview findings, provides accurate baseline information on examiner perceptions of the system and its impacts on their specific practice. Study findings are also congruent with research in the United Kingdom on computer use by physicians in the consulting room in which both the time required to gather more explicit data and concerns over depersonalization of the patient encounter have surfaced [5,6,7]. In addition, this project begins an exploration of the relationship between a system that enforces thoroughness and aids in diagnosis and the stress clinicians may feel from the uncertainty inherent in patient care. The implementation arrangement in the setting under study also had an impact on examiners' willingness to use the system. The later phases of this longitudinal project will use a variety of evaluation methods to address these issues as the study examines long-term impacts of the system on patients, clinicians, and the organization as a whole.

* Designed by Fuzzy Logic, Inc., La Jolla, CA.

ACKNOWLEDGEMENTS

This project was supported by a research grant from the Kaiser-Permanente Medical Care Program.

Reference

[1]. R.M. Bernstein., G.R. Hollingworth., G. Viner., J. Lemelin. Family Practice Informatics: Research Issues in Computerized Medical Records. Proceedings of the Seventeenth Annual Symposium on Computer Applications in Medical Care. Washington DC: IEEE Computer Society Press, November 1993:93-97.

[2]. C.J. McDonald., W.M. Tierney., J.M. Overhage., D.K. Martin., G.A. Wilson. The Regenstrief Medical Record System: 20 Years of Experience in Hospitals, Clinics, and Neighborhood Health Centers. *M.D. Computing* 1992; 9:206-217.

[3]. G.M. Hayes. Computers in the Consultation: The UK Experience. Proceedings of the Seventeenth Annual Symposium on Computer Applications in Medical Care. Washington DC: IEEE Computer Society Press, November 1993:103-106.

[4]. I.N. Purves. Implications for Family Practice Record Systems in the USA; Lessons from the United Kingdom. Proceedings of the American Medical Informatics Association 1993 Spring Congress, pg. 54. St. Louis, MO.

[5]. G. Herzmark., G. Brownbridge., M. Fitter., A. Evans. Consultation Use of a Computer by General Practitioners. *Journal of the Royal College of General Practitioners* 1984; 34: 649-654.

[6]. G. Brownbridge., M. Fitter., M Sime. The Doctor's Use of a Computer in the Consulting Room: An Analysis. *International Journal of Man-Machine Studies* 1984; 21:65-90.

[7]. G. Brownbridge., R. Lilford., S. Tindale-Biscoe. Use of a Computer to Take Booking Histories in a Hospital Antenatal Clinic. *Medical Care* 1988; 26:474-187.

[8]. M.S. Gerrity., R.F. DeVellis., J.A. Earp. Physicians' Reactions to Uncertainty in Patient Care. *Medical Care* 1990; 28:724-736.

[9]. V.J. Felitti. *Patient Entry into a Large, Multispecialty Medical Group.* Unpublished report, Kaiser-Permanente Medical Care Program, San Diego,.

[10]. C.E. Aydin., V.J. Felitti. *Health Appraisal: Why Do They Really Come?* Unpublished report, Kaiser-Permanente Medical Care Program, San Diego, 1993.

[11]. C.E. Aydin. Survey Methods for Assessing Social Impacts of Computers in Health Care Organizations. In J.G. Anderson., C.E. Aydin., S.J. Jay (Eds.), *Evaluating Health Care Information Systems.* Sage Publications, Thousand Oaks, CA, 1994, pp. 69-115.

[12]. C.E. Aydin., R.E. Rice. Bringing Social Worlds Together: Computers as Catalysts for New Interactions in Health Care Organizations. *Journal of Health and Social Behavior* 1992; 33:168-185.

[13]. J.G. Anderson., S.J. Jay., H.M. Schweer., M.M. Anderson. Why Doctors Don't Use Computers: Some Empirical Findings. *Journal of the Royal Society of Medicine* 1986; 79:142-144.

[14]. W.J. Doll., G. Torkzadeh. The Measurement of End-User Computing Satisfaction. *MIS Quarterly* 1988; 12:259-274.

[15]. R.L. Schultz., D.P. Slevin. Implementation and Organizational Validity: An Empirical Investigation in R.L. Schultz, D.P. Slevin (Eds.), *Implementing Operations Research/Management Science.* New York: American Elsevier, pp. 153-182.

[16]. C.E. Aydin., R.E. Rice. Social Worlds, Individual Differences, and Implementation: Predicting Attitudes Toward a Medical Information System. *Information and Management* 1991; 20:119-136.

[17]. K.H. Kjerulff., M.A. Counte., J.S. Salloway., B.C. Campbell. Understanding Employee Reactions to a Medical Information System. Proceedings of the Fifth Annual Symposium on Computer Applications in Medical Care. IEEE Computer Society Press, Los Angeles, CA, pp. 802-805.

[18]. J.G. Anderson., S.J. Trajkovski., R. Campbell., A. Haley., M.M. Anderson. Determining Clinical Practice Styles from Computer-Based Data. Proceedings Medinfo 92, 7th World Congress on Medical Informatics, Geneva, Switzerland, 6-10 September, 1992.

Obstacles and Approaches to Clinical Database Research: Experience at the University of California, San Francisco

Thomas B. Newman, MD,MPH
Andrew Brown MD, MPH
M. Janet Easterling

Department of Laboratory Medicine, University of California, San Francisco, CA

With increasing availability of clinical data in machine-readable form, and decreasing cost of storing and manipulating that data, retrospective research using clinical databases has become more feasible. Nonetheless, much of the potential for clinical research using these data remains unrealized. Obstacles to clinical database research include difficulty accessing data, difficulty using retrospective data to draw valid inferences about medical tests and treatments, and a shortage of investigators trained and interested in using a clinical database to answer their questions. At the University of California, San Francisco, we have developed a Clinical Database Research Program (CDRP) to try to overcome these obstacles. The CDRP maintains a relational database of patient data obtained from diverse sources and a small staff dedicated to providing such data to researchers. The CDRP staff also provides support for design and analysis of studies using the database--the development of methods for such studies is our primary research interest. Finally, to increase the number of investigators using the database for research, we are integrating training in clinical epidemiology and clinical research methods into residency and fellowship training, and offering an elective in clinical database research for trainees who wish to undertake a specific project.

As more and more patient care activities generate data in machine readable form, and available hardware and software improve, there is increasing potential for using routinely collected clinical data for research [1-3]. However, considering the vast stores of clinical data theoretically available to potential investigators, the actual amount of clinical research therefrom has been quite modest. In this paper, we will review some obstacles to clinical database research and the approaches the University of California, San Francisco (UCSF) Clinical Database Research Program (CDRP) is taking to overcome them.

OBSTACLES

Difficulty Accessing Data

Data are dispersed. At UCSF, there is a wide variety of clinical data already in machine-readable form. However, as at many medical centers [4], the data are dispersed in separate systems that have evolved independently of one another. Independent computer systems have been implemented in the clinical laboratory, medical records, the pharmacy, radiology, the emergency department, and so on. Some of these systems provide data to the medical center's clinical display system (STOR), which allows retrieval of data on a particular patient at the point of care. However, what is sent to the clinical display system is often a free text report. Coding and data structure present in the original database are not generally preserved. In addition, many data are currently not reported to STOR. Thus, at UCSF useful data are difficult to obtain because of the number of different platforms and personnel involved.

Competition between research and patient care. That relevant data are scattered throughout the medical center is not necessarily an insurmountable obstacle to clinical researchers. For many research questions, data from only one or a few sources might be enough. However, simply finding the data is not sufficient--the personnel familiar with the systems involved have to agree to provide it (in suitable format, with appropriate documentation) to potential investigators. These personnel often do not view provision of data for research as their highest priority. Furthermore, clinical database research is often an iterative process. Thus, the first (and second and third) request for data may need to be revised after some initial analyses. This process is difficult if the personnel involved do not view provision of research data as an important part of their job. In addition, the competition is not just

0195-4210/94/$5.00 © 1994 AMIA, Inc.

for personnel, but for computer time. In order to avoid slowing down clinical systems, research queries may need to be run as batch jobs late at night, diminishing the possibility of interactive data requests.

Scientific Problems with Retrospective Studies

Data collected as a part of patient care are less suitable for answering many types of research questions than data collected prospectively, either for an observational study or for part of a clinical trial [5]. For example, whereas most guidelines for designing or interpreting studies of diagnostic tests specify that a "gold standard" test must be uniformly and blindly applied to all the subjects, in clinical practice results on one test often affect the decision to order subsequent tests, as well as their interpretation. Similarly, retrospective studies of treatments are difficult because the intensity of treatment for a particular disease is likely to be correlated with a worse outcome from that disease simply because patients with more severe disease are treated more intensively. These scientific problems with retrospective studies limit the types of questions that can be addressed with a clinical database, and tend to be discouraging to potential investigators, particularly those without advanced training in epidemiology or statistics.

Underutilization of data

Research is time consuming. Even when the data collection phase is abbreviated by accessing existing data, considerable effort is required to review the literature, design a study, analyze the data, write the paper and get it published. Thus, if only investigators closely associated with a clinical database are mining it for research purposes, it is likely to be underutilized. To realize the full potential of clinical databases for research, the number of investigators using them should be maximized.

There are, however, a number of obstacles to attracting investigators to this type of research. In academic medical centers, tradition, funding availability, and prestige all tend to focus investigators' efforts on becoming an expert on a narrow topic. For any particular topic, the amount that one can learn from a clinical database is limited. The promise of clinical database research is a small (but significant) amount of information about a multitude of different topics, rather than the great depth of study about a particular topic that is helpful for long-term funding and academic success. Thus one of the problems in attracting investigators to clinical database research is that faculty see it as unlikely to advance their careers.

APPROACHES

Facilitating Access: the CDRP Database

An obvious solution to dispersed data is integration. Other investigators have reported systems for integration of heterogenous databases that involve querying the component databases nightly [4], or at the time of a query [6]. At UCSF we took a different approach, dictated by different goals and limited resources. We wanted to allow interactive access to the database while avoiding competition for personnel or computing time between research and clinical care. In addition, because the primary purpose of our database is retrospective research, efficient access to a large store of historical data was more important to us than immediate access to data that are current or even several months old. We therefore obtained data, usually in the form of formatted ASCII text, from a variety of computers on campus, and placed the data into a separate relational database that can be queried interactively for research. We update each of the various components of the database about twice a year from dumps from the computers on which the current data reside.

An overview of the most important current contents of the database, together with approximate space requirements, is provided in the Table. Most of the data are numerical or coded, but some laboratory results are free text. To facilitate retrieval of laboratory data, we used a fourth generation language (4GL) to add unique admission numbers and binary flag fields for maximum, minimum, first, and last for each inpatient test result to identify those results most likely to be of interest from a particular admission.

In spite of not doing any primary data collection ourselves, creation of the database has been labor intensive. The current database, which includes about 5.5 years of data, has taken about two person-years to assemble. Most of this has been programming time, but identifying data sources and getting the personnel involved to provide the data dumps is also time-consuming. In

Table: Major tables in the UCSF-CDRP database, as of August, 1994.

Source of Data Table	# Records	Storage Space	Example fields
Clinical laboratory			
Results	31,000,000	3,200 Mb	Unit number, date, test number, result text, numeric result, admit number, maxflag (see text)
Microbiology			
Specimens	549,000	250 Mb	Unit number, specimen number, source, date
Isolates	163,000	13 Mb	Specimen number, organism, count
Medical records			
Patients	239,000	37 Mb	Name, unit number, sex, date of birth
Admissions	175,000	30 Mb	Admit number, admit date, drg
Diagnoses	688,000	52 Mb	Admit number, ICD-9 diagnosis code
Procedures	388,000	35 Mb	Admit number, ICD-9 procedure code
Obstetrics	29,000	6 Mb	Maternal age, delivery date, type of delivery, gestational age, birth weight
Cardiology			
Echocardiograms	280,000	17 Mb	Unit number, procedure number, procedure date, result code, admit number
Treadmill tests	37,000	8 Mb	

addition, to assure the completeness and quality of the data we have performed regular comparisons with written medical records. However, now that this considerable amount of ground work has been accomplished, we will be able to turn increasing attention to adding data from new sources, to facilitating retrieval with graphical interfaces, and to recruiting and assisting investigators (see below).

Rigorous Retrospective Studies

Although there are many questions that cannot be answered using retrospective data, there are many that can. Because our database is particularly rich in diagnostic data, we have focussed on study designs for assessing diagnostic tests.

Most guidelines on design or interpretation of studies of diagnostic tests are aimed at protecting against falsely concluding that a diagnostic test is helpful when it is not. This is because traditionally, many more research studies (and papers) have been directed at identification of new diagnostic tests than at evaluation of existing tests. The times, however, are a changin'. In the era of managed care, there is increasing interest in identifying existing diagnostic tests that are *not* useful. Luckily, it is easier to show that a test is *not* useful than that it *is* useful. For a diagnostic test to be clinically useful, it must be abnormal at least some of the time, these abnormalities must not be readily predictable from other available data, abnormalities must affect management, and the management decisions must lead to a better outcome. A study that calls into question any one of these necessary but not sufficient criteria can suggest that a diagnostic test is not useful.

One study design that lends itself well to clinical database research is what we have called a *Diagnostic Yield Study*. This design is appropriate for examining tests for diseases that are often sought and seldom found. (Such tests seem to be done frequently at academic centers.) In a diagnostic yield study, a group of patients of interest is identified based on their having had a particular laboratory test. In many cases, this group can be made more homogenous with respect to clinical indications for the test by including or excluding patients based on results of other tests, previous discharge diagnoses, and so on. Results on the test for the whole group of subjects are obtained, but only those with abnormal results are studied further. The questions such a study can answer are: how often is the test abnormal? When it is abnormal, could the abnormality have been predicted from other tests? Was management affected by the abnormal result? What was the outcome?

For example, we used the database to study the diagnostic yield of direct bilirubin levels in jaundiced newborn babies [7]. From about 5000 determinations of direct bilirubin, we identified those whose results were above the 95th percentile. In most cases we could see from the database that the result was not clinically significant because the elevation was temporary and was not accompanied by any other tests or discharge diagnoses suggestive of hepatobiliary disease. In the relatively few cases in which there was any doubt, we reviewed medical records. All of the infants who appeared to have had clinically significant direct hyperbilirubinemia had other signs or laboratory evidence of illness before the direct bilirubin elevation was noted. We recommended that direct bilirubin levels be ordered much more selectively in jaundiced infants.

We have done similar studies (with similar results) on the other laboratory tests commonly done to evaluate jaundice in newborn babies [8]. Other examples of diagnostic yield studies that have identified unnecessary or over-used tests include a study of IgM levels as a screening test for congenital infection in small-for-gestational-age newborns [9], and a University of Pennsylvania study of stool cultures for hospital-acquired diarrhea [10].

A variant of the diagnostic yield study is a study of *diagnostic redundancy*. In this design, results of two or more tests ordered together are compared to identify how often they give discrepant results. (When both are normal or both are abnormal, it presumably was not necessary to do both tests.) Medical records of the small subset with discrepant results can then be reviewed to see which test (apparently) gave the right answer. Even in cases where no "gold standard" is available, records can be reviewed to determine which test was *believed* by the treating physicians, and whether specific circumstances can be defined in which one test or the other is more likely to be helpful.

For example, at UCSF a "liver panel" included determinations of aspartate amino transferase (AST), alkaline phosphatase, and total bilirubin. However, using the database we found that there were very few instances in which the bilirubin was high when both the AST and alkaline phosphatase were normal, and that these instances seldom reflected liver disease [11]. As a result, bilirubin was removed from the liver panel.

Similarly, a Clinical Scholar is using our database to determine how often Lactate Dehydrogenase (LD) isoenzymes provide information beyond that available from creatinine kinase (CK) isoenzymes in the diagnosis of acute myocardial infarction. By selecting patients in whom CK and LD isoenzymes are ordered on the day of admission, patients in whom the goal is to rule-out (or in) a myocardial infarction (MI) can be readily identified. In most such patients, results of both CK and LD isoenzymes are congruent--either both normal or both abnormal. In the minority in whom there is a discrepancy, discharge diagnoses can be reviewed, to determine which result was believed. (Although our database includes discharge diagnoses, our experience is that they are not abstracted reliably enough to use as an outcome variable, so they must be obtained from the medical record for a study of this design.) If circumstances in which LD is believed over CK can be identified (e.g., when the duration of symptoms before admission is longer or when, based on other studies, the CK seems to be falsely negative), we can generate recommendations for more selective ordering of that test.

Recruiting and Training Investigators

A major challenge for those interested in use of clinical databases for research is attracting investigators to use the data. Creation and maintenance of a clinical database are expensive. To justify this investment, the number of questions the database is used to answer must be maximized. This means, for the most part, maximizing the number of people using it.

The first step in encouraging investigators to use a clinical database for research is to assemble a database that includes data items of sufficient interest. At present, the richest, most reliable data in the UCSF CDRP are data from the clinical labs. Our strategy is to obtain additional data according to the interests of potential investigators. We obtained cardiology and obstetrics data because we had fellows interested in using them. Our next two additions to the database are likely to be mortality data and pharmacy data. These will greatly expand the range of possible studies that can be done with the database.

As discussed above, a major obstacle for investigators is that many of the studies for which use of a clinical database is most feasible are relatively small clinical studies, not likely to attract extramural funding. On the other hand, ready availability of data for modest studies is very helpful for trainees. Using a clinical database to do one's own research project is a great way to learn about clinical research. Thus one large group of potential users includes medical students, residents, and fellows who are interested in clinical research. The possibility that, if they think of a good question, they can design and begin a study in one month, and possibly finish in another provides strong motivation. We are developing an elective in clinical database research that will help lead trainees through the steps involved - from identification of a research question to writing up the results.

CONCLUSION

Clinical database research has great potential, not just for answering clinical questions, but as a tool for training residents, fellows, and faculty in clinical research. Centralizing patient data in a relational database that allows interactive queries, providing a staff knowledgeable in study design and analysis, and facilitating clinical database research by trainees seem to be promising ways to realize more of this potential.

References

1. Pryor DB, Califf RM, Harrell F Jr., et al. Clinical data bases. Accomplishments and unrealized potential. Med Care 1985;23:623-47

2. Tierney WM, McDonald CJ. Practice databases and their uses in clinical research. Stat Med 1991;10:541-57

3. Safran C. Using routinely collected data for clinical research. Stat Med 1991;10:559-64

4. Marrs KA, Steib SA, Abrams CA, Kahn MG. Unifying heterogeneous distributed clinical data in a relational database. Proc Annu Symp Comput Appl Med Care 1993;644-8

5. Mantel N. Cautions on the use of medical databases. Stat Med 1983;2:355-62

6. Kamel MN, Zviran M. Heterogeneous databases integration in a hospital information systems environment: a bottom-up approach. Proc Annu Symp Comput Appl Med Care 1991;363-7

7. Newman TB, Hope S, Stevenson DK. Direct bilirubin measurements in jaundiced term newborns. A reevaluation. Am J Dis Child 1991;145:1305-9

8. Newman TB, Easterling MJ. Yield of reticulocyte counts and blood smears in term infants. Clinical Pediatrics 1994;33:71-6

9. Mahon BE, Yamada E, Newman TB. Problems with serum IgM as a screening test for congental infection. Clinical Pediatrics 1994;33:142-6

10. Siegel DL, Edelstein PH, Nachamkin I. Inappropriate testing for diarrheal diseases in the hospital. JAMA 1990;263:979-82

11. Brown AN, Sheiner LB, Cohen SN. Evaluation of bilirubin in a liver screening panel [letter]. JAMA 1992;268:1542

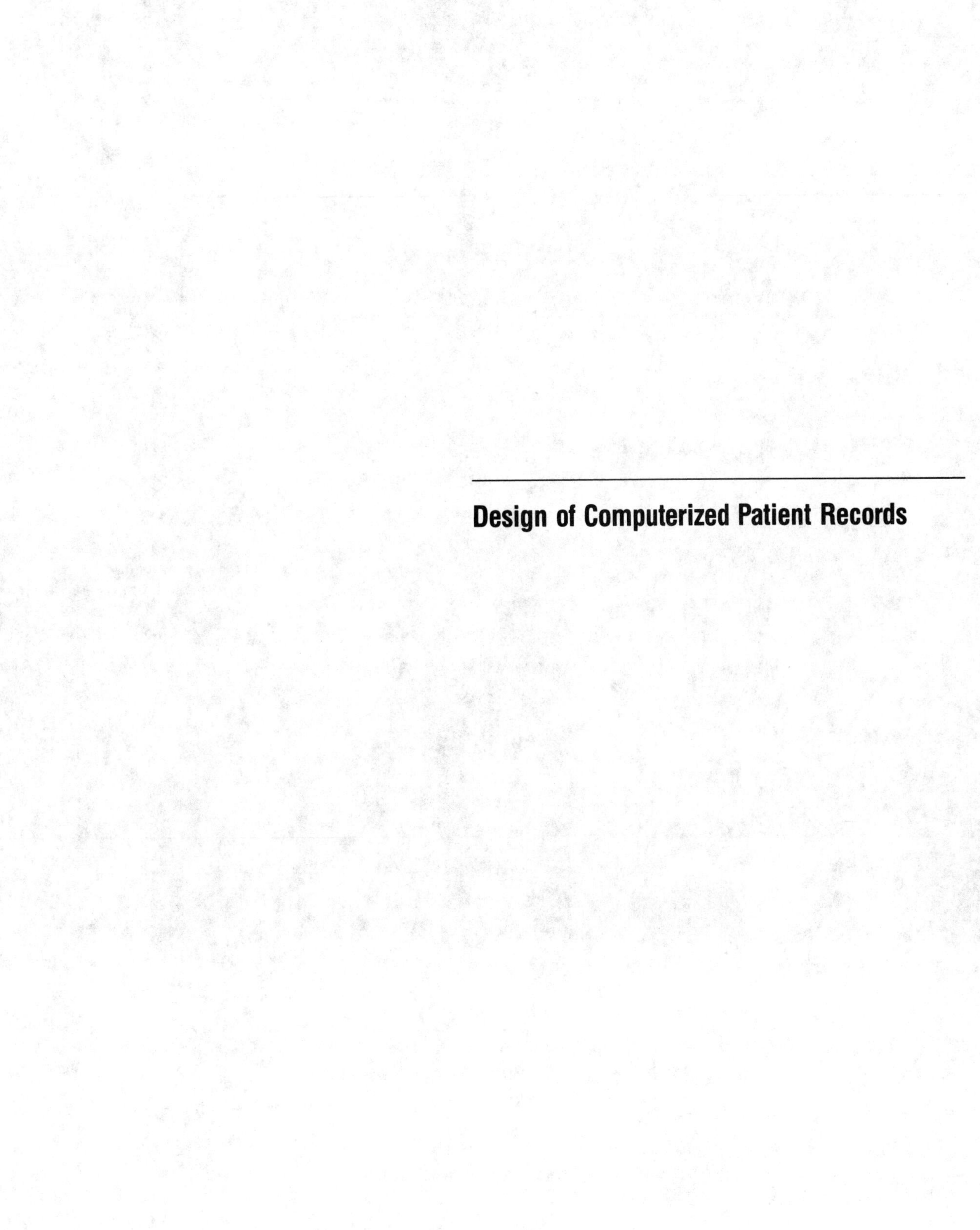

Design of Computerized Patient Records

Traditional Medical Records as a Source of Clinical Data in the Outpatient Setting

Paul C. Tang, MD, Northwestern University School of Medicine, Chicago, IL
Danielle Fafchamps, PhD, Hewlett-Packard Labs, Palo Alto, CA
Edward H. Shortliffe, MD, PhD, Stanford University School of Medicine, Stanford, CA

ABSTRACT

We conducted an observational study at a university hospital clinic to determine the success with which physicians find patient information using traditional hospital records as the source of data. We recorded 168 consecutive patient cases presented to attending physicians by internal medicine residents, and analyzed the transcripts to identify questions indicating that the physicians could not find patient information in the medical record. In 81 percent of the cases, physicians could not find all the patient information that they desired during a patient's visit. We performed thematic analysis to generate a set of 15 prototypical questions asked by physicians regarding patient information. The multi-authored medical record system we studied did not provide effective access to patient information for physicians making clinical decisions in an outpatient setting. Improved methods for addressing prototypical questions arising in routine practice are needed.

INTRODUCTION

All physicians have experienced the frustration of fruitlessly seeking a piece of patient information in a bulky medical record. The traditional document that began as a personal record, maintained by the family physician to keep track of an individual's health over a lifetime, has evolved into a multi-authored creation that is intended to serve many purposes: "to recall observations, to inform others, to instruct students, to gain knowledge, to monitor performance, and to justify interventions."[1] Physicians accordingly realize the central role that medical records play in supporting efficient and effective delivery of healthcare at reasonable cost, and we routinely see comments in the literature reflecting growing concerns that our traditional record system is no longer suited to serving the roles for which they were originally intended [2-6]. Despite these concerns, few empiric studies have characterized the shortcomings in ways that can usefully guide future improvements. Most physicians appear resigned to accepting the time-consuming process of foraging for data in the record, and later recording observations – tasks that may consume up to 38 percent of the physician's time associated with an outpatient visit [7]. With mounting pressures on physicians to improve the cost- and time-efficiency of patient-care encounters, tasks that often consume more than one third of the physician's time are logical targets for analysis and improvement.

The Institute of Medicine (IOM) completed an extended study of patient-record systems, motivated by precisely this sense that our bulky medical records of the past are hindering the quality and efficiency of the healthcare enterprise [8,9]. Although the IOM study found ample published evidence of dissatisfaction with current approaches to medical records, empiric data documenting and characterizing the extent to which paper-based patient record systems satisfy the practitioner's need for patient information could not be found. In this paper we seek to correct this deficit.

We used ethnography, an observational method employed in anthropology [10,11], to determine whether physicians were able to find patient information when relying on the current medical record system. Although difficulty finding desired information may occur either because data are missing from a chart, or because the data are present but cannot be located in reasonable time, our ethnographic observational approach did not distinguish between these two circumstances. Instead, we identified information needed to make decisions during a given patient visit. We also identified prototypical questions posed by physicians seeking information to make patient-care decisions, the answers to which were not found in the medical record. One goal of our study was to gain insight into the kinds of tools that could support answering these prototypical questions and thus better prepare physicians to make optimal patient-care decisions. To the extent that some data were simply missing from the chart, we recognize that tools to facilitate the capture and organization of necessary information are also required. Such tools, however, were not the focus of this study.

METHODS

Studies in medicine [12] and in other disciplines [13] have established that observational studies provide more complete details of work practice than do those based on subjects' recall as elicited in interviews or questionnaires. One of us (D. F.) developed the ethnographic design and carried out the data collection. Observations of actual outpatient visits formed the context for analyzing physician work in our study.

The study was approved by the institutional review board and conducted in the internal medicine clinic (IMC) of a university hospital. All clinic health-care professionals (27 internal medicine residents, 13 faculty physicians supervising residents, 3 nurses, and 4 clerical staff) agreed to participate. The residents were evenly divided among first, second, and third year post-doctoral physicians. In addition to the hospital record, the clinic maintains shadow records, containing copies of IMC progress notes, for all patients seen within the last 18 months. Both the patient's hospital record and clinic shadow record are requested by clinic staff in preparation for each patient visit. Computer terminals in the IMC allow health-care providers to retrieve laboratory-test results and radiology reports. Lab-test results are stored for 30 days in the computer. The residents discuss all patient cases with a faculty physician. During 16 afternoon clinic sessions, we recorded on audio tape three types of discussions: (1) residents' case presentations to attending physicians, (2) telephone and face-to-face conversations among clinic staff related to patient visits, and (3) physicians' verbal answers to brief interviews immediately following the patient visit regarding type of visit, availability of documents (both hospital record and shadow record), the list of active problems, problem acuity, missing patient data (laboratory-test results, medications, radiology reports, etc.), and diagnostic or therapeutic plans. We did not enter patient examining rooms, nor did we study interactions between patients and their providers.

As soon as one case was completed, the observer began recording the next available case. Our goal was to record as many verbal interactions as possible for a given patient visit. For example, if we recorded a resident's case presentation for a patient visit, we then recorded all follow-up interactions of the physician with other sources of patient information regarding that patient's care (e.g., a physician's telephone calls to ancillary departments, interactions with nurses concerning that patient, and calls to other physicians who had participated in the patient's care).

Medical transcriptionists translated the 35 hours of tape recordings into 502 pages of text. All patient names or other identifying information was deleted from the transcripts prior to analysis.

Data Analysis

We reviewed transcripts for evidence that physicians could not find patient information that they felt they needed. We analyzed only cases of return patients (visits by patients who had been seen previously in the institution). If a physician could not find a patient datum in the record, this was considered one data-deficit unit (DDU). As mentioned earlier, our observational study design did not include having the investigator thoroughly review patients' charts to distinguish between the case where a patient datum was actually in the chart, but the physician could not find it, from the case where the datum was not recorded in the chart. We felt this distinction was not relevant for the purpose of this study, since the effect on clinical practice was the same – data were not able to be found when physicians looked for them in order to make clinical decisions on a patient during a given patient visit.

We performed a systematic analysis of similarities and differences across data-deficit units, using thematic analysis. We grouped data-deficit units into categories via an iterative refinement process by looking for similarities in the questions physicians asked as they searched for missing patient information. For example, the following illustrates a data-deficit unit:

> Attending: <u>Did anyone do an echo?</u> Or do we have any evidence of that?
>
> Resident: Um, well it would be nice to know if he had an echocardiogram or not done while he was in the house. But, unfortunately...we don't know.

This text extract was subsequently grouped with other data-deficit units in a category typified by the question: "Has a specific diagnostic test ever been performed on this patient?" We formulated a *prototypical question* for each category of data-deficit units.

RESULTS

In 136 of the 168 (81%) case presentations, physicians did not have all the information they would have liked to have available in order to make patient care decisions during the current visit. We found 538 data-deficit units (mean number per case 3.7, range 1-20) in the 136 cases where some patient data was missing. Of the 538 data-deficit units, 370 (69 percent) data items were generated at our own study institution and could have been expected to appear in the hospital chart. The other 168 units involved data regarding patient-care encounters at other institutions or practices where the patient had been seen.

Difficulty Finding Patient Information in the Record

Clinic shadow records or hospital records were available to the physicians in 95 percent of patient visits. Despite the general availability of the record, however, physicians could not locate all the information they sought within the record, since 82 percent of the data deficit units occurred when the record was available. Eighteen percent of the DDUs arose in the 5 percent of visits where no records were available during the patient visit. Foraging through the record to extract relevant information often required more time than providers were willing to invest.

Types of Patient Data Affected

We identified the following categories of data-deficit units: laboratory-tests/procedures (36 percent), medications/treatments (23 percent), history (31 percent), and other (10 percent). The last category included deficit units such as insurance constraints that affect decision making during that visit.

Physicians' Strategies for Coping with Missing Patient Data

Physicians used three coping strategies to deal with missing patient data: (1) searching alternate sources of patient information, (2) making clinical decisions without the desired information, and (3) relying on the patient or family members to report the missing information.

To find patient information not readily available in the record, providers searched alternate sources of patient data (e.g., checking the clinical laboratory-test results on a computer terminal, rummaging through laboratory-test report bins, or calling another provider) in 42 percent of data-deficit units. In the remaining cases, the providers relied on patient or family reports in 26 percent, and made do without the information they were seeking in 32 percent. The preceding statistics sum to 100% because they reflect the final strategy used (in cases where more than one strategy was employed) by each provider to cope with the problem of missing information. We did not assess the reliability of patients' reports, which sometimes can be problematic, as illustrated in the following excerpt:

> Resident: She was started on tetracycline, but she was told that it was yeast. It doesn't make sense.

When physicians were not able to obtain all the desired information to make decisions, they sometimes deferred those decisions to a follow-up visit. In the interim, they requested the missing information again, reordered some diagnostic tests, and in some cases made decisions without having all the available information.

Prototypical Questions Concerning Patient Information

We analyzed the three most important categories of frequently missing patient information (results of tests and procedures, medications and treatments, and active problems or past medical history) to develop prototypical questions that physicians ask regarding patient information. These questions and their relative frequencies within the four DDU categories are listed in Table 1.

DISCUSSION

Physicians studied in our hospital-based practice setting could not find relevant patient information in 81 percent of outpatient visits. Part of the problem is caused by absent charts, but we also discovered that physicians had difficulty finding information even when the charts were available.

By observing practicing physicians and their use of available information to make decisions regarding care of specific patients, we were able to assess the adequacy of the medical record system as the primary source of patient data. Other observational studies have looked at physicians' needs for domain information [12] and at physicians' information requests for (broadly defined) information during clinical teaching rounds [14]. In the latter study, 52 percent of the questions asked during teaching rounds pertained to individual patients. Our study quantified the prevalence of failing to find patient information in the medical record, and characterized, in the form of prototypical questions, the type of information sought in the outpatient setting.

Review of the prototypical questions which arose during decision making in actual practice revealed a need for more than simple access to patient data; physicians sought data in its clinical context. For example, when asking about a patient's past experience with antihypertensive medications, the physician is not just interested in a list of medications (access to simple data), but rather is also interested in how the patient's blood pressure responded and whether the patient had any adverse effects or complications from the therapy (data in a clinical context). The traditional record is ill-suited to provide answers to prototypical questions, such as: "Has this patient ever been on medication X? If so, when, for what reason, and with what response?" Yet, these are precisely the types of questions posed routinely during clinical decision making, demonstrating a need for improved access to patient information. Methods for integrating and analyzing patient information are needed in order to answer many of the prototypical questions we recorded.

At the institution where we conducted our study, laboratory-test results were not kept on-line past 30 days, after which printed results were assumed to be available in the hospital chart. The relatively short time that lab test results were available on the computer contributed

Table 1: Distribution of Prototypical Questions

Categories of questions (percent of total questions)	Questions	Percent of data-deficit units within category
Results of tests and procedures (36%)	What were the results of a specific diagnostic test or procedure?	36%
	What tests or procedures were done by other providers? Why were they done?	20%
	Was there adequate follow-up?	14%
	What was the trend of the laboratory-test results?	11%
	Has a specific diagnostic test ever been performed on this patient?	10%
	What is the status of routine health-care maintenance for this patient?	9%
Medications and treatments (23%)	What medications have been prescribed for this patient? By whom? For what reasons?	54%
	What responses to medications have been observed in the past?	32%
	What medications and dosages has the patient been taking?	15%
Active problems and past medical history (31%)	What was done by another provider?	49%
	What past problems has this patient had?	19%
	What active problems does this patient have?	9%
	What evidence led to the diagnosis of a specific disease?	9%
	What symptoms and signs of a specific problem have been documented in the past?	8%
	What medication allergies does this patient have?	6%
Other (10%)		

to the relatively high number of laboratory-test results that were unavailable to clinicians during the outpatient visits. Furthermore, many departmental test results were not available through the laboratory terminals, such as results from electrocardiograms, treadmill tests, echocardiograms, pulmonary function tests, arterial blood gases, nuclear medicine tests, and others.

Although we studied only a single clinic and a single institution's medical record system, it is reasonable to assume that the data provided here would be typical of those for other hospital-based clinics, particularly in academic settings where care is often distributed over a large number of providers who share a single patient chart. Compared to patients in the university medical center clinic where we conducted our study, patients seen by small group practices are more likely to see the same physician consistently. In another study, however, physicians found that their own entries in the medical record were as difficult to read as was information entered by others[2]. Furthermore, failure to find information from consultants' reports would be a prevalent problem in either setting. Also, demographics of group practice are changing rapidly, with more providers practicing in larger groups where multiprovider care (and charts) are the rule, as they were in our study group.

Our results raise questions that require further investigations. What are the cost and quality implications of making decisions without the results of tests that were ordered and performed, but whose results cannot be found? How do we justify the cost or risk of a diagnostic test, if clinical decisions are then made without knowledge of the results? How many tests are ordered because the results of a previous test cannot be found? What are the risks of changing a patient's medication without an accurate medication history? Since we did not follow the course of individual patients, we could not determine the actual impact of decisions having been made without specific information. Only a longitudinal study could provide formal data on how missing data or limited access to information affect patient-care outcomes. However, our data justify concern that the current medical record system is negatively affecting both the costs and quality of health care. Organizations and agencies interested in these issues should consider the effect of the medical record on the quality and cost of clinical decision making.

Information can be unavailable because the chart is missing, or because either the data were not recorded in the chart or the physician could not find the data in the chart. In the latter case, there are several reasons why a physician may not find the information, including a lack of time, a lack of ability, or a lack of motivation. Although we cannot guarantee that a more meticulous search for a longer period of time would not have allowed the physicians to uncover more information, the purpose of the study was to determine how successful physicians are when attempting to find the patient information for which they expressed a need when discussing a patient's case with an attending physician in routine clinical practice. Practical considerations certainly limit the physician's ability to gather data. The residents were evenly divided among first, second, and third year post-doctoral physicians and thus had varying levels of expertise and experience coping with data limitations. One might consider that the extra time residents have to see a patient (60 or 30 minutes, depending on whether the patient is new to the clinic or returning to a familiar provider) might compensate for less developed coping strategies for finding information. Alternatively, it is possible that residents are better at finding information than attendings (since they use the chart more extensively due to their intensive clinical work), but such distinctions were not the point of our study and we have no data to support their discussion. Although we did not review the medical records to distinguish between cases where physicians could not find the information (for whatever reason) when it was in the chart, from those cases when the data were not recorded in the chart, the impact of not having the information when decisions were made was the same. Any plans to improve upon this situation must consider both these possibilities, and tools are needed to alleviate both causes for missing information.

Even though our study identifies a problem without documenting a solution, the prototypical questions we derived do suggest that information-management methods which help practitioners find relevant information contained in the medical record may address some of the weaknesses of current record-keeping systems. The Institute of Medicine's Study on Improving the Patient Record concluded that the computer-based patient record is an essential technology for health care [8]. The report stressed, however, that their notion of a computer-based record system was more than simply an electronic version of the paper-based record. It should provide tools to manipulate, format, and display information in flexible ways to support physicians making clinical decisions on their patients. Certainly, automatic capture of data which already exist in electronic form (e.g., pharmacy data, discharge summaries) would help computer-based patient records to be more complete in terms of these types of data. Furthermore, with careful attention to the user interface, it may be possible to have physicians enter information in the computer-based record that is not currently recorded in the paper chart, such as reasons for prescribing a certain medication. For the cases where the primary data originate from another institution, regional or even nationally linked records will be required.

The results of our study show that physicians have great difficulty finding relevant patient information using traditional, multi-authored records. Methods to retrieve patient data and tools to put data in their clinical context will be required to answer effectively the prototypical questions we identified. Improving the patient record system will ultimately have a profound effect on health care, as the record is central to clinical decision making.

Acknowledgments

We thank the faculty, residents, nurses, and clerks who graciously gave us their permission to record their discussions on tape. We thank Jaap Suermondt for his helpful discussions and his technical help with the data analysis. We thank Blackford Middleton for his helpful comments on drafts of this paper. We are also grateful for editorial assistance from Lyn Dupré.

Reference

1 Reiser SJ. The clinical record in medicine; Part 1: Learning from cases. Ann Intern Med. 1991; 114:902–7.

2 Zimmerman J. Physician utilization of medical records: preliminary determinations. Med Inform. 1978;3:27–35.

3 Tufo HM, Speidel JJ. Problems with medical records. Med Care. 1971;9:509–17.

4 Zuckerman ZE, Starfield B, Hochreiter C, Kovasznay B. Validating the content of pediatric outpatient medical records by means of tape-recording doctor–patient encounters. Ped. 1975;56:407–11.

5 Dawes KS. Survey of general practice records. BMJ. 1972;3:219–23.

6 Romm FJ, Putnam SM. The validity of the medical record. Med Care. 1981;19:310–5.

7 Mamlin JJ, Duke HB. Combined time-motion and work sampling study in a general medicine clinic. Med Care. 1973;11:449–56.

8 Institute of Medicine. Committee on Improving the Patient Record. The Computer-Based Patient Record: An Essential Technology for Health Care. Washington, DC: National Academy Press; 1991.

9 Shortliffe EH, Tang PC, Detmer DE. Patient records and computers [Editorial]. Ann Intern Med. 1991;115:979-81.

10 Ellen RF (ed.). Ethnographic Research. Academic Press, London, 1984.

11 Fafchamps D. Ethnographic workflow analysis: specifications for design. In: Bullinger HJ; ed. Human Aspects in Computing: Design and Use of Interactive Systems and Work with Terminals. Amsterdam: Elsevier; 1991; 709-15.

12 Covell DG, Uman GC, Manning PR. Information needs in office practice: are they being met? Ann Intern Med. 1985;103:596–9.

13 Sheil BA. Coping with complexity. Office Tech People. 1983;1:295–320.

14 Osheroff JA, Forsythe DE, Buchanan BG, Bankowitz RA, Blumenfeld BH, Miller RA. Physicians' information needs: analysis of questions posed during clinical teaching. Ann Intern Med. 1991;114:576–81.

The Patient Care Component: Patient-Centered Horizontal Integration in a Vertical World

A. Clayton Curtis, M.D., Office of Health Program Research and Development, Indian Health Service, Tucson, Arizona

This paper describes the structure and operational properties of the Patient Care Component, a patient care data system developed by the Indian Health Service to support primary care in a multi-site, decentralized, health care organization. Sharing the same technology base as the Department of Veterans Affairs Distributed Hospital Computer Program, the system requires a minimal level of investment in technology compared to alternative approaches and is in operation at 140 sites. The Indian Health Service and historical aspects of the system are described briefly; the paper focuses on the design objectives for the system and lessons learned from development and several years of operational experience.

BACKGROUND

The Indian Health Service (IHS) is part of the U. S. Department of Health and Human Services and is, like the National Institutes of Health and the Centers for Disease Control, an agency of the U. S. Public Health Service. It is responsible for providing comprehensive health care to approximately 1.2 million American Indians and Alaskan Natives, often from birth to death, in rural and generally remote regions of the country. This is accomplished through a system of IHS direct care facilities (47 hospitals and 122 outpatient centers), IHS-funded tribal programs (another 7 hospitals and 149 outpatient sites), and services contracted for from the private sector. The organization has approximately 15,000 employees and a budget of about 1.7 billion dollars. Its programs range from installation of basic sanitation infrastructure, such as water and sewer systems, to dental and medical care delivered in facilities, communities, schools, and homes.

Efforts to bring information systems support to primary care in the IHS began in 1968 with development of the Health Information System (HIS), which used clinically-oriented encounter forms to capture a wide range of patient data in ambulatory care settings. The HIS was mainframe-based, written in COBOL, and did not use a database management system (DBMS). A later version, the Patient Care Information System (PCIS) [1,2], expanded on the HIS while retaining its essential nature. These systems eventually served the Sells Service Unit (in Southern Arizona) in an on-line mode, and the Billings (Montana) and Alaska Areas through microfiche. While advanced for their time, their reliance on mainframe and non-DBMS technology made the HIS and PCIS too expensive and inflexible to be attractive for widespread implementation, and constant targets for cutbacks.

In 1983, the IHS decided to decentralize its information systems to deliver computing capacity and control of data management to points of patient care and program management in the field. As a result of previous experience, vendor independence and portability across hardware platforms were major considerations. At the same time, there was considerable pressure on IHS by its parent agencies to purchase commercial systems for cost accounting and any clinical applications. During the market survey carried out in response to these directives, which was markedly unsuccessful, IHS became aware of the Department of Veterans Affairs Distributed Hospital Computer Program (DHCP). In 1984, the IHS decided to adopt DHCP's underlying technology as the basis for development of the Resource and Patient Management System (RPMS) and to make selective use of DHCP applications while converting clinical applications such as the PCIS (as the Patient Care Component, or PCC) to operate in the DHCP setting to support ambulatory and longitudinal care.

This paper presents experience with implementing PCC as a patient-centered data system and introducing PCC into the DHCP as a vehicle for integration of data from vertical applications.

THE VA DISTRIBUTED HOSPITAL COMPUTER PROGRAM

With 171 medical centers, approximately 200,000 employees, and a budget for medical programs of some 12.5 billion dollars, the Veteran's Health Administration is a large operation by any standard. Its major information system is the DHCP, whose basic goal is to provide automation support for both clinical and administrative activities. Historically, despite significant opposition from the commercial sector, emphasis has been placed on:

- Self-directed evolution, in-house development, and dedication to user-driven specification and design.
- A high degree of vendor independence and platform portability.

- Standardization in the areas of programming language (MUMPS), data exchange protocols (HL7), and graphics standards (X-Windows)

These considerations have had significant impact on every phase of DHCP, from application design through hardware and software procurement.

Initial DHCP releases focused on rapid-payoff vertical departmental applications. Now, more than ten years after its inception, DHCP is beginning to provide direct support for front-line providers. Applications in this category include ones developed *de novo* by the VA as well as ones which borrow from their IHS counterparts. The infrastructure provided by existing, widely deployed, departmental systems is an asset.

A strong technology focus differentiates the VA's approach to computational support for patient care from that of the IHS. Major initiatives currently underway across the VA system include imaging, intelligent workstations, and point-of-care data collection and verification. These have significant implications both in terms of resource requirements and impact on future application design strategies. In addition, the VA explicitly espouses the goal of a complete electronic medical record.

THE IHS PATIENT CARE COMPONENT

The PCC is a product of a mixed heritage, melding functional attributes of its predecessor, PCIS, and technology drawn from the DHCP. Its objectives are surprisingly similar to those set down twenty-five years ago, although the circumstances of implementation have changed dramatically.

Common barriers to the delivery of comprehensive health care faced by the IHS include:

- Patient mobility, partly as a result of a hierarchy of health care facilities.
- Distance to health care, and the related opportunity cost of not taking full advantage of the patient's visit.
- Limited time with the patient, perhaps as little as six to ten minutes.
- Provider turnover, typically on the average of every two to five years.
- Difficulty of keeping track of periodically performed tasks.

As a consequence of these motivators, the goals of the PCC are to:

- Support providers of front-line primary care with generic capabilities as well as specialty-oriented applications.
- Meet the comprehensive needs of longitudinal care and ambulatory settings.
- Integrate patient data from multiple disciplines and sources, even across sites.
- Record core aspects of every encounter of a patient with the health care system, whether services are provided directly or through external contracts.
- Provide managerial and administrative data as a byproduct of the patient care process.

Clinical data systems have developed in the IHS primarily as a result of grass roots interest rather than through top-down management direction or as a follow-on to the automation of ancillary systems. Thus, the PCC evolved in a climate which emphasized ways to improve the quality and effectiveness of direct patient care in a setting characterized by small rural sites, a mobile patient population, and community-based public health.

From an organizational perspective, this has meant establishing design guidelines and operational policies which emphasize:

- Independence of clinical data from data management policies of ancillary departments.
- Accommodation of data originating outside the site.
- Patient-centered data organization.
- Access to data along multiple axes.
- Minimizing ownership and control issues characteristic of vertical applications.

To date, the IHS has not aspired to a complete electronic record, viewing the PCC as a summary and index of the traditional record rather than an eventual replacement; this has had a strong influence on application design. However, major emphasis is placed on PCC's role as a focal point for communication and data sharing among members of the health care team, even in the face of security and confidentiality constraints.

The IHS has had to approach the development of information systems in general, and medical systems specifically, from a much lower level of technology than the VA. Beyond geographical remoteness of facilities, as well as a generally lower level of resources for development of computing infrastructure, this is a reflection of the disparity in size of facilities, a consequently lower level of clinical services offered, and extraordinary difficulty in recruiting and retaining competent IRM staff. While working toward increased sophistication in the long run, IHS has traditionally had to develop less technology-intensive approaches to problems such as data capture in ambulatory care settings (e.g., using clinically-oriented encounter forms rather than direct provider-system interaction).

THE PCC AS A FOCUS FOR PATIENT-CENTERED DATA INTEGRATION

Technical integration

PCC was designed specifically to integrate tightly with DHCP. This relationship is represented schematically in Figure 1, which illustrates major PCC and DHCP files (squared and rounded rectangles, respectively) and the sharing of core DHCP files (patient file, drug file, etc.) by PCC through pointer linkages. As can be seen, the PCC file structure is patient- and visit-centered, and designed for ease of access along axes of patient, visit, time, or class of data. For example, the patient-specific Health Summary follows links from patient file to data file, population-based epidemiological reports follow links from visits to data, and program-specific reports (such as immunization statistics) focus on individual data files. The flat, normalized structure combines aspects of both relational and network database models, and simplifies addition of new data classes.

Like all RPMS applications, PCC relies on the VA Kernel for services such as database management, menuing, messaging, etc. Unlike another notable comprehensive system, the Department of Defense Composite Health Care System (CHCS), RPMS and PCC are designed specifically to coexist with DHCP. This has made it possible to attempt bi-directional transfer of technology between IHS and VA [3]. The PCC is currently in test at the VA medical center in Tucson, and has required only minimal adaptation to cope with VA-specific health care practices.

Operational integration

In operation, the PCC supports three major types of integration:

Cross-application As shown in Figure 2, the PCC receives data from a number of sources, including active links from both VA and IHS applications (e.g., lab, pharmacy), entry of encounter form data supplied by providers, and automated external data sources. This repository structure isolates clinical data from dependencies on data management policies of ancillary systems and provides the ability to store data arising from other sites without contaminating data used for workload measurement, etc. in ancillary packages. In addition, it allows generic tools, such as the PCC query manager (QMAN) and the clinical reminder system to access data without issues of ownership or complex data structures [4].

Cross-discipline Health care in the IHS is truly a multi-disciplinary activity, involving a spectrum of staff including physicians, nurses, community health workers, etc. The PCC is the team's system, rather than a "physician's system" or a "nurse's system".

Cross-facility As noted above, the PCC database houses patient care data regardless of the site at which it was delivered. This has been exploited in the IHS multi-facility integration project (MFI).[5], which uses electronic mail to route transactions reflecting clinical activity and alteration of demographic data to all sites at which the patient has records.

Achievements

Resources for formal evaluation of PCC have been non-existent. However, outcomes observed as a result of site reports and surveys of provider perceptions include improvements in:

- integration of patient information across sources;
- communication among health care team members;
- follow-up of high-risk patients;
- provision of preventive services;
- performance of tasks related to chronic conditions.

The PCC has proven its value in production use as a system which is patient centered from the perspective of front-line providers, but which is simultaneously capable of supporting views of the database focused on cohorts or selected data classes for purposes of quality assurance and program management. Beyond its clinical roles, PCC has replaced earlier statistical data collection systems with clinically-relevant data capture, and now provides the basis for third-party billing -- an increasingly important aspect of patient care in the current fiscal climate.

FUTURE CHALLENGES

To remain a long-term success, the PCC must successfully address a number of critical issues:

- requirements for storage of additional types of data as interests and priorities change -- e.g., health status and risk factors, radiology, microbiology.
- requirements for new modes of integration with specialty systems -- e.g., maternal and child health, which imposes a strong programmatic framework on a constellation of independent classes of data (such as procedures, anatomic path, and pharmacy).
- incorporation of decision support capabilities -- e.g., enhanced clinical reminders and surveillance, which entails development of more powerful inferencing facilities with tighter integration into mechanisms through which data enters the system.
- complexities of inter-site data exchange -- e.g., inter-facility transfer, and installation in the database, of patient data; for IHS this currently means adaptation of the MFI project to HL7 as a part of working with the VA.
- position and funding limitations impacting the use of clerical-based data entry, which may dictate shifting data entry workload to clinicians.

The common factor underlying all of these matters is the requirement to adapt to changing circumstances. This need for flexibility was anticipated early on, and PCC was designed with an open architecture. This has enabled it to accommodate changes such as the recent addition of microbiology results, tests in a live DHCP environment at a VA medical center, and -- perhaps the ultimate role shift -- use as a "patient" information system in a veterinary school!

CONCLUSIONS

The PCC has been in operation in the IHS for six years, expanding from the initial sites of development and testing to support daily patient care at some 220 hospitals and clinics; in fiscal year 1993 (the most recent period for which statistics are available) approximately 2,912,500 ambulatory visits were recorded in PCC at 85 IHS direct care sites. For contrast, the Tucson VA medical center pilot project captured data at that single facility from some 186,200 visits in PCC in the twelve months beginning February 1993. The system has also had an impact outside IHS: it is the basis of the VA's PCE (Patient Care Encounter) application, now in the early stages of release within the VA DHCP system. PCC forms the outpatient component of the hospital system of Saipan, and has informally been reported to be in operation as far away as Siberia.

The PCC and its predecessor systems represent a quarter-century of experience in pragmatic support of primary care providers in busy, low-technology, ambulatory care settings. Many of the lessons learned can be distilled into three observations:

1. It's more important to first establish an appropriate repository for clinical data (i.e., in terms of data representation and scope) than to expend significant resources on developing sophisticated approaches to data capture. While the latter is a necessity in the long run, operational success and clinical acceptance is impossible without functional relevance to care providers, and that is primarily an outcome of managing data which is useful in direct patient care.

2. It's vital to avoid "analysis paralysis" and get systems into the field where real-world experience can be used to test acceptance and define the need for future enhancements. This is particularly true in large, multi-site organizations where practical limitations on large scale testing are bound to bias initial designs.

3. It's easier to talk about integration than to achieve it (or "Integration is fine as long as I don't have to do anything"). In addition to workable technical approaches, a mind set is required which places high value on integration of information systems -- as well as their intimate involvement in the health care process, to the ultimate benefit of the patient -- and accepts the necessity of cooperation from the numerous groups of interest which comprise the medical milieu. This mind set has to be fostered in development centers, ancillary services, and (ironically) the provider community.

Despite its "school of hard knocks" flavor, the PCC experience provides evidence that technology integration can be successful given the right circumstances, and that an integrated, patient-centered clinical database can play an important role in an environment of sophisticated vertical applications.

REFERENCES

[1] A. Garratt An Information System for Ambulatory Care. In: *Proceedings of the Third Symposium on Computer Applications in Medical Care (SCAMC 79).* Dunn R (ed). Washington: IEEE Computer Society Press, 1979

[2] G. Brown The Patient Care Information System: A Description of its Utilization in Alaska. In: *Proceedings of the Fourth Symposium on Computer Applications in Medical Care (SCAMC 89).* O'Neil J (ed). Washington: IEEE Computer Society Press, 1980

[3] A. Curtis Portability of Large Scale Medical Information Systems: the IHS-VA Experience. In: *Proceedings of the Fifth International Congress on Medical Informatics (MEDINFO 86).* Salamon R, Blum B, Jorgensen M (eds). Amsterdam: North Holland, 1986

[4] A. Curtis Knowledge-Based Systems in an Imperfect World: Data-Based Decision Support Systems in Ambulatory Care. In: *Proceedings of the Sixth International Congress on Medical Informatics (MEDINFO 89).* Barber B, Cao D, Qin D, Wagner G (eds). Amsterdam: North Holland, 1989

[5] A. Curtis Multi-Facility Integration: An Approach to Synchronized Electronic Medical Records in a Decentralized Health Care System. In: *Proceedings of the Seventh International Congress on Medical Informatics (MEDINFO 92).* Lun K, Degoulet P, Piemme T, Rienhoff O (eds). Amsterdam: North Holland, 1992

The opinions expressed in this paper are solely those of the author, and not necessarily those of the Indian Health Service or the U. S. Government.

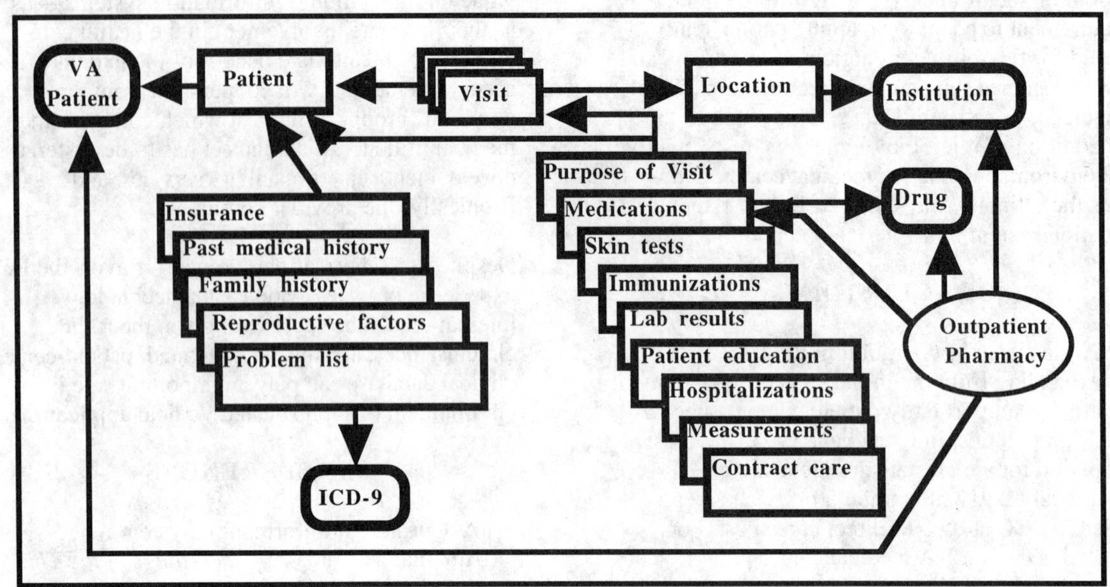

Figure 1
Relationship of PCC and DHCP

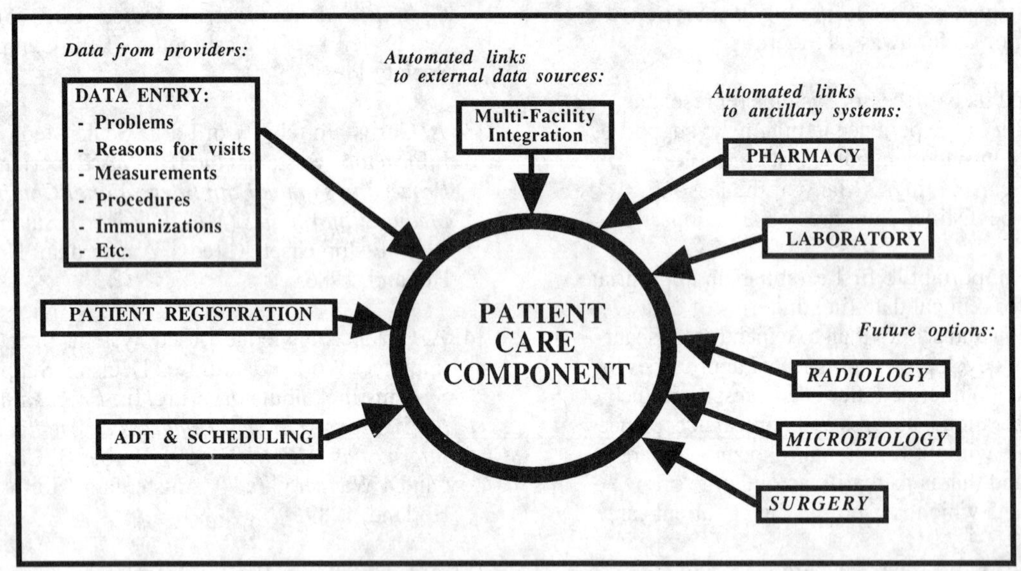

Figure 2
PCC as an integrating focus

A Practice-Based Information System for Multi-Disciplinary Care of Chronically Ill Patients: What Information Do We Need?

William P. Moran, MD, MS,[1] Catherine Messick, MD, MS,[1] Paula Guerette, PhD,[1] Roger Anderson, PhD,[2] Douglas Bradham,. DPH,[2] James L. Wofford, MD, MS,[1] Ramon Velez, MD, MSc,[1] and the Community Care Coordination Network Database Group

[1]Departments of Internal Medicine and [2]Public Health Sciences, Bowman Gray School of Medicine of Wake Forest University and [1]Reynolds Health Center, Winston-Salem, North Carolina

Primary care physicians provide longitudinal care for chronically ill individuals in concert with many other comunity-based disciplines. The care management of these individuals requires data not traditionally collected during the care of well, or acutely ill individuals. These data not only concern the patient, in the form of patient functional status, mental status and affect, but also pertain to the caregiver, home environment, and the formal community health and social service system. The goal of the Community Care Coordination Network is to build a primary care-based information system to share patient data and communicate patient related information among the community-based multi-disciplinary teams. One objective of the Community Care Coordination Network is to create a Community Care Database for chronically ill individuals by identifing those data elements necessary for efficient multi-disciplinary care.

INTRODUCTION

Approximately 35 million Americans have chronic severe disability, and more than 9 million Americans are unable to perform a major activity of daily living, disproportionately affecting low income and elderly individuals [1,2]. Historically the acute care hospital has been the focus of health care for chronically ill patients and the traditional medical record has served as a repository for patient data as well as provided for continuity of care and exchange of information among the many participating disciplines [3]. Shorter hospital stays have resulted in patients returning to the community earlier in the course of illness and resulted in the provision of many health care and support services to the community. Furthermore, many individuals with disabling chronic diseases are able to maintain independent community living only with the assistance of community health care and social service agencies. Some patients may even require care or services from several agencies, and the number, intensity, and types of service may vary over time.

Most communities have developed an array of community-based health care and social services such as in-home professional services, personal care services, transportation, adult day care and respite care. These services are often highly fragmented with many service providers operating a number of different programs with varying eligibility criteria. Information systems to provide accessible patient clinical data and expedite information exchange, analogous to the traditional medical record, have not kept pace with the development of community-based health and social services. In addition, the current health care delivery system does not promote the routine collection of patient and caregiver psychosocial data to support the delivery of formal and informal health and social services to chronically ill individuals. Even when community-wide information systems have been implemented by social service agencies to help coordinate community-based services [4], the information system cannot be used to identify patients in need of services, but only serve patients who have been referred by health care providers. Finally, social service-based systems may not be designed to facilitate communication between agencies and the primary care providers.

The primary care physician must play a critical role in development and application of innovative information systems to facilitate the timely, effective and efficient delivery of these services to chronically patients living in the community [2]. The primary care physician participates in all levels of care: identifying chronic conditions which lead to impairment and disability; maintaining contact with chronically ill and disabled

0195-4210/94/$5.00

patients as they move through the continuum of care; deciding about the need for hospitalization; authorizing almost all formal home and community care services. Therefore, the primary care physician is particularly well positioned to actively participate in the development and use of community-based health and community service information systems.

Clinical management computer systems have been developed and implemented within some primary care practices for tracking both chronic illness and preventive care procedures [3-7]. These systems may also be an effective tool for the primary care physician to improve the care of chronically ill and disabled patients. The Community Care Coordination Network (CCCN), a project funded by the Robert Wood Johnson Foundation, will use such an existing clinical information system at Reynolds Health Center (RHC), a large urban community health center, to link health center primary care providers, community service providers and hospital personnel.

Two interventions within the CCCN will be studied in a factorial design, randomized, controlled trial. One intervention is the development of a network-based "Community Care Alert" which will serve to identify patients whose functional status and needs may have changed by "alerting" providers to the occurrence of sentinel diagnoses or health care events, such as emergency department visits or hospitalizations. This "alert" is intended to mobilize members of a multi-disciplinary team to address patient needs in response to changes in health and functional status. The other CCCN intervention is the development of a community care database, containing data necessary for multi-disciplinary, inter-agency care coordination. The database will target patient, caregiver and health care system factors which have been shown to influence health care and community service delivery as well as patient quality of life and caregiver burden. Secure off-site access to the database from the two acute care hospitals and the limited number of participating community health and service providers will be available using a dial-in, dial-back process. Eligible patients must consent to participate in the CCCN study, and agree to release health care data to the hospitals and agencies participating in the CCCN.

A goal of the CCCN is to reduce the rates of unmet community service needs, unnecessary emergency department visits, hospitalization, total health care costs. A more important goal is to improve patient and caregiver quality of life. The project is in the first year, and we present the process of database development, and database elements included in the CCCN database.

METHODS

Setting and Population The Med/Track (Clinical Software Systems Inc., Hingham, MA) system implementation and data elements have been described in the past [7], copntaining data elements presented in Table 1. Mark-sense forms and optical scanning are currently employed for rapid, inexpensive data entry of encounter data at RHC, and will be employed for CCCN questionnaires and forms. To standardize data collection, trained interviewers will administer all patient questionaires. The caregiver questionaires will be self-administered. The CCCN data will be linked to the traditional patient files and displayed in supplemental user-defined datasets within the RHC clinical information system.

Table 1. "Traditional" data elements in the RHC database.

Patient Demographics
Primary Care Provider
Diagnoses
Medications
Allergies
Preventive Care
Visit History

The study population for the CCCN are one thousand chronically ill patients with functional impairments. Patients will be identified by searching the database (over 57,000 patient records) for patients with diagnoses associated with a high prevalence of functional impairment. Patients will be screened for deficits in activities of daily living (ADL) and instrumental activities of daily living (IADL); those with 3 or more IADL impairments or any ADL impairment will be eligible for the study.

Database Development Process Several strategies were employed to determine which data elements would be collected within the CCCN. First, the literature was reviewed for data elements which have been shown to be predictors of health service utilization, hospitalization, prolonged length of stay, or the need for community-based health or social services. Next, a group of community-based health and service providers (physicians, nurses, hospital and agency social workers, home care administrators) gathered and analyzed the data collection instruments currently used by their agencies. The group determined that the bulk of information collected by agencies was required by third party payers for reimbursement, and the remainder supported the clinical care plan. There was a large degree of heterogeneity in format and content of currently collected information, both across agencies and among third party payers. The group suggested collecting information of clinical benefit in supporting multi-disciplinary care but not currently collected by agencies or required by third parties.

The group then reviewed a series of standardized data collection instruments derived from the literature, and chose instruments which reflected their data needs, and satisfied third party requirements. Previouly validated medical and psychosocial screening and data collection instruments were chosen for the CCCN database when available to accomplish data collection. When several data collection tools were possible (eg. depression screens), instruments specifically validated in the target population (chronically ill, predominantly elderly patients) were selected. Data elements duplicated in screens and instruments were removed. Finally the investigators added research-related and generic health quality measures necessary for analysis of the trial.

RESULTS

The CCCN database consists of a variety of data elements, organized into three general components: patient-centered data, caregiver data (ie. informal support) and professional and community service data (ie. formal support). Patient-centered data include a range of information about patients' physical function, cognitive function, sensory impairment, affect and personal health care decisions. These data represent a combination of standardized instruments and measures developed specifically for the CCCN. For example, a standardized assessment of the patient's ability to perform daily activities (OARS) will be supplemented by a more detailed assessment of the types of personal assistance and assistive devices used, as well as a patient assessment of the degree to which a daily activity need is met [8]. The Center for Epidemiologic Studies-Depression Scale (CES-D) and nutritional screen [9] were incorporated because of the exceedingly high prevalence of depression among chronically ill individuals [1,10]. The short form of the Mini-Mental State Exam (MMSE) is included because cognitive impairment is a major determinant of the need for formal and informal community services, and a major source of caregiver stress [11]. Table 2 presents the patient-centered data elements.

Table 2. Patient-centered assessments in the CCCN database.

Functional Status (OARS)
Social Support
Cognitive Function (MMSE)
Depression Screen (CES-D)
Vision/Hearing Screens
Assistive Devices/Aids
Nutrition Screen
Home/Environmental Screen
Advanced Directives

The professional and community service data component provides detailed information not typically found in a medical record, but determined by the focus group to be important in the provision of appropriate community-based care This information includes a listing of the types of health and community services used (eg. Home Health, Meals on Wheels) the names, addresses and phone number of formal caregivers, and important hospital and pharmacy data. Table 3 presents the professional and community services data elements.

Table 3. Professional and community service data

Professional Services
Hospital Discharge Plans
Professional Care Plans
Personal Care Services
Type
Frequency
Duration
Pharmacy Name and phone

The availability of information about the social support and informal caregiver status was also identified by the focus group as extremely important in the care of chronically ill patients. The database will include extensive information about the extent of the patients' informal caregiving and social network, and will indicate risk factors for social isolation [12]. In addition, patient's primary caregiver data will include functional assessment, affect screen, and level of caregiver burden and stress; information which could help identify patient/caregiver pairs who need additional services. Table 4 presents the social support data elements.

In pilot testing, the interviewers required between one and one-half to two hous to complete the entire patient battery. The caregiver self-administered survey, at approximately a seventh grade reading level, required approximately 30 to 45 minutes to complete.

Table 4. Caregiver data elements in the CCCN database.

Demographics
Functional Assessment
Social Support
Perceived Need for Services
Self-reported Health Status
Depression Screen (CES-D)
Health Quality of Life (SF-36)
Caregiver Burden
Caregiver "Hassles" Index

DISCUSSION

The central hypothesis of the CCCN study is that a multi-disciplinary database, coupled with improved communication between community care personnel and primary care physicians may improve patient care outcomes and prevent unnecessary use of emergency services or hospital admission [13]. Even during exacerbations of illness when hospital services are needed, a community-based computer system could facilitate data exchange between hospital and health care and community service providers, assuring hospital personnel that needed post-discharge services and follow-up will be provided. Finally, a practice-based information system may aid physicians in identifying patients in need of services, match patients to available services [4], and reduce duplication and fragmentation of health care and community services [14].

To alter the current health service utilization among chronically ill patients and improve patient and caregiver quality of life, Community Care Database must contain data which supports health and social service providers in addressing the needs of chronically ill, functionally impaired patients and their caregivers. These data are qualitatively distinct from the traditional medical database, and must focus less on diagnoses and medications and more on the functional impairment resulting from chronic illness, patient environment and social support and caregiver needs and social support. These data must detail, and indeed justify, the professional and physical resources necessary to maintain the individual in the community.

A major concern in designing the database is the use of widely accepted and validated instruments. For many home care agencies, data collection has been determined as much by the requirements for reimbursement as to support clinical decision-making. Thus, patient data collected by various agencies, although similar, is not directly comparable. Importantly, data comparability may facilitate the provision of services to individuals who may not otherwise be identified simply on the basis of functional status. For example, the needs of a functionally impaired individual living alone may be dramatically different from an individual with an extensive social support network. Nonetheless, the standardized instruments must satisfy agencies' financial reporting requirements to prevent duplicate data collection. The CCCN database attempts to address these requirements.

In order to generalize to the practice of health professionals in the community, the database content must reflect data of diagnostic or prognostic significance across the range of chronic disease diagnoses. Thus the CCCN database incorporates screening measures for important, high prevalence co-morbidities such as cognitive impairment and depression. However, the amount of time required to collect data must not be prohibitive so shortened instruments (GDS, MMSE) have been incorporated when available. A shortcoming of the database is the lack of an extensive assessment of patient health care preferences beyond the solicitation of advanced directives and health care power of attorney. The standardized collection of these data could have a significant impact on the primary CCCN outcome measures such as emergency room visits, hospital readmissions, length of stay, and total health care charges.

The CCCN database includes extensive data on informal caregiving and on formal community services. One effort within the CCCN will be to relate these support systems in such a way that care managers in the CCCN may anticipate the formal service needs of patients in response to changes in patient or caregiver status [15]. Unfortunately, the CCCN cannot at present automatically link patient (care recipient) and caregiver health care data since many caregivers may receive primary care in other settings.

Finally non-medical outcome measures such as quality of life and life satisfaction must be incorporated into the CCCN database since traditional measures such as return to work, morbidity and mortality are not the most discriminating outcome measures in chronic disease management, and cannot measure effects of health and service provision on caregivers. In managing chronic illness, maintaining function, maximizing independence and preserving patient autonomy become the goals of treatment, and the multi-disciplinary team must work in concert to support these goals. The CCCN database potentially provides a common infrastructure from which to coordinate these efforts.

Acknowledgements: The authors wish to thank the CCCN database working group: Forsyth Memorial Hospital and Home Care Services, NC Baptist Hospital and Home Care agency, Forsyth County Department of Social Services, Olsten Kimberly Quality Care, Primary Health Concepts Inc/ Home Health Professionals, and Senior Services of Forsyth County Inc. We also thank the clinicians and staff of the Reynolds Health Center for their enthusiastic support. This project is supported by grants from the Robert Wood Johnson Foundation Program "Building Health Systems for People with Chronic Illnesses" and the Kate B. Reynolds Poor and Needy Trust.

References

[1]. Pope AM, Tarlov AR (eds). Disability in America: Toward a National Agenda For Prevention. Washington, DC: National Academy Press, 1991.

[2]. US Department of Health and Human Services: Public Health Service. Healthy People 2000: National Health Promotion and Disease Prevention Objectives. Boston: Jones and Bartlett Inc., 1992.

[3]. MacAdam M, Capitman J, Yee D, Prottas J, Leutz W, Westwater D. Case Management for Frail Elders: The Robert Wood Johnson Foundation's Program for Hospital Initiatives in Long-Term Care. Gerontol 1989; 29,6:737-744.

[4]. Johnson SC, Withers L. TIME: Tracking Information for Maintaining the Elderly. QRB 1988; 14:341-344.

[5]. Frame PS. Can Computerized Reminder Systems Have an Impact on Preventive Services in Practice? J Gen Intern Med 1990; 5(suppl):S112-115.

[6]. Carey TS, Thomas D, Woolsey A, Proctor R, Philbeck M, Bowen G, Blish C, Fletcher S. Half a Loaf is Better than Waiting for the Bread Truck: A Computerized Mini-Medical Record for Ambulatory Care. Arch Intern Med 1992; 152:1845-1849.

[7]. Moran, WP, Wofford JL, Hamrick V et al. Implementing Computerized Tracking at a Community Health Center: Challenges and Solutions. Proceedings of the Seventeenth Annual Symposium on Computer Applications in Medical Care. New York: McGraw-Hill Inc., 1993; 139-143.

[8]. Multi-dimensional Functional Assessment: The OARS Methodology, A Manual (2nd Edition) 1975. Center for the study of Aging and Human Development, Duke University, Durham, NC.

[9]. The Nutrition Screening Initiative, 2626 Pennsylvania Ave., NW. Ste. 301, Washington, DC 20037.

[10]. Coulehan JL, Schulberg HC, Block MR, Janosky JE, Arena VC. Medical Comorbidity of Major Depressive Disorder in a Primary Medical Practice. Arch Intern Med. 1990;150:2363-2367.

[11]. Braekhus A, Laake K, Engedal K. The Mini-Mental State Examination: Identifying the Most Efficient Variables for Detecting Cognitive Impairment in the Elderly. J Amer Geriatr Soc. 1992;40:1139-1145.

[12]. Sherbourne C, Stewart A. The MOS Social Support Survey. Soc Sci Med. 1991;32:705-714.

[13]. Boult C, Boult L, Murphy C, Ebbitt B, Luptak M, Kane RL. A Controlled Trial of Outpatient Geriatric Evaluation and Management. J Am Geriatr Soc. 1994;42:465-470.

[14]. Barnett GO. The Application of Computer-Based Medical-Record Systems in Ambulatory Care. N Engl J Med. 1984; 310:1643-1650.

[15]. Council on Scientific affairs, American Medical Association. Physicians and Family Caregivers: A Model for Partnership. JAMA. 1993;269:1282-1284.

A Cooperative Model for Integration in a Cardiology Outpatient Clinic

Ronald Cornet[1], Erik M. van Mulligen[1,2], Teun Timmers[1]
[1]Dept of Medical Informatics, Erasmus University Rotterdam, The Netherlands
[2]University Hospital Dijkzigt, Rotterdam, The Netherlands

ABSTRACT

With the increasing amount of digitally stored patient information, such as images and findings, the possibility and need arise for a system which is able to both store and display this information in a structured, user-friendly way. In the common situation where different information systems are used within one department, this means that the various information systems have to be integrated. However, integration requires more complex management of data, processes and windows. This management can be handled by a Workspace Manager, which controls inter-application tasks, and interaction with the user. Furthermore, this Workspace Manager supports the user with the definition of complex tasks such as collecting problem-related patient information from the various remote systems.

In an outpatient clinic for cardiology this architecture is used to achieve cooperative integration of an open Computer Patient Record with a range of information-specific services.

INTRODUCTION

Currently, much research is directed towards the development of a Computer Patient Record (CPR) [1,2]. In general, this leads to a stand-alone application that communicates only with various existing systems for data retrieval [3]. The disadvantage of such an approach is the lack of reusability of CPR functionality for different medical domains. Reusablity is highly desired for sharing of, e.g., modules for history taking, and display facilities for various kinds of signals, images, and data. Without reuse of components, a new CPR must be developed from scratch and no structural approach to improve reusability in an existing system is known. Another disadvantage of such an approach is the inability to easily integrate existing commercial solutions and new software developments within the CPR.

Other research in medical informatics has introduced reusable components as building blocks for a medical workstation, thereby using various mechanisms [4,5]. In this paper, we present an architecture that allows reuse of components in order to realize a CPR for a cardiology outpatient clinic. The functionality included in these components is either developed locally or supplied by commercial vendors. Beyond this, the architecture provides a powerful mechanism to anticipate new developments, such as digital image display, image analysis and clinical decision support.

In order to make a reusable-components based system act like a single application to the clinical end-user, the following architectural features are required (Figure 1):

(1) *standard communication* supporting the exchange of data and procedure calls between the components;

(2) *integration* supporting uniform access from one workstation to remote components as if they all reside on the same host;

(3) *cooperation* automating interaction between the components and serializing components for a user task;

(4) *user interfacing* for interaction with the user and presentation of data.

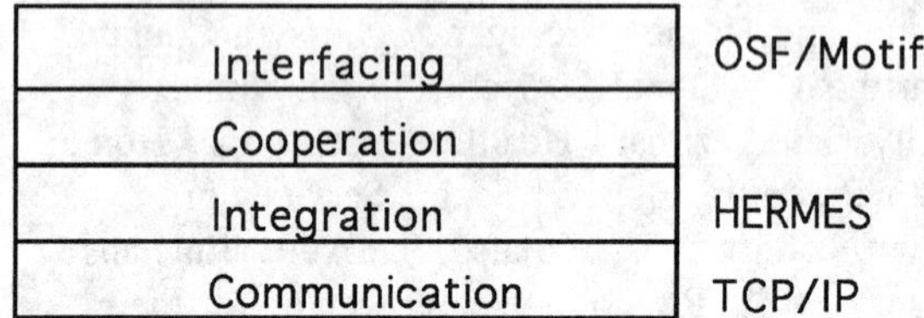

Figure 1: *Architectural features of a cooperative and interface-integrated system.*

Communication and integration are provided by the HERMES kernel architecture which was developed at the Department of Medical Informatics. This client-server-based kernel supports the integration of existing applications in a uniform way and provides a message language both for data exchange and remote procedure calling [6,7]. It promotes the development of reusable components as autonomous services in a network. The system runs on HP9000 /700 series workstations under UNIX with MOTIF. Together with the HERMES kernel, a set of basic services for access to commercial databases, to a Hospital Information System, and to a Departmental Information System is available. In a data model service additional information about the data is stored; this data model forms the bridge to a HERMES environment suited for clinical data analysis [8].

In this paper, we first explore the notion of cooperation as the next level of integration. Then preliminary results on the prototype of a Workstation for the cardiology outpatient clinic will be described.

COOPERATION: the next level of integration

On top of the HERMES integration layer, we have designed a new layer for cooperation. This layer, the Cardiological Workspace Manager (CWM), controls the operation of the components by means of the HERMES integration kernel. The reference model for this architecture is shown in Figure 2.

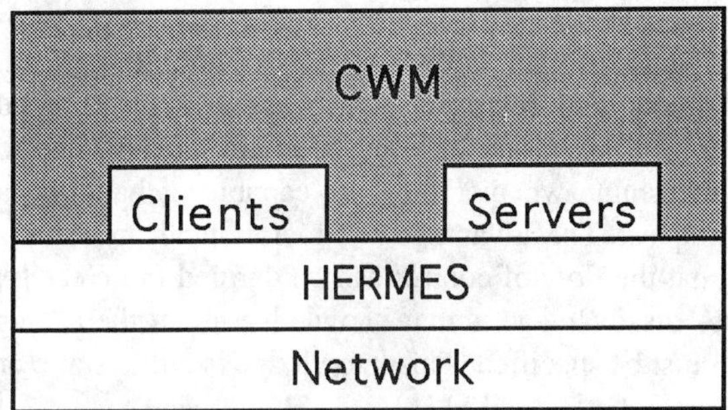

Figure 2: *A reference model showing the HERMES layers on top of the network.*

Requirements

The aim of a cooperative system such as our CWM is to support tasks that go beyond the scope of a single component, such as (1) decomposition of a user task into calls to the various components, (2) automation of the data- and command flow between components, and (3) a watchdog function to guard consistency and completeness of data.

Other requirements for the cooperative environment are its capability to include seamlessly new components, such as clinical decision support and literature access server components, and possibilities to modify and add tasks flexibly. The cooperative environment also has to provide functionality to anticipate multi-processing, i.e., to serialize and activate components concurrently that run on different hosts in a network with different response times.

This range of tasks requires an environment that supports the representation of procedural, event-driven and data-driven flows. In principle, one can choose from the following approaches to such an environment:

- *callback-based* (event-driven and procedural); environments using this mechanism associate events with callback procedures that on their turn can activate other callback procedures. When an event occurs, the system activates a callback automatically.
- *rule-based* (data-driven); in a rule-based system pre-conditions are expressed in terms of data. A rule can modify data, possibly causing other rules to be activated. As a consequence, one cannot implement a procedural flow.
- *object-based* (event-driven); each object is a combination of local data and methods. Methods can be activated by sending an event to an object, which in its turn can send events to other objects.
- *agent-based* (data-driven and procedural); an agent can be seen as an autonomous object; i.e. it contains a processor and incorporates its own data repository, logic and knowledge to reason about its environment. Methods can be called to manipulate data and delegate tasks to other agents.

As will be explained below, we have chosen for the agent-based model. The CWM has four classes of tasks:

User interaction tasks

The CWM provides the user-interface with a number of user tasks specific for the cardiology outpatient clinic. These user tasks include, e.g., support of consultation, review of patients, and generation of referral and discharge letters.

The CWM provides a mechanism to separate tasks in sequences of sub-tasks. Eventually, the sub-tasks open sessions with the appropriate services.

Window management tasks

A potential drawback of having many different components, each having its own windows for interaction with the user, is an uncoordinated appearance of the user interface. The CWM contains window management tasks that embed the server component windows in an overall user-interface that automatically positions, sizes, and (un)maps the windows.

Two modes for controlling the appearance of windows of the servers can be discerned:

- Reparenting; the window hierarchy (X11) is modified in such a way that a server window becomes a child of a window of the CWM. The window management tasks of the CWM operate through the parent of the server window.
- Communication; the CWM sends requests to the servers for positioning or hiding windows.

Which control mechanism is used depends on the server. Control by communication can be realized only for modifiable or new applications.
Display of the windows of the servers can happen in 3 different ways:

- A desktop metaphor; one window at a time is shown, the user can select windows by turning over "pages" of an imaginary notebook.
- Task-oriented window management: from a menu-bar, various types of information can be selected, and each source of information has its own area on the screen.
- Intelligent positioning: the CWM determines which information must be shown and where windows should be positioned.

Although flexibilty is decreased, window management is essential to avoid cluttering the screen with too many windows.

Inter-operation tasks

Since the CWM contains knowledge about the state of the servers, it can take care of a number of tasks considering information which is shared by the various servers.

- Clinical context: the CWM keeps track of the currently used domain and notifies the servers of the consequences of this domain.
- Synchronization:
  - of tasks: if a task consists of a number of steps, the CWM takes care of the correct sequence of sub-tasks.
  - of data: if another patient (or another global item) is selected by a server, the CWM notifies the other servers of the change.
  - of time frame: the CWM can handle a time-related user request, e.g. to display the first angiogram after the last PTCA.
- Communication: the CWM functions as a daemon to inform existing systems when data is stored or modified in one of the other systems [9]. For example, when an angiogram is stored in the angio-database, this is reported to the CPR.

Watchdog tasks

The data that is collected in the CPR will generally not only be used for patient care, but also for clinical data analysis. This brings up the need for a mechanism that checks data completeness and consistency. This will partly be done by the servers, but where the checks go beyond the scope of one application, this will be done by the CWM. Such a watchdog mechanism may also be used for educational purposes, to check if a user performs certain actions before making a decision.

WORKSTATION ARCHITECTURE

Cooperation mechanism

The mechanism we have chosen to achieve cooperation is the one of agents. The advantage of an agent-mechanism is that it is dynamic and that new agents can be incorporated easily into the system. This is in contrast with a rule-based or event-driven system, which leads to a static system with a large number of rules or triggers.
The agents can be organized in a hierarchical or a flat structure [10]. In a hierarchical structure meta-agents contain knowledge about the lower-level agents, and determine which agents are addressed for certain tasks. In a flat structure, agents need to determine whether they are capable of handling a request. The advantage of a hierarchical structure is that the flow of control can be defined more easily. A disadvantage is that knowledge about the agents must be specified. This knowledge is either static or it can be learned [11].

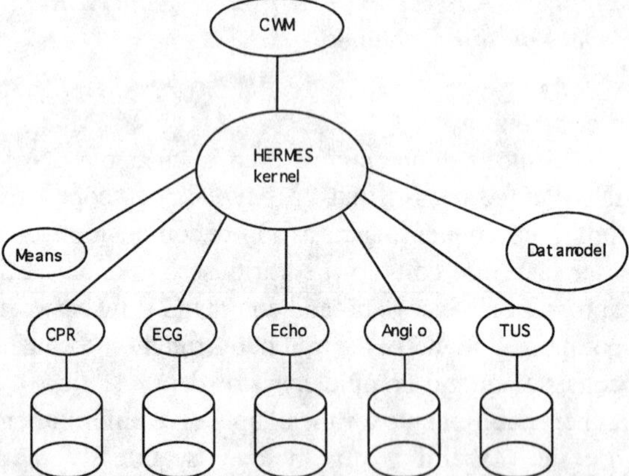

Figure 3: *The Cardiological Workspace Manager as a clinician's view to a number of information systems.*

Components for a cardiology outpatient clinic

Figure 3 shows the components of the cardiological workstation as it is currently developed. Other servers which will be included are X-ray image and UMLS-servers, and a connection to Medline.

The following independent components will be connected in the near future.
Hermes Kernel: in use at various locations since September 1993.
Open CPR: The Computer Patient Record is adapted to the HERMES environment, according to the specifications as described in [1].
Angio: A CathLab database system has been developed during the last year.
ECG: The department of cardiology is currently considering which ECG-management system to use. Openness is a decisive requirement.
MEANS: An ECG-analysis module which has been developed at the department of Medical Informatics.
Echo: This year a VingMed image server on a SUN platform will be installed.
TUS: A MUMPS PC-networked Departmental Information System containing laboratory data, appointments, and other alphanumerical patient data.
Datamodel: The CPR consults this service for information on, e.g., the datatype, thesauri, and possible and plausible datavalues.

Local Database
Since all components are located at different hosts, the network load may be high, decreasing the speed

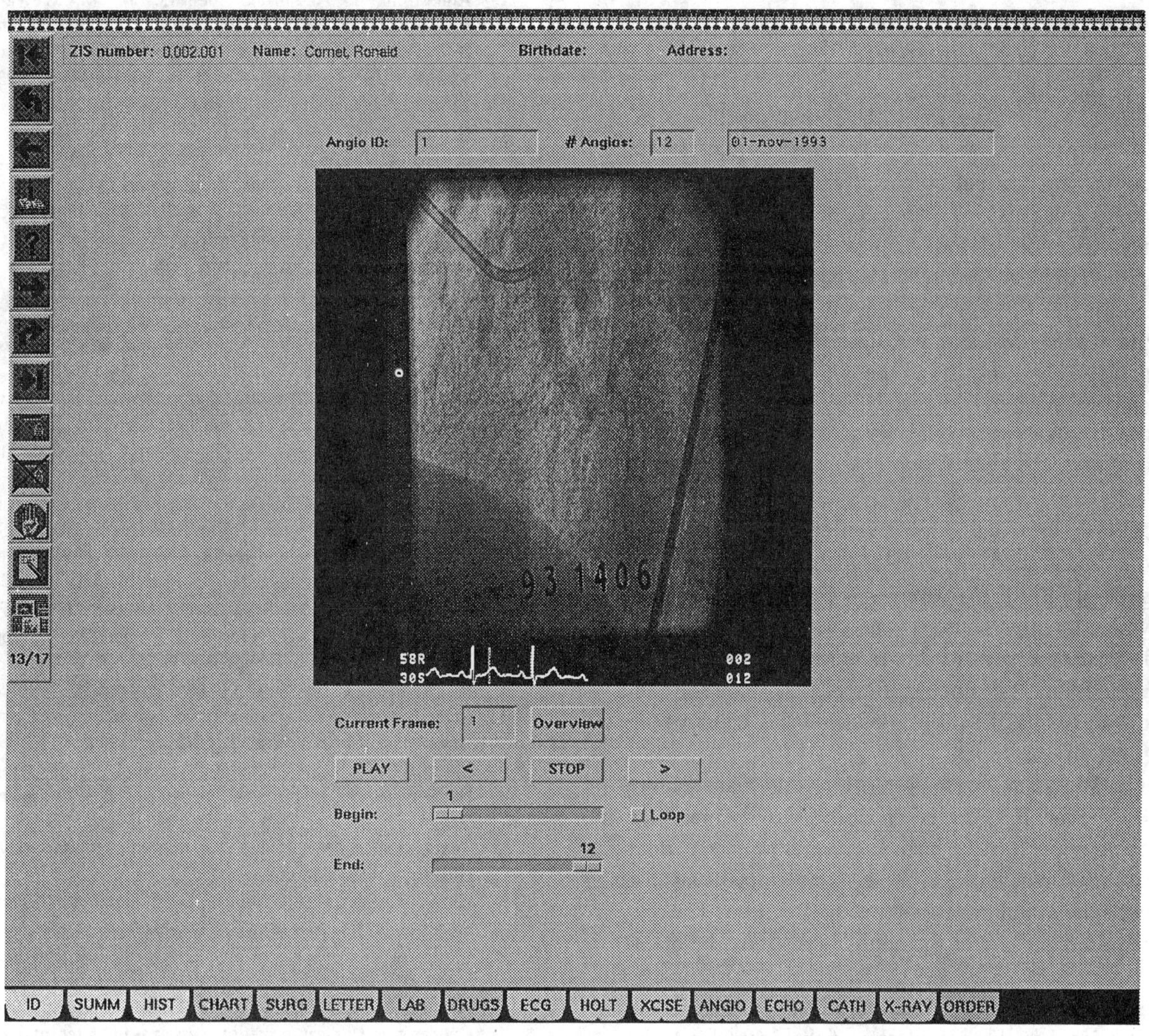

Figure 4: *An example of integrating the interface of a server into the Cardiological Workspace Manager: an angiogram is displayed as one of the pages of a notebook, being the desktop metaphor of the Patient Record. The user can select the type of information through the tabs at the bottom of the screen. With the buttons on the left hand side the user can navigate through the "notebook".*

of the system. Therefore, the use of a local database must be considered for storage of pre-fetched data. Agents, being active in the background in a transparent way, may provide an ideal solution to the problem of synchronization of the information in remote components. In particular, an agent can generate alerts where an existing, not open legacy system is not able to do that.

Sample screen

Figure 4 shows a sample screen of the prototype workstation. Currently, the following server components have been included: appointments, vital signs, letters, laboratory-data, ECG-signals with interpretation, angiograms, and echograms.

When the CWM is started, connections are opened with each individual server. Then, the agenda is shown, from which a patient is selected. The user can then turn over the pages of the CWM, which selects the information to be shown on this page.

A request is sent to the appropriate server, containing patient-number, whether the selected page contains an index or an image, and an identification of the window in which the server should display. The result is that the user views the information (e.g. an angiogram) as if it is part of the CWM desktop. As described above, this is achieved by reparenting the windows of the servers to the CWM.

CONCLUSION

Earlier, we have adopted a client-server model for the integration of heterogeneous systems and software [6,7]. However, in a clinical environment, where many sources and kinds of data and information are to be integrated, this level of integration is not sufficient, as control and management of actions, dataflow and windows are necessary as well.

The Workspace Manager offers this management. Its power lies in its capability to define inter-application tasks, such as window- and data-management, but also more complex tasks such as collecting data from different applications. The only requirement is that the applications must be open.

Several important issues are still open to research. One issue is the granularity of the agents and how their functionality is defined [12].

The proper balance must be found between pre-structuring user-interfaces and allowing maximum flexibility. Related to this is the question of how and to what extent one can tailor the behaviour of the interface to a particular user.

Finally, the pervasive problem of correctly mapping data in existing systems into the CPR remains. The additional features of the datamodel service may play an important role in this.

References

[1] Ginneken AM van, Stam H, Duisterhout JS. A Powerful Macro-model for the Computer Patient Record. Accepted for *Symposium on Computer Applications in Medical Care*. Washington, DC: 1994.

[2] McDonald CJ, Barnett GO. Medical record systems. In: Shortliffe EH, Perreault LE, eds. Medical Informatics: Computer Applications in Health Care. Reading MA: Addison-Wesley, 1990:181-218.

[3] Suermondt HJ, Tang PC, Strong PC, Young CY, Annevelink J. Automated Identification of Relevant Patient Information in a Physician's Workstation. In: *Proceedings Symposium on Computer Applications in Medical Care*. Washington, DC: McGraw-Hill, Inc., 1993: 229-232

[4] Greenes RA. Promoting productivity by propagating the practice of "plug-compatible" programming. In: Miller RA, ed. *Proceedings of the 14th Annual Symposium on Computer Applications in Medical Care.* Washington DC. Los Alamitos: IEEE Computer Society Press, 1990:22-6

[5] Degoulet FJ, Coignard J, Scherrer JR et al.. The Helios European Project on Software Engineering. In: Timmers T, Blum BI (eds.) *Software Engineering in Medical Informatics*. Amsterdam: Elsevier Scientific Publishers. 1991:125-37

[6] Van Mulligen EM, Timmers T, Van Bemmel JH. A new architecture for integration of heterogeneous software components. Methods of Information in Medicine 1993;32:292-301

[7] Van Mulligen EM, Timmers T, Brand J, Cornet R, Van den Heuvel F, Kalshoven M, Van Bemmel JH. HERMES: a health care workstation architecture. J of Bio-Medical Computing 1994;34:267-275

[8] Timmers T, Van Mulligen EM, Van den Heuvel F. Integrating clinical databases in a medical workstation using knowledge-based modeling. In: Lun KC, Degoulet P, Piemme TE, Rienhoff O, eds. *Proceedings of the Seventh World Congress on Medical Informatics*. Geneva. Amsterdam: North-Holland Publ Comp, 1992:478-82

[9] Marrs KA, Steib SA, Abrams CA, Kahn MG. Unifying Heterogeneous Distributed Clinical Data in a Relational Database. In: *Proceedings Symposium on Computer Applications in Medical Care*. Washington, DC: McGraw-Hill, Inc., 1993: 644-648

[10] Giroux S, Senteni A, Lapalme G. Adaptation in Open Systems. Reflection as a backbone. In: *International Conference on Intelligent and Cooperative Information Systems*, 1993:114-123

[11] Namatame A, Tsukamoto Y. Learning Agents for Cooperative Hyperinformation Systems. In: *International Conference on Intelligent and Cooperative Information Systems*, 1993:124-133

[12] Mylopoulos J, Rose T, Woo C. Task-Oriented Development of Intelligent Information Systems. In: *International Conference on Intelligent and Cooperative Information Systems*, 1993:206-219

Section V

Support for Clinicians

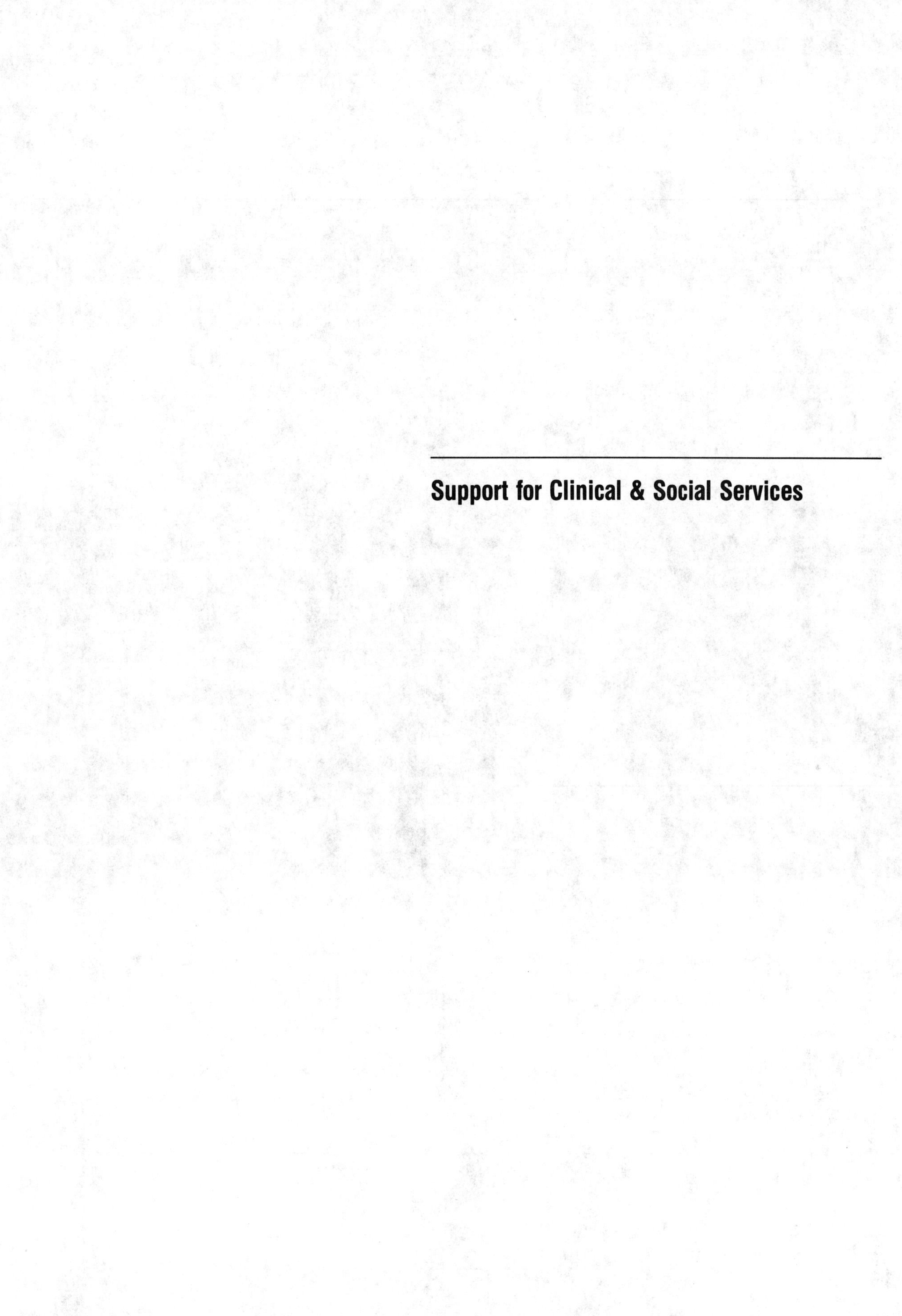

Support for Clinical & Social Services

CHESS: An Interactive Computer System For Women With Breast Cancer Piloted With An Under-Served Population

Fiona M. McTavish[1], David H. Gustafson[1], Betta H. Owens[1], Meg Wise[1], Jean O. Taylor[1], Funmi M. Apantaku[2], Haile Berhe[1] and Brian Thorson[1]

[1]Center for Health Systems Research and Analysis
University of Wisconsin
Madison, Wisconsin
[2]National Black Leadership Initiative on Cancer
University of Illinois
Chicago, Illinois

ABSTRACT

The Comprehensive Health Enhancement Support System (CHESS) is an interactive computer system containing information, social support and problem solving tools. It was developed with intensive input from potential users through needs-assessment surveys and field testing. CHESS had previously been used by women in the middle and upper socio-economic classes with high school and college education. This article reports on the results of a pilot study involving eight African-American women with breast cancer from impoverished neighborhoods in the city of Chicago. CHESS was very well received, extensively used and produced feelings of acceptance, motivation, understanding and relief.

INTRODUCTION

A diagnosis of breast cancer often creates a crisis for women and their families [1,6]. According to crisis theory, people often experience depression, fear, guilt, and helplessness during a health crisis because their former coping strategies are no longer effective [2,9]. Research indicates that information and emotional, social and spiritual support play a key role in helping patients cope [1,3,5,11]. This can lead to more accurate expectations [4], improved physical health, and improved survival rates [1,5,11]. Information and support also improve the physical and emotional health of breast cancer patients and their primary caregivers [6].

With the increased pressure to contain health care costs, more effective ways of providing information, support, decision and problem solving tools for patients are critical. While health care providers inform patients about their diagnoses and possible treatments, they have limited time to convey the necessary information. Patients are asking for more information, given in a way that is easily understood and in increments that are not overwhelming. Access to the information and social support needed to cope with breast cancer can be difficult to obtain. Geographical barriers, limited accessibility to existing services, limited financial resources, and the complexity of the disease and its treatment hinder women from getting the information, problem-solving tools and social support systems they need. The Comprehensive Health Enhancement Support System (CHESS) was designed to overcome these barriers [7].

OVERVIEW OF CHESS

CHESS is an interactive computer-based system designed on the premise that successful response to a medical crisis requires information, social support, and decision-making and problem-solving skills. People have different needs and learning styles and therefore seek different ways to solve their problems throughout the crisis[13,14]. CHESS' user friendly interface addresses the research findings that information and support is most valuable when it meets the following criteria: it is convenient, comprehensible, affordable, timely, non-threatening, anonymous, and controlled by the user [1,9-12]. For instance, some people prefer structured decision-making help that leads them through analysis of options, decision criteria, values and perceptions. Others read the literature, or interact with other women who have made similar decisions. CHESS is a flexible system offering a wide variety of mechanisms to meet the needs of people in a health crisis. CHESS modules have been developed for Breast Cancer, AIDS/HIV Infection, Substance Abuse, Sexual Assault, and Academic Crisis. A brief description of the components and services of the CHESS Breast Cancer Module follows.

Information Components:

Questions and Answers (QA) is a compilation of brief answers to many common questions about breast cancer. Users have the option to link to more in-depth information within the CHESS Instant Library.

Instant Library (IL) is a collection of over 100 articles drawn from scientific journals, newsletters, brochures, pamphlets and the popular press on breast cancer and related issues.

Ask an Expert (AE) allows users to anonymously ask questions about breast cancer and receive an answer within 48 hours.

Getting Help/Support (GH) is a tutorial that helps users understand how to find a good provider and how to be an effective consumer. The tutorial also provides sample wordings of how to set up an appointment or talk with a health care provider.

Social Support Components:

Discussion Groups (DG) provides a non-threatening place to communicate anonymously with other women affected by breast cancer. Discussion groups are available for women with breast cancer, partners of women with breast cancer, and other special groups.

Personal Stories (PS) are real accounts of women affected by breast cancer. Our research team interviewed patients, partners, and adult children for personal descriptions of their experiences and how they coped with breast cancer. These stories represent a wide range of experience and background.

Problem Solving Components:

Decisions and Conflicts (DC) uses utility theory to help people think through difficult decisions such as what surgery to have and whether to take adjuvant chemotherapy or tamoxifen treatment. Users can read a description of each option or read an excerpt from the personal story of a woman who chose that option. They can read about criteria other women considered in making the choice, why each may be an important consideration for them, what research says about their choices, and how each concern affects each criterion.

Action Plan (AP) combines statistical decision theory and change theory to help users think through how to implement a decision they have made. It is one thing to decide to adopt a low fat diet, and yet another to implement a decision in the face of ingrained habits or family pressures. This program asks users thirteen questions about their plan to implement a decision. Using the results, it predicts the likelihood of success in the implementation of the plan. It also identifies ways the user can strengthen her prospects for successful implementation.

CHESS is reviewed and updated biannually. Our system allows us to post particularly newsworthy or significant information at any time. In the recent case of falsified data regarding lumpectomy and mastectomy surgery, we updated CHESS immediately and kept people informed of the latest findings and reports. This easy update feature allows users access to the most recent information and discoveries about breast cancer and can ease the fears and concerns that can arise from uncertainty.

CHICAGO PILOT STUDY

Our most recent pilot study of the CHESS breast cancer module consisted of eight African-American women in impoverished neighborhoods of inner city Chicago. Through the efforts of the Midwest National Black Leadership Initiative on Cancer, Cook County Hospital agreed to participate in this study. This study took place between 10/1/93 to 1/15/94. All of the women were stage I or stage II breast cancer patients. They were contacted by a patient advocate from Cook County Hospital and asked if they would be willing to participate in a pilot study of CHESS. This was strictly voluntary, with no financial compensation for the participants.

Twenty women were offered CHESS, thirteen agreed to have it in their home (65% acceptance rate). However, five women changed their minds and decided not to take part in the study between the time of their original agreement to participate and when they were contacted to schedule a time to place the computer in their home. This recruitment rate (40%) is much lower than what we have experienced in other pilot studies (over 80% acceptance rate). We believe this may be due to a four to six week delay between the time the women initially agreed to be in the study and scheduling computer installation in their home. In previous studies once the woman agreed to participate the computer was placed in her home within one week.

The age of the women ranged from 36 to 66 years old. Six of the eight women were 55 or younger. All of the women were single (either divorced, separated, widowed or never married) at the time of the study. Half had never completed high school and only three of the eight women had any prior computer experience. All of the women were on public assistance. Five of the women had had lumpectomies and two had had mastectomies within the past year (5 had surgery in the past six months). Only one woman had CHESS prior to deciding what surgery to have.

A computer was installed in the home of each woman by a CHESS staff member, who gave approximately one hour of instruction and orientation. Use data was automatically collected by the computer and one survey was mailed to each participant.

CHESS was used 886 times within the 15 week access period (Table 1). "Use" was defined as an entry lasting at least a minute into a CHESS service. On average, each woman used CHESS 7 times per week and was on the system for more than one hour per week.

Table 1: Cook County Study: Use of CHESS Services

Service	# of Uses	Minutes
Discussion Group	442	5046
Ask an Expert	227	1487
Questions & Answers	83	617
Personal Stories	43	504
Instant Library	48	341
Decisions & Conflicts	20	208
Getting Help/Support	18	76
Action Plan	5	48

In the Chicago Pilot Study involving 8 African-American women, 55% of the total time of use was in the Social Support Components (Discussion Group, Personal Stories), 41% in the Information Components (Ask an Expert, Instant Library, Questions and Answers, Getting Help/Support), and 4% in the Problem Solving Components (Decisions & Conflicts and Action Plan).

The use patterns of a previous CHESS pilot study involving 20 Caucasian women from the University of Wisconsin Hospital and Clinics diagnosed with stage I or stage II breast cancer indicates that 67% of their use was in the Social Support Components, 31% in the Information Components and 2% in the Problem Solving Components of CHESS (Table 2).

Table 2: Usage of CHESS Components, by Percentage of Total Uses, of Two Study Populations

CHESS Component	Cook County	UW Hospital
Social Support	55 %	67 %
Information	41%	31%
Problem Solving	4 %	2 %

As in previous studies involving HIV+ men who used CHESS, African Americans tend to use the Support Component of CHESS less than the Caucasian participants, while using the Information Components more[7]. It is unclear at this point what accounts for this difference. Further study of various ethnic populations' use patterns of CHESS are needed to determine what accounts for the difference and if specialized adaptations of CHESS are required to meet the differing needs of various populations.

In the follow up survey from the Chicago Pilot (returned by 5 of the 8 women) the women indicated that they felt acceptance, motivation, understanding, and relief while using CHESS (all over 5.0 on a 7 point scale). They experienced low levels of negative emotions such as stress, boredom, fear, sadness, indifference, helplessness and anger (all less than 3.0 on a 7 point scale). Elation and empowerment were low (2.25 and 2.2), while anxiety was relatively high (4.5). This finding is opposite what we have found in previous studies, where women felt empowered and their anxiety level was low (Table 3). Many of the written comments by the African-American women seem to agree with our previous studies however, leading us to believe that the term 'empowerment' and 'empathy' may have been misunderstood.

Table 3: Emotions Felt While Using CHESS

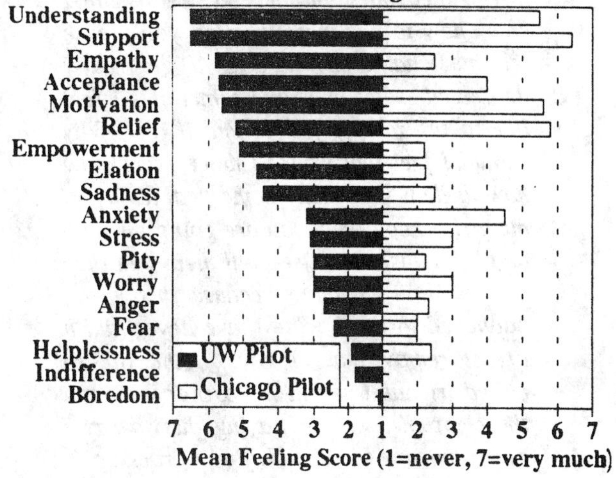

Questions regarding the value and ease of use of CHESS were rated on a 1-7 scale (7 being very valuable or very easy to use). The overall value of CHESS was rated 7.00, with only three of the services being rated below 7.00. Action plan was rated the lowest at 6.50.

Action plan was also rated the lowest in terms of ease of use (4.80), however overall CHESS was rated 5.80. Six of the eight CHESS services were rated above 6.00 in ease of use. Despite the relatively lower ease of use score of Discussion Groups (5.25), this service was used more extensively than any other CHESS service (Table 4). CHESS appears to be extremely user-friendly and lack of computer experience is not a barrier to use. Five of the eight women in this pilot had never used a computer prior to CHESS.

Table 4: Ease of Use & Value (0 - 7 scale)

Service	Ease of Use	Value
CHESS Overall	5.80	7.00
Questions & Answers	6.75	7.00
Instant Library	6.75	7.00
Getting Help/Support	6.00	6.75
Personal Stories	6.60	7.00
Ask an Expert	7.00	7.00
Discussion Groups	5.25	7.00
Decisions & Conflicts	6.75	6.67
Action Plan	4.80	6.50

Other results indicate that there has been a reduction of depression and isolation. The following message was left in the CHESS Discussion Group by a woman in the Chicago Pilot Study using the code name Barbara:

> *"I feel sad and lonely a lot and all my so-called friends that I thought I had have all turned their backs on me. So I really don't know how to deal with it. Can you please tell me what I should do? I get really depressed sometimes and sometimes I feel like taking my life just to end it all. Why should I feel that way? I don't even know how to deal with this. Some people say to me girl, I know what you are going through and I get upset because I tell them that they do not know anything because this hasn't happened to them. They have never had a breast removed but I have. And the so called friends I had in my corner were not there for me. So I'm saying this to say I need someone to talk to before I crack up."*

Within 24 hours Barbara received four messages from other women in the pilot test as well as the discussion group facilitator. While not all women experienced the depth of pain Barbara felt, many had similar experiences of isolation and misunderstanding by those close to them.

The women who had CHESS became change agents in their community. As they learned more about breast cancer, they began to talk to others in their community and became a resource for them. There were also 10 known secondary users (family members, friends, or neighbors) in the Chicago pilot. The use data of these secondary users is not included in this paper.

CHESS provided an opportunity to get information, support and problem-solving tools to this under-served population in the convenience of one's own home. The following quotes are from two of the Chicago pilot study participants:

> *"I learned more about my cancer from CHESS. It was very informative. I also learned that there are people who care about others."*

> *"I had a computer that I could take my time with and get answers."*

The barriers (geographic location, cost, child care...) that had prevented these women from accessing information and support were easily overcome by their in-home use of the CHESS computer.

CONCLUSION

This pilot study confirmed that a computer system is a viable option for an under-served population. In a health care system which is desperately trying to contain cost, CHESS can help ease the load of doctors and patient advocates, while allowing women to take back control of their lives. CHESS can allow health care providers (patient advocates, doctors, nurses...) to more efficiently track patients, maintain better communication, and make better use of their time.

While these results are only preliminary and with a limited number of users, we are very encouraged. These results reinforces the need for more extensive studies to determine CHESS' effectiveness in meeting the decision, information, and emotional needs of women diagnosed with breast cancer in under-served populations.

References

1. Nelles,W.B., McCaffery, R.J., Blanchard, C.G., & Ruckleschel, J.C. (1991). Social Supports and Breast Cancer: A Review. *Journal of Psychosocial Oncology*, 9(1), 21-34
2. Aguiler, D. (1990). *Crisis intervention: Theory and methodology* (6th ed.). St. Louis, MO: C.V. Mosby.
3. Blanchard C., Labraque, M., Ruckleschel, J., & Blanchard, E. (1990). Physician Behaviors, Patient Perceptions, and Patient Characteristics as Predictors of Satisfaction of Hospitalized Cancer Patients. *Cancer*, 65, 186-192.
4. Johnson, J.E. (1973). Effects of Accurate Expectations about Sensory and Distress Components of Pain. *Journal of Personality & Social Psychology*, 27, 261-275.
5. Ward, S., Leventhal, H., Easterling, D., Luchterhand, C., & Love, R. (1991). Social Support, Self Esteem and Communication in Patients Receiving Chemotherapy. *Journal of Psychosocial Oncology*, 9(2), 95-116.
6. Waxler-Morrison N., Hislop, T.G., Mears, B., & Kan, L. (1991). Effects of Social Relationships on Survival for Women with Breast Cancer: A Prospective Study. *Social Science & Medicine*, 33, 177-138
7. Boberg, E.W., Gustafson, D.H., Hawkins, R.P., Peressinni, T., Chan, C., Bricker, E., Pingree, S., Berhe, H., (1994). Development, Acceptance and Use Patterns of a Computer-Based Education and Social Support System for People Living with AIDS/HIV Infection. *Computers in Human Behavior*, (in press)
8. Gustafson, D.H., Wise, M., McTavish, F., Taylor, J., Wolberg, W., Stewart, J., Smalley, R., Bosworth, K.. (1993). Development and pilot evaluation of a computer-based support system for women with breast cancer. *Journal of Psychosocial Oncology*, 11(4), 69-93.
9. Breemhaar, B., van den Borne, H.W. (1991). Effects of Educational and Support for Surgical Patients: The Role of Perceived Control. Patient Education and Counseling, 18, 199-210
10. Moos, R.H., Schaeffer, J. (1984). The Crisis of Physical Illness: An Overview and Conceptual Approach. In Moos (Ed.), *Coping with Physical Illness II: New Perspectives*. New York: Plenum Medical Book Company, 3-25.
11. Speigal, D., Kraemer, H., Bloom, J., Gottheil, E. (1989). Effect of Psychosocial Treatment in Survival of Patients with Metastatic Breast Cancer. *The Lancet*, 8668(2), 888-891.
12. Cawley, M., Kostic, J., Cappello, C. (1990). Informational and Psychosocial Needs of Women Choosing Conservative/Primary Radiation for Early Stage Breast Cancer. *Cancer Nursing*, 13, 90-94
13. Lehman, C., Rimer, B., Bkuumberg, B., Cristinizio, Z., Engtrom, P., MacElwee, N., O'Connor, K., & Seay, V. (1990). Effects of Coping Style and Relaxation on Cancer Chemotherapy Side Effects and Emotional Responses. *Cancer Nursing*, 13, 308-315.
14. Miller, S., Magnum, C. (1983). Interacting Effects of Informational and Coping Style in Adapting to Gynecologic Stress: Should the Doctor Tell All?. *Journal of Personality & Social Psychology*, 45, 223-236.

The Use and Impact of a Computer-Based Support System for People Living with AIDS and HIV Infection

David H. Gustafson, Robert P. Hawkins, Eric W. Boberg, Earl Bricker, Suzanne Pingree and Chien-Lung Chan

Center for Health Systems Research and Analysis
University of Wisconsin
Madison, Wisconsin

ABSTRACT

CHESS (the Comprehensive Health Enhancement Support System) is an interactive, computer-based system to support people facing AIDS/HIV Infection and other health-related crises or concerns. CHESS provides information, referral to service providers, support in making tough decisions and networking to experts and others facing the same concerns. CHESS is designed to improve access to health and human services for people who would otherwise face psychological, social, economic or geographic barriers to receiving services.

CHESS has been evaluated in a random-assignment study with over 200 men and women living with AIDS and HIV infection. When CHESS was placed in subjects' homes for 3-6 months, use of CHESS was extremely heavy, with the average subject using CHESS 138 times for 39 hours. Compared with a control group which did not receive CHESS, subjects who used CHESS reported significantly higher quality of life in several dimensions, including social support and cognitive functioning. Users also reported significant reductions in some types of health care costs, especially inpatient services (hospitalizations).

All segments of the study population used and benefited from CHESS, including women, minorities and those subjects with lower levels of education. Thus, CHESS appears to be an effective means of delivering education and support to the diverse populations which are affected by AIDS and HIV infection.

INTRODUCTION

CHESS, the Comprehensive Health Enhancement Support System, is a multi-service system supporting HIV infected people, as well as people facing other major life crises [1,2]. CHESS runs on a personal computer, typically placed in the home for three to six months; it can also be installed in health care settings or community sites. CHESS' nine services offer a range of information, social and emotional support, and problem-solving tools for people in health crises. The Information Services offer answers to commonly asked questions (***Questions and Answers***), detailed articles (***Instant Library***), communication with medical experts (***Ask an Expert***), and a tutorial on finding and using resources effectively (***Getting Help/Support***). The Support Services include programs that allow patients to communicate with each other (***Discussion Group***) and read personal accounts of people who have coped with the same crisis (***Personal Stories***). The Problem-Solving Services include programs to help people understand their lifestyle risks and patterns (***Assessment***), decision aids (***Decision Analysis***), and a guided program to implement decisions(***Action Plan***). CHESS is now offered for six topics: AIDS/HIV, early stage breast cancer, acquaintance rape, academic failure (focusing on African American males), adult children of alcoholics, and stress management.

CHESS was conceived following our experience with the BARN (Body Awareness Resource Network) system [3]. BARN is a widely-used, computer-based health promotion/behavior change system for 6th- to 12th-grade students, with information and skill-building activities on AIDS, alcohol and other drugs, body management, human sexuality, smoking and stress management. Compared with BARN, CHESS provides more in-depth information, additional decision- and behavior-support services, and a communications link to other users. CHESS design has been further shaped by various aspects of crisis [4,5] and change [6,7] theories. In situations fraught with irrationality and emotion, CHESS is designed to provide: (1) an organized and systematic way for people in crisis to obtain good information, tailored to their needs, and delivered in an educationally sound way; (2) help in making and implementing decisions; and (3) social support from peers and professionals. People in crisis use CHESS to anonymously ask potentially embarrassing questions of experts and communicate with people sharing the same problem. They can get the information and support they need at any time of the day.

0195-4210/94/$5.00 © 1994 AMIA, Inc.

The variety of services in CHESS allows people to use it selectively to best meet their needs. Some use the expert systems for guidance in thinking through difficult issues. Others think through issues by exploring CHESS databases of information. Still others seek advice from experts and peers through CHESS computer mediated communication systems. Many will use all CHESS services as they explore one particular issue. Regardless of how they use it, CHESS is designed to reduce the asymmetry of knowledge between patients and health care providers, to increase patient and family sense of control, and to empower patients to be more active participants in their clinical care.

CHESS has been developed over the last four years by a team of decision, information, education, communication, and medical scientists from the University of Wisconsin-Madison under a grant from the W.K. Kellogg Foundation. The AIDS/HIV module was evaluated with a grant from the Agency for Health Care Policy and Research.

THE RESEARCH DESIGN

The purpose of this research was to assess the impact of CHESS on: (1) health status and quality of life; (2) risk behaviors and (3) health service utilization, of HIV-infected people. CHESS was evaluated in a randomly-assigned experiment with 204 HIV-infected people from Madison and Milwaukee, Wisconsin. The 107 experimental subjects (who were given CHESS for three or six months) and 97 control subjects, answered a pre-test and two or three post-tests; the first given two months after installation and the last given three months after removal of CHESS. An additional nine women participated in the first cohort as a pilot test and were not randomly assigned. In addition to the outcome variables mentioned above, we also examined use of CHESS and cost of operating CHESS.

The computers used in this study were IBM-compatible personal computers assembled by local manufacturers, and had 386sx16 microprocessors (CHESS will run acceptably on 286 machines), 40 MB hard drives, 1MB RAM, 3.5" floppy disk drives, color VGA monitors and 2400-baud modems. Communications were transmitted via modem to a central "host" computer (also a 386sx PC) with multiple modem connections. The computers were installed in subjects' homes by the project director, who also gave a 45-minute tutorial on CHESS use. Whenever possible, the computers were locked down to immovable objects using a cable and padlock. No computers were lost or stolen from homes during this study. Equipment failure was very rare. Only 3 units needed to be replaced during the study. Most other service questions were handled over the phone by the project director or programming staff.

The content of the AIDS/HIV module was initially developed in 1990-1991. Prior to the initiation of each cohort, the content was reviewed and updated to insure that the information was accurate and up-to-date. Late-breaking information was posted in Discussion Group. CHESS content continues to be reviewed and updated annually.

RESULTS

CHESS Use

Use of CHESS was heavy. The 116 subjects (including the nine non-randomly assigned women) used CHESS 15,966 times, an average of 138 uses per person (more than once per day on average) with a duration of 39 hours each. These figures do not include use of Health Charts (a program which users were required to use which routinely collects health status and health concerns data) or the Dictionary function (intended to help people understand complex medical terms). Nor does it include uses of less than one minute in duration. Over 34% of CHESS uses occurred between 9:00 p.m. and 7:00 a.m., a time when most other sources of information and support are not available.

Social Support services accounted for 79% of all uses, 73% in ***Discussion Group*** alone. Information services accounted for 17% of all uses and Problem-Solving services just 4%. Subjects considered all services to be important, arguing that all but Social Support services could accomplish their goals with just one use. Even so, these findings raise important questions about the role and relative importance to the user of Information and Problem-Solving components in a support system of this type.

While making about as much overall use of CHESS as whites, minorities allocated their use somewhat differently among CHESS services. Minorities used ***Discussion Group*** a smaller proportion of their total use (68% versus 78%) than whites, while using Information services more (22% versus 15%) and Problem-Solving services more (6% versus 3%). Women used CHESS 13% more frequently than men. In particular they were more likely to use the Information services, especially ***Ask An Expert***.

Other demographics were also important predictors of use. People who had not yet developed AIDS symptoms used CHESS more frequently, in particular the ***Discussion Group*** and ***Personal Stories***. Younger people used CHESS more frequently, especially ***Questions and Answers***, ***Personal Stories***, and ***Discussion Group***. Thus, the results suggest possible reversals of traditional information use patterns that increase knowledge gaps between races, genders, etc. [8]

Quality of Life

Quality of life analyses, after the first two months of installation, found CHESS users significantly higher on five of eight dimensions, and lower on none. CHESS users reported improved cognitive functioning, an increased sense of social support, and leading a more active life, while controls stayed steady or got worse on each of these variables. CHESS users also reported greater improvement than controls in actively participating in their health care, and they reported decreased levels of negative emotions while controls stayed the same. There were no significant differences at any time between the groups for depression, physical functioning, or reported level of energy.

If CHESS was left in place only three months, its positive effects mostly disappeared once it was removed. However the results were more encouraging when CHESS is left in the home for six months. Figure 1 portrays the average quality of life score as a percent of maximum for the Madison subjects over the four time periods. Even with a smaller sample size (30 experimental and 28 control), the positive effects of CHESS were significant at five months (when CHESS was still in the home) for active life, social support and participation in health care. And non-significant but still positive trends continued for cognitive function and negative emotions.

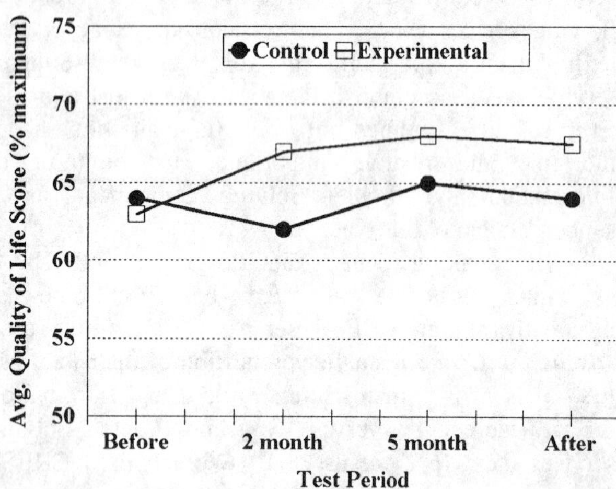

Figure 1. Average Percent Maximum Quality of Life Score -- Madison Cohort Only

Moreover, three months after CHESS was removed from the longer-term (six month) implementation, CHESS continued to have significant positive effects on social support and participation in health care. Non-significant positive trends continued in cognitive functioning and negative emotions but disappeared for active life. These results suggest a longer than 3-month implementation not only continues the beneficial effects CHESS has while it is in the home, but also has carryover effects after CHESS is removed.

Risk Attitudes and Behaviors

CHESS did not significantly change sexual risk behavior, but the six month implementation did, after CHESS was removed, improve attitudes toward risk behavior and toward disclosure of HIV status to potential partners, compared to pre-test.

Health Services Utilization

CHESS users self-reported number of visits to health care providers, time spent with providers, satisfaction with visits, number of admissions to hospitals and length of stay. We examined CHESS effect on the reported utilization of health services and then monetized that effect by using average Madison area charges for the relevant health services.

Outpatient services There were no significant CHESS effects on number of visits to various ambulatory care providers while CHESS was in the home, although the number of phone contacts increased in the experimental group compared to the controls. Using an average charge figure for each service, the total charges for ambulatory care was reduced by 17% in the CHESS group compared to a reduction of 7% in the control group, but this effect was also not statistically significant.

However, three months after removing CHESS, the experimental group had (compared to pre-test) significantly fewer visits to dentists, primary care and alternative care providers, while the significant CHESS effect on number of calls disappeared.

CHESS had a statistically significant effect on the time spent with providers when a visit did occur. While CHESS was in the home, significant reductions occurred (compared to the control group) in time spent with primary care, HIV and mental health providers. The experimental group's total time spent with non-emergency providers decreased 8% while control group time increased 13%. This difference was also significant. Hence, while it may not show in charges, since those figures are not based on time spent, the intensity of resource utilization was significantly lower in the CHESS group, both during and after the period of CHESS use.

Inpatient services CHESS also had significant effects on in-patient care. While CHESS was in the home, the average probability of admission in the control group increased 42% versus 16% in the CHESS group. In the three months after CHESS removal, the probability of admission increased another 25% in the control group while it decreased 2% in the CHESS group. These results were not statistically significant.

However changes in length of stay were significant. If a person was admitted to the hospital, there was 61%

increase in average length of stay in the control group and a 29% reduction in the CHESS group. After CHESS was removed, average length of stay continued to be 35% higher than pre-test levels in the control group and 26% lower in the experimental group. As it turned out, there were pre-test differences between control and experimental groups that make the analysis of this data challenging. The analysis did take these differences into account as covariance. However, there is no way to completely remove the effect those differences have.

By combining admission rate and average length of stay it is possible to estimate the effect of CHESS on the costs of inpatient care. One way to analyze the data would be to argue that while they had CHESS, the experimental group costs went down $148 at the same time that the control group costs went up $457, for a total difference of $605, a difference maintained (at a slightly lower level) even after CHESS was removed (Figure 2A).

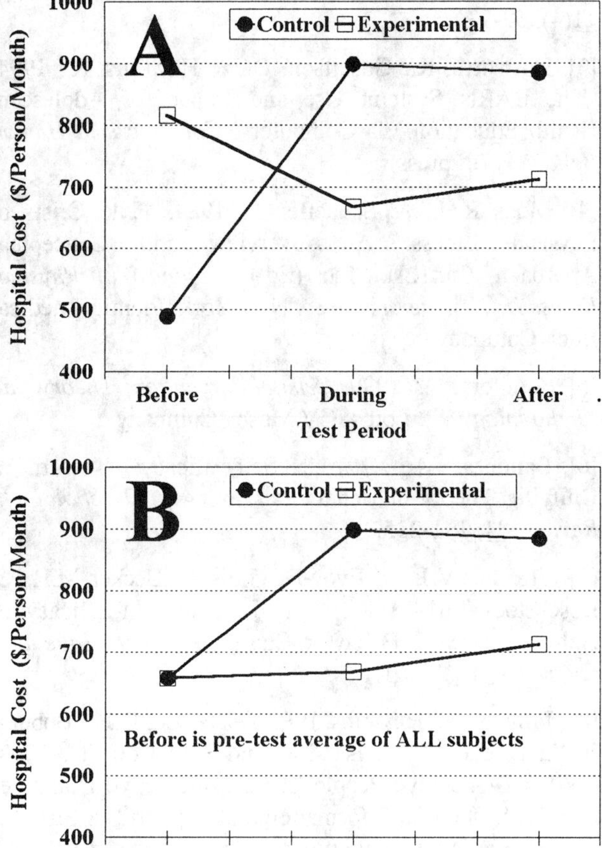

Figure 2. Average Hospital Cost Per Person Per Month

Because of the pre-test differences, a more conservative approach would be to average the pre-test costs of all subjects, and use this as a basis to compare post-test differences between the two groups (Figure 2B). Using this approach, pre-tests costs of $658 per person per month increased during the period of CHESS use by $240 for the controls, but only $10 for the CHESS group, a difference of $230 (which decreased slightly to $174 after CHESS was removed).

At pre-test, approximately 30% of our subject population had AIDS, 35% symptomatic HIV infection, and 35% asymptomatic HIV infection. Using data obtained in the AIDS Cost and Service Utilization Study [9] on the average monthly costs for inpatient services for people at various stages of HIV infection, we calculated that our population would be expected to have an average monthly cost for inpatient services of $685 per person per month, a value similar to the average we obtained for pre-test costs of all subjects in this study. The difference in inpatient costs between control and experimental subjects during the period of CHESS use was thus at least 33% of the average total inpatient costs. Inpatient costs would be expected to account for about 60% of total health care costs in this population [9].

Effects of CHESS on Minority Subjects

Thirty nine minority subjects were involved in the CHESS study. At pre-test, we found that minorities were much more depressed than whites. Also, their utilization of health services was higher for primary care, HIV care, emergency care and dental care, but lower for mental health and other non-HIV specialty care.

Separate outcome analyses for minorities were hampered by the small sample size. However, interactions of experimental condition with minority group status and educational level were not significant. That is, CHESS effects were not significantly larger or smaller for minorities than for whites.

In absolute numbers, although not significant, the experimental group of minorities showed a reduction (relative to the control group) in number of visits to dentists, primary care, mental health, and emergency care while CHESS was in the home. The total number of visits for non-emergency care dropped 17% in the experimental group and increased 8% in the control, while CHESS was in the home. After removal, the reduction compared to pre test was 42% for the experimental group and 3% for the control group.

CONCLUSION

The results of this evaluation are very encouraging. HIV-positive individuals (including minorities) used CHESS frequently over a period of several months. CHESS was highly valued by subjects as indicated in unsolicited letters of support as well as in formal evaluation. CHESS improved quality of life and made use of health services more efficient. No significant effects were detected on risk behaviors.

Additional research should examine the effects of CHESS in greater detail. One study should compare CHESS against other non-technology-based interventions costing about the same. We also need to conduct studies on the specific utility of various CHESS components (i.e., which CHESS services make the most difference, for whom, and under what conditions?). In addition, further study of CHESS impact on costs of care is needed. The pre-test differences in length of stay between control and experimental groups, as well as the self-report nature of the data make further study of health service use desirable. Toward that end, a study has been funded by the Agency for Health Care Policy and Research to further examine effects of CHESS on costs of care. This study will include aspects of care not addressed in this study (drugs and home care) and will supplement self reports with data from medical and billing records.

Of course, CHESS has important implications for crises other than AIDS. CHESS currently has programs addressing breast cancer, rape, adult children of alcoholics, academic failure and stress management. New programs are planned on diabetes, depression, and substance abuse. Some of these programs (e.g. diabetes) are likely to have positive effects on costs and quality of life. The primary benefit of others may center on quality of life. The effect of CHESS on these other areas deserves careful evaluation.

In addition to studying the impact of CHESS, work is needed to identify the most cost-effective means for its deployment. CHESS computers could be loaned by clinics and HMO's, CHESS could be placed in the National Information Infrastructure (the "Information Superhighway"), or made available through interactive television systems. These efforts are particularly important if CHESS is to reach populations and providers that do not have access to personal computers.

Finally, the potential of CHESS for collecting data means that a wide array of research issues can be addressed. The decision analysis program collects data on the importance people place on different decision criteria and the utility they assign to different options. Hence, we have an almost unique means of analyzing data on the values and perceptions of people in crisis. The dialogue taking place in the discussion groups can offer us important insights into the group dynamic of computer mediated communication systems and can also help us understand the issues being faced by people in crisis. The CHESS use data offers an opportunity to learn how CHESS has its effects, by telling us not only what services are being used, but also the styles or patterns with which people seek help, and even (for instance) what article in the Instant library is being read most frequently. These are just a few of the examples of the rich data that are available to give us new insights into crisis and the means to address it.

References

[1]. Gustafson, D.H., Bosworth K., Hawkins R.P., Boberg E.W., & Bricker E., 1992, "CHESS: A Computer-Based Support System for Providing Information, Referrals, Decision Support and Social Support To People Facing Medical and Other Health-Related Crises," *Proceedings of the 16th Annual Symposium on Computer Applications in Medical Care*, 16, 161-165.

[2]. Gustafson, D.H., Wise, M., McTavish, F., Taylor, J.O., Wolberg, W., Stewart, J., Smalley, R.V., & Bosworth, K., 1994, "Development and Pilot Evaluation of a Computer Based Support System for Women with Breast Cancer," *Journal of Psychosocial Oncology*, 11(4), 69-93.

[3]. Bosworth, K., Gustafson, D., & Hawkins, R., 1994, "The BARN System: Use and Impact of Adolescent Health Education Via Computer," *Computers in Human Behavior*, (in press).

[4] Moos R.H., & Schaeffer J., 1984, "The Crisis of Physical Illness: An Overview and Conceptual Approach," In: R.H. Moos (Ed.)., *Coping With Physical Illness II: New Perspectives*. New York: Plenum Medical Book Company.

[5] Aguilera, D., 1990, *Crisis Intervention: Theory and Methodology*. St. Louis: CV Mosby Company.

[6] Bandura, A., 1977, "Self-Efficacy: Toward a Unifying Theory of Behavioral Change," *Psychological Review*, 84, 191-215.

[7]. Strecher V.J., McEvoy-DeVellis B., Becker M.H., & Rosenstock I.M., 1986, "The Role of Self-Efficacy in Achieving Health Behavior Change," *Health Education Quarterly*, 13, 73-91.

[8]. Pingree, S., Hawkins, R.P., Gustafson, D.H., Boberg, E.W., Bricker, E., Wise, M., and Tiillotson, T., 1993, "Will HIV-Positive People Use an Interactive Computer Support System for Information and Support? A Study of CHESS in Two Communities," *Proceedings of the 17th Annual Symposium on Computer Applications in Medical Care*, 17, 22-26.

[9]. Hellinger, F., 1993, "The Lifetime Cost of Treating a Person With HIV," *Journal of the American Medical Association*, 270(4), 474-478.

The Development of a Client Application for the Collaborative Social and Medical Services System

Dwight M. Moore, Hillary S. Gilson, Ph.D.,Yizhen Li, M.S., Risa B. Bobroff, M.S., Cynthia A. Petermann, M.S., Dennis R. Moreau, Ph.D., J. Robert Beck, M.D., Gregory J. Buffone, Ph.D.

Medical Informatics and Computing Research Program
Baylor College of Medicine
Houston, Texas

ABSTRACT

This paper describes the design and implementation of a client application for the Baylor College of Medicine Teen Health Clinics. The application is the front end to the Collaborative Social and Medical Services System (CSMSS) under development by Baylor's Medical Informatics and Computing Research Program [8]. The application provides distributed access to an underlying object oriented database system. A process driven and patient centered design will provide staff members with a complete set of services, including forms for data entry and viewing, query, and access management to facilitate efficient and effective delivery of services. Role-specific interfaces will be supplied for clerks, nurses, nurse practitioners, physicians, and social workers. The client application is being designed using object oriented methodologies and technologies with the C++ programming language, and will operate within a Microsoft Windows operating environment utilizing Object Linking and Embedding for application interoperability.

INTRODUCTION

There is an appropriate and increasing desire in the United States to integrate social service activities with medical care, so that the whole person and the entire suite of problems he or she presents can be treated in a coordinated fashion. Parochial systems of health care, community development, family services, and job training too often produce fragmented support for the poor and the disadvantaged. We believe medicine as well as social services can benefit from improved communication and information management made feasible by high performance communications and computation across a network [1].

An integrated social service and medical care environment has been created within the Teen Health Clinics of the Baylor College of Medicine [8]. These clinics are staffed through the collaborative efforts of the Department of Obstetrics and Gynecology at Baylor, the Population Program within the College, and the Harris County Hospital District (HCHD), the fourth largest health services agency in the nation. There are five Teen Clinic sites currently dispersed throughout the city of Houston, Texas.

This work is based in part on our experience with a protoype application called the Virtual Chart System [3]. Like the BHCHP homeless project [4] and SuperChart [6], we use the client-server paradigm to support distributed communication. Like the patient-tracking system of the UCLA Children's Health Center [9], we use an object-oriented approach to the development of flexible user interfaces. Because our development effort is focused on support for both social and medical services in the Teen Health Clinics, we must support differing technological frames for different classes of users. The thrust of the project is to enhance clinical care and social service with products and systems that can be assembled using currently available technologies. A system with these goals must offer a spectrum of services to meet our end users' needs - allowing them to perform their job function more efficiently and with higher quality. This entails addressing issues such as data model design [2], data security mechanisms [5], and the client architecture.

This paper presents a scenario of how the CSMSS Client Application will be used in the clinic environment. We present a description of the methodologies and processes involved in the client specification, design, and implementation. The paper closes with a description of our outstanding technology issues.

SCENARIO

Nurse Jones arrives at the clinic, places her lunch in the refrigerator, pours a cup of coffee, and sits down at her desk. She logs into the CSMSS, checks her e-mail, notes the all-staff meeting in her personal appointment scheduler, and is ready to begin her work for the day.

The first activity of the day involves auditing yesterday's charts. Nurse Jones selects a patient from a list of all of the patients seen at this clinic on the previous work day for chart review. The patient's chart appears on the screen, with the summary of the last patient visit displayed. After scanning the summary page, Nurse Jones pages through the patient's chart, examining the data collected. It is apparent that Clerk Smith forgot to scan in the patient's immunization form. She creates an annotation that will appear with the patient's chart indicating the omission, and the responsible person. The message is automatically forwarded to Clerk Smith.

The telephone rings and interrupts Nurse Jones. The lab is calling with some test results for another patient. Nurse Jones locates the patient's name in the patient list and selects it for lab results entry. A form appears on the screen with the patients pending lab tests. Nurse Jones enters the results on the form. Since the lab result was positive, Nurse Jones sends a form letter, using her word processor, to the patient asking her to call the clinic as soon as possible.

Nurse Jones takes a pen-based computer with her to see the patient in the exam room. She scans the patient's chart summary, which is already displayed on the screen, and notes that the patient is here for a 3 month oral contraceptive check-up. Nurse Jones notices that the patient's weight seems high, so she requests a tabular summary of the patient's weight and blood pressure over time. Nurse Jones then starts a "3-month follow up" session with the system.

Nurse Jones enters the exam room and asks the patient about how she feels and if there are any side effects related to use of oral contraceptives. With the pen, she checks off these observations on the form displayed on the screen. During the conversation, Nurse Jones notices a bruise on the patient's arm, and asks her about it. The patient seems worried, and reluctant to talk about the bruise. Nurse Jones will send an appropriate electronic mail message to the social worker, after the session is concluded.

Nurse Jones reviews her observations and upon completion her orders/services form is displayed. She checks off the review and records that she counseled the patient on weight control and proper use of the oral contraceptives. She schedules a 6 month follow-up, using the appointment scheduler. She then makes an appointment for the patient to see the social worker, prints a new appointment card for the patient, and continues seeing patients.

METHODOLOGY & CURRENT SPECIFICATION

A combination of object oriented methodologies have been used in the analysis and design of the CSMSS Client Application. A number of investigations were conducted to obtain the requirements. The investigations were accomplished by interviewing staff members, observing the clinics' operation, examining patient charts, analyzing the clinic Medical Protocols document, and holding focus group meetings with subsets of the clinic staff.

Based on the information obtained through the investigation described above, the following roles were established: clerk, nurse, nurse practitioner, physician, and social worker. Within each role we listed the operational tasks each user might perform. By specifying the tasks, we were able to establish a work flow process. For example, a nurse might audit charts or record a patient's medical history. Each patient specific task was further broken down by patient problem. For example, a sickle cell anemia test is only listed during a patient's first visit and tests for gonorrhea and chlamydia are listed as options whenever a patient comes in for a pregnancy test.

The CSMSS is designed to be extensible in order to accommodate changes in health care and social services delivery as well as evolving software standards and technology. The application has been subdivided into modules, each of which provides a unique service, thereby reducing the amount of functional coupling. As a result, future services can be added to the application without affecting existing services. This ability to "drop in" new modules at any time plays an important role in the extensibility and ultimate longevity of the CSMSS Client Application.

Currently, the client application consists of a Session Manager, a Form Manager, a Patient Browser, and an Access Manager, all of which operate within the Integrated Desktop Environment, as described below. Each module communicates with the CSMSS Server Application by way of the Client Protocol Framework, depicted in Figure 1. In addition, the modules communicate with the Session Manager which maintains the desktop environment.

Integrated Desktop Environment

The integrated desktop is a computer based working environment for the CSMSS user. It provides an operating environment for both third party applications and the CSMSS Client Application, as well as a fundamental set of services. The goal of the desktop environment is to integrate the CSMSS with third party applications by providing an efficient and intuitive interface. To achieve this goal, we identified applications needed by the user, basic services needed by the desktop environment, and CSMSS tools needed in the desktop environment.

Applications. Third party applications include a word processor, a spreadsheet, an electronic mail system, and a scheduling system.

Basic Services. A set of "basic services" was defined for the desktop environment which includes folders, a wastebasket, an access control mechanism, and a search utility.

The folder is merely a container of desktop objects, including other folders. It offers the ability to organize or group a collection of objects.

The wastebasket supports the disposal of desktop objects. It manages the lifetime of disposed objects, i.e., should they be disposed of immediately, should they live in the wastebasket for some time, or should they be returned to the desktop environment. It is important to understand that the wastebasket does not remove objects from the CSMSS Server Repository, it only supports the removal of objects from the desktop.

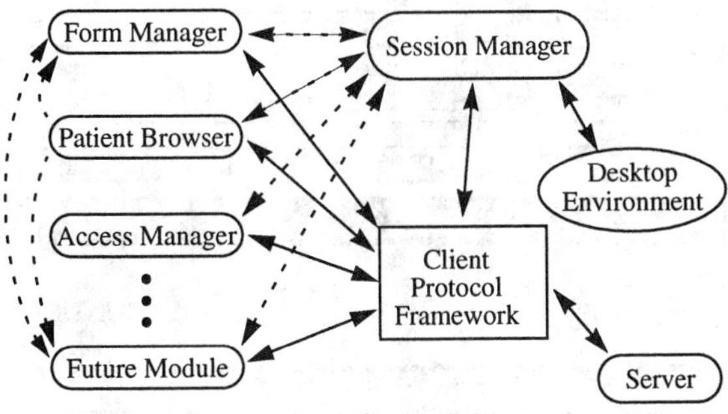

Figure 1. The CSMSS Client Architecture

The access control mechanism provides security for the desktop environment. It prevents unauthorized use of the desktop by requiring users to log into and out of the environment. This mechanism also enables/disables certain system features on a per user/role basis, by requesting authentication from the CSMSS Server Application [8].

A search utility provides the desktop environment with a search capability. It is utilized to locate desktop objects within the desktop environment.

Tools. A set of tools needed in the desktop environment include the Session Manager, Form Manager, Patient Browser, and Access Manager.

Session Manager - provides the user with the initial interface to the CSMSS. Presentation of the interface is based on a user role. The Session Manager is responsible for logging users into and out of the CSMSS, launching various client modules, and storing all CSMSS specific desktop objects.

When a user logs into the desktop environment, the Session Manager is launched, and connects the user to the CSMSS Server Application. This process includes retrieving user specific configuration information, restoring the desktop to its previous state, and presenting the user with any pending notices that need to be addressed.

When a user logs out of the system, the Session Manager stores the current state of the desktop environment, cleans off the desktop, and terminates all connections with the CSMSS Server.

Form Manager - provides a process driven (task oriented) mechanism for entering and viewing patient data which is entered into or viewed from a form. Access to the patient data is provided via a query mechanism built into the form. The Form Manager provides two basic types of forms including the View Form and Report Form.

The View Form supports patient data entry, viewing and query by example. Data entry includes typed input from a keyboard or hand written input from an electronic pen & pad device. Type checking and range validation services are also provided. Data viewing and query are complementary operations. To view data a query is executed explicitly by the user or implicitly by the system based on a user action or the current process. The results of a query are displayed in the current form or a new form depending on the context.

The Report Form provides "fill in the blank" queries. This type of form allows the user to perform more powerful queries than the example based queries possible with the View Forms by providing access to aggregate information, result sorting, and report layout customizing.

Instantiation of the Form Manager is provided by the Session Manager. The Session Manager provides the Form Manager with a patient object and the current process (if needed). The Form Manager presents the user with a list of the forms needed for the process and by default opens the first form in the list. The user has the flexibility to override the current process if needed.

An example is shown in Figure 2. The user has selected "Initial Visit" from the Session Manager. This action prompted the Session Manager to instantiate a Form Manager. There is no patient context for the Form Manager since the patient has not been defined in the system. The current task or process is presented to the user by way of a list of forms (defined in the process "Initial Visit"). The Form Manager presents the first step of the process by opening the Patient Registration form.

Patient Browser - provides access to patient lists (see Figure 2). The primary patient list is the Master Patient Index (MPI) maintained by the CSMSS Server. The MPI is available to all CSMSS users who have access to the Patient Browser. Users may access the MPI to create any number of private lists of patients. If necessary, users may search the MPI for patients using demographic information as search criteria. The Patient Browser also offers access to patient registration and patient chart information.

Access Manager - provides an interface to the CSMSS Access Management Facility [5].

FUTURE WORK

Future work on the CSMSS Client Application includes the investigation of a combination of data entry techniques and offering new services to the user to enhance the current CSMSS. Data acquisition and providing for user mobility are the two most challenging aspects of application development in this domain. Two data entry methods currently being investigated include voice input and hand written input.

Voice input will allow hands off operation. Currently, there are several commercial systems with vocabular-

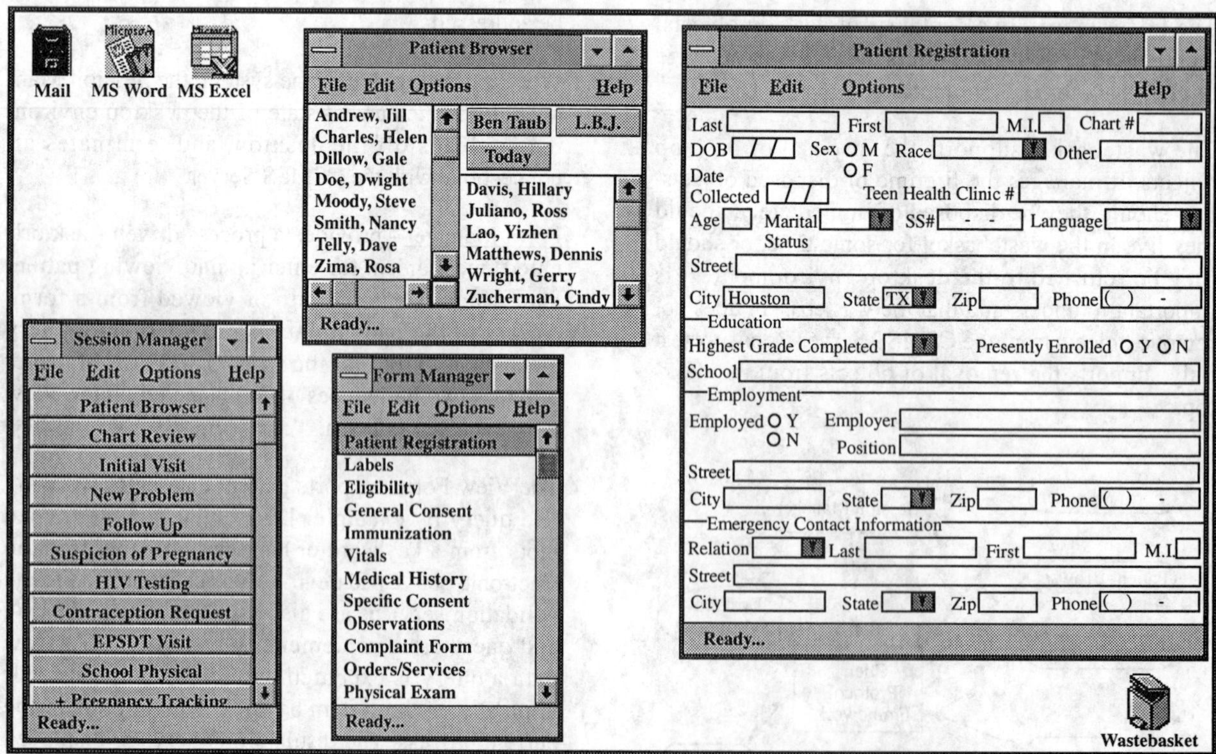

Figure 2. The Collaborative Social and Medical Services System's Client Application Desktop Environment

ies exceeding 50,000 words [7]. Handwriting recognition offers a comparable challenge. While voice will enable the hands off computing, in some instances, speech is not appropriate or even possible. For example, while a patient is being interviewed by a physician, a physician may need to communicate information to both the computer and the patient. Thus, writing with an electronic pen device may be an appropriate alternative. Both voice recognition and handwriting recognition technologies are improving rapidly and represent significant potential for future development.

Additions required for CSMSS Client Application evolution include an Object Browser and a Forms Creator. The Object Browser will provide ad hoc browsing of objects defined in the CSMSS Data Model [2] (e.g., Patients, Encounters, and Problems). Users will be able to choose a root object from which to start browsing. For example, a user will be able to select a patient object. From the patient object, the user will be able to explore patient data by traversing links between component objects. The Forms Creator will offer users the ability to create forms that meet their specific needs. They will be able to define processes by establishing a sequence of forms to be displayed, and they will be able to assign access to a given form.

CONCLUSION

The CSMSS Client Application utilizes current technologies and standards to provide an integrated solution to support social services and clinical care. By taking advantage of high speed computing and communications across networks we are able to provide a complete set of services allowing our users to perform their job more efficiently and with higher quality. Our design has emphasized on abstractions that increase the flexibility of the system, permitting quick development and enhancement of user interfaces, and allowing users to develop their own views of data; at the same time preserving the integrity of patient medical data in a distributed, collaborative environment.

Acknowledgments

The work reported here was supported (in part) by grant LM04905 from the National Library of Medicine.

The authors would like to thank the staff of the Baylor College of Medicine Teen Health Clinics for their help in this project.

References

[1]. Beck, JR, Buffone GJ, Burger AM, Petermann CA. "At Last: Integrated Diagnostic Images, Medical Records, and More - Networked". *Advanced Imaging*, Vol. 8, No. 11, November 1993.

[2]. Bobroff, RB, Petermann CA, Beck JR, Buffone GJ. Analysis, Requirements, and Development of a Collaborative Social and Medical Services Data Modal. *Proceedings of the Eighteenth Annual Symposium on Computer Applications in Medical Care*, Washington DC, November 1994.

[3]. Buffone, GJ, Petermann, CA, Fowler, J, Long, KB, Gilson, HS, Li, Y, Gorry GA, Beck, JR. The virtual chart system: Decentralized electronic medical data management. *AMIA Spring Congress*, 1993.

[4]. Chueh, HC, Barnett, GO. Client-server, Distributed Database Strategies in a Health-care Record System for a Homeless Population. *Journal of the American Medical Informatics Association*, Vol. 1, No. 2, March/April 1994.

[5]. Dargahi, R, Classen DW, Bobroff RB, Petermann CA, Moreau DR, Beck JR, Buffone GJ. The Development of a Data Security Model for The Collaborative Social and Medical Services System. *Proceedings of the Eighteenth Annual Symposium on Computer Applications in Medical Care*, Washington DC, November 1994.

[6]. Fiacco, PA, Winthrop, HR. Incorporating Client-Server Database Architecture and Graphical User Interface into Outpatient Medical Records. *Proceedings of the Fifteenth Annual Symposiium on Computer Applications in Medical Care*, Washington, DC, November 1991.

[7]. Meisel, WS. "Talk To Your Computer". *BYTE*, Vol. 18, No. 11, October 1993.

[8]. Petermann, CA, Bobroff, RB, Moore, DM, Gilson, HS, Li, Y, Fowler, J, Dargahi, R, Classen DW, Moreau DR, Beck JR, Buffone GJ. Collaborative Social and Medical Services System. *Proceedings of the Eighteenth Annual Symposium on Computer Applications in Medical Care*, Washington DC, November 1994.

[9]. Wilton, R. User-Specific Interfaces for Clinical Data-Management Systems: An Object-Based Approach. *Proceedings of the Sixteenth Annual Symposiium on Computer Applications in Medical Care*, Washington, DC, November 1992.

Collaborative Social and Medical Service System

Cynthia A. Petermann, MS, Risa B. Bobroff, MS, Dwight M. Moore, Hillary S. Gilson, PhD, Yizhen Li, MS, Ross Dargahi, David W. Classen, Jerry Fowler, MS, Dennis R. Moreau, PhD, J. Robert Beck, MD, and Gregory J. Buffone, PhD

Medical Informatics and Computing Research Program
Baylor College of Medicine
Houston, Texas

ABSTRACT

This paper describes the Collaborative Social and Medical Services System, a robust information infrastructure for integrated social and medical care. The Collaborative Social and Medical Services System design and architecture address the primary goals of creating a readily extensible social and ambulatory care system. Our initial step toward reaching this goal is the delivery of an application supporting the operations of the Baylor Teen Health Clinics. This paper discusses our protoype experiences, system architecture, components, and the standards we are addressing.

INTRODUCTION

Information required for patient care has traditionally been assembled in a paper chart format from a variety of sources by a team of providers including physicians, nurses, therapists and clerical staff. A recent review by the Institute of Medicine highlights the limitations and resultant impediments to efficient and effective health care created by the perpetuation of a paper-based record as the primary medical information repository[1]. Despite its limitations, the paper-based record provides the current communication and information management "workstation" for health care providers.

Information system applications that support technical services (diagnostic imaging, laboratory, etc.) and nursing have been available for several years and are being improved or supplemented by new entries into the field. To date, clinical workstation applications and computer-based patient records have focused on text and numeric data, with some recent systems beginning to incorporate static images[2,3]. Overall, these applications have demonstrably improved the efficiency of health care delivery when appropriately fitted to the target institutions' information systems strategy. However, many difficulties have impeded the common use of applications that address the requirements of physicians and other direct providers of health care. Such difficulties include the complexity of the functional requirements and the mobility of the user population, to name only a few. Nevertheless, computerization of clinical data is essential to containing or reducing cost while maintaining quality.

Clinical medicine is not the only discipline that may benefit from the application of computer-based technologies. There is an increasing need in our society today to have integrated systems of health care, community development, family services, and job training as a support structure for the poor and the disadvantaged.

To address the information management needs of such collaborative services, we are designing and implementing the Collaborative Social and Medical Services System (CSMSS). The CSMSS is a new health and human services system designed to address the general domains of social and primary clinical care as well several long term strategic issues which include; the need for an application architecture that is capable of extension and adaptation to changes in technology (e.g., multimedia, human-computer interfaces such as voice-to-text) and the need for a data model capable of supporting "generic" ambulatory services for collaborative medical and social services.

BAYLOR TEEN HEALTH CLINIC DOMAIN

We are creating an architecture and application framework to support integrated social services and primary medical care with the Teen Health Clinics (THC) of the Baylor College of Medicine as an initial test of our systems architecture[4]. These clinics are staffed through the collaborative efforts of the Department of Obstetrics and Gynecology at Baylor, the Population Program within the College, and the Harris County Hospital District (HCHD), the fourth largest health services agency in the nation.

The target population includes adolescent boys and girls 19 years of age and under, who reside primarily in the Houston, Texas inner city. Patients receive services such as family planning, sexually transmitted disease screening and treatment, perinatal care, case management (i.e., social work), counseling, and support services. Adolescents may receive services at any clinic site at no cost to the adolescent or family members.

Current management practices, which are heavily constrained by the use of paper based records, result in inefficiency of care due to delayed access to information or the inability to conduct research on THC's patient population. According to the statistics developed by the Clinic staff, the inability to effectively coordinate the various patient care priorities and schedules is a significant barrier to good care. For example, a counselor providing case management will often need to balance school schedules, clinic visits, well baby follow-up, and the Best Friends Program for a new mother. In addition, the lack of ready access to patient information impairs clinical and social service staff ability to provide continuity of care. In fact, some dropout from the program is attributable to the difficulty in coordinating the records and schedules for clinics and other programs provided by the THCs. The paper charting system used by the THCs today inhibits any outcomes, utilization review, and quality improvement research based on large volumes of patient data. There is no way to measure the impact of having the ability to conduct these types of research would have on their abilities to provide better overall care.

Beyond the current needs of the THCs it is essential that one basic architecture and data model also address requirements which may be imposed on this system in the future as it is applied to other clinical and social services domains.

Changing demands arise from an inability to predict patterns of health care delivery, the evolving nature of the integration of health care and social services, the transitory nature of emerging information systems standards, and the rapidly expanding volume and types of information that can reasonably be expected to become part of the patient record. All of these issues mandate an architecture capable of adapting to these challenges.

THE VIRTUAL CHART SYSTEM - A PROTOTYPE

We constructed a "proof of concept" prototype, called the Virtual Chart System (VCS) to aid in refining project specifications in light of the THC requirements and our long term strategic goals[5,6].

The prototype was constructed using the Virtual Notebook System (VNS) technology for collaborative work developed at Baylor College of Medicine[7].

We found the VNS "notebook" metaphor and underlying system architecture are fundamentally inadequate to support the development of comprehensive clinical information systems. A combination of VNS code and TCL/TK scripts were required to obtain the desired prototype application functionality[8]. We also found that the proposed system would require -

- a highly structured yet generalized data model to support clinical and social domains
- a provision for schema evolution in the database implementation strategy
- enforced structured data entry
- "write-once", read-only data entry
- an integrated facility for efficient and reliable data retrieval
- a multi-threaded server design for achieving system performance necessary to support a clinical application
- a security model capable of providing for the complex access policies necessitated by conflicting privacy and access requirements

The deficiencies noted in the prototype and subsequent reviews and comments by clinical users are substantial enough to warrant the development of a new architecture designed from the outset to support robust and highly-functional collaborative medical and social services applications.

CHARACTERISTICS OF THE CSMSS ARCHITECTURE

Data model and database

The data model must be capable of significant evolution over time without major redesign or major changes to the associated applications. For example, the support of multimedia capabilities within the patient record will allow the incorporation of more complete and more detailed documentation of the context in which medical care and social services decisions are made. Additionally, incorporation of multimedia capabilities in the broader system design will allow support of expanded services and capabilities including educational, conferencing, and telemedicine applications using the same server infrastructure. Thus, there is a need for rapid adjustment to and design of alternative data models which may be integrated with the original model as needed. For this reason, we have chosen an Object-Oriented Data Base Management System (OODBMS) as the foundation for our server architecture[9].

Client/Server

To provide for the dynamic nature of technology evolution we have chosen to modularize our system design at a high level by defining robust interfaces that should survive these changes. The client application depends only on the protocol between the client and the server to support access to patient data[4]. Building new clients based on other platforms under new operating systems will not require changes to the server architecture. The server, likewise, can be ported without changes to clients as long as the protocol is preserved[10]. We have abstracted the services provided by the OODBMS into a virtual interface that is supported by our broker layer. This insulates our server from depending on any particular OODBMS inherently. The intent of these design decisions is to make components of our design as portable, survivable, and maintainable as possible.

Access Control

The medical care delivery setting in general, and the outpatient clinic setting in particular, demand extraordinary flexibility from any access control mechanism associated with an underlying patient record system. The reasons for this needed flexibility include the following:

- Clinics need local control of their staff rosters since personnel rosters can change dynamically for a variety of reasons. This requirement implies the need for establishing access for individuals on that roster for access appropriate to their assigned role. If role definition (job function) is also in the hands of the end user, the access control must be specified in terms understandable by the clinic system administrator (probably not the terms of internal data model components or widgets).
- The nature of health care delivery requires a preemption mechanism which gets the security mechanism "out of the way" in emergency circumstances. Accountability requires that this action be backed by an authenticated audit trail.
- The changing nature of access control policies and their inherent complexity require flexibility. Most existing access control models (e.g. ACLs, C-LISTS) have difficulty supporting certain simple access management requests[11]. For example, the request "Revoke all access to patient records for Mr. Jones" is very difficult to accomplish in an ACL-based system and the request "Revoke all access to Mr. Presley's patient record" is very difficult in a C-List-based system.

Our approach utilizes an extended access matrix model to allow flexible policy enforcement while being manageable by clinic staff[10].

Data Entry Methods

The informational needs of the THCs will necessarily change over time, establishing significant justification for any system to be adaptive to these inevitable changes. We will provide an interactive mechanism for user definition of forms for data collection to support user driven adaptation of the application over time and in response to emergent requirements. We will also provide a mechanism for controlling the sequence and conditions under which forms are presented to users, thereby allowing user driven definition of the workflow process.This process is currently controlled by manually issued standing orders.

We recognize that system acceptance and utilization depends greatly upon the ease of data entry in the system. We are investigating the potential uses of voice and handwriting recognition input technologies integrated with mobile computers to enhance data acquisition.

CSMSS COMPONENTS

All of the CSMSS components are based on object oriented software engineering methodologies. Figure 1 depicts a high level view of the architecture of the CSMSS system. The application is based on a Client-Server model and supports geographically distributed clinic operations. Communication between client and server will occur via T-1 lines for Phase I, and subsequently on higher performance communications facilities, e.g. ATM, as multimedia and conferencing features become part of the environment.

Applications running on the client workstation communicate using Microsoft's Object Linking and Embedding (OLE) 2.0 facilities, allowing "drag and

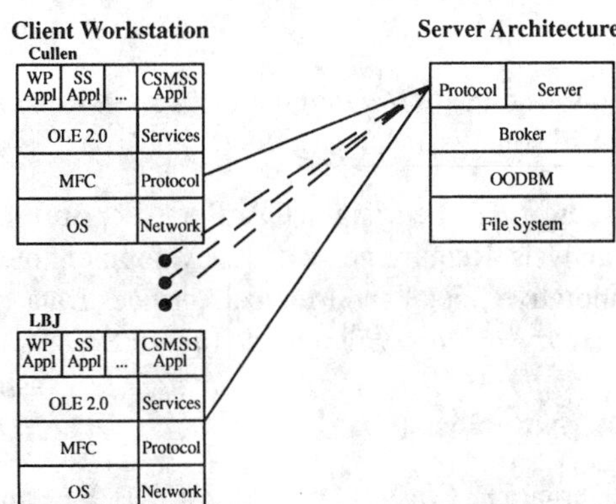

Figure 1. Collaborative Social and Medical Services System Architecture

drop" activation with highly flexible sharing of data between applications. The CSMSS Client application requests Server information through a basic services interface which generates the appropriate protocol requests to be transmitted over the network to the server.

The server receives protocol requests and translates them into service requests administered by agents. These services are cast in terms of a virtual OODBMS independent of any specific OODBMS and are mapped into requests specific to a particular OODBMS in the broker layer. The specific OODBMS supports navigation of the data model and finally makes file system requests that allow access to the text, imagery, bitmaps, and eventually digital voice and video that will comprise the electronic version of a patient-centered medical record.

STANDARDS

The CSMSS is being developed with attention to emerging standards. Adherence to systems standards will support portability and long term viability of CSMSS in the face of rapidly evolving software and hardware technologies. Provision for supporting medical messaging standards will allow effective data interchange and support integration of CSMSS within broader scale medical information contexts.

The systems standards that CSMSS will support are: ANSI C++ as our application development language, the Microsoft Foundation Classes (MFC) as our standard class library, Microsoft OLE for standard application communication and interoperability, Berkeley sockets for application access to network capabilities, Kerberos for standard authentication and encryption services[4,10].

The CSMSS will provide a Health Level 7 (HL7) interface for acquiring information from other hospital information systems. The specification operational guidelines and reminder/event notification rules will be provided using the ASTM E1460 (Arden Syntax). Finally, the data model at the core of CSMSS is based on the ANSI/HISPP MSDS JWG (IEEE P1157) for a Common Data Model[9].

CONCLUSION

Applications that address the requirements of physicians or other providers are not in common use due to the complexity of the functional requirements and the absence of a robust application infrastructure for the facilitation of the development of social and outpatient services applications. The focus of the CSMSS development activities have been twofold: first, to establish just such an infrastructure for supporting the collaborative social and medical services applications, and second, to develop a domain specific application using this infrastructure focused on supporting the activities of the THCs.

The CSMSS project schedule spans 3 years with a 3 phase development and deployment schedule. Our first phase, which we will deliver to the THCs January of 1995, will be the electronic version of the current THC's paper charting system with native interfaces to other hospital systems. Phases 2 and 3 will include the ability for the user to define data forms, multimedia capabilities and an integrated HL7 interface to other hospital information systems.

The Medical Informatics and Computing Research Program will continue to enhance, evaluate and evolve CSMSS as a foundation for exploring the development of innovative information systems across an expanding number of applications areas.

ACKNOWLEDGMENT

The work reported here was supported (in part) by grant LM04905 from the National Library of Medicine. We thank the staff of the Baylor College of Medicine Teen Health Clinics for their help in this project.

REFERENCES

[1]. Dick RS, Steen EB. The Computer-Based Patient Record: An Essential Technology for Health Care. National Academy Press, Washington DC, 1991.

[2]. Essin DJ. Intelligent processing of loosely structured documents as a strategy for organizing electronic health care records. Meth Inform Med, August 1993, 265-8.

[3]. Dick and Steen, pp. 56-80.

[4]. Moore DM, Gilson HS, Li Y, Bobroff RB, Petermann CA, Moreau DR, Beck JR, Buffone GJ. The Development of a Client Application for the Collaborative Social and Medical Services System. *Proceedings: Eighteenth Annual Symposium on Computer Applications in Medical Care*, Washington DC, November 1994.

[5]. Beck JR, Buffone GJ, Burger AM, Petermann CA. "At Last: Integrated Diagnostic Images, Medical Records, and More - Networked". Advanced Imaging, Vol. 8, No. 11, November 1993.

[6]. Buffone GJ, Petermann CA, Fowler RG, Long KB, Gilson HS, Li Y, Gorry GA, Beck JR. The virtual chart system: Decentralized electronic medical data management. AMIA Spring Congress, 1993.

[7]. Gorry GA, Long KB, Burger AM, Jung CP, Meyer BD. The virtual notebook system -- an architecture for collaborative work. J Org Comput 1991; 1: 233-5.

[8]. Ousterhout, J K *Tcl and the Tk Toolkit*. Reading, MA: Addison-Wesley, April 1994.

[9]. Bobroff RB, Petermann CA, Beck JR, Buffone GJ. Analysis, Requirements and Development of a Collaborative Social and Medical Services Data Model. *Proceedings: Eighteenth Annual Symposium on Computer Applications in Medical Care*, Washington DC, November 1994.

[10]. Dargahi R, Classen DW, Bobroff RB, Petermann CA, Moreau DR, Beck JR, Buffone GJ. The Development of a Data Security Model for The Collaborative Social and Medical Services System. *Proceedings: Eighteenth Annual Symposium on Computer Applications in Medical Care*, Washington DC, November 1994.

[11]. Orr, G.A., Brantley, B.A., "Development of a Model of Information Security Requirements for Enterprise-Wide Medical Information Systems", *Proceedings of the Sixteenth Annual Symposium on Computer Applications in Medical Care*, Baltimore, MD, November 1992.

Clinician-Directed Systems: Design, Implementation & Enhancement

A Simple Inpatient Psychiatric Clinical Information System Designed and Developed by Clinicians

T. Bradley Tanner, MD
Peter Murray, MD
Maureen Allen, RN

University of Pittsburgh/Western Psychiatric Institute and Clinic
3811 O'Hara Street, Pittsburgh, PA 15213

ABSTRACT

Objective: The growth of computer technology allows clinicians to develop a separate information system to replace inefficient paper-based approaches to documenting clinical care. Methods: A clinician team developed a system to replace standard paper forms using computer software running on 486 PC computer. Clinicians, directing the project at every step, refined handwritten forms to create a complete word processor application merging information from an individual database. Results: A system developed outside the traditional hospital information system simplifies the generation of a variety of required inpatient documents (treatment plans, progress notes, patient lists, and treatment summaries). A wide variety of clinicians converted from a traditional paper-based approach to the computer system. Conclusions: Computer technology allows the local development of an information system oriented toward clinical needs. Hospital clinical information systems will benefit from the input of clinicians with experience designing a computerized solution.

INTRODUCTION

Many sites are developing an electronic medical record incorporating on-line information entry and retrieval. Such systems clearly represent the future of health care delivery and documentation. Clinicians waiting for such systems to evolve are still saddled with repetitive, inefficient, paper-based approaches to clinical care. This is especially true for providers of care to psychiatric patients. This paper describes a clinical information system designed and developed by clinicians to aid the process of inpatient psychiatric treatment.

Many currently available computerized medical information systems require clinicians alter their treatment to fit a more structured approach [1-4]. Other systems focus on reducing costs rather than saving time [5]. Such software is typically not developed and altered by numerous clinicians who work daily with patients and the information system. Clinicians typically function as consultants to a non-clinician (or single clinician) software development team. Once developed such software is not usually altered except in minor ways.

Significant clinician involvement improves the functionality of a system [6, 7]. A clinician team (medical students, residents, attending physicians or nurse clinical coordinators) started the project because of their interest in improving the process of providing psychiatric care and their belief that a computer would be an essential tool. They believed that clinicians working with the software in a clinical setting and empowered to change the system would generate an even higher quality product than the above more traditional model.

Older computer technology might not have allowed true clinician based prototyping because of cost and complexity. Advances in hardware and software technology, however, allow clinicians to investigate the potential benefits of computer technology without depending on an information specialist [8, 9].

The initial clinician team identified the most burdensome and repetitive aspect of patient care: preparation of documentation. The developers attempted to replace paper-oriented tasks with a computerized approach. The team chose the latest and simplest technology (graphical word processing software running on Windows™) to improve the chances for long-term acceptability.

This project strove to develop the software incrementally over a 1 year period by allowing the users to develop the software. Clinicians completely guided and developed the system and insured the system remained focused on the needs of clinicians.

Users joined the development and altered the system to make it easier and more functional. This project can serve as model upon which information specialists can build.

METHODS

System Environment

The project used four standard PC-compatible computers incorporating 486 processors and high quality SuperVGA monitors. Each machine had Windows for Workgroups™ installed. Microsoft Word™ managed the creation of paper documents, entry of data and printing of documentation. One of the computers stored template documents and patient information files that were made available to all other computers. This computer also coordinated requests to print to a laser printer.

Work Environment

A 30 bed inpatient psychiatric unit served as the test site. The university based unit primarily treats patients with Schizophrenia, Schizoaffective and Bipolar disorders. At a given time, users of the system include two attendings, four residents, a chief resident, and six to eight medical students.

Installation

All computers arrived with Windows installed. Staff installed word processing software, upgraded Windows to the version supporting file and printer sharing, and connected the four computers together with standard coaxial cabling. A non-public room requiring a special clinician key for access housed the four computers and printer.

Development

The standard computer configuration was chosen based on the experience of the first author (TBT). Because the system would be further designed and maintained by computer novices, common and easily supported software was selected. All later decisions were made by users of the system at a given point in time (described below as members of the team).

The team changed every three months as a new set of attending and resident physicians joined the unit. Users typically had either no typing experience or minimal computer skills such as an understanding of a DOS-based word processor. The first author assumed responsibility for keeping the project focused and maintaining a common interface for all users.

The team first altered standard treatment plans to convert them to a word processor format. Over a two month interval, the team optimized the template to provide information in a more pleasing and useful format while still conforming to the purpose of the documentation. The medical records committee approved the altered treatment plan form. The team similarly altered the daily progress notes and medication reorders.

If forms required similar information, the team altered the forms to allow them to share common information. For example, "Observations" on the progress note roughly correlated to "Progress Toward Goals" on the treatment plan. "Problems" on the progress notes was identical to "Identified Problems" on the treatment plan.

The following areas fully covered the process of documenting care.

Patient name (e.g., Doe, John)
ID # - The hospital unique identification number
Demographics - Age, Marital Status, Race, Sex
(e.g., 36yo SBM)
Admission date
Legal Status (Voluntary or type of commitment)
Next date for commitment hearing

Problems
Strengths
Findings/Observations
Primary diagnosis
Assessment
Medications
Plan

Minimum discharge criteria
Planned discharge date
Follow-up arrangements (Date, Time, Clinic)
Follow-up clinician and physician

The above categories formed the framework for a simple mail-merge database. A mail-merge database is essentially a table where columns represent the data items (as above) and there is one row per patient.

The system did not interfere with the process of entering information. It did not correct data entry errors or verify data (such as checking to insure that dates were valid). The system allowed free text and did not require the data be encoded (e.g., use of a diagnostic code or clinician ID number). The development team decided that such additions would not add sufficient value to the system and would potentially lead to a more complex system requiring additional training and effort. They decided to keep the project focused on simplifying the process of documenting the provision of care.

Because the system focuses on replacing handwritten documentation, retaining information after discharge was unnecessary. The hospital chart remained the sole repository of clinical reports generated by the system. The development team rejected the possible benefit of extending the system to store information after discharge. Storing information saved only a small amount of time if a patient required readmission. The more complex design and difficulty of protecting confidentiality outweighed the potential time-savings.

The team continually updated the documentation system to improve legibility and clarity. They also continued to identify repetitive data entry and make necessary changes to the mail merge database structure and the documentation forms. The top priority remained ease of use.

Enhancement

The team investigated additional applications of the database that might improve care and reduce paperwork time commitments. A resident typically organizes him or herself by creating lists of the most significant patient information as well as *to do* lists. Creating and organizing these lists requires significant time expenditure. The clinician team produced a simple *patient information sheet* by pulling required data from the mail-merge database. The mail-merge database already included essential historical information such as problems and medications. A resident's *To do* items were best placed in the *Plan* area of the database. The new information sheet created a useful list of essential information for each patient without requiring additional effort.

An additional use of the software was identified when physicians covering the unit on a weekend mentioned a desire for more information. They noted they did not have enough information to answer some questions such as queries about discharge planning. The team created a *covering attending progress note* to address this limitation. These forms were printed Friday afternoon by the residents and detailed the problems, medications, and discharge plan. The note left space for weekend attendings to write their findings, assessment and plan. Access to essential clinical information allowed covering attendings to spend more time interviewing patients and less reviewing charts.

Deployment

In a one year period, approximately 50 clinicians on the inpatient unit used the system. All covering attendings use the weekend progress notes. Users included psychiatry residents, attending physicians, medical students, nurses and a psychology intern. Training occurred via a hands-on approach. In the later stages of the project, the head nurse (previously a novice computer user) assumed responsibility for proper training.

RESULTS

Clinicians working on the unit readily accepted the system designed above. With the exception of a one hour introduction from the head nurse, new users learned the system from experienced users. All users became proficient enough at typing to use the system.

At the end of a one year period all residents, attendings, and medical students were using the system to generate progress notes. All treatment planning documentation changed from handwritten to almost completely typewritten.

Attendings covering the unit on the weekend successfully converted from dictated or handwritten notes to the new weekend progress note system. Attendings noted a decrease in time dedicated to paperwork, and more importantly, a better understanding of patients' problems, treatments, and discharge plans.

More legible documentation has led to easier chart reviews, identification of problems and communication between treatment providers. Residents and medical students have noted that the system allows them to keep track of a greater number of problems. They also note their knowledge of the problems is more detailed. Residents who subsequently worked on inpatient units that do not use the mail-merge system have commented on the difficult readjusting to the old handwritten system. Residents note that the handwritten system wastes time by requiring them to rewrite similar information for different forms. They also mentioned an inability to maintain as full and complete of a problem list without the benefit of automation.

There have been no reports of breaches of confidentiality or inappropriate use of the computer.

DISCUSSION

We have developed a system that simplifies the process of providing and documenting patient care without creating a complicated information structure. This clinician driven system solves clinician needs based solely on clinician input.

The acceptance of the system on the part of numerous residents and attendings is a testament to the success of the system. The change in documentation from handwritten to typewritten should also be seen as a significant change.

It is difficult to quantify the impact of the new system. In the hectic inpatient environment, measurement of time spent documenting is difficult. Full evaluation of the new database system would require a control group using the old handwritten system. Clinicians are reluctant to revert to the old handwritten system - a system seen by most users as inadequate.

The successful protection of patient confidentiality is due to the placement of computers in a secure area, the limitation of the system to the generation of documentation, and the deletion of patient information after discharge.

The product of this design process has some significant weaknesses. The clinician driven system lacks error-checking, encoding, or other standard approaches to collecting data. The lack of structure makes it impossible to analyze trends or collect summary data. Nonetheless, the system has outlined the essential clinical information and defined computer-generated reports which satisfy medical record requirements.

No formal relational database is used and the system is unconnected to a more comprehensive information system. Such a system may be able to further reduce time spent documenting treatment by eliminating the need to enter data already collected elsewhere. A true client/server database is currently being developed. The database developers are building upon the success of the clinician-designed system.

CONCLUSIONS

The project demonstrates that clinicians can take the first step toward reducing paperwork, improving documentation, aiding communication and clarifying the treatment plan. This project created a system that satisfied clinicians and was enthusiastically implemented by them.

Although it is possible to wait for a better solution to come along, it is prudent to use the technology available today to improve patient care. A clinician designed system provides a template for designers of more complete medical information systems.

Clinicians with an understanding of the benefits of computerization will hold further development to a high standard. Clinicians with experience using a system designed for their purposes will be more active in the process of designing the electronic medical record. Their involvement is essential to developing a comprehensive system that actually improves the quality of medical care.

ACKNOWLEDGMENTS

Implementation and support has been provided by the unit's head nurse, Noreen Fredrick, M.S.N. The Schizophrenia Treatment and Research Center and Western Psychiatric Institute and Clinic have provided an innovative and supportive environment allowing us to test this new concept of clinician driven software development.

REFERENCES

[1]. Modai I, Rabinowitz J. Why and how to establish a computerized system for psychiatric case records. Hospital & Community Psychiatry 1993 Nov;44(11):1091-5.

[2]. Smith GC, Clarke DM, Herrman HE. Establishing a consultation-liaison psychiatry clinical database in an Australian general hospital. General Hospital Psychiatry 1993 Jul;15(4):243-53.

[3]. Weiss KM, Chapman HA. A computer-assisted inpatient psychiatric assessment and treatment planning system. Hospital & Community Psychiatry 1993 Nov;44(11):1097-100.

[4]. Rabinowitz J, Modai I, Valevski A, Zemishlany Z, Mark M. Benefits of a structured format for paper and computerized psychiatric case records. Hospital & Community Psychiatry 1993 Nov;44(11):1095-7.

[5]. Tierney WM, Miller ME, Overhage JM, McDonald CJ. Physician inpatient order writing on microcomputer workstations. Effects on resource utilization.. JAMA 1993 Jan 20;269(3):379-83.

[6]. Siders AM, Peterson M. Increasing Patient Satisfaction and Nursing Productivity Through Implementation of an Automated Nursing Discharge Summary. Fifteenth Annual Symposium on Computer Applications in Medical Care. 1991: 136-140.

[7]. McKinnie DB. Design and Implementation of a Microcomputer Based Student Health Center System. Fourteenth Annual Symposium on Computer Applications in Medical Care. 1990: 849-853.

[8]. Hausam RR, Klimczak JC, Hahn AW. Computerized medical records--new opportunities. Missouri Medicine 1993 Nov; 90(11):705-6.

[9]. Hausam RR, Balas EA. Computerized medical records. Dream or reality?. Missouri Medicine 1993 Oct; 90(10):649-52.

The author can be reached via the internet at Tanner+@pitt.edu

Implementing a Physician's Workstation using Client/Server Technology and the Distributed Computing Environment

Thuan Q. Pham, M.S.[1], Charles Y. Young, Ph.D.[1], Paul C. Tang, M.D.[2], Henri J. Suermondt, Ph.D.[1], Jurgen Annevelink, Ph.D.[1]

[1]Hewlett-Packard Laboratories, Palo Alto, CA
[2]Northwestern Memorial Hospital, Chicago, IL

Abstract

PWS is a physician's workstation research prototype developed to explore the use of information management tools by physicians in the context of patient care. The original prototype was implemented in a client/server architecture using a broadcast message server. As we expanded the scope of the prototyping activities, we identified the limitations of the broadcast message server in the areas of scalability, security, and interoperability. To address these issues, we reimplemented PWS using the Open Software Foundation's Distributed Computing Environment (DCE). We describe the rationale for using DCE, the migration process, and the benefits achieved. Future work and recommendations are discussed.

INTRODUCTION

The objective of the Physician's Workstation (PWS) project [1] is to investigate and develop a comprehensive and highly integrated set of information management tools for use by physicians in ambulatory care. We successfully developed and deployed an experimental prototype using an open systems architecture [2] based on HP's broadcast message server (BMS) [3]. Although the prototype works well in the context of a small work group, it has several limitations due to the characteristics of the BMS framework: scalability is limited due to the narrow bandwidth of the BMS; security is limited; and interoperability is limited to only a few hardware platforms. To overcome these limitations, we redesigned and reimplemented PWS's distributed computing framework using the Distributed Computing Environment (DCE) [4] from the Open Software Foundation (OSF).

This paper describes the design and implementation of the new PWS prototype. In particular, we illustrate our leveraging of DCE's technologies and services to make PWS a more scalable, secure, robust, and open distributed application.

In the following sections, we first describe the original architecture of PWS and discuss its limitations with respect to scalability, security, and interoperability. We then present the new client/server architecture and DCE-based implementation which overcome those limitations. Finally, we conclude with a vision of future work with regard to the emerging distributed computing technologies.

BACKGROUND: ORIGINAL PWS ARCHITECTURE

The original PWS architecture, illustrated in Figure 1, uses a message server as a backbone for both communication and data integration. The strength of this architecture is that, using the simple string-based message protocol, new applications could be developed independently and integrated easily into the PWS environment. As a result, the original prototype achieved the desirable openness and integration among application components.

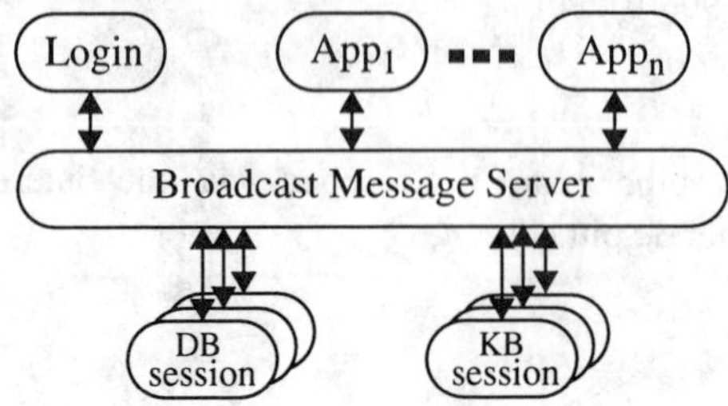

Figure 1: Original architecture of PWS that relies on BMS for communication and integration.

However, the architecture's total dependence on the broadcast message server has some undesirable consequences. Due to the limited capabilities of the BMS, the prototype lacked the scalability, security, and hardware interoperability needed for robust distributed applications. We address these issues in the following subsections.

Scalability

The scalability limitation of the original prototype is a result of the total reliance on the BMS as an all-purpose software bus for sending both control messages and large chunks of patient data among applications. All software components of PWS are dependent on one message server for all message distribution and data exchange. As more and more applications or sessions come on-line, the message server quickly becomes the bottleneck that degrades performance.

Security

The BMS environment does not provide any security services. Without a security service, an application cannot verify the identity or trust the intention of other applications. There is no provision in the BMS environment to prevent unauthorized users from receiving data that are placed on the bus, since anyone can subscribe to, receive, and monitor any and all bus traffic.

Furthermore, BMS messages are broadcast in plain text. Data encryption is needed, but it requires a security service component to authenticate and/or broker the encryption keys. Although it could be possible to implement a BMS-based security service, such effort would require a significant amount of work and would likely result in a non-standard implementation.

Interoperability

Currently, all PWS applications run on one hardware platform. To deploy the system on a much larger scale, PWS components will have to operate on a variety of hardware platforms, many of which may not support BMS.

NEW PWS ARCHITECTURE

Applications in the BMS environment can take on a client or server role in their behavior, but strictly speaking, these applications are peers that communicate by broadcasting on the BMS. From our experience in using PWS, we observe that most messages are one-to-one communications or data exchanges between two components. A more effective architecture would allow application components to communicate directly with each other, while using the message server to broadcast important events and shared information.

Thus, the fundamental goals of our new PWS architecture are to: use client/server technology to facilitate the direct communication between program components, use the event service mechanism for global control and event notification, and leverage DCE services to make PWS a robust, scalable, and secure distributed application.

What is DCE?

Developed by the Open Software Foundation (OSF), DCE is a framework and environment for building distributed applications in a heterogeneous computing environment. DCE provides both a development and a runtime environment for distributed applications. This includes the interface definition language (IDL) and compiler, remote procedure calls (RPC) [5,6], threads, directory and security services, distributed file system (DFS), distributed time service (DTS), and an application programming interface (API).

Why DCE?

The move to DCE enables us to leverage its distributed computing services and infrastructure to build robust distributed applications. For example, DCE's IDL allows us to define the interface between client and server applications; RPC makes a remote server's service appears like a local procedure call, greatly simplify networking; directory, timing, and security services are essential to any distributed system; and the emerging DCE standard and compliance ensure interoperability across many hardware platforms, ranging from workstations to personal computers.

PWS Client/Server Architecture

Figure 2 illustrates the new architecture of PWS, in which each application is either a client, a server, or both (since a server application can be a client of another). The interactions between programs are mostly in the form of a client invoking a service of a remote server using an RPC.

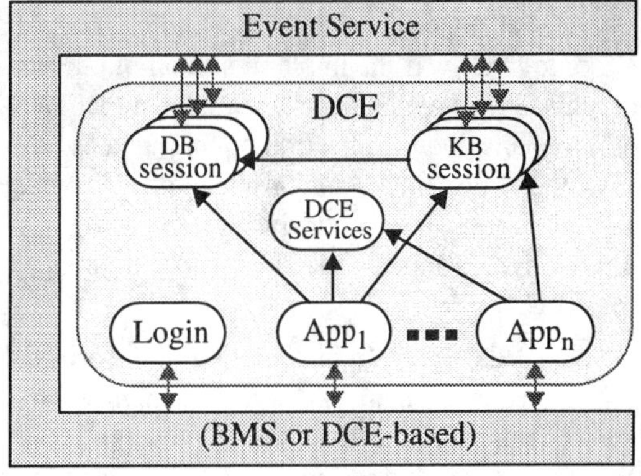

Figure 2: DCE-based client/server architecture of PWS

With RPC facilitating the direct data exchange between client and server applications, the event service is used effectively to handle control messages, such as broadcasting shared states and event notifications. For example, when a user logs in to PWS, the *Login* application creates a database session server, and broadcasts the server's full path name in the DCE environment to all interested application components. Using this name, applications can go to the DCE's cell directory service (CDS) to find and establish their own direct connections to the server. With a much lighter work load, the event service now has sufficient processing capacity to handle many more processes.

IMPLEMENTATION

Interface Definition

The first step in our implementation was to identify operations to be supported by server applications. From these, we defined the server interface using the IDL. The IDL compiler then generated the stub code for client and server modules. These stubs, when linked into the respective programs, enabled server and client applications to communicate with each other using the defined interface and RPC.

Server Implementation

To implement the server applications, we first implemented the server functionality as defined in the interface. Then, we wrote the server initialization and clean up routines so that the servers properly registered and unregistered themselves with DCE directory service. In addition, we set up an exception handling mechanism in each server so that it could remove itself from the DCE environment should an exception occur.

Client Implementation

The step that required the most work in our port of PWS onto DCE was the implementation of client programs. There are many applications in the PWS prototype, and each application communicates with many others. For each client application, we replaced an asynchronous, interrupt-driven program logic with a simpler synchronous, procedural program logic, using RPC.

In other words, to obtain information in the original architecture, each client application asynchronously posted one or more messages to the message server. When some other component provided an answer, the client application received the message from the message server, matched it with the originating request, and called some predefined functions to process the result. In the new architecture, most communications are point-to-point between the client and server components, in the form of (synchronous) remote procedure calls. With RPC, the results are available immediately when the call completes, removing the complexity of matching results with requests in the asynchronous mode of communication.

In addition, we enhanced our client applications by using multiple threads to implement parallel control. The use of threads in conjunction with RPC is significant because threads allow client applications to execute many RPC calls independently and concurrently. Hence, if an RPC call running in one client application thread is waiting for a server to produce the result, other threads in the client application can still proceed with their execution. Furthermore, by dispatching threads to carry out a user's requests, the main application thread is always under the user's control, thereby increasing the application's responsiveness.

For example, two of the most lengthy operations in PWS are the queries of a patient's detailed history of problems and medications, which involve the database server. When the provider first selects a patient to review, the display application must fetch patient information from the database while performing other tasks. To improve performance, we devised two job queue data structures, DxQueue and RxQueue, and assigned each queue to be processed by a thread. When the display application needs to fetch a patient's drug information or diagnosis, it simply places the query statements in the respective queue, and continues to handle more user requests. Meanwhile, for each query placed in the queue, the thread managing the job queue makes an RPC to get the results from the database.

Encapsulation of Non-DCE Components

In a new system, there may be a need to integrate legacy components. For this, DCE servers can be used to interface DCE components with non-DCE components. For example, the DCE/DB interface component in Figure 3 is actually a DCE server process that handles requests for data from a non-DCE database.

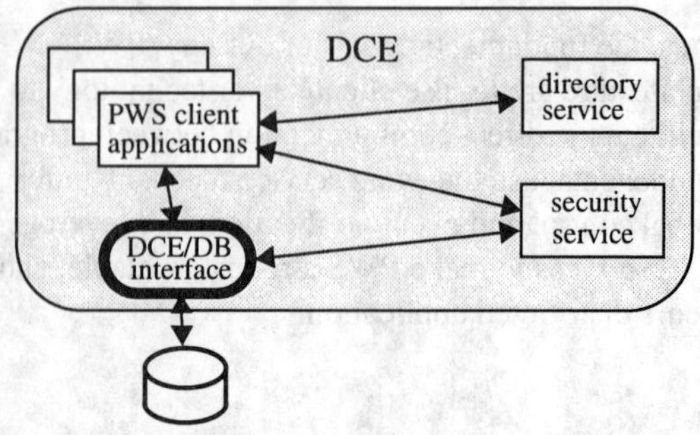

Figure 3: interfacing with non-DCE components

In our current implementation, we use a DCE server process as an interface to an object oriented database. When the DCE/DB interface server receives an RPC requesting information from a client, it queries the database. The query results are then returned to the calling process via an RPC return argument. Interface components such as this enables the integration and continued support of legacy systems.

DISCUSSION

The benefits of our migration to DCE are numerous. First of all, the new prototype is more scalable and robust. By allowing application programs to interact with one another directly, we removed the bottleneck from the broadcast message architecture. By using RPC to transmit data between client and servers, we achieved better efficiency and data privacy. By using the DCE directory service and RPC facility, we allowed client applications to interact with server applications without having to know their dynamic physical location in a distributed environment, and without having to handle the complex networking details. With DCE's RPC and services, accessing a server process running across the country was no more difficult than accessing one running on a local machine.

Furthermore, once ported, PWS applications immediately benefited from the security mechanism provided by DCE. These benefits include authentication, access control, and encryption.

The move to DCE also presented some challenges. First and foremost, the DCE environment requires system administration skills much like that of a Unix workstation (e.g., add new user account and security credential, setup user profile, etc.). The current lack of DCE system administration tools continues to make this task tedious and laborious.

In addition, DCE server processes are usually several megabytes in size and require much computing resources to run with adequate performance. In every DCE environment, there is an overhead of computing resources to run the essential DCE services such as security service, directory service, distributed time service, and various other essential DCE daemons.

DCE is a large and complex system. The DCE's architecture, facilities, capabilities, and application programming interface (which includes over several hundred functions) required some time to master.

To port an existing application to DCE, a change in the program's design is sometimes necessary. This is particularly true for applications that use asynchronous communication. Although RPC alleviates the problem of matching replies with requests, it is a synchronous communication protocol. Used serially, RPC takes away the program's ability to perform other work while the request is being processed by some server. This is unnecessarily restrictive and inefficient. Thus, to use RPC and still preserve the efficiency of asynchronous programs, we needed to redesign programs to use a combination of threads and RPC. In effect, we had to write multithreaded programs.

Lastly, although DCE is being accepted by more and more companies as the platform to implement open, distributed heterogeneous computing [7], its technology is still young. Early commercial implementations of DCE may still be a bit unstable and inefficient.

FUTURE EXTENSIONS

During the development of this PWS prototype, we identified a number of potential areas for further investigation.

Reduced Development Cost

Although building a robust DCE application is a complex job, the task is highly repetitive, and template driven. For example, a DCE server basically needs some initialization routines, clean-up routines, exception handling threads, and access control mechanism. After developing the first robust server, the task of implementing the basic structure of additional servers became routine.

OODCE [8], a C++ class library that encapsulates many DCE facilities, has been developed. This library offers much promise in reducing development cost and time. For example, an OODCE's server class object includes a full implementation of an exception handler, an access control list (ACL) manager, and some value-added facilities such as an object factory and activation mechanism. We would like to employ OODCE to help improve any future development.

Improved Fault-tolerance

As the system scales up to handle more and more processes, the reliance on a single message server creates a single point of failure. To address this, we can replace the message server with a hierarchy of DCE-based event services, which can be replicated to improve fault tolerance. Furthermore, such a DCE-based event service mechanism can interoperate with client programs from all DCE environments, making the system even more open.

Object Interoperability

The objects and distributed computing community is currently proposing a distributed object model that provides interoperability between different software platforms. For example, with such a model, an object in a Smalltalk application can interact with another object in a C++ application.

Specifically, the object model being adopted by the industry is the Common Object Request Broker Architecture (CORBA) [9,10] by the Object Management Group (OMG). To this extent, we ported a database interface component from DCE IDL to CORBAL IDL, and ported an application component, the drug formulation browser, of PWS to access the drug formulation server using the CORBA model. This work begins to establish a migration path from DCE to CORBA should we need to migrate in the future.

SUMMARY

We started this paper with a description of the original PWS architecture which relied on the asynchronous, broadcast message server as an integration framework for both interprocess communication and data exchange. In the discussion, we enumerated the architectural limitations that were learned through our use of PWS.

To overcome the limitations of the original architecture, we presented a new PWS design. The new architecture combines an efficient mix of synchronous, point-to-point client/server communication for data exchange, and asynchronous, broadcast messaging for event notification and operational synchronization. By using each communication model for its strength, the new PWS prototype is more efficient and scalable.

The scalability, security, and interoperability of a distributed application depend not only on the architecture, but also on the framework on which it is implemented. Using DCE, the new PWS prototype is able to leverage the distributed system technologies and services to achieve these properties.

ACKNOWLEDGMENTS

We would like to thank our colleagues Mike Higgins, Mark Gisi, Danielle Fafchamps, Phil Strong, Philippe De Smedt, and the reviewers for their insightful comments on previous drafts of this paper.

References

[1] P.C. Tang, J. Annevelink, D. Fafchamps, W.M. Stanton, and C.Y. Young. Physician's Workstations: Integrated Information Management for Clinicians. In: P. Clayton, ed., Proceedings of the Fifteenth Annual Symposium on Computer Applications in Medical Care. McGraw-Hill, New York, 1991, pp. 569-573.

[2] C.Y. Young, P.C. Tang, and J. Annevelink. An Open Systems Architecture for Development of a Physician's Workstation. In: P. Clayton, ed., Proceedings of the Fifteenth Annual Symposium on Computer Applications in Medical Care. McGraw-Hill, New York, 1991, pp. 491-495.

[3] M. Cagan. The HP Softbench Environment: an Architecture for a New Generation of Software Tools. Hewlett-Packard Journal, June 1990, pp. 36-47.

[4] OSF DCE Application Development Reference, Open Software Foundation, Revision 1.0, Prentice-Hall, Englewood Cliffs, New Jersey, 1993.

[5] B.J. Nelson. Remote Procedure Call. Technical Report CSL-81-9, Xerox Palo Also Research Center, 1981.

[6] A. Birrell and B.J. Nelson. Implementing Remote Procedure Calls. Technical Report CSL-83-7, Xerox Palo Also Research Center, 1983.

[7] Mary Hubley. Achieving Interoperability. Datapro Information Services Group. CW Custom Publications, Framingham, MA, 1994.

[8] John Dilley. Object-Oriented Distributed Computing with C++ and OSF DCE. International Workshop in DCE, October, 1993.

[9] Object Management Group. Common Object Request Broker Architecture and Specification. Document Number 91.12.1, Revision 1.1, 1991.

[10] Digital Equipment Corporation, Hewlett-Packard Company, Hyperdesk Corporation, International Business Machines Corporation, NEC Corporation, and Open Software foundation. Joint Submission on Interoperability and Initialization. OMG TC Document 94-3-5, March, 1994.

Adoption of Information Technology Enabled Innovations by Primary Care Physicians: Model and Questionnaire Development

David R. Dixon[1], MD and Bradley J. Dixon[2], MBA
[1]Faculty of Medicine - Department of Family Medicine; [2]Western Business School
University of Western Ontario, London, Ontario, Canada
[1]D4Dixon@WBS.Business.UWO.CA

A survey instrument was developed based on a model of the substantive factors influencing the adoption of Information Technology (IT) enabled innovations by physicians. The survey was given to all faculty and residents in a Primary Care teaching institution. Computerized literature searching was the IT innovation studied. The results support the role of the perceived ease of use and the perceived usefulness of an innovation as well as the intent to use an innovation as factors important for implementation. The model and survey instruments developed show significant potential to enhance our understanding of the process of implementing IT innovations such that Physicians will adopt them.

INTRODUCTION

Computers are information management tools that can allow a physician to more efficiently manage information from a patient's chart and additional resources. Information technology (IT) also allows a means to easily manipulate information for other uses, such as preventive care and patient education. There are many other ways that IT can enable innovations in the use of information in providing health care.

An American study [1] found possible benefits to hospitals from increased utilization of computers include increased quality of care, decreased transcription errors, decreased reliance on clerical staff, and the possibility of attracting new physicians to hospitals. In one hospital, when a computerized pharmacy reminder system was introduced, they found medication changes were implemented 20 hours sooner than with a traditional paper-based system [2]. Currently there is a low utilization of information systems by physicians [1], although a 1988 study of family (primary care) physicians [3] found that 45% had computers in their office with 17% maintaining partial medical records and 2% maintaining full records on an information system. It is predicted that by the year 2000, 75% of hospitals will have computerized patient lists and facesheets, and 35% will have fully computerized documentation [1]. Unless physicians are willing and prepared to use information technology, it will be difficult to realize these benefits.

Research has been performed investigating the factors affecting individuals' use of innovations, including IT enabled innovations[4], [5]. Some key factors identified are the perceived usefulness of an innovation, as well as the perception of how easy it is to use [6]. Perceived usefulness refers to the perceptions of how useful a skill or technology would be to that person [7], [8]. This can be either a concrete or abstract benefit, or a way to avoid negative outcomes. Perceived ease of use refers to the perceptions of how much effort is involved in learning new skills and putting those new skills to use. The Technological Acceptance Model (TAM) developed by Davis [6], [7] found that perceived usefulness and, to a lesser extent, perceived ease of use both affected a person's attitude to adoption of an IT enabled innovation. The person's attitude leads to behavioral intentions, which in turn lead to actual behavior, such as computer use.

In a self-report survey [11], Smith and Zastrow found that physicians viewing computers as easier to use or more useful were more likely to favour adoption. In another study [12], it was found that computer systems providing value to physicians will have greater utilization. A case study of computerized ambulatory care records performed in the early 1990s [13] found that clinic staff accepted the information technology. They also noted that physician acceptance of the system increased with increased ease of use.

Recent research [9], [10] has found that a person's sophistication will also affect his or her choice to adopt a new technology. End-User Sophistication (EUS) is a measure of how many areas of knowledge a person has, the amount of knowledge in each area, and how well they can apply their knowledge. These characteristics are known, respectively, as breadth, depth, and finesse. It was found that if the fit between the individual's sophistication and the capabilities required by the innovation matched, the individual was likely to have success in adopting the innovation [9], [10].

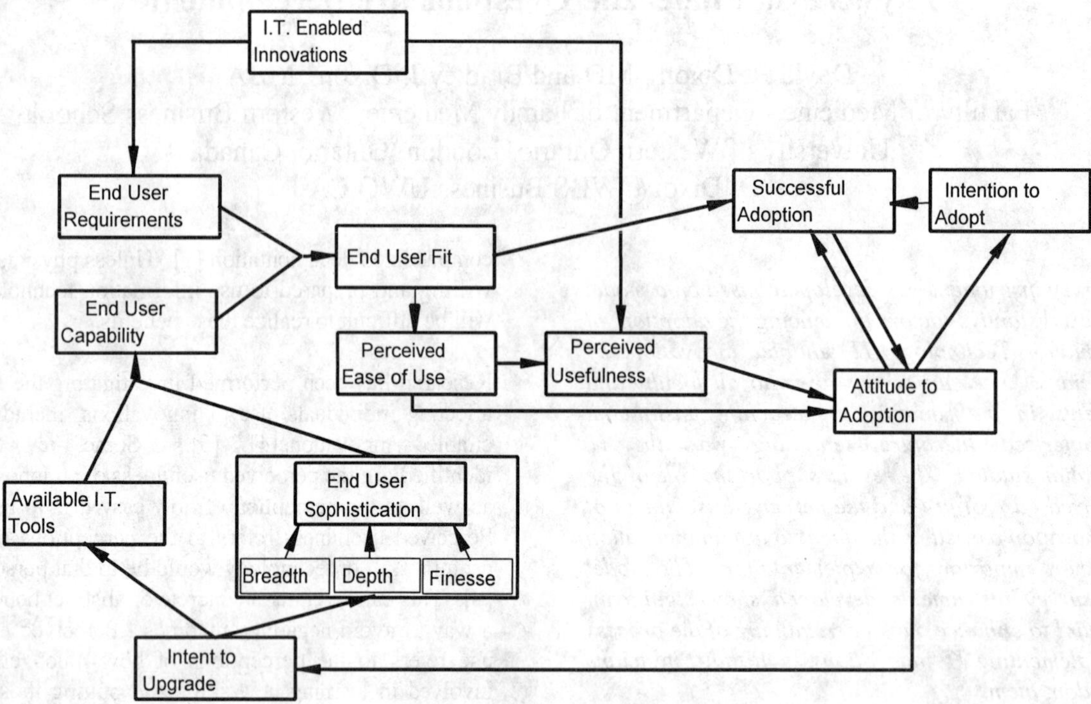

Figure 1: Proposed Model for the Adoption of Information Technology (IT) Enabled Innovations

Building upon the TAM and the EUS research, figure 1 shows the model developed. Each IT enabled innovation, for example a computer application like on-line literature searching, provides benefits and requires resources. The benefits influence the perceived usefulness, while the resources required determines the end user requirements. The end user requirements include the skills and competencies as well as the IT tools needed by the user to use the innovation. The tools and the skills of the user define the user's capabilities. The capabilities, when compared to the requirements determine the fit. If the requirements exceed the capabilities, there will be a decrease in the perceived ease of use of the innovation. As the deficit of a user's capabilities compared to requirements decreases, the fit increases as does the perception that the innovation is easier to use. Perceived usefulness is affected by the perceived ease of use and the characteristics of the innovation. These characteristics are both internal and external to the innovation. Internal factors include the task performed, effort required, and information provided. External factors involve pressures or requirements to adopt, benefits such as promotion or job security gained from adopting, and personal satisfaction.

Both perceived ease of use and perceived usefulness will influence the attitude towards adoption; The more the innovation is perceived as useful and easy to use the attitude towards innovations becomes more favourable. With a positive attitude, an intention is formed to either adopt the innovation or upgrade the skills or tools needed to allow the adoption of the innovation. If the innovation is adopted, success will be enhanced both by a good end user fit, as well as a positive attitude. Successful adoption will also enhance the attitude towards further adoption or upgrading.

End user sophistication is determined by a person's breadth and depth of knowledge as well as their finesse at using that knowledge. Their sophistication can be increased by education, training, and practical experience. Increased sophistication will increase the user's capabilities and ultimately the user's success.

This study was undertaken to develop a survey instrument to test the hypotheses underlying the model presented in Figure 1. We focussed on three hypotheses: 1) perceived usefulness is directly related to favourable intentions to adopt or upgrade skills, 2) perceived ease of use is directly related to favourable intentions, and 3) end user fit is directly related to favourable intentions. The innovation used to test this model was Computerized Literature Searching.

METHODS

The instrument was developed using questions from several sources. Attitude questions were modified from a scale developed for clinical psychologists [14]. Perceived ease of use and usefulness questions were generated from guidelines found to yield reliable questions [15]. Sophistication was measured across many areas that a family physicians may be exposed to in a standard practice setting. These questions were developed based on Marcolin et al. [9], [10]. Intent questions were created specifically for this questionnaire. Questions were constructed for both computerized literature searching and computers in general. Demographic information was also acquired.

Knowledge endpoints on the scales were defined as novice and expert. Novice "indicates that the person can perform basic functions, but require assistance to perform more advanced functions." Expert "indicates that the practitioner is skilled in basic and advanced functions and is able to provide assistance while uncommonly requiring assistance themselves." To ask about expected knowledge, the respondent was asked to "indicate the level of knowledge that you feel an average general or family practitioner should attempt to acquire in the next few years to most effectively practice medicine." Usage was scaled as yearly, monthly, weekly, more than once per week, daily, and more than once per day. There were no definitions given for the computer applications, although examples of common programs were provided. The survey instrument also contains items addressing a number of different types of IT applications. A copy of the survey instrument is available from the authors.

The survey was directed to residents and full time physician faculty members in the Department of Family Medicine at the University of Western Ontario. All nineteen faculty members and all 69 residents in the family medical centres from January 1993 to August 1993 were surveyed.

RESULTS

There was a response rate of 95% (18/19) for full time physicians on faculty and 84% (58/69) of residents. The total response rate was 86% (76/88). One faculty member and two residents declined to complete the questionnaire. No response was received from the remaining nine residents.

As a measure of scale reliability, Cronbach's alphas were calculated for all scales, and are summarized in Table 1. A scale was judged to have sufficient internal reliability for continued investigation if its reliability coefficient (alpha) was greater than 0.70. Only the attitude scale did not meet these criteria.

Scale Description	Alpha
Attitudes	.68
Perceived Ease of Use - Computers	.83
Perceived Usefulness - Computers	.92
Intent - Computers	.76
Perceived Ease of Use - Lit Search	.76
Perceived Usefulness - Lit Search	.91
Intent - Lit Search	.76
Finesse	.94

Table 1: Scales and reliability coefficients for the instrument.

Figure 2 shows use and knowledge of computerized literature searching. Faculty and residents rated their usage (from yearly (1) to more than once per day (6)) and knowledge (from none (0), and novice (1) to expert (7)). Usage and knowledge, both current and expected were not significantly different between faculty and residents. Faculty showed slightly more usage and knowledge of literature searching systems than residents.

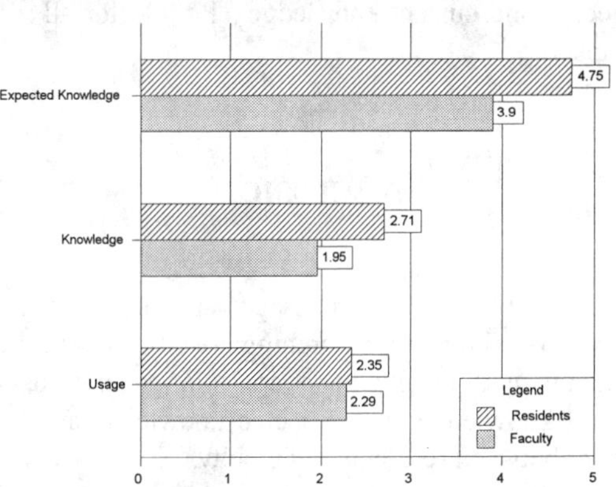

Figure 2: Physician knowledge and usage of computerized literature searching. Usage shown is yearly (1) to more than once per day (6). Knowledge is novice (1) to expert (7).

Figure 3 compares current and expected knowledge of computerized literature searching. The knowledge gap is the difference between what people currently know and what they believe they need to know, their capabilities and requirements respectively. The knowledge gap represents the non-technological component of end-user fit. There is a clear knowledge gap expressed by both residents and faculty with respect to computerized literature searching (p<.000).

Correlations were calculated between the knowledge gap and usefulness, showing significant positive correlations for computerized literature searching (r=.41, p<.001). There was no significant correlation found between knowledge gap and perceived ease of use (r=-.09). Intentions of adopting computerized literature searching were significantly correlated with perceived usefulness (r=.26, p<.05) and perceived ease of use (r=.32, p<.01).

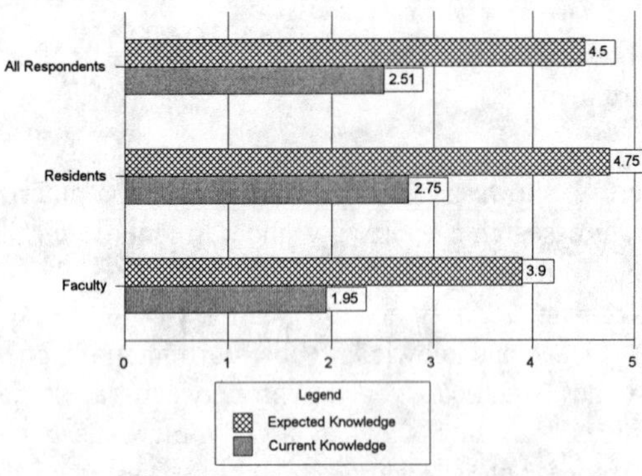

Figure 3: Knowledge gap for computerized literature searching - the difference between expected and current knowledge. P<.000 for all groups.

DISCUSSION

It is notable that both usage and knowledge of computerized literature searching are quite low for both residents and faculty members. In general, usage, current knowledge, and expected knowledge are quite similar between residents and faculty.

The most striking differences are seen in Figure 3. This shows the knowledge gap that currently exists. Faculty and residents feel they need more knowledge about computerized literature searching than they currently have. As expected, the knowledge gap was strongly correlated to the perceived usefulness of literature searching. Computerized literature searching appears to be an ideal area to focus on implementation at present. There is a significant knowledge gap identified by both faculty and residents, and computerized literature searching is readily available, and relatively easy to use. Also, many physicians have had occasion to use paper-based literature searching facilities, which require much of the same knowledge. Eventually, this gap will decrease with successful implementation and other innovations will be the focus of our research.

The model presented in Figure 1 is generally supported by the results from this study. It is unclear why the knowledge gap did not correlate with the measures for perceived ease of use, although it was correlated with perceived usefulness. Possibly, end user fit acts directly on perceived usefulness. The small sample size precludes the use of advanced statistical techniques like structural modelling (e.g., LISREL) needed to adequately test this model. Another limitation of the current research is the use of self-report measures of usage. Methods to objectively capture use were not available, but are being developed.

The contribution of this model to Medical Informatics research is to develop tools to provide insight into the implementation of IT innovations, specifically how to entice physicians to use computers. From figure 1, the key areas are perceived usefulness, perceived ease of use, and sophistication. Sophistication is build partially by experience, and partially by education. Perceived usefulness is affected by education as to the costs and benefits of a computer innovation, sophistication, and the persons own needs. Perceived ease of use is affected by a person's capabilities, which is related to their sophistication, and the tools available to them. As people gain experience, their sophistication should increase, leading to an increased perception of the ease of using other related innovations. Education can increase both a person's sophistication and their perceptions of the usefulness of a new program, leading to a more successful adoption. Also, by adding rewards or requiring behaviours, the usefulness of an innovation will increase to gain the reward or satisfy the requirements.

Future Research Directions

As this survey is further validated and refined, it can be sent to community physicians to allow a rational development of continuing medical education programs and computer resources to facilitate the implementation of information technology in physicians' offices. This survey can also be used to examine the needs of undergraduate medical students. It may provide a basis for integrating computer instruction in the undergraduate curriculum and training in the Department of Family Medicine.

The underlying causal relationships in the model are better explored using a longitudinal research design. Using these scales as pre- and post- intervention measures during an IT implementation will provide a significant opportunity to test the model's hypotheses further. The similarity of our results obtained in a medical setting to the results obtained in Management Information Systems research, where the components of this model have been drawn from, provide the support to pursue our research agenda further.

The role of IT in health care is increasing dramatically, and understanding how physicians develop their attitudes towards IT is critical to successful implementations. We believe that this survey instrument, and the model upon which it is based, is a useful tool to gain insight about implementing IT innovations.

References

[1]. Remmlinger E, Grossman M. Physician Utilization of Information Systems: Bridging the Gap Between Expectations and Reality. In: Proceedings of the 1992 Annual HIMSS Conference. Chicago: Healthcare Information and Management Systems Society, AHA, 1991:119-123.

[2]. Rind DM, Safran C, Phillips RS, et al. The Effect of Computer-Based Reminders on the Management of Hospitalized Patients with Worsening Renal Function. SCAMC 1991; 28-32.

[3]. Schmittling GT. Computer use by family physicians in the United States. Journal of Family Practice 1989; 29:198-200.

[4]. Mathieson K. Predicting User Intentions: Comparing the Technology Acceptance Model with the Theory of Planned Behavior. Information Systems Research 1991; 2(3):173-191.

[5]. Goldman L. Changing Physicians' Behavior: The Pot and the Kettle. NEJM 1990; 322(21):1524-1525.

[6]. Davis FD, Bagozzi RP, Warshaw PR. User Acceptance of Computer Technology: A Comparison of Two Theoretical Models. Management Science 1989; 35(8):982-1001.

[7]. Louie B, Reid R. Building a Decision-Support System. Leadership 1992; May/June:18-23.

[8]. Davis FD. Perceived Usefulness, Perceived Ease of Use, and User Acceptance of Information Technology. MIS Quarterly 1989; September:318-340.

[9]. Marcolin B, Huff SL, Munro MC. End User Sophistication: Measurement and Research Model. ASAC 1992; 108-120.

[10]. Marcolin BL, Huff SL, Compeau DR, Munro MC. End User Sophistication: A Multitrait-Multimethod Analysis. ASAC 1993; 110-121.

[11]. Smith WR, Zastrow R. What are the Sources of Physician Resistance to Adoption of the Computerized Patient Record [poster]. SCAMC 1993; 17:906-906.

[12]. Clayton PD, Pulver GE, Hill CL. Physician Use of Computers: Is Age or Value the Predominant Factor. SCAMC 1993; 17:301-305.

[13]. O'Dell DV, Tape TG, Campbell JR. Increasing Physician Acceptance and Use of the Computerized Ambulatory Medical Record. SCAMC 1991; 848-852.

[14]. Farrell AD, Cuseo-Ott L, Fenerty M. Development and Evaluation of a Scale for Measuring Practitioners' Attitudes Toward Computer Applications. Computers in Human Behavior 1988; 4:207-220.

[15]. Moore GC, Benbasat I. Development of an Instrument to Measure the Perceptions of Adopting an Information Technology Innovation. Information Systems Research 1991; 2(3):192-222.

User Comments on a Clinical Event Monitor

George Hripcsak, Paul D. Clayton
Columbia-Presbyterian Medical Center

Columbia-Presbyterian Medical Center's health care providers have access to alerts and interpretations generated by an Arden Syntax-based clinical event monitor. They have the opportunity to send comments to the clinical information services staff. Over a period of 26 months, they sent 126 comments. The comments were analyzed using the critical incident technique, resulting in a hierarchy of categories that summarizes user concerns. The majority of comments (65) indicated that the messages were actually (8) or at least potentially useful (57). A minority (28) indicated that they were unhelpful (27) or actually harmful (1). Another group (27) made suggestions or asked questions. The comments have been very helpful for the maintenance of Medical Logic Modules (MLMs) and the clinical event monitor itself.

INTRODUCTION

Clinical event monitors, reminder systems, and other forms of automated decision-support systems are experiencing increasing visibility, trust, and use [1]. Such systems improve provider compliance with accepted guidelines [2-4], but response is generally less than 100%, and often as low as 20 to 40%. Finding out what causes health care providers not to follow a guideline is critical to improving event monitors and the guidelines that they implement. Potential causes include: incorrect, outdated, or controversial guidelines; incorrect guideline implementation; confusing, inappropriate, or untimely presentation; extenuating or unusual patient circumstances; etc.

Questionnaires have been used to ascertain the attitude of providers toward automated decision-support systems. Rind and co-authors mailed questionnaires to 622 physicians who had received computer-generated reminders [5]. They reported that 53% of respondents (of 288 who offered an opinion) found the reminders helpful, and 31% (of 312) found the reminders annoying; respondents also judged the appropriateness of reminder criteria. Teach and Shortliffe used questionnaires to assess physicians' general attitudes toward automated decision-support systems [6]. Henderson and co-authors compared providers' compliance with "correct" versus "incorrect" computer-generated instructions and with active versus passive instructions [7]. Other groups have analyzed physicians' assessment of computer-generated consultation advice [8-9].

We took a more open-ended approach. Health care providers at Columbia-Presbyterian Medical Center (CPMC) have access to computer-generated alerts and interpretations on their patients [10]. We set out to obtain feedback (in the form of electronic comments) from providers about the alerts and interpretations, in whatever form and on whatever aspect the provider desired. The goal was to obtain information about what concerned the providers, without biasing their responses with our preconceptions. We then used the critical incident technique [11] to organize their responses into a logical framework. The technique has been used in other contexts, including the analysis of the use of MEDLINE for clinical problem solving [12].

METHODS

CPMC provides automated decision-support through its clinical event monitor [10], which is based upon the Arden Syntax for Medical Logic Modules [13]. Clinical events in the medical center (e.g., admissions, laboratory results) trigger pertinent rules called Medical Logic Modules (MLMs). Each MLM reads data from the clinical database, evaluates medical criteria, and, if appropriate, generates a message. Alert messages warn of emergent situations. For example, one MLM warns of new or worsening renal insufficiency. Alerts are presented to providers when they sign onto the clinical information system to review a patient's data. Interpretation messages convey passive information. For example, one MLM calculates the creatinine clearance from blood and urine laboratory values. Interpretations are presented with their corresponding data values.

During the study, providers reviewed messages on screens like the one in Figure 1. If they wanted to send a comment, they pressed the F6 key. They were then presented with a comment screen, which instructed them to:

> Enter your comments about the computer-generated message, and press F3 when you are finished. They will be forwarded to Clinical Information Services.

The comments were forwarded to the Clinical Information Services staff and logged. Comments were collected from the time the system was turned on for clinical care (March, 1992) to the present (May, 1994).

Comments were analyzed using the critical incident technique [11]. This technique has been used to determine the reasons for success or failure of a process involving human beings, based upon narrative answers to open-ended questions. By categorizing the answers, the technique produces a framework from which one can better grasp the issues involved. In this study, we used the open-ended request on the comment screen (quoted above).

Comments were analyzed one by one. Comments that addressed similar issues were grouped into categories and given descriptive phrases. As each new comment was reviewed, it was placed into an existing category, or a new category was created for it. Occasionally, the descriptive phrase was altered slightly to accommodate a new comment. Categories themselves were grouped into higher level categories, thus creating a hierarchy. Whenever a category was added or changed, the number of comments analyzed so far was recorded. These data were later used to assess the reliability of the categories. Comments were ordered randomly to avoid biasing the category definitions due to temporal trends.

RESULTS

From March, 1992 to May, 1994, an average of 20 alert messages were generated per day. Interpretations did not begin until March, 1993; after that, 2000 interpretation messages were generated per day. MLMs were based upon laboratory results, demographics, admit-discharge-transfer data, and discharge diagnoses.

A total of 126 comments were collected during the study period from physicians (97), nurses (19), and medical students (10). The comments were instigated by both alerts (77) and interpretations (49). Comments addressed the computer-generated messages themselves, patient status, and decision-support systems in general. Only 0.5% of alerts led to comments, although they were more numerous when the system was first turned on (2%). Even fewer (0.01%) interpretations led to comments; this is not surprising, since interpretations are passive whereas alerts are active.

The categories generated by the analysis are shown in Table 1. The comments in category 1 indicated that MLMs are at least potentially useful. All eight reports of benefit (1a) involved detection of a missed laboratory abnormality, with a consequent early work up or change in plan. No comment provided proof that a patient outcome was actually improved due to the message. Nevertheless, one comment reported the early placement of a ureteral stint in the setting of acute urinary obstruction; what would have happened if the message had not been sent or if the stint had not been placed as quickly remains unclear. Comments in category 1b focused more on the patient than on the message itself (e.g., "The patient's potassium was repleted. Thank you."). They indicated that the MLMs' advice was appropriate but not specifically that the message made a difference for the patient. Category 1c, which contains simple expressions of gratitude (e.g., "thank you"), was the largest. Users did not specify whether the message actually helped a specific patient.

The comments in category 2 indicated that MLMs are not useful. There was one harmful episode due to a message (category 2a). The physician read an alert that warned of renal insufficiency and called the patient to come into the emergency room for a follow-up creatinine test. The blood test was obtained, and the value had not worsened further. The physician later reviewed the previous creatinines and realized that the MLM had detected a six month increasing trend; there was no need for emergent follow-up. This message did not cause physical harm, but it did incur a cost in patient worry, patient time, emergency room charges, and physician time. Category 2b indicated that the message was not useful for a particular patient (e.g., "Patient is no longer taking digoxin."). Category 2c contained six general statements that MLMs were not useful or helpful.

Categories 3 and 4 contained a number of useful suggestions and comments that led to changes in the MLMs, fixes to the system, and new MLMs. Similarly, six comments from category 2 led to changes in MLMs' behavior. One comment warned that a tuberculosis alert appeared to be incorrect. The laboratory had changed its vocabulary without alerting the clinical database administrator, and an MLM called "positive_TB_culture" generated 93 inappropriate alerts in 20 minutes. The problem was uncovered, and the inappropriate alerts were inactivated before most were seen. Sometime later, another alert by the same MLM reported a "positive tuberculosis culture" based upon finding the organism M. chelonei. A user comment indicated that this was not generally a pathogen, and therefore the culture was not really positive. It was still desirable to send the alert, but the message was rephrased to read, "tuberculosis culture result." The logic of an MLM that detects renal insufficiency based upon serum creatinine was modified to account for serum ketones because of a user comment. A bug in a central database retrieval program was uncovered by another user comment. Occasionally, comments requested changes in formatting, such as altering spacing or using lowercase letters. Several users commented on the misspelling of |supersede,| which was actually spelled correctly. Some criticisms were difficult to remedy. For example, medications had to be inferred from blood level tests, since pharmacy data were not yet available. Therefore, these MLMs were unreliable. Overall, the comments were very useful for the maintenance of MLMs.

Category 5, which contained comments about other applications, reflected the lack of a suggestion box elsewhere in the clinical information system, and the fact that users see the event monitor as integrated with the rest of the clinical information system. Category 6 contained what appeared to be aborted comments (e.g., word fragments).

First-level categories (1-6) and second-level categories (a-d) underwent no further changes after the 45th comment (out of 126) was analyzed. This implies that adding more comments would probably not change them much. Therefore, the categories appear to be qualitatively representative of user comments. Third-level categories ("subcategories") were altered or added through the 112th comment (out of 126). The subcategories of 2b enumerate reasons why a message was not useful. Since the subcategories evolved through the end of the analysis, there are probably other reasons that are not listed; more comments are needed. Other second-level categories were not divided into subcategories because their comments were either homogeneous or too disparate to group logically.

There was no correlation between type of user (physician, nurse, or medical student) and category of comments.

DISCUSSION

The qualitative categories generated by the analysis are representative of user concerns, based upon the fact that categories remained stable after 45 out of 126 comments were analyzed. Nevertheless, the proportion of comments in each category is likely to be severely biased. For example, one would expect to see more comments from users who were very happy or very unhappy with the messages. Since a small number of messages instigate comments, any differential will be amplified in the result. It is interesting, however, that the proportion of users who found messages useful versus those who found messages not useful corroborates Rind's findings (53% found reminders helpful and 31% found reminders annoying) [5].

It is notable that how few users sent comments. To encourage comments one could alter the screen flow so that it becomes inconvenient *not* to send a comment. This would provide a more accurate picture of how many users hold each opinion, and it might uncover additional reasons for MLM failures (more 2b subcategories), but users might find it intrusive. A limitation of the current mechanism is that comments are biased toward users who feel comfortable enough to write text on a screen. Furthermore, users who do not even look at alert or interpretation messages will not enter the screen flow necessary to send a comment.

The reports of benefit (category 1a) and the reports of potential usefulness (1b and 1c) are heartening, but they are tempered by the report of harm (2b). The possibility of the latter outcome must be recognized whenever such systems are studied or installed. Hopefully, such episodes will be minimized by MLM revisions spurred by user comments.

Providing users with the ability to comment freely on the decision-support system has allowed us to analyze their concerns and helped us to adjust MLMs and the clinical event monitor to suit their needs. The open-ended approach has supplied a broad range of information although it may not reflect the proportion of users with each opinion accurately. While they have been very useful, user comments should not be seen as a replacement for a formal evaluation. In the future, the clinical event monitor will be used to implement care plans and practice guidelines, and user comments will be an integral part of the system.

ACKNOWLEDGMENT

This work was supported by the International Business Machines Corporation and by a grant from the National Library of Medicine LM04419 (IAIMS).

REFERENCES

[1] Johnston ME, Langton KB, Haynes RB, Mathieu A. Effects of computer-based clinical decision support systems on clinician performance and patient outcome. Ann Intern Med 1994;120:135-42.

[2] McDonald CJ, Wilson GA, McCabe GP. Physician response to computer reminders. JAMA 1980;244:1579-81.

[3] Barnett GO, Winickoff RN, Morgan MM, Zielstorff RD. A computer-based monitoring system for follow-up of elevated blood pressure. Med Care 1983;21:400-9.

[4] Pestotnik SL, Evans RS, Burke JP, Gardner RM, Classen DC. Therapeutic antibiotic monitoring: surveillance using a computerized expert system. Am J Med 1990;88:43-8.

[5] Rind DM, Safran C. The development and evaluation of computer-generated alerts in an inpatient setting. In: Lun KC, et. al., editors. Proc. 7th World Congress on Medical Informatics (MEDINFO 92). Amsterdam: North Holland, 1992; 249-254.

[6] Teach RL, Shortliffe EH. An analysis of physician attitudes regarding computer-based clinical consultation systems. Comput Biomed Research 1981;14:542-58.

[7] Henderson SE, Crapo RO, East TD, Morris AH, Wallace CJ, Gardner RM. Computerized clinical protocols in an intensive care unit: how well are they followed? In: Miller RA, editor. Proceedings of the Fourteenth Annual Symposium on Computer Applications in Medical Care; 1990 Nov 4-7; Washington, D.C. New York: IEEE Computer Society Press, 1990: 284-8.

[8] Bankowitz RA, McNeil MA, Challinor SM, Parker RC, Kapoor WN, Miller RA. A computer-assisted medical diagnostic consultation service. Ann Intern Med 1989;110:824-32.

[9] van der Lei J, Musen MA, van der Does E, Man in't Veld AJ, van Bemmel JH. Comparison of computer-aided and human review of general practitioners' management of hypertension. Lancet 1991;338:1504-8.

[10] Hripcsak G, Cimino JJ, Johnson SB, Clayton PD. The Columbia-Presbyterian Medical Center decision-support system as a model for implementing the Arden Syntax. In: Clayton PD, editor. Proceedings of the Fifteenth Annual Symposium on Computer Applications in Medical Care; 1991 Nov 17-20; Washington, D.C. New York: McGraw-Hill, Inc., 1992; 248-52.

[11] Flanagan JC. The critical incident technique. Psychological Bulletin 1954;51:327-58.

[12] Lindberg DAB, Siegel ER, Rapp BA, Wallingford KT, Wilson SR. Use of MEDLINE by physicians for clinical problem solving. JAMA 1993;269:3124-9.

[13] Hripcsak G, Ludemann P, Pryor TA, Wigertz OB, Clayton PD. Rationale for the Arden Syntax. Comput Biomed Res, in press.


```
Computer-Generated Alert Display

 Name: PATIENT, TEST                Sex: M  Birthdate: 10/03/934   MRN: 3131313
 MLM: CREATININE_MONITOR                                 Date: 93/10/27  05:27
 ------------------------------------------------------------------------------
    This message is computer-generated; your own clinical judgment must
    supersede.  Press F1 for more information.  Press F6 to send comments.

 The patient's serum creatinine level (1.4 mg/dl on 27 Oct 1993 at 04:44) may
 signify new or worsening renal insufficiency.

 This analysis was based upon the following recent creatinines (the time
 intervals between successive creatinines are not necessarily equal):

 (0.9, 0.7, 0.8, 0.9, 1.4)









 Help=F1  Alert List=F3  Comment on Alert=F6  Scroll Up/Down=F7/F8   Signoff=F11
 Print=F10    Prev Alert=F9    Next Alert=ENTER    Census=F2    CIS Main Menu=F1
```

Figure 1. Alert display screen. The user presses F6 to send a comment.

Total (126)

1. Indications that MLMs are useful (65)
    - a. reports of benefits to a specific patient due to an MLM (8)
    - b. statements that MLM advice was followed for a specific patient, without indicating whether actions would have been different without the MLM message (13)
    - c. general expressions of gratitude ("thank you") and general statements that MLMs are useful (44)
2. Indications that MLMs are not useful (28)
    - a. reports of harm to a specific patient due to an MLM (1)
    - b. statements that an MLM message was not pertinent to or useful for a specific patient (21)
        - i) complicating condition (7)
        - ii) medication discontinued (6)
        - iii) duplicate message (2)
        - iv) laboratory error (1)
        - v) missing message that should have been sent, reported under another message (1)
        - vi) not noted (4)
    - c. general statements that MLMs are potentially wasteful or harmful (6)
3. Suggestions and questions about MLMs (16)
    - a. suggestions and requests for new MLMs (8)
    - b. suggestions for additions to existing MLMs (4)
    - c. suggestions for changes to MLM message wording or spelling (3)
    - d. neutral questions about how an MLM works (1)

        (questions that implied that the user thought the MLM was in error were counted in category 2)
4. Comments about the user interface for messages (6)
    - a. suggestions for improvements to display screens (3)
    - b. reports of bugs in display screens (3)
5. Comments about other systems (5)
    - a. clinical information system (1)
    - b. laboratory system (4)
6. Unintelligible responses (6)

Table 1. Comment categories with number of comments in parentheses.

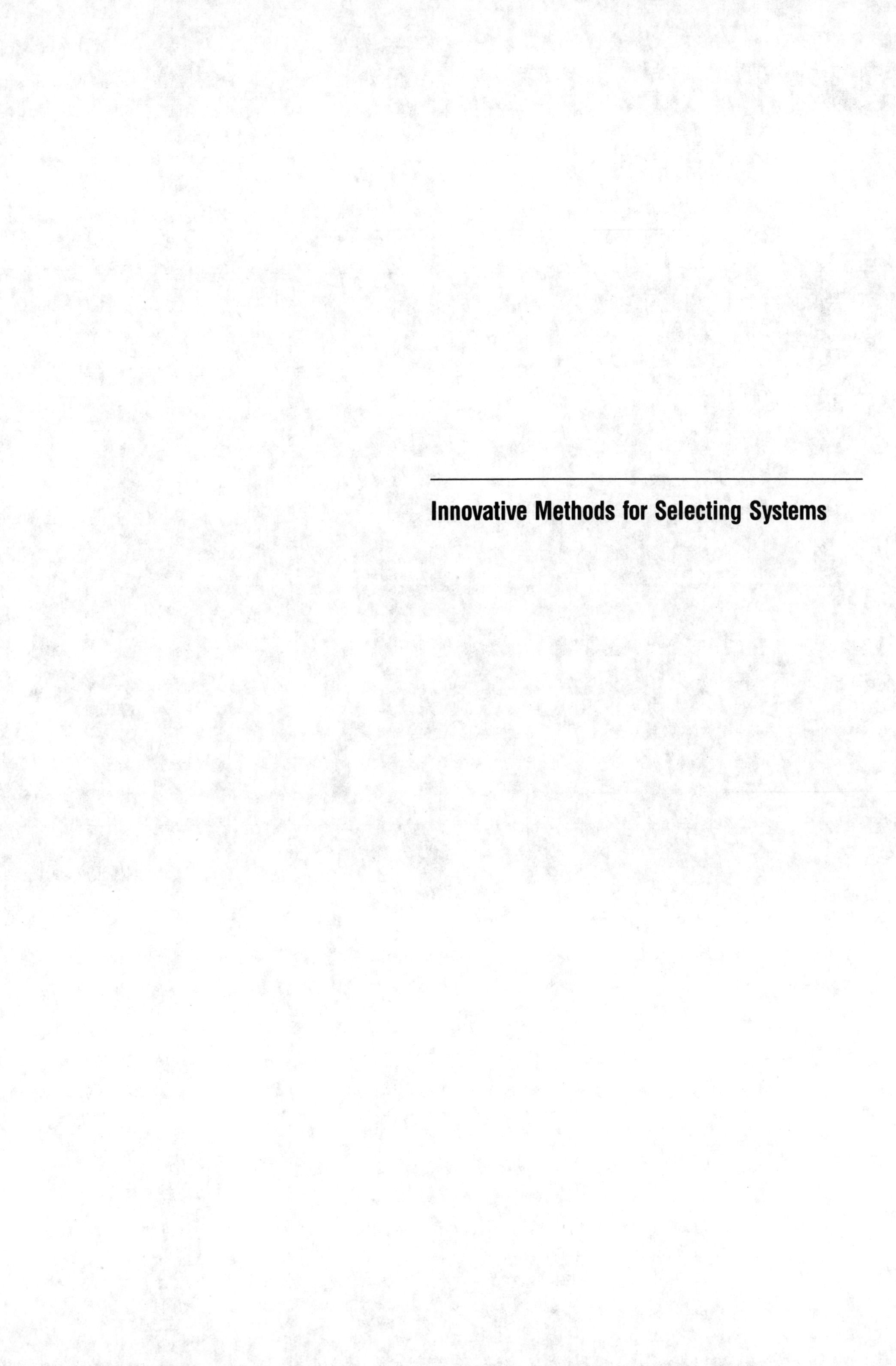

Innovative Methods for Selecting Systems

The Use Of A Clinical Case Study In A Clinical Information System Selection Process

C. Martin Harris, M.D., M.B.A. and Kathleen W. Scanlon, M.S., R.N.,

Office of Information Systems and Technology
University of Pennsylvania Health System
Philadelphia, PA 19104

ABSTRACT

The University of Pennsylvania Health System recently underwent an extensive selection process for a new clinical information system. In addition to a traditional system selection approach, a clinical case study was utilized during our selection process. This was done in an effort to better prepare the clinicians involved in the selection process, as well as to help identify key operational issues that the institution would need to resolve, related to the design and implementation of a new clinical system. We will describe here the reasons this approach was chosen, how the case study was utilized, and provide an assessment of its usefulness.

INTRODUCTION

Healthcare reform will be one of the major public policy initiatives for the decade of the 1990's. The combination of legislative initiatives and healthcare marketplace evolution will result in a changing delivery system for patient care services. Provider organizations will be required to provide detailed information on cost and quality to payors and patients. Clinical information systems which support orders management, results management, clinical documentation, clinical decision support and access to external expert information will be the basis for delivering cost effective patient care while enhancing the quality of clinical services. In response to these demands many provider organizations will be implementing clinical information systems during this decade. Optimal benefits from these systems can be best accomplished if collaborative practice paradigms are developed and extensive clinician utilization is achieved. To select a clinical system which will support integrated practice it is important that provider organizations use evaluation tools during the selection process that identify their clinical processes. Traditionally healthcare institutions have used lists of functional and technical requirements to assess information system capabilities. To more accurately identify clinical process requirements, The University of Pennsylvania Health System (UPHS) utilized a clinical case model to assess its clinical information system needs.

BACKGROUND

Much has been written in the last decade about the need to involve clinicians in the clinical information systems selection and implementation process. In a study that elicited over 600 physician's attitudes toward computer use, Anderson et al. (1) concluded that direct physician involvement in the design and implementation of clinical systems is essential to successful system implementation and utilization. Kovner et al. (2) advises in a recent review of project outcomes of the New Jersey Department of Health Nursing Incentive Reimbursement Awards (NIRA) that nurses selecting information systems should thoroughly investigate potential systems and be cautious about vendor's promises. There has, however, been very little written in the literature to provide clinicians with a model to guide their clinical system selection process.

In reviewing nursing's involvement in the design and implementation process of a medical information system at the Clinical Center of the National Institutes of Health (NIH), Romano (3) recommends that the healthcare professionals who will be using the system identify required system functions, as well as general system characteristics. She goes on to identify some of the functionality that clinicians typically need to have. Thompson (4), in an evaluation of a selection process of a Hospital Information System (HIS), reports that Manfredi and Peterson (5) consider the acquisition of software for a hospital as a matter of life and death because of the critical nature of the operations involved. They uphold that the selection process must be done in a clear and organized manner. Ginsburg and Caretta (6) maintain that the development of a checklist of system requirements should play a major part in the selection planning process. Groom and Harris (7) utilize the concept of a clinical case study in their discussion on clinical operations automation, which focuses on the selection of data acquisition devices to support clinical operations. While they use a case study concept to help highlight the operational needs, they fall short in not recommending that such an approach can drive the system selection process.

The Case Study Development Process

APPROACH

The decision to use a clinical case study approach in the system selection process at UPHS was driven by two primary objectives. The first was to ensure that the clinical system vendor demonstrations adequately and fairly represented each clinical system being presented by the vendors. This was important because of the lack of clinical systems experience amongst the clinicians at UPHS. It was necessary to make sure that the clinical users would be able to make a fair comparison between each vendor system. The second objective in using a case study approach was to begin educating the clinical users in understanding what a clinical information system was, and to begin identifying the operational changes that would result from the process of implementing a clinical system. In order to achieve these objectives a clinical case study that represented a typical day at the medical center was developed.

The case study begins early one morning with an attending physician in his office printing out his inpatient census from the clinical information system. Before he leaves for the hospital, the physician proceeds to view the most recent clinical data on his patients, including laboratory and radiology results, and current medication orders.

Meanwhile, at the hospital, nurses are using computer generated printouts from the clinical system in their morning report. After report, the nurse manager on one unit goes to the clinical system to check the unit census. Another nurse accesses the system to enter an admission assessment on a new patient. On arrival at the hospital the physician enters a number of orders in the clinical system on a patient who has suddenly deteriorated. During this process the physician is alerted by the clinical system of a drug allergy that the patient has, and of the need to get clearance by the Infectious Disease service for a restricted antibiotic. The nurse caring for the patient receives the printout of new orders before the physician arrives on the unit and begins to act upon them. On arrival to the unit the physician confers with the resident on his service about the patient's condition and additional studies that are indicated. The resident then proceeds to access the clinical system and enters a procedure note for a lumbar puncture he has performed. At the same time, the nurse caring for the patient enters a transfer note in the system, since a decision has been made to transfer the patient to the ICU. The attending goes on to see a new patient who was admitted during the night, first reviewing on-line the diagnostic studies that were performed, and the orders that were entered for the patient.

The clinical case study continues to follow patients and clinicians in the medical center throughout the remainder of the day. The overall intention being to help the clinicians evaluating the clinical systems gain an understanding of what they could and could not expect from a clinical information system. Particularly, with regard to the implications it would have in their daily practice.

IMPLEMENTATION

Three clinical information systems vendors were selected to demonstrate their system at UPHS. Several weeks prior to the scheduled demonstrations, each of the vendors were given copies of the clinical case study and specific instructions regarding the functionality they would be expected to demonstrate, as well as the output documents their system would need to generate. UPHS personnel met with vendor representatives from each of the vendor companies to review the demonstrations they had developed, and to make certain they understood the desired outcome. The expectation set forth by UPHS required that each vendor begin their system demonstration with the UPHS case study. The system features and functions they used for the case study had to exist as currently available products. If they completed the case study demonstration within the allotted timeframe the vendor could then go on and show other functionality or future system enhancements. This helped to ensure that the UPHS evaluators saw the same situations demonstrated by each vendor, and could then evaluate each from the same frame of reference.

ASSESSMENT

Most system selection processes involve an approach whereby identified functional requirements are presented to the vendor in a request for proposal (RFP) document. The vendor responds back to the institution indicating the degree to which their system can meet the requirements. While such an approach can be very helpful in determining the functionality within a given system and in comparing functionality between two or more systems, it does little to help identify the operational issues that the institution will need to resolve. For example, at UPHS a traditional RFP process was also used in addition to the clinical case study. Functional requirements were compiled for the nursing, physician and ancillary components of the systems. Review of each vendor's responses revealed very little difference between the systems and did nothing to help illustrate potential operational changes that implementing a clinical information system would necessitate.

The clinical case study, however, when demonstrated by each system vendor helped to point out differences in functionality between vendor systems, as well as bringing to light some potentially significant operational issues. One such example involved the entry of orders into the systems. All three of the vendor RFPs stated that this functionality was available in their system. The clinical case study, however, helped to identify capabilities which support the entry of defined order sets. The case study in turn helped us to define the institutional processes that are required to develop order sets supportive of collaborative practice.

In demonstrating the entry of orders that are necessary prior to a procedure being performed (prep orders), it became evident that one vendor system had a limitation of four prep orders per procedure, while the other vendors had no such limitation. Operationally this limitation was unacceptable and without the use of the case study probably would not have been identified in a standard vendor demonstration process.

Another operational issue that the case study identified involves the need to ensure that data is entered into the system in a timely manner, this is particularly true with regard to medication charting. It became clear through the use of the case study that clinicians need to be assured of being able to access accurate information within a reasonable timeframe, otherwise, their incentive to use the system will be greatly diminished.

Through the use of the case study we were able to see the impact that on line medication charting could have on a nurse's productivity. One system allowed for access to multiple patients, including being able to retrieve just those patients the nurse was assigned to, while documenting medications. In another system medication charting could only be done by individual patient, which had the potential to significantly increase the time spent when charting on multiple patients.

CONCLUSION

The selection of a clinical information system is not an easy task. The traditional RFP process can be very helpful in defining a system's functional features, and has contractual value later during the vendor negotiation process. It is essential, however, that key operational issues be identified as early as possible in the system procurement process. Early issue identification can influence the final system decision, as well as provide opportunities in the system design and development phases to develop either technical or operational solutions. The use of a clinical case study in the clinical information system selection process can greatly facilitate the challenge of identifying the key operational issues within an institution. Issues that will significantly impact upon the ultimate success and acceptance of the system.

References

[1]. Anderson, J.G., Jay, S.J., Schweer, H.M., and Anderson, M.M., Why Doctors Don't use Computers: Some Empirical Findings. The Journal of the Royal Society of Medicine. 79 142-144, March 1986.

[2]. Kovner, C.T., Hendrickson, G., Knickman, J.R. & Finkler, S.A. Changing the Delivery of Nursing Care - Implementation Issues and Qualitative Finding's. JONA. 23 (11) 24-34, 1993.

[3]. Romano, C.A., Development, Implementation and Utilization of a Computerized Information System for Nursing. Nursing Administration Quarterly,

10 (29) 1-9, 1986.

[4]. Thompson, A.M., An Evaluation of the Selection Process of Hospital Information Systems. Journal of Medical Systems. 14 (5): 245-282, 1990.

[5]. Manfredi, M.J. & Peterson, D.M., Software: A Team Approach to Investigating the Options. Journal of Healthcare Financial Management. 43 (3): 68-80, 1989.

[6]. Ginsburg, D.A., & Caretta, W., Selecting an Automated Patient Accounting System. Journal of Healthcare Financial Management. 42 (6): 58-62, 1986.

[7]. Groom, D.A. and Harris, J.W., Evaluation and Selection of Systems for Automating Clinical Operations. Biomedical Instrumentation and Technology. 5: 173-185, 1991.

Selecting a Commercial Clinical Information System: An Academic Medical Center's Experience

E. Tin Wong, Ph.D.
Thomas W. Abendroth, M.D.

Center for Information Technology
The Milton S. Hershey Medical Center
The Pennsylvania State University

Abstract

Choosing a commercial clinical information system to meet the information needs of patient care, research, education, administration, finance, and ongoing changes of the healthcare system of an academic medical center is a challenging task. For the past six months, The Milton S. Hershey Medical Center undertook this task through (i) establishing a task force, (ii) assessing end-user information needs, (iii) understanding future institutional development and strategies, (iv) conceptualizing the ideal system, (v) identifying a short list of vendors, (vi) sending RFIs to vendors, (vii) visiting vendors' headquarters, (viii) technical review, (ix) reference calls, (x) using consultation services, (xi) on-site demonstration, and (xii) visiting the vendor's clients.

Introduction

The Study Group on Information Sciences of the Association of Academic Health Centers suggested that academic health centers may not be able to maintain their quality patient care, education, and research if integrated information systems are not implemented during the 1990s [1]. A recent study estimated that about 40 percent of existing hospitals will be out of business by the year of 2000 due to inefficiencies and the inability to compete [2]. For the past few years, many community hospitals and academic medical centers, which strive for survival and competitiveness, turn to clinical information management systems as one of many strategic measures [3, 4]. Zinn and DiGiulio have summarized the tangible qualitative and quantitative benefits of clinical information systems [5]. More importantly, use an integrated clinical information system properly could translate into financial gain and competitive advantage [4].

Choosing a commercial clinical information system for an academic medical center is a challenging task. The selected system has to meet the information needs of patient care, research, education, administration, finance, and ongoing changes in healthcare. In addition, many well developed clinical information systems are available in the current market. Each system has its strengths and weaknesses in terms of functionality, hardware and software architecture platforms, and uses of emerging technologies. Furthermore, commercial clinical information systems are costly.

The Milton S. Hershey Medical Center has committed to implement an integrated clinical information management system in the next two to three years. For the past six months, the Medical Center undertook a selection process and chose a commercial clinical information system.

Institutional Environment

The Penn State's Milton S. Hershey Medical Center, consisting of the University Hospital, Children's Hospital, and College of Medicine, is a 500-bed tertiary care teaching hospital and ambulatory care complex. Currently, there are several stand-alone clinical systems, including Clinical Laboratory, Pharmacy, and Radiology. There is no data exchange among these systems. All clinical patient data are communicated between departments by paper and managed manually. Although a fiber optic data backbone network exists throughout major campus buildings [6], there is no method for clinicians to review patient information and place orders on-line.

Overview of the Selection Process

Before undertaking the selection of a clinical information system, the Medical Center carefully considered previous experiences and advice of other institutions that had successfully selected and implemented clinical information systems [7 - 9].

Establishing a Task Force

A 24-member task force representing most end-user constituencies was established. The charge of the task force was to select a commercial clinical information system that will integrate with existing

0195-4210/94/$5.00 © 1994 AMIA, Inc.

departmental systems, provide on-line patient data review, allow physician order entry, and create a centralized clinical data repository. Table 1 shows the departments represented on the task force. The diverse background of the task force reflected the Medical Center's belief that the selected system would have to meet various demands. The task force members met every week for one to two hours to plan, discuss, and execute the selection process. Average attendance was about 75 percent.

Assessing End-User Information Needs

Identifying end-user information needs is a major determinant of success in implementing a new information system. Prior to the current task force, several individuals spent more than 100 hours to conduct an institutionwide end-user needs assessment [10]. The assessment revealed the needs of end-users in the following areas:

- patient data retrieval,
- order entry,
- nursing automation,
- a centralized clinical data repository, and
- a research data repository.

Understanding Future Institutional Development and Strategies

Understanding and incorporating future institutional development and strategies into the selection process will maximize the investment and benefits of the selected clinical information system. For instances, the following events are inevitable in the near future for the Medical Center:

- increase in outpatient volume,
- increase in off-site practice,
- tracking capitated patients' costs,
- analyzing contracts,
- performing case management,
- installing a wireless communication network, and
- using handheld devices to capture clinical data at points of need.

The system must accommodate such future information needs without major reconfiguration.

Conceptualizing the Ideal System

Once the current and future information needs were assessed, the task force conceptualized the ideal system that would match the requirements of the Medical Center. Such an ideal system would feature:

- open architecture,
- industry standards such as TCP/IP, SQL, and HL7,
- scalability in both hardware and software,
- fault tolerance,

Table 1

Departments with Which the CIS Task Force Members are Associated

Admissions/Registration/Scheduling
Biostatistics and Epidemiology
Health Information Services
Hospital Administration
Hospital/Health Finance Management
Information Systems
Physicians from:
Anesthesia
Clinical Laboratory
Medicine
Pediatrics
Radiology
Rehabilitation
Surgery
Nursing Administration
Outpatient Services
Pharmacy Services
Professional Billing

- complex ad hoc query handling,
- acceptable response time,
- multi-platform workstations accessibility,
- data exchange with remote sites,
- multiple security levels,
- flexible tools for customization and development, and
- decision support capability.

These features were used as part of the evaluation criteria in the selection process.

Identifying a Short List of Vendors

To ensure an efficient and effective selection process, the task force focused on five outstanding vendors. This list of vendors was obtained through communications with colleagues and consultants, and observations of vendor demonstrations at conferences such as SCAMC and HIMSS.

Sending RFIs to Vendors

The five vendors were informed and a Request For Information (RFI) was sent to each vendor. The RFI served two main purposes – allow task force members to understand each system in detail and to provide a starting point for further investigations. The creation of the RFI was based on our conceptual ideal system and Campbell and his associates' suggestions [7]. In addition, a summary of the Medical Center was included in the RFI. The vendors were requested to limit their responses to 30 pages and return their responses in about six weeks.

Visiting Vendors' Headquarters

With the returned RFIs, there were still many unanswered questions about the vendors and their products. A group of task force members spent a full day in each vendor's headquarters to get acquainted with their products and leadership through personal contacts, presentations, and demonstrations. These vendor headquarters visits specifically emphasized the clinical evaluation criteria and vendor information in the RFI (see Table 2). The group used an assessment form, similar to Table 2, to comment and rate the vendors on a scale of 1 (low) to 5 (high).

The results of these visits were reported to the task force. On the basis of the RFIs and site visits, two out of five vendors were eliminated because they could not meet the identified criteria.

Technical Review

A team of technical task force members visited each of the remaining three vendors for two full days to develop an in-depth understanding of the hardware and software platforms, database management, interfacing with existing departmental systems, networking, flexibility for future modification and development, and planning and installation approaches. This review indicated that one of the three vendors was slightly preferable to the other two, but all three were feasible from a purely technical perspective.

Reference Calls

Meanwhile, several task force members conducted telephone interviews of four to five clients of each vendor. The survey was based on the reference call questions suggested by Campbell et al. [7], with emphases on vendors' services and support, customer satisfaction, implementation problems, and system integration.

The survey results revealed that all except two clients would recommend their vendors to others. In addition, all interviewed clients expressed a certain degree of dissatisfaction in services and support, especially the clients of fast-growing vendors. On the other hand, clients having partnerships with their vendors expressed higher satisfaction. Most clients expressed moderate satisfaction with their implementation processes and the integration of their legacy systems and the newly installed systems.

Based on the technical review and reference calls, the task force had placed one of the three vendors on indefinite hold.

Using Consultation Services

Seeking outside help was another measure of the task force to ensure an unbiased selection. For a minimal fee, the task force obtained vendor profiles compiled by an independent consultant. Each vendor profile included product descriptions, company history, strengths and weaknesses, system pricing, assessment, and references. These documents were used as supplementary information to the task force.

Table 2

An Outline of Request for Information

An Outline of Request for Information
Clinical Evaluation Criteria
Review of patient information
Order communication
Source data capture
Confidentiality and security
Other resources to support patient care
Secondary uses of clinical data
Multi-function clinical workstation
Maximizing system availability and benefits
Exchange of data with remote sites
Technical Evaluation Criteria
Networking
Database
System management
Interfacing with other systems
Local enhancements and extensions of system functions
Vendor Information
Company history
Product information
Product use
Product sales
Key competitive features
Approach to installing products
Clients' input into product development
Future product plans
Clients list
Proposed cost

On-Site Demonstration

The task force invited each of the remaining two vendors to the Medical Center for a three-day on-site demonstration. These demonstrations were conducted about three weeks apart. Each vendor scheduled ten different demonstration sessions with different emphases for top leadership, departmental administrators, task force members, nurses, physicians, and general audiences. All sessions included a basic demonstration of the proposed system. The purposes of these demonstrations were to (i) allow the task force members who had not seen the systems before to evaluate each system firsthand; (ii) let the top management and departmental administrators understand what could be expected from the selected system; and (iii) educate the end-users about the objectives, capabilities, and usefulness of clinical information systems. Participants were asked to rate the systems on a scale of 1 (low) to 5 (high) in the following categories:

- overall impression,
- patient information review,
- nursing care,
- physician order entry,
- registration and scheduling,
- response time, user-friendliness, and
- usefulness to your work.

Overall, both systems were well received by the participants and scored 4 or above in all but two categories (nursing care, and registration and scheduling). The on-site demonstration also provided the task force an opportunity to compare the two systems very closely and understand the responses from end-users.

Visiting the Vendors' Clients

A group of task force members spent a full day at live installation sites to learn about the approaches, experiences, and problems of its planning, implementation, and operation of the clinical information system. These sites were chosen because of their similarity to the Medical Center in size, practice environment, and installed systems.

Final Decision

Based on all the evaluation criteria, the responses from RFIs, series of demonstrations, and all available information, one of the two vendors was chosen by task force members through secret ballots to implement an integrated clinical information system for the Medical Center.

Discussions

The Medical Center will start to implement an integrated clinical information system within six months of contract negotiation. A critical element in the success of the selection process was the strong support from both the top leadership and end-users institutionwide. As a result, the task force members were able to make a well informed and carefully considered judgment. On the other hand, the process was time-consuming and expensive. A physician spent 50 percent of his time to guide, coordinate, and implement the process. Additionally, about 950 person-hours were spent in meetings, and 148 person-days and $50,000 on traveling. Although this selection process might be unique to the Medical Center, there were a few lessons worth mentioning.

Not one system in the market will exactly match the information needs of an institution. Future in-house customization and development of the selected system are necessary. Consequently, the task force closely examined each product's application development tools and flexibility.

The selection process was quite complex due to the many factors considered and the sheer volume of information collected for each vendor. It was very difficult to determine which factors were most important during the final decision process. Therefore, prioritization of these factors at an early stage of the search process, based on the institution's needs, is helpful. The tremendous amount of vendor information caused confusion among task force members. Since the task force members were volunteers with busy work schedules, they were overwhelmed by all the information collected for each vendor. To address this, a summary of the vendors and their products was presented to the task force before the final decision was made. Other alternatives to avoid information overload may include cutting down the number of vendors to two quickly and keeping the search period as short as possible.

Each vendor has strengths in certain products and weaknesses in others. For instance, a vendor may have a good order entry module but not a nursing care system; whereas another vendor has a good nursing care system but not an order entry module. Defining the requirements and priorities of the system well at the beginning and focusing on it throughout the selection process will help to differentiate multiple systems.

Creating a long term, mutually beneficial partnership with the chosen vendor is important. Examples of such a partnership include: developing new products together, being an alpha or a beta site for the vendor's new product(s), and being a showcase or a visiting site of the vendor. Clients of different vendors claimed that many benefits could be achieved through a good partnership. These benefits included receiving preferential services and support, free products, and substantial discounts on new products.

Finally, documenting in the contract the required services and support from the vendor during and after the implementation of the CIS was consistently advised during the reference calls.

Acknowledgment

E. Tin Wong is supported by the Medical Informatics Fellowship Training Program at The Penn State's Milton S. Hershey Medical Center.

References

[1] A report titled "Integrated Information Management Systems in Health Care." Prepared by the Study Group on Information Sciences of the Association of Academic Health Centers, Washington, DC, 1991.

[2] Eckstein MG. EDI Tactics to Implement President Clinton's Healthcare Reform Strategy. EDI World, pp. 45-49, Dec 1993.

[3] Moriarty DD. Strategic Information System Planning for Health Service Providers. Health Care Management Review, 17(1), pp. 85-90, 1992.

[4] Morrissey J. Spending More on Computers to Help Keep Costs in Line. Modern Healthcare, pp. 63-70, Feb 14, 1994.

[5] Zinn TK, DiGiulio LW. Actualizing System Benefits - Part I. Computers in Healthcare, pp. 32-34, Mar 1988.

[6] Meier JH. A Guide to the Hershey Medical Center Data Network. CIT Document: IT.000103.PSC, Aug 1993.

[7] Campbell JR, Bahensky JA, Rejda E, Gleser M. Tutorial 5: Contract Development Issues for an Integrated Computerized Patient Record Addressing Institution of Medicine Criteria, 17th SCAMC, 1993.

[8] Person MM, III. The Smart Hospital: A Case Study in Hospital Computerization. Carolina Academic Press, Carolina, 1988.

[9] Bloom C. Selection & Installation Activities: Integrating System Implementations - By the Numbers. Healthcare Informatics, pp. 26-32, Feb 1994.

[10] Abendroth TW. End-user Participation in the Needs of Assessment for a Clinical Information System. In: Clayton PD, ed. Proc 15th SCAMC, pp. 233-237, McGraw Hill, New York, 1991.

Dimensions Associated With Successful Implementation of a Hospital Based Integrated Order Entry System

Charlene Weir, Ph.D., Mike Lincoln, M.D., David Roscoe, R.N., M.Ed., Charles Turner, Ph.D., and Gordon Moreshead, Director, SLCISC

Salt Lake City Veteran's Affair Information Systems Center
Salt Lake City, Utah

ABSTRACT

Implementation of an integrated electronic medical record requires direct physician order entry. This application involves multi-level changes in the whole system of care, from physicians attitudes to interdepartmental relations. This study reports the results of the first round of a modified Delphi, where a diverse group of individuals were asked to identify the most important facilitating and impeding factors associated with implementation of an order entry application. From a Q-sort of their responses, we identified 20 systemic, behavioral, and attitudinal dimensions perceived to be causal factors in successful implementation. We also explored how these dimensions may influence success by comparing successful with unsuccessful hospitals in terms of the frequency with which these dimensions were differently mentioned by respondents. We found that although available functionality was the most commonly mentioned factor by all participants, hardware availability, physician involvement, administration support, and medical administration involvement were more often mentioned by successful hospitals than by less successful hospitals. These results suggest that these factors were not present in the less successful hospitals.

We also found that the frequency of responses within each category varied depending on the institutional role of the individuals responding. Those involved in support tended to see organizational variables as more important than those in clinical positions, whereas clinicians viewed administrative support and involvement of the chief as more important. These findings support the notion that the changes involved in instituting a physician order entry system are system wide and involve individual as well as organizational factors.

INTRODUCTION

The Salt Lake City Information Service Center of the Veteran's Administration (SLC ISC) released their order entry system, Order Entry/Results Reporting 2.5 (OE/RR 2.5), to the field in March, 1993. OE/RR 2.5 integrated several clinical packages (e.g., pharmacy and lab) and provided a single environment where clinicians can enter clinical orders and obtain clinically relevant patient information. Response to the package has varied widely across institutions. A series of studies were planned to identify factors that discriminate successful from non successful implementation of OE/RR 2.5 in order to prepare for the next version. This paper reports on the first study of the series.

A fully integrated hospital information system is essential in order to maximize quality management activities, cost control, and clinical decision support. Full acceptance and implementation of an electronic medical record is often viewed as a direct function of physician change as these professionals must make radical changes in their everyday work [1,2,3]. However, the literature on physician change indicates that such change is difficult to achieve and often not long lasting [4]. Yet physician behavior change actually occurs in the context of a larger institutional setting. As work in Total Quality Management has illustrated, individuals are rarely the barriers to change [5]. Rather, it is often system level factors interacting with individuals that cause failures. The purpose of this study is to simultaneously identify both individual and institutional level variables associated with successful adoption by physicians of an integrated order entry system.

Specifying the causal variables of a multidetermined event, such as the successful change to on-line order entry, is difficult because people often do not have accurate access to the causes of their behavior [6]. Participants perceptions of a changing system will vary depending on whether the implementation was successful [7], and whether they had direct involvement in the process [8]. In addition, different cognitive and behavioral variables are important at different stages of change [9]. Individuals already committed to a change focus more on issues surrounding actual implementation, whereas those still contemplating the change are more concerned with the pros and cons [10]. Furthermore, each category of individuals has their

0195–4210/94/$5.00

own perspectives. Physicians will have their own unique perception of the value of an electronic medical record, one that is different from those developing the software, and different again from those in charge of implementing and supporting the change. No particular point of view or point in time may provide the complete picture.

In this first study, salient dimensions were derived from open-ended responses of people directly involved in implementation attempts of a direct order entry system. An effort was made to have participants represent all of the varied hospital departments that would be involved in such an implementation attempt. Physician representation included administrators, nominated opinion leaders [11], and randomly selected users. The results from this first study will allow the development of a questionnaire based on the identified dimensions in a second study.

METHODS

Two sets of hospitals were identified based on their relative success at implementing OE/RR 2.5 and their participation as either beta sites or with early implementation. The first set consisted of three hospitals judged to be successful at implementing order entry 2.5 and the second set consisted of three relatively unsuccessful hospitals. Success was defined two ways. The first consisted of nomination by OE/RR 2.5 software engineers working at the SLC ISC, and secondly by the percentage of providers directly using order entry at each institution as reported by participants of the study. The percentage of providers using order entry differed significantly between hospital sets [$F(1,37) = 34.97$; $p = .00$; Means: success = 74.4%; failure = 15.3%].

A questionnaire was mailed to the following individuals from each institution: 1) Medical Administration Staff, such as chiefs of staff and directors of bed services; 2) Administrators, including the director of the Information Resource Management department (IRM) which provides hardware and software support, Nursing, and Medical Records; 3) Support staff, such as the computer support staff from pharmacy and lab who had been assigned to assist with the implementation of OE/RR, specifically designeted coordinators responsible for training and implementing OE/RR 2.5, and IRM staff; 3) Users, including ward clerks, physicians, and nurses; and 4) Physician opinion leaders nominated by a random selection of 5 physicians from each institution. Over the 6 hospitals, ninety-two individuals received a questionnaire.

Fifty seven percent (n = 52) responded. Of those fifty-two, twelve reported that they did not know enough to answer the questions. This left a sample size of forty. Twenty responded from the predefined successful hospitals and twenty responded from the less successful hospitals. The response rate did not differ significantly by institution.

The questionnaire consisted of five questions:

1) What proportion of physicians, nurse practitioners, and physician assistants at your institution enter most of their orders directly using OE/RR 2.5?;
2) What proportion nurses directly use OE/RR 2.5?
3) How well do you think OE/RR 2.5 meets the clinical needs of practitioners? This question is answered on a 1 (not at all) to 5 (very well) scale?;
4) Please list 6 to 10 of the most significant facilitating factors for implementing OE/RR 2.5 at your institution?;
5) Please list 6 to 10 of the most significant barriers impeding the implementing OE/RR 2.5 at your institution?

To identify valid dimensions, the open-ended responses to the above questionnaire were sorted independently into categories by two clinicians (author 1 and author 3) working at the ISC using a modified Q-sort. The sorting was done separately for facilitating factors and for barriers. Neither the number of categories nor their content was specified a priori. One author produced 10 categories and another 14 for both facilitating factors and barriers. Two categories across both sorters had greater than 80% overlap in content and the remaining differences were essentially the inclusion of two categories in one by the third author. After discussion between sorters, the categories were agreed upon. Individual response items were then coded into these categories by two independent raters. Initial agreement between raters was acceptable with 78% of the items coded in the same category.

RESULTS

Identification of Dimensions

Table 1 and 2 list the identified categories in the order of frequency of response. Totals are greater than the number of respondents as some people mentioned items from the same category more than once. These are the categories that reflect the causal factors perceived to be most salient by the respondents. Functionality was an important factor for all respondents. This category had the most items for both facilitating factors and barriers. In addition, many of the categories of the facilitating factors are the inverse of the barriers. In other words, there were only twenty unique categories overall. For example, the presence of supporting administration is a facilitating factor and the absence of a supportive administration is cited as a barrier.

The actual ranking of categories, however, differed between facilitating factors and barriers. Perceived benefits and helpful, experienced support support were most frequently mentioned as facilitating factors, whereas hardware and uncooperative physicians were mentioned as the next most common barriers.

Table 1: Number of times each facilitating factor dimension identified by respondents within success (S), Failure (F) groups and total sample (T)

DIMENSIONS FACILITATING FACTORS	S	F	T
Functionality (i.e. health summaries, discharge summaries)	20	24	44
Knowledgeable, cheerful support from IRM, on-line help	15	17	32
Perception of many potential benefits	14	7	21
Ability to customize software to meet physician needs	8	8	16
**Supportive administration, chiefs of staff, and attending	14	1	15
**Direct involvement of physicians, provider open-mindedness	13	2	15
Good working relationship with developers	10	5	15
An interdisciplinary, effective, implementation group	8	6	14
Good implementation strategies (e.g. good PR, bring all services)	4	7	11
**Support by medical administration and other allied fields.	7	1	8
**Implementation mandatory	6	0	6
Sufficient number of people hired to implement and train users	3	3	6
**Adequate Hardware, terminals, etc.	10	1	11
*Good training and instruction	4	0	4

Note: A single asterisk (*) indicates significance at the p < .05 level; two asterisks (**) indicate significance at the p = .01 level between successful and less successful hospitals using X^2 (39) .

Table 2: Number of times each barrier dimension identified by respondents within success (S), Failure (F) groups and total sample (T)

BARRIERS	S	F	T
Functionality not sufficient, software is not working well	17	22	39
Uncooperative or computer phobic attitude of physicians	18	15	33
*Insufficient terminals, system too slow, nonportable screens	21	8	29
System not user friendly, inadequate interface	13	15	28
Program takes too much time, too labor intensive	9	12	21
Inadequate training, insufficient material, residents rotations	11	8	19
Inadequate pharmacy application which interfaces with OE/RR	9	5	14
Poor implementation, e.g.. location where first introduced	5	6	11
Bureaucracy prevents change; Interdepartmental conflict	5	5	10
**Inadequate administration application, also interfaces with OE/RR	8	2	10
Lack of effective, cheerful IRM support	7	2	9
Non supportive section chiefs /Chief of Staff	3	5	8
Providers don't know how to type	5	3	8
Insufficient personnel to adequately implement and train	4	1	5

Note: A single asterisk (*) indicates significance at the p < .05 level; two asterisks (**) indicate significance at the p = .01 level between successful and less successful hospitals using X^2 (39).

Variables differentiating hospital group

To identify which variables differentiated successful from the less successful hospitals, a chi-square analysis was performed for each category comparing the number of individuals from each hospital group mentioning an item within that category. Those that were significantly different are note by asterisks in the table. Several categories differentiated the two hospital groups. Significantly more people from the successful hospital group reported supportive administration and supportive heads of medical sections as facilitating success. In addition, significantly more people from the successful hospital group mentioned that direct involvement of physicians, mandatory implementation, adequate training, and sufficient hardware facilitated success. In terms of barriers, only inadequate hardware and lack of ability to easily do patient transfer and advance admission orders (medical records package) differentiated the two groups and in both cases the item was mentioned more frequently by the successful hospitals.

The two hospital groups also differed in terms of two other variables. Individuals responding from the successful hospitals had higher ratings of the clinical value of OE/RR 2.5 than those from the less successful hospital [$F(1,37) = 10.76$; $p = .002$; Means: success = 3.33; failure = 2.22].

Respondent Role

To determine the impact of an individual's role, two groups were created from the full participant list. The first group consisted of support personnel and included directors of resource management, who are responsible for providing support for hardware, customization of software, and training needs, and individuals hired specifically for support in specific departments or overall for OE. The second group consisted of clinicians and included users, opinion leaders, and medical administration. For each dimension, the number of individuals from each group reporting items was compared using a chi-squared analysis. The results of this analysis are represented in Table 3. This table only reports those dimensions found to be significantly different.

TABLE 3: Percentage of people in the support (S) and clinician (C) groups identifying each category for both facilitating factors and barriers.

DIMENSION	S	C
Facilitating Factors		
Organized, interdisciplinary implementation group	50	5
Support of Chiefs of Staff and medical administration	21	63
Mandatory Implementation	0	33
Sufficient personnel	50	10
Barriers		
Bureaucracy, such as interdepartmental infighting	50	17
Pharmacy package did not meet clinician needs	75	4

Note: Cell entries refer to the percent of respondents endorsing each item.

As can be seen from the table, the support personnel were more sensitive to institutional variables, such as the presence of an interdisciplinary implementation group, the resistance of the VA bureaucracy to change, and the availability of sufficient personnel for training and support. The one exception was the factor, "mandated implementation", which refers to the administrative policy of requiring physicians to enter orders. This factor was only mentioned by clinicians (and only in the success hospitals), suggesting that the clinician respondents felt that encouraging full participation by all physicians was important to success. This is reasonable if a fully electronic medical record is to evolve from a physician order entry system. The support personnel also mentioned the difficulty of the interface with the pharmacy application, significantly more than the clinicians. This finding is most likely a function of the role of support in maintaining that interface.

DISCUSSION

The results from this study support the finding of others that a major factor in successful implementation of physician order entry is the patterns of organizational policy development and implementation[3]. Commitment from top leaders and administrators is essential to making the necessary cultural and social changes required for physicians to evolve into the necessary roles and to adopt the needed practice patterns. Measurement of the influence of different variables, therefore, must be done within the complete context of implementation, using the perspectives of all participants in order to capture each individual's unique contribution. The differing perspectives of the respondents illustrates the importance of taking a system level approach.

For the most part, the pattern of responses reflected the more in-depth experience that the more successful hospitals had with implementing a new application. The impact of problems with hardware, training, and support from medical administration are issues that become apparent as implementation unfolds. However, the impact of involved physicians, committed administration, and mandated implementation are factors more likely present prior to the decision to implement and thus are system variables predictive of success.

The importance of involvement of physicians at all levels was also identified more frequently by successful hospitals than less successful hospitals and this finding is also congruent with other work[8]. The support and interest of medical administrators, the existence of at least a small group of interested and active physicians, and the mandating of order entry for all physicians are individual and system factors that all point to a great deal of physician involvement. It is also important to note that how valuable OE/RR 2.5 was perceived differed depending on the success or failure experience of the institution.

REFERENCES

1. Lundsgaarde, H.P. Evaluating medical expert systems, Soc. Sci. Med. 24: 805-819, 1987
2. Massaro TA. Introducing physician order entry at a major academic medical center: I. Impact on organizational culture and behavior. Acad Med. 1993;68:20-5.
3. Sittig DF, and Stead W.W. Computer-based Physician Order Entry: The Sate of the Art. J. of Am. Med. Infor. Ass. 1994;1:108-123.
4. Hodge MH. Direct use by physicians of the TDS medical information system. In Blum BI, Duncan K (eds). A History of Medical Informatics. New York: ACM Press. 1990: 345-56.
5. Williamson, J. Medical quality management systems in perspective, pp 23-72. In Couch, JB (ed.) . Health Care Quality Management, Tampa, Florida:Hillsboro Printing, 1991.
6. Nisbett, R. W., & Wilson, T. D. (1977). Telling more than you can know: Verbal reports on mental processes. Psychological Review, 84, 231-259.
7. Hirt ER, Zillmann D, Erickson GA, Kennedy C. Costs and benefits of allegiance: Changes in fans' self-ascribed competencies after team victory versus defeat. JPSP, 1992: 63; 724-738
8. Eisenberg JM. Doctor's Decisions and the Cost of Medical Care. Health Administration Press: Ann Arbor, Mich. 1986.
9. Bandura A. Social foundations of thought and action: A social cognitive theory. Englewood Cliffs, NJ: Prentice-Hall. 1986.
10. Gollwitzer, P. M. Action Phases and Mind Sets. In E. T. Higgins and R. M. Sorrentino (Eds.), Handbook of motivation and cognition: Foundations of social behavior . 1990: 53-92. New York: Guilford Press.
11. Lomas J, Endin M. Anderson G. Opinion leaders versus audit and feedback to implement practice guidelines: Delivery after previous cesarean section JAMA, 1991; 265(1): 2202-2207.

PURSUING USABLENESS AND EFFECTIVENESS IN THE DEVELOPMENT OF A SHARED PATIENT CENTERED INFORMATION SYSTEM

M.Cristina Mazzoleni[1] and Franco Galli[2]
[1] Medical Informatics Service, [2] Hemodialysis Unit, Clinca del Lavoro Foundation, IRCCS, Medical Center of Pavia, Italy

ABSTRACT

Our experience supplying a shared patient centred information system is here described, pointing out some of the critical aspects underlying usableness and effectiveness.
Between and within unit integration, together with providing each professional role with added value and the special attention to adjust input and information retrieval to the actual needs (often identified only by an assiduous frequentation), has proved to be the essential point.
A study case is presented.

INTRODUCTION

As regards patient care, our Centre had been characterised for a long time by islands of automation, with little or no transfer or condivision of information from one system to another.

Purchased, internally developed and general purpose integrated packages were often used by physicians to achieve specific results.
The efforts, in terms of data entry, to support these fragmentary systems were often charged to personnel with no direct incomes. The burden of making data available to all these separate purposes was too great.
Dissatisfaction was growing.

The reasons for the failures were quite note. The problem was how to effectively impact on the clinical structure, assuring quality improvement for both patient care and daily practice.

From such an experience, it was beyond doubt that:
- the need for a centralized, comprehensive information system existed
- information sharing was critical
- it had to be a tool supporting the hospital daily activities
- maintenance must be relatively easy, semplifying the existing process

Users had become quite skilled in managing personal computers, and some important advances in networking and database management technologies occurred. This scenario made a (re)organisation feasible.
Under the care of four people of the internal group of medical informatics, a few years ago the SIO project was begun. The activities of SIO were to develop an integrated, shared patient centred information system, tailored to the basic needs of the users, while paying special attention to providing the distinct healthcare professionals with unique system functionality.
As the enterprise was - and continues to be - quite difficult, we decided to describe here our experience as a study case. Since generalisation and abstraction are often obscure, a module for a hemodialysis unit is presented to show the adopted approach in concrete form.

PRIMARY AIMS OF THE PROJECT

Most of our patients collect a long series of contacts with our structure, both hospitalisation and medical examinations, often with many tests. The generic patient is treated, inside the Centre, by many physicians, each for a specific aspect, but all of them need to know the past and present situation of the patient.
The most important aim hence is to make a complete clinical patient history available everywhere, whenever, and in the most useful form it is needed, in order to evaluate the patient condition better.
Other expectations are:
- availability of a tool for the monitoring of clinically interesting parameters
- possibility of population selections for clinical research
- time reduction of routine activities
- facilitation in supplying more exhaustive documentation, including diagnostic iter, to the general practitioner who takes care of the patient once discharged.

GENERAL ASPECTS

One of the first questions was whether to develop the information system within the medical informatics group or to purchase it. Considering the variability of physician requirements, the support and improvement such systems require, internal development was chosen.

As regards hardware architecture, since modularity was a mandatory guide-line, the solution of a network with a database (Informix on-line) server (HP9000/827) and client PC (386xx, 4Mb) was adopted.
Windows environment was preferred both for strictly technical reasons and because of the personnel habit of using graphical interfaces (Macintosh and Windows). Powersoft Power Builder object oriented development system was also used.
In the following some critical aspects are pointed out.

Data share
As already stated [1], the principal function of a patient centred information system is the communication of information. To provide this fundamental added value, sharing a common data base is the most effective solution. Two aspectsneeded to be considered:

1- many typically divisional data had no interest for other physicians, while the outcome that the specialist draws from the data is the information needed. The efforts to achieve uniform data structure among units are often out of proportion to the potential benefits.
It seemed opportune to discriminate between public and divisional information, defining as "public" all that concerns:

- patient identification and demographic data
- anamnesis (updated, along the several contacts of the patient , with new events, and diagnosis and therapy for hospitalisation)
- outcomes

and "divisional"That which is used or collected for clinical, organisational or scientific aim of each division or unit in a division.

2- some areas, for example laboratories, often use specific software, with particular file management, and historical deepness of the archives depending only on the workload.
The only link to a clinical information system is the patient identifier. Interfacement, more then integration, may be convenient.

The system we are setting up is mainly an aggregation of integrated modules with few interfacements (with transfer into the common database of the data) to laboratory packages purchased from different vendors.

Data completeness and reliability
A patient's clinical history is written by different people in distinct moments. It is useful only if it is complete and reliable.
To achieve completeness we have carried out the following steps:

1- attribution of an event to a patient is accomplished only by personnel who either has the elements to discriminate among namesakes, or works on scheduled (pre identified) patients.

2- carrying out automatic processes to maintain the basic structures of the patient history

3- data input: up to now, generally, data are first written on paper form, and afterwards transferred to a computer. In our Centre no clerical worker is devoted to clinical data entry, with the exception of the radiology service. People, independently from the professional role, input data and information that they have personally collected or elaborated upon, and that will be at least personally useful in order to complete or more effectually perform their assigned work [2,3].

To achieve reliability, the fact that each one has to input , or at least to sign, his or her own data may be a good assurance. This can be strengthened through the use of the inputted data shortly afterwards.

Strategies of capabilities assignment are needed as in any other information system.

Interface and system behaviour
Competition with a consolidated and often well fitting daily practice and patient data organisation is sometimes difficult.
The interface and system behaviour are critical sides of the system, as regards both data entry and dialogue for information retrieval.

Two extreme, typical scenarios:
- the management of events whose frequency is high, and in which the involved information is typically predefined
- the data investigation following a free schema aimed to extemporary problems

Within the powerful and user-friendly Windows environment we have adopted, task orientation through accelerators to directly point to optimised paths has been preferred for the first case. For the second one, free navigation through the time scale and the different data structures (public and divisional) has proved to be suitable.
Moreover, other benefits in terms of usableness came from :
- designing data input screens as similar as possible to the paper form used to collect data previously.
- facilitating item selection from long lists partitioning it into a suitable number of subtypes, on the bases of both a generally accepted affinity criteria and frequency of use.
- making intensive usage of drop down list boxes.
In accordance with [4] dialogue features are: error tolerance, auto-explication, and user controllability.

Automation planning
A hospital is an aggregation of mainly data suppliers (laboratories, services) and data users (wards, clinical units); each one strictly bound to the others.
The more automation can proceed side by side, the stronger the impact and effectiveness may be. Moreover, in our opinion as in [5] , carrying out basic procedures for many users is to be preferred, especially in the early stage, postponing the additional specific options.

Software life cycle
Exhaustive interviews and group discussions on data flow diagrams with users often were not sufficient to learingall the user recording activities and the information requirements. Prototyping and subsequent use for a real patient sample are necessary tools to make users focus the system real behaviour, and evaluate the achievement of the aims.

HEMODIALYSIS SUBSYSTEM

Context
Generally , a patient arrives at the hemodialysis unit after, at least, one hospitalisation and subsequent discharge, and keeps on being subjected to hemodialytic therapy,on average, three times a week, until transplant or other events occurs. From that time on, the patient is charged to the physicians of the unit for any clinical problem.

Dialytic population is divided into 4 groups, as 2 shift of sessions a day are performed. Nurses, technicians and physicians work on shifts respectively to administer the 4-hour dialytic therapy and manage the patients, to prepare the machines, to evaluate patient state, and consequently balance the treatment.

Mainly nurses are interested in what may happen during a session, while the physician looks at several sessions, together with lab tests, to draw a trend and to produce, monthly, a synthesis.

All the other clinical problems that may arise are worked out concurrently. Often hospitalisation and other events occur during the dialytic life of a patient.

The system
According to the discrimination stated above, the patient is known to the system , and the following information are available to the physician accepting the patient inside the unit:

private data: name, date of birth, address, etc.

anamnesis: it is composed of
- the history told by the patient himself at the admission to the ward
- the reason for the hospitalisation
- the diagnosis and the therapy at the discharge from the ward (this is due to the fact that the outcome of an hospitalisation is necessary the anamnestic connection for any following contact)

outcomes: typically textual reports of diagnostic test and data from lab tests collected during the hospitalisation

Divisional data (in this case ward data) such as hospitalisation length, particular classifications of the patient, etc. are not generally available .

Within the unit other departmental information is needed (mainly structured):

patient-bound: - clinical, such as specific coded diagnosis, risk factors, vascular access, etc.
- aimed to patient management such as shift, conveyance, etc.

pharmacological and substitutive treatment-bound: types of treatment, characteristic of treatment as filter, optimal session duration , dry weight, therapy, etc.

While the first group of information is quite steady, the treatment-bound ones are variable and have historical value.

Once the treatment is started, session-bound information, treatment changes, and lab tests continue to be collected . This is the information core on which the patient care is performed.

For each session the patient's sheet is printed (fig.1). It is composed of two sections.

The right one (B) refers to the current session and represents the data collection form. Shaded fields are the ones subjected to input by an identical mask. It is used by the nurse to record physiological parameters such as blood pressure, weight, heart rate, symptoms (at every hour of the session), and technical information such as types of the needles used and the presence of difficulties connected to the vascular access, etc. The session sheet is used by the physician too (during rounds), to notify treatment changes and the need of extemporary controls. As physicians, and also nurses, alternate in taking care of the patient, continuity must be assured.

The bottom most part of (B) is aimed at communication of clinical notes: the last recorded ones are listed to let anyone know the recent past conditions and to make the patient realise that his situation is under control, independently from the person whom he has spoken with.

The left section (A) refers to the previous 6 sessions

(A)

Date	LUN 25.04		MER 27.04		VEN 29.04		LUN 02.05		MER 04.05		VEN 06.05	
Real sess. length	5:00		4:30		4:00		4:30		4:30		5:00	
Dry weight	58.0		58.0		58.0		58.0		58.0		58.0	
Excess from dry weight	3.0	OK	2.0	OK	3.0	0.5	4.0	OK	2.5	1.0	4.0	OK
	Start	End	Start	End	Start	End	Start	End	Start	End	Start	End
BA	120/80	110/70	100/80	90/70	120/80	100/70	140/90	120/70	120/80	120/80	140/100	120/80
HR	70	60	100	80	80	80	90	70	80	80	90	70
QB	300	300	300	300	300	300	300	300	300	300	300	300
Access	AA16		AA16		AA16		AA16		AA16		AA16	
Hypotension			3									
Collapse					3;4							
Cramp			1									
Hypertension												
Praecord.												
Arrhythmia							1;5				3	
Short QB												
Shudders/Temp												
Other events												
Notes												

Current Session Program

Session Therapy. Last review date : 03.12.1993

Epo2000 scx3 - Rocefin 1g

Therapy in progress. Last review date: 03.12.1993

Nitrodur 20cm - INSULINA - ROCEFIN 1 gr.

Type of dialytic treatment. Last review date: 29.09.1993

Tipo dialisi : Bicarbonato Bagno : Softpac S 195 + Bicart
Filtro : Gambro Lundia Alpha 500 K : 1.5 Ca : 1.75 Na : 140 HCO3 : 34
Infusato : Portata (l/h) :

Characteristic of treatment. Last review date : 30.11.1993

Eparinizzaz. cont. - Unità/h : 900 per ore : 4.5 QB attac.(ml/min) : 150 Peso secco teorico : 58
Calo orario Max. (Kg) : 0.7 Durata teor. (h) : 4.5 N° sedute sett. : 3

(B)

Fondazione Clinica del Lavoro - Divisione di Nefrologia ed Emodialisi - Prof. A. Salvadeo

Centre Pavia via Boezio Shift : MON-WED-FRI morning Session : Regolare Ambulatoriale

CHIARA ERMINIA - 09.05.1994 Monitor n° : 10

	Start time : 7.30	1 hour	2hour	3 hour	4 hour	5 hour	End Time : 11.55
Weight	62	61.3	60.8	60	59.2		58.3
BP	110/80	110/80	100/75	100/70	110/70	/	100/70
HR	70	80	70	65	70		65
Ven.Press. Shortage	130		120		120		
QB	250						250
Events*		A			B		

(*) I = Hypotension K = Collapse C = Cramp H = Hypertension S = Praecord. A = Arrhythmia F = Short QB B = Shudders/Temp. E = Other events

ACCESS : Single needle [M] Needles [AA16] Catheter [C] Single needle next time [ ]

Reason for difficult access

Reason for treatment interruption Reason for post dialysis hospitalisation

Program Performed Programming Urgent tests [E]

Notes

[N]

Summary of last session clinical notes

29.04 Asthenia from a week. Ht going down
02.05 Suspicious feverish event
04.05 Rheumatologic examination. Bodily therapy

Feverish in the weekend

Treatment changings

Ca; 2.0

Nurse Physician Sheet 7

Fig. 1 : Session sheet.

and to the present type and characteristics of the treatment. It is used mainly by nurses to compare the present session course with the previous ones, in terms of parameter values, occurrence of symptoms and access modality and by the physician to balance substitutive treatment and therapy on the basis of the previous weeks. The inspection of the recorded data 2 days after the input, has resulted in a certain amount of corrections.

Automatic order entries for lab tests are available. The data from laboratories come back to be merged together with other information specifying the particular circumstance in which withdrawal has been performed (i.e. pre or post dialysis). Periodical evaluation of data draws to a textual synthesis automatically updating the patient anamnestic history.

Output/added value

For nurses:

- faced with the input of at most 22 data pointsper patient (meanly a 2 minute per patient operation in a task oriented manner), on the left side (A) of the session sheet as described above. Before system installation they used a pamphlet from which, among all the other information, they extracted what they needed out
- order entries and labels for test tubes
- worksheets for the machine management
- administrative reports.

For physicians:

- faced with a variable data entry, depending on the patient conditions, predefined analytical flowsheets and composite synthetical documents are produced. Free navigation lets physicians investigate all the other public and departmental information to support them in evaluations and making decisions
- population selections on the basis of condition matching both on (up to now) a few departmental structured information, and on lab tests.
- other outputs aimed at routine procedures.

CONCLUSION

Routinely usage of the system over a one year period has shown:

- within unit integration is a necessary condition to attain the minimum usableness level . Most the personnel used the system even before laboratory interfacements were in place.
- between unit integration represents an unavoidable step to prevent from dangerous, partially manual and partially automated, compromise solutions that could bring back to a fragmentary situation.
- tuning of the system on the real needs underlying a consolidated daily practice is obtainable only through the real usage of the system and assiduous frequentation of the clinical units. Session sheet composition and layout have been modified many times to let personnel use it as the only tool to carry out session activities.
- when data input continuity is mandatory, time relief in routine activities may become a sufficient condition to assure data completeness. Nurses , whom most of the daily input effort is charged to, do not complain of being overburdened.

Moreover, as the development of the entire system is on going , we remember that a focus on achieving a high level of usableness may force us to spend time for improvements that are not sometimes proportionally appreciated.

REFERENCES

[1]. Howard L. Bleich, Warner V. Slack. Designing a hospital information system: a comparison of interfaced and integrated systems. Yearbook of Medical Informatics, 1993.

[2]. K. E. Campbell, K. Wieckert, L. M. Fagan, M.A. Musen. A computer-based tool for Generation of Progress Notes. Proceedings of the Seventeenth Annual Symposium on Computer Applications in Medical Care. (pp. 284-288).

[3]. P.D. Clayton, G.E. Pulver, C.L. Hill. Physician use of computers: Is age or value the predominant factor?. Proceedings of the Seventeenth Annual Symposium on Computer Applications in Medical Care. (pp. 301-305).

[4]. M.F. Sanz, E.J. Gomez, I. trueba, P. Cano, M.T. Arredondo, F. del Pozo. A Pen-Based System to Support Pre-Operative Data Collection Within an Anaesthesia Department. Proceedings of the Seventeenth Annual Symposium on Computer Applications in Medical Care. (pp. 321-325).

[5]. N.K. Roderer, A.C. Long, P.D. Clayton. IAIMS at Columbia-Presbyterian Medical Center : accomplishments and challenges. Yearbook of Medical Informatics, 1993.

[6]. R.S. Pressman. Software Engineering: A Practitioner's Approach - Second Edition. McGraw-Hill, Inc. New York,1989.

[7]. P. Coad, E. Yourdon. Object - Oriented Analysis Second Edition. Prentice Hall, Inc. New Jersey, USA, 1991.

PAGES 663 THROUGH 668
WERE DELIBERATELY LEFT BLANK.

Section VI

Support for Clinical Decision Making

Approaches to Development of Clinical Expert Systems

A Case-Based Assistant for Clinical Psychiatry Expertise.

Isabelle Bichindaritz

Université René Descartes
UFR de mathématiques et informatique
LIAP-5
45 rue des Saints-pères
75006 Paris, France
tél : (+33) 1 44 55 35 63
email : bici@math-info.univ-paris5.fr

Université René Descartes
Faculté de Médecine Cochin-Port Royal
Hôpital Sainte-Anne, CMME
service of professor Samuel-Lajeunesse
100 rue de la santé
75014 Paris, France

Abstract. *Case-based reasoning is an artificial intelligence methodology for the processing of empirical knowledge. Recent case-based reasoning systems also use theoretic knowledge about the domain to constrain the case-based reasoning. The organization of the memory is the key issue in case-based reasoning. The case-based assistant presented here has two structures in memory : cases and concepts. These memory structures permit it to be as skilled in problem-solving tasks, such as diagnosis and treatment planning, as in interpretive tasks, such as clinical research. A prototype applied to clinical work about eating disorders in psychiatry, reasoning from the alimentary questionnaires of these patients, is presented as an example of the system abilities.*

1 INTRODUCTION

Case-based reasoning proposes an artificial intelligence methodology for the processing of empirical knowledge. By definition, a case is a set of empirical data. It may often be presented to the system as an instance of a certain type or concept, in problem-solving as well as in classification. The mainspring of case-based reasoning is to use one or several already met cases to process a new case. The processing of a new case may belong to an analysis task, such as solving a diagnostic problem [1] or planning [2], or to a synthesis task, such as concept learning [3].

A case-based reasoning system uses a knowledge-base containing a set of previously met cases, which is enriched each time a new case is processed. The case knowledge-base is similar to a memory. Reasoning involves organizing this memory to make possible the comparison of a new case with the numerous memorized cases. An indexed memory is partitioned by means of indexes, which are the elements of the cases representation retained as significant regarding the task to realize.

Moreover, case-based reasoning systems permit to build knowledge-bases automatically by case-based learning. This learning process may be conducted through the guidance of an expert, such as in [1], or unsupervised.

In the system presented here, the memory structures are twofold. First, cases represent specific, contextualized experiences, and second concepts represent general knowledge. The problem of the evolution of the structures from the accumulation of numerous cases to the incremental concept learning is the key problem addressed in this paper. This memory organization gives the system the ability to perform, in a unified framework, analytic tasks, such as diagnosis or treatment planning, and synthesis tasks such as assistance to clinical research.

The motivation for this work is that clinical expertise is not uniform. On the contrary, it assumes, for the same clinician, many skills, such as diagnosis, therapy and research.. So these facets must not be conceived as separated, but as the result of the growth, thru experience, of a unique competence, presented here as the discerning organization of the memory.

The second section presents important issues in case-based reasoning, such as its emergence and its evolution. The third section studies the case-based reasoning tasks addressed here. The fourth section deals with the memory organization. The fifth section proposes the example of a prototype for the system that studies the alimentary questionnaires of eating disordered patients. Finally, the sixth section brings out the conclusion.

2 CASE-BASED REASONING EVOLUTION

2.1 Emergence

The original research on case-based reasoning emerged from work in natural language understanding. Schank proposed a knowledge representation, scripts [4], and a memory organization, memory-organization packets or MOPs [5], allowing to known parts of the texts to understand to be efficiently retrieved. Later, the organization of the knowledge in a structured network, with high-level and low-level knowledge, appeared, jointly with the ability to learn. The design of memories to learn, such as GBM [6], aimed at the acquisition of knowledge from textual data, and were implementations as faithful as possible to the theory of dynamic memory [5]. They were followed by the first case-based reasoning systems, and progressively applied to the various tasks they presently cover.

2.2 Evolution

Later, researchers in case-based reasoning realized the importance of using a model of the domain to constrain the reasoning process. Some researchers proposed that ossified cases and paradigmatic cases should be integrated to the memory [7]. Others used case-based reasoning to short-cut a causal model of heart-failure disease [8]. Yet others used a causal physio-pathological model to constrain the case-based reasoning [9]. This model simulates the expert's reasoning, and is a heuristic guiding the case-based reasoning, which is the central process performed by the system. Case-based and model-based reasoning systems complement each other well, partly because of the type of knowledge representation they share : large chunks of knowledge rather than fragmented parts as rule-based reasoning systems [10].

In weak-theory domains, such as psychiatry, case-based reasoning is a main reasoning, and can give results where model-based and rule-based reasoning systems cannot be constructed. Moreover, a case-based reasoner can also use case-based reasoning as a heuristic. The system presented here, as most case-based reasoning systems, operates in a weak-theory domain. It differs from the systems presented above by the variety of the types of tasks it performs : analytic tasks such as diagnostic problem solving or treatment planning, and synthesis tasks such as concept learning. Concept learning is an assistance for clinical research, by facilitating the formulation of research hypotheses.

3 CASE-BASED REASONING TASKS

3.1 Analysis tasks

A task can be defined by an input space, a processing, often involving several steps, and a solutions' space. An analytic task is characterized by a limited solutions' space. Diagnoses for instance are solutions to the diagnostic problem, which are well-known by the clinician. Treatment planning, when the number of possibilities for each elementary treatment and for their combinations, is not too important, can be considered as an analytic task, as well as most problem-solving tasks. Furthermore case-based reasoning provides a means of transforming non analytic tasks into analytic tasks, by choosing among a set of previously solved cases, and of adaptation and combination heuristics.

Analytic tasks take advantage of the domain knowledge. When it is incomplete, ambiguous, or fastidious, case-based reasoning can perform such tasks advantageously.

3.2 Synthesis tasks

A synthesis task is a task the solutions' space of which is potentially unlimited. Most interpretive tasks, dealing with the interpretation of data, are synthesis tasks. In particular, clinical research is a synthesis task : among the numerous possible interpretations of clinical data, some must be chosen and studied. One of the aspects of clinical research this system focuses on is concept learning. Concept learning is a learning task that groups a set of empirical descriptions of instances in classes also called concepts [11]. Each concept has a particular characterization, generally expressed by a set of attributes, with numerical or symbolical values, and by relations between these attributes. Moreover, the concepts are organized in a hierarchy. More formally [12]:

1. Given: a set I of instances to be presented sequentially, and their descriptions $d_i : I = \{ d_i \}$;
2. Find: conceptual classes C_j that group those instances in categories ;
3. Find: an intentional definition for each category that characterizes the class D_j ;
4. Find a hierarchy H that organizes these classes.

An incremental concept learning system incorporates new instances one at a time to the concepts learnt from the previously processed instances. A good example of these systems is COBWEB [13]. It was then improved in CLASSIT [12].

Case-based systems, which are inherently incremental, are naturally adapted to this kind of concept learning. UNIMEM [3] is a case-based reasoning system for incremental concept learning. In the hierarchy it builds, each concept is linked to more general concepts by generalization links, and to less general ones by specialization links. New cases can be classified in several concepts at a time, giving that concepts can be added, modified or deleted after a time.

All the incremental concept learning systems presented so far are unsupervised. They don't take advantage of domain knowledge, either in knowledge bases, or in experts.

PROTOS [1], an exemplar-based classifier, is a supervised concept learning system. The main difference with the preceding systems is that it learns the categories it uses from the expert, and cannot learn new categories from the examples.

Nevertheless, PROTOS organization of cases and concepts are grounded on psychological research about concepts. For [14], concepts are organized around theories : only theories, and the structure they provide, can give concepts a cohesion, through explanations, possibly combining several levels of abstraction. Thus, the search for concepts cohesion is an important quality criterion for an incremental concept learning system.

3.3 Architecture

The reasoning process passes through several steps, which are the same for analysis and synthesis tasks :

1. The interpretation of the new case input data in order to determine potential indexes ;
2. The identification and retrieval of memorized cases, candidates to the processing of the new case : potential candidates are selected for their proximity to the new case, according to a certain *point of view*, filtering the significant description elements ;
3. The establishing of relations of correspondence between the potential candidates and the new case ; generally, these relations are quantified by a matching score, measuring the similarity between cases : this step leads to the selection of the best candidate, also called the best analogue ; it can be a memorized case or concept ;
4. The knowledge transfer from the best analogue to the new case, eventually including the adaptation of the memorized process of the best analogue ;

5. The explanation of the adaptation : it builds explanations from all the knowledge it possesses, that contained in the domain model, available from the beginning, and that in the indexed memory of cases ; this explanation process is detailed in [15] ;
6. The updating of the memory : if the modifications of the concepts are judged significant enough, the memory is updated, and the new case is stored under the modified concepts.

An important detail is that here, a candidate is a concept ; but it can also be a case if the match is closer. It then leads to the generation of a new concept.

In this system, the reasoning process is guided by a model of the domain, as in 2.2. Its role is to constrain the reasoning process whenever it is sensible, as can be seen on the schema of the architecture of the system (Figure 1).

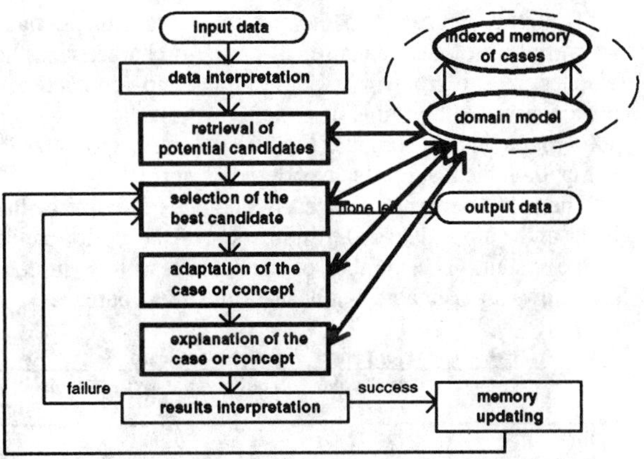

Figure 1. Schema of the architecture of the system.

The most important difference with a classical case-based reasoning system is in the adaptation step. The system adds to the regular adaptation step of case-based reasoning systems, an explanation step.

4 ORGANIZATION OF THE MEMORY

The organization of the memory is close to that of GBM [6]. Cases are sets of <attribute, value> pairs. Concepts are sets of quadruplets <attribute, value, positive counter, negative counter>. They are organized in a hierarchy, where the nodes are concepts. Each node is linked to the more general nodes above it in the hierarchy, and to the more specialized nodes under it, as well as cases directly indexed under it.

Each new case presented to the system entails, during the search through the memory, the updating of all concepts sharing enough <attribute, value> pairs with the new case. If the difference (positive counter - negative counter) goes down under a certain threshold (a parameter of the system), the corresponding attribute is withdrawn from the concept. If a concept has no attribute left, it is withdrawn. At the same time, if the new case shares enough <attribute, value> pairs with a concept, new generalizations, and new concepts, may be created. A generalization is constituted with all the common <attribute, value> pairs of the cases or concepts that are indexed under it. A concept is a generalization and the explanation generated for it. So, whenever a new case is processed, all related memorized concepts are updated, some eventually suppressed, and new concepts are sought for.

The organization of the memory has been improved, in particular for dealing with the problem of the dependence of concepts upon the order of presentation of instances. In this application, the small number of cases makes it compulsory to remedy for this situation. The search for the closest cases in memory, and for the concepts to which they belong, leads to the adaptation of the concept hierarchy so that the closest cases fall under the same concepts. This change permits to recover from hazardous concept formations.

Thus the classification obtained is dynamic, which meets an objective of ability to evolve. The threshold parameter permits to adapt the fineness of the classification. The usefulness of the classification is addressed by the model of the domain through the explanations provided for each concept : concepts are enriched with knowledge shared by all sub-concepts and cases depending on them. Besides, the explanation of the concepts also meets the objective of cohesion of the concepts.

So the memory is a dynamic memory containing both general concepts and specific cases.

5 PROTOTYPE EXAMPLE

5.1 Presentation

Psychiatry is a complex real-world domain, and a weak-theory one. In such domains, case-based reasoning is an advantageous AI methodology provided that cases are available [10]. In the eating-disorders' domain of psychiatry, the *Clinique des Maladies Mentales et de l'Encéphale* is a service active in clinical research, with well-documented patients' cases.

The aim of the system is to assist clinical expertise in the service, by learning thru experience [17]. The prototype presented in this section is applied to the study of the alimentary questionnaires of 61 in-patients. It proposes, for each new case presented to it, a diagnosis, a treatment plan, and at the same time, updates the concepts already in memory, thus serving clinical research.

5.2 Cases

The patients are 31 restrictive anorexics and 30 bulimic anorexics (according to the DSM-III-R criteria [16]). In this system, a case is a patient alimentary questionnaire, filled by the patient him or herself ; it is composed of a list of 232 foods, and 3 types of response per food :

1. The appreciation of the food by the patient, which can range between 3 values : "I appreciate it", "I'm indifferent to it" and "It disgusts me", respectively coded "1", "2" and "3" ;
2. The avoidance of the food by the patient, which can take the values "I avoid it", or "I don't avoid it", coded "0" and "1" ;
3. The reason of the possible avoidance of the food by the patient: it consists of one or two sentences hand-

written by the patient, such as "Too much fat.", "I don't eat meat.", "It makes me feel sick.". The reasons of avoidance are coded into 22 values ranging from "1" to "22" (in particular "9" means "fat", and "7" means "calories").

An example of a case is the following :

```
<Apricot-appreciation, 2>
<Apricot-avoidance, 1>
<Sausage-appreciation, 3>
<Sausage-avoidance, 0>
<Sausage-reason, 9>
<Banana-appreciation, 3>
<Banana-avoidance, 0>
<Banana-reason, 7> ...
```

The cases in memory are not all pathological. The case-base is composed of 61 patients' cases, and 36 control cases (see [5] for a discussion of the importance of the control case-base).

Another type of knowledge in memory is theoretical knowledge about foods. In this prototype, it represents the description of 572 foods, including alimentary category, composition in 35 elements such as water, mineral salts, vitamins ..., and aspect. The representation of a food takes the form <attribute, numerical value, qualitative value>, where qualitative value may take 5 values ranging from "very low" to "very high". For example, the food *low fat fish* is represented that way :

```
<calories, 112.0, very-low>
<water, 70.0, high>
<proteins, 24.0, very-high>
<plant-proteins, 0.0, very-low>
<animal-proteins, 24.0, very-high>
<glucides, 0.0, very-low> ...
```

5.3 Clinical problem-solving

The two clinical problems studied are diagnosis and treatment planning.

Here, the best analogue case serves as a model for solving the new case. Its diagnosis is proposed for the new case, and the treatment planning it had is also proposed for the new case. Concerning the alimentary questionnaires, the treatment planning is the list and sequence of the foods to be reintroduced. It is adapted to the new patient because not all the foods avoided are the same between the patients. Moreover, the order of reintroduction in the memorized case was elaborated with the patient after sometimes several hours of discussions with the clinicians. This order is a consensus between the patient and the clinicians, and is carefully prepared.

An example of this reasoning is the following :

```
The most similar patient in memory is
Ms MMM. This patient is a restrictive
anorexic, so I propose this diagnosis for
 the new patient Mrs XXX.

Important differences I have noted are
that the patient XXX appreciates more
kinds of meat (chicken and turkey) than
Ms MMM, which should make the treatment
less difficult.

The foods reintroduction I propose is:

1st week : salmon,
           veal,
           white rice
           orange.
2nd week : lamb,
           pasta,
           chocolate ...
```

5.4 Clinical research

Eating disorders are severe mental diseases, most of the time long-lasting, if not ever-lasting. The diagnosis is stated by simply matching the DSM-III-R criteria. A difficulty in diagnosis is that the diagnostic categories change over the life-time, and often several times, so that it is more exact to speak about the dominant symptomatology at a given time. This diagnostic instability leads to question the foundations of the diagnostic categories. Thus, it is an interesting subject to study the differences related to food choices, if any, between the diagnostic sub-groups.

The study must group the patients according to their answers to the questionnaire, in order to characterize the diagnostic sub-groups, to determine and characterize homogeneous sub-groups of patients within the diagnostic sub-groups, and to compare them to a control group of 36 non-pathological subjects considered as normal.

The results are summarized if Table 1 : the size of the input and output data is an indication of the performance of the system. The number of concepts learnt is limited, and shows a reasonable synthesis of the questionnaires.

Table 1. Performances of the concept learning.

	restrictive anorexics	bulimic anorexics	control subjects
Number of subjects	31	30	36
Number of concepts	52	55	30
Index size	2458	2528	1746

An example of a concept learnt, grouping 19 restrictive anorexics, is the following :

```
<prawn-appreciation, 1, 19, 2>
<tripes-appreciation, 3, 20, 1>
<potted-mince-appreciation, 3, 21, 2>
<dry-sausage-appreciation, 3, 21, 2>
<bacon-appreciation, 3, 22, 1>
<French-beans-appreciation, 1 , 28, 1>
<courgette-appreciation, 1, 30, 1>
<low-fat-fish-appreciation, 1, 31, 0>
<milk-chocolate-avoidance, 0, 25, 1>
<French-fries-avoidance, 0, 25, 1>
```

It is the eighth larger concept learnt from the restrictive anorexics with number of patients regrouped (19 of 31).

A short form of the explanations generated by the system contains the following elements :

```
The foods appreciated share :
   <calories, very-low>
   <water, high>
   <glucides, very-low>
   <lipids, very-low>
   <magnesium, very-high>
   <potassium, high>
   <lipids, very-low>
   <vitamin-B6, normal> ...

They are also appreciated by the control
subjects, in the same proportion for {French-
```

```
beans,courgette,low-fat-fish},    but   in   a
higher proportion (90%) for {prawn}.
They can be separated in 2 sub-groups, with:
group 1 = {prawn, low-fat-fish}
   <proteins, very-high>
   <sodium, high>
   <cholesterol, very-high>
   <phosphorus, very-high> ...
group 2 = {French-beans, courgette}
   <proteins, very-low>
   <sodium, very-low>
   <cholesterol, very-low>
   <phosphorus, very-low> ...
The foods in disgust share : ...
```

The content of the results is interesting for the application domain. It was found that the hierarchy constructed for the restrictive anorexics is very different from that of the bulimic anorexics, and that the two pathological hierarchies are very different from the control one. For instance, the simplest result is that the restrictive anorexics all appreciate and don't avoid low-fat fish, and only that food, and the system gave an explanation for this: low-fat fish is rich in animal proteins, and very poor in lipids and glucides : it is an optimized choice for a restrictive person. As for the bulimic anorexics, the food appreciated by 27 of them is melon, for which interesting explanations were proposed.

Subgroups were more complex, but it was found that the explanations given by the system permitted to characterize them in a meaningful way for the expert clinicians. The evaluation of the discrepancies and the similarities between the pathological subjects, and the control ones is an interesting measure of psychopathology.

6 CONCLUSION

The system presented here is a case-based assistant for clinical psychiatry expertise.

As recent case-based reasoning systems, it uses domain knowledge to guide the reasoning process. In a domain such as psychiatry, where empirical knowledge, by the study of control and patients' cases, is as important as theoretical knowledge, both types of knowledge are essential to the reasoning process.

The organization of the memory including two structures in close interrelationships, cases and concepts, gives the system a double ability : for problem-solving tasks, which are essentially analytic tasks, such as diagnosis and treatment planning, and for interpretative tasks, which are essentially synthetic tasks, such as assisting the formulation of hypotheses for clinical research.

The prototype presented is currently enriched with the numerous other data collected from the patients : biological, behavioural, psychological and anamnestic, and comparisons with other formalization methodologies, statistical or data analytic, traditionally used in the domain, is also a present topic of research.

Acknowledgments

I would like to thank professor Samuel-Lajeunesse, doctor Mirabel-Sarron (M.D.) and Magali Volery (dietician) for sharing ideas and work in eating disorders research.

References

[1] Ray Bareiss, *Exemplar-Based Knowledge Acquisition.* Academic Press Inc., San Diego, California, (1989).

[2] Kristian J. Hammond, 'Case-Based Planning : A Framework for Planning from Experience'. *Cognitive Science* 14, 385-443, (1990).

[3] Michael Lebowitz, 'Experiments with Incremental Concept Formation : UNIMEM'. *Machine Learning,* vol. 2, 103-308, (1987).

[4] Roger C. Schank and R.P. Abelson, *Scripts, Plans, Goals and Understanding.* Lawrence Erlbaum Associates, Hillsdale, New Jersey, (1977).

[5] Roger C. Schank, *Dynamic Memory : a Theory of Learning in Computers and People.* Cambridge University Press, (1982).

[6] Michael Lebowitz, 'Concept learning in a rich input domain.' In : *Machine Learning : An Artificial Intelligence Approach*, Volume II. R.S. Michalski, J.G. Carbonell, T.M. Mitchell, Morgan Kaufmann Publishers, Inc., Los Altos, California, 193-214, (1986).

[7] Christopher K. Riesbeck and Roger C. Schank, *Inside Case-based Reasoning.* Lawrence Erlbaum Associates, Hillsdale, New Jersey, (1989).

[8] Phyllis Koton, 'Reasoning about Evidence in Causal Explanations'. In : *Proceedings of the American Association for Artificial Intelligence*, 256-261, (1988).

[9] Isabelle Bichindaritz and Brigitte Séroussi, 'Contraindre l'analogie par la causalité'. *Technique et Sciences Informatiques*, volume 11, N° 4, 69-98, (1992).

[10] Janet L. Kolodner, *Case-Based Reasoning*, Morgan Kaufmann Publishers, Inc., San Mateo, CA, (1993).

[11] André Thaysé et al., *Approche logique de l'intelligence artificielle*, Tome 4. Dunod informatique, Paris, (1992).

[12] John H. Gennari, Pat Langley and Doug Fisher, 'Models of Incremental Concept Formation', *Artificial Intelligence* 40, 11-61, (1989).

[13] Douglas H. Fisher, 'Knowledge Acquisition Via Incremental Conceptual Clustering', *Machine Learning* 2, 139-172, (1987).

[14] Douglas L. Medin, 'Concepts and Conceptual Structure'. *American Psychologist*, Vol. 44, N° 12, 1469-1481, (1989).

[15] Isabelle Bichindaritz, 'A Case-Based Reasoning System Using a Control Case-Base', *European Conference in Artificial Intelligence*, Amsterdam, 38-42,(1994).

[16] American Psychiatric Association., *Diagnostic and statistical manual of mental disorders, Third Edition, Revised (DSM-III-R)*, American Psychiatric Association, Washington DC, (1987).

[17] Janet L. Kolodner and Robert M. Kolodner, 'Using Experience in Clinical Problem Solving: Introduction and Framework', *IEEE Transactions on Systems, Man, and Cybernetics*, Vol. SMC-17, N°. 3, 420-431, (1987).

XNEOr: Development and Evaluation of an Expert System to Improve the Quality and Cost of Decision-Making in Neuro-Oncology

Bernard L. Maria, M.D., Ferose A. Lambay, Douglas Dankel II, Ph.D., Sharma Chakravarthy, Ph.D., Suleyman Tufekci, Ph.D., Robert Marcus, M.D., Amos Kedar, M.D., University of Florida, Gainesville, FL.

The treatment of brain tumors requires a large team of medical experts. However, the process of medical decision-making for these patients is hampered by the frequent inaccessibility of the experts because of conflicting scheduling, inconsistencies in the management of different patients, and the fact that multiple experts often yield multiple opinions. The goals of this work were (1) to develop and validate an expert system to assist the medical team deliver efficient, quality care to children with recurrent medulloblastoma, a common type of pediatric brain tumor, and (2) to determine if the expert system can be used as an educational tool. The results of our study indicate that residents enjoy learning by using XNEOr, the brain tumor expert system. XNEOr enabled residents to order appropriate ancillary tests for patients and to make fewer incorrect treatment decisions. The potential net effect of residents using XNEOr may be increased patient and family satisfaction and decreased probability of medical liability. At a time of important changes in our health care system, novel expert systems hold promise as tools to reduce medical costs, improve the quality of multi-expert medical care, and advance health care education.

INTRODUCTION

The management of brain tumors is complex because of the required involvement of specialists from multiple medical disciplines including neurosurgery, neurology, radiation oncology, hematology-oncology, neuropsychology, and rehabilitation medicine [1]. This complexity has lead some to claim that pediatric brain tumors cannot be approached algorithmically [2]. However, advances in computer and information technology can provide physicians and other allied health professionals with expert systems that transform complex clinical knowledge into efficient management and educational tools [3,4]. Medulloblastoma is one of the most common brain tumors in the pediatric age group [5]. The tumor produces symptoms such as headache, nausea and vomiting, and gait imbalance. Magnetic resonance imaging (MRI) of the brain provides valuable information on the tumor's size and degree of involvement of the brain. Once the tumor is detected with MRI, the patient undergoes an operation to remove as much of the tumor as possible. Because of the propensity of medulloblastoma to grow back (recur) following surgery alone, the patient is then treated with radiotherapy and chemotherapy. The medical team meets to develop a proposed treatment plan that is established based on the risk that the tumor will recur and the risk that therapy will produce unacceptable side effects. The risk that a medulloblastoma will recur can be estimated by considering a variety of factors including tumor size, extent of brain involvement, degree of spread in the spinal fluid spaces, and extent of the surgical resection. Brain tumor referral centers including the one at the University of Florida hold multi-expert conferences and clinics to develop comprehensive treatment options for patients.

The multi-expert decision-making process in brain tumor referral centers is costly, time consuming, and complicated by the following factors: (1) experts are often inaccessible owing to conflicting scheduling, (2) junior members of the team are reluctant to propose management strategies because of the presence of more senior physicians, the so-called "upward ripple paranoia", (3) management decisions in patients with similar clinical risk factors are not consistent over time, and (4) multiple experts often yield multiple opinions. In addition, physicians in residency training are in need of educational tools that capture the decision-making skills of multiple experts.

The absence of a system to develop truly cohesive and consistent management strategies for patients can reduce the quality of care and increase medical costs. Uncertainties about patient management can increase the number of unnecessary ancillary tests ordered by residents. Moreover, the risk of medical liability increases for physicians making less than optimal patient management decisions. We designed *XNEOr*, an expert system that corrects many inefficiencies in managing children with brain tumors.

Previous Work

During the past decade, medical expert systems have been developed for diagnosis (INTERNIST-1/CADUCEUS, NEUROLOGIST-1, NEUREX, ANGY, CENTAUR), diagnosis and therapy (MYCIN, CASNET/GLAUCOMA, EMERGE, IRIS, ARAMIS), and monitoring and therapy (BABY, ANNA, MED-1, ONCOCIN) [6-19]. Most of these expert systems were engineered from single medical domains such as neurology, oncology, and pediatrics.

We previously developed and tested a radiation oncology expert system (single medical domain), *XNEOn*, for managing patients with newly-diagnosed medulloblastoma [20]. We asked the following question: can *XNEOn* be designed to correctly select radiation treatment doses, fractions and volumes for patients with newly-diagnosed medulloblastoma? Knowledge was extracted from radiation oncologists and represented in decision rules in the expert system shell *Exsys Pro*. *XNEOn* was tested for accurate decision-making in 11 hypothetical clinical cases. *XNEOn* found the correct treatment plan in 9 cases (82%). In two cases, the rules had been constructed incorrectly in that they specified radiation treatment for all patients at diagnosis, including infants (which can produce untoward effects on the developing brain of the infant). Success with the modified version of *XNEOn* motivated the development of *XNEOr* for recurrent medulloblastoma, a significantly more complex clinical problem. We used an incremental approach to building *XNEOr* because there is considerably more uncertainty about the value of various combinations of surgery, radiotherapy and chemotherapy than for newly-diagnosed medulloblastoma. We modularized the knowledge representation to provide users of the new system with a good explanation facility and interface in managing patients.

System Development

XNEOr was developed by using several of the classical stages of software engineering including specification, conceptualization, formalization, prototyping, implementation, validation and verification, and modification. Knowledge acquisition and representation was intricate: firstly, several independent decision trees were designed for each treatment modality; secondly, the detailed knowledge extracted from each of the experts was coalesced and modeled into extensive flow charts, and integrated into 92 decision rules (production rule format) with 30 optimal treatment solutions. During the initial development stages, the clinical decision trees were modified frequently by the experts. The final design has two levels in the depth of the knowledge within the decision trees. The first level provides for the correct selection of the treatment modalities (surgery, radiotherapy, chemotherapy) and the second level enables the user to select a detailed radiation plan including radiation dose, fraction size, treatment schedule, and treatment volume. In addition, *XNEOr* is designed to provide an explanation to the user of why a particular treatment is selected. For example, if the user of *XNEOr* selects the treatment modality "radiotherapy" in a very young child, *XNEOr* will specify that children younger than three years of age should not be given radiotherapy because of the risks of injuring the developing nervous system.

The following clinical case illustrates an interaction with *XNEOr*. A two and one half year old girl was diagnosed with medulloblastoma and the tumor was surgically removed. She was then treated with chemotherapy without complications for 12 months. The chemotherapy was discontinued at that time since there was no evidence of residual tumor. At five years of age, she has developed headache, weakness and vomiting. MRI of the brain shows a 3 cm recurrent medulloblastoma in the cerebellum. MRI of the spine is normal. The spinal tap is positive for tumor cells. The 111 Indium CSF study is normal. The family is eager to carry on with any therapy recommended by the team of medical experts. In this example, all the *XNEOr* prompts and output are shown in plain type, the resident's input in **bold**, and comments about the interaction are shown in the parentheses:

• Enter the age of the patient in months:
60 months (the patient is 5 years old at the time of tumor recurrence)...
• Is the tumor symptomatic or asymptomatic ?
Symptomatic (headache, vomiting and weakness)...

• Was there any prior radiation ?
No (because of the child's young age at diagnosis, radiotherapy was not administered; she had received chemotherapy)...
• Is this recurrence localized or disseminated?
Disseminated (MRI of spine is negative but spinal tap shows the presence of tumor cells)...
• Is there gross spinal disease ?
No (MRI of spine is negative)...
• How was the previous chemotherapy tolerated?
Good tolerance...
• Is the 111 Indium CSF study normal?
Yes...
• Are there any socio-economic factors or other factors that preclude additional therapy?
No...

The output of the system is given as follows: Give radiation therapy (NOTE: Give cranio-spinal irradiation (CSI) with boost to any gross metastatic disease with standard dose comprising of CSI : 2500 to 3600 cGy, posterior fossa : 5500 cGy; No Neurosurgery (NOTE: Since the disease is disseminated, neurosurgery is not recommended); Consider intrathecal chemotherapy via an Ommaya Reservoir.

Validation and Verification

Ten hypothetical clinical cases of recurrent medulloblastoma were prepared by one of the co-authors (BLM) who is knowledgeable about this disease and its clinical manifestations. The hypothetical patients had a broad range of symptoms, physical examination findings and laboratory results so as to reflect the diversity of clinical manifestations of medulloblastoma. The same 10 cases were then executed on *XNEOr* and the experts determined that *XNEOr*'s treatment selections (levels I and II) were correct in the 10 cases.

Five of eight radiation oncology residents familiar with the workings of the multidisciplinary brain tumor group of experts at the University of Florida were randomly selected for participation in the study comparing their performance in managing the 10 cases with and without the aid of *XNEOr*. All five residents consented to participate. They were instructed to request as few or as many tests as necessary to prescribe a correct overall treatment plan (level I) and the correct radiation treatment parameters (level II), when appropriate. They were asked to be cost effective and to order only those ancillary tests required to prepare a treatment plan.

Each resident studied the 10 cases independently. In each case, the resident ordered tests to formulate a treatment plan. The experts had pre-determined what tests were required for correct treatment decisions. When an appropriate test was ordered by the resident, the results of the test were provided by the examiner. When an unnecessary test was ordered, the residents were told that the results were pending. The residents were unaware of whether the results of pending tests would be provided to them during the interaction. The residents were then asked whether the patient should have surgery, radiotherapy and chemotherapy. When radiotherapy was selected, the radiation oncology residents were asked to provide details on radiation dose, schedule, fraction size and volume. After specifying overall management and treatment decisions in all 10 cases, each resident then conducted an interactive consultation with *XNEOr* on the same 10 cases. In all, 50 independent trials were conducted by the five residents with 10 trials each. The radiation treatment decisions were reviewed by an expert radiation oncologist amongst the authorship (RM) and scored as (C) correct and agrees with *XNEOr*, (I) incorrect but still within acceptable standards of radiation oncology care, (D) dangerous or serious, and (L) potentially life-threatening. We then determined (1) if the correct treatment modalities (surgery, radiotherapy, chemotherapy) were selected, (2) if the correct radiation dose, schedule, fraction and volume were selected, (3) if the appropriate medical tests were ordered, and (4) how the residents rated their interactions with *XNEOr*.

RESULTS

Before using *XNEOr*, the residents collectively ordered a total of 46 unnecessary tests including computed tomograms of the head, complete bone scans, bone marrow aspirations, and single photon emission computed tomographies. The residents failed to order a total of 59 tests required for decision-making including lumbar punctures for analysis of the cerebrospinal fluid and MRI.

The residents correctly selected all three treatment modalities of surgery, radiotherapy and chemotherapy in 32 ± 7% (95% CI = 18-46%) of cases (Table 1). They selected the correct radiation dose, schedule, fraction and volume in 50 ± 7% (95% CI = 22-78%) of cases (Table 2); 28 ± 4% of the radiation oncology residents radiation treatment decisions were scored as dangerous or life-threatening by the radiation oncology expert.

With *XNEOr*, the residents ordered the appropriate tests and selected the correct therapy in 100% of cases tested. Five of five residents said they would use *XNEOr* for learning and in their future clinical practice (Table 3). One of the five residents rated the explanation facility of *XNEOr* as fair and requested that literature citations be used to support underlying decision-rules. One of the five residents had considerable *a priori* experience with advanced user interfaces. This resident rated the user interface as "fair".

Table1. Overall Treatment Decisions.

Subject No.	*3 of 3*	*2 of 3*	*1 of 3*
1	0.4	0.4	0.2
2	0.3	0.3	0.4
3	0.3	0.6	0.1
4	0.3	0.3	0.4
5	0.3	0.6	0.1
Mean	0.32	0.44	0.24
Sample SD	0.05	0.067	0.078
Binomial SD	0.07	0.07	0.06
95% CI	18,46	30,38	12,36
Std. error	3%	3%	3%

Table 2. Radiation Treatment Decisions.

Subject No.	*C*	*I*	*D*	*L*
1	0.6	0.2	0.1	0.1
2	0.4	0.4	0.2	0
3	0.4	0.1	0.5	0
4	0.4	0.2	0.4	0
5	0.7	0.2	0.1	0
Mean	0.5	0.22	0.26	0.02
Sample SD	0.06	0.049	0.08	0.02
Binomial SD	0.07	0.044	0.06	0.02
95% CI	22,78	12,32	10,42	0,6
Std. error	3.13%	2.20%	3.60%	1%

Table 3. Feedback on use of *XNEOr*.

Criteria	1	2	3	4	5
Use in Practice	yes	yes	yes	yes	yes
Explanations	ok	ok	ok	good	fair
User Interface	ok	ok	good	fair	good
Tutoring	good	good	good	ok	good

DISCUSSION

Diagnostic reasoning is used in many areas including debugging software programs, fault localization in electronic circuits, and automobile engine failure. Medical diagnostics uses abductive inferencing as a problem-solving methodology. A diagnostician identifies one or more significant diseases that may cause a subset of symptoms by associating causal relationships. If a set of symptoms and clinical findings (manifestations) suggests increased intracranial pressure in a child (headache, vomiting, weakness), a physician identifies, through hypothesis generation, a set of diseases (differential diagnosis) that can account for the manifestations. Then, certain laboratory tests including an MRI of the head will be ordered to more clearly define the underlying problem. The results of this study suggest that, while complex, pediatric brain tumors can be approached algorithmically and their management can be modeled in rule-based expert systems.

Patients with medulloblastoma must have access to more than one medical expert to receive quality care. Medical decision-making in such patients is complex and time-consuming. We developed *XNEOr,* an intricate rule-based expert system that improves the efficiency of decision-making by residents in children with recurrent medulloblastoma. While the data presented on evaluation of *XNEOr* in five residents must be considered preliminary, the system may offer important cost-savings. *XNEOr* may potentially (1) reduce the time required by residents or primary care providers to interact with multiple experts, (2) reduce the number of inappropriate laboratory tests ordered, and (3) reduce the variability (and cost variance) in the assessment and treatment of patients. In building *XNEOr*, we captured the skills and heuristics of professionals in neurosurgery, radiation oncology, and hematology/oncology. Thus, *XNEOr* may be a valuable educational resource in other institutions and centers where residents are learning to evaluate and treat children with brain tumors.

XNEOr will need regular updating, validation and verification. We will research how changes in the medical management of medulloblastoma can be incorporated into *XNEOr* in a cost effective manner. We will need to determine if residents learn from*XNEOr* and if the system has limitations in handling an even broader range of clinical cases. Our experience in designing *XNEOr* would suggest that expert systems using production rules and an algorithmic approach can mimic complex decision-making involving multiple experts.

Future Research

Many current database applications in engineering, manufacturing, communications and medicine demand some reasoning in their processing activities. There is an explicit need to provide a database management system (DBMS) to store data and manage the *XNEOn* and *XNEOr* expert systems. However, such applications require more sophisticated control mechanisms than simple value matching. Conventional DBMS fail to meet the requirements of the brain tumor domain because they are passive in nature whereas our expert systems require database support to react to a variety of situations defined over the state of the system and specific events that demand immediate actions. Thus, Active Databases may therefore be required to provide support to our expert systems.

In conclusion, expert systems like *XNEOr* will undoubtedly benefit patients by enhancing the management of brain tumors. The potential net effect of *XNEOr* may be increased patient and family satisfaction, increased empowerement of health care professionals, and decreased probability of medical liability. At a time of important changes in our health care system, novel expert systems that confront the challenges of multi-expert decision-making hold promise as tools to reduce costs, improve the quality of care, and advance health care education.

References

[1] S.J. Barrer, L. Schut, L. N. Sutton and D.A. Bruce. Re-operation for recurrent brain tumors in children. Child's Brain, 11:375-386, 1984.

[2] M.E. Cohen. Why a Neuro-oncologist?. Journal of Child Neurolcgy, 8:287-290, October,1993.

[3] P. Krause, J. Fox, M. O'Neil and A. Glowinski. Can we formally specify a medical decision support system?. IEEE Expert, pp. 56-60, June 1993.

[4] P.R. Schloeffel. A personal computer database system for head and cancer records. Journal of Medical Systems, 12(1): 43-55, 1983.

[5] F.H. Tomlinson, B.W. Scheithauer, F.B. Meyer, W.A. Smithson, E.G. Shaw, G.M. Miller and R.V. Groover. Medulloblastoma I: Clinical, Diagnostic and Therapeutic Overview. Journal of Child Neurology, 7:142-155, April 1992.

[6] H.E. Pople, Jr. Knowledge-based expert systems: the buy or build decision. W. Reitman (editor) Artificial Intelligence Applications for Business, Norwood, N.J.: Ablex, 1984.

[7] Z. Xiang, S.N. Srihari, S.C. Shapiro and J.G. Chutkow. Analogical and propositional representations of structure in neurological diagnosis. Proceedings of the First Conference on Artificial Intelligence Applications, IEEE Computer Society, December 1984.

[8] J.A. Reggia. A production rule system for neurological localization. Proceedings of the Second Annual Symposium on Computer Applications in Medical Care, IEEE, November 1978.

[9] S.A. Stansfield. ANGY: a rule-based expert system for identifying and isolating coronary vessels in digital angiograms. Proceedings of the First Conference on Artificial Intelligence Applications, IEEE Computer Society, December 1984.

[10] J.S. Aikins. Prototypical knowledge for expert systems. Artificial Intelligence, 20:163-210, 1983.

[11] E.H. Shortliffe. Computer-based medical consultations: MYCIN. New York: Elsevier, 1976.

[12] S.M. Weiss and C.A. Kulikowski, Saul Amarel and Aran Safir. A model-based method for computer aided medical decision-making. Artificial Intelligence, 11:145-172, 1978.

[13] D.L. Hudson and M.E. Cohen. EMERGE: a rule-based clinical decision-making aid. Proceedings of the First Conference on Artificial Intelligence Applications, IEEE Computer Society, December 1984.

[14] M. Trigoboff and C.A. Kulikowski. IRIS: a system for the propagation of inferences in a semantic net. Proceedings IJCAI-77, pp.274-280, 1977.

[15] J.F. Fries and D. McShane. ARAMIS: a national chronic disease data bank system. Proceedings of the Third Annual Symposium on Computer Applications in Medical Care, IEEE, pp. 798-801, 1979.

[16] L.E. Rodewald. BABY: an expert system for patient monitoring in a newborn intensive care unit. M.S. thesis, Computer Science Dept., University of Illinois, Champaign-Urbana, 1984.

[17] H. Silverman. A digitalis therapy advisor. MIT Technical Report TR-143, December 1974.

[18] F. Puppe and B. Puppe. Overview on MED1: a heuristic diagnosis system with an efficient control structure. Report SEKI-83-02. Fachbereich Informatik, Universitat Kaiserslautern, West Germany, 1983.

[19] E.H. Shortliffe, A.C. Scott, M.B. Bischoff, A.B. Campbell, W. van Melle and C.D. Jacobs. ONCOCIN: an expert system for oncology protocol management. Proceedings IJCAI-81, pp. 876-881, 1981.

[20] B.L. Maria, F.A. Lambay, S. Chakravarthy, D.D. Dankel II, S.Tufekci, N. Mendenhall and W.R. Lee. *XNEOn* : a diagnostic expert system for pediatric neuro-oncology. Proceedings of the Fourth International Conference on Management of Technology, IIE, University of Miami, February 1994.

[21] F.A. Lambay. Management of Recurrent Brain Tumors: Using an Artificial Intelligence Approach. M.S. thesis, Industrial and Systems Engineering Dept., University of Florida, Gainesville, Florida, 1994.

Computerized Detection of Nosocomial Infections in Newborns

Beatriz H.S.C. Rocha [1], M.D.; John C. Christenson [1,2], M.D., FAAP;
Andrew Pavia [1,2], M.D.; R. Scott Evans [1,3], Ph.D.; Reed M. Gardner [1,3], Ph.D.
(1) University of Utah, Salt Lake City, UT 84112
(2) Primary Children's Medical Center, Salt Lake City, UT 84112
(3) LDS Hospital, Salt Lake City, UT 84143

Hospital-acquired infections are responsible for an increase in patient mortality and costs. Their detection is essential to permit better infection control. We developed an expert system specifically to detect infections in pediatric patients. The expert system is implemented at LDS Hospital that has a level three newborn intensive care unit and well baby units. We describe how the knowledge base of the expert system was developed, implemented, and validated in a retrospective study. The results of the system were compared to manual reviewer results. The expert system had a sensitivity of 84.5% and specificity of 92.8% in detecting hospital-acquired infections when compared to a physician reviewer. The Cohen's kappa between the expert system and the physician reviewer was 0.62 (p<.001).

INTRODUCTION

Hospital-acquired infections (HAIs) are a major health problem nowadays [1]. They are responsible for increased mortality and costs [2,3]. HAIs are a leading cause of death in the United States, responsible for at least 30,000 deaths each year [2,3]. Furthermore, HAIs cause an increase in the length of hospital stay by 5 to 10 days. The cost to treat HAIs in the USA has been estimated to be between 5 and 10 billion dollars annually [2].

The detection of HAIs is essential for enabling prompt treatment, reduce transmission, and enabling preventive interventions. The current detection methods usually involve manual surveillance that is not only time consuming and expensive, but typically produces results only after the patient is discharged. The ideal detection system would detect the infection immediately after the patient had any positive results indicating an infection. Such an early detection system would permit earlier interventions and could potentially reduce the morbidity and mortality of the disease.

Computers have been used to speed up the infection detection process [4-7]. One successful example of an automated surveillance is the Computerized Infectious Disease Monitor (CIDM) [4,5]. CIDM was designed to detect HAIs primarily in adult patients. However, to our knowledge, little work has been done in the area of pediatrics to improve the detection of HAIs using a computer.

Based on our group's previous experience, we developed an expert system to detect HAIs in pediatric patients. The system is currently implemented at LDS Hospital, Salt Lake City, Utah. LDS Hospital is a tertiary care hospital with a level three (most severe) newborn intensive care unit and well baby units.

Our goal was to determine if an expert system using Boolean logic could improve the detection of HAIs in the pediatric patients. We developed a rule-based expert system and tested its performance in a retrospective study against the newborn patient data stored in the hospital database for a period of two years. In the following sections, we describe the development of the expert system's knowledge base, its implementation, and its validation.

METHODS

The development of the expert system can be divided in three main phases: development of the knowledge base, its implementation, and validation.

Development of the Knowledge Base

The first step in the development of our expert system was the medical knowledge acquisition to create the knowledge base (KB) to detect HAIs. This knowledge was acquired through medical knowledge engineering sessions [8].

Medical knowledge acquisition was necessary to create the rules for detection of HAIs. Review of published literature [9,10] and experts' experience were fundamental in the knowledge acquisition process. During the knowledge acquisition process, the principal author interacted with experts in the field of pediatric infectious disease to acquire the knowledge necessary to build the system. The principal author and two medical experts adapted published rules for detecting hospital-acquired infections to a pediatric setting, and created new rules when necessary.

The rules for detect patients with hospital-acquired infections were developed through knowledge engineering sessions over a period of two years which involved over 100 hours of interaction. During these knowledge engineering meetings, methods of detecting and managing the infections were also discussed. These sessions were of one hour duration and were audio taped. After each meeting, the knowledge obtained was organized into Boolean rules by one of the authors (BHSCR). At the beginning of each knowledge engineering session, the rules from the previous session were presented and reviewed. Corrections and additions were made and then a new infectious disease topic was discussed. From these knowledge engineering sessions, 154 rules were created.

These rules obtained during the knowledge acquisition form the knowledge base of our computerized expert system. Examples of rules used in the expert system are shown in Figure 1.

Figure 1: Two examples of the rules in the knowledge base

If there is a positive blood culture for Escherichia coli, ***then*** give an alert for definite bacteremia.
If there is a positive tracheal aspirate culture for Enterococcus, ***then*** give an alert for possible lower respiratory infection.

Implementation of the Knowledge Base

After the knowledge engineering process, the second phase of the project was to implement the knowledge base. The knowledge base was developed in frames using the programming language PAL (PTXT Application Language), that was developed in house. The HELP (Health Evaluation through Logical Processing) Hospital Information System (HIS) was the platform used for the development of the expert system [11,12]. HELP is a comprehensive HIS with clinical modules, such as, pharmacy, laboratory, radiology, etc.. All information is stored in an integrated patient database in a coded format. This clinical database is continuously available. The HELP system also has a long term patient database, which contains clinical information stored for the past ten years.

The HELP system has the ability to be both "data" and "time" driven. "Data" driven is the capability of the HELP system to activate the expert system frames each time data required by the system's knowledge base is stored in the patient database. For example, every time a positive microbiology culture result is stored in the patient database, the expert system is activated and determines if the patient has an infection. Examples of the types of data that activate the expert system are positive microbiology culture results, cerebral spinal fluid (CSF) study results, and bacterial antigen detection assays results. "Time" driven is a capability of HELP system that activates the knowledge base at specific times. For example, a program to print the reports with the results for the infectious disease department is "time" driven and activated once each day at 1:00 PM.

Figure 2, is a block diagram schematic showing how the expert system is implemented. As soon as the microbiology results or other results are available, they are entered in the hospital's laboratory computer system. This computer immediately transfers the coded results to the HELP patient database, where they are stored. When the data is stored in the patient database, the program to detect HAIs is automatically "data" driven. Using the rules in its knowledge base, the system determines if the patient has an infection. Positive results generated by the expert system are called alerts. When an alert is generated, it is immediately stored in an alert file. From this file, the alerts can be printed as a report, or presented on a bedside terminal. The whole process just described takes less than five minutes.

There are three types of alerts for HAIs: definite, probable, or possible infections. A "definite" alert means that there is a 100% chance that the patient has an infection. For example, a positive cerebral spinal fluid culture for Neisseria meningitidis would be a "definite" infection. "Probable" alert means that there is about a 75% chance, or in other words, a high probability that the patient has an infection. For example, a positive antigen detection in stool specimen for Rotavirus would be a "probable" infection. A "possible" alert means that there is about a 50% chance that the patient has an infection, for example, one positive tracheal aspirate culture for Aspergillus would indicate a "possible" infection. Each infection is also classified as hospital-acquired or not, depending on when the infection was detected.

Our expert system was developed to detect eight common types of hospital-acquired infections. These are bacteremia, central nervous system infections, conjunctivitis, diarrhea, lower respiratory tract infections, surgical or wound infections, urinary tract infections, and viral infections.

The rules of the expert system were improved by analyzing the data for all newborn patients, who were in LDS Hospital for a 20 months period (Jan. 92 to Aug. 93). The expert system determined if the patient had an infection or not. The results produced by the expert system were reviewed by the knowledge engineers and necessary corrections or modifications to the rules were done in this phase.

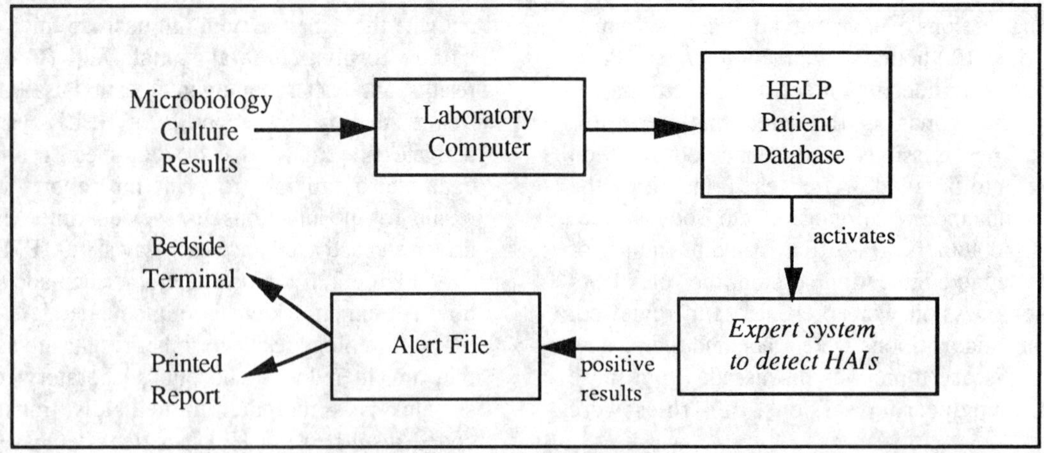

Figure 2: System functioning

Validation of the Knowledge Base

Finally, to validate the KB of the expert system and to test our hypothesis - that an expert system was able to detect HAIs in pediatric patients - we tested the expert system against a different set of patients. The system analyzed the data of all newborn patients in the hospital between Jan. 90 and Dec. 91 (24 months).

One physician expert in pediatric infectious diseases (AP), reviewed only the patients with some information that might indicate an infection and that was used by the expert system's knowledge base. This consisted of all patients with a positive microbiology culture result, with cerebral spinal fluid (CSF) study results, and with bacterial antigen detection assays results. The reviewing physician did not know the rules used by the knowledge base. He estimated the chance of the patient having an infection, as "definite", "probable", "possible", or "no infection", without knowing the results generated by the computer. The results produced by the manual reviewer were compared to the results produced by the expert system. The physician reviewer was considered to be the "gold-standard".

RESULTS

The expert system analyzed all newborns admitted to the LDS Hospital for the 24 months, period from January of 1990 through December of 1991. The positive and negative results, as well as the data and rules used to reach these results, were stored in a computer file. The number of newborn patients admitted to the hospital during this period was 5,201 (Table 1). For these patients, the computer system was activated 605 times; 514 were activated by positive microbiology cultures and 91 for CSF analysis results. Since the information of the CSF analysis was not complete in the database for this period of time, it could not be analyzed. Therefore, the results produced by the expert system and the physician reviewer for CSF analysis are not reported in this study. During this period, 92 alerts were generated (by positive microbiology cultures), which corresponds to 17.9% of the total number of times the system was triggered by microbiology results (Table 1).

Table 1: Population analyzed

• Total of patients admitted: 5,201
• No. of times the expert system was activated: 605 - by positive microbiology cultures: 514 - by CSF analysis: 91
• Number of alerts generated by microbiology cultures: 92 (17.9 %)

The results produced by the expert system and the physician reviewer are presented in Table 2 and Table 3. Classifying alerts by type, there were 13 alerts for "definite" infections, 15 alerts for "probable" infections, and 64 alerts for "possible" infections generated by the expert system (Table 2). The most common alert generated by the expert system was "possible" conjunctivitis infection, issued 35 times (Table 3). The physician reviewer classification

Table 2: Number of alerts generated by the expert system (ES) and physician reviewer (MD).

		MD				
		definite	probable	possible	no inf.	total
ES	def.	13	0	0	0	13
	prob.	8	5	2	0	15
	poss.	0	2	30	32	64
	no inf.	0	1	10	411	422
	total	21	8	42	443	514

	Definite inf.		Probable inf.		Possible inf.		Total	
	ES	MD	ES	MD	ES	MD	ES	MD
bacteremia	13	18	7	1	7	9	27	28
lower respiratory tract infection	0	1	4	3	14	19	18	23
central nervous system infection	0	2	2	0	3	3	5	5
urinary tract infection	0	0	0	0	4	7	4	7
surgical or wound infection	0	0	1	2	1	0	2	2
conjunctivitis	0	0	1	2	35	4	36	6
Total	13	21	15	8	64	42	92	71

Table 3: Number of alerts by type of infection generated by the expert system (ES) and physician reviewer (MD).

generated 21 "definite" infections, 8 "probable" infections, and 42 "possible" infections (Table 2).

The results comparing the expert system to the physician reviewer ("gold standard") are presented in Table 4. To create the contingency table, the "definite", "probable" and "possible" classifications were considered to be a positive infection and the classification "no infection" was considered to be a no infection. The sensitivity of the expert system was 84.5% and the specificity was 92.8%.

Table 4: Contingency table comparing expert system to physician reviewer

True positive rate:	84.5 % (sensitivity)
False negative rate:	15.5 %
False positive rate:	7.2 %
True negative rate:	92.8 % (specificity)

The Cohen's kappa (coefficient of agreement) [13] between the alerts given by the expert system and the physician reviewer's classification was 0.62 (p<.001). Agreement occurred when the physician reviewer gave the same classification ("definite", "probable", "possible", or "no infection") as the expert system did.

DISCUSSION

The main difference when comparing our expert system with the existent ones [4-7], was that our system was specifically developed to detect HAIs in pediatric patients. Other systems were developed to do HAIs surveillance in populations composed primarily of adults, applying the same rules when a pediatric patient was encountered. Pediatric patients are different from other age groups. They have very specific types of infections requiring specific rules to detect them. Another difference was that our system was developed not only to detect infections based on positive cultures, but also give alerts for other types of exams, such as cerebral spinal fluid chemical analysis.

Our expert system when tested with newborns patients had performance similar to other expert systems [4-6] in sensitivity and specificity. Overall, the expert system had a good sensitivity and a high specificity. The system was unable to detect only 11 infections identified by the physician reviewer. There was only one "probable" infection and 10 "possible" infections undetected. This number is less than three percent of all the times the system was activated. These false negatives were spread among the different types of infections. We plan to improve the expert systems' performance in this area by adding new rules to the knowledge base, and by correcting some of the existing ones. Some inappropriate alerts were generated, but in a very reasonable amount. There were 32 false positive alerts and all of them were generated by the same rule used in the detection of "possible" conjunctivitis. Correction to this rule would avoid all false positives. In general, the rules developed were able to detect infections very well.

Other expert systems classify only if an infection is present or not [4-6]. However, an infection can be present in different degrees of probability. For example, a positive CSF culture result for Enterococcus is definitely an infection, while a positive tracheal aspirate culture for Bacillus cereus may or may not be an infection. The capability of the expert system to classify the infections as "definite", "probable", or "possible" is very useful. This feature is very helpful when reviewing the results and analyzing the patient data. Normally, physicians and nurses reason with a certain degree of uncertainty, and these classifications can help them in their reasoning. The presence or absence of an infection is not always clear, and these classifications can help the user interpreting the alert.

The comparison between the physician reviewer ("gold standard") and the expert system resulted in a significant Cohen's kappa of 0.62, meaning that there was good agreement between the two. The physician reviewer agreed with all 13 "definite alerts" given by the expert system. The system proved to be sensitive and highly specific for these infections. None of the "definite" infections according to the physician reviewer were classified as "no infection" by the expert system. The infections classified as "definite" by the physician reviewer, and that were not classified as "definite" infection by the expert system, were classified as "probable" infections by the computer.

There was a lower agreement for both the "probable" and "possible" infections. The physician reviewer disagreed with the results of two rules to detect "probable" infections (one for bacteremia and one for central nervous system infection), and considered all these infections to be "definite" infections as discussed above. The great majority of disagreements for the "possible" infections were caused by one rule, the one that caused all the false positives. With changes in the two "probable" rules and removal of the "possible" rule that caused the problems, the Cohen's kappa would increase to 0.84. The agreement for "no infections" was very high, showing that the false negatives were small. This characteristic is important since the false negatives should be avoided in the case of an infection.

From these results, it seems possible for an expert system to help with the surveillance and detection of hospital-acquired infections in newborns. Despite these good results, the system needs to be tested in a prospective study. We plan to verify its performance and effect in daily use. The expert system is currently operational at LDS Hospital and will soon be implemented at Primary Children's Medical Center, Salt Lake City, Utah. We plan to do a prospective study during which the results of the expert system will be compared with the manual surveillance done by the Infectious Control Nurses. The system will also be tested for other age groups (older children) that were not available at LDS Hospital. If the system proves to be successful, the effect of the alerts on physicians behavior will be tested. We plan to present the alerts directly to the attending physician through bedside terminals. We want to determine if giving the alerts directly to the attending physicians, can reduce the time to intervention and reduce the morbidity and mortality of the infection.

Acknowledgment

Beatriz H.S.C. Rocha is supported by a scholarship from the National Council for Scientific and Technological Development (CNPq), Secretary for Science and Technology, Brazil.

Reference

1. Haley RW, Culver DH, White JW, Morgan WM, Emori TG. The nationwide Nosocomial Infection Rate - A new need for vital statistics. American J of Epidemiology 1985; 121(2):159-167.

2. Wenzel RP, Streed SA. Surveillance and use of computers in hospital infection control. J of Hospital Infection 1989; 13:217-229.

3. Gentry LO. Future developments in nosocomial infections: the perspective in the United States. J of Hospital Infection 1990; 15 Suppl A:3-12.

4. Evans RS, Gardner RM, Bush AR, Burke JP, Jacobson JA, Larsen RA, Meier FA, Warner HR. Development of a Computerized Infectious Disease Monitor (CIDM). Computers and Biomedical Research 1985; 18:103-113.

5. Evans RS, Larsen RA, Burke JP, Gardner RM, Meier FA, Jacobson JA, Conti MT, Jacobson JT, Hulse RK. Computer Surveillance of Hospital-Acquired Infections and Antibiotic Use. JAMA 1986; 256(8):1007-1011.

6. Kahn MG, Steib SA, Fraser VJ, Dunagan WC. An Expert System for Culture-Based Infection Control Surveillance. Proceedings of Seventeenth Annual Symposium on Computer Applications in Medical Care 1993; 171-175.

7. Mertens R, Jans B, Kurz X. A Computerized Nationwide Network for Nosocomial Infection Surveillance in Belgium. Infection Control and Hospital Epidemiology 1994; 15(3):171-179.

8. McGraw KL, Harbison-Briggs K. Knowledge acquisition: Principles and Guidelines. Englewood Cliffs, New Jersey: Prentice-Hall, 1989.

9. Garner JS, Jarvis WR, Emori TG, Horan TC, Hughes JM. CDC definitions for nosocomial infections, 1988. American J of Infection Control 1988; 16(3):128-140.

10. The SENIC Project. Appendix E. Algorithms for diagnosing infections. American J of Epidemiology 1980; 111(5):635-643.

11. Pryor TA, Gardner RM, Clayton PD, Warner HR. The HELP System. J of Medical Systems 1983; 7(2):87-102.

12. Kuperman GJ, Gardner RM, Pryor TA. HELP: A Dynamic Hospital Information System. Springer-Verlag, 1991.

13. Cohen J. A coefficient of agreement for nominal scales. Educational and Psychological Measurement 1960; 20(1):37-46.

Instantiating and Monitoring Treatment Protocols

Serdar Uckun, MD, PhD

Rockwell International Science Center

444 High St., Palo Alto, CA 94301

ABSTRACT

This paper presents a system for protocol-based treatment planning, plan execution, and execution monitoring. The approach, named SPIN, is developed as a component of the Guardian system. Guardian is an experimental architecture for intelligent patient monitoring and control. The paper describes and illustrates SPIN in a clinical scenario.

1. INTRODUCTION

Protocol-based treatment plays a major role in critical care and emergency care. Since crisis situations are commonly encountered and are often associated with time pressure in these environments, there is usually no time for inventive thinking or decision making based on first principles. In a crisis situation, protocol-based treatment can ensure that all possible actions are considered by the clinician no matter how chaotic the situation. Examples are protocols for Advanced Cardiac Life Support (ACLS) [1] and anesthesia crisis management [2].

We are developing an intelligent agent architecture for patient monitoring and control applications named Guardian [3]. Guardian is designed to perform a variety of reasoning tasks in a critical care environment. These tasks range from data reduction and abstraction to higher-level cognitive skills such as diagnosis and therapy management. We recently developed a new therapy management component for Guardian which takes advantage of readily available treatment protocols by instantiating and executing skeletal treatment plans. In this article, we describe the method in detail, exemplify its use in a clinical scenario, and discuss the strengths and weaknesses of the representation and the execution framework.

2. METHODS

Our approach to therapy management is named SPIN, for **S**keletal **P**lan **In**stantiation. In this approach, we define a *skeletal plan* as a hierarchical plan which outlines *all* management options for a given disorder. Each skeletal plan is recursively composed of finer-granularity plans. A hierarchy of plans terminates at actions which represent basic management steps. Skeletal plans and actions are instantiated at runtime according to the current context (i.e., patient status and the internal state of the agent). Instantiation involves parameterization of actions and all execution decisions including branching. Figure 1 shows a conceptual hierarchy of treatment plans which may be individualized as a skeletal plan in SPIN.

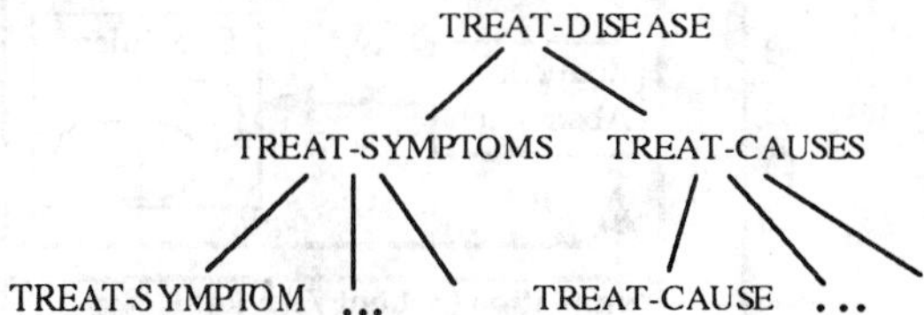

Figure 1. A conceptual hierarchy of treatment plans and actions.

2.1. Architecture

SPIN is a component of Guardian. However, rather than discussing Guardian in detail, we identify the functional requirements of a sufficient software environment for SPIN:

- A facility for continuous real-time monitoring of physical and physiological parameters, and abstraction and interpretation of these parameters into concepts such as clinical signs and diseases.
- A cache for all active plans and actions.
- An event-driven scheduler for plan execution monitoring (the "events" in question are either observations or changes in the status of active plans and actions).
- Another scheduler (ideally, with faster cycle time) for closed-loop control of actions.
- Three temporal databases to record interpreted values and planning activities (one timeline each for observations, intentions, and expectations).

Figure 2 illustrates the Guardian architecture from the perspective of planning skills.

2.2. Control Schemas

Each plan controls and monitors the execution of all its constituent plans and actions based on a control sentence named *control schema* (see Table 1). Plans are executed under the provision that control is local and hierarchical; that is, each plan can only control the execution of subplans and actions declared in a hierarchy rooted at that plan.

The simple syntax of the control schema is surprisingly powerful in capturing various orderings of actions and subplans under a master treatment plan. Further control on the execution of individual subplans and actions is exerted recursively by subplans and actions themselves.

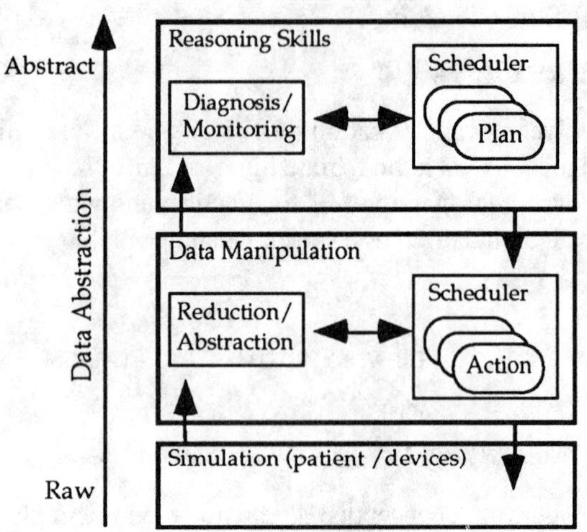

Figure 2. Planning in Guardian.

```
EXP ::= (op [plan|action|EXP]+)
op ::= execute | one-of | all-of

plan: pointer to another plan
action: pointer to another action
execute: all subsequent plans, actions, and
expressions are to be executed in the pro-
vided sequence.
one-of: only one of the listed plans, ac-
tions, or expressions is to be instantiated
(in order of preference).
all-of: all plans, actions, or expressions
in this phrase are to be instantiated si-
multaneously.
```

Table 1. Syntax and semantics of control schemas.

2.3. Local Control of Plans and Actions

Each plan and action has three attributes which have Lisp expressions as their values. These expressions query the temporal database in order to assess whether certain conditions hold. The results of expression evaluation trigger state transitions for plans and actions.

- preconditions specify the conditions under which a plan or action can be executed. Preconditions are evaluated when a plan or action is in *standby* state; successful evaluation results in a transition to *active* state.
- goal-conditions specify the situations under which a plan or action may be terminated successfully. Thus, goal-conditions are only evaluated for active plans or actions. When evaluation is successful, a state transition to the *terminated* state takes place.
- discontinuation-conditions are conditions under which an active plan or action should be aborted before its goal conditions are satisfied. When these conditions hold, an active plan or action transitions to *discontinued* state.

Any state transition in a subplan causes its parent plan to transition to a *modified* state. Any plan which is in *modified* state reevaluates its control schema. This is how SPIN steps through active plans and performs plan execution monitoring.

2.4. Action Execution

The Guardian architecture supports two kinds of actions: support actions in the form of recommendations to the user, or closed-loop control actions[1]. In other to equip an action with closed-loop control capability, two additional attributes need to be declared:

- dosage-function: a Lisp function which returns the new value of a controlled parameter based on current readings of related parameters.
- control-interval: specifies the period of the control loop, that is, how frequently the dosage-function should be reevaluated.

Three types of actions are possible in the closed-loop mode: actions that execute only once (e.g., one-time administration of a drug), actions that execute periodically (e.g., periodic administration of a drug), and continuous actions (e.g., controlling an infusion pump or O_2 administration). These categories only differ in the way they are handled by the action controller.

The action controller maintains a list of all active closed-loop actions. At each cycle (typically once every few seconds), the controller evaluates any action due for reevaluation based on its control-interval. Unless the goal-conditions or the discontinuation-conditions of a scheduled action is satisfied, the controller executes the dosage-function and propagates any prescribed changes to therapy parameters. If the action is terminated or discontinued, all active plans that relate to this action are notified. Subsequently, control schemas of all related plans are reevaluated.

3. MISMATCH RECOGNITION

SPIN does not make the assumptions that actions will be performed as requested, or that actions and plans will always result in desired or expected effects. Instead, it monitors the execution of plans and senses

[1]Guardian is a proof-of-concept system which currently works on a simulated patient. We realize that significant issues such as legal aspects and safety have to be challenged and resolved before closed-loop control of therapy could become a reality in critical care.

any divergence from intentions and expectations and records its findings on three parallel timelines.

Information posted on the *observed* timeline includes actual parameter readings, values of clinical signs and symptoms, diagnostic hypotheses, and status information on treatment plans and actions. Intentions are the desired goals of treatment plans, and are posted on the *intended* timeline when a plan is activated. As one might expect, however, complete satisfaction of intentions is not a realistic expectation for every treatment plan. Some plans serve to remedy the adverse conditions slightly but cannot provide full recovery; others have significant side effects. Therefore, we record the expected effects of an activated plan in the *expected* timeline. The expectations of a plan are the sum of all expectations posted by its constituent actions. Figure 3 illustrates possible time courses of observations, intentions, and expectations for a hypothetical case of myocardial infarction. In this example, neither the treatment produce its expected results nor the intentions of the plan are realized. Subsequently, mismatch recognition may step in and attempt to reason about the situation. The mismatch recognition component of SPIN is under development.

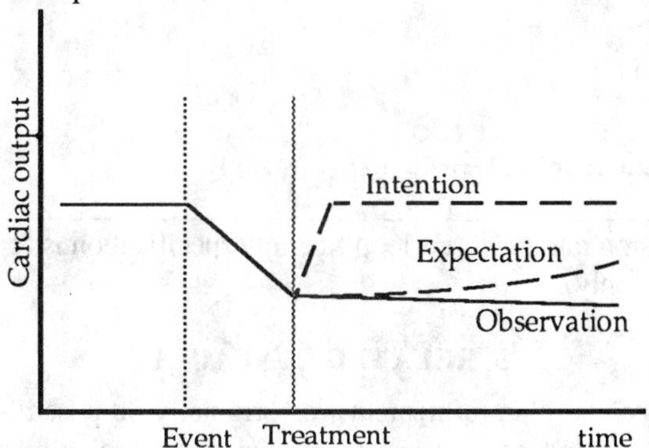

Figure 3. Intentions, expectations, and observations.

Observation-expectation mismatches may be used to 1) force plan revision in anticipation that a more effective treatment path might be chosen; 2) flag noncompliance to treatment and force reconsideration of relevant diagnostic hypotheses if all efforts fail; and 3) detect user compliance with treatment requests and to generate alerts when necessary. Inter-expectation mismatches may be used to identify potentially conflicting or redundant actions. These include actions prescribing different doses of the same drug, or actions neutralizing each other's effects. Intention-expectation mismatches may be used for plan optimization and revision by comparing the expectation–intention "distances" of possible treatment paths. Similarly, observation–intention mismatches may be useful in situation assessment, i.e., determining the distance of the current patient state from a desired recovery state.

4. AN ILLUSTRATIVE EXAMPLE

We believe that SPIN offers considerable flexibility and strength in representing, executing, and monitoring treatment protocols. In this section, we exemplify the approach using a simple treatment scenario. Consider the following protocol:

> *In response to an acute bleeding episode, the clinician needs to monitor blood pressure, central venous pressure, heart rate, and hematocrit closely. Severe hypotension may be treated with IV bolus of vasopressor which may be repeated as necessary to maintain acceptable blood pressure. Blood volume should be restored using crystalloids. Blood transfusion should be used when blood or packed red blood cells are available, if bleeding cannot be controlled soon, and if hematocrit is too low (summarized and modified from [2]).*

Table 2 illustrates part of the plan declaration for the management of bleeding. Table 3 shows the subplan for restoring blood volume, and Table 4 exemplifies a closed-loop control action which regulates the infusion of a crystalloid solution (normal saline). Due to space limitations, declarations as shown do not include all representational details.

We can represent vasopressor administration with a periodic closed-loop action. In this case, the control-interval will specify the frequency at which vasopressor administration should be reconsidered, the preconditions will specify the necessary conditions for repeated administration (possibly an assessment based on vital signs such as blood pressure and heart rate), and the dosage function will titrate the medication according to body weight and the intensity of desired effect.

The use of blood transfusion or packed red blood cells (RBCs) may be represented in a disjunctive phrase in the plan for restoring blood volume. In this case, both actions should be conditionalized on the availability of the related blood product and a low level of hematocrit. In addition, both preconditions may observe the duration of the bleeding episode and not authorize the action until the episode is long enough to warrant a transfusion. If both preconditions hold, packed RBCs will be preferred over whole blood according to the order specified in the ONE-OF phrase. Finally, both actions should have discontinuation conditions monitoring a transfusion reaction.

```
;; a plan to manage bleeding
;; CARDIAC is the name of the knowledge base
(def-bb1-object CARDIAC.manage-bleeding
  :attributes ((preconditions t)
               (control-schema
                      (ALL-OF CARDIAC.monitor-vital-signs
                              CARDIAC.manage-hypotension
                              CARDIAC.restore-blood-volume))))
```

Table 2. Partial declaration for a plan to manage bleeding.

```
;; a plan to restore blood volume
(def-bb1-object CARDIAC.restore-blood-volume
  :attributes ((preconditions t)
               (control-schema
                      (ALL-OF CARDIAC.infuse-normal-saline-high-rate
                              (ONE-OF CARDIAC.transfuse-packed-RBCs
                                      CARDIAC.transfuse-blood)))))
```

Table 3. Partial declaration for a plan to restore blood volume.

```
;; a closed-loop action to control fluid infusion
(def-bb1-object CARDIAC.infuse-normal-saline-high-rate
  :attributes ((preconditions t)
               (control-interval 60)  ;; once every minute
               (dosage-fn
                (let* ((weight (current-value-of-parameter 'body-weight))
                       (base-rate (weight * 1.0)) ;; ml/kg/min
                       (cvp (current-value-of-parameter 'central-venous-pressure)))
                  (cond ((> cvp 16)  (* 0.8 base-rate))
                        ((< cvp 8)   (* 1.6 base-rate))
                        ((< cvp 12)  (* 1.2 base-rate))
                        (t base-rate))))
               (goal-conditions
                 (> (current-value-of-parameter 'mean-arterial-pressure) 90.0))
               (discontinuation-conditions nil)))
```

Table 4. Partial declaration for an action which controls an infusion rate in closed-loop (therapy specification is for illustration purposes only).

In the case of an adverse reaction, the discontinuation condition assures that the transfusion is aborted immediately.

When the overall treatment plan is instantiated, the action for a high-rate normal saline infusion will also be triggered. Since we expect an ICU patient to receive a saline infusion at all times, there will already be a previously-activated saline infusion action. In this case, SPIN will detect a potentially redundant instantiation and choose the high-rate infusion over the maintenance infusion. The maintenance infusion will be suspended until the high-rate infusion has accomplished its goals.

The failure of a plan step is not detrimental to the execution of SPIN. Assuming that the overall plan considers all possible outcomes of treatment, another remedial action will be chosen when the plan is reevaluated upon failure of one of its steps.

5. RELATED RESEARCH

Skeletal plan refinement was originally proposed by Friedland as a means to reduce the complexity of planning [4]. Similar ideas were exploited later in the PROTEAN [5] and PROTEGE/EON systems [6]. Instead of planning in an unconstrained search space, the skeletal plan refinement method relies on available abstract (or skeletal) plans which were refined in the context of a particular problem. SPIN further simplifies skeletal plan selection by caching top-level skeletal plans with each disorder. Thus, search is limited to local search and instantiation within a plan skeleton. In addition, SPIN merges plan instantiation and execution steps. As such, it integrates planning and replanning.

There are major differences between SPIN and traditional AI planners such as SIPE [7]. SPIN does not synthesize new plans using its knowledge of the domain. SPIN does not need to replan during execution either since all plan steps are already defined in the protocol. In most classical planners, actions are instantaneous and execution follows a sequential thread. However, actions and plans are durative in SPIN and they are typically executed concurrently. As a consequence, SPIN actions and plans are interruptable and continuable since they execute over time intervals. SPIN also shares some features with intelligent agents which integrate high-level planners with low-level reactive controllers, such as PRS [8].

The DRIPS system uses abstraction hierarchies of actions selects optimal plans using a decision-analytic approach [9]. However, the selection depends on static features of the world and cannot be influenced by runtime events such as plan failure.

Finally, SPIN expands earlier medical AI efforts in protocol-based therapy such as ONCOCIN [10]. ONCOCIN is an expert system which supervises cancer chemotherapy protocols. It does not maintain state at runtime and its plans are difficult to maintain. In contrast, plans in SPIN are modular and easy to extract and represent in the form of protocols. In our experience, we had little difficulty representing treatment plans in SPIN even where protocols were not readily available in structured form.

6. DISCUSSION

6.1. Future Research

A major limitation in SPIN is in the control of plan and action selection. Disjunctive choices (ONE-OF) are resolved by trial-and-error in sequential order. This approach may be acceptable in an experimental setting, but in the real world of clinical medicine it is deficient. Future enhancements to SPIN should include decision-theoretic measures for selecting among conjunctive plans. These measures may include value, side effects, consequences, and cost. Reasoning about resource availability (e.g., personnel, devices) is another important target for SPIN.

6.2. Conclusions

In this paper, we present an architecture for skeletal plan instantiation, execution, and execution monitoring. This architecture operates in a highly uncertain environment where actions are durative and goal satisfaction is not always a reasonable expectation. Since actions may be taken on the basis of uncertain information, diagnosis tasks closely interact with treatment tasks and vice versa. Finally, plan construction is not only time consuming and difficult but also unnecessary in this domain since treatment protocols are already available in textbooks. Such features of the domain require a different approach to plan generation and execution than can be achieved with classical AI planners. SPIN is the end result of these considerations.

We successfuly used SPIN in the Guardian system on a number of simulated clinical scenarios. Further studies and improvements are underway. More rigorous assessments of the performance and representational adequacy of SPIN will be undertaken in a further study which involves comprehensive cognitive experiments.

Acknowledgments

This research was performed at the Knowledge Systems Laboratory at Stanford University. The Guardian project is sponsored by NASA contract NAG 2-581 under ARPA order 6822 and by a grant from the Whitaker Foundation administered by NSF. Barbara Hayes-Roth, David Gaba, John Drakopoulos, and Karl Pfleger provided helpful comments during the development of SPIN.

References

1. American Heart Association, *Textbook of Advanced Cardiac Life Support*. 1990, Dallas, TX.
2. Gaba, D.M., K.J. Fish, and S.K. Howard, *Crisis Management in Anesthesiology*. 1994, Churchill Livingstone, New York, NY.
3. Hayes-Roth, B., R. Washington, D. Ash, R. Hewett, *et al.*, *Guardian: a prototype intelligent agent for intensive-care monitoring*. Artificial Intelligence in Medicine, 1992. **4** (2): 165–185.
4. Friedland, P.E., *Knowledge-based experiment design in molecular genetics*. PhD dissertation, Stanford University, 1979.
5. Hayes-Roth, B., B. Buchanan, O. Lichtarge, M. Hewett, *et al. PROTEAN: deriving protein structure from constraints*, in *Proc. AAAI-86*, Philadelphia, PA, pp. 904–909.
6. Musen, M.A., S.W. Tu, and Y. Shahar. *A problem-solving model for protocol-based care: from e-ONCOCIN to EON*, in *Proc. MEDINFO-92*. 1992. Geneva, Switzerland, pp. 519–525.
7. Wilkins, D.A., *Domain-independent planning: representation and plan generation*. Artificial Intelligence, 1984. **22**: 269-301.
8. Georgeff, M.P. and A.L. Lansky. *Reactive reasoning and planning*, in *Proc. AAAI-87*. 1987. Seattle, WA: Morgan Kaufmann, pp. 677-682.
9. Haddawy, P. and M. Suwandi. *Decision-theoretic refinement planning using inheritance abstraction*, in *Proc. AIPS-94*. 1994. Chicago, IL: AAAI Press, pp. 266-271.
10. Langlotz, C.P., L.M. Fagan, S.W. Tu, B.I. Sikic, *et al.*, *A therapy planning architecture that combines decision theory and artificial intelligence techniques*. Computers and Biomedical Research, 1987. **20**: 279–303.

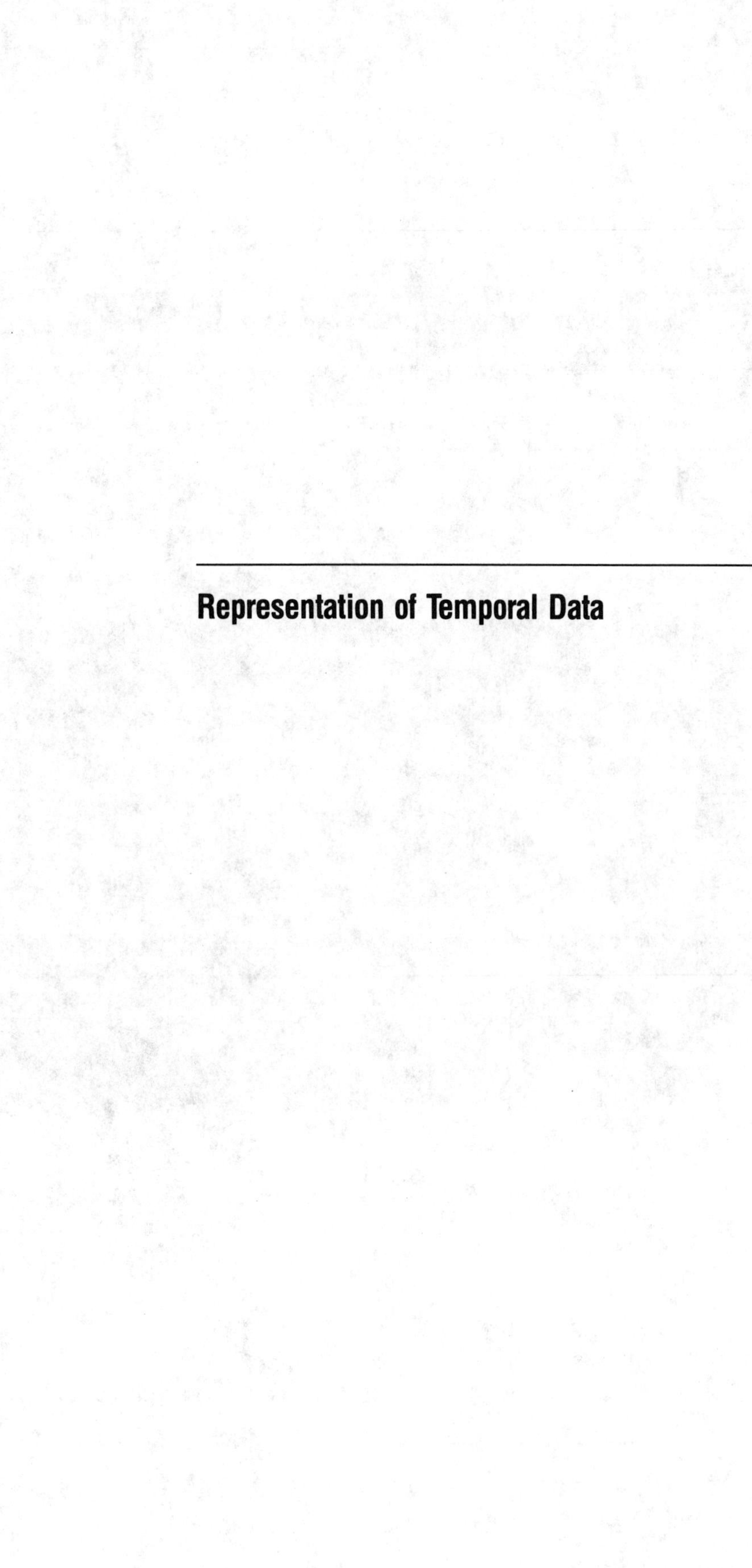

Representation of Temporal Data

Knowledge-Based Temporal Abstraction for Diabetic Monitoring

Yuval Shahar, Amar K. Das, Samson W. Tu, Frederic B. Kraemer, Mark A. Musen

Section on Medical Informatics, Stanford University School of Medicine
Stanford, CA 94305-5479

Abstract

We have developed a general method that solves the task of creating abstract, interval-based concepts from time-stamped clinical data. We refer to this method as knowledge-based temporal-abstraction (KBTA). In this paper, we focus on the knowledge representation, acquisition, maintenance, reuse and sharing aspects of the KBTA method. We describe five problem-solving mechanisms that solve the five subtasks into which the KBTA method decomposes its task, and four types of knowledge necessary for instantiating these mechanisms in a particular domain. We present an example of instantiating the KBTA method in the clinical area of monitoring insulin-dependent–diabetes patients.

1. THE TEMPORAL-ABSTRACTION TASK

Clinical data, such as blood-glucose values, are typically gathered over time within the scope of one or more interpretation contexts (e.g., a healthy person, an insulin-dependent diabetes patient, pre-breakfast periods, regular insulin therapy). The **temporal-abstraction (TA) task** accepts as input time-stamped parameters (e.g., blood glucose values) and events (e.g., NPH insulin injections), and returns as output interval-based, context-specific parameters at the same or at a higher level of abstraction. The process of summarizing large amounts of clinical data over time supports a physician assessing a patient's condition by creating abstract concepts (e.g., 2 weeks of LOW pre-breakfast blood glucose and HIGH pre-supper values) from raw numerical data (e.g., pre- and post-prandial blood glucose values).

The goal of the TA task is to evaluate and summarize the state of the patient over a time interval, to identify various possible problems, to assist in a revision of an existing therapy plan, or to support a generation of a new plan. In addition, generating clinically meaningful interval-based concepts supports the task of explaining a decision-support system's plans and actions to different users (e.g., a resident physician, a nurse, an experienced clinical expert). Finally, clinical guidelines can represent goals and policies as temporal patterns to be achieved or avoided.

Several issues need to be handled by a method solving the TA task: (1) the arriving input or the queried output parameter values might be of different types (e.g., numbers, symbols) and abstraction levels (e.g., BLOOD GLUCOSE LEVEL = 64 mg%; GLUCOSE STATE = LOW); (2) input data might arrive out of temporal order, and existing interpretations should be revised accordingly; (3) several alternate interpretations might need to be maintained and followed over time; (4) from the knowledge-representation aspect, **acquisition** of necessary knowledge from domain experts should be facilitated, as well as **maintenance** of that knowledge. **Reusing** the domain-independent abstraction knowledge for solving the TA task in other domains should be possible, as well as **sharing** some of the domain-specific knowledge with other tasks in the same domain.

2. THE KNOWLEDGE-BASED TEMPORAL-ABSTRACTION METHOD

Generalizing our previous work [1,2], we have defined a domain-independent problem-solving method [3] for interpreting data in the time-oriented, knowledge-intensive domains common to clinical applications. We propose a highly modular approach, with semantics clearly defined for both the problem-solving method and the domain-specific knowledge needed by it. The **knowledge-based temporal-abstraction (KBTA)** method decomposes the TA task into five parallel subtasks (Figure 1): (1) **temporal-context restriction**: creation of relevant interpretation contexts crucial for focusing and limiting the scope of the inference, (2) **vertical temporal inference**: inference from contemporaneous propositions into higher-level concepts, (3) **horizontal temporal inference**: inference from propositions of similar type, attached to intervals that cover different time periods,

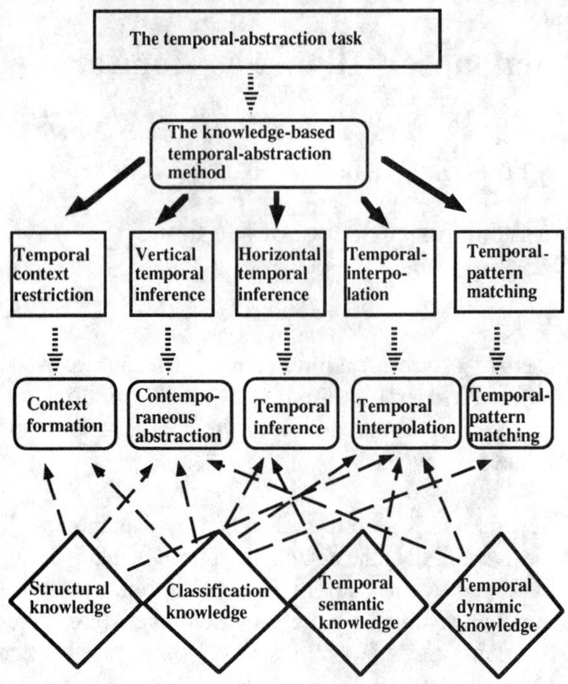

Figure 1: The knowledge-based temporal-abstraction method and its mechanisms. ▭ = task; ⬭ = method or mechanism; ◇ = knowledge type; ➞ = DECOMPOSED-INTO relation; ⇣ = SOLVED-BY relation; – –➞ = USED-BY relation.

(4) **temporal interpolation**: bridging gaps between disjoint points or intervals, associated with propositions of similar type, to create longer intervals, and (5) **temporal-pattern matching** (creation of intervals by matching of patterns over disjoint intervals, associated with propositions of various-types). An analysis of most existing temporal-reasoning systems in clinical medicine supports this decomposition [3].

The five subtasks that the KBTA *method* poses are solved, respectively, by five lower-level temporal-abstraction **mechanisms** (computational modules that cannot be decomposed further). The mechanisms include three basic TA mechanisms which we described previously [1, 2], a mechanism for matching temporal patterns, and a mechanism for creating relevant temporal interpretation contexts. Types of output abstractions include **state** (e.g., LOW) **gradient** (e.g., INCREASING) **rate** (e.g., FAST) or **pattern** (e.g., CRESCENDO). The **contemporaneous abstraction** mechanism abstracts one or more parameters and their values, attached to contemporaneous time points or time intervals, into a value of a new, abstract parameter. The **temporal inference** mechanism infers specific types of interval-based logical conclusions, given interval-based propositions, using an extension of Shoham's temporal semantic properties [4]. Temporal inference also determines the domain value of an abstraction created from two joined abstractions (e.g., DECREASING and SAME might be concatenated into NONINCREASING). The **temporal interpolation** mechanism bridges gaps between temporal points or intervals, using domain-specific dynamic-change knowledge about the parameters involved. In particular, it uses local (forward and backward, around a time point or interval) and global (between 2 time points or intervals) **truth-persistence** functions to model a belief in the value of a <*parameter*, *value*, *context*> proposition [3]. Global persistence functions are represented as maximal-temporal–gap thresholds that can be bridged. The **temporal-pattern–matching** mechanism matches predefined or online queries for temporal patterns that are defined in terms of the interval-based abstractions, at any level of abstraction, created by the other TA mechanisms. The output is a higher-level parameter of the pattern abstraction type, such as REBOUND HYPERGLYCEMIA. The **context-forming** mechanism creates temporal **interpretation-context intervals** that are a temporal frame of reference for interpretation, and thus enable a TA mechanism to conclude abstractions relevant to that and only that context. The relation between an interpretation context or subcontext and its generating task, event, abstraction or supercontext can be any of Allen's 13 temporal-interval relations [5]. Thus, contexts generated by events and by abstractions also enable anticipation of future complications and interpretation of past findings in the light of the present interpretation. Creating contexts requires knowledge about the structure of clinical tasks, events, and abstractions.

3. DOMAIN-SPECIFIC KNOWLEDGE: ONTOLOGIES

To be useful for a particular clinical domain, the TA mechanisms require instantiation with domain-specific knowledge. This domain-specific knowledge, mostly declarative, is the *only* interface between the KBTA method and the knowledge engineer or the domain expert. Thus, the development of a TA system particular to a new domain relies only on creating or editing a predefined set of knowledge categories. As shown in Figure 1, we distinguish among four domain **knowledge types** used by the TA mechanisms: (1) **structural knowledge** (e.g., IS-A and PART-OF relations in the domain); (2) **classification knowledge** (e.g., classification of blood glucose value ranges into HYPOGLYCEMIA, LOW, NORMAL, HIGH); (3) **temporal semantic knowledge** (e.g., the relations among propositions attached to intervals and their subintervals); and (4) **temporal dynamic knowledge** (e.g., persistence of the value of a parameter over time).

The domain-specific knowledge required by the TA mechanisms is represented as a **parameter-properties ontology**—a theory that represents the raw and abstract parameters in that domain (e.g., blood glucose value and state abstractions), their temporal properties, and the relations among them (e.g., IS-A, ABSTRACTED-INTO) [2]. The parameter-properties ontology is used by all the TA mechanisms. The context-forming mechanism refers also to an ontology of **events** such as insulin administration, and an ontology of **interpretation contexts**.

4. THE RÉSUMÉ SYSTEM AND THE DIABETES DOMAIN

We have developed a software system, **RÉSUMÉ**, that implements the temporal-abstraction method [2]. A simple TA pattern-matching language queries the internal temporal fact base for particular predefined temporal patterns or for online interaction with the user. More complex queries can be answered by a relational database temporal-query system, **Chronus**, that is an extension of the temporal pattern-matching mechanism [6]. The TA mechanisms do not operate in a fixed order; they are activated by the currently available data and the previously derived abstractions. In addition, an underlying truth-maintenance system updates the temporal-interval conclusions, since these are by nature **nonmonotonic** and therefore **defeasible**, that is, their validity depends on primitive data that might be modified when more past or present data are known. The control structure implemented in the RÉSUMÉ system is specialized to the TA task, and allows several levels of task-specific control (e.g., desired output types and abstraction classes, which TA mechanisms to use, the relevant temporal contexts). It is thus both a data- and a goal-driven task-specific control.

We applied the RÉSUMÉ methodology to the area of treating insulin-dependent **diabetes mellitus** (**DM**) patients. One of us (F.B.K) is a diabetologist, and was the domain expert for this experiment. We created a parameter-properties ontology (Figure 2), an event ontology (Figure 3), and a context ontology (Figure 4). Acquiring the three initial core ontologies required two meetings of 2 hours each. Administrations of regular insulin and of isophane insulin suspension (**NPH**) are *events*, generating different insulin-action *interpretation*

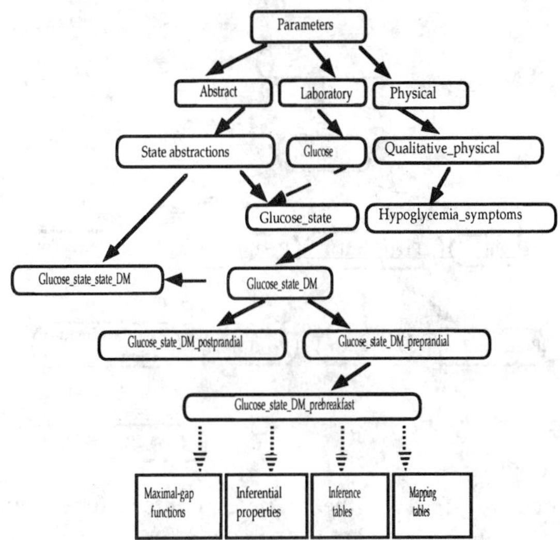

Figure 2: Part of the diabetes parameter-properties ontology. (oval) = class; (rectangle) = property; (arrow) = IS-A relation; (striped arrow) = PROPERTY-OF relation; (dashed arrow) = ABSTRACTED-INTO relation.

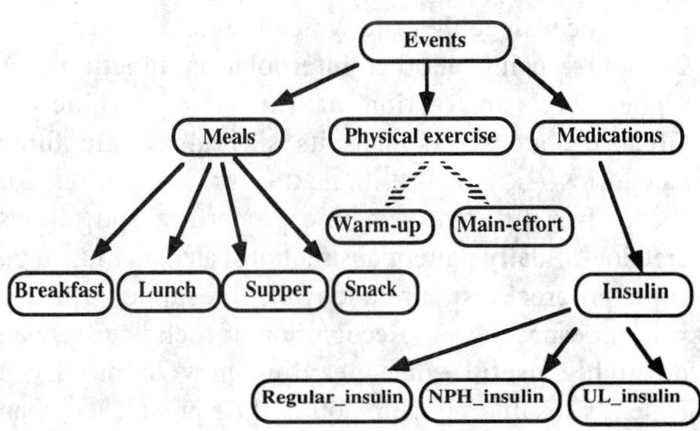

Figure 3: Part of the diabetes event ontology. (oval) = class; (arrow) = IS-A relation; (dashed arrow) = PART--OF relation.

contexts that are *subcontexts* of the DM *interpretation context*. Meal events create pre- and post-prandial contexts—Glucose_state_DM_prebreakfast values [See Figure 2] can thus be inferred regardless of absolute time. The Glucose_state abstract parameter has six values that correspond to the ranges used by the domain expert (`HYPOGLYCEMIA`, `LOW`, `NORMAL`, `HIGH`, `VERY HIGH`, `EXTREMELY HIGH`). These values are sensitive to the context in which they are generated; for instance, postprandial values allow for a higher range of the normal value. Glucose_state value propositions in the same DM context have the semantic property of being **concatenable** into propositions holding over longer intervals [4]; *same-day* values between different

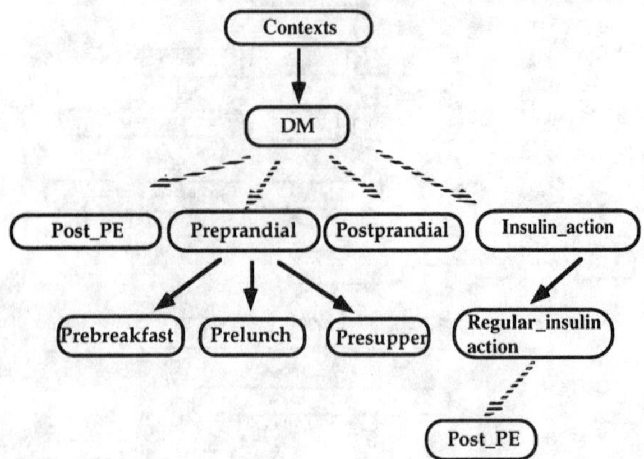

Figure 4. Part of the diabetes context ontology. ⬭ = class; ⟶ = IS-A relation; - - -▶ = SUBCONTEXT relation.

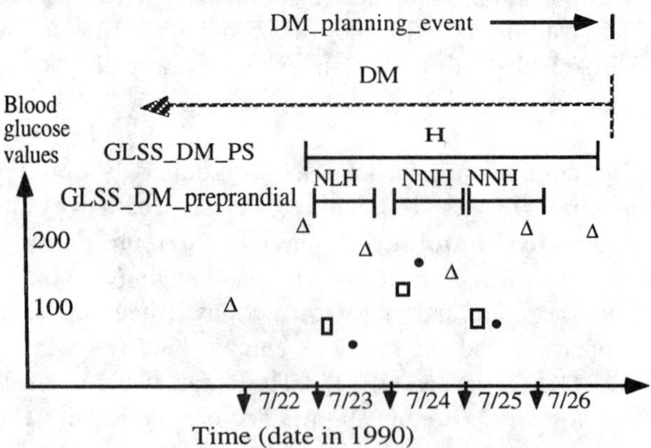

Figure 5: An example of abstraction by the RÉSUMÉ system of data from patient 3. ├- - -▶ = (open) context interval; ├─┤ = abstracted interval; ❐ = prebreakfast glucose; • = prelunch glucose; Δ = presupper glucose; `GLSS_DM_PS` = Glucose_state_state abstraction in the DM and pre-supper context; `GLSS_DM_PREPRANDIAL` = Glucose_state_state abstraction in the DM and preprandial context.

preprandial phases can be bridged up to 6 to 8 hours apart (defined by a truth-persistence interpolation function). *Same-phase* parameters such as Glucuse_state_DM_prebreakfast have longer global persistence, since they are typically bridged over 24 to 28 hours, using another interpolation function. A higher-level abstraction of the state of glucose, Glucose_state_state, maps its six values into three categories (`LOW`, `NORMAL`, `HIGH`, or `L`, `N`, `H`, for short), has different semantic properties, and allows creation of daily pattern abstractions such as `LLH` (e.g., from prebreakfast, prelunch and presupper glucose values, respectively). Recognition of such patterns can be highly useful when deciding how to modify a patient's insulin regimen; noting their prevalence is an important step in determining if the pattern is a common one for the patient. Asserting anywhere in the temporal fact base an event named `DM_planning` initiates the reasoning by generating a retrospective `DM` interpretation context for the preceding 2 weeks (this time window is used by the domain expert in practice and is modifiable) that enables creation of the DM domain abstractions.

We applied the RÉSUMÉ system to electronic data from insulin-dependent–diabetes patients. The input to RÉSUMÉ included both the diabetes ontology (figures 2 through 4) and the patient-specific raw data. A sample of the results is shown in Figure 5. In this particular time window, two significant findings are highlighted: The Glucose_state_state parameter in the presupper context had the value `HIGH` for a period of more than 3 days, and a diurnal pattern of `NORMAL` or `LOW` blood glucose levels at morning and lunch, and `HIGH` pre-supper glucose levels (e.g., `NNH`, `NLH`) appeared at least three times in the same week. The combined pattern suggests an adjustment of the intermediate-acting insulin (e.g., NPH). The pattern can be predefined as an internal pattern-type parameter or can be noted in response to an external online query for state abstractions of the Glucose_state parameter.

5. DISCUSSION

The truth-maintenance system in RÉSUMÉ resembles Russ's **temporal control structure (TCS)** system [7]. However, TCS leaves all domain-specific temporal reasoning to the user-created procedures. In contrast, the RÉSUMÉ domain-independent (but specific to the TA task) TA mechanisms perform all of the TA, given the declarative representation of the domain's ontology.

The **TrenDx** system of Haimowitz and Kohane [8] builds on Kohane's constraint-satisfaction **temporal-utilities package** [9], and defines domain-specific patterns called **trend templates (TTs)**. TrenDx is useful in detecting that the data is consistent with one or more TTs, including TTs of which only a part is observed. The goal of TrenDx is different from that of RÉSUMÉ. TrenDx does not create any intermediate abstractions, since its goal is not to abstract, summarize, or answer queries about the data, as it is in the TA task, but rather to match data efficiently against a set of predefined patterns. Data can only be accepted at the lowest level; thus, no input of intermediate-level abstractions is possible. No explicit domain ontology of parameters and events exists, and a constraint (e.g., significant change in a parameter) might be repeated with the same implicit role in different TTs and even at different parts of the same TT. Like RÉSUMÉ, TrenDx assumes implicitly an ill-defined domain that cannot be modeled easily numerically, and therefore requires detection of essentially associative temporal patterns.

Kahn's **TOPAZ** system (10) integrates a quantitative physiological model and a symbolic model for aggregation of clinically significant intervals. TOPAZ can associate interpretation methods with an interval representing a *context* of interest. RÉSUMÉ extends this capability by the context-forming mechanism, which uses an explicit context ontology to enable creation of context-specific abstractions and activation of specific functions, but does not limit generated interpretation contexts to the temporal extent of the parent event, allowing any desired relation between the generating interval and the generated context. Lehmann's **AIDA** system [11] is a diabetes-treatment decision support prototype system, whose underlying model attempts to reflect the (patho)physiology of insulin action and carbohydrate absorption in quantitative terms. Note that systems such as TOPAZ and AIDA assume a precise underlying mathematical model of the domain; most clinical domains defy complete quantitative modeling.

It might be desirable to detect patterns defined by *events*, such as insulin use, and not only by *parameters*, such as glucose states. Such patterns might generate more meaningful interpretation contexts. Such work has been described by Kahn and his colleagues [12] with encouraging results for an algorithm combining clinical and temporal considerations.

Acknowledgments

Dr. M. G. Kahn of the University of Washington, St. Louis, supplied the data. This work has been supported in part by grant HS06330 from the Agency for Health Care Policy and Research, by grants LM05157 and LM05305 from the National Library of Medicine, and by a gift from Digital Equipment Corporation. Dr. Musen is a recipient of National Science Foundation Young Investigator Award IRI-9257578.

References

[1]. Shahar, Y., Tu, S.W., and Musen, M.A. (1992). Knowledge acquisition for temporal-abstraction mechanisms. *Knowledge Acquisition* **4**, 217–236.

[2]. Shahar, Y., and Musen, M.A. (1993). RÉSUMÉ: A temporal-abstraction system for patient monitoring. *Computers and Biomedical Research* **26**, 255–273.

[3]. Shahar, Y. [1994]. *A Knowledge-Based Method for Temporal Abstraction of Clinical Data.* Ph.D. Dissertation, Program in Medical Information Sciences, Stanford University, CA.

[4]. Shoham, Y. (1987). Temporal logics in AI: Semantical and ontological considerations. *Artificial Intelligence* **33**, 89–104.

[5]. Allen, J.F. (1984). Towards a general theory of action and time. *Artificial Intelligence* **23**, 123–154 .

[6]. Das, A.K., and Musen, M.A. (in press). A temporal query system for protocol-directed decision support. *Methods of Information in Medicine.*

[7]. Russ, T.A. (1989). Using hindsight in medical decision making. *Proceedings, Thirteenth Annual Symposium on Computer Applications in Medical Care* (L. C. Kingsland, Ed.), pp. 38–44, Washington, D.C: IEEE Comput. Soc. Press.

[8]. Haimowitz, I.J., and Kohane, I.S. (1993). An epistemology for clinically significant trends. *Proceedings of the Tenth National Conference on Artificial Intelligence*, pp. 176–181, Menlo Park, CA: AAAI Press.

[9]. Kohane, I.S. (1987). Temporal reasoning in medical expert systems. *Technical Report 389, Laboratory of Computer Science, Massachusetts Institute of technology*, Cambridge, MA.

[10]. Kahn, M.G. (1991). Combining physiologic models and symbolic methods to interpret time-varying patient data. *Methods of information in Medicine* **30**, 167–178.

[11]. Lehmann, E.D., Deutsch, T., Carson, E.R., and Sonksen, P.H. (1994). AIDA: an interactive diabetes advisor. *Computer Methods and Programs in Biomedicine* **41**, 183–203.

[12]. Kahn, M.G., Abrams, C.A., Cousins, S.B., Beard, J.C., and Frisse, M.E. (1990). Automated interpretation of diabetes patient data: Detecting temporal changes in insulin therapy. *Proceedings, Fourteenth Annual Symposium on Computer Applications in Medical Care* (R. A. Miller, Ed.), pp. 569–573, IEEE Comput. Soc. Press, Los Alamitos.

Intelligent Diagnostic Monitoring Using Trend Templates

Ira J. Haimowitz, Ph.D., Corporate Research and Development,
General Electric Company, Schenectady, NY*

ABSTRACT

In previous work we have defined our *trend template* epistemology for clinically significant trends and we have illustrated and tested a program *TrenDx* that monitors time-ordered process data by matching the data to trend templates. Our initial application domain was pediatric growth monitoring. In continuing work we have explored monitoring hemodynamic and respiratory parameters of intensive care unit patients. This application has highlighted the needs for advances in our representation and monitoring algorithms. In particular, we have added reasoning with uncertainty to the trend template epistemology, and a new control structure allowing numerical ranking of competing trend templates. Furthermore, intelligent monitoring in any medical domain requires a coherent framework for diagnostic monitoring. In this paper we show how TrenDx can be extended to a framework including sending alarms, changing clinical context, and filtering data streams. [1]

INTRODUCTION

Trend Templates and TrenDx

In previous work [1, 2] we have defined our *trend template* epistemology for clinically significant trends, consisting of *landmark points* representing events in a process and *intervals* representing phases of that process. Below is part of a trend template for normal pediatric growth in boys. This partial template includes two landmark points, representing birth and the onset of puberty, which is at temporal distance 10 to 13 years from birth. The two intervals, representing periods of a child establishing height and weight centiles and of pre-pubertal growth, also have temporal uncertainty as indicated.

Notice also that the two intervals are represented as *consecutive phases,* so that the endpoint of the first interval is infinitesimally before the begin point of the second interval. Also attached to each interval are *value constraints* that restrict the value of relevant parameters that occur in data during the intervals. In particular, these value constraints place limits on the Z-scores (number of standard deviations from the population mean) of the normal growth patient's heights and weights.

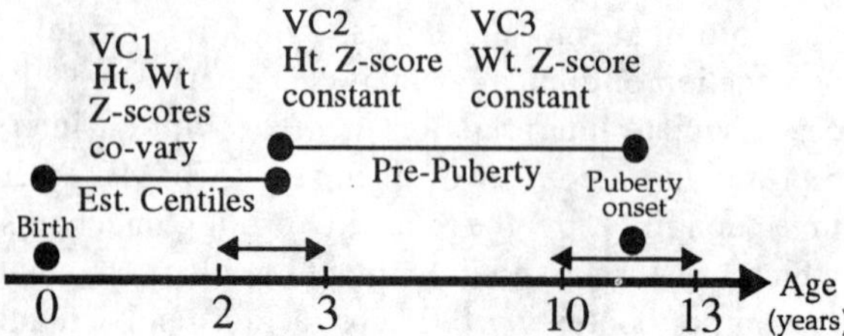

Figure 1 Partial trend template for normal pediatric growth.

We have illustrated and tested a program *TrenDx* that monitors time-ordered process data by matching the data to trend templates. The program branches to consider alternate temporal chronologies of how the process data has evolved.

Previous Work in Pediatric Growth Monitoring

General pediatricians that monitor their patients' growth suffer from data overload in that they have insufficient time per patient to investigate the entire time-series of growth data (heights, weights, and bone ages). Our goal in that domain was to develop a screening tool for general pediatricians that could examine growth chart data and suggest a possible disorder.

As described in [2] we conducted a preliminary clinical trial using 30 consecutive growth records from the endocrinology clinic at Boston Children's Hospital. The results were encouraging in that TrenDx showed promise in reaching the same diagnosis as a panel of experts, at a time no later than the experts, in most of the cases. The trial was also useful in uncovering some representational issues that needed further research. We are currently planning a larger scale trial using hundreds of clinical cases where will we compare TrenDx monitoring performance to humans of various expertise: medical students, general pediatricians, and pediatric endocrinologists.

Intensive Care Unit Monitoring

We have attempted to apply our approach to the domain of intensive care unit (ICU) monitoring. Here there is also data overload: eight or more patients are in an ICU, and each patient is monitored with dozens of hemodynamic and respiratory variables sampled

1. This work has been supported (in part) by grants NIH R01 LM 04493, 1T15LM07092, NICHHD 5T32 HD07277-9.

* This research was performed at the Laboratory for Computer Science, Massachusetts Institute of Technology,

several times per minute. It is impossible for nurses to steadily monitor even minutes worth of continuous data from an individual patient. Our goal in ICU monitoring is developing context-sensitive monitors whose use will significantly reduce the high false positive rates typically produced with single-variable threshold monitors. TrenDx can potentially monitor the adequacy or failure of external interventions on ICU patients, and the normality or abnormality of physiological mechanisms in these patients. Interventions and mechanisms may display a characteristic multivariate pattern over several phases. An automated monitor must apply specific filters and value constraints appropriate for each phase of the intervention or mechanism.

In Figure 2 are one hour of ICU data from an 8 month old girl with adult respiratory distress syndrome [3]. Four signals are plotted from 12:00 a.m. to 1:00 a.m.: heart rate taken from the electrocardiogram (ECG), mean arterial blood pressure, oxygen saturation, and fraction of inspired oxygen (FIO_2). Data were compressed by reporting values only upon changes. Usually, the patient received oxygen via the ventilator, FIO_2 at 50%. Approximately once every two hours, the patient was ventilated by the nurse squeezing a hand bag filled with 100% oxygen, so that a bronchodilator could be delivered in aerosol form. One handbagging session was from 12:22 a.m. until 12:31 a.m. As illustrated in the figure, the change to hand-bagging was marked by an immediate rise of FIO_2 from 50% to 100%, remaining at 100% during hand bagging. Within a minute after hand-bagging began, O_2 saturation rose sharply to 100%. These two changes are expected in such a handbagging session. During such hand-bagging it is preferable that the patient's hemodynamics remain stable. However, in this patient mean arterial blood pressure dropped from about 12:26 a.m. to 12:31 a.m, and ECG-measured heart rate rose steadily from approximately 12:27 until 12:30 a.m. These two changes are not usually expected. This pattern in these four parameters occurred during each of the six hand-bagging sessions for this patient over a twelve-hour period.

One possible explanation for this hemodynamic fault is that the oxygen handbagging increased pressure in the chest cavity. This could have depressed the patient's vena cava and compromised her venous return to the heart, resulting in the falling blood pressure. The heart rate increase may have been a normal baroreceptor reflex to the falling heart rate. Whatever the explanation, this hemodynamic fault is worthy of a clinician's attention.

Framework for Intelligent Diagnostic Monitoring

In order to achieve robust monitoring performance in multiple domains, we have extended our trend detection algorithm TrenDx to a broader framework for intelligent diagnostic monitoring. This framework includes a means of representing significant multivariate trends with multiple phases, and methods of detecting those trends from data. Also included are means for generating reliable alarms, displaying and explaining significant trends, and changing the clinical context. More complete details of the framework are in the author's dissertation [4].

REPRESENTING SIGNIFICANT TRENDS

Regression-Based Trend Templates

To advance our original work we needed a trend representation with robust matching, and allowing ranking of competing trend hypotheses. We modified trend template value constraints to be parameterized statistical models describing variation in data assigned to an interval. More precisely, let hyp be a TrenDx hypothesis consisting of a trend template TT; *hyp* assigns data to the intervals of TT. Let *I* be an interval of TT and let

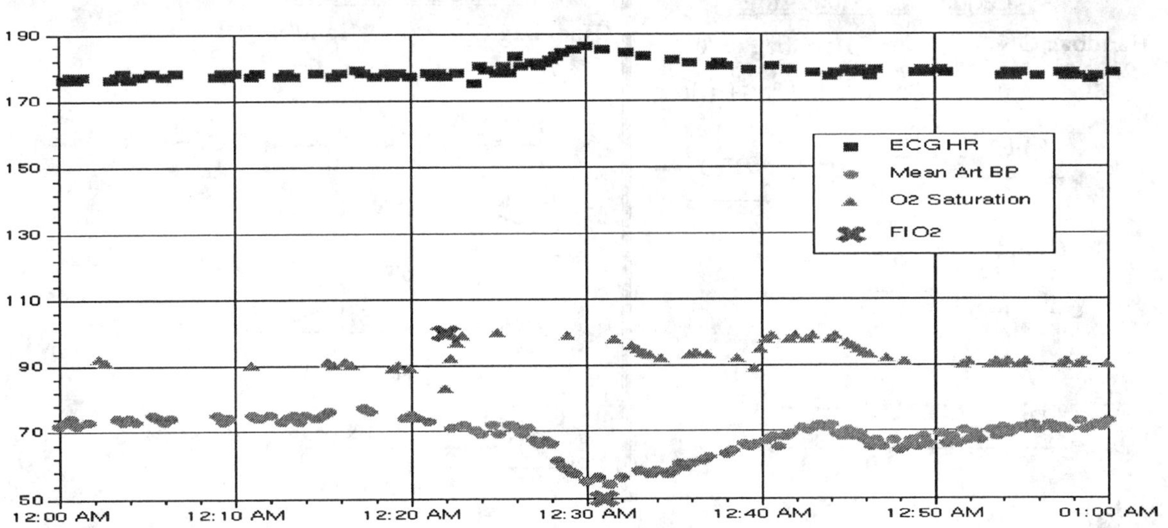

Figure 2: One hour of four signals plotted from an intensive care unit patient.

D(I, hyp) be the data assigned to I in hyp. Each value constraint consists of two main components:

1.a function F that maps the data D(*I*, *hyp*) to a time-indexed real-valued sequence $\{Y_t\}$.

2.a linear regression model describing the pattern of $\{Y_t\}$.

The primary set of linear regression models used in this research are polynomials of degree 0, 1, and 2, with qualitative or quantitative constraints on some subset (perhaps empty) of the polynomial coefficients. A *qualitative constraint* is a member of the set {+, -}, representing that the parameter is positive or negative.[2] A *quantitative constraint* is either a single numerical value or a numerical range `[min max]` of values. There are seven qualitatively distinct elementary regression models used in value constraints. These seven models are sufficient to roughly distinguish between different types of behaviors.

Constant models with quantitative parameter constraints can be used to represent steady states. An interval of normal human temperature may constrain temperature to be constant at 37 degrees Celsius. A constant model without a numerical estimate represents quiescence at an unknown level.

Linear models with quantitative slope constraints can help distinguish clinically distinct trends. For example, blood pressure loss due to handbagging may have a slope in the range -1 mm Hg to -3 mm Hg per minute, whereas blood pressure loss due to internal hemorrhaging may have a slope in the range -10 mm Hg to -20 mm Hg per minute. Linear models with qualitative slopes constraints can roughly distinguish responses.

Quadratic models with qualitative constraints are useful for representing trends having a sharp increase or decrease followed by a stabilization. They can better fit data showing a nonlinear response than can a linear model. When qualitative or quantitative constraints on quadratic coefficients are not derivable, a knowledge engineer may better characterize a quadratic trend with qualitative constraints on the first and second derivatives.

Monitor Sets

A *monitor set* is a set of trend templates forming a clinical context. The trend templates within a monitor set are viewed as a partition of trends that may occur in a particular clinical context. The members of a monitor set are concurrently matched against the same patient data by TrenDx.

In a diagnostic setting one trend template within a monitor set is the *expected* or *normal model*; the other trend templates are *fault models*. The fault models are those that if matched well warrant attention by the person or system observing the device.

Monitor Set for Oxygen Handbagging

In Figure 3 are two trend templates comprising a monitor set of patient response to 100% oxygen handbagging. One trend is expected and the other suggests a fault.

The hemodynamic fault trend template consists of eight intervals. The changes in four parameters are each represented in a pair of intervals. Temporal relations between these intervals establish a pattern that is fairly specific to this particular population response. The top two intervals denote that, during handbagging, the fraction of inspired oxygen (FIO_2) remains con-

2. In this research a parameter estimate of 0 is considered a quantitative estimate.

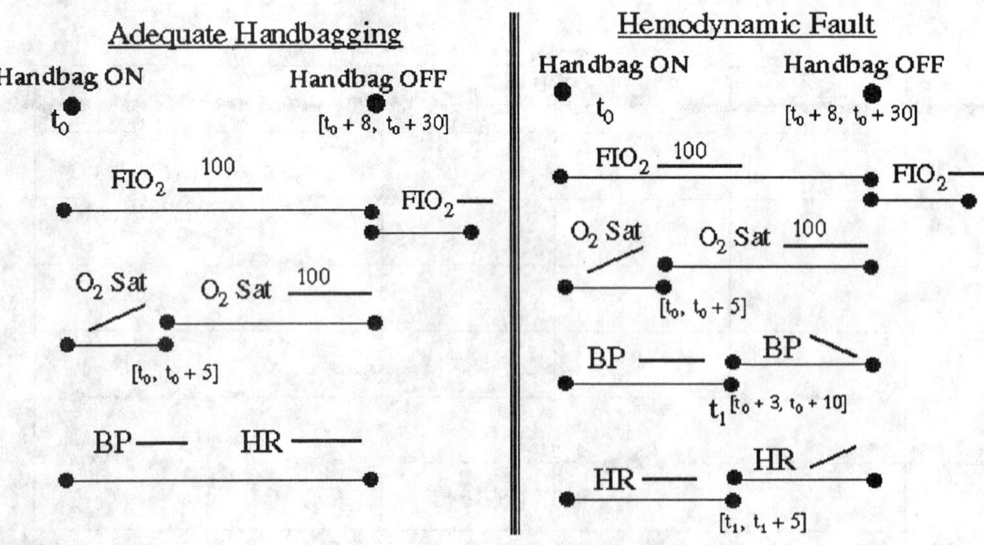

Figure 3: Competing trend templates for oxygen handbagging.

stant at 100 percent, and that for three minutes after handbagging, FIO_2 is constant at some unspecified value. Given the time of `Handbag On` for a particular patient, the trend detection program TrenDx can use these two intervals to estimate that patient's time of `Handbag Off`. TrenDx estimates based on when FIO_2 has changed from 100 percent. The next two intervals describe the rise and stabilization of oxygen saturation of hemoglobin. During `saturating Hb`, O_2 saturation is linear and increasing; during `saturated Hb`, O_2 saturation is constant at 100 percent. The two other pairs of intervals constrain the responses of blood pressure and heart rate. Each parameter first has a steady phase, beginning at the same time as `Handbag On`. During these phases, both parameters are constant. A second phase of decreasing BP, beginning 3 to 10 minutes after `Handbag On`, constrains BP to be linear and decreasing. This phase ends at `Handbag Off`. A second phase of increasing HR, beginning 0 to 5 minutes after the begin point of `decreasing BP` constrains HR to be linear and increasing. The temporal relations between these intervals insure that as TrenDx matches process data early in the template, the program constrains the expected match to data in the future.

The trend template for adequate handbagging contains the same landmark points and the same response intervals for FIO_2 and O_2 Sat. The adequate handbagging trend template differs in its trends for BP and HR, both of which are constrained to be constant in a single interval whose length is the handbagging period.

MATCHING DATA TO TREND TEMPLATES

The trend diagnosis program TrenDx matches patient data to the regression-based trend templates in each monitor set. TrenDx instantiates the trend templates for a particular patient by anchoring a landmark point of a trend template to an event in the patient history. In this ICU example, the landmark point `handbag on` is anchored to the time of a special datum generated by a switch on the ventilator noting that the ventilator no longer supplies oxygen. In principle instantiation could also proceed via the results of a strong match to a preliminary trend template.

The goodness of fit of value constraint *vc* for the hypothesis *hyp*, denoted by Fit*(vc, hyp)*, is the <u>mean absolute percentage error</u> (MAPE) between sequence values $\{Y_t\}$ and regression model estimations $\{\hat{Y}_t\}$:

$$Fit(vc, hyp) = \frac{\sum_t \left| \frac{\hat{Y}_t - Y_t}{Y_t} \right|}{N - p} \qquad \text{(EQ 1)}$$

where N is the number of values within the interval, and p is the number of parameters that are estimated. MAPE is particularly useful for comparing the goodness of fit between models of different variables of possibly different measurement scales.

The goodness of fit of a hypothesis to the data assigned to the intervals of its trend template is a weighted average of the fits to the individual value constraints. The weights may be defined by experts; by default the weights are the (N-p) used as the denominators of value constraint scores. For each trend template, which has temporal uncertainty, TrenDx optimizes over all temporal distances to find the best matching hypothesis to the data.

TrenDx matched the trend templates in Figure 3 to four signals of data between 12:22 and 12:31 a.m. during which the patient received oxygen via a handbag. Several intensive care unit physicians agreed the patient was experiencing some hemodynamic fault during this period. TrenDx also matched the same monitor set to five other periods of handbagging in this patient during the same day. The results were similar enough that we only show results of matching to the first handbagging session.

Figure 4 shows the four signals of ICU data and results of TrenDx matching to this data. Note that the outlying heart rate between 12:24 a.m. and 12:25 a.m. caused a jump in the match scores to both trend templates. Had that outlier been removed or smoothed by filtering, the error scores for both trends would have remained lower.

The best matches of each trend template stay close in score until 12:27:21 a.m., when the percentage error for the adequate handbagging trend template rises while that for the compromised venous return stays level. The difference between these two, plotted at the bottom of the graph, rises steadily for the duration of the handbagging episode. This difference, if judged significant, may be used as a means for sending an alarm.

JUDGING TREND SIGNIFICANCE

Generally, TrenDx matches to a monitor set by computing for each time slice of data the best matching score for the normal trend template and for each competing fault. Throughout this section we denote the sequence of best scores for the normal template $\{TT_n\}$ and the sequence for each fault template $\{TT_{fi}\}$. High values in these sequences indicate a poor match to data. We denote by $\{TT_n - TT_{fi}\}$ the sequence of score differences some fault model and the normal model. High values in this sequence indicate that the fault model matches better than the normal model.

We now must devise a scheme for answering the following questions:

- When has the normal model become a significantly poor match to the data to require attention? The answer is a property of the sequence $\{TT_n\}$.

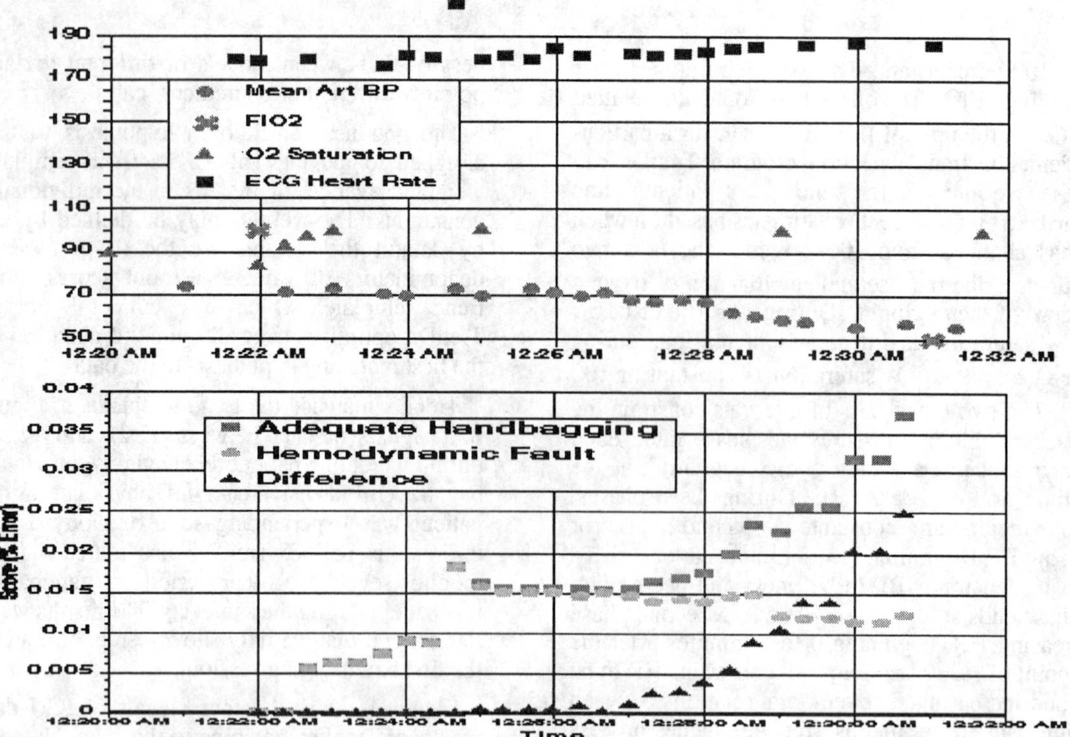

Figure 4: TrenDx results of monitoring ICU data during handbagging.

- When is a fault model a significantly better match to the data than the normal model?

  The answer is a property of the sequence $\{TT_n - TT_{fi}\}$.

There are many possible means to answer these questions. In fact, trying to answer them uncovers another monitoring problem. Notice that each of the TrenDx result plots in Figure 4 is in fact a time-ordered sequence of data, and we wish to detect particular types of trends in these sequences. Does this mean we are back to square one of diagnostic monitoring? Not really, for we have significantly reduced the complexity of our monitoring task in two respects, First, we no longer must represent the *relevant diagnostic categories*, which requires extensive domain knowledge. Instead, we must represent the *relevant monitoring strategies*, which depend less on the progress of disorders but more on the monitoring environment. Second, we have also reduced the dimension of the relevant temporal patterns we seek. No longer are we finding multivariate patterns measurements, but instead we seek univariate patterns in either the time-sequence of best scores $\{TT_n\}$, or the time-sequence of difference in best scores $\{TT_n - TT_{fi}\}$, for some fault model.

In principle, we may use any univariate trend detection scheme available, including TrenDx. We illustrate a few straightforward methods, based on thresholds and accumulation of differences over time.

Thresholds

The simplest method of determining whether the score for of $\{TT_n\}$ or $\{TT_n - TT_{fi}\}$ is significant is establishing a threshold over which the matching score triggers an alarm. A threshold for a high score of $\{TT_n\}$, denoted by TT_n^*, is best determined by experience from training cases. Let $\overline{TTn}$ denote the average value of $\{TT_n\}$ over time for a normal patient case (contiguous data set). We presume $\overline{TTn}$ is normally distributed.[3] We recommend a two-stage supervised learning procedure. In the first stage, run a set of normal cases through TrenDx matching to the normal trend template and compute unbiased estimates of the mean and standard deviation of $\overline{TTn}$. In the second stage, run both normal and abnormal cases through TrenDx using different levels of TT_n^* for sounding an alarm. Select a value of TT_n^* producing satisfactory sensitivity and specificity. If the normality assumption was a close approximation, then choosing TT_n^* as two estimated standard deviations above the mean of $\overline{TTn}$ will yield a sensitivity of better than 0.95.

A significant threshold for $\{TT_n - TT_{fi}\}$ may be learned similarly: first estimate the distribution using

3. This presumption is based on intuition rather than a statistical result. Because $\{TT_n\}$ is non-negative, there may be some skew. With sufficient cases one can test an empirical distribution for normality [5, page 322].

faulty cases, then optimize sensitivity and specificity from normal and faulty cases. One may also find a threshold by relying on intuition, based on a TrenDx score giving a mean percentage error in explaining the data. $\{TT_n - TT_{fi}\}$ being above a threshold p means that the normal trend template is p percent more erroneous than the fault model. One may also consider judging a faulty trend as significant using a threshold for the *percentage better match* of the fault model: $\frac{TT_n - TT_f}{TT_n} = 1 - \frac{TT_f}{TT_n}$.

Accumulators

More reliable sensitivity and specificity may be achieved by accumulating features of $\{TT_n\}$ or $\{TT_n - TT_{fi}\}$ than by mere comparison of a single value to a threshold. Various accumulators are used in *statistical process control* [6, chapter 5]. We re-label the sequences of interest to include their time stamp t: $\{TT_{n,t}\}$ and $\{TT_{n,t} - TT_{fi,t}\}$. Any of the accumulators below may yield satisfactory performance:

- *Runs:* Alarm if R successive values are over a threshold K.
- *Duration:* Alarm if all values within some time range are over a threshold K.
- *Cumulative sum (CUSUM):* Alarm if the accumulated sum of values over a threshold K exceeds another threshold M.
- *Exponentially weighted moving average (EWMA):* Alarm if a geometrically weighted sum of W_t exceeds a threshold K:

  $$W_t = r\left(TT_{n,t} - TT_{fi,t}\right) + (1-r)\,W_{t-1}\,;\; W_0 = 0;$$

  r between 0 and 1.

Just as when using threshold tests for significant trends, one should test any of these accumulation techniques on training data to choose parameter estimates yielding acceptable sensitivity and specificity.

TRIGGERING ALTERNATE MONITOR SETS

Monitor sets represent the set of competing trends in a diagnostic context. The significance of a fault trend may be a sign that the diagnostic context has changed. This in turn may warrant triggering of an alternate monitor set.

The monitor set representation may be supplemented to include rules of the following form:

> If fault trend template TT_f is significant, then trigger monitor set M_j. The temporal distance between point P of TT_f and the anchor point Q on each trend template of M_j is the range $[t_b, t_e]$.

The significance test may be determined via any of the means in the previous section. TrenDx can apply these rules to monitor trends in a changing diagnostic context. Then each of the trend hypotheses in the new context are temporally anchored to process the new data within the appropriate intervals.

GENERATING ALARMS

Having information that a fault trend is significant at time T_0, an automated monitor can send an alarm to operators or clinicians caring for the process. The alarm can state the name of the trend template and the time T_0. Additional text may include descriptions of important value constraints or intervals. The text for these trend template components come fairly naturally from the knowledge representation and from the qualitative temporal interval relations. For example, the text for an alarm of a handbagging hemodynamic fault may read:

> Handbagging hemodynamic fault was detected at 12:27:21 a.m. A phase of decreasing blood pressure proceeded a phase of increasing heart rate.

An alarm may also display some or all of the data in the fault intervals for the best matching fault hypothesis at time T_0.

An automated monitor may wish to alarm based on a boolean combination of significant trends. Forward chaining of a set of production rules may follow any of the significance methods of the previous section.

A more thorough method for deciding whether to send an alarm at time T_0 is evaluation of a *decision model* weighing the costs and benefits of sending the alarm versus not sending the alarm. The utility of alarming is based on:

- estimated probabilities of the normal and abnormal trends, and
- probabilities, costs, and benefits of each action a clinician may take upon seeing the alarm.

The utility of not alarming is based on the trend probabilities as well as

- probabilities, costs, and benefits of each action a clinician may take upon not seeing the alarm.

Considered as a single decision to made at time T_0, one can encode this decision model straightforwardly as a decision tree. This decision is more accurately made in the context of the time progression of the patient, partially as reflected by the best matching trend templates at each time. A critical review of *dynamic decision modeling* techniques is in [7].

DATA VISUALIZATION

Operators in monitoring environments with multiple channels of high frequency data may have extreme difficulty tracking all of this data for significant trends. An intelligent trend detector such as TrenDx may be used to intelligently filter this data to show the operator only that data corresponding to an important component of a faulty process. This display can be driven by rules of the following form:

If fault trend template TT_f is significant, then display data of parameter P_i during the time specification T_i (for i from 1 to some integer k).

The significance test may be determined as previously discussed. Rules may be specific to the monitored process and the operator observing the data.

Each time specification T_i is a Boolean combination of temporal intervals, and may be expressed in a temporal query language such as the time-line language of [8]. Intervals of trend templates can be the time intervals over which data should be displayed.

Rule: If hemodynamic fault significant, then display BP during decreasing phase and a minute before.

BP BP 00:27:21 To DISPLAY

Figure 5: Filtering a data stream using TrenDx results.

An example intelligent display appears in Figure 5. The rule states that when the trend for a handbagging hemodynamic fault is significant, the display should show the blood pressures assigned to the decreasing phase of the trend template and a minute before. The optimal hypothesis for this fault trend is used for sending some data to the display. Thus this high frequency data stream has been filtered. This filtering technique is part of a broader data visualization effort [9].

RELATED WORK

Our work is compatible with time series analysis and signal processing [10]. When applied without context these techniques may produce high false positive rates and redundant alarms. These should lessen if such methods are used within trend template value constraints, which provide an appropriate temporal context.

Others have investigated monitoring using knowledge-based temporal patterns. Keravnou and Washbrook [11] have built a temporal model for diagnosing skeletal dysplasias. Their representation is more limited than trend templates in that time points cannot be fully flexible, and symptoms are limited to tokens for qualitative states. Chemical engineers [12, 13] have used qualitative descriptions of temporal trends in terms of first and second derivatives of single variables. Using rules with temporal patterns in antecedents, they have had promising results monitoring data streams similar to an ICU. These representations are limited in only handling univariate trends over fixed time slices.

REFERENCES

[1] Haimowitz, I. J. and I. S. Kohane. "Automated Trend Detection with Multiple Temporal Hypotheses." IJCAI-93, Chambery, France, 146-151, 1993.

[2] Haimowitz, I. J. and I. S. Kohane. "An Epistemology for Clinically Significant Trends." AAAI-93, Washington, DC, 176-181, 1993.

[3] Nichols, D. G., J. J. McCloskey and M. C. Rogers. "Adult Respiratory Distress Syndrome." In *Textbook of Pediatric Intensive Care*. Baltimore, MD, Williams and Wilkins, 1993.

[4] Haimowitz, I. J. *Knowledge-Based Trend detection and Diagnosis.* Doctoral thesis, Massachusetts Institute of Technology, May 1994.

[5] Sachs, L. *Applied Statistics*. New York, Springer-Verlag, 1984.

[6] Ryan, T. P. *Statistical Methods for Quality Improvement*. Wiley Series in Probability and Mathematical Statistics. New York, Wiley, 1989.

[7] Leong, T.-Y. "Dynamic Decision Modeling in Medicine: A Critique of Existing Formalisms," SCAMC-93, Washington, D.C., 478-484, 1993.

[8] Cousins, S. B. and M. G. Kahn "The Visual Display of Temporal Information." *Artificial Intelligence in Medicine,* **3:** 341-357, 1993.

[9] Fackler, J. and Kohane, I. "Hypothesis-Driven Data Visualization: SmartDisplay," SCAMC-94.

[10] Priestly, M. B. *Spectral Analysis and Time Series.* New York, Academic Press, 1981.

[11] Keravnou, E. T. and J. Washbrook. "A Temporal Reasoning Framework Used in the Diagnosis of Skeletal Dysplasias." *Artificial Intelligence in Medicine,* **2:** 239-265, 1990.

[12] Cheung, J. T.-Y. and G. Stephanopolous. "Representation of Process Trends - Part II. The Problem of Scale and Qualitative Scaling." *Computers in Chemical Engineering,* **14**(4): 511-539, 1990.

[13] Konstantinov, K. B. and T. Yoshida. "Real-Time Qualitative Analysis of the temporal Shapes of (Bio)process Variables." *AIChE Journal,* **38**(11): 1703-1715, 1992.

ACKNOWLEDGMENTS

Peter Szolovits, Isaac Kohane, Howard Shrobe, James Fackler and Milos Hauskrecht have supplied valuable comments on this work. Phillip Phuc Le has continually provided programming support and sound ideas.

A temporal analysis of QMR: abstracted temporal representation and reasoning and initial assessment of diagnostic performance trade-offs

Constantin F. Aliferis, M.D., Gregory F. Cooper, M.D., Ph.D., and Richard Bankowitz, M.D.*
Section of Medical Informatics & Intelligent Systems Program
University of Pittsburgh, Pittsburgh PA
*University Hospital Consortium, Oak Brook, IL

ABSTRACT

Explicit temporal representation and reasoning (TRR) in medical decision-support systems (MDSS) is generally considered to be a useful but often neglected aspect of system design and implementation. Given the great burden of explicit TRR both in knowledge acquisition and computational efficiency, developers of general-purpose large-scale systems typically utilize implicit (i.e., abstracted) forms of TRR. We are interested in understanding better the trade-offs of not incorporating explicit TRR in large general-purpose MDSS along the dimensions of system expressive power and diagnostic accuracy. In particular, we examine the types of abstracted TRR employed in QMR, a diagnostic system in the domain of general internal medicine, and the high-level effects of such an implicit treatment of time in the system's diagnostic performance. We present our findings and discuss implications for MDSS design and implementation practices.

INTRODUCTION

In a review of TRR in MDSS, Kahn [1] proposes an empirical classification which separates systems in two main categories, one based on *temporal ignorance*, and one on explicit representation and utilization of temporal concepts. More specifically he demonstrates how the earlier systems overrode the need for explicit Knowledge Representation and Reasoning (KRR) by incorporating temporal information into ordinary atemporal formalisms. For instance, the INTERNIST-I system would ask questions of the type "did the patient have a history of disease x?", that clearly correspond to an *implicit* or *abstracted* form of TRR. It is obvious that the systems' developers were operating on the assumption that the user of the system would abstract relative data from historical observations and provide it to the program.

Explicitness in TRR practically entails the existence of two main components. First we need a model of time (i.e., a description of temporal primitive entities from which time is composed, plus a set of properties of time, as for example linearity and finiteness). Second, we need an association of entities (objects and relations) to the model of time, such that we can reason about them in one or more temporal contexts, and represent/infer useful temporal knowledge. For all but the most trivial medical domains the use of temporal ignorance is a heuristic approximation to modelling time explicitly. It was applied in a number of influential systems like MYCIN, PIP, DxPlain, CASNET, and ABEL [2]. This way, the developers of MDSS were able to avoid explicit reasoning about temporal concepts, an area within which AI was not well developed in the 70's, or even the early 80's.

On the other hand, a well-known problem in KRR is what Levesque and Brachman call the "fundamental trade-off in KRR" [3]: *more expressive power generally means less computational tractability (and the opposite)*. Given the extensive burden of TRR in terms of efficiency, as well as knowledge acquisition, we believe that any effort to incorporate explicit TRR in large-scale MDSS should be well-justified in terms of expected gains in system performance and/or knowledge engineering (i.e., expressivity of a temporal model vs the atemporal one). In other words, we need to examine *why* and *how* important is the ability to reason explicitly (as contrasted to an abstracted manner) about temporal processes and entities. The importance of TRR has been considered more or less "obvious" and thus has been inadequately explored in the medical AI and medical informatics (MI) literature, especially with respect to *quantifying* its importance.

The basic arguments that have been offered in favor of the necessity of explicit TRR in medical DSSs are :

(a) The *epistemological argument*: observations of physicians diagnostic and therapeutic problem-solving suggest that temporal models of normal and abnormal processes are used, intricate temporal abstractions are created and used to generate and validate or rule-out competing hypotheses. Additionally, physicians are able to utilize temporal planning for either diagnosis (e.g., "watchful expectancy") or therapy [4].

(b) The *linguistic argument:* analysis of discharge summaries and other medical texts indicate an impressive amount of TRR [5].

(c) *Pragmatics argument #1*: certain medical domains

are based on the premise of a time-evolving process, and TRR is fundamental for them (characteristic examples include the protocol-based therapy management, ICU real-time monitoring and intervention, signal processing as in EKG and EEG interpretation) [6,7].

(d) *Pragmatics argument #2*: evaluation of DSSs diagnostic performance shows that some failures to reach the proper diagnosis is attributed to lack of TRR capabilities [8,9].

By carefully examining these arguments, we can make the following remarks: the epistemological and linguistic arguments are purely *descriptive* and do not justify directly the importance of TRR. The first pragmatics argument is certainly true, but refers to a clearly defined, limited subset of DSSs with few or no implications for the majority of systems that perform diagnosis/treatment selections in wide areas of medicine such as INTERNIST-I, MYCIN, etc. These latter systems' need for TRR could be substantiated by the second pragmatics argument, in the sense that, ceteris paribus, if TRR accounts for a substantial number of diagnostic failures and the problems can not be fixed in a reasonable way (i.e., by respecting KA and efficiency constraints), then we can conclude that TRR is indeed necessary.

Unfortunately, support for the second pragmatics argument comes in the form of anecdotal evidence rather than from planned experiments designed to prove or disprove the validity of this hypothesis. One famous example is the 1982 NEJM evaluation of INTERNIST-I (one of the most often cited instances of the second pragmatic argument), which on the basis of 3 cases (out of a total of 19 diagnostic problems) supposedly indicates that explicit TRR is indeed necessary. But the 99% confidence limits of 3/19 (16%) are between 2 and 47%, suggesting that no strong conclusion can be reached from this data regarding the effects of TRR. Even more importantly, the cases were not representative of the average encountered clinical case, since they were CPC cases that were selected on the basis of being very challenging [8].

The previous discussion indicates the need for further investigation and quantitative analysis of the importance of TRR in general-purpose DSSs. It should be clear on the other hand, that for a variety of DSS domains this need is well justified by the nature of the domain (i.e., the nature of the entities represented is so deeply temporal, that either we can not reason about it without taking into account time, or it is grossly ineffective to utilize some implicit/abstracted form of KRR). These domains/tasks include:

- Protocol therapy management,
- Biomedical signal processing,
- "Deep" causal models of diseases/physiology which are grounded on dynamic systems.
- Intensive care unit (ICU) decision-support.

Additionally, it might be more parsimonious and/or natural to represent some normal or abnormal processes in temporal terms (for instance hormonal cycles or compartmental models [6,7,9-11]).

The research presented here intends to investigate the following hypothesis: *In systems operating as aids to clinicians (as opposed to systems that are fully automated) the human operator of the system can provide the necessary abstraction reasoning from temporal entities to the system's atemporal knowledge representation language, such that the system would not have to explicitly incorporate TRR to achieve equal levels of performance as in the temporally explicit case.*

There are a number of additional interesting questions associated with this conjecture:

(i) What constitutes an appropriate collection of abstracted (atemporal) knowledge representations, corresponding to the domain to be modelled?

(ii) Are there specific temporal entities that are crucial to DSS performance? What is the proper level of description of those entities?

(iii) How would these results be useful for systems that operate in automated mode?

In the following sections, we investigate this hypothesis and the related questions by means of an analysis of QMR, a well known MDSS, operating in the domain of diagnosis for general internal medicine, along the dimensions of :

- expressive power (what types of abstracted TRR can be handled by the system)
- performance degradation due to temporal complexities of patient cases.

METHODS

1. Temporal analysis of QMR's terms

We devised a series of variables that correspond to what previous theoretical and empirical work suggests are important temporal reasoning and representation attributes [12-17]. These were used by the first author to classify each finding in QMR as temporal or not based on the following criterion. A QMR finding is temporal if *any* of the following is true: *explicit* reference to either time points/intervals or units, temporal relationships/reasoning, events or facts described in some temporal context, processes occurring over time (explicitly static/evolving, or in sequence/overlapping), or patterns (temporal or spatio-temporal).

We additionally recorded the QMR type (history, physical, simple-inexpensive lab, intermediate lab, advanced-expensive lab) and importance (the "import" value of QMR indicating "need for a finding to be explained if found" [8]), for all findings, regardless of temporal nature. Temporal types (I and II), ontology, and temporal reasoning were created empirically in an incremental fashion, and refined as new QMR findings were examined. Temporal types-II correspond to simple abstractions over QMR findings. A temporal type-I provides a way to describe covariation of variables (i.e., it is a temporal pattern). In essence it is an abstraction over temporal types-II. Reasoning types, on the other hand, denote fundamental relations and other properties that can be put together to form temporal types I&II (for examples of temporal types, and reasoning types see results sections 1.2-1.4). To ensure consistency in the categorization of temporal QMR findings (according to temporal type, and reasoning type) the following procedure was followed: first temporal findings were identified. In the next step values for the variables for *each temporal type*-II were assigned. Due to the limited number of types-II (<120), consistency checks (with previously established temporal types-II) were easier and less error-prone to carry out than the full set of temporal QMR findings. After the types-II had been characterized, individual findings were categorized as belonging to any of specific temporal types-II. As a consequence, each finding would inherit the variable value assignments of the corresponding abstract type-II. As a final step, each individual finding was examined for differences with the type-II it belonged to (due to the abstraction process), and the necessary adjustments were made to the deviating attributes of the individual findings. Then, temporal types-I and temporal reasoning types were abstracted and classified empirically. Standard descriptive statistics were computed for all variables. Bivariate associations were examined with Likelihood Ratio (G^2) tests of independence, Kendall's tau and the gamma coefficient (for ordinal variables). Multivariate relations were examined with the previous statistics controlling for possible confounders [18].

2. Effects of lack of explicit TRR on diagnostic performance

Ideally we would like to test the following (null) statistical hypothesis: *Lack of explicit TRR in QMR does not cause decreased diagnostic performance, (compared to the case where explicit TRR is employed).* Figure 1 presents an idealized experiment built around a post-test design [19] in which the same group of cases is presented to the system. Assuming that the diagnostic system has explicit TRR and that it can be turned on and off at will, diagnoses are performed twice, once with TRR being active and once with TRR being inactive. The performance in the first case is compared to the second one. Obviously this best-case experiment is unattainable. There is no MDSS employing explicit TRR that operates with a scope comparable to that of general internal medicine. Nor is TRR typically implemented in a manner that can be turned on and off, leaving the system reliability intact.

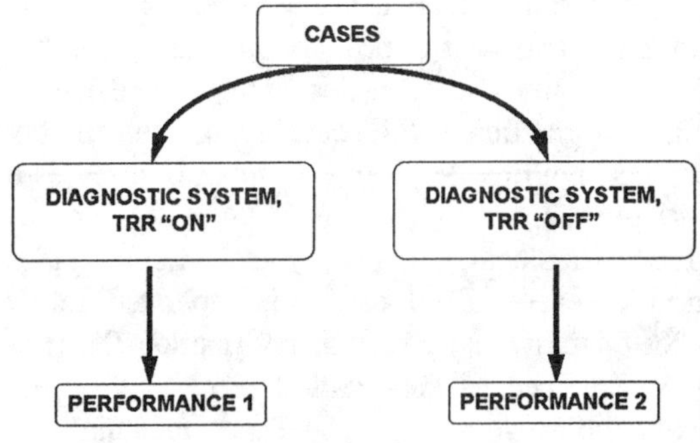

Figure 1: An idealized experiment

Since modifying QMR to incorporate an explicit TRR model is equally infeasible for the purposes of this study, we designed a modified version of the previous experiment, represented in figure 2.

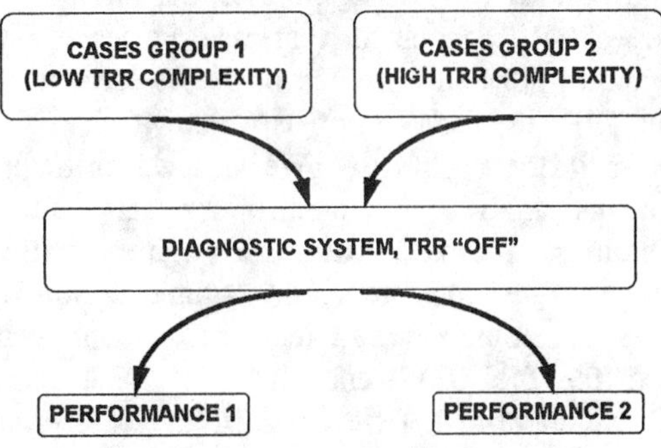

Figure 2: A modified experiment

In this second design two groups are presented to the system. The two groups are similar in every aspect that we would expect to affect performance, except for temporal content. We would like to compare the performance of the system in the two groups. All other things being equal, one would attribute any diagnostic performance discrepancy to the temporal content of the cases (and equivalently to the lack of explicit TRR by QMR). Note that it is important to maintain a prospective design, to avoid a case-control setup (and the associated potential biases with respect to identifying the risk factor, and establishing case-control comparability) [20]. Important considerations in the execution of this design are:

(a) Selection of a representative sample of actual patient cases. We used 105 cases from the latest formal evaluation of QMR (each consisting of history, physical, initial laboratory tests, and discharge summary and diagnoses). The third author (R.B.) is the primary investigator in that study. The coding of the patient information was done by experienced

QMR users, and the cases are considered to be representative of the cases admitted to a large university hospital.

(b) Potential confounders: We considered, and controlled for analytically, several potential confounders (rareness of primary diagnosis, length of case, uncertainty in the description of evidence, spatial information references, causal information references, multiple levels, and number of diseases in true diagnosis).

(c) TRR assessment: The history and physical (H&P) portion of each patient case was separated into a number of individual pieces of information (POI). A POI was defined as the smallest piece of clinically relevant information that could be meaningful if stated in the given document context (thus a POI could be either a stand-alone statement or a qualification of a previously established statement). Each POI was characterized as temporal or not based on the criteria described for QMR findings. For each POI the values of the confounder attributes were assessed. The percentage of temporal POIs divided by the total number of POIs in the case, constituted our measure of TRR content for that case. For each POI the temporal attributes utilized in the assessment of explicit TRR (methods section 1) were evaluated and summarized for each case. We utilized principal components analysis to identify summary linear combinations of those measures as more detailed metrics of the case temporal content. Similar measures of complexity and temporal content were assessed for the QMR encodings for each case. Finally we identified TRR types in the cases that exceeded the expressive capacity of the QMR abstractions (these are discussed in [21]). The temporal attributes' value assignments (for both cases and QMR inputs) were blinded with respect to the case outcome.

(d) Performance assessment: Our criterion was the percentage of cases for which QMR found the primary diagnosis. The following matching criterion was used:

- A match occurred iff the gold standard (GS) primary diagnosis is clinically *equivalent* to one of the q (%) first diagnoses in the QMR differential diagnosis (DD) list. The primary discharge diagnosis (ICD9 primary diagnosis) was considered to be the GS.

- q is defined to be a percentage of diagnoses from QMR's differential diagnosis list. As discussed later in the results section, we chose a q that gave us a mathematically convenient diagnosis rate in the assessment of the effects of TRR content of each case.

- Equivalence is one of the following: *identity, synonymy,* or a *close match.*

- Close match was taken to mean a significantly overlapping disease category or a disease which is at most one level down or up in a recognized clinical classification as those found in major textbooks of medicine (e.g., Harrison's or Cecil's textbook of medicine etc.).

Cases with no established true diagnoses were excluded. When the first (primary) diagnosis in the GS differential was asserted, or given as a finding in QMR, or was not in QMR's KB, the next diagnosis would be the primary one (with a recursive application of the exclusion and skipping rules).

(e) Analysis: All variables associated potentially with diagnostic performance were descretized (based on their 50th percentile as a single cutoff point). Odds-ratios of correct diagnoses were computed between the explanatory variable categories [18].

Logit models (using the continuous variable versions and a standard statistical package) and Bayesian models (through the application of the K2 inductive learning algorithm) were built to assess quantitatively the impact of TRR in the cases to the system's diagnostic accuracy. The interrelations of TRR content and the rest of the explanatory variables were also examined with respect to diagnostic accuracy [18,22].

RESULTS

1. Temporal analysis of QMR's terms

1.1. Ontology

It was found that QMR utilizes the following temporal ontology to express temporal findings.

(a) Entities :

(i) Generic: disease, syndrome, finding, symptom, laboratory value, test result, medical procedures, drugs, causal factors, diagnostic factors.

(ii) Temporal: periods, points of time, seasons, parts of the day, disease intervals, EKG - related intervals, systolic/diastolic periods, units of time.

(b) Relationships/Properties: History of, during, before, after, coincides with, repeating, properties (frequency, speed, rhythm, regularity).

Also Boolean combinations of the above are used to derive more complex propositions.

1.2. Temporal types-I

Forty-nine different TRR types-I were found (and combinations of those). Table 1 presents the most frequent ones, with frequencies.

1.3. Temporal types-II

A total of 116 temporal types-II were found to be employed by QMR within its findings. Table 2 presents the most frequent ones, together with frequencies (% of total number of temporal findings).

1.4. Temporal reasoning

A total of 20 different temporal reasoning types were identified (as well as combinations of those). Table 3 presents the most frequent ones, and their frequencies, together with the relation that they correspond to.

Table 1: Most frequent of temporal types-I (higher level of abstraction over QMR findings)

(1) Hx of disease prior to current one [19.5%]
(2) Hx of event/factor exposure/finding before disease [15.8%]
(3) Event/factor exposure/finding before disease [13.0%]
(4) Hx of remote event/factor exposure/finding before disease [8.2%%]
(5) Finding during period [5.6%]
(6) Finding/disease after drug/medical procedure [4.8%]
(7) Increase/decrease in measurement [4.5%]
(8) Finding at onset/early/middle/late period (e.g., season) [3.5%]
(9) Hx of recurrent/chronic symptom/disease/ finding [2.7%]
(10) Abrupt onset [2.1%]

Table 2: Most frequent of temporal types-II (lower level of abstraction over QMR findings)

(1) Hx of syndrome/disease [11.2%]
(2) Hx of drug administration prior to current illness [8%]
(3) Improvement/worsening of function after/during test/medical procedure/state [7.3%]
(4) Hx of familial disease/behavior [7.2%]
(5) Abnormal/normal finding/syndrome after drug/medical procedure [4.4%]
(6) Hx of exposure to animals/factors [3.6%]
(7) Hx of recent medical procedure [3%]
(8) Hx of recent exposure to factor environment /food/behavior [2.7%]
(9) Increased/decreased rhythm/rate/speed [2.4%]
(10) Measurement per unit of time > C [2.3%]

Table 3: Most frequent temporal reasoning types (in parentheses the fundamental relation each type corresponds to)

(1) Hx of [42.6%] *(before)*
(2) Hx of recent [12.7%] *(before with qualitative distance)*
(3) Finding during period [8.5%] *(during)*
(4) Finding after or during event [8%] *(after or during)*
(5) Properties (e.g., duration etc.) of a temporal primitive [7.7%] *(arbitrary property)*

Figure 3 depicts a multiple-inheritance hierarchical classification of temporal types I & II that captures their main features. A similar classification was developed for temporal reasoning (not shown here).

1.5. Frequency and importance of temporal entities

Of all 4431 QMR findings 17.5% were classified as temporal. Table 4 presents frequency distributions for some of the findings attributes.

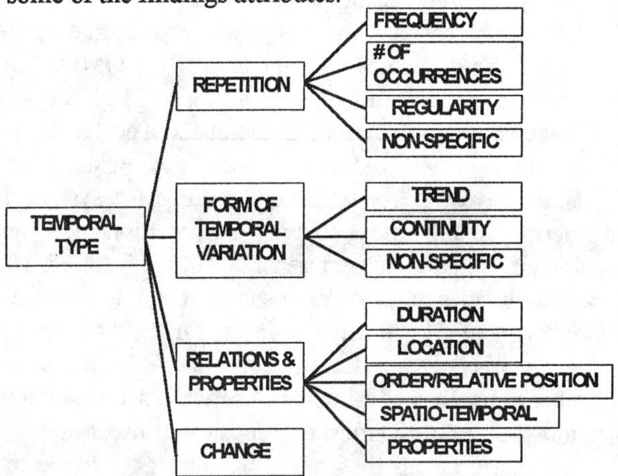

Figure 3: Temporal type (I & II) abstraction

Interesting associations include: Findings that reference temporal units have higher importance (G^2 $p<.0001$, gamma=-.51 with t-value=-3.6). Similarly when we have explicit reference to procedures or patterns, the importance is higher (G^2 $p=.015$ and G^2 $p=.0005$, gamma=.64 with t-value=3.44 respectively). Overall, however, temporal findings have less import than non-temporal ones (G^2 $p<.0001$, gamma=.65 with t-value23.2). Symptoms and signs had less import than more advanced lab findings (G^2 $p<.0001$, tau=0.11 with $p<.0001$). At the same time though, temporal findings are characterized by smaller values in the QMR TYPE scale of diagnostic sophistication (see methods) (G^2 $p<.0001$, tau=.49 with $p<.0001$). When we control for QMR TYPE, the relationship between temporality and importance vanishes.

Table 4: Frequency distributions for main attributes

Among all findings:
TEMPORAL : yes 17.5%, no 82.5%
QMR TYPE : history 11.5%, symptom 5 %, sign 25.4%, lab simple 6.5%, lab intermediate 30.7%, lab expensive/invasive 20.9%
IMPORT : low 2.3%, medium-low 15.8%, medium 35.5% medium-high 32.4%, high 14%
Among temporal findings only:
TIME PRIMITIVES : implicit 93.3 %, explicit points 0.3%, explicit intervals 6.4%
TIME UNITS : yes 5.5%, no 94.5%
TEMPORAL UNCERTAINTY : no 97%, yes 3%
PROCESSES : yes 45.9%, no 54.1%
REPEATING PATTERNS : yes 22.5%, no 77.5%

2. Effects of lack of explicit TRR on diagnostic performance

Based on our diagnostic success criteria, we had to discard a number of patient cases, for any of the following reasons: the diagnosis was a finding in QMR, the diagnosis was not part of the QMR's KB, the cases did not represent a straightforward diagnostic problem (but a therapeutic or "rule-out" problem), QMR did not produce a diagnostic list, diagnoses were asserted (i.e., given to the system as fact), or all the necessary information was not available in the patient record. Thus 35 out of 105 cases were excluded from subsequent analyses. We experimented with various values for the q parameter (see methods), and decided to use q=100% to provide a better balance of sample size between successful and non-successful diagnostic groups (as it turns out, our results are insensitive to this parameter for the tested range of 20 to 100%).

From the examined confounding variables, most were characterized by a small worsening of diagnostic performance (odds ratios were between .54 and .74). TRR content had an odds ratio of .7, which means that the odds of getting a correct diagnosis versus an incorrect one in the high TRR complexity group, was 70% the odds of a correct diagnosis in the low TRR complexity group. Unfortunately, our modest sample size did not allow for tight confidence limits (95% c.l. = .27 to 1.83), and all the associations examined were not statistically significant (at the .05 level), so they must be interpreted as indicative only. Finally, we built a Bayesian Network model utilizing the K2 algorithm. In the most probable model found for this data (as shown in Figure 4), diagnostic correctness is determined jointly by TRR content, uncertainty, diseases number, and spatial information.

This model provides an interpretation of the dependency of diagnostic performance on TRR content and the rest of the variables in the form of a conditional probability distribution:

p(correct-diagnosis | diseases, uncertainty, spatial info, TRR-content)

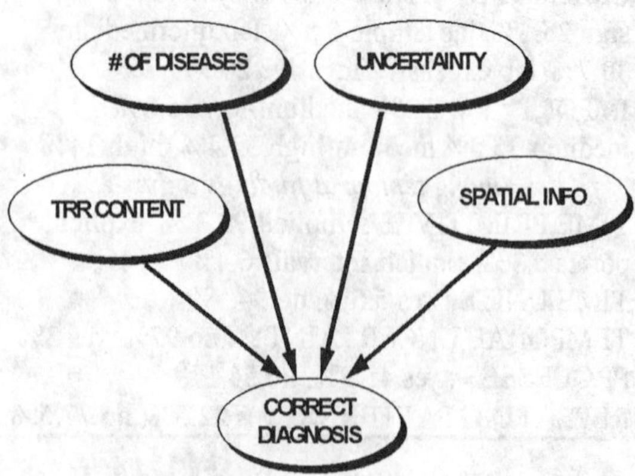

Figure 4: Determinants of diagnostic accuracy

By examining this distribution we concluded that no clear form of covariation exists between TRR content and successful diagnosis, when the rest of the explanatory variables are taken into account. For instance, high TRR content is associated with low probability for correct diagnoses (p=.17) when the other three predictors take the value 'high', while high TRR content is associated with high probability for a correct diagnosis (p=.8) when number of diseases=high and uncertainty=low. Other interesting observations have to do with holding the values of the rest of the three variables constant and observing the probabilities of successful diagnosis: sometimes the probability of a correct diagnoses increases, other times it decreases, when we go from low to high TRR content (depending on the set values of the confounders). Utilizing the principal components - derived measures of TRR case content yielded similar findings. Although the interpretation of these results is complicated and should be viewed with caution in light of the modest sample size, it suggests that *TRR content per se is not a very strong indicator of the diagnostic performance of QMR, in the context of this study, which is evidence in favor of our initial hypothesis.*

DISCUSSION

In this paper we presented an initial analysis of QMR's implicit TRR both in terms of expressive power and performance. At the knowledge-engineering level we were surprised to find out that the QMR knowledge base contains an impressive array of different temporal types, which we identified and classified. The various temporal types are composed of a small number of primitives. We identified this ontology. We additionally abstracted specific temporal patterns and types of temporal reasoning employed, and examined their importance. We believe that the identification of these temporal entities offers three potential benefits:

(a) It *explains the ability of the system* to cope with the rich temporal nature of most patient cases, since it shows an abundance of TRR structures which can be mapped to patient-specific information. In few cases, the patient records were found to contain TRR types that were not in the QMR lexicon [21]. Naturally, this success is highly dependent on the human users of the system, who perform the abstraction from the patient record to the program.

(b) In cases where the system is expected to function independently from human users, it suggests the *types of temporal abstraction mechanisms (and thus intelligent temporal data pre-processors)that should be in place* for the system to function properly. These abstractions complement the set of suggested mechanisms offered by other researchers who have presented well-defined temporal abstraction mechanisms, aimed at having general applicability [14,16]. In contrast to those mechanisms, the abstractions from QMR can be used independently of specific problem-solving methods and software tools. The expected gains are flexibility and speed of development, whereas the trade-off is in clarity of specification and possibly in domain-independent applicability.

(c) In an exploratory sense, it is a starting point for identifying *important TRR requirements for the design of formal MDSS models employing explicit TRR* (for example, among other things, they raise interesting questions about the proper temporal granularity of representing disease-finding relations).

In the second part of the experiments described in this paper, we focused at the performance level. We found that *TRR content has a fairly small, and statistically non-significant, effect on the diagnostic performance of QMR.*

Although we demonstrate satisfactory heuristic power for the QMR system/domain with respect to the temporal robustness of its heuristic, implicit handling of time, we believe that by conditioning the diagnostic performance of the system on a set of a well-specified temporal criteria [23], we will be able to gain further insight into the limits of implicit TRR. Such an analysis can be greatly facilitated by using a formal language for TRR. We plan to pursue this direction of research. Finally it should be kept in mind that our findings are specific to the QMR system and domain. We hope that these results will stimulate similar analyses for other medical systems and domains, so that eventually MDSS developers will be able to make more conscious and informed choices when it comes to selecting among explicit and implicit TRR methods, given their operational constraints and domain of application.

ACKNOWLEDGEMENTS

The first author is indebted to Prof. B.G. Buchanan, and Dr. R.A. Miller for their invaluable guidance throughout the design, implementation, and interpretation of the research described in this paper. The authors would also like to thank Dr. N. Giuse for her assistance with the utilization of the QMR diagnostic performance patient cases in this paper, as well as for useful comments.

Reference

(1) Kahn MG "Modelling time in medical decision-support programs" Med Dec Making 1991;11:249-264.

(2) E. Shortliffe and L. Perreault (eds.): Medical Informatics: Computer applications in Health Care. Addison-Wesley 1990.

(3) Levesque HJ, Brachman RJ. A fundamental tradeoff in knowledge representation and reasoning. In: *Readings in Knowledge Representation*. Levesque HJ, Brachman RJ (eds.) Morgan Kauffman Publishers 1985, 42-70.

(4) Kassirer J. Kopelamn R "Learning clinical reasoning" Williams and Wilkins 1991.

(5) Sager N "Medical language processing: computer management of narrative data" Reading Mass: Addison-Wesley 1987.

(6) Fagan LM "VM: representing time-dependent relations in a medical setting" Doctoral dissertation, Stanford 1980.

(7) Ackerman E, Gatewood L "Mathematical models in the health sciences" Univ. of Minnesota Press, 1979.

(8) Miller RA, Pople HE, Myers JD. INTERNIST-I, an experimental computer-based diagnostic consultant for general internal medicine. N Engl J Med 1982; 307: 468-476.

(9) Long W, Naimi S, Criscitielo M "Development of a knowledge base for diagnostic reasoning in cardiology" Comput Biomed Res 1992;25: 292-311.

(10) Stefanelli M "Therapy planning and monitoring" (editorial) Artificial Intelligence in Medicine 1992;4: 189-190.

(11) Chandrasekaran B, Wong T, Pryor T " 'Deep' models and their relation to diagnosis" Artificial Intelligence in Medicine 1989;1: 29-40.

(12) Allen JF, Hayes PJ "A common sense theory of time" IJCAI proceedings 1985:528-531.

(13) Berzuini C, Bellazi R, Quaglini S, Spiegelhalter D "Bayesian networks for patient monitoring" Artificial Intelligence in Medicine 1992;4: 243-260.

(14) Shahar Y Musen MA "RESUME: a temporal-abstraction system for patient monitoring". Comput Biomed Res 1993; 26: 255-73

(15) Das A, Tu S, Purcell G, Musen M "An extended SQL for temporal data management in clinical decision-support systems" SCAMC 1992:128-132.

(16) Kohane I. "Temporal reasoning in medical expert systems" MEDINFO 1986: 170-174.

(17) Shoham Y "Temporal logics in AI: Semantical and ontological considerations " Artificial Intelligence 1987;33: 89-104.

(18) Agresti A "Categorical data analysis" Wiley 1990.

(19) Spector P "Research designs" Sage 1981.

(20) Colton T "Statistics in Medicine" Little, Brown 1974.

(21) Aliferis CF, Cooper GF, Buchanan BG, Miller RA, Bankowitz R, Giuse N "Temporal reasoning abstractions in QMR" Report SMI-94-03, 1994.

(22) Cooper GF, Herskovits E "A Bayesian method for the induction of probabilistic networks from data" Machine Learning, 1992; 9: 309-347.

(23) Aliferis CF, Miller RA "On the heuristic nature of Medical Decision Support Systems" Report SMI-94-05, 1994.

Incorporating Temporal and Clinical Reasoning in a New Measure of Continuity of Care

S. Andrew Spooner, M.D.
Division of Medical Informatics, Department of Internal Medicine
Washington University School of Medicine, St. Louis, MO 63110

Previously described quantitative methods for measuring continuity of care have assumed that perfect continuity exists when a patient sees only one provider, regardless of the temporal pattern and clinical context of the visits. This paper describes an implementation of a new operational model of continuity—the Temporal Continuity Index—that takes into account time intervals between well visits in a pediatric residency continuity clinic. Ideal continuity in this model is achieved when intervals between visits are appropriate based on the age of the patient and clinical context of the encounters. The fundamental concept in this model is the expectation interval, which contains the length of the maximum ideal follow-up interval for a visit and the maximum follow-up interval. This paper describes an initial implementation of the TCI model and compares TCI calculations to previous quantitative methods and proposes its use as part of the assessment of resident education in outpatient settings.

INTRODUCTION

Continuity of medical care has been operationally defined as "the extent to which the same provider is seen during a sequence of visits" [1]. Previously described quantitative methods for measuring continuity of care have assumed that perfect continuity exists when a patient sees only one provider, regardless of the temporal pattern and clinical context of the visits; but even a patient who sees the same provider 100% of the time may have poor continuity if the visits are inappropriately timed. This paper describes an implementation of a new operational model of continuity that takes into account some temporal and clinical factors and applies it in measuring continuity of care for well visits in a pediatric residency continuity clinic.

Continuity of care is an essential component of primary care [2]. Patients consider continuity an important determinant of the quality of their health care [3, 4], and health care providers regard continuous care as the ideal [2, 5, 6]. Evidence exists from outcomes studies that health care delivery systems which allow continuity result in lower health care costs [7, 8], more efficient identification of problems [9], better compliance with drug regimens and appointments [10-13], and improved job satisfaction of health care workers [11, 12, 14]. Medical educators consider continuity of care to be an essential, albeit elusive, goal in outpatient medical education [15-17] since continuous care provides students and residents with a more complete picture of the natural history of disease and well care. An objective measure of continuity of care would be of great use to medical educators as they attempt to ensure high quality educational experiences in increasingly outpatient-oriented training programs.

Traditional measures of continuity of care, which have been reviewed elsewhere, have considered continuity from the point of view of a patient, a visit, or a provider [3, 18, 19]. The most frequently used patient-based measure, Usual Provider Continuity (UPC [20]) is the ratio of the number of visits to a patient's "usual" provider to the total number of visits for that patient. A patient-based measure that uses temporal information is Sequential Continuity (SECON [18]), which views a series of clinical encounters as pairs of consecutive visits; SECON is the ratio of the number of pairs with the same provider to the total number of pairs. Visit-based measures compute continuity based on the visits that occurred during a fixed interval prior to the visit in question. A visit-based measure that uses temporal information is *discounted fraction-of-care continuity* (f_τ) [21]. f_τ is a modification of UPC which uses weights based on how recent a previous visit is relative to the present visit. This measure is said to be visit-based because it assigns a number to a visit; one computes a score for the patient by combining all of the patient's visit scores. Provider-based methods combine the results from patient-based or visit-based methods for each provider. Implicit in all these measures is an assumption that one provider per patient represents perfect continuity.

While measures like SECON and f_τ take some temporal aspects of continuity into account, no continuity measure takes clinical context into account. For example, if a patient sees a physician for two well visits spaced nine months apart, the continuity that this pattern of visits represents can be good or bad, depending on the patient's age and clinical problems. If the initial visit was for a newborn, then this pattern represents poor continuity. If the initial visit was for a two year old, then a nine-month interval may represent good continuity.

Hoekelman and Peters [22] modified the Well Baby Visit index of Barron and Mindlin [23] to create a Health Supervision Index (HSI) that could be applied to a pattern of well visits in the first two years of life. This measure divides the first two years of life into periods during which at least one well visit must occur. For the first six months of life, the periods are one month long; during the second six months, two months; and for the second year of life, three months. This partitioning of the first two years corresponded to the prevalent American Academy of Pediatrics recommendations [24] at the time. While HSI addresses the temporal nature of a certain kind of medical care, it is not generally applicable to all ages and clinical problems.

TEMPORAL CONTINUITY INDEX

Assumptions

In the Temporal Continuity Index (TCI) model, it is assumed that there is an ideal interval between visits and that continuity decreases and eventually vanishes altogether as this ideal interval is exceeded. Thus, to achieve maximal continuity, it is not enough to see just one provider; ideal continuity in this model is achieved when intervals between visits are appropriate based on the age of the patient and clinical context of the encounters. These intervals vary with the age of the patient and the clinical problems addressed in the visits. In this model, each visit receives a continuity score, the Temporal Continuity Index (TCI_v), between 0 and 1; continuity for patients (TCI_{pt}) and providers (TCI_{pr}) may be computed by averaging the TCI_v for each relevant visit. It is assumed that the primary data represent ambulatory visits between identifiable patients and providers, and that the time for each visit and basic diagnostic coding for each visit is available.

Expectation Intervals and Closing Criteria Model

The fundamental concept in this model is the *expectation interval*, which contains the length of the maximum ideal follow-up interval for a visit (t_i), and the maximum follow-up interval (t_m). Each visit has an expectation interval and a set of closing criteria. *Closing criteria* define which future visits may close a prior visit v_0; for example, only those subsequent visits with diagnoses similar to v_0 may close v_0. If v_0 is closed by a subsequent visit before t_i, maximal continuity for that visit is achieved. If it is closed between t_i and t_m, then v_0 receives a continuity score less than maximal, depending on the position of the closing visit within the interval. Closing visits after t_m result in a minimal continuity score for the visit. Each time a visit is recorded, (whether it closes another visit's interval or not) its expectation interval is computed and attached to the visit. The model intentionally omits the concept of the minimal ideal follow-up interval, since to specify a minimal interval would tend to penalize providers for seeing a patient earlier than expected.

Figure 1 illustrates a visit which is associated with an expectation interval and a set of closing criteria. Closing visits (visits which meet the closing criteria) must occur before t_m or the expectation interval will time out spontaneously, which results in a TCI_v of 0 for the visit. The linear taper between t_i and t_m represents the decreasing continuity if a closing visit occurs between t_i and t_m. In most situations, closing visits must involve the same provider; this need not be the case, however: for instance, one may want to allow different providers but require they be in the same practice group.

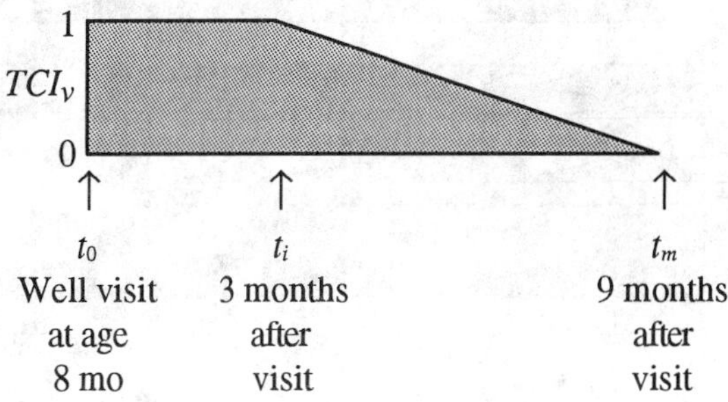

Figure 1: Expectation interval for a visit. For this well visit in an eight-month old, t_i is 3 months and t_m is 9 months after the visit.

Clinical Reasoning

The length of expectation intervals vary with the clinical problem. Age of the patient at a well visit affects expectation intervals; follow-up for well care in a teenager allows much longer intervals than follow-up for well care in infants. Diagnoses at non-well visits would also affect expectation intervals; for example, follow-up for tinea capitis is of longer duration than for an asthma exacerbation, because the natural history of one disease episode is longer than the other.

Not all visits require follow-up, so lack of a follow-up visit for certain types of visits need not imply a penalty for the provider's continuity score. For instance, most acute illnesses resolve without complications, so no closing visit is necessary. Well visits, on the other hand, are expected to be followed by an appropriately timed follow-up well visit. Thus, well visits are classified as *penalty visits*; there is a penalty to the continuity score if there is no follow-up of these visits. Visits associated with other diagnoses may be penalty visits depending on the clinical context. In the TCI model, the TCI_v of a penalty visit is included in the average for the provider whether it is zero or non-zero. The TCI_v of non-penalty visits is omitted from the computation of TCI_{pr} if it is zero.

The specification of closing criteria requires clinical knowledge to determine which visits close which others. An visit may close a prior well visit if it involved the same patient, the same physician, and is itself a well visit. For other diagnoses, these criteria may be more complex.

Figure 2 illustrates the pattern of visits for four patients over eight months. TCI computations for patients A, B, and C are shown in Table 2.

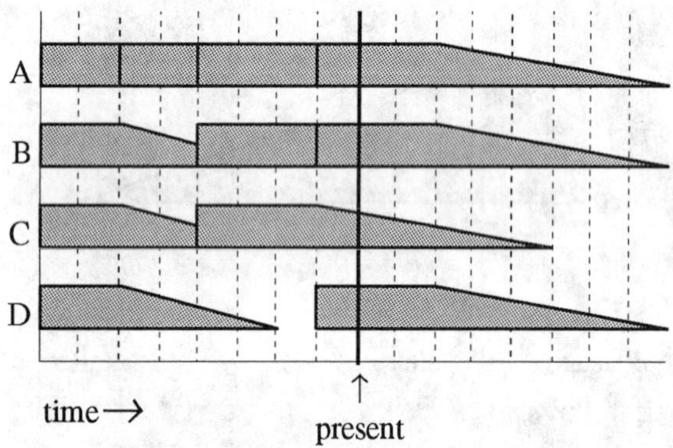

Figure 2: Pattern of visits for four patients. Patient A has ideal intervals among the four visits and thus has maximal continuity. Patients B, C, and D have progressively worse continuity, since the expectation interval between visits is closed after the magnitude of TCI_v begins to taper.

IMPLEMENTATION OF THE MODEL

Program Design

A program was written in the Common Lisp Object System (Macintosh Common Lisp, Apple Computer, Cupertino, CA) to store residents' experience data and to perform continuity of care calculations according to the Temporal Continuity Index model. Relational tables from the Resident Group Practice continuity clinic database (patient identifiers, resident identifiers, and diagnostic data) in the Department of Pediatrics at Washington University School of Medicine were used as input to construct objects in three classes (resident, patient, and visit). Since the objective of this program was to provide an index of continuity for each resident, the program did not produce continuity scores for each patient.

Resident Object

Resident objects contain an identifier and an indicator of the resident's level of training. To each resident object is attached two lists of visit objects: a *pending* visit list and a *final* visit list. New visits enter the pending list to await closure. As soon as all possible closing visits have occurred (if any), the visit is moved to the final list. The final list contains visits which have been closed by another visit or which have spontaneously timed out because no closing visit occurred. The chief reason for maintaining two separate lists is to decrease the number of visits to consider closing each time a new visit enters the system.

Patient Object

The patient object contains patient identifiers, demographic information, and a list of diagnoses with which the patient has been associated.

Visit Object

Each visit object carries identifiers for the relevant resident and a patient, along with the date, diagnosis codes, state of the visit (open or closed), closing criteria, closing penalty (to indicate whether there is a penalty for not explicitly closing the visit), and the expectation intervals t_i and t_m. The visit also holds the maximum TCI_v for the visit. The state of the visit (open or closed) refers to the absence or presence of a closing visit, respectively; a closed visit may stay on the resident's open list until the possibility of out-of-order entry of further closing visits has passed.

Derivation of Expectation Intervals

The American Academy of Pediatrics publication *Guidelines for Health Supervision II* [25] was used to establish the best times at which children should be seen by their primary care provider for health supervision. Based on these times, maximal ideal time intervals for a follow-up well visit (t_i) were established for each age range (Table 1). The breakpoint for each age range is the midpoint of the interval between the last two ages recommended by the AAP guidelines for the corresponding ideal follow-up interval. Maximum meaningful follow-up intervals (t_m) were established for each age range by multiplying the ideal interval by three.

Derivation of Closing Criteria

In this implementation a closing visit for a well visit was defined as another well visit of the same patient to the same physician within the appropriate time interval. Visits for acute illnesses did not count as closing visits for well visits.

Computing TCI for a Provider (TCI_{pr})

TCI_{pr} for each resident is taken as the mean TCI_v for each visit associated with that resident for which TCI_v can be calculated. From the pending list, only those visits for which a TCI_v have been computed are used to calculate the mean. From the final list, all visits except non-penalty visits with TCI_v of zero are used to compute the mean.

Table 1: Follow-up intervals for well care based on AAP guidelines. Current AAP guidelines recommend a newborn visit, a visit at 2-4 weeks, and visits at 2, 4, 6, 9, 12, 15, and 18 months, followed by an annual visit until age 6 and then every two years until adulthood.

Age Ranges	Ideal Follow-up Interval (t_i)	Maximum Follow-up Interval (t_m)
0-5 mo	2 mo	6 mo
5-16.5 mo	3 mo	9 mo
16.5-21 mo	6 mo	18 mo
21 mo-5.5 yr	1 yr	3 yr
≥ 5.5 yr	2 yr	6 yr

Table 2: Continuity calculations involving three patients with different patterns of well care. Computations are as of 11/1/94. Patient A has the optimal pattern of well care. f_τ (discounted fraction of continuity) and SECON (sequential continuity) are included for comparison to TCI scores.

Patient	M.D.	Visit	Date	Patient Age	TCI Computation				f_τ score	*SECON* score
					Ideal F/U (t_i)	Max F/U(t_m)	Closed by	TCI_v		
Patient A: Ideal Situation										
A	1	A-1	3/1/94	2 mo	2 mo	6 mo	A-2	1	N/A	N/A
A	1	A-2	5/1/94	4 mo	2 mo	6 mo	A-3	1	1	1
A	1	A-3	7/1/94	6 mo	3 mo	9 mo	A-4	1	1	1
A	1	A-4	10/1/94	9 mo	3 mo	9 mo	N/A	N/A	1	1
Mean for Patient A								1	1	1
Patient B: Missed 4 mo appointment										
B	1	B-1	3/1/94	2 mo	2 mo	6 mo	B-2	0.5	N/A	N/A
B	1	B-2	7/1/94	6 mo	3 mo	9 mo	B-3	1	1	1
B	1	B-3	10/1/94	9 mo	3 mo	9 mo	N/A	N/A	1	1
Mean for Patient B								0.75	1	1
Patient C: Ideal timing, alternating providers										
C	1	C-1	3/1/94	2 mo	2 mo	6 mo	C-3	0.5	N/A	N/A
C	2	C-2	5/1/94	4 mo	2 mo	6 mo	C-4	0.25	0	0
C	1	C-3	7/1/94	6 mo	3 mo	9 mo	N/A	N/A	0.47	0
C	2	C-4	10/1/94	9 mo	3 mo	9 mo	N/A	N/A	0.33	0
Mean for Patient C								0.38	0.27	0
Mean for M.D. 1								0.83	0.73	0.63

COMPARISON TO PREVIOUS METHODS

In Table 2 is a schedule of visits for three patients, which represents the continuity clinic activity for one resident (M.D. 1) from 3/1/94 to 11/1/94. Patients A, B, and C all begin attending the continuity clinic at age 2 months on 3/1/94. Patient A keeps the recommended schedule of appointments. Patient B misses the four-month well visit, and patient C alternates visits between two residents.

The TCI_{pr} for M.D. 1 as of 11/1/94 is the mean of TCI_v for visits A-1, A-2, A-3, B-1, B-2, and C-1. The other visits have not yet closed or are with another physician, so they do not count in the TCI_{pr} calculation yet. So TCI_{pr} is 0.83 for this resident based on these data on 11/1/94. This reflects the less than perfect sequence of visits for the three patients the resident saw. To use UPC to calculate a continuity score for the resident requires calculating UPC for each patient the resident saw and then averaging the values. In this case UPC for patients A and B is 1.0, regardless of the fact that patient B missed an appointment. UPC for patient C is 0.5, since that patient saw the usual provider half the time, so the UPC-based continuity score for the resident is 0.83.Averaging discounted fraction of continuity (f_τ) for the eight visits for which it is possible to compute an f_τ yields a value of 0.73. The problem with patient B remains, though; patient B's continuity was maximal by the f_τ method despite the inadequate temporal pattern of visits. SECON is included in Table 2 to illustrate the problem of underestimating the continuity of a patient who alternates providers.

FUTURE PLANS

The next step in this work on continuity measurement is to extend the TCI score to include clinical visits with illness diagnoses. Work is underway to collect expert opinion from the practicing pediatricians in the Community Outpatient Practice Experience Program on intervals for the most common ambulatory pediatric diagnoses. To handle non-well diagnoses, the model described here will need to take into account visits in which multiple diagnoses are listed. Closing criteria for such visits are more complex, since a follow-up visit may not have diagnostic coding identical to the original visit. Further extensions of the model may also need to consider a *minimal* ideal continuity interval.

Other future work includes the establishment of norms of continuity (TCI_{pr})based on clinical encounter data collected from practicing pediatricians. These norms should allow the use of TCI as a standard for residents in their continuity clinic experience. Ultimately this work will lead to a large scale database implementation of continuity of care measurement in the ongoing pediatric residency program, for which we are now constructing the data model. As residency programs increasingly use outpatient settings for resident education, measures such as the Temporal Continuity Index will help to assure adequate preparation for primary care physicians.

ACKNOWLEDGMENTS

I would like to thank Michael G. Kahn, M.D., Ph.D., Chief, Division of Medical Informatics, Department of Internal Medicine at Washington University School of Medicine for his persistent guidance. Thanks also to Mark E. Frisse, M.D., Associate Dean and Director, School of Medicine Library, for his mentorship in this fellowship. I would also like to thank Kimberlee C. Recchia, M.D., Director of the Community Outpatient Practice Experience program at St. Louis Children's Hospital for access to data on residents' clinical experiences.

Dr. Spooner is an American Academy of Pediatrics Fellow of the Pediatric Scientist Development Program of the American Medical School Pediatric Department Chairmen, Inc.

Reference

[1] Eriksson EA, Mattsson LG. Quantitative measurement of continuity of care: Measures in use and an alternative approach. Med Care 1983; 21:858-75.
[2] Institute of Medicine. A Manpower Policy for Primary Health Care. Washington, DC: National Academy of Sciences, 1978.
[3] Shortell SM. Continuity of medical care: conceptualization and measurement. Med Care 1976;14:377-91.
[4] Mindlin RM, Densen PM. Medical care of urban infants: Continuity of care. Am J Public Health 1969; 59:1294-301.
[5] McWhinney IR. Continuity of care in family practice: Part 2. Implications of continuity. J Fam Pract 1975; 2:373-4.
[6] Alpert JJ, Charney E. The Education of Physicians for Primary Care. Washington, DC: US Government Printing Office, 1973.
[7] Alpert JJ, Robertson LS, Kosa J, Heagerty MC. Delivery of health care for children: Report of an experiment. Pediatrics 1976; 57:917-30.
[8] Wasson JH, Sauvigne AE, Mogielnicki P, et al.

Continuity of outpatient medical care in elderly men. JAMA 1984; 252:2413-7.

[9] Starfield BH, Simborg DW, Horn SD, Yourtee RN. Continuity and coordination in primary care: their achievement and utility. Med Care 1976; 14:625-36.

[10] Charney E, Bynum R, Eldredge D, et al. How well do patients take oral penicillin? A collaborative study in private practice. Pediatrics 1967; 40:188-95.

[11] Becker MH, Drachman RH, Kirscht JP. Predicting mother's compliance with pediatric medical regimens. J Pediatr 1972; 81:843-54.

[12] Becker MH, Drachman RH, Kirscht JP. A field experiment to evaluate various outcomes of continuity of physician care. Am J Public Health 1974; 64:1064-70.

[13] Boethius G. The treatment of hypertension: an analysis of drug prescription data. Acta Med Scand (suppl.) 1976; 602:120-3.

[14] Caplan EK, Sussman MB. Rank order of important variables for patient and staff satisfaction with outpatient services. J Health Hum Behav 1966; 7:133-7.

[15] Ruane TJ, Brody H. Understanding and teaching continuity of care. J Med Educ 1987; 62:969-73.

[16] Moore L, Busing N. Continuity of care in the family medicine residency. Can Fam Physician 1993; 39:531-34.

[17] Zones SZ, Schroeder SA. Evolving residency requirements for ambulatory care training for five medical specialties, 1961 to 1989. West J Med 1989; 151:676-8.

[18] Steinwachs DM. Measuring provider continuity in ambulatory care. Med Care 1979; 17:551-65.

[19] Smedby Ö, Eklund G, Eriksson EA, Smedby B. Measures of continuity of care: a register-based correlation study. Med Care 1986; 24:511-8.

[20] Breslau N, Reeb KG. Continuity of care in a university-based practice. J Med Educ 1975; 50:965-9.

[21] Smedby B, Smedby Ö, Eriksson EA, Mattsson LG, Lindgren Å. Continuity of care: An application of visit-based measures. Med Care 1984; 22:676-80.

[22] Hoekelman RA, Peters EN. A health supervision index to measure standards of child care. Health Serv Reports 1972; 87:537-43.

[23] Barron BA, Mindlin RL. An index of infant health supervision. Pediatrics 1969; 43:892-4.

[24] Council on Pediatric Practice. Standards of Child Health Care. Evanston, IL: American Academy of Pediatrics, 1967.

[25] Committee on Psychosocial Aspects of Child and Family Health. Guidelines for Health Supervision II. Elk Grove Village, IL: American Academy of Pediatrics, 1988.

Computer-Based Approaches to Knowledge Acquisition

Automated Medical Knowledge Acquisition: A Study of Consistency

Gwendolyn C. Murphy, Ph.D. and Charles P. Friedman, Ph.D.
University of North Carolina at Chapel Hill

ABSTRACT

Knowledge bases are more representative of the population of medical experts if they are constructed by a group of individuals, rather than one practitioner. However, one runs into problems with consistency when information is elicited from a group without a consistent format and terminology. This study examines the consistency of relatively unconstrained computer-elicited medical knowledge using the computer program, KSSO. The results of this study show that the group of ten general internists were somewhat consistent in the diagnoses they listed for a patient presenting with chest pain. They were much less consistent in the findings they listed to differentiate between the diagnoses they had listed. The mean number of subjects listing each diagnosis was 3.3 $\pm$2.7 while the mean for findings was 2.0 $\pm$ 1.5. The implications of these data are discussed.

INTRODUCTION

Until recently, development and maintenance of many knowledge bases (KBs) has been a task that required the services of a knowledge engineer to translate the elicited data into machine language [1]. Most knowledge bases have been constructed by having one expert develop one disease profile at a time. The disease profile is then evaluated and modified by a group of experts [2]. Because it has been so time-consuming a task, only a small group of people has usually been involved. Rarely are multiple experts asked to develop a profile for the same disease [3]. Consequently, the acquired knowledge may reflect representations particular to the small group of authors. To increase the generalizability of the KB, it could be based on the collaboration of many different groups of individuals. Automated knowledge acquisition is now making this possible.

Several computer programs have been developed to facilitate knowledge acquisition by different individuals working on the same project [1,4, 5, 6]. The validity and reproducibility of such an approach is beginning to be documented [3]. One program that was designed to elicit knowledge from individuals in an unconstrained way and without the need for a knowledge engineer is Knowledge Support System Zero (KSS0). KSS0 is an "implicit", problem-solving program because the user does not need to understand how the program works [7]. A program of this type provides a method to build a representation of the subject's conceptual structure without direct elicitation. Instead, the subject provides examples within the domain of interest and then states in concrete terms how to distinguish between the examples [8]. Shaw and Gaines have developed the program KSS0 and have used it to elicit and compare information from multiple experts [9]. According to Shaw, hierarchical and spatial cluster analysis of the gathered data can be used to develop the conceptual structure for that subject [10].

KSS0 is based on personal construct psychology of Kelly [11]. Kelly proposed that individuals use their experience to develop constructs, which are defined as abstract qualities that one uses to model reality. As each person tests these constructs against reality, s/he revises them. Kelly hypothesized that each person evolves a finite number of constructs and attributes that go along with those constructs. The constructs and attributes are related in such a way that a grid, called a repertory grid, can be produced from the elicited data and an hierarchical classification can be developed from the grid.

A major problem that has been encountered with multi-center knowledge acquisition is consistency of the product. Medicine is such a complex field that there are usually several possible ways to approach any problem. As a result, it is difficult to find an agreed upon standard. Instead, standards of care vary from region to region, and sometimes even from practitioner to practitioner. This study answers the question of how consistent is a group of general internists in how they describe the diagnosis of a patient who presents with chest pain. Specifically, what diagnoses are on their differential, and what findings (history, physical, and laboratory) do they use to distinguish between the diagnoses?

PROCEDURE

The subjects were ten relatively young,

faculty-level physicians, each of whom had finished three years of residency training and was board certified in internal medicine. They had been in practice an average of 5.3 years (range 1-11 years). These physicians were all participants in a Faculty Development Fellowship in General Internal Medicine at the University of North Carolina at Chapel Hill, but they came from ten different academic institutions from across the mid-Atlantic region. Eight of the ten subjects estimated they had encountered one hundred to one thousand patients presenting with chest pain. Two of the subjects estimated they had seen over a thousand such patients.

The program, KSS0, asks the subject to generate a list of constructs (diagnoses in this study) and attributes (findings in this study). The diagnoses and findings were to be applicable to a patient presenting with chest pain. The subject then entered the list of diagnoses into the computer. For this portion, subjects were limited to a maximum of 15 diagnoses because that was the most that could fit on the computer screen simultaneously. In some cases the subjects had to reduce their initial list of diagnoses. They were told to choose the most likely and/or important diagnoses.

Next, the subject was directed to enter a finding (history, physical exam, or laboratory test) by specifying the result and its opposite (e.g., febrile--afebrile). The computer positioned the finding and its opposite at either end of a line. The subject then placed each of the previously listed diagnoses where it seemed to belong on a line between the finding and its opposite. For example, if the finding was febrile-afebrile, pneumonia would likely be at the febrile pole, and angina would likely be at the afebrile pole. See Figure 1.

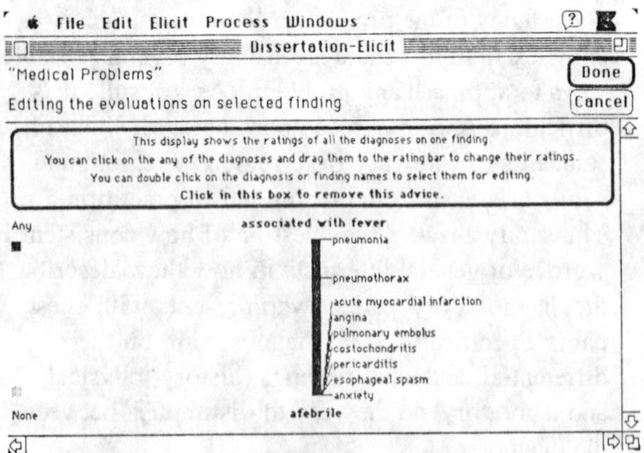

Figure 1
Rating the diagnoses on one finding

The subject placed all the diagnoses on the scale where s/he thought they belonged. Once the subject had moved all the diagnoses to their desired position, the subject could proceed to the next screen for the next finding. This process continued until the subject had entered all the findings s/he could. For each finding, the program recorded a number from 1-9 to denote the position of the diagnosis on the finding. KSS0 used these values to construct a repertory grid of the diagnoses by findings. See Figure 2.

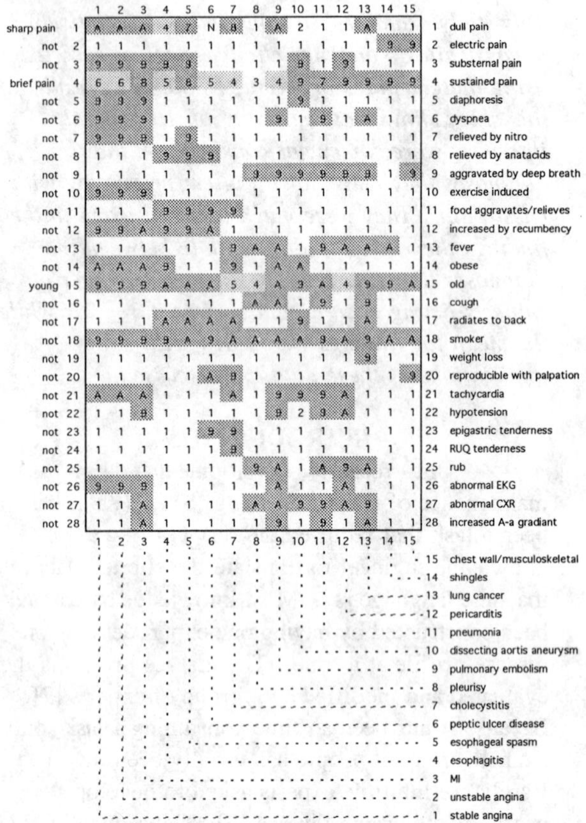

Figure 2
Example of a repertory grid

The repertory grids provide a large amount of data. Terms that were synonymous (such as shortness of breath and tachypnea) were merged by the first author and verified by an experienced family physician. Any question of whether they were synonymous resulted in them not being merged. The diagnoses and findings were sorted by the number of subjects listing each. The mean and standard deviation was calculated for the number of subjects listing each diagnosis or finding. The degree of overlap in diagnoses or findings can be summarized by a coefficient of consistency (CC) in which the number of elements listed by two or more subjects is divided by the number of entries listed after merging synonymous terms.

$$CC = \frac{E_c}{E_m}$$

CC=coefficient of consistency
Ec= the number of consistent elements listed
Em=number of merged elements

This coefficient can vary between one (if all of the subjects list the same elements) and zero if there are no elements in common. The results are presented below.

RESULTS

The data from this study are based on a single session with each subject. The terms used by the subjects to express diagnoses varied between general terms and very specific ones. For example, for musculoskeletal diseases, some subjects listed "chest wall--musculoskeletal" while others listed "rib fracture" or "costochondritis". All or nearly all of the subjects had one or more diagnoses in the areas of musculoskeletal, cardiac, pulmonary, and gastrointestinal disease. Several diagnoses were listed by seven or more subjects, including angina, pneumonia, pulmonary embolus, chest wall/musculoskeletal, myocardial infarct, pericarditis, and pleurisy. There were 14 diagnoses listed by only one subject. The findings listed showed much more variability than did the diagnoses. There were 78 findings listed by only one subject, and only two findings listed by seven or more subjects. The mean number of physicians listing each diagnosis and finding was 3.3 and 2.0 respectively. The coefficient of consistency for the diagnoses and findings was .60 and .40 respectively. See Table 1 below for the means, standard deviations, and coefficients of consistency.

Table 1
Means, standard deviations and coefficients of consistency for diagnoses and findings

Type of Entry	# MDs/entry mean ± s.d.	CC
Diagnoses	3.3 ± 2.7	.60
Findings	2.0 ± 1.5	.40

The frequencies of diagnoses and findings are shown by Figures 3 and 4.

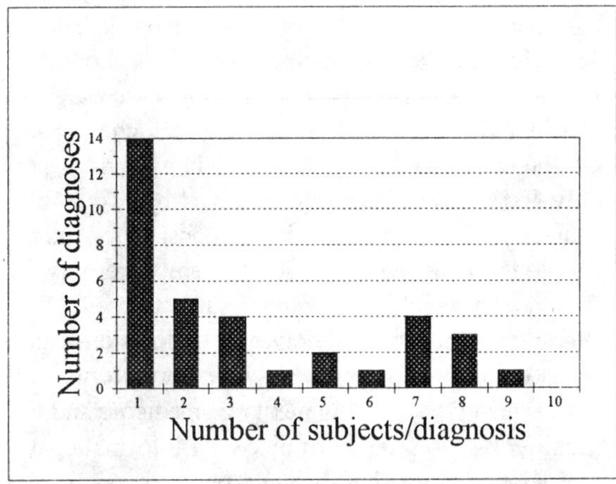

Figure 3: Frequencies of diagnoses listed
Number of subjects listing the same or a synonymous diagnosis using KSSO

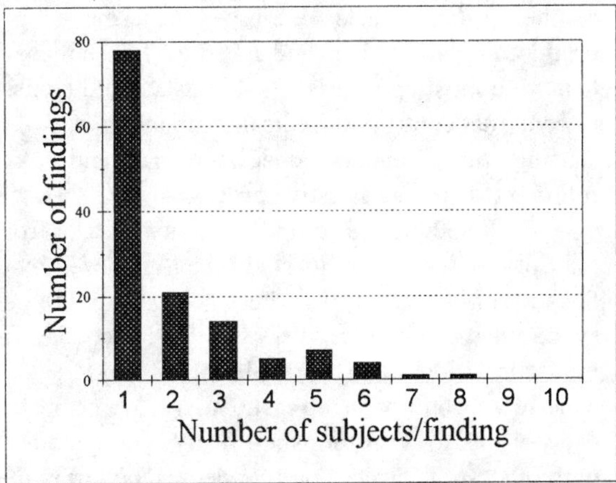

Figure 4: Frequencies of findings listed
Number of subjects listing the same or a synonymous finding using the program KSSO

DISCUSSION

KSSO is a knowledge acquisition tool that offers a relatively unconstrained graphical interface with which the user interacts directly. The question being answered in this study was how consistent a group of general internists was in the diagnoses and findings they used to describe the diagnosis of a patient who presented with chest pain. The results show that when there are few constraints put on the format or terminology to be used, the subjects were somewhat consistent in the diagnoses they listed, and much less consistent in the findings they listed.

A coefficient of consistency (CC) is defined and calculated. It can be interpreted as the percentage of the entries listed by two or more subjects. The CC for diagnoses was .60, or 60% of the diagnoses were listed by two or more subjects. This figure indicates that the physicians showed a fair degree of consistency in the diagnoses they considered for a patient presenting with chest pain. On the other hand, the CC for findings was .40, or only 40% of the findings were listed by two or more subjects. This shows much less consistency than was found with the diagnoses. There were only 18 findings on which four or more subjects used synonymous terms, and only two findings on which seven or more subjects used synonymous terms. However, given the complexity of medicine and considering the number of pieces of information a physician could gather during a patient session, perhaps a coefficient of .40 shows reasonable consistency. It must also be remembered that the subjects were allowed only one iteration of data elicitation. More consistency would probably have resulted if the subjects were given the terms produced by all of them and asked to choose those that were most appropriate. This data could be used to construct controlled medical terminologies, starting with an unconstrained vocabulary and refining it using an iterative process.

KSS0 allows for the collection of data from multiple subjects. In this study the terms used by the subjects were merged when they appeared to be synonymous. The person responsible for condensing the information into a workable format and a concise vocabulary has to make a large number of decisions as to what terms are really synonymous with others. The more one condenses the terms the higher the degree of consistency that is achieved. Effort was made to merge only those terms that were clearly synonymous. But, because of the subjectivity that is possible in this step, it must be considered a weakness in the methods. A second weakness was the restriction of subjects to no more than 15 diagnoses. This would tend to increase the degree of consistency by forcing subjects to choose only the 15 most likely or important. The data collected might be further strengthened by allowing the subjects to choose the best diagnoses and findings from the merged list and to have them use KSS0 a second time using their revised diagnoses and findings. Overall, the method used was a reasonable one, but could be strengthened.

CONCLUSIONS

Expert knowledge acquisition and representation are crucial elements in the production of an expert system knowledge base or a standardized protocol for use in clinical practice. The elicitation of inter-related medical information from an expert takes a great deal of time. Because of the time involved, knowledge is usually elicited from only one expert, with verification of that knowledge by a group of experts. However, a knowledge base would be more representative of medical expertise if it were constructed by a group of experts rather than by one expert.

There are problems with eliciting knowledge from multiple medical experts, not the least of which is inconsistency in the elicited information. Medical knowledge is not a stable and agreed upon set of facts. Instead, it is a rapidly changing body of knowledge that has regional and individual variation. In the past, the format and terminology have often been standardized prior to elicitation of knowledge [12,13,14]. This forces the subject to modify his/her understanding to fit the format. Cognitive research argues that in constraining the format, one changes the elicited knowledge to the point where it may no longer conform to the knowledge the subject generally uses [15]. Perhaps, rather than standardizing the format and terminology prior to knowledge elicitation, it would be more valid to elicit knowledge in a relatively unconstrained format and then determine the most appropriate format. The data presented here offer a first step toward that end.

Acknowledgements
We would like to thank Mark Musen M.D., Ph.D. for his guidance during the preparation of this paper.

References

1. Giuse, N.B., Giuse, D.A., & Miller, R.A. Computer assisted multi-center creation of medical knowledge bases. In *Proceedings of the Twelfth Annual Symposium on Computer Applications in Medical Care,* pages 583-90. IEEE Computer Society Press, Washington, D.C., 1988.

2. Giuse, N.B., Bankowitz, R.A., Giuse, D.A., Parker, R.C., Miller, R.A., Medical knowledge base acquisition: the role of the expert review process in disease profile construction. In *Proceedings of the Thirteenth Annual Symposium on Computer Applications in Medical Care,* pages 105-9, IEEE Computer Society Press, Washington, D.C., 1989.

3. Giuse, N.B. et. al., Evaluating consensus among physicians in medical knowledge base construction. *Methods of Information in Medicine* 32: 137-45, 1993.

4. Kingsland, L.C. III, Lindberg D.A.B. The criteria form of knowledge representation in medical artificial intelligence. MEDINFO 86 Proceedings pages 12-16, North-Holland, Amsterdam, 1986.

5. Miller, P.L., Blumenfrucht, S. J., Rose, J.R., et. al., Expert system knowledge acquisition for domains of medical workup: An augmented transition network model. In *Proceedings of the Tenth Annual Symposium on Computer Applications in Medical Care,* pages 30-35. IEEE Computer Society Press, Washington, D.C., 1986.

6. Weiss, S. M.,Politakis, P.G., & Ginsberg, A. Empirical analysis and refinement of expert system knowledge bases. In *Proceedings of the Tenth Annual Symposium on Computer Applications in Medical Care,* pages 53-60. IEEE Computer Society Press, Washington, D.C., 1986.

7. Musen, M.A .*Automated generation of model-based knowledge-acquisition tools.* San Mateo, CA: Morgan Kaufmann Publishers, Inc., 1989.

8. Shaw, M.L.G., & Gaines, B.R. KITTEN:Knowledge initiation and transfer tools for experts and novices. *International Journal of Man-Machine Studies* 27:251-280, 1987.

9. Shaw, M.L.G., & Gaines, B.R. Comparing conceptual structures: consensus, conflict, correspondence and contrast. *Knowledge Acquisition* 1:341-363, 1989.

10. Shaw, M.L.G. *On becoming a personal scientist: Interactive computer elicitation of personal models of the world.* London: Academic Press, 1980.

11. Kelly, G.A., *The psychology of personal constructs.* N.Y.:Norton, 1955.

12. Bouhaddou, O., Warner, H.R., Yu, H., Lincoln, M.J. The knowledge capabilities of the vocabulary component of a medical expert system. In Miller, R.A. (ed) *Proceedings of the Fourteenth Annual Symposium on Computer Applications in Medical Care,* pages 655-60, IEEE Computer Society Press, Washington, D.C., 1990.

13. Cimino, J.J. Representation of Clinical laboratory terminology in the unified medical language system. In *Proceedings of the Fifteenth Annual Symposium on Computer Applications in Medical Care,* pages 199-203, IEEE Computer Society Press, Washington, D.C., 1991.

14. Masarie, F.S.,Jr., Miller, R.A., Bouhaddou, O, Giuse, N. B., & Warner, H. R. An interlingua for electronic interchange of medical information: using frames to map between clinical vocabularies. *Computers and biomedical Research* 24:379-400, 1991.

15. Adair, J.G. & Spinner, B. Subject's access to cognitive processes: Demand characteristics and verbal report. *Journal of the theory of social behavior* 11:31-52, 1981.

Improving Prediction of Preterm Birth Using a New Classification Scheme and Rule Induction

Jerzy W. Grzymala-Busse
Department of Electrical Engineering and Computer Science
University of Kansas
Lawrence, KS 66045
E-mail: jerzy@cs.ukans.edu

Linda K. Woolery
School of Nursing
University of Missouri
Columbia, MO 65203
E-mail: nurswool@mizzou1.missouri.edu

Abstract. *Prediction of preterm birth is a poorly understood domain. The existing manual methods of assessment of preterm birth are 17% – 38% accurate. The machine learning system LERS was used for three different datasets about pregnant women. Rules induced by LERS were used in conjunction with a classification scheme of LERS, based on "bucket brigade algorithm" of genetic algorithms and enhanced by partial matching. The resulting prediction of preterm birth in new, unseen cases is much more accurate (68% – 90%).*

1. INTRODUCTION

Many healthcare providers collect data on pregnant women for assessment of preterm birth risk. Current technology makes possible collection of a plethora of data, yet a perinatal healthcare provider has no access to a general, reliable and valid method of preterm birth assessment [1]. Preterm birth is defined ambiguously in the literature on the subject. In our work we will assume that preterm delivery is before the 36th week of gestation and fullterm starts from the 36th week.

In the United States the rate of preterm birth has been between 8 and 12% for the last two decades [9]. Preterm birth is the most common cause of low birthweight and perinatal mortality and it causes almost 70% of all neonatal deaths [16]. At the same time, preterm infants are 40 times more likely to die than infants born at term. Moreover, surviving preterm infants are at increased risk of lifelong handicaps including cerebral palsy, respiratory diseases, blindness and deafness [9]. Accurate assessment of preterm birth permits intervention with appropriate educational programs, bedrest, and early symptom identification. Tocolyting drugs may be used to suppress preterm labor.

Most existing methods to assess preterm birth are based on risk scoring, done manually. These methods are between 17% and 38% predictive in determining preterm birth [9]. This range of accuracy is obviously not satisfactory. Some authors conclude that—in general—manual risk screening tools are not sufficient to be used in the prediction of preterm labor [3, 8]. Our research shows that performance of computer-based methods for prediction of preterm birth is significantly better than performance of manual methods.

2. MACHINE LEARNING

The exact causes for initiation of uterine contractions leading to delivery are mostly unknown. Since this domain is poorly understood, our hypothesis was that AI methods, which usually work well under these circumstances, should be applied. The task is to identify regularities hidden in large datasets characterized by many attributes containing information about pregnant women. In this work the chosen methodology was of machine learning from examples. Classification rules for prediction of preterm birth were induced using machine learning program LERS (Learning from Examples based on Rough Sets), developed at the University of Kansas. System LERS may work with imperfect data, e.g., with missing attribute values, continuous attributes, or inconsistencies in input data. The system handles inconsistencies using rough set theory [4–6, 12, 13, 18]. Other machine learning systems that are use rough set theory include Datalogic/R [19], and RoughDAS and RoughClass [17].

A machine learning system looks for regularities in a data set. In most of these systems, such regularities are expressed as rules in the following format:

if (attribute_1, value_1) **and** ···
and (attribute_n, value_n) **then** (decision, value).

Table 1. Decision Table—Training Examples

Example	Attributes			Decision
	Risk_factor	Infant_sex	Age	Delivery
1	smoking	male	31–45	preterm
2	smoking	female	31–45	fullterm
3	none	female	<20	fullterm
4	none	male	20–30	fullterm
5	smoking	male	20–30	preterm
6	none	female	31–45	fullterm
7	none	male	<20	preterm

Input data for system LERS may be presented in the form of a decision table, where *examples* (e.g., patients) are characterized by *attributes* (e.g., *Risk_factor*, *Infant_sex*, *Age*, etc.) and a *decision* (e.g., *Delivery*). An example of a very simple decision table is presented in Table 1. This table is presented here only for illustration. The actual decision tables will have many more variables and examples. The current version of system LERS can handle more than one hundred attributes and many thousands of examples. The decision table from Table 1 has six examples, named 1, 2,..., 6. In machine learning from examples, a *concept* is understood as the set of all examples having the same value for a decision. Patients 1, 2, and 3 all belong to the same concept of *Delivery* having the value *preterm.*

In this work algorithm LEM2 of LERS has been used [6]. This algorithm induces rules in their simplest form. The first criterion in looking for attribute-value pairs, candidates for the left-hand side of a rule, is relevancy of the attribute-value pair to the concept described by the right-hand side of the rule.

Rules, induced by LERS, are more general than information contained in the original decision table

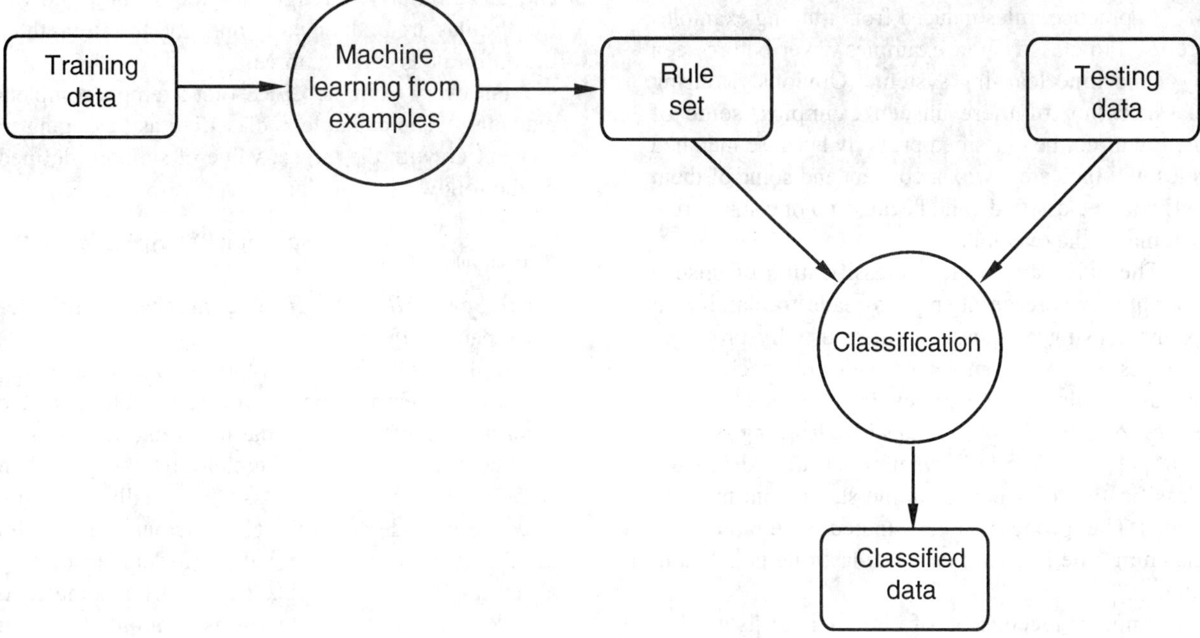

Fig.1 Machine learning from examples and classification

Table 2. Decision Table—Unseen Examples

Examples	Attributes			Decision
	Risk_factor	Infant_sex	Age	Delivery
8	smoking	female	20–30	preterm
9	none	female	20–30	fullterm
10	none	male	31–45	preterm

representing input data, since—in general—more new examples may be correctly classified by rules than may be matched with examples from the original decision table.

All rules, induced by LEM2 from Table 1, are:

(Infant_sex, male) & (Risk_factor, smoking) ->
(Delivery, preterm),

(Age, <20) & (Infant_sex, male) ->
(Delivery, preterm),

(Infant_sex, female) -> (Delivery, fullterm),

(Age, 20-30) & (Risk_factor, none) ->
(Delivery, fullterm).

3. CLASSIFICATION

In practice, rules induced from training examples are used to classify new examples never before seen by a machine learning system. Obviously, during classification of these unseen examples, some of them will not be classified properly because matched rules will indicate a wrong concept and some of them will not be classified at all because no one single rule will match the example.

The naive approach to classification of unseen examples, where an attempt is made to classify an example using all possible rules, usually produces poor results. Some more sophisticated mechanisms of classification have been developed. One of them is a *decision list* [15], used in machine learning systems CN2 [11] and C4.5 [14], where rules are ordered and classification of a new example starts from the first rule. The process is terminated when the first matching rule is identified. The last rule is a default rule.

Another mechanism of classification is used in AQ15 [10]. In AQ15, first the *complete matching* is examined, in which all attribute-value pairs of a rule must match all values of the corresponding attributes for the example. If complete matching is impossible, a partial matching is done, where some attribute-value pairs of a rule match the values of corresponding attributes. The choice of the best rule is made on the basis of estimates of probabilities.

In LERS yet another approach was used, similar to the "bucket brigade algorithm" of *genetic algorithms* [2, 7]. Every rule is equipped with a number of correctly classified examples during training, called *strength*. In our example, this number is equal to two for the first rule:

(Infant_sex, male) & (Risk_factor, smoking) ->
(Delivery, preterm),

because this rule correctly classifies two examples: 1 and 5. Similarly, strengths of the second and the fourth rules are both equal to one, and the strength of the third rule is equal to three.

For every example LERS first attempts complete matching. The example is classified as belonging to concept C with the largest value of support, defined by the following formula:

$$\sum_{\text{matching rules } R \text{ describing } C} \text{Strength}(R) * \text{Specificity}(R),$$

where *Specificity* (R) is the total number of attribute-value pairs of the rule R.

In the bucket brigade algorithm partial matching is not considered to be worth the trouble. On the other hand, LERS uses partial matching because it is a successful addition to complete matching. When complete matching is impossible partially matching rules are considered, with some attribute-value pairs of a rule matching the values of corresponding attributes for the example. For a partially matched rule R, the additional factor is computed, called *Matching_factor* (R), the ratio of the number of

Table 3. Experimental Results

	Dataset 1	Dataset 2	Dataset 3
Number of Training Examples	1654	1218	6608
Number of Unseen Examples	1593	1218	6608
Number of Attributes	13	73	67
Number of Rules	178	170	1133
Prediction Rate: Naive Classification Scheme	72.69%	44.66%	35.43%
Prediction Rate: New Classification Scheme	89.96%	72.00%	67.99%

matched attribute-value pairs of the rule *R* to the total number of attribute-value pairs of the rule *R*. In partial matching, the example is classified as belonging to the concept *C* with the largest value of support defined by

$$\sum_{\text{partially matching rule } R \text{ describing } C} \text{Matching\_factor}(R) * \text{Strength}(R) * \text{Specificity}(R).$$

The classification mechanism of LERS will be illustrated using examples from Table 2.

Example 8 is completely matched by the rule

(Infant_sex, female) -> (Delivery, fullterm),

with the strength equal to 3. This is the only rule that completely matches the example, hence the decision is (Delivery, fullterm). That is inconsistent with the value of *Delivery* for example 8 from Table 2, so this example is incorrectly classified. Example 9 is completely matched by two rules

(Infant_sex, female) -> (Delivery, fullterm),

(Age, 20-30) & (Risk_factor, none) -> (Delivery, fullterm),

with strength equal to 3 and 1, respectively. Both rules support the same value *fullterm* of the decision. In this case the value *fullterm* is consistent with the value of decision for example 9 from Table 2, so this example is correctly classified. Example 10 cannot be matched completely by any rule. However, it is partially matched by the following three rules

(Infant_sex, male) & (Risk_factor, smoking) -> (Delivery, preterm),

(Age, <20) & (Infant_sex, male) -> (Delivery, preterm),

(Age, 20-30) & (Risk_factor, none) -> (Delivery, fullterm).

All three rules have the same *Matching_factor* equal to 0.5. Pair (*Delivery, preterm*) has support 0.5 * 2 * 2 + 0.5 * 1 * 2 = 3, while pair (*Delivery, fullterm*) has support 0.5 * 1 * 2 = 1, so the final decision is (*Delivery, preterm*), consistent with the value of *Delivery* for example 10 from Table 2. Thus, this example is correctly classified.

4. EXPERIMENTAL RESULTS

Experiments were done on three large datasets. Each of the datasets was split in half; half of the data were used for machine learning using system LERS, while the other half of the data were used for validation of the rule sets using two approaches: a naive approach for complete matching of every example with all possible rules and the classification scheme of LERS. As follows from Table 3, the prediction rate (or accuracy) for the classification scheme of LERS for all three datasets was much higher than for manual methods.

5. CONCLUSIONS

The experimental results show that the prediction rate of rule sets with appropriate classification scheme is much higher (68% – 90%) than the traditional manual methods (17% – 38%). All of these rule sets were induced from raw data. Only the examples with the most obvious errors such as maternal weight equal to 10 or 700 pounds or systolic pressure of 14,000 were removed. There was an attempt to validate rules through inspection by experts in the area; however, diagnosticians were not prepared to interpret rules, in spite of the fact that the rules were written almost in plain English. Further research is necessary to include additional attributes, such as stress, sexual activity, or nutritional status that were not taken into account.

Acknowledgment. The authors are grateful for datasets provided by: St. Luke's Regional Perinatal Center (Kansas City, MO), Healthdyne Perinatal Services (Marietta, GA), and Tokos Corporation (Santa Anna, CA).

References

[1] G. Alexander, J. Weiss, T. Hulsey, E. Papiernik. Preterm birth prevention: an evaluation of programs in the United States. *Birth* 18, 1991, 160–169.

[2] L. B. Booker, D. E. Goldberg, J. F. Holland. Classifier systems and genetic algorithms. In *Machine Learning. Paradigms and Methods*. J. G. Carbonell (ed.), The MIT Press, 1990, 235–282.

[3] R. Creasy. Preventing preterm birth. *New England J. of Medicine* 325, 1991, 727.

[4] J. W. Grzymala-Busse. Knowledge acquisition under uncertainty—a rough set approach. *Journal of Intelligent & Robotic Systems* 1, 1988, 3–16.

[5] J. W. Grzymala-Busse. *Managing Uncertainty in Expert Systems*. Kluwer Academic Publishers, 1991.

[6] J. W. Grzymala-Busse. LERS—A system for learning from examples based on rough sets. In *Intelligent Decision Support. Handbook of Applications and Advances of the Rough Sets Theory.* R. Slowinski (ed.), Kluwer Academic Publishers, 1992, 3–18.

[7] J. H. Holland, K. J. Holyoak, R. E. Nisbett. *Induction. Processes of Inference, Learning, and Discovery*. The MIT Press, 1986.

[8] J. McGregor, J. French, R. Richter, A. Franco-Buff, A. Johnson, S. Hillier, F. Judson, J. Todd. Antenatal microbiologic and maternal risk factors associated with prematurity. *Am. J. Obstet. Gynecol.* 163, 1990, 1465–1473.

[9] M. McLean, W. Walters, R. Smith. Prediction and early diagnosis of preterm labor: a critical review. *Obstet. Gynecol. Surv.* 48, 1993, 209-225.

[10] R. S. Michalski, I. Mozetic, J. Hong, N. Lavrac. The multi-purpose incremental learning system AQ 15 and its testing application to three medical domains. *Proc. of the 5th Nat. Conf. on AI*, 1986, 1041–1045.

[11] T. Niblett, I. Bratko. Learning decision rules in noisy domains. *Proc. of the Expert Systems '86, the 6th Annual Technical Conference of the British Computer Society*, 1986, 25–34.

[12] Z. Pawlak. Rough sets. *Int. J. Computer and Information Sci.* 11, 1982, 341–356.

[13] Z. Pawlak. *Rough Sets: Theoretical Aspects of Reasoning about Data.* Kluwer Academic Publishers, 1991.

[14] R. Quinlan. *C4.5: Programs for Machine Learning.* Morgan Kaufmann Publishers, 1993.

[15] R. L. Rivest. Learning decision lists. *Machine Learning* 2, 1987, 229–246.

[16] M. Rosen, I. Merkatz, J. Hill. Caring for our future: a report of the expert panel on the content of prenatal care. *Obstet. Gynecol.* 77, 1991, 782–787.

[17] R. Slowinski, J. Stefanowski. 'RoughDAS' and "RoughClass' software implementations of the rough set approach. In *Intelligent Decision Support. Handbook of Applications and Advances of the Rough Sets Theory.* R. Slowinski (ed.), Kluwer Academic Publishers, 1992, 445–456.

[18] L. Woolery, J. W. Grzymala-Busse, S. Summer, A. Budihardjo. On the use of LERS-LB knowledge acquisition for expert system development in nursing. *Comput. Nurs.* 9, 1991, 227–234.

[19] W. P. Ziarko. Acquisition of control algorithms from operation data. In *Intelligent Decision Support. Handbook of Applications and Advances of the Rough Sets Theory.* R. Slowinski (ed.), Kluwer Academic Publishers, 1992, 61–75.

Turning Medical Data into Decision-Support Knowledge

[1]Bohren, Benjamin F. and [1,2]Hadzikadic, Mirsad
[1]Carolinas Medical Center and [2]UNC-Charlotte

Advances in information collection and analysis are reaching the point of providing physicians with the help of computer-based assistants. These systems will provide rapid second opinions to physicians in a clinical setting as well as assist them in the analysis of large sets of patient descriptions for research purposes. This paper presents INC2.5 as such a decision-support system. INC2.5 extracts information from databases of previously seen patients to build a decision tree which is used to predict the outcome of new patients on a chosen variable. The concept of matching new patients with the most similar previously seen patient, on which INC2.5 is based, can be easily understood by its users. Further adding to INC2.5's ease of use is its flexibility in allowing users to customize decision trees to their liking. In order to convey the uncertainty of the environment, INC2.5 presents all decisions with a confidence factor.

INTRODUCTION

Doctors are faced with the process of making critical decisions everyday. While years of experience can help them be more efficient and accurate in their diagnoses, automated decision support tools can add an extra measure of confidence. However, their usefulness will extend only as far as the user's trust. This trust can be achieved by providing accurate results over an extended period of time. The clinical advantage of such systems will extend well beyond helping one doctor make better decisions. Eventually they will facilitate the spread of knowledge to institutions with fewer resources.

For the physician involved in research, a decision support system should be able to assist him/her in finding correlation's amongst large quantities of data. Additionally, the system should be able to decipher which predictor variables appear to be most relevant to the selected predictive variable. With such information, the physician could minimize the number of tests required for an accurate diagnosis, thereby reducing the cost of care.

INC2.5

INC2.5[6] is a general classification system capable of uncovering patterns of relationship amongst records stored in databases. INC2.5, similarly to COBWEB[1], CLASSIT[2], CYRUS[3], UNIMEM[4], and CLUSTER/2[5], works in an incremental manner, incorporating new knowledge one experience at a time. This is similar to the way humans learn over time and can be viewed as analogous to the physicians pattern of seeing one patient at a time. Hereafter, the term *patient* will be used to replace experience when referring to a single encounter.

INC2.5 differs from other classification systems in several key issues: (a) evaluation function, (b) tree-building operators, and (c) classification and prediction algorithms. First, INC2.5 uses a similarity-based patient evaluation function which optimizes patient's predictive variable only with respect to the *most similar* group of previously seen patients rather than with respect to all available patients. Second, INC2.5 uses unique tree-building operators, pull-in and pull-out, to reverse unwarranted decisions made Early in the classification process when less information was available. Finally, the classification and prediction algorithms are designed to maximize predictive performance of the system in the presence of noise.

Classification

INC2.5 uses the evaluation function to classify and group patients based on similarities and dissimilarities found in their patient descriptions[6,7]. Each patient description contains a list of information the physician deems possibly relevant to the diagnosis in question. This list contains information ranging from patient age to specific test results and hereafter will be referred to as the patient's *variables*. Each group of patients within the decision tree, will be referred to as a *category*.

0195-4210/94/$5.00

The process of building the decision tree is known as *classification.* Each new patient is classified into the branch of the tree which maximizes the *evaluation function.* The evaluation function can be broken into two components, similarity and cohesiveness. Similarity is used for both classifying previous patients and predicting the class membership of new patients. Cohesiveness calculates the average similarity of all pairs of patients contained in a category.

The similarity of two patients is based on the comparison between the two sets of variables. The function is derived from the contrast model[8], which defines similarity as a linear combination of common and distinctive variables. The following equations review the similarity function **s(A,B)** where **A** and **B** denote descriptions of patients or categories **a** and **b**, respectively; **c(A,B)** represents the contribution of **a**'s and **b**'s common variables; and **d(A,B)** introduces the influence of the variables of **a** not shared by **b**.

$$s(A,B) = \frac{sim(A,B) + sim(B,A)}{2}$$

$$sim(A,B) = \frac{c(A,B) - d(A,B)}{c(A,B) + d(A,B)}$$

The degree of similarity between **A** and **B** ranges from -1.0 to +1.0. In an extreme case where **A** and **B** are identical then **c(A,B)** would have a value, while **d(A,B)** and **d(B,A)** would equal zero, yielding the similarity measure equal to 1.0. Conversely, if they are completely dissimilar all the values will be in **d(A,B)** and **d(B,A)** while **c(A,B)** equals zero, yielding -1.0.

The cohesiveness measures also ranges from -1.0 to +1.0 and reflects the similarity between all member patients within a given category. A category will have a cohesiveness measure of 1.0 if and only if all member patients are identical. On the other hand, a category in which member patients are completely opposite would have a cohesiveness measure of -1.0.

Prediction

Prediction follows classification and works on the same principle. INC2.5's goal is to maximize the similarity score between the patient in question and one of the patients in the decision tree. This is efficiently achieved by only searching the branches which maximize similarity, thus providing an effective method of indexing decision trees. Once the system has searched the appropriate branches, the outcome of the most similar patient will be used as the prediction for the new patient. Furthermore, the system will report the similarity score which is in essence the degree of confidence INC2.5 has in the prediction.

Customization of Decision Trees

INC2.5 is flexible enough to allow physicians to build custom decision trees. The easiest way to customize a decision tree is to build it using a selected group of patients, patient variables, or both. For example, a physician may wish to have only his/her patients included in the tree. While this might limit the variety of patients, it could ensure that all data was collected more consistently.

Besides changing the input data, INC2.5 allows the user to adjust *certainty* (CT) and *variable* (VT) thresholds which can be used to fine tune a decision tree to be most effective within a given domain. The certainty threshold is used to determine if there is enough evidence to support a prediction. In order for INC2.5 to make a prediction, the similarity score of the closest match must exceed the certainty threshold. With the default value, CT = -1, INC2.5 will always make a prediction. At higher degrees of certainty, it is possible that no patient will be found with a similarity greater than the required certainty. In this case any number of methods could be used to provide the user feedback including the use of prior probability or stating that no prediction is possible with the given information.

The variable threshold requires a greater understanding of INC2.5. This threshold attempts to weed out patient variables which are inconsistent with those of other patients within the same category. Inconsistent values can occur either in variables which are less relevant to the diagnosis or via data entry errors. When comparing a patient with an existing category, the category will have multiple values for each variable representing the union of all member patient's values for the variable in question. The patient is said to have this variable in common if the category has the same value for the variable. For example, assume a category consists of eight red and two blue members. In this situation if

VT = 0, the default value, all objects with either red or blue color would have the color variable in common. On the other hand, if the threshold value is greater than the percentage of blue objects, VT > 0.2, any new object with the color blue will NOT have the color variable in common with this category. Consequently, the higher the incidence of a variable in a given category, the higher its relevance to the category description.

In general, INC2.5 is a flexible decision support system whose results can be used in a clinical setting as a second opinion or in a research setting for data analysis.

TEST DATABASE

The medical database used for testing INC2.5 include breast cancer, general trauma, and low back pain. While INC2.5 performed consistently across all domains, we will restrict our discussion to the widely available breast cancer database[1] which was retrieved from the machine learning repository at University of California at Irvine. It consists of 699 patients with two ideal classes, YES and NO. YES means the patient had a recurrence of breast cancer within five years, and NO means there was no recurrence during the five year period. Within the database, 458 of the patients are benign, NO, and 241 are malignant, YES. For each patient there are nine associated variables.

TESTING METHODOLOGY

INC2.5 results, presented in the following section, show performance for various tree sizes and threshold settings. Each point in the graphs represents an averaged performance over a series of ten runs. For each run, a classification set and prediction set of patients were randomly selected from the database so that no patient appeared more than once in the union of the two sets. The classification set was then used to build the decision tree subsequently utilized to predict the outcome variable, YES/NO reoccurrence, for each patient in the prediction set.

The outcome variable is only used once a match has been found, at which time INC2.5 predicts the same outcome for the new patient. In other words, the outcome variable neither influences the classification process nor guides the prediction process.

PERFORMANCE ANALYSIS

This section will perform a step by step analysis of the database. The steps presented here are just a guideline to follow. Tests can be performed in any order once a user is familiar with INC2.5.

Initial Learning Curve

Step one is to build a learning curve using default values for both thresholds. A learning curve will answer two important questions: (1) Is INC2.5 predicting significantly better than random guessing, i.e. 50% for two category domains? (2) What is the optimal tree size required to maximize accuracy while minimizing time? As demonstrated in Figure 1, the initial learning curve (CT = -1) is performing significantly better than random guessing.

When comparing the tree size to its performance the learning curve grows as expected by gradually improving with the size of the tree. It flattens just past the tree size of 100 patients. This would indicate that a random sample of 100 patients is sufficient to distinguish amongst the various outcomes. In other words, patient samples greater than 100 added no additional knowledge to the decision tree.

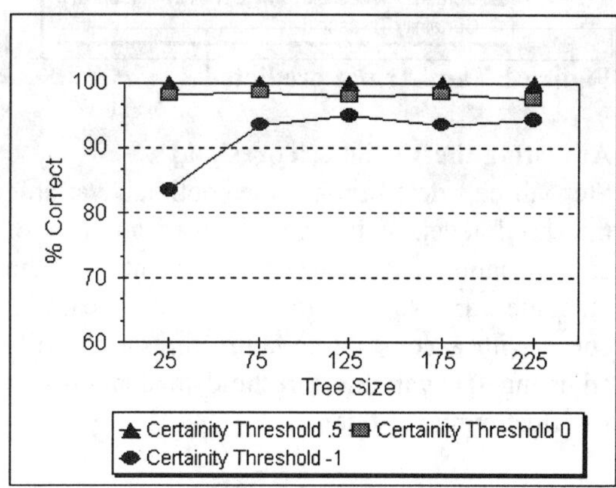

Figure 1 Breast cancer learning curves

Adjusting Certainty Threshold

Step two is to adjust the certainty threshold (CT), thereby increasing the desired level of confidence for each prediction. Figure 1 shows that when CT = 0, meaning at least half of the variables are identical, the performance of INC2.5 is consistently better than that obtained

[1]The breast cancer database was obtained from Dr. William H. Wolberg at the University of Wisconsin Hospitals, Madison.

with CT = -1. Increasing the threshold to 0.5 improves performance to almost flawless prediction.

On the down side, Figure 2 shows the number of patient diagnoses INC2.5 was unsure about. At the original threshold, CT = -1, INC2.5 will always give a prediction, thus the flat curve at zero patients not predicted. Moving up to a zero threshold, the domain shows a curve with a negative slope indicating, as one would expect, with a larger classification set INC2.5 is able to find good matches for more patients in the prediction set. The outcome remains consistent with expectations at the 0.5 threshold level as well.

By evaluating Figures 1 and 2 we can conclude that INC2.5 will perform well in both small and large data sets, but with a degree of confidence directly proportional to the tree size.

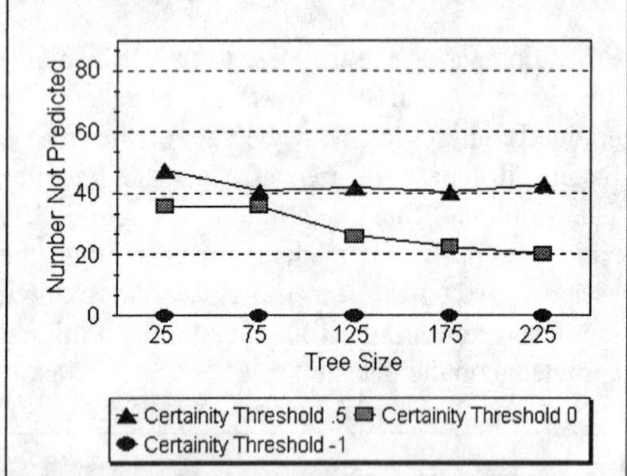

Figure 2 Number not predicted

Adjusting the Variable Threshold

Step three, determining the optimal variable threshold level, will give the user an idea of each variable's usefulness in the prediction of the outcome variable. Figure 3 displays a learning curve with a constant certainty threshold while adjusting the variable threshold to demonstrate its effect on the test domain.

The variable threshold has the most effect on databases with little consistency amongst variable values. In these cases, a high threshold would eliminate many variables thereby narrowing information used to make decisions.

When set properly, the threshold will eliminate the infrequent variable values which cloud the decision process, thereby maximizing the ability to find good matches in the tree. For example, Figure 3 demonstrates how the threshold worked effectively for the tree of twenty-five patients improving performance as the system eliminated a greater number of variables.

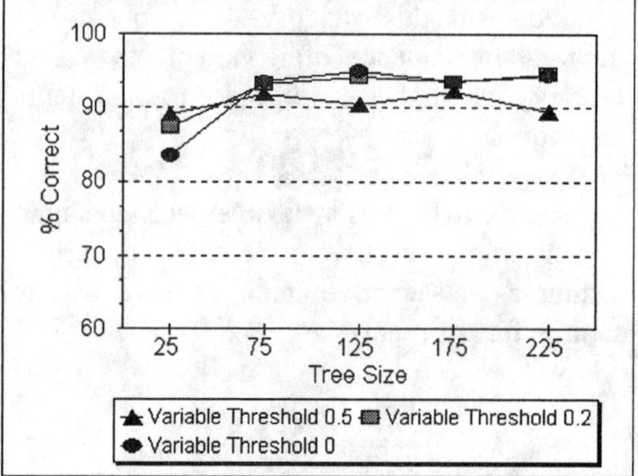

Figure 3 Effects of the variable threshold

Notice for larger patient sets the highest threshold caused a drop in performance. This indicates that too many variables were eliminated from the decision process. The 0.2 threshold neither improved nor hurt performance on the larger patient sets while helping the decision process in the smallest patient set. Therefore, for the breast cancer database 0.2 would be the optimal threshold.

Determining Variable Relevance

Step four, attempting to reduce the number of variables required for the decision process can produce two major benefits: (1) a reduced set of attributes which would make statistical analysis easier and (2) if proven to be effective, many costly tests could be eliminated during the diagnosis process. The variable reduction process assumes INC2.5 has been successful at forming a tree with categories containing a majority of patients having the same outcome. In that case, the variables common to most patients are good predictors of the outcome, while variables which vary widely over the category are not relevant to the outcome.

For this test a tree of one-hundred patients was built using all provided variables. Then INC2.5 systematically reduced the number of relevant variables by incrementing the relevancy measure. The relevancy measure is an experiential indicator sensitive to the depth of the tree as well as the frequency and distributions of variable values. Figure 4 shows prediction results plotted against the number of variables used during training and prediction. The same training and prediction sets were used for all runs thereby making the variables used the only varying factor.

During this test, the relevancy measure is incremented one percent at a time and new prediction results are generated at each percentile where one or more variables drop out.

Figure 4 shows that the number of variables can often be dramatically reduced without significant loss in performance. In this example, the prediction rate was maintained while the number of variables dropped from nine to one, that being uniformity of cell size.

The benefits of reducing the amount of information required for accurate diagnosis will be reaped in both research and clinical terms. Researchers will save precious resources during future data collection. Clinical staffs will save time and money by eliminating unnecessary tests which in turn could have a positive effect on controlling the cost of health care.

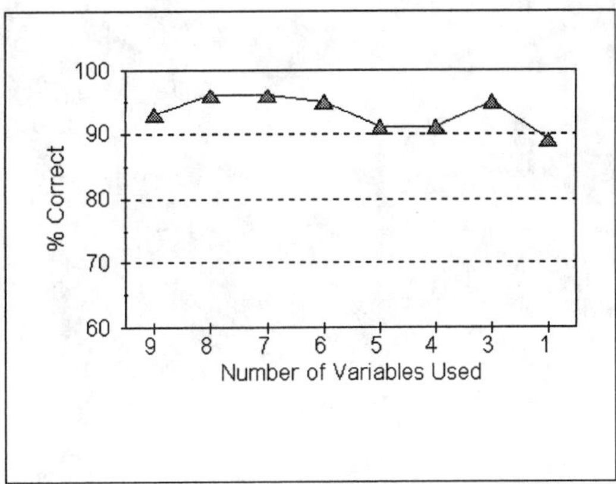

Figure 4 Effects of reducing the variables used during classification and prediction.

CONCLUSION

INC2.5 has the ability to look at sets of patients and provide quality information concerning the predictability of an outcome variable as well as the relevance of patient variables with respect to the outcome. Once the user has formed general characteristics of the data, he/she can fine tune INC2.5 for optimal performance. Increased performance can be achieved via three basic methods:

1. adjusting certainty threshold
2. adjusting variable threshold
3. eliminating irrelevant variables

The certainty threshold is easiest to use and generally yields the greatest improvement in accuracy. The variable threshold requires a greater understanding of the analysis process, thus making it more difficult to find an optimal value, but it adds to the accuracy of the prediction results. Finally, eliminating variables can preserve the quality of the output while reducing the cost of data acquisition.

Future work will concentrate on providing the ability to evaluate linear variables and enabling INC2.5 to read XBase data storage format.

ACKNOWLEDGMENT

The authors would like to thank Amber Harrington for her constant support and encouragement as well as her proof-reading of this manuscript.

Reference

[1] Fisher, D. H. Knowledge Acquisition Via Incremental Conceptual Clustering. In *Machine Learning*, **2**, 2 (1987) 139-172.

[2] Gennari, J. H., Langley, P., and Fisher, D. H. Models of Incremental Concept Formation. In *Artificial Intelligence*, **40**, 1-3(1989) 11-59.

[3] Kolodner, J. L. Retrieval and Organizational Strategies in Conceptual Memory: A Computer Model, Lawrence Erlbaum Associated, Publishers, London, 1984.

[4] Lebowitz, M. Experiments with Incremental Concept Formation: UNIMEM. In *Machine Learning*, **2**, 2 (1987) 103-138.

[5] Michalski, R.S., and Stepp, R.E. Learning From Observation: Conceptual Clustering. In Machine Learning: An Artificial Intelligence Approach, R.S. Michalski, J.G. Carbonell, and T. M. Mitchell (eds.), Morgan Kaufman Publishes, Inc., Lao Altos, CA, 1983.

[6] Hadzikadic, M., Automated Design of Diagnostic Systems. *Artificial Intelligence in Medicine Journal*, **4** (1992a) 329-342.

[7] Hadzikadic, M. and Bohren, B. F., INC2.5: A Concept Formation System. Technical Report 008-1994, UNCC, 1994.

[8] Tversky, A. Features of Similarity. *Psychological Review*, **84** (1977) 327-352.

Application of Fuzzy Logic & Neural Networks to the Clinical Domain

Detecting Dysfunctional Behavior in Adolescents: The Examination of Relationships Using Neural Networks

John C. Reid, Ph.D., Satish S. Nair, Ph.D., Javad H. Kashani, M.D., and Venkatesh G. Rao
University of Missouri, Columbia, MO

We describe a neural network that models the effect of personality, social, and environmental variables on hopelessness in adolescents. A sensitivity analysis suggests the effect that variation in each of the input variables will have on the output. Clinical implications are that health professionals can focus their attention on the variables most likely to impact upon the outcome.

INTRODUCTION

Several researchers have discussed the relationship of hopelessness with depression and other psychiatric disorders. The topic is of interest particularly in adolescents because of the association between hopelessness and suicidal tendency [1-6]. Additionally, hopelessness is also related to other kinds of psychopathology in children and adolescents [7-10].

To assist in identifying these relationships, neural networks seem particularly appropriate, as they can quantify complex mapping in a compact and elegant manner [11-12]. Neural networks have been used in general psychiatry in a broad range of problems. They have modeled brain functioning in schizophrenia [13], have classified PET scans [14], and have modeled humans on a continuous performance task under CNS stimulants [15].

The purpose of this study was to identify the most important mental health variables from a set of personality, family support, and social support variables that related to hopelessness by modeling these relationships using a neural network. We desired to see which variables made the greater contributions and determine how changing them affected hopelessness.

METHOD

Sample

One hundred fifty adolescents were selected from a systematic sample of over 1700 high school students in a midwestern town, stratified a priori to obtain equal numbers of males and females at each of three ages: 14, 15, and 16 [16]. One hundred forty-two were white, six were black, and two were oriental. Data from seven were discarded due to missing information. There were no differences in social class, age, or family status between those who participated in the study and those who did not.

Instruments

Instruments included the Millon Adolescent Personality Inventory (MAPI) [17]; the Diagnostic Interview for Children and Adolescents (DICA) [18]; the Parental Bonding Questionnaire [19]; the Social Support Questionnaire [20], and the Hopelessness Scale for children [4].

We included the following Millon personality scales: Cooperative, Forceful, Personal Esteem, Sensitive, Social Tolerance, Family Rapport, Impulse Control, and Societal Conformity. The rest of the Millon scales were omitted from the analysis because they were judged to be less relevant to the problem at hand. The following descriptions of the personality scales are excerpted from the Millon Adolescent Personality Inventory Manual [17]. In the Cooperative scale, higher scores suggest being soft-hearted and sentimental. In the Forceful scale, higher scores denote being strong-willed, tending to lead and dominate others. High scores in Personal Esteem mean greater struggle by the individual for social approval. In the Sensitive scale, higher scores denote discontentment and pessimism. In addition to the personality scales, the Millon also has scales of expressed concerns. In the Social Tolerance scale, higher scores mean more pathology, and are associated with such items as being alone rather than being sociable, and taking advantage of people. Higher scores in Family Rapport mean more pathology and are characterized by such items as wanting to be away from home and destructive criticism from parents. Higher scores on the Impulse Control scale indicate more compulsive behavior. In the Societal Conformity

0195-4210/94/$5.00

scale, higher scores mean more pathology, less adjustment, and more aggressiveness. The parental bonding and social support questionnaires provided the following scales : Parental Care and Parental Overprotection, and Social Support (number of supportive people) and Satisfaction as being probable factors in hopelessness. The binary DICA diagnosis scales included were: oppositional disorder, conduct disorder, anxiety, major depression and dysthymic disorder, combined, and alcohol and drugs, combined. We also included a Psychosocial Stress scale from the DICA.

Neural network modeling and analysis

We trained a multilayer back propagation neural network with the responses of the adolescents, and subsequently performed a sensitivity analysis. Back-propagation is a mapping network that learns an approximation to a nonlinear function, y = f(x), from sample (x,y) pairs by propagating the errors successively back through the layers. The equations for a back-propagation network have been derived by Rumelhart & McClelland [21]. The back propagation network learns by changing its weights to minimize the sum of squared errors between its output and the supplied target data. We also validated the training process to ensure that the network mapped the relationships well. The network that modeled the complex relationships between the variables in the study had 19 inputs, 1 output, and 20 and 10 neurons each in the two hidden layers. The inputs were the responses of 143 adolescents to the MAPI, DICA, Parental Bonding Questionnaire, and the Social Support Questionnaire. The output was the Hopelessness score from Kazdin's Hopelessness Scale for children. The adolescents' responses to the various variables formed 143 training "patterns" for the neural network. All the required code was developed in-house using the C programming language. The data were normalized before training the neural network. The errors dropped rapidly during training and were less than 10% in prediction of the Hopelessness score for each of the 143 adolescents after 4,000 epochs. Though further training allowed reduction of error to less than 0.1%, this was avoided to prevent a phenomenon called "overtraining" which affects the ability of the neural net to capture general trends in the data.

After being trained in the manner described above, a neural network acts as an expert for predictions. If a new case is presented to the network, it should be able to predict the hopelessness score for that adolescent, based on the training that it has received, as an expert would do. While an expert would probably have problems drawing inferences from such a large number of variables, a neural network handles the complexity easily. In addition, the neural model can describe the relative importance of each input variable, which may be a difficult problem for an individual expert.

Sensitivity

The network was presented with the "case history" of each adolescent, and one aspect of the "case history" was perturbed at a time by a fixed amount to observe the change in the network's output, thus quantifying the sensitivity of the system. The result represents the change in hopelessness for a specified change in any of the input variables. For instance, the percentage change in hopelessness (output) can be estimated if family support (input) is doubled. The methodology thus quantifies the relative importance of each of the personality and support variables on hopelessness.

The sensitivity analysis revealed the dominant factors that affect hopelessness. We perturbed each of the Millon, the DICA diagnoses, Parental Bonding, and Social Support scales to study their effect on the Hopelessness scale. The sensitivity analysis considers one variable at a time, keeping the remainder constant. Each variable was perturbed across its range for each adolescent and a rate of change of hopelessness, i.e., a measure of sensitivity, was computed for each variable. The rate of change was then averaged over all the cases.

Statistical comparison

We also compared our results to a linear statistical model, with hopelessness as the dependent variable and the 19 input variables as independent variables. However, because multicollinearities inflate the variances of predicted values and of parameter estimates, we did a principal components regression, using principal components as the independent variables in the model.

RESULTS

Table 1 lists the slopes for each variable at a

representative point, the "unperturbed" value, of the output across the range of the input variable. These slopes have been normalized by multiplying by the range of the input variable.

Referring to the values in Table 1, the following variations are relatively large and are therefore of special significance. High scores on Forceful imply greater pathology and are associated with aggressiveness and domination. Thus a forceful person is less likely to be hopeless.

Higher scores in Sensitive and Social Tolerance are associated with greater pathology, and were related to greater hopelessness. Higher scores in Impulse Control are also associated with greater pathology, but Hopelessness decreased as Impulse Control increased, perhaps because Impulse Control is associated with aggressiveness. Similar to forceful, Conduct Disorder was also negatively related to hopelessness. The use of alcohol and drugs tended to be related to an increase in hopelessness.

Table 1: Input Slopes

Forceful	-10.8
Sensitive	8.2
Social Tolerance	6.2
Impulse Control	- 4.2
Conduct Disorder	- 3.6
Alcohol & drug	3.0
Family Rapport	2.9
No. of Supportive People	- 2.5
Societal Conformity	2.3
Cooperative	- 1.9
Oppositional	- 1.9
Depression (MDD & DD)	1.9
Personal Esteem	- 1.3
Parental Overprotection	1.0
Satisfaction Rating	- 1.0
Sex	- 0.9
Psychosocial Stress	- 0.3
Parental Care	0.2
Anxiety	0.1

Validation study

To test the efficacy of the network training, 80% of the adolescents were randomly selected for "training" the network, and the remaining 20% were used for validation. The network predictions agreed with the actual Hopelessness score within 25% for 79% of the adolescents and within 50% for 93% of the adolescents.

Statistical analysis

A principal components analysis of the 19 variables yielded one eigenvalue accounting for 33% of the variance, and a second accounting for 11%. A scree test (involving the graphic display of eigenvalues) suggested that eigenvalues beyond two would be less important. Variables with large weights on the first eigenvector included Forceful, Sensitive, Family Rapport, Impulse Control, and Societal Conformity. Variables with large weights on the second eigenvector included Anxiety, Cooperative, Forceful, and Personal Esteem.

A regression analysis on the 19 components had significant tests of regression parameters on seven of the components; the first two parameters were significant at the .001 and .01 levels, respectively.

Social Tolerance, which had the third largest weight in the neural network analysis was not identified as important by this statistical analysis. Conduct Disorder and Alcohol were in the fourth component, whose regression parameter was also significant.

The regression analysis identified Anxiety as important to hopelessness, whereas findings from the neural network analysis would suggest that clinician attention to anxiety would be unproductive in reducing hopelessness.

DISCUSSION

These results imply that hopeless adolescents should be more assertive, should be more sociable, and should be less sensitive. The magnitudes of the slopes describe the relative importance of the input variables on the output variable.

This investigation and model validation demonstrate that the application of artificial neural networks is useful in adolescent psychiatry. This approach enhances the clinician's and the researcher's ability to study and handle multivariate problems, and enables us to see how a change in one input variable may potentially affect the outcome. It is not known whether certain personality traits predispose the individual to hopelessness or the opposite. We also present further evidence of the impact of the environment on the youth. Studies using larger numbers of subjects would have greater accuracy of responses. Although a specific study pertaining to hopelessness is reported in this paper, the sensitivity approach outlined for determining the relative importance of factors that cause or affect a certain phenomenon or property using neural networks has more general applicability.

References

[1]. Dyer, J. A. T. & Kreitman, N. (1984), Hopelessness, depression and suicide intent in parasuicide. Br. J. Psychiatry, 144:127-133.

[2]. Asarnow, J. R., Carlson, G. A. & Guthrie, D. (1987), Coping strategies, self-perceptions, hopelessness, and perceived family environments in depressed and suicidal children. J. Consult. and Clin. Psychol., 5: 361-366.

[3]. Asarnow, J. R. & Carlson, G. (1988), Suicide attempts in pre-adolescent child psychiatry inpatients. Suicide Life Threat. Behav., 18: 129-136.

[4]. Kazdin, A. E., French, N. H., Unis, A. S., Esveldt-Dawson, K. & Sherick, R. B. (1983). Hopelessness, depression, and suicidal intent among psychiatrically disturbed inpatient children. J. Consult. and Clin. Psychol., 51:504-510.

[5]. Kazdin, A. E., Rodgers, A. & Colbus, D. (1986), The hopelessness scale for children: Psychometric characteristics and concurrent validity. J. Consult. and Clin. Psychol., 54:241-245.

[6]. Asarnow, J. R. & Bates, S. (1988), Depression in child psychiatric inpatients: cognitive and attributional patterns. J. Abnorm. Child Psychol., 16: 601-615.

[7]. Kashani, J. H., Reid, J. C. & Rosenberg, T. K. (1989). Levels of hopelessness in children and adolescents: a developmental perspective. J. Consult. and Clin. Psychol., 57: 496-499.

[8]. Kashani, J. H., Dandoy, A. C. & Reid, J. C. (1992), Hopelessness in children and adolescents: An overview. Acta Paedopsychiatr., 55:33-39.

[9]. Kashani, J. H., Soltys, S., Dandoy, A. C., Vaidya, A. F. & Reid, J. C. (1991), Correlates of hopelessness in psychiatrically hospitalized children. Compr. Psychiatry, 32:330-337.

[10]. Kashani, J. H., Dandoy, A. C., Vaidya, A. F., Soltys, S. M. & Reid, J. C. (1990), Correlates of severe psychiatric disorders of inpatient children. Am. J. Psychiatry, 47:750-784.

[11]. Hopfield, J. J., (1982), Neural Networks and Physical Systems with Emergent Collective Computational Abilities. Proc. Natl. Acad. Science, 79:2554-58.

[12]. Mistry, S. I. & Nair, S. S. (1993), Nonlinear HVAC Computations Using Neural Networks. ASHRAE Transactions, 99-1: 775-784.

[13]. Hoffman, R. E. & McGlashan, T. H., (1993), Parallel distributed processing and the emergence of schizophrenic symptoms. Schizophr. Bull., 19:119-140.

[14]. Kippenhan, J. S., Barker, W. W., Pascal, S., Nage, J., Duara, R. (1992), Evaluation of a neural network classifier for PET scans of normal and Alzheimer's disease subjects. J. Nucl. Med., 33:1459-67.

[15]. Servan-Schreiber, D. & Cohen, D. (1992), A neural network model of catecholamine modulation of behavior. Psychiatric Annals, 22:125-130.

[16]. Kashani, J. H., Hoeper, E. W., Beck, N. C., Corcoran, C. M., Fallahi, C., McAllister, J., Rosenberg, T. J. K., & Reid, J. C. (1987), Personality, psychiatric disorders, and parental attitude among a community sample of adolescents. J. Am. Child Adol. Psychiatry, 26:879-885.

[17]. Millon, T., Green, C.J., & Meagher, R. B. Millon Adolescent Personality Inventory Manual. Interpretive Scoring Systems, Minneapolis, 1982.

[18]. Herjanic, B. & Reich, W. (1982), Development of a structured psychiatric interview for children: Agreement between child and parent on individual symptoms. J. Abnorm. Child Psychol., 10:307-324.

[19]. Parker, G., Tupling, H. & Brown, L. B. (1979), A parental bonding instrument. Br. J. Med. Psychol., 52: 1-10.

[20]. Sarason, I. G., Levine, H. M., Basham, R. B., et al. (1983), Assessing social support: The social support questionnaire. J. Pers. Soc. Psychol., 44: 127.

[21]. Rumelhart, D., & McClelland, J. (1987), Parallel Distributed Processing: Explorations in the Microstructure of Cognition. MIT Press: Cambridge, MA.

HYCONES II: a tool to build Hybrid Connectionist Expert Systems

Beatriz de F. Leão , MD, PhD(1), Alex Guazzelli, MSc(2), Eneida A. Mendonça, MD (1)
(1)Institute of Cardiology RS, Porto Alegre RS, Brazil
(2)Institute of Informatics, Federal University of Rio Grande do Sul, Porto Alegre, RS, Brazil

This paper describes HYCONES II - a tool to enable the construction of hybrid connectionist expert systems to solve classification problems. HYCONES II offers to the knowledge engineer a hybrid knowledge base that integrates frames with three different neural network models: the combinatorial neural model - CNM, the Fuzzy ARTMAP and the Semantic ART - SMART models. The latter is a new model, introduced by this paper, based on a combination of the two previous models. The validation section compares the performance of these three neural models to solve diagnostic problems in two medical domains. This paper also presents HYCONES II knowledge representation features, built in the symbolic component of its hybrid knowledge-base, to deal and represent fuzzy medical variables. Finally, the present status and future developments of the project are presented.

INTRODUCTION

Hybrid connectionist expert systems solve well-known problems of conventional expert systems, such as knowledge acquisition and learning. Although this is still a new technology, hybrid systems are being successfully used in several application areas [1]. HYCONES first version integrated frames with the combinatorial neural model - CNM [2]. The system showed a good performance: 31 out of 33 congenital heart disease diagnoses were correctly pointed out by HYCONES, when using its hybrid knowledge base (HKB) automatically trained from scratch, using a case database [3]. Because of this promising results, it was decided to progress to HYCONES II - a tool to build hybrid systems, offering to the knowledge engineer options to choose different neural models to work with and features to facilitate domain knowledge representation when dealing with fuzzy variables.

This paper gives an overview of HYCONES II, comparing the performance of the different neural networks models now available, when solving diagnostic problems in two different domain areas in medicine.

THE FUZZY ARTMAP MODEL

The Adaptive Resonance Theory (ART) deals with a system involving self-stabilizing input patterns into recognition categories, while maintaining a balance between the properties of plasticity and stability. ART models are being successfully used to recognize characters [4]. ART includes a series of different connectionist models: Fuzzy ARTMAP, Fuzzy ART, ART 1, ART 2, and ART 3. Among them, the Fuzzy ARTMAP one stands out for being capable of learning analogical patterns, using two basic ART modules. The Simplified Fuzzy ARTMAP model is a simplification of the Fuzzy ARTMAP neural network. Contrasting with the first model, the new one is capable of learning analogical patterns using only one ART module. A description of this model can be found in [5]. The presence of a single ART module does not hamper the Simplified Fuzzy ARTMAP model. The same performance levels are attained when the latter one runs without the second ART module. This is certified by the match-tracking strategy, that jointly maximizes generalization and minimizes predictive error.

Due to the powerful features of recognizing categories inherent to the ART model, it was decided to incorporate it in HYCONES II and validate its performance to solve medical diagnostic problems, comparing it to the CNM version of HYCONES. The goal was to offer more options to the knowledge engineer. As it will be described below, the Fuzzy ARTMAP model, although reported as excellent to recognize categories, concluded as much as CNM for the right diagnoses, but the semantic content of the activated neural networks was inadequate to be used in the explanatory module of HYCONES. This lack of semantics was investigated and, finally, a new neural model was proposed - the Semantic ART - SMART. The next sections describe how this was accomplished.

0195-4210/94/$5.00 © 1994 AMIA, Inc.

HYCONES' II ARCHITECTURE

HYCONES II keeps the basic architecture of its prior version, adding the other two neural networks (NN) models: Fuzzy ARTMAP and Semantic ART (SMART) and their respective learning algorithms: **(1) the Hybrid Knowledge Base (HKB)** - consisting of a combination of a frames mechanism with the three NN models: CNM, Simplified Fuzzy ARTMAP and Semantic ART (SMART); **(2) the Inference Machine** - controlling the inference process through the activation of the NN. Whenever the evidence is not enough for the NN to reach a conclusion, the inference process carries on with the pattern-matching mechanism in the symbolic part of the knowledge-base; **(3) the Learning Machine** - responsible for: the inductive and deductive learning features of the CNM algorithm; the Fuzzy ARTMAP algorithm and, finally, the SMART learning algorithm that is an adaptation of the CNM method; **(4) the Case Database** - responsible for the storage of all correctly solved classification problems. These correct classifications are used by the learning machine as the training examples for the HKB refinement. A description of HYCONES' architecture, its integration between frames and NN and the CNM learning algorithm can be found in [2,6,7].

The first step in the development of HYCONES II was, then, the incorporation of the Fuzzy ARTMAP model in the connectionist component of the HKB. This implied in a complete modification of the learning process, as it was implemented for CNM. Learning in Fuzzy ARTMAP is based on the creation of recognition categories in response to an arbitrary order of input cases. This process is regulated by a vigilance parameter, which is a number in a range from zero to one. The vigilance parameter defines the networks' level of generalization and specialization. When the parameter is set to zero, the network assumes maximum generalization; when it is set to one, the network assumes maximum specialization.

VALIDATION

Two medical domains were chosen to validate HYCONES' II performance: congenital heart diseases (CHD) and renal syndromes. This domain selection was only due to the case database availability. To build up the CHD case base, 66 medical records were extracted from the cardiac surgery database of the Institute of Cardiology RS (ICFUC-RS). These records cover the period extending from January 1986 to December 1990 and describe 22 cases of *Atrial Septal Defect* (*ASD*), 29 of *Ventricular Septal Defect* (*VSD*), and 15 of *Atrial-Ventricular Septal Defect* (*AVSD*), the three most frequent congenital heart diseases. For validation purposes, 33 additional cases, from the same database and period mentioned above, were also extracted. From these cases, 13 report *ASD*, 10 mention *VSD* and 10 refer to *AVSD*. This database is exactly the same used to validate HYCONES' first version [3]. To build the renal syndromes case base, 381 medical records from the database of the *Paulista School of Medicine* were analyzed and 58 evidences were semi-automatically extracted, covering the patients' clinical history and physical examination data. From the total number of selected cases, there are 136 occurences of *Uremia*, 85 of *Nephritis*, 100 of *Hypertension*, and 60 of *Calculosis*. From the 381 cases analyzed, 245 were randomly chosen to build the training set, while the remaining ones were used to build the testing set.

To validate HYCONES II, 46 versions of the HKB with congenital heart diseases were built; for the renal domain, another set of 46 HKB versions were constructed. For both medical domains, the HKBs were automatically generated from the training databases. From these 46 versions, one operates with the CNM model and the other 45 deal with the two ART models. These ART versions are divided in three groups: 15 versions were built using the Simplified Fuzzy ARTMAP model; 15 used the Simplified Fuzzy ARTMAP model without the normalization of the input patterns, and 15 used the Semantic ART model (described below). These 45 ART versions were grouped in three sets of five, according to the vigilance parameter used: 0.0; 0.7; and 0.9. Like other ART architecture, Fuzzy ARTMAP performance depends on the order of the input cases. For this reason, the cases were given in five different random orders, originating five different HKB versions for each distinct value of the vigilance parameter. Therefore, fifteen distinct versions of the trained HKB were created. For validation purposes, these fifteen versions were grouped into three sets, according to their correspondent vigilance, named **ART0, ART7** and **ART9,** respectively. The results shown in TABLE I below compare the CNM version with the best result obtained with Simplified Fuzzy ARTMAP model for both medical domains.

TABLE I - HYCONES II FUZZY ARTMAP VALIDATION

Diagn	CNM CHD N (%)	ART7 CHD N (%)	CNM Renal N (%)	ART7(*) Renal N (%)
Correct	31 93.9	29 87.9	95 74.8	108 85.0
Wrong	0 -	4 12.1	10 7.9	19 15.0
Not enough evidence	2 6.1	0 -	22 17.3	0 -
Total	33 100	33 100	127 100	127 100

(*) $p<0.05$ under the $\chi 2$ test, when compared to the CNM version.

HYCONES II - Simplified Fuzzy ARTMAP and HYCONES - CNM similarly performed for the CHD domain. The first one pointed out correctly to 29 of the 33 testing cases (87.9%), while the second one indicated correctly 31 of the same cases (93.9%). In the renal syndromes domain, however, the performance of HYCONES II - Simplified Fuzzy ARTMAP was superior to the one exhibited by CNM ($p < 0.05$). Both versions pointed out correctly, respectively, to 108 (85%) and 95 (74.8%) diagnoses of the 127 testing cases presented to the system.

HYCONES II - Simplified Fuzzy ARTMAP, therefore, displayed a satisfactory performance. However, the semantic contents of the neural nets it generated made no medical sense and could not be used to explain the system reasoning. Also, these contents were completely different from the ones stemming from the CNM networks, which were very similar to the knowledge graphs elicited from experts in CHD. In fact, the Simplified Fuzzy ARTMAP version used evidence that represented the complementary coding of the input pattern, to reach a diagnosis. This coding, inherent to the Simplified Fuzzy ARTMAP model, duplicates the input pattern, generating a new one depicting the evidence observed (*on-cell*) and, at the same time, the absent evidence, in relation to the total evidence employed to represent the input cases (*off-cell*).

The next step taken was to improve the semantic contents of the Simplified Fuzzy ARTMAP model. To achieve this, the complementary coding process was removed and the modified model was, then, revalidated through the same testing sets as above described. In the CHD domain, the performance of HYCONES II - Simplified Fuzzy ARTMAP, without complementary coding, proved to be inferior to the one presented by CNM ($p < 0.05$). In the renal syndromes domain, the performances of HYCONES II - Simplified Fuzzy ARTMAP, without complementary coding, and HYCONES - CNM were similar. The first pointed out correctly to 98 of the 127 testing cases (77.2%), while the second one pointed out correctly to 95 of the same cases (74.8%).

However, the recognition categories formed by this modified Simplified Fuzzy ARTMAP still presented quantitative and qualitative differences in their contents, when compared to the networks activated by CNM and to the knowledge graphs elicited from experts. This discrepancy, although smaller than the one observed in the original Fuzzy ARTMAP model, still restrained HYCONES' explanation mechanism.

THE SEMANTIC ART MODEL

The Semantic ART model (SMART) was, then, proposed. Its goal was to improve the semantic contents of ART recognition categories. To build this new model, the Simplified Fuzzy ARTMAP architecture was preserved, while its learning algorithm was replaced by the CNM inductive learning mechanism (the punishments and rewards algorithm, associated with the pruning mechanism) [8]. A new validation phase was, then, performed over the same testing sets, as depicted in TABLE II.

TABLE II - HYCONES II SMART VALIDATION

Diagn	CNM CHD N (%)	SMART CHD N (%)	CNM Renal N (%)	SMART Renal (*) N (%)
Correct	31 93.9	29 87.9	95 74.8	108 85.0
Wrong	0 -	4 12.1	10 7.9	19 15.0
Not enough evidence	2 6.1	0 -	22 17.3	0 -
Total	33 100	33 100	127 100	127 100

(*) $p<0.05$ under the $\chi 2$ test, when compared to the CNM version.

For the CHD domain, the performance comparison among SMART and CNM versions showed similar results. The first one pointed out correctly to 29 of the 33 testing cases (87.9%), while the second one singled out correctly 31 of the same testing cases (93.9%).

For the renal syndromes domain, the performance of HYCONES II - SMART was superior to the one presented by the CNM version ($p < 0.05$), and equal to the performance presented by the Simplified Fuzzy ARTMAP version. SMART and Simplified Fuzzy ARTMAP singled out correctly 108 of the 127 testing cases (85%), while the CNM version pointed out correctly 95 of the same 127 testing cases (74.8%).

Finally, it was observed that the NN generated by HYCONES II - SMART were similar in content to the networks generated by CNM and to the knowledge graphs elicited from multiple experts.

DEALING WITH FUZZINESS

It is well known that humans can operate with and decide upon fuzzy or uncertain data. Usually, to describe what is observed in the real world, human beings create categories to qualify the real objects. For example, someone's height is usually described as tall, medium or small. The fuzzy sets theory deals with that through the definition of membership functions in fuzzy spaces. These functions take each individual domain value and figure out the respective membership possibilities in each fuzzy space. In this example the fuzzy spaces are: tall, medium and small and the domain value is the individual height measurement. To build HYCONES II application to support the treatment of patients submitted to cardiac surgery, a case database was used and an expert was interviewed, invoking a knowledge acquisition methodology based on knowledge graphs [9]. Very frequently, the expert came up with graphs that used categories to qualify the medical finding. For example, it was mentioned by him that the hemodynamic parameter cardiac output is categorized as *adequate, inadequate or marginal*. The same approach was used to describe other hemodynamic parameters or lab data. As the knowledge acquisition phase proceeded, it became clear that the expert, whenever dealing with quantitative data, instead of reasoning upon the raw data, used categories or linguistic variables that defined fuzzy spaces, as they are named in the fuzzy sets theory. It became then evident that the concepts of the fuzzy sets theory were necessary to represent this knowledge in HYCONES II HKB. The next step was to ask the expert to submit the information about the compatibility (membership) functions used to define the semantics of the linguistic variables. As this line of questioning had never been tried before with the expert, there was, initially, the belief that he would find it difficult to explicit this knowledge. Surprisingly, he defined these functions very easily and promptly, either as a graphic or a table. Even though most of the time he drew a trapezoid function, in some cases the morphology of the pertinence function was unusual, as shown in FIG 1, where the finding systemic vascular resistance is described as: *low*, *normal* and *high*.

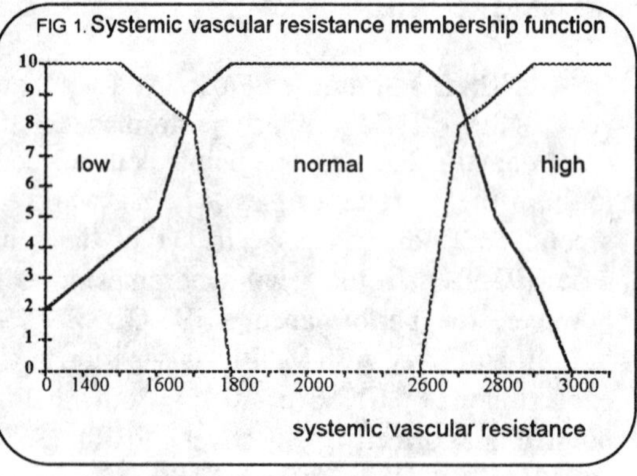

FIG 1. Systemic vascular resistance membership function

To represent these fuzzy variables in the symbolic component of HYCONES II HKB, the domain knowledge was divided into two sub-classes: one representing those findings where linguistic variables had been used (*fuzzy_findings*) and another to describe *non-fuzzy* ones (*non_fuzzy_findings*). In addition, an object to describe the linguistic variables was created - *language_var*. A semantic link connects these two objects. A simple and direct method to figure out the value of the membership functions was implemented. Whenever a case is being entered, either in the creation of the case database or in the consultation mode, HYCONES II verifies if the given finding is a fuzzy one. If so, instead of giving to the inference process (NN) the raw data, a transformation is made, in order to offer to the NN a finding described by its corresponding linguistic variables, together with the values of the membership function that the raw data can be mapped into.

In addition to the system intended to support post-operative treatment of cardiac surgery patients, HYCONES II fuzzy features are also being used in the development of the *Pharmacy* system. This system is intended to support the hospital pharmacist. It will be integrated in the hospital information system to check the medical prescription, issuing warnings whenever necessary.

CONCLUSION

There are several contributions to single out in this paper: the design, implementation and validation of the Simplified Fuzzy ARTMAP and SMART models. The latter one, however, stands out for its learning mechanism, which provides a higher semantic value to the recognition categories, when compared to the categories formed by conventional ART models. This important enhancement is obtained through the incorporation of specificity and relevance concepts to ART's dynamics. The original ART algorithm mainly considers the frequency of occurrence of the given evidence to create its recognition categories. Sensitivity is, however, only one of the factors considered by experts. Previous work has already shown that experts are able to identify not only what is more frequent, but rather, what is more relevant and specific while solving a diagnostic problem [9]. CNM's learning algorithm intends to imitate this behavior. CNM dynamics allows for a smooth learning curve, leading to an almost *intuitive* recognition of environmental patterns. By rewarding those pathways showing higher frequency and specificity, and punishing those less frequent, CNM algorithm guarantees the identification of the essential features of each category. Fuzzy ARTMAP's performance was increased when the CNM learning algorithm was incorporated into its dynamics and, what is more important, the newly created recognition categories presented a semantic content similar to knowledge graphs elicited from experts and also similar to CNM's trained networks.

HYCONES II, thus, offers to the knowledge engineer the choice among three different neural networks: CNM, Semantic ART and Simplified Fuzzy ARTMAP, all of which display good performance. Indeed, the first and second models, contrasting with the third one, support the context in a semantic way. In addition to the new neural models, HYCONES II is now able to describe and represent fuzzy medical findings.

Finally, this paper describes an additional contribution of an on-going research project on Artificial Intelligence in Medicine, led by the Medical Informatics Group of the Institute of Cardiology RS Medicine Graduate Program, in cooperation with the Federal University of Rio Grande do Sul Graduate Program in Computer Science. This research effort already led to two M.Sc. dissertations and some additional publications [3,5,7,8,10]. Presently, other two M.Sc. dissertations are invoking HYCONES II.

Reference

[1] Kandel A, & Langholz G. edts. Hybrid Archictectures for Intelligent Systems. CRC Press, Boca Raton, 1992.

[2] Machado R.J. & Rocha A.F. The Combinatorial Neural Network: a Connectionist Model for Knowledge-Based Systems. In: Proc of the Third Intern. Conf. on Information Proces. and Management of Uncertainty in Knowledge-Based Systems, Paris, 9-11, 1990

[3] Leão B.F & Reátegui E. B., HYCONES: a Hybrid Connectionist Expert System, In: Proceed.of the 17th Annual Symp. on Computer Applications in Medical Care, Washington, 461-465, 1993.

[4] Carpenter G.A., Grossberg S. Markuzon N., Reynolds J.H. and Rosen D. B., Fuzzy ARTMAP: a neural network architecture for incremental supervised learning of analog multidimensional maps. IEEE Trans. on Neural Networks, 3, 698-713, 1992.

[5] Guazzelli A., Barone D.A.C. and Filho E.C.B.C., A Simplified ARTMAP Architecture for Real-Time Learning, In: Proceedings of the International Workshop on Artificial Neural Networks, Sitges-Barcelona, 255-259, 1993.

[6] Reátegui E. B. Um modelo para sistemas especialistas conexionistas híbridos. Master of Science Dissertation, Computer Science Graduate Program, Federal University of RGS, Porto Alegre, Brazil. p.126, August 1993.

[7] Reátegui E.B. & Leão B. F., Integrating Neural Networks with the Formalism of Frames, Proceedings of the First World Congress on Neural Networks, Portland, 1993.

[8] Guazzelli, A. & Leão B. F., Incorporating Semantics to ART. In: Proceedings of the IEEE International Conference on Neural Networks, Volume III, p. 1726-31, Orlando, 1994.

[9] Leão B. F. & Rocha A.F. Proposed Methodology for Knowledge Acquisition: A Study on Congenital Heart Disease Diagnosis. Methods of Information in Medicine, 29, 30-40, 1990.

[10] Guazzelli A. Aprendizagem em Sistemas Híbridos. Master of Science Dissertation, Computer Science Grad. Program, UFRGS, Porto Alegre, Brazil. p.146, May 1993.

Advanced Clinical Monitoring: Considerations for Real-Time Hemodynamic Diagnostics

Julian M. Goldman, MD*, Marc J. Cordova, MSEE+

Dept. of Anesthesiology*, University of Colorado School of Medicine, Denver, CO, 80222
Dept. of Electrical Engineering+, University of Colorado at Boulder, Boulder, CO, 80309

ABSTRACT

In an effort to ease staffing burdens and potentially improve patient outcome in an intensive care unit (ICU) environment, we are developing a real-time system to accurately and efficiently diagnose cardiopulmonary emergencies. The system is being designed to utilize all relevant routinely-monitored physiological data in order to automatically diagnose potentially fatal events. The initial stage of this project involved formulating the overall system design and appropriate methods for real-time data acquisition, data storage, data trending, waveform analysis, and implementing diagnostic rules. Initially, we defined a conceptual analysis of the minimum physiologic data set, and the monitoring time-frames (trends) which would be required to diagnose cardiopulmonary emergencies. Following that analysis, we used a fuzzy logic diagnostic engine to analyze physiological data during a simulated arrhythmic cardiac arrest (ACA) in order to assess the validity of our diagnostic methodology. We used rate, trend, and morphologic data extracted from the following signals: expired CO_2 time-concentration curve (capnogram), electrocardiogram, and arterial blood pressure. The system performed well: The fuzzy logic engine effectively diagnosed the likelihood of ACA from the subtle hemodynamic trends which preceded the complete arrest. As the clinical picture worsened, the fuzzy logic-based system accurately indicated the change in patient condition. Termination of the simulated arrest was rapidly detected by the diagnostic engine. In view of the effectiveness of this fuzzy logic implementation, we plan to develop additional fuzzy logic modules to diagnose other cardiopulmonary emergencies.

INTRODUCTION

The morbidity of life threatening events may be adversely affected by any delay in the institution of corrective measures. Therefore, many patients are intensively monitored in the ICU in order to facilitate the rapid and early diagnosis of these events.[1] Diagnostic delays may be the result of insufficient nurse:patient staffing ratios, dependency upon unsophisticated patient monitor diagnostic and alarm algorithms, and the lack of the capability of current monitoring systems to display the relevant physiologic history.

Usually, critically ill patients are intensively monitored, and it would be ideal if the available physiological signals could be analyzed to provide early detection of impending problems. However, because of the nature and complexity of medical diagnosis, accurate diagnoses are difficult to make using typical computer models. Furthermore, the simplistic signal processing algorithms in general use do not actively exclude noise and other artifact from signal averages, and frequent false alarms are the result. Not only are displayed signal values frequently incorrect, but the erroneous data cannot be used to formulate accurate medical diagnoses. Ideally, we should be able to make more reliable diagnoses by simultaneously monitoring several physiologic signals[2] and implementing newer, more powerful algorithms such as neural networks and fuzzy logic. An advanced comprehensive monitor could be used as a tool to heighten the skills of medical personnel, not merely act as an extension of their skills.[3]

Some currently-used physiologic signal processing techniques have been effective. For example, several physiologic monitor manufacturers successfully employ conventional signal processing techniques to analyze the ECG. However, when reliably-analyzed signals are not available, we have successfully used neural networks to accurately analyze real-time physiologic waveform data. The neural network method of signal analysis can identify and eliminate artifactual waveforms from the time series, thereby improving the validity of

0195-4210/94/$5.00

the data stream and potentially improving the diagnostic reliability of the system.[3,4] Furthermore, a characterization of the waveform morphology can serve as a reliable input into an advanced comprehensive monitoring system.

METHODS

Design Considerations

In order to create a comprehensive monitor capable of performing reliable patient diagnoses, we have a functional set of criteria that must be met by the system. First and foremost, our system must be able to physiologically adapt to individual patients with unique conditions. We cannot realistically expect to use some "normal" baseline as a relative measure of a patient's condition. Therefore, the monitor needs to be informed of the application context (patient age, sex, and medical conditions). Second, if we analyze the signals over multiple time-frames, we can broaden the applicability of the system to disorders which vary in their time course. For example, a given drop in mean blood pressure would have a different diagnostic meaning if the decrease occurred over thirty seconds or thirty minutes. Third, our monitor would need to incorporate an "omniscient" awareness of all signals available. This omniscience allows us to detect the presence of all physiologic signals which are available as inputs, intelligently select the optimal signal sources by eliminating redundant or noisy signals, and optimize the selection of appropriate fuzzy rules in order to exclude the subsets of rules which are dependant on unavailable data. Fourth, performing multiple signal analysis allows us to determine the monitoring context (for example, detection of patient movement artifact). Knowledge of this context then provides us the opportunity to refine the diagnosis. For example, as a patient moves about in bed, movement artifact may distort the ECG waveform and generate an erroneous single-signal diagnosis e.g. ventricular tachycardia. However, simultaneous evaluation of the other available signals (e.g. pulse oximeter plethysmograph, arterial blood pressure waveform) may detect the presence of a normal state. Finally, the monitor needs to record the physiologic history preceding a significant medical event. This historical perspective allows for a more accurate differential diagnosis and subsequently a more effective treatment.

Before design began on the control system, we looked at the dynamics of several diagnoses strictly from a clinical point of view. We selected five specific potentially fatal cardiopulmonary emergencies to generate the system design. The conditions were:

1. arrhythmic cardiac arrest (e.g. ventricular fibrillation)
2. tension pneumothorax (air surrounding and compressing a lung)
3. pericardial tamponade (fluid surrounding and compressing the heart)
4. venous air embolism (air in the right ventricle and pulmonary artery)
5. exsanguination (severe blood loss)

These five conditions were chosen because they are important, testable, and maximally stress the diagnostic limitations of the system. All of these conditions result in a similar clinical picture of cardiovascular depression which may be difficult to discriminate between. Each of these events can be difficult to diagnose (for a physician, let alone a computer) without constantly and carefully watching all of the physiologic trends. The varying time course of these trends provides diagnostic clues.

Before design began on the control system, we looked at the dynamics of each diagnosis strictly from a clinical point of view. Each of the five medical events were evaluated by examining all of the information that would normally be electronically acquired from each patient, and which could contribute to the diagnosis. For example, a blood pressure monitor can give us mean blood pressure, systolic and diastolic pressure, and heart rate. Other monitored signals include ECG, central venous and pulmonary artery pressures, oxygen saturation by pulse oximetry, airway pressure, systemic arterial pressure, and capnography. Aside from the instantaneous information, an accurate diagnosis depends upon a closer examination of trends which can be assembled from the data. This includes the rate of change for all of the provided information and a classification of each waveform's morphology. For example, from our blood pressure signal we could determine how fast the mean blood pressure was changing (and the direction of change), as well as a waveform classification into categories such as normal, line flush, noise, or damped. We then created a matrix that related the five diagnoses to all of the processed data to help us assess the necessity for each calculated signal value, and to investigate the rule structure required to diagnose each event. We found that not all of the information is necessary for each diagnosis and each event can have several variations during its onset depending on a patient or environmental context.

Knowing what the system expectations were, we evaluated several types of decision systems to find the most effective and efficient. A traditional rule-based expert system was ruled out because of the known limitations of these systems (discussion below), and the difficulty of changing the rule structure to add additional diagnoses later on.[6] Neural networks would appear to be ideal to recognize these data patterns, however it is difficult (if not impossible) to generate adequate examples to train the network. Fuzzy logic on the other hand, gives us the flexibility to meet all of our initial objectives.[7]

Fuzzy logic is ideal for analyzing rapidly changing variables and classifying data into more than one category. For example, if we look at a classical rule system, a rule could state that if a patient's systolic blood pressure (BPS) is greater or equal to 100 mmHg, then we could classify this pressure as "NORMAL". If BPS was less than 100 mmHg, then we would classify it as "LOW." Now if a person has a BPS of 99 mmHg, then according to the strict rules this person would be classified with "LOW" BPS. In reality, we see that this patient has the characteristics of a pressure that is somewhat low and somewhat normal. This will help us to more accurately describe the true medical condition. Rather than using a classical ruled structure, we can implement a fuzzy logic-based system in order to classify elements into more than one category.[7] This gives us a realistic approach to making a medical diagnosis. With this characterization tool, we can set up a fuzzy logic system to reliably analyze various physiologic trending patterns. We can classify all of our inputs according to ranges from very low to very high and then present our output in the form of a likelihood for the event (e.g. not, somewhat, or very likely). For example, if we wanted to detect ACA, one of our fuzzy rules might look like this: "IF mean blood pressure is Very Low and heart rate is Zero and end tidal CO_2 is Very Low THEN the Likelihood of ACA is Very Likely." (Fig. 1 and 2) These rules are not as complex to derive because *we created our diagnostic matrix as the foundation for these rules.*

Experimental Diagnosis of Simulated ACA

A data file was hand-generated using anticipated physiological values consistent with the development ACA in an adult patient. The data set was created for three monitors: ECG, systemic arterial blood pressure, and the capnograph. In addition to the signal amplitude and rate information, a characterization of waveform morphology was generated. ECG complexes were described as "lethal" or "non-lethal". (Lethal ECG complexes are defined for the purpose of this experiment as complexes inconsistent with the maintenance of life-sustaining cardiac output.) Capnograms and blood pressure waveforms were described as "normal morphology", "abnormal morphology", or "absent".

The data set began with all signals in the normal range, and progressed to a modest decrease in BPS accompanied by the abrupt appearance of a lethal ECG morphology. Exhaled CO_2 concentration decreased more slowly than BPS as might occur with a mechanical ventilator set to deliver a low minute ventilation. Blood pressure-derived heart rate dropped almost instantaneously to a very low value, whereas the ECG-derived heart rate changed erratically to simulate the ECG monitor's unpredictable analysis of heart rate during ventricular fibrillation. Subsequently, all values approached zero to simulate untreated ACA. After maintaining all values near zero for several seconds, all values were rapidly increased to their low-normal range.

The ACA diagnostic capability of the fuzzy logic rule set was evaluated by reading the prepared data set. The data set was read into a custom Visual Basic program (version 3.0, Microsoft Corp., Redmond, WA) which used a dynamic linked library fuzzy logic tool (CubiCalc RTC version 1.20, Hyperlogic Corp., Escondido, CA) and displayed a graphical representation of the likelihood of ACA over time. The trend of CO2 concentration, BPS, and ECG-derived heart rate were similarly graphed. The relationship of the likelihood of ACA ("not likely", "somewhat likely", or "very likely") was assessed relative to the onset and amount of change of the three input variables.

RESULTS

Detection of the onset of ACA, evidenced by a transition from "not likely" to a high degree of "somewhat likely", occurred immediately after the onset of the lethal ECG complex and hypotension. Progression to "very likely" occurred just prior to the nadir of all of the signals and remained in that state until restoration of the circulation. The transition back to a state of "not likely" occurred rapidly: ACA "not likely" was diagnosed as soon as the physiological signals *started* to normalize. Of note was the rapid detection of the onset of ACA, and the smooth transition of the likelihood indicator throughout the event. The performance of the experimental system exceeded our expectations, mainly because of the rapid recognition capabilities.

CONCLUSION

We have formulated the architecture of a prototype comprehensive cardiopulmonary monitoring system. The system utilizes all available relevant signals from routinely-monitored ICU patients to diagnose and trend the onset and resolution of adverse cardiopulmonary events. Raw signals may be processed by conventional or neural network algorithms to provide reliable data for analyses by fuzzy logic rules. The performance and capabilities of neural network physiologic waveform analysis was evaluated previously[3], and now the capabilities of utilizing fuzzy logic to analyze this preprocessed data has been studied.

In view of the performance of the ACA-detection module, we plan to continue our development of additional diagnostic modules and perform invivo studies to further evaluate the concepts proposed here. Initial invivo development will require refining the data trending structures, formulating additional fuzzy rules, and evaluating performance of the system on real data. Eventually, system development will require the long-term collection of ICU patient data in order to capture and analyze adverse events.

REFERENCES

1. Bradshaw KE et al: Physician Decision Making: Evaluation of data used in a computerized intensive care unit, in Decision Support Systems in Critical Care, ed. Shabot MM and Gardner RM, Springer-Verlag, 1994.

2. Phelps EB, Goldman JM: Automated Situational Analysis for Operating Room Anesthesia Monitoring. Biomedical Sciences Instrumentation, V28, 111-16, 1992.

3. Bradshaw KE et al: Development of a Computerized Laboratory Alerting System, in Decision Support Systems in Critical Care, ed. Shabot MM and Gardner RM, Springer-Verlag, NY, NY, 1994.

4. Goldman JM, Dietrich BD: Artificial Neural network Analysis of Respiratory Waveforms: Data input and system design considerations. Journal of Clinical Monitoring, 7:119, 1991.

5. Goldman JM, Dietrich BD: Artificial Neural network Analysis of Physiologic Waveforms. Proceedings of the Annual International Conference of the IEEE EMBS, V13:No.4, 1660-1661, 1991.

6. Barber R: BONES: an expert system for diagnosis with fault models, Ellis Horwood Ltd., Chichester, West Sussex, England, 1992.

7. Kosko B: Neural Networks and Fuzzy Systems, Prentice Hall, Englewood Cliffs, NJ, 1992.

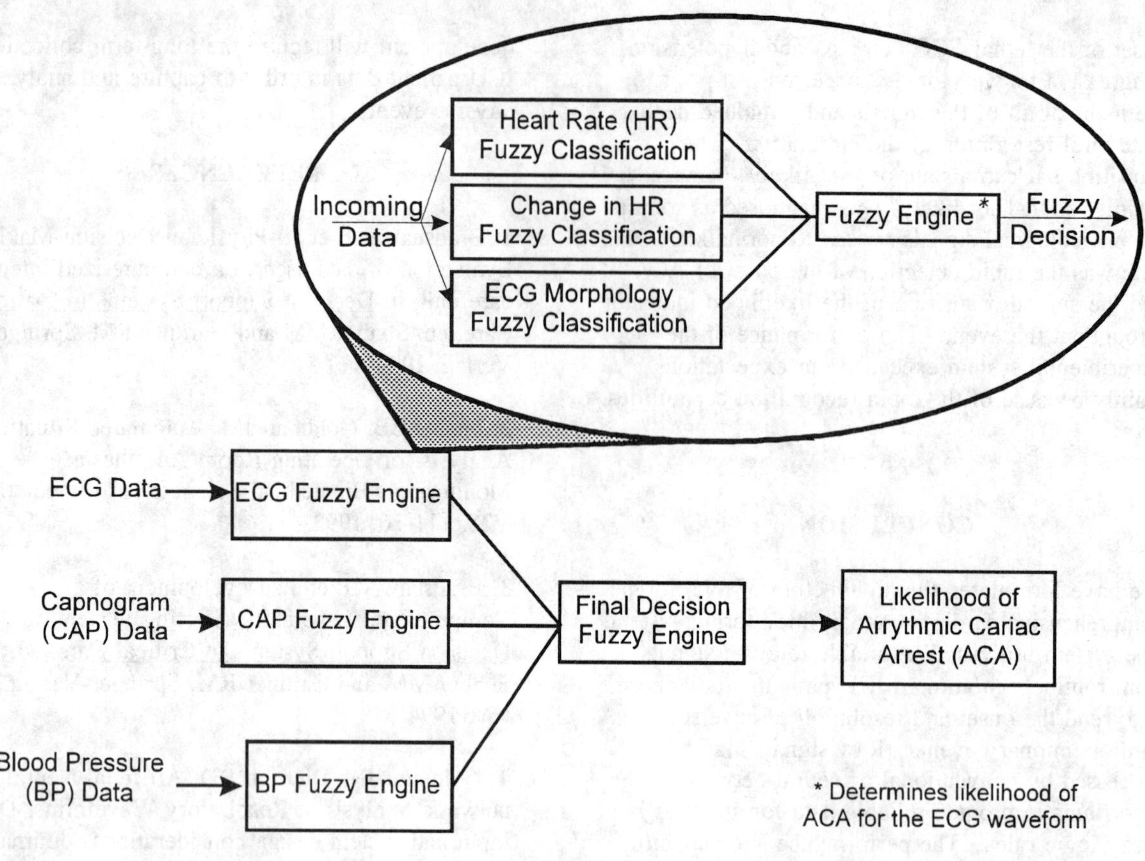
Heart Rate (HR)
Fuzzy Classification
Incoming
Data
Change in HR
Fuzzy Classification
ECG Morphology
Fuzzy Classification
Fuzzy Engine *
Fuzzy
Decision
ECG Data
ECG Fuzzy Engine
Capnogram
(CAP) Data
CAP Fuzzy Engine
Blood Pressure
(BP) Data
BP Fuzzy Engine
Final Decision
Fuzzy Engine
Likelihood of
Arrythmic Cariac
Arrest (ACA)
* Determines likelihood of
ACA for the ECG waveform

Fig. 1

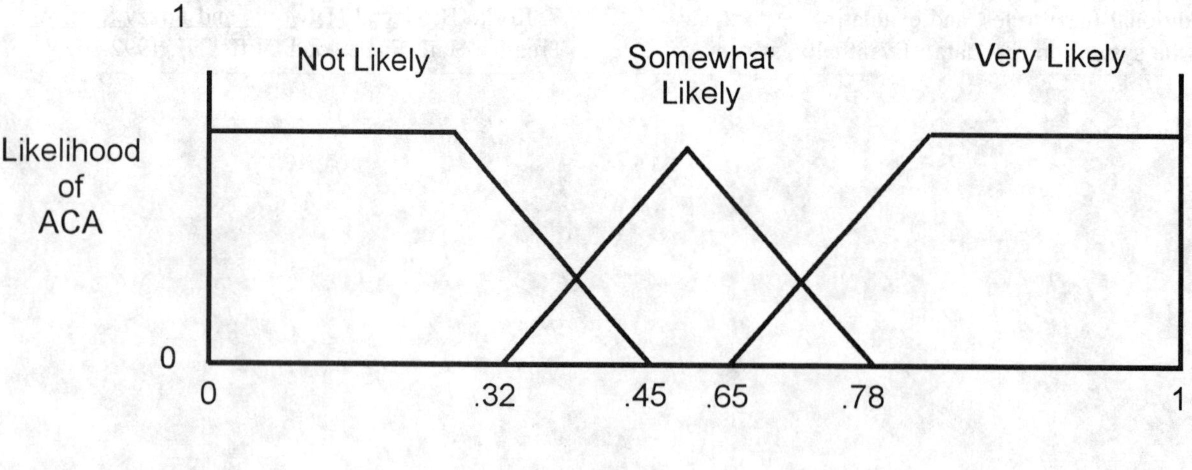
1
Not Likely
Somewhat
Likely
Very Likely
Likelihood
of
ACA
0
0
.32
.45
.65
.78
1

Fig. 2

Fuzzy Logic Assisted Control of Inspired Oxygen in Ventilated Newborn Infants

Yao Sun MD, Isaac Kohane MD, PhD, Ann R. Stark MD
Children's Hospital, Harvard Medical School, Boston, MA

The control of oxygen delivery to mechanically ventilated newborn infants is a time intensive process that must balance adequate tissue oxygenation against possible toxic effects of oxygen exposure. Investigation in computer assisted control of mechanical ventilation is increasing, although very few studies involve newborn infants. We have implemented a fuzzy controller for the adjustment of inspired oxygen concentration (FIO2) in ventilated newborns. The controller utilizes rules produced by neonatologists, and operates in real-time. A clinical trial of this controller is currently taking place in the neonatal intensive care unit (NICU) of Children's Hospital, Boston, MA.

INTRODUCTION

Oxygen toxicity plays a role in the development of chronic lung disease in newborn infants requiring mechanical ventilation. [1,2] In premature infants, inadequate maintenance of tissue oxygenation is implicated in the development of retinopathy of prematurity. [3] In order to avoid the effects of too much or too little oxygen, control of oxygen delivery to ventilated newborns has become a priority in neonatal intensive care.

Among the many ventilator parameters that affect patient respiratory status, the inspired oxygen concentration (FIO2) is most frequently manually adjusted on an acute basis to control oxygen delivery and maintain patient hemoglobin oxygen saturation levels. Manual control of the FIO2, however, may lag the clinical condition of the patient. That is, a patient may have an increased oxygen requirement as demonstrated by a lower oxygen saturation, but the manual increase of FIO2 may be delayed by human response times (i.e. a clinician may not be present to respond immediately). Conversely, a patient may have a decreased oxygen requirement as clinical conditions improve, yet the amount of oxygen delivered may not be immediately decreased. The latter scenario may be more common because of the perception that a patient with high oxygen saturation is "doing well" and does not require immediate intervention.

We have designed a microcomputer based system to help control the FIO2 delivered to mechanically ventilated newborn infants. This system utilizes a fuzzy logic controller based on "rules" generated by neonatologists who routinely provide care for ventilated infants. The goal of this control system is to maintain patient oxygenation (measured by oxygen saturation using pulse oximetry) at a target level set by the physician.

Instead of controlling the ventilator directly, the system currently operates by displaying suggested FIO2 changes to the physician, who then decides whether to execute the recommended change. This ensures medical safety until the system is fully tested for clinical efficacy. A clinical trial of the FIO2 control system is currently taking place in the neonatal intensive care unit (NICU) of Children's Hospital, Boston, MA.

BACKGROUND

Computer Assisted Ventilation

Investigation into computer-controlled or computer-assisted mechanical ventilation is expanding. One form of computer assistance is an "expert system" designed to advise the clinicians about ventilator management. Some recent examples include: VentPlan, a ventilator management advisor that interprets patient physiologic data to predict the effect of proposed ventilator changes [4]; WeanPro, a program designed to help wean post-operative patients from ventilators [5]; and KUSIVAR, a program which describes a comprehensive system for respiratory management during all phases of pulmonary disease. [6] Although many such expert systems have been described, few have been tested in clinical patient care.

Other investigators have studied direct computer control of specialized aspects of ventilator management. In adults for example, studies of computer-controlled optimization of positive end-expiratory pressure, and computerized protocols for management of adult respiratory distress syndrome have been explored by East. [7] A computerized ventilator weaning system for post-operative patients has been tested by Strickland. [8]

Experience in computer controlled ventilation in infants, however, is limited. In one of few reports available in the literature, Morozoff and Evans showed that their computerized FIO2 controller could maintain the hemoglobin oxygen saturation (SaO2) of a ventilated newborn infant for approximately 1 hour periods with results comparable to manual FIO2 control. [9]

0195-4210/94/$5.00

Morozoff and Evans describe their FIO2 controller as a "differential-feedback" controller. Other investigators have described similar FIO2 controllers for adults based on the "proportional-integral-derivative" (PID) design. [10] For best response, most PID controllers and feedback-loop controllers need to have their control parameters optimized for the system in which they are used. This may lead to degradation of performance if the system changes (e.g. if the patient's physiologic status changes, or the controller is switched to a new patient). Yu addressed this problem in FIO2 control by using multiple controllers that dynamically adapted by selectively utilizing the controller that best matched the system response at any given point in time. [11]

Fuzzy logic controllers

Since Zadeh first published his seminal paper on fuzzy sets in 1965 [12], applications utilizing fuzzy logic have proliferated rapidly. Mamdani's development of fuzzy controllers in 1974 [13] gave rise to the utilization of these controllers in ever expanding capacities, particularly in Japan where many industrial processes now employ fuzzy control. [14] In addition, fuzzy control techniques have recently been applied to various medical processes, such as pain control [15]and blood pressure control. [16]

When compared to classical control theory, a fuzzy logic approach to control offers the following advantages: [14,17]

1) It can be used in systems which cannot be easily modeled mathematically. In particular, systems with non-linear responses that are difficult to analyze may respond to a fuzzy control approach.
2) As a rule-based approach to control, fuzzy control can be used to efficiently represent an expert's knowledge about a problem.
3) Continuous variables may be represented by linguistic constructs that are easier to understand, making the controller easier to implement and modify. For instance, instead of using numeric values, temperature may be represented as "cold, cool, warm, or hot".
4) Fuzzy controllers may be less susceptible to system noise and parameter changes, thus making them more robust.
5) Complex processes can often be controlled by relatively few logic rules, allowing a more understandable controller design and faster computation for real-time applications.

In the context of FIO2 control in the newborn infant, a fuzzy logic approach can simplify the many complex factors and interactions that determine patient oxygenation. For example, a ventilated infant may exhibit decreased oxygen levels in the blood (as measured by SaO2) for many different reasons, including: failure to make respiratory effort, an obstructed endotracheal tube, or an increase in pulmonary shunting. Each cause may require differing changes in FIO2 to maintain target SaO2 levels, and many other factors may influence oxygenation. At different times, the same magnitude of change in FIO2 may result in completely different oxygenation states, even within the same patient.

FIO2 control in the newborn thus demonstrates some of the previously mentioned features which make classical control techniques difficult to apply: the system to be controlled is complex with many factors and interactions, it is very difficult to model mathematically, and system responses to FIO2 changes are often non-linear and unpredictable.

SYSTEM DESCRIPTION

FIO2 Controller

We chose SaO2 as our measurement parameter and FIO2 as our control parameter for the operational model of maintaining patient oxygenation.

SaO2 as measured by pulse oximetry is a well established method of monitoring patient oxygenation status. Its advantages over direct measurement of blood oxygen levels include rapid equilibrium with changes in blood oxygen levels, continuous monitoring, and noninvasive sampling. We used the error between the patient's SaO2 and the target SaO2 (ΔSaO2), and the slope of SaO2 (SaO2-slope) as the specific inputs to the fuzzy controller.

Although many ventilator parameters affect patient oxygenation (e.g. mean airway pressure, ventilatory rate, tidal volumes, etc.), the FIO2 is used to maintain the desired oxygenation status when the patient's overall respiratory status has been stabilized.

The design of the fuzzy controller then follows standard methods, with fuzzification of the input parameters, construction of fuzzy inference rules, and defuzzification or calculation of a "crisp" output value that represents the controller's action.

To fuzzify the input parameters, the values of ΔSaO2 and SaO2-slope were divided into fuzzy regions, with 7 regions chosen for ΔSaO2 and 5 regions chosen for the SaO2-slope. Triangular membership functions were assigned to each region, as illustrated in Figure 1.

Slope SaO2

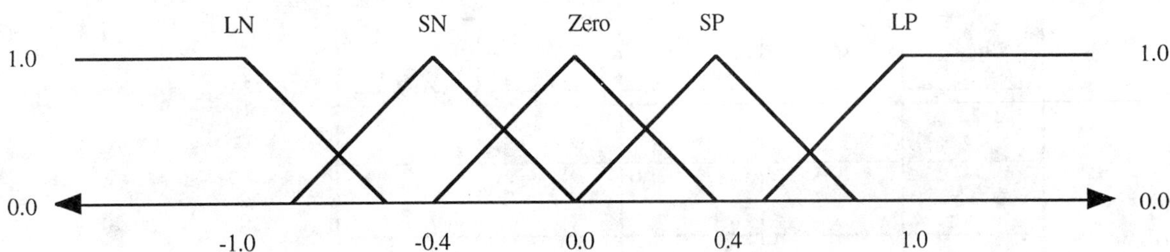

ΔSaO2

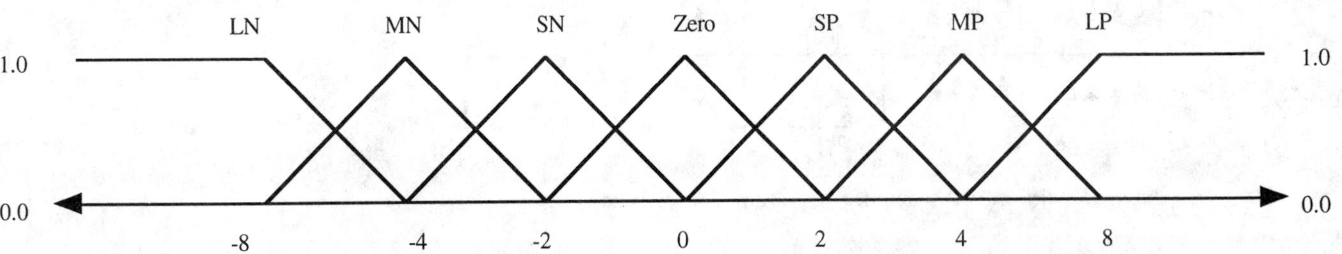

Figure 1
Membership Functions of Input Parameters
LN: large negative, MN: medium negative, SN: small negative
SP: small positive, MP: medium positive, LP: large positive

Using the fuzzy input parameters, the inference rules that form the body of the controller were constructed in the standard declarative form: IF situation THEN action . The combination of 7 ΔSaO2 fuzzy regions and 5 SaO2-slope fuzzy regions yields 35 rules. The logic of these inference rules are based on the expert knowledge of the neonatologists. Some example rules follow:

Rule: IF the ΔSaO2 is small-negative
AND the SaO2-slope is medium-negative
(situation)
THEN increase the FIO2 by a
medium-positive amount.
(action)

Rule: IF the ΔSaO2 is large-negative
AND the SaO2-slope is large-negative
THEN increase the FIO2 by an
extremely-large-positive amount.

Rule: IF the ΔSaO2 is small-negative
AND the SaO2-slope is small-positive
THEN do nothing.

All 35 rules are summarized in Table 1.

For any pair of ΔSaO2 and SaO2-slope inputs, we apply each of the inference rules in turn. Each rule will yield an action value. The defuzzification step then involves choosing a method to combine all the action values into a final value (a "crisp" value) that represents the controller output. We used the weighted mean of all the rule outputs to produce a single output value, in this case a change in the FIO2. [18]

Although there are relatively few fuzzy inference rules, continuously calculating the crisp output in real-time may not always be feasible. To help minimize time-delays, we compiled the fuzzy inference rules into a look-up table at runtime. Thus, during actual fuzzy control operation, evaluating the inputs becomes a simple and fast table look-up producing the controller output.

The FIO2 controller operates as follows:

1) SaO2 values are obtained for the patient every 1-2 seconds.
2) Every 10 seconds, the ΔSaO2 and the SaO2-slope are calculated.
   ΔSaO2 = (ave. SaO2 values over last 10 seconds) - target SaO2
   SaO2-slope = least squares regression of SaO2
3) The calculated ΔSaO2 and SaO2-slope are used as

ΔSaO2 \ SaO2-slope	LN	SN	ZERO	SP	LP
LP	0	0	↓↓	↓↓↓	↓↓↓↓
MP	↑	0	↓↓	↓↓	↓↓↓
SP	↑	0	↓	↓	↓↓
ZERO	↑↑	↑	0	↓	↓↓
SN	↑↑↑	↑↑	↑	0	0
MN	↑↑↑↑	↑↑↑	↑↑	↑	0
LN	↑↑↑↑↑	↑↑↑↑	↑↑↑	↑↑	0

Table 1

Inference rules for FIO2 control, given fuzzified ΔSaO2 and SaO2-slope

indices for the compiled fuzzy controller look-up table. A suggested FIO2 change is returned as the controller output.

System Components

The FIO2 fuzzy control system is implemented on an Apple Macintosh and is programmed in Macintosh Common Lisp. The SaO2 data is obtained from a Nellcor N-200 pulse oximeter through a RS-232 serial port on the back of the oximeter.

CLINICAL STUDY

Study Design

In order to test the FIO2 control system in a medically safe manner, the computer did not directly control the ventilator oxygen delivery. Instead, suggestions for changes in FIO2 were displayed for the physician to execute according to his/her best medical judgment. The computer system was programmed to record automatically all recommended and actual FIO2 changes.

The clinical trial protocol was approved by the Clinical Investigations Committee of Children's Hospital, Boston, MA., and informed consent was obtained from the parents of patients entered into the study. Patients were eligible if they were newborn infants admitted to the NICU and required mechanical ventilation. Patients were excluded if they had demonstrated intracardiac shunting of blood from right to left, or if they required vasoactive pressor medications to maintain blood pressure.

Each infant was studied for a 6 hour period of time. The initial 2 hours served as a control period during which the computer system collected SaO2 and FIO2 data. No interventions were made during this time. For the subsequent 2 hour experimental period, the system made recommendations for FIO2 changes in addition to acquiring data. The investigator manually carried out the recommended FIO2 changes if they were consistent with his/her clinical judgment. Finally, another 2 hour control period of data gathering (without recommendations for FIO2 change) completed the study period for the patient.

All clinical care activities proceeded as usual, and the NICU medical and nursing staff were not prevented from manually adjusting the FIO2 at any time during the trial.

Preliminary Study Results

Patient #1: target SaO2 = 93%

	Ctrl-1		**Expt**		**Ctrl-2**	
	FIO2	SaO2	FIO2	SaO2	FIO2	SaO2
Ave:	26	96	25	94	26	94
SD:	0	1.6	6.0	1.9	2.6	3.0

Patient #2: target SaO2 = 95%

	Ctrl-1		**Expt**		**Ctrl-2**	
	FIO2	SaO2	FIO2	SaO2	FIO2	SaO2
Ave:	27	95	26	95	29	94
SD:	4.6	3.2	6.1	2.6	8.5	5.1

(Ctrl: control period, Expt: experimental period, Ave: average, SD: standard deviation)

SUMMARY

Controlling oxygen exposure in newborn infants is a delicate balance. The infants must receive enough oxygen to ensure adequate tissue oxygenation and to prevent hypoxemia. Conversely, too much oxygen may produce toxic effects.

The FIO2 fuzzy controller shows promise in the preliminary trials to control patient oxygen saturation levels, and was able to maintain a target SaO2 better than routine manual control. Further clinical trials will test the actual clinical efficacy of this FIO2 controller, and additional patient data will allow more fine tuning of the fuzzy control parameters (e.g. the shape of the membership functions and the choice of fuzzy regions).

The ease of implementing this fuzzy controller illustrates some of the advantages of this approach. No complex mathematical models were required, the simple rule-based nature of the controller is easy to understand and modify, expert knowledge about the problem is utilized, and the controller was easily designed for non-linear system responses.

Current research in fuzzy control include combining it with other techniques such as neural networks and genetic algorithms [19,20], and adaptive or self-modifying fuzzy control. [18,21] As more medical processes become candidates for computerized control, the numerous options offered by these approaches will enhance the ability to produce a safe and clinically efficacious control system.

REFERENCE

[1]Saugstad, O. Oxygen toxicity in the neonatal period. *Acta Paediatr Scand* **1990**, *79*, 881.

[2]Wispe, J.; Roberts, R. Molecular basis of pulmonary oxygen toxicity.*Clin Perinatol* **1987**, *14*, 651-66.

[3]Avery, G.; Glass, P. Retinopathy of prematurity: what causes it?*Clin Perinatol* **1988**, *15*, 917-28.

[4]Rutledge, G.; Thomsen, G. Ventplan: a ventilator-management advisor.*Proc Annu Symp Comput Appl Med Care* **1991**, 869.

[5]Tong, D. Weaning patients from mechanical ventilation. A knowledge-based system approach.*Comput Methods Programs Biomed* **1991**, *35*, 267.

[6]Rudowski, R.; Frostell, C.; Gill, H. A knowledge-based support system for mechanical ventilation of the lungs. The KUSIVAR concept and prototype.*Comput Methods Programs Biomed* **1989**, *30*, 59.

[7]East, T.; Bohm, S. A successful computerized protocol for clinical management of pressure control inverse ratio ventilation in ARDS patients.*Chest* **1992**, *101*, 697.

[8]Strickland, J.; Hasson, J. A computer-controlled ventilator weaning system.*Chest* **1991**, *100*, 1096.

[9]Morozoff, P.; Evans, R. Closed-loop control of SaO2 in the newborn infant.*Biomed Instrum Technol* **1992**, *26*, 117.

[10]O'hara, D.; Bogen, D.; Noordergraaf, A. The use of computers for controlling the delivery of anesthesia.*Anesthesiology* **1992**, *77*, 563.

[11]Yu, C.; He, W. Improvement in arterial oxygen control using multiple-model adaptive control procedures.*IEEE Trans Biomed Eng* **1986**, *34*, 567.

[12]Zadeh, L. Fuzzy Sets.*Inf. Control* **1965**, *8*, 338-53.

[13]Mamdani, E. Application of fuzzy algorithms for control of simple dynamics plant. *Proc. IEEE* **1974**, *121*, 585-8.

[14]Mamdani, E. Twenty years of fuzzy control: experiences gained and lessons learnt.*Proceedings of the Second IEEE International Conference on Fuzzy Systems* **1993**, 339-44.

[15]Carollo, A.; Tobar, A.; Hernandez, C. A rule-based postoperative pain controller: simulation results.*Int J Biomed Comput* **1993**, *33*, 267-76.

[16]Ying, H.; McEachern, M.; Eddleman, D. W.; Sheppard, L. C. Fuzzy control of mean arterial pressure in postsurgical patients with sodium nitroprusside infusion. *IEEE Transactions on Biomedical Engineering* **1992**, *39*, 1060-69.

[17]Mamdani, E. H.; Østergaard, J. J.; Lembessis, E. In *Advances in fuzzy sets, possibility theory, and applications*; P. P. Wang, Ed.; Plenum Press: New York, 1983.

[18]Glorennec, P. Y. In *Fuzzy Logic*; R. Lowen and M. Roubens, Ed.; Kluwer Academic Publishers: Dordrecht, The Netherlands, 1993; pp 541-551.

[19]Nauck, D.; Klawonn, F.; Kruse, R. Combining neural networks and fuzzy controllers In: *Fuzzy Logic in Artificial Intelligence. 8th Austrian Artifical intelligence Conference, FLAI '93*. E. P. Klement and W. Slany. Linz, Austria: Springer-Verlag, 1993:35-46.

[20]Takagi, H.; Lee, M. Neural networks and genetic algorithm approaches to auto-design of fuzzy systems. In: *Fuzzy Logic in Artificial Intelligence. 8th Austrian Artifical intelligence Conference, FLAI '93*. E. P. Klement and W. Slany. Linz, Austria: Springer-Verlag, 1993:68-79.

[21]Nowé, A.; Vepa, R. A reinforcement learning algorithm based on 'safety' In: *Fuzzy Logic in Artificial Intelligence. 8th Austrian Artifical intelligence Conference, FLAI '93*. E. P. Klement and W. Slany. Linz, Austria: Springer-Verlag, 1993:47.

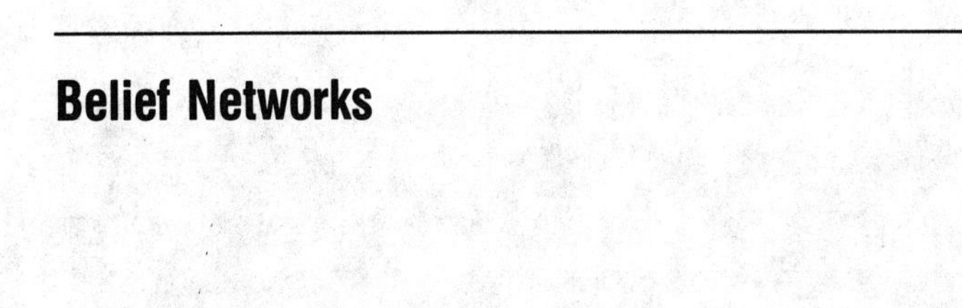

Belief Networks

Automated Transformation of Probabilistic Knowledge for a Medical Diagnostic System

Yu-Chuan Li, MD, Peter J. Haug, MD, Homer R. Warner, MD, Ph.D.
Department of Medical Informatics, University of Utah, Salt Lake City, Utah

Iliad is a large medical diagnostic system that covers more than 2000 diagnoses and 9000 findings. Due to the size and the complexity of this system, a robust knowledge representation is essential to consistently and efficiently model the medical knowledge involved. In this paper, we describe the knowledge representation currently used in Iliad and a probabilistic representation based on the Bayesian network formalism which can be derived using the information that the Iliad knowledge base contains.

1. INTRODUCTION

Iliad is a medical diagnostic support system developed at the University of Utah by Warner et al. [1]. Though it began as a system designed to help diagnose diseases in the Internal medicine area, it has grown to cover knowledge domains including Obstetrics/Gynecology, Dermatology, and Psychiatry. Currently, its knowledge base (KB) comprises of 2300 diseases and intermediate diagnoses and 9000 relevant findings. These findings include sociodemographic data, medical history, medications, physical examinations, laboratory test results, and pathological and radiological findings.

Iliad operates in three different modes: consultation, critiquing and simulation [2]. It has been proven to be a useful tool in teaching medical students diagnostic skills [1, 3, 4] and is currently used for that purpose in several medical schools in the United States. The expansion and refinement of the KB has been one of the most important aspects of this project. Due to the size and complexity of knowledge encompassed by this system, a robust knowledge representation (KR) is essential.

The KR that is currently used in Iliad will be referred to as the Iliad-KR in the following text. In addition to the Iliad-KR, we are currently exploring an alternate probabilistic representation based on Bayesian networks. In this paper, we discuss the weakness and strength of both KRs and similarities that have led to the development of a computer program that can automatically transform any KB expressed in the Iliad-KR into a Bayesian network.

2. THE ILIAD KNOWLEDGE REPRESENTATION

Instead of using heuristic scores like earlier diagnostic expert systems [5, 6], Iliad was designed around a multi-membership Bayesian model. This choice was based on the potential benefits associated with probabilistic formulations and on local experience with Bayesian medical decision systems [7, 8, 9]. Diagnostic medical knowledge is encoded in self-contained modules called frames. Each frame contains a list of findings associated with the disease that the frame represents. The TPR (true positive rate) and FPR(false positive rate) of each finding for a given disease is also included to facilitate the Bayesian calculation. During the early effort at knowledge engineering, the researchers discovered that multi-membership Bayes alone was not able to model all of the medical knowledge they intended to capture for two reasons: (1) The assumption of conditional independence of findings seldom held true for all findings associated with a disease, and (2) some medical diagnosis are routinely described using deterministic decision logic. Three mechanisms were devised to amend the multimembership model. These are referred to as "clustering", "OR sets" and "deterministic frames". "Clustering" and "OR sets" were used to address the problem of conditionally dependent findings, while "deterministic frames" were used to capture the Boolean logic sometimes used by physicians to describe a diagnosis.

2.1 The Deterministic Frames

As opposed to the frames that contain TPR/FPR, which we call probabilistic frames, a deterministic frame contains a list of relevant findings, Boolean decision logic, and the expected base frequencies for each of the findings in an inpatient population. The value of the frame is then determined by a heuristic algorithm that combines the truth status of the Boolean logic and the frequencies of the findings [10].

2.2 The Clusters and the OR sets

Clusters are frames (either deterministic or probabilistic) which contain a set of related findings that represent intermediate pathophysiologic states or syndromes [11]. These states or syndromes are then used as findings in the probabilistic frames that represent diseases or higher-level concepts (which can also be clusters). A deterministic frame does not contain clusters in the Iliad-KR.

Findings that are considered conditionally dependent but do not constitute an intact intermediate concept can be assigned as an OR set . Findings in an OR set are treated as mutually exclusive. When more than one finding in an OR set are instantiated (known to be true or false), only the finding with the most information will be active. A multi-membership, Bayesian formalism, together with these complimentary mechanisms make up the current Iliad knowledge representation.

2.3 The Algorithms Used to Reason in the Iliad-KR

In order to reason within this complex KR and obtain posterior probabilities for likely diagnoses, several algorithms were implemented in addition to the standard multi-membership Bayes' calculation. These algorithms include (1) a heuristic algorithm that propagates probabilities from clusters to higher-level frames, and (2) an algorithm that evaluates deterministic frames and returns probabilistic interpretations. Detailed descriptions of these algorithms can be found in [10].

3. BAYESIAN NETWORKS AND THE ILIAD-KR

3.1 Similarity Between the Two Knowledge Representations

Bayesian networks have been vigorously studied in the last few years as a normative knowledge representation in domains involving probabilistic dependencies. Possible applications in medical decision-support systems have also been enthusiastically explored [12-14]. We found the Bayesian network appealing because of its consistent representation of probabilistic dependencies among variables (also referred to as "nodes" in the following text) and the mathematical characteristics it embodies [15].

Further examination of the Iliad-KR and Bayesian networks provided us insight into the similarity between these two KRs. We found that the causal relations which need to be specified (as arcs) in Bayesian networks can be identified in the Iliad-KR: (1) The Iliad-KR uses frames to represent the relation between the diseases (or intermediate states) and the findings. These relations are, in most cases, direct causal relations. For example, variant angina is implemented as a finding in the frame "coronary artery spasm", this can be easily translated into a causal link from the "coronary artery spasm" node to the node that represents variant angina. (2) The clusters in the Iliad-KR can be treated as intermediate nodes caused directly by the diseases nodes that are their parents. Each cluster links, in turn, to a set of finding nodes. (3) The OR sets in the Iliad-KR imply hidden intermediate causes that can be added as an intermediate node in Bayesian network terms.

The need for exponential number of conditional probabilities has been criticized as one of Bayesian networks weakness. This requirement becomes problematic when a node has multiple parents or predecessors. Then, the number of probabilities required is $2^{(\text{number of parents})}$. A common approach to managing this requirement is through the "noisy OR gate model." Using this model reduces the probabilities needed for any node to one conditional probability of that node given each of its predecessors. The noisy OR gate model is based on the assumptions that (1) an event is presumed false if all of its listed causes are false (accountability) and (2) each exception to a normal causal relation between variables acts independently (exceptional independence) [15]. If these assumptions hold true, a complex conditional probability can be decomposed into simple ones using formula(6) below.

In the Iliad-KR, these simple conditional probabilities are explicitly assigned in the probabilistic frames. In the deterministic frames, the probabilistic relationship is actually implied in the Boolean logic of each frame. As a highly simplified example, if C causes <u>A and B</u>, conditional probabilities P(A|C) and P(B|C) are both 1. If C causes <u>A or B</u>, the conditional probabilities P(A|C) and P(B|C) are both 0.5. Formula (3) and (4) show the general form of this derivation.

3.2 Weakness and Strength of the Two Knowledge Representations

The Iliad-KR has given us an efficient and workable system capable of providing useful probabilities. Domain experts and knowledge engineers have created thousands of frames using this KR. The simplicity of the calculations associated with this KR, has made it possible to do any diagnostic inference in seconds on a personal computer. However, the heuristic components in the Iliad-KR calculations make the probabilities generated by the system mathematically unsound. In addition, the multi-membership basis of Iliad-KR also relies on the false assumption that all diseases are completely independent. This has resulted in the generation of less discriminative and overly confident posterior probabilities by the system [16].

On the other hand, Bayesian networks provide a mathematically sound representation with extensive expressiveness. Our experience with a renal mass diagnostic KB suggests that Bayesian network models demonstrated better reliability and discriminating ability than the current Iliad model [16]. Nonetheless, the price for this theoretically sound solution is the demand for combinatorially increasing numbers of probabilities and the use of NP-hard inference algorithms. Although the number of probabilities needed can be dramatically decreased by using a noisy OR gate model, this is only appropriate when the assumptions of the noisy OR gate model are not violated.

The most serious drawback to a Bayesian network model may be its inference algorithms: Both exact and approximate probabilistic inference in general Bayesian networks have been proven to be NP-hard [17, 18]. This means that for some Bayesian networks, the computation time needed to reach a solution will grow exponentially with the size of the network. Researchers in this area have not clearly characterized the classes of Bayesian networks that require exponential running time. Yet there has been significant work to restrict the topology and the conditional probabilities of the network to guarantee polynomial running time for approximation algorithms [19, 20]. For Bayesian networks with arbitrary topology, empirical evaluation is often useful to gain insight into the computation time needed [21].

4. THE TRANSFORMATION ALGORITHMS

Based on the similarity between Bayesian networks and the Iliad-KR discussed above, we have developed a set of algorithms to facilitate a transformation from the Iliad-KR to a Bayesian network.

Most of the findings in a frame can be transformed directly into the successors of the node that represents the frame itself. Some exceptions are nodes that represent age, sex and risk factors. Although they are used in the Iliad KB as findings of a disease, age and sex are obviously not caused by the diseases. In another example, cigarettes smoking is considered a finding under the frame "lung cancer", yet it is not caused by "lung cancer". Under these conditions, we have chosen to reverse the causal relationship by applying a Bayesian calculation

$$P(d^+|r^+)=\frac{P(r^+|d^+)P(d^+)}{P(r^+|d^+)P(d^+)+P(r^+|d^-)(1-P(d^+))}$$

...... (1)

where D is the disease node and R is the node to be reversed. Because TPR, FPR and prior probabilities for disease are readily available in the Iliad KB, $P(r^+|d^+)$, $P(r^+|d^-)$ and $P(d^+)$ can be obtained to calculate the conditional probability of D given R, i.e., the right hand side of equation (1). Since R now becomes a root node, we estimated its prior probability $P(r^+)$ by using formula (2) where n is the number of the original parents of R.

$$P(r^+)=\frac{\sum_i^n P(r^+|d_i^+)P(d_i^+)+P(r^+|d_i^-)(1-P(d_i^+))}{n}$$

...... (2)

In deterministic frames, a joint probability distribution is implied by the Boolean logic embedded in each frame. Let $f_1 \ldots f_n$ be the findings in a deterministic frame X, this joint probability distribution can be represented by formula (3). However, the causal relationship implied by this formula (X is dependent on $f_1 \ldots f_n$) is inconsistent with the causal semantics that are modeled throughout the Iliad-KR (X causes $f_1 \ldots f_n$). In order to have consistent causal semantics, we asserted that $f_1 \ldots f_n$ should be children of X and derive the conditional probabilities $P(f_i^+|x^+)$ by using formula (4) where f_i is the ith finding in X.

$$P(x,f_1,\ldots,f_n)=P(x|f_1,\ldots,f_n)\prod_i P(f_i) \text{.....(3)}$$

$$P(f_i^+|x^+)=\frac{P(x^+,f_1,\ldots,f_i^+,\ldots,f_n)}{P(x^+,f_1,\ldots,f_n)} \text{...........(4)}$$

In the right hand side of formula (3), $P(x|f_1,\ldots,f_n)$ can be easily obtained from the Boolean logic and $P(f_i)$ is the frequency of the finding f_i embedded in Iliad's deterministic frames.

To accommodate the OR set heuristic in the Iliad-KR, we insert a synthetic intermediate node between the frame and the findings in an OR set. The TPR for the most important finding in the OR set is used as the conditional probability for the link between the synthetic node and the node that represents the frame. The conditional probability between this finding and the synthetic node will then be assigned 1 and the conditional probabilities for the rest of the findings are normalized accordingly. This implementation is intended more to maintain the correct semantics of the resulting Bayesian network than to simulate the OR set heuristic, although it does act similarly whenever the most important finding in the set is instantiated.

All the transformation algorithms were developed under the noisy OR gate model. As we describe in Section 3.1, this model is only valid when the assumptions of accountability and exceptional independence hold true. Although the exceptional independence assumption does hold true in the Iliad-KR most of the time, the accountability assumption is violated if the list of causes for a node is not exhaustive. To accommodate this assumption, we have added a parent node labeled as "Other causes" to each non-cluster findings [12]. Each of the "Other-causes" node was assigned a prior probability of 1 and a conditional probability derived from calculating its lower bound:

$$P(f^+)\leq\sum_i P(f^+|d_i^+)P(d_i^+)+P(f^+|c^+)P(c^+)$$

$$P(f^+|c^+)\geq\frac{P(f^+)-\sum_i P(f^+|d_i^+)P(d_i^+)}{P(c^+)} \text{......(5)}$$

where d_is are the listed causes of finding f, and c is the "Other-causes" node. Thus, $P(f|c)$ is the conditional probability for the link between c and f. $P(c^+)$ is by definition 1. The equal sign only holds when the d_is and c are mutually exclusive and exhaustive. All the information on the right hand side of formula (5) is either stored in the Iliad KB or derivable from it.

Using the noisy OR gate model, we can decompose a complex conditional probability into simple ones. For example, assuming d_1 and d_2 are parents of f, the probability of f conditioned on both d_1^+ and d_2^+ can be derived from formula (6).

$$P(f^-|d_1^+,d_2^+)=P(f^-|d_1^+)P(f^-|d_2^+) \text{..............(6)}$$

Thus all the complex conditional probabilities needed for Bayesian networks can be derived from the probability of f conditioned on each of its parents.

5. THE RESULTING BAYESIAN NETWORK

By utilizing the algorithms described above, we have developed a computer program that can read directly the Iliad KB and transform it into a Bayesian network. The result is a multiply connected Bayesian network consisting of 11,406 nodes which has a multi-level structure as deep as 36 levels. The nodes are heavily interconnected and common findings are shared by as many as 62 parents. The size and complexity of this Bayesian network makes exact algorithms impractical for its inference. Among the existing approximation algorithms, we have chosen to use the likelihood weighting algorithm as our first inference algorithm because of its simplicity in implementation [22]. We are also investigating other weighting algorithms as well as various Markov sampling techniques [23, 24].

The initial results based on the forward simulation algorithms have been encouraging. We observed a trend of convergence when we increase the number of iterations for the simulation. On a synthesized case with 12 pieces of evidence, this Bayesian network consistently generated reasonable results after 40,000 iterations. However, under the likelihood weighting algorithm that we are using, the rate of convergence could degrade if the evidence occurred on nodes with extreme conditional probabilities (close to 0 or 1). We have found that the reversal of age, sex and risk factor nodes actually contribute to a better convergence rate. Many of the reversed nodes, are root nodes and are frequently present as part of the evidence.

6. DISCUSSION

The restricted assumptions associated with earlier probabilistic models like simple Bayes and multi-membership Bayes have limited their applications to narrow medical domains [9]. Bayesian networks eliminate many of these restrictions. In addition, the expressiveness of Bayesian networks can be especially advantageous in building large, broad-spectrum diagnostic systems where numerous intermediate pathophysiologic states may be present and shared by many diseases. However, it is a tremendous effort to build a comprehensive diagnostic system from scratch. One way to prevent the duplication of a knowledge engineering effort is to convert an existing system to a Bayesian network. Shwe and Middleton et al. have demonstrated this approach by reformulating Internist-I into a Bayesian network [12]. Their new system called QMR-DT showed a diagnostic accuracy comparable to the original Internist-I, despite the many approximations that were used in the conversion processes. However, because of the inherent two-level structure of the Internist-I KB, the resulting Bayesian network did not take advantage of this formalism's ability to express the multi-level structure of diagnostic reasoning.

Iliad was constructed using a KR that accommodates intermediate pathophysiologic states and conditionally dependent findings. We have found that, by utilizing the set of algorithms described above, most of the parameters needed by a Bayesian network can be derived from this KR. A program has been developed to automatically transform the Iliad-KR into a Bayesian network. Several advantages are associated with this approach: (1) Whenever the Iliad KB is updated, we only need to rerun this program once to include the updated knowledge into the Bayesian network. (2) This program allows us to explore different options in the transformation processes. For example, the conditional probability between a finding and the "Other-causes" node was derived by calculating the lower bound of its value. We can run this program multiple times with different values of this probability to generate Bayesian networks with different emphasis on "Other-causes".

We have also found that not all the probabilities in the Iliad KB are consistent with the clinical setting we are trying to model. This is partly because many of the probabilities have been tested and adjusted under the system's own inference heuristics. Converting to a well defined, mathematically consistent model has highlighted some of these questionable probabilities. Where appropriate, we are replacing them with estimates derived from data in the HELP clinical database [25].

Computation time has always been an issue in large Bayesian networks. Given the size and complexity of the Bayesian network derived from the Iliad KB, no existing inference algorithm can guarantee a response time suitable for interactive consultation although many are highly parallelizable. A more likely scenario is to integrate the inference engine into a health information system, process the data in the background once they are available, and provide the results when needed. We have potential applications which we are exploring include quality assurance for medical care [26], and medical free text processing [27].

* This publication is supported in part by grant number 5 R01 LM05323 from the National Library of Medicine.

References

[1]. Warner HR, Haug PJ, Bouhaddou O, Lincoln MJ, Warner HRJ, Sorenson D, Williamson JW, Fan C. Iliad as an expert consultant to teach differential diagnosis. In: Proceedings of the 12th Symposium on Computer Applications in Medical Care (SCAMC), IEEE Computer Society Press 1988:371-376.

[2]. Warner HR Jr. Iliad - Moving medical decision-making into new frontiers. In: Proceedings of International Symposium of Medical Informatics and Education. Salamon R, Protti D, Moehr J. eds. University of Victoria, B.C., Canada, 1989:267-70.

[3]. Cundick R, Turner CW, Lincoln MJ, Buchanan JP, Anderson C, Warner HRJ, and Bouhaddou O. Iliad as a patient case simulator to teach medical problem solving. In: Proceedings of the 13th Symposium on Computer Applications in Medical Care (SCAMC), IEEE Computer Society Press. 1989:902-6.

[4]. Turner CW, Williamson JW, Lincoln MJ, Haug PJ, Buchanan JP, Anderson C, Grant M, Cundick R, Warner HR. The effects of Iliad on medical student problem solving. In: Proceedings of the 14th Symposium on Computer Applications in Medical

Care (SCAMC), IEEE Computer Society Press. 1990:478-81.

[5]. Barnett GO, Cimino JJ, Hupp JA, Hoffer EP. DXplain: An evolving diagnostic decision-support system. JAMA 1987;258:67-74.

[6]. Miller RA. Pople HEJ, Myers JD. Internist-I: An experimental computer-based diagnostic consultation for general internal medicine. N Engl J Med 1982;307:468-76.

[7]. Ben-Bassat M, Carlson RW, Puri VK, Davenport MD, Schriver JA, Latif M, Smith R, Portigal LD, Lipnick EH, Weil MH. Pattern-Based Interactive Diagnosis of Multiple Disorders: The Medas System. IEEE Transactions on Pattern Analysis and Machine Intelligence, Vol.PAMI-2, No.2, March 1980.

[8]. Warner HR, Olmsted CM, Rutherford BD. HELP - A program for medical decision making. Comp Biomed Res 1972; 5:65-74.

[9]. Warner HR, Toronto AF, Veasy LG. Experience with Bayes' theorem for computer diagnosis of congenital heart disease. Ann N.Y. Acad Sci 1964; 115:558-67.

[10]. Sorenson DK, Cundick RM, Fan C, Warner HR. Passing Partial Information among Bayesian and Boolean Frames. In: Proceedings of the 13th Symposium on Computer Applications in Medical Care (SCAMC). Kingsland LC, ed. Los Alamitos, CA: IEEE Computer Society Press. 1989:50-54.

[11]. Turner CW, Lincoln MJ, Haug PJ, Warner HR, Williamson JW, Whitman N. Clustered disease findings: aspects of expert systems. In: Proceedings of International Symposium of Medical Informatics and Education. Salamon R, Protti D, Moehr J. eds. University of Victoria, B.C., Canada, 1989:259-63.

[12]. Shwe MA, Middleton B, Heckerman DE, Henrion M, Horvitz EJ, Lehmann HP, Cooper GF. Probabilistic Diagnosis Using a Reformulation of the INTERNIST-1/QMR Knowledge Base I and II. Meth Inf Med 1991; 30: 241-67.

[13]. Olesen KG, Kjaerulff U, Jensen E, Jensen FV, Falck B. Andreassen S, Andersen SK. A MUNIN network for the median nerve - a case study on loops. Appl Artif Intell 1989; 3:384-404.

[14]. Heckerman DE, Horvitz, Nathwani BN. Update on the Pathfinder project. In: Proceedings of the 13th Symposium on Computer Applications in Medical Care (SCAMC). Kingsland LC, ed. Los Alamitos, CA: IEEE Computer Society Press. 1989:203-7.

[15]. Pearl J. Probabilistic Reasoning in Intelligent Systems: Networks of Plausible Inference. Morgan Kaufman, San Mateo, CA, 1988.

[16]. Li YC, Haug PJ. Evaluating the quality of a probabilistic diagnostic system using different inferencing strategies. In: Proceedings of the 17th Symposium on Computer Applications in Medical Care (SCAMC), Washington DC, 1993:471-477.

[17]. Cooper GF. The Computational Complexity of Probabilistic inference using Bayesian Belief Networks. Artificial Intelligence 1990; 42:393-405.

[18]. Dagum P, Luby M. Approximating probabilistic inference in Bayesian belief networks is NP-hard. Artificial Intelligence 1993; 60:141-153.

[19]. Heckerman DE. A tractable inference algorithm for diagnosing multiple diseases. In: Proceedings Fifth Conference on Uncertainty in Artificial Intelligence, Windsor, Ont, 1989:174-81.

[20]. Henrion M. Search-based methods to bound diagnostic probabilities in very large belief nets. In: Proceedings Seventh Workshop on Uncertainty in Artificial Intelligence, Los Angeles, CA, 1991.

[21]. Shwe M, Cooper GF. An empirical analysis of likelihood-weighting simulation on a large, multiply connected belief network. In: Proceedings Sixth Conference on Uncertainty in Artificial Intelligence, Boston, MA, 1990:498-508.

[22]. Fung R, Chang KC. Weighting and Integrating Evidence for Stochastic Simulation in Bayesian Networks. In: Machine Intelligence and Pattern Recognition: Uncertainty in Artificial Intelligence 5,Vol 10. Henrion M, Shachter R, Kanal LN, Lemmer JF. eds. Elsevier, Amsterdam, 1990:209-20.

[23]. Henrion M. An introduction to algorithms for inference in belief nets. In: Machine Intelligence and Pattern Recognition: Uncertainty in Artificial Intelligence 5, Vol 10. Henrion M, Shachter R, Kanal LN, Lemmer JF .eds. Elsevier, Amsterdam, 1990:129-38.

[24]. Shachter RD, Peot M. Simulation Approaches to General Probabilistic Inference on Belief Networks. In: Machine Intelligence and Pattern Recognition: Uncertainty in Artificial Intelligence 5, Vol 10. Henrion M, Shachter R, Kanal LN, Lemmer JF .eds. Elsevier, Amsterdam, 1990:221-31.

[25]. Pryor TA, Gardner RM, Clayton PD, Warner HR. The HELP system. J Medical System 1983; 7:87-102.

[26]. Lau LM, Warner HR. Performance of a Diagnostic System (Iliad) as a Tool for Quality Assurance. In: Proceedings of the 15th Symposium on Computer Applications in Medical Care (SCAMC), IEEE Computer Society Press. 1991:1005-10.

[27]. Haug PJ, Ranum DL, Frederick PR. Computerized Extraction of Coded Findings from Free-Text Radiologic Reports. Radiology 1990; 174:543-48.

Generating Explanations and Tutorial Problems from Bayesian Networks

Peter Haddawy, Ph.D., Joel Jacobson, Charles E. Kahn, Jr., M.D.
Department of Electrical Engineering and Computer Science, University of Wisconsin–Milwaukee;
Section of Information and Decision Sciences, Department of Radiology, Medical College of Wisconsin,
Milwaukee, Wisconsin

We present a system that generates explanations and tutorial problems from the probabilistic information contained in Bayesian belief networks. BANTER is a tool for high-level interaction with any Bayesian network whose nodes can be classified as hypotheses, observations, and diagnostic procedures. Users need no knowledge of Bayesian networks, only familiarity with the particular domain and an elementary understanding of probability. Users can query the knowledge base, identify optimal diagnostic procedures, and request explanations. We describe BANTER's algorithms and illustrate its application to an existing medical model.

INTRODUCTION

Bayesian networks have become the representation of choice for building decision-making systems in domains characterized by uncertainty, and have been applied to several medical domains [1-5]. The models currently available and under development provide a wealth of detailed knowledge that can be used for educational purposes as well as clinical decision support. Unfortunately, the information contained in these models is not easily intelligible; tools are needed to make this information comprehensible. The availability of shells for performing inferences over Bayesian network models [6,7] and the recent development of explanation generation algorithms [8,9] have made building such a tool possible.

This report presents BANTER (Bayesian Network Tutoring and Explanation), a generic Bayesian-network shell that provides decision support and tutors users in diagnosis and in selection of optimal diagnostic procedures. BANTER can be used with any Bayesian network containing nodes that can be classified as hypotheses, observations, and diagnostic procedures. The system is designed so that the user need know nothing about Bayesian networks in order to interact with it effectively. In fact, none of the system's dialogs with the user indicates that the system is using a Bayesian network to perform its reasoning. The user needs only some knowledge of the particular domain and an elementary understanding of probability.

BANTER computes the posterior probability of a diagnosis, determines the best diagnostic procedure to affirm ("rule in") or exclude ("rule out") a diagnosis, quizzes the user on the selection of optimal diagnostic procedures, and generates explanations of its reasoning. It can generate story problems and quiz the user on diagnoses and selection of optimal diagnostic procedures. Almost all of the system's reasoning is driven by the Bayesian network knowledge base; setting up the system for a new network requires minimal effort.

METHODS

System Environment

BANTER is implemented in C* and runs on top of the HUGIN Bayesian network inference system [6]. HUGIN performs all probability computations using a belief network specified in HUGIN's network definition format. The HUGIN interface consists of a set of functions from the HUGIN libraries, which are used to load and compile a belief network, instantiate and uninstantiate nodes, propagate changes in individual nodes throughout the network, and obtain probability values for nodes. BANTER's graphical interface is written using the Xaw graphics tool kit of the X11 public-domain windowing package; the widespread popularity of this package makes the interface highly portable.

System Configuration

BANTER is easily configured for new networks. To set up a new network model, BANTER requires a HUGIN network definition file, a BANTER definition file, and a story template file. For medical models, the BANTER definition file contains a list of nodes grouped as HISTORY, PHYSICAL FINDINGS,

---

* The software is available at *ftp//ftp.cs.uwm.edu/pub/tech_reports/ai/BANTER.tar.Z.*

DISEASES, and DIAGNOSTIC PROCEDURES. Each node is of the type FLOAT, INTEGER, STRING, or BOOLEAN.

Generating Tutorial Problems

The story template file is used to create the text for randomly generated story problems. The system generates a story problem by randomly choosing a set of values for the patient history and physical findings, randomly choosing a disease of interest, and expressing these choices by instantiating the story template. The template contains the following types of directives:

{*label*: $text_1$:$text_2$: ... :$text_{n+1}$}

Print the text for the corresponding state of node *label*: $text_1$ corresponds to the first state (as listed in the HUGIN definition file), $text_2$ for the second, and $text_{n+1}$ for the UNKNOWN state. A percent sign ("%") in the text stream indicates where the node's value will be inserted; for nodes of type FLOAT, one can specify the number of printed digits (e.g., "%.%%").

<BOOLEAN:$text_1$:$text_2$>

Pick a random boolean value, and print $text_1$ if TRUE or $text_2$ if FALSE.

[*class*]

Print the names of nodes of the specified *class* (for medical models: HISTORY, PHYSICAL-FINDINGS, or DISEASES), excluding those that have been selected already. If a node is BOOLEAN, its name will be included only if its current state is TRUE. For nodes of other types, the name and value will be displayed.

(*class*)

Print the names of nodes of the specified *class*, excluding those that have been selected already. If a node is of type BOOLEAN, its name will be included only if its current state is FALSE. For nodes of other types, the name and value will be displayed.

Determining the Best Test

The best test to rule in or rule out a hypothesis is determined by positively and negatively instantiating each test outcome and determining the posterior probability of the hypothesis given the test outcome and the patient's history and physical findings. The best test to rule in the hypothesis is the one that results in the highest post-test probability and the best test to rule out the hypothesis is the one that results in the lowest post-test probability.

Generating Explanations

Following Suermondt's INSITE method [8], BANTER generates explanations in two steps. The first step identifies the evidence that has the most influence on the given hypothesis. The second step identifies the strongest and most comprehensible paths linking the influential evidence with the hypothesis. Both algorithms are used to explain the current belief in a disease: we first identify those nodes among the specified history and physical findings that were most influential in producing the reported posterior probability of the disease and then find the paths along which that influence flows. To explain the selection of the best test, only the second algorithm is used: here we only need to find the paths of influence from each test outcome to the disease.

Identifying Influential Evidence. To identify the most influential pieces of evidence, we first determine the influence of each evidence node on a hypothesis by performing a sensitivity analysis. We remove all evidence from the network and then instantiate each evidence node individually and record the posterior probability of the hypothesis. We then filter out all evidence nodes that do not influence the hypothesis in the direction of its posterior probability given all the evidence. For the remaining nodes, the posterior probabilities are then normalized so that they fully span the range 0 to 1; call this the importance of each node. We define important nodes to be ones with an importance value greater than some threshold. The threshold is selectable by the user and is currently set to 0.7. We normalize the posterior probabilities since we are interested in identifying pieces of evidence with relatively strong influence on the probability of the hypothesis. This is not determined by the absolute value of the posterior probability but rather by the value relative to the prior probability of the hypothesis and the posteriors for the other pieces of evidence.

Our algorithm differs from that of Suermondt [8]. Rather than instantiating each piece of evidence individually, Suermondt removes each piece of evidence individually and computes the posterior probability of the hypothesis without that piece of evidence. An influential piece of evidence is one for which the posterior probability without the evidence is significantly lower than with the evidence. While our approach will identify each piece of evidence that is individually significant, Suermondt's approach will not flag a piece of evidence as significant if it does

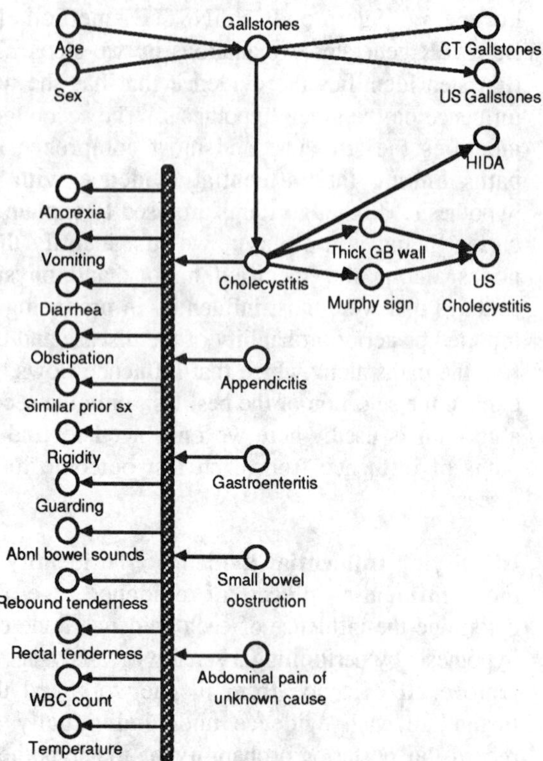

Figure 1. Bayesian network model of gallbladder disease. (The vertical bar simplifies the illustration: all input nodes influence all output nodes.)

not increase the probability of the hypothesis in the presence of other pieces of evidence. For example, if two pieces of evidence each raise the probability of the hypothesis to one, neither will be flagged as significant since when each is removed the probability of the hypothesis is still one. Suermondt further discusses using his technique on all possible subsets of the set of evidence in order to identify sets of evidence that may be collectively significant but for which no single element is individually relevant.

Identifying Paths of Influence. To determine the paths along which an evidence node influences a hypothesis node, we first identify all paths along which evidence can flow based on d-separation [10]. This set often will be too large for meaningful explanation, so we limit the explanation to five paths, ranked by strength and length. Our foremost objective is to tell the user how the evidence influences the hypothesis. For the explanation to be accurate, BANTER needs to identify the strongest paths; for it to be concise, we choose the shortest paths among those that are equally strong. The method of identifying paths of influence is described in greater detail elsewhere [11].

RESULTS

We applied BANTER to a Bayesian network model of acute gallbladder disease (Figure 1) [5]. The two principal diagnoses are gallstones and cholecystitis; appendicitis, gastroenteritis, small bowel obstruction, and abdominal pain of unknown cause serve as alternative diagnoses. The remaining nodes represent a patient's history, physical findings, and test results. Using the story template file (Figure 2), BANTER generates a story problem (Figure 3).

Querying the Knowledge Base

The user queries the knowledge base by setting up a scenario. A scenario is created by specifying a set of known values for the history and physical findings, as well as a set of diseases of interest. This is done by clicking on nodes in windows displaying for history, physical findings, and diseases of interest. The user now can ask the system to compute the posterior probability of the selected diseases or to determine the best tests to rule in and rule out the selected

```
{SEX:Mr. Jones:Mrs. Jones:The patient}
{AGE:is % years old, and} presents with [HISTORY], and denies (HISTORY).
{SEX:His:Her:The patient's} {TEMPERATURE:temperature is %.%.}
{SEX:His:Her:The patient's} {WBC-COUNT:WBC count is %.%.}
Physical examination reveals [PHYSICAL-FINDINGS], and no evidence of (PHYSICAL-FINDINGS).
What is the best test to <BOOLEAN:rule in:rule out> [DISEASE]?
```

Figure 2. Story template for gallbladder-disease model.

```
Mrs. Jones is 41 years old, and presents with ANOREXIA, and denies VOMITING, DIARRHEA,
     OBSTIPATION, SIMILAR-SX-PREVIOUSLY.  Her WBC count is 12.6.  Physical examination reveals
     GUARDING, and no evidence of RIGIDITY, REBOUND-TENDERNESS, ABNORMAL-BOWEL-SOUNDS.

What is the best test to rule out GALLSTONES?
```

Figure 3. Story problem generated by BANTER.

diseases.

Requesting an Explanation
The user can obtain an explanation of the reasoning that lead the system to select these tests (Figure 4). The system starts by explaining how the known history and physical findings influence the probability of gallstones. Having explained how the pretest probability of gallstones was arrived at, the system continues by explaining each possible test further influences the probability of gallstones.

Quizzing the User
In addition to asking the system to perform computations, the user can ask to be quizzed in the selection of optimal diagnostic procedures. This can be done in two ways. The user can specify a scenario and choose the test he or she thinks best to rule in or rule out the selected disease. If an answer is incorrect, the system tells the user which tests are preferable to the one selected and can explain its reasoning. The second way the user can be quizzed is by selecting the "story" action. In this mode, the system randomly selects a patient history, a set of physical findings, and a disease of interest, and presents the scenario to the user in English (Figure 3). The user can select an answer from the quiz menu and continue as described above.

DISCUSSION

BANTER transforms the information contained in a Bayesian network into an easily intelligible form for medical education and clinical decision support. BANTER quizzes and tutors users on the evaluation of diagnoses and optimal selection of diagnostic procedures. Since almost all the system's reasoning is performed using the Bayesian network knowledge base, configuring the system to work with a given network requires little effort. On the other hand, since nothing in the system's functionality indicates that it is using a Bayesian network for its reasoning, the complex details of the representation are hidden from the user.

Future research will focus on (1) explanations in extremely large networks, (2) more informative explanations, and (3) rigorous evaluation. In the newly emerging models that contain thousands of nodes, inference will become too slow to provide acceptable interaction and the explanations produced by the current algorithm will become too lengthy. For a given problem, typically only a portion of a given network model will be relevant. We have developed a technique for specifying a Bayesian network as a collection of rules in probability logic and generating that portion of the network relevant to a given computation [12]. Integrating this technique

```
Before presenting any evidence, the probability of GALLSTONES being present is 0.128.
The following pieces of evidence are considered 'important' (in order of importance):
  Presence of GUARDING results in a post-test probability of 0.175 on GALLSTONES.
  AGE of 41 results in a post-test probability of 0.172 on GALLSTONES.

Calculating chains. .
Their influence flows along the following paths:
  GUARDING is caused by CHOLECYSTITIS, which is caused by GALLSTONES.
  AGE influences GALLSTONES.
Presentation of the evidence results in a posterior probability of 0.227 for the presence of
    GALLSTONES.

The best tests to rule in GALLSTONES (in order):
  A positive CT test results in a probability of 0.987 on GALLSTONES.
  A positive ULTRASOUND FOR GALLSTONES test results in a probability of 0.601 on GALLSTONES.
  A positive HIDA test results in a probability of 0.406 on GALLSTONES.
  A positive ULTRASOUND FOR CHOLECYSTITIS test results in a probability of 0.344 on
    GALLSTONES.

Calculating chains. .
Their influence flows along the following paths:
  GALLSTONES are seen by CT.
  GALLSTONES are seen by ULTRASOUND FOR GALLSTONES.
  GALLSTONES causes CHOLECYSTITIS, which is detected by HIDA
  GALLSTONES causes CHOLECYSTITIS, which causes SONOGRAPHIC MURPHY SIGN, which is detected by
    ULTRASOUND FOR CHOLECYSTITIS
  GALLSTONES causes CHOLECYSTITIS, which causes ULTRASOUND THICK GB WALL, which is detected
    by ULTRASOUND FOR CHOLECYSTITIS
```

Figure 4. Explanations generated by BANTER.

into BANTER will significantly reduce the complexity of inferences in very large networks.

BANTER provides more informative explanations by associating semantic information with Bayesian networks. Instead of displaying paths of influence with arrows, we indicate how each node influences its successor with terms like "causes" or "detects." Including abstraction information may make explanations more informative and more concise. Rather than explain only the current scenario, one could explain a more general scenario, of which the current one is an instance. For example, in the case of cholecystitis elevating temperature, one could additionally tell the user that any inflammatory disease, of which cholecystitis is an instance, has the tendency to elevate temperature.

We currently are evaluating BANTER's explanatory content and style in tests with physicians at various levels of training. In addition to the model of gallbladder disease described above, we are applying BANTER to belief-network models for diagnosis of liver lesions by magnetic resonance imaging [4] and echocardiographic diagnosis (Díez FJ, personal communication).

Because of its generality and ease of use, BANTER can be used in a wide variety of settings where belief networks models have been formulated. Its ability to quiz users and provide explanations – without explicit reference to a belief network model – makes the system useful for clinical decision support and medical education.

Acknowledgments

We thank Dr. Finn V. Jensen and the HUGIN group at Aalborg University for generously providing us the use of HUGIN for this work. This work was supported in part by NSF grant IRI-9207262 (PH) and the 1993 American Roentgen Ray Society Scholarship (CEK).

References

[1] Andreassen S, Woldbye M, Falck B, Andersen SK. MUNIN — a causal probabilistic network for interpretation of electromyographic findings. In: Proceedings of the International Joint Conference on Artificial Intelligence. Menlo Park, CA: AAAI Press, 1987: 366-372.

[2] Shwe MA, Middleton B, Heckerman DE, et al. Probabilistic diagnosis using a reformulation of the INTERNIST-1/QMR knowledge base. I. The probabilistic model and inference algorithms. Methods Inf Med 1991; 30:241-255.

[3] Andreassen S, Jensen FV, Olesen KG. Medical expert systems based on causal probabilistic networks. Int J Biomed Comput 1991; 28:1-30.

[4] Tombropoulos R, Shiffman S, Davidson C. A decision aid for diagnosis of liver lesions on MRI. In: Safran C, ed. Proceedings of the Seventeenth Annual Symposium of Computer Applications in Medical Care. New York: McGraw-Hill, 1993: 439-443.

[5] Haddawy P, Kahn CE Jr, Butarbutar M. A Bayesian network model for radiological diagnosis and procedure selection: work-up of suspected gallbladder disease. Med Phys 1994; 21:1185-1192.

[6] Andersen SK, Olesen KG, Jensen FV, Jensen F. HUGIN — a shell for building Bayesian belief universes for expert sytems. In: Proceedings of the Eleventh International Joint Conference on Artificial Intelligence. Menlo Park, CA: AAAI Press, 1989: 1080-1085.

[7] Srinivas S, Breese J. IDEAL: a software package for analysis of influence diagrams. In: Proceedings of the Sixth Conference on Uncertainty in Artificial Intelligence. San Mateo, CA: Morgan Kaufmann, 1990: 212-219.

[8] Suermondt HJ. Explanation in Bayesian Belief Networks [Ph.D. thesis]. Medical Information Sciences, Stanford University, 1992.

[9] Suermondt HJ, Cooper GF. An evaluation of explanations of probabilistic inference. Comput Biomed Res 1993; 26:242-254.

[10] Pearl J. Probabilistic Reasoning in Intelligent Systems: Networks of Plausible Inference. San Mateo, CA: Morgan Kaufmann Publishers, 1988.

[11] Haddawy P, Jacobson J, Kahn CE Jr. An educational tool for high-level interaction with Bayesian networks. In: Proceedings of the 6th IEEE International Conference on Tools with Artificial Intelligence. New Orleans, LA: IEEE Press, 1994: (in press).

[12] Haddawy P. Generating Bayesian networks from probability logic knowledge bases. In: Uncertainty in Artificial Intelligence: Proceedings of the Tenth Conference. San Mateo, CA: Morgan Kaufmann, 1994: 262-269.

Experimental Analysis of Large Belief Networks for Medical Diagnosis

Malcolm Pradhan*, Gregory Provan, Max Henrion
Institute of Decision Systems Research
4984 El Camino Real, Suite 110, Los Altos, CA 94022
*also Section on Medical Informatics, MSOB X-215
Stanford University, CA 94305

We present an experimental analysis of two parameters that are important in knowledge engineering for large belief networks. We conducted the experiments on a network derived from the Internist-1 medical knowledge base. In this network, a generalization of the noisy-OR gate is used to model causal independence for the multi-valued variables, and leak probabilities are used to represent the nonspecified causes of intermediate states and findings. We study two network parameters, (1) the parameter governing the assignment of probability values to the network, and (2) the parameter denoting whether the network nodes represent variables with two or more than two values. The experimental results demonstrate that the binary simplification computes diagnoses with similar accuracy to the full multivalued network. We discuss the implications of these parameters, as well other network parameters, for knowledge engineering for medical applications.

ISSUES IN BUILDING LARGE NETWORKS

There is increasing interest in Bayesian belief networks and influence diagrams as representations for medical knowledge that are soundly based on the principles of probability and decision theory. However, questions remain about their practicality for building very large knowledge bases. The work we describe here is part of a long term project to explore and evaluate techniques for knowledge engineering and inference with very large belief networks (BNs). Like any large knowledge-engineering project to encode medical expertise, building a large BN is a lot of effort, and issues of network complexity and the required precision of the probabilities are critical. Presumably, a larger, richer network with more precise probabilities can support more accurate diagnosis. But, what kind of relationships are there between representation and performance?

In this paper, we report some initial experimental results as part of an attempt to help answer these questions. We emphasize that these experiments are not an external validation of the diagnostic accuracy of the network. Here, we focus on two issues: First, what are the effects of alternative ways of expressing the probabilities? We start with frequency integers—0, 1, 2,...,5—to express the links between variables, and compare various mappings from frequencies to conditional probabilities. Second, how much difference does it make to express variables as two-valued or binary (for example, a disease may be present or absent) instead of four-level (for example, a disease may be absent, mild, moderate, or severe). Using four levels should create a more accurate representation and should lead to better diagnosis, but the improvement in performance may not be worth the additional knowledge engineering and computational effort.

Our experimental results demonstrate that the binary simplification computes diagnoses with similar accuracy to the full multivalued network. In addition, the frequency to probability mappings may significantly affect the overall accuracy of the diagnoses.

CPCS: KNOWLEDGE BASE TO BELIEF NETWORK

The Quick Medical Reference–Decision Theoretic (QMR-DT) project seeks to develop practical decision-analytic methods for large knowledge-based systems. The first stage of the project converted the Internist-1 knowledge base [4] (QMR's predecessor) into a binary, two-layered BN [3,12]. In the second stage of the QMR-DT project we are creating a multilayer BN with multivalued variables, and developing efficient inference algorithms for the network.

To create a large multilevel, multivalued BN we took advantage of a rich knowledge base, the Computer-based Patient Case Simulation system, developed over two years by R. Parker and R Miller [7] (CPCS–PM) in the mid-1980s as an experimental extension of the Internist-1 knowledge base. The CPCS–PM system is a knowledge base and simulation program designed to create patient scenarios in the medical sub domain of hepatobiliary disease, for use in medical education. Unlike that of its predecessor Internist-1, the CPCS–PM knowledge base models the pathophysiology of diseases—the intermediate states causally linked between diseases and manifestations. The original CPCS–PM system was developed in FranzLisp. Diseases and intermediate pathophysiological states (IPSs) were represented as Lisp frames [5].

To construct the BN we converted the CPCS–PM knowledge base to CommonLisp and then parsed it to create nodes. We represented diseases and IPSs as four levels of severity in the CPCS BN—absent, mild, moderate, and severe. Predisposing factors of a disease or IPS node were represented as that node's predecessors, and findings and symptoms of a disease or IPS node as the successors for that node. In addition to the findings, CPCS contained causal links between disease and IPS frames, we converted these links into arcs in the BN. Frequency weights [11] from the CPCS–PM ranged from 0 to 5 and were mapped to probability values, as described in the next section.

We generated the initial CPCS BN automatically from the knowledge base, we did manual consistency checking using domain knowledge to edit the network. Because the CPCS–PM knowledge base was not designed with probabilistic interpretations in mind, we had to make numerous minor corrections to remove artifactual nodes, to make node values consistent and to confirm that only mutually exclusive values were contained within a node.

As we checked the validity of the resulting network it became clear that in the original CPCS–PM used frequency weights to represent frequencies *and* to control inference in the system. In the initial version of the CPCS BN we have identified, but not corrected, these inconsistencies. We will explore the effects of further knowledge engineering on the performance of the network in future work.

The resultant network has 450 nodes and over 900 arcs. Seventy-four of the nodes in the network are predisposing factors and required prior probabilities; the remaining nodes required *leak* probabilities (described in the *Network Implementation* section) assessed for each of their values. We thus had to assess almost 600 probabilities to specify the network fully.

For our experiments we used a subset of the full network comprising 110 nodes, which is the set of all ancestor and predecessor nodes of three disease nodes—ascending cholangitis, acute viral hepatitis, and alcoholic hepatitis—shown as heavy outlined nodes in Figure 1. Because the complexity of a BN rises exponentially with the size of the network, inference in a sub network can be accomplished in reasonable time, which is not possible for the full CPCS BN.

MEDICAL IMPLICATIONS OF THE NETWORK PARAMETERS

We varied the mapping and domain-size parameters to assess their effect on this BN representation. The first parameter studied was the frequency to probability mapping. In converting the CPCS–PM knowledge base to a BN, we make the assumption that the frequency weights used in the Lisp knowledge base can be mapped to probability values. The default mapping, called *standard*, is based on the interpretation of frequency weights from the original work to convert the Internist-1 knowledge base to a two-level network [11]. The standard mapping used

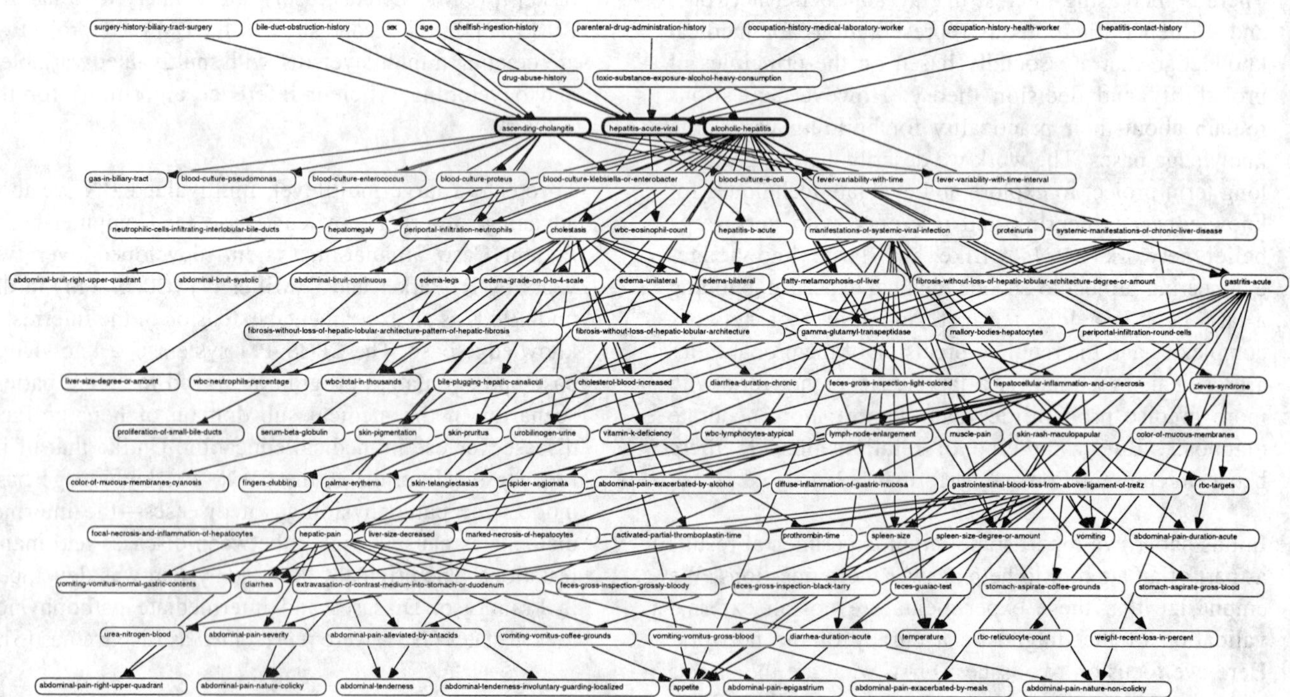

Figure 1. We performed experiments on this 110-node subset of the full 450-node CPCS BN. We chose the subset by including all ancestors and predecessors of the disease nodes ascending cholangitis, acute viral hepatitis, and alcoholic hepatitis—shown as dark outlined nodes in row three.

in the two-level BN had a diagnostic performance comparable to the QMR program [3]. We also used two other mappings, *categorical* and *curvilinear*, as shown in Table 1.

There are two reasons to vary the mappings. First, doing so allows us to test whether the interpretation of the standard mappings is accurate. Second, varying the mappings lets us test the sensitivity of a large BN to the probability values. This latter point has an implication for knowledge engineering—when data cannot be found easily it is much easier for experts to assess probabilities in orders of magnitude, say, than as exact values. For example, the categorical mapping interprets the frequency weights as follows: 0 to 3 are small probabilities, and 4 to 5 are high. We empirically determined the cutoff of 3 based on the frequencies already assigned in the network. The curvilinear mapping was determined to be consistent with the frequency values in the network by a domain expert.

Table 1. Mappings used to represent frequency weight from the original CPCS knowledge base as probabilities in the CPCS BN.

	Frequency					
Mapping	0	1	2	3	4	5
standard	0.0025	0.025	0.2	0.5	0.8	0.985
categorical	0.001	0.001	0.001	0.001	0.999	0.999
curvilinear	0.0001	0.001	0.01	0.1	0.9	0.99

The second parameter studied was the domain size of variables. We converted the disease and IPS nodes (which have the four values absent, mild, moderate, and severe) in the original network to nodes with the binary values absent, and present. The domain size influences knowledge engineering: the size of the conditional probability tables grows exponentially with the number of values. The assessment task for experts is also more difficult for multivalued variables compared to binary variables.

NETWORK IMPLEMENTATION

In this section we describe the network used for the experiments, outline the experiments conducted, and discuss the techniques used to analyze the data.

Assumptions

The CPCS network is a multilevel BN in which a *noisy-OR* representation [1,8,9] is used to model the arcs between nodes. The noisy-OR is a simplified BN representation that requires far fewer parameters than does the full conditional probability matrix. The noisy-OR is defined over a set of *binary*-valued variables. Consider an effect variable x, which has n cause variables or predecessors, $d_1,...,d_n$. The noisy-OR can be used when (1) each d_i has a probability p_i of being sufficient to produce the effect in the absence of all other causes, and (2) the probability of each cause being sufficient is independent of the presence of other causes [2].

The noisy-OR gate is commonly used in binary-valued networks to model causal independence. In the CPCS BN, however, disease nodes may have four values (absent, mild, moderate, severe). To accommodate this requirement in the CPCS BN, we use a generalization of the noisy-OR gate called the *noisy-MAX*. Like the noisy-OR, the number of probabilities required to specify the noisy-MAX grows linearly, in contrast to the exponential space requirements of the full specification of conditional probabilities in the network. The specification of a complete conditional probability matrix for a node m with s_m values and n predecessors requires the assessment of $(s_m - 1)\prod_{i=1}^{n} s_i$ probabilities, where s_i is the number of values of predecessor i (for a binary network this reduces to 2^n). In contrast, the causal independence assumption in the form of a noisy-gate reduces this assessment task to $\sum_{i=1}^{n}(s_m - 1)s_i$ probabilities.

Like any other knowledge representation scheme, the BN representation suffers from incompleteness, in that it typically cannot model every possible case. A *leak variable* represents the set of causes that are not modeled explicitly. A *leak probability* is assigned as the probability that the effect will occur in the absence of any of the causes $d_1,...,d_n$ that are modeled explicitly. If the leak variable is modeled explicitly, then it can be treated like any other cause. In this representation the leak node is always assumed to be on; that is, p(*l*=*true*) = 1.0.

Explicitly representing leak nodes in the CPCS BN would almost double the size of the network, so we represent leaks implicitly in the probability tables of the nodes. We developed Netview [10], a graphical tool for visualizing and knowledge engineering belief networks, to facilitate the maintenance and editing of large networks and the associated leak probabilities.

Noisy-MAX implementation

Consider a generalization of the noisy-OR situation in which each variable is allowed to have a finite discrete state space (rather than just a binary state space). This generalization was first proposed by [2], but he did not describe the algorithmic details. In developing this generalization, we assume that we have a set D of predecessor variables $d_1,...,d_n$. Consider first the case where we have a variable x with a subset D_I of D that are present, with the predecessors indexed by $i,j,...,q$.

The variable domains in CPCS BN are all partially ordered, for example, {absent, mild, moderate, severe}, and it turns out that such a partial ordering is necessary for all variable domains. In the remainder of this paper we assume that all variables have ordered domains.

We denote by starred superscripts the state taken by each variable: $i^*, j^*, \ldots, q^*$. The value x^* of variable x is given by $x^* = \max\{i^*, j^*, \ldots, q^*\}$ [2]. In other words, x^* takes on as its value the maximum of the domain values of its predecessors, given that the predecessors are all independent. The unconditional probability with leak node L of maximum value λ and multiple predecessors each with probability η_i is

$$P(x \le x^*) = P(L \le \lambda) \prod_{i:d_i \in D_I} [\eta_i P(x \le x^*) + (1-\eta_i)]$$

and the unconditional probability is given by

$$P(x = x^*) = P(x \le x^*) - P(x \le x^* - 1).$$

Using this approach, we can compute the value $P(x = x^* \mid D_I)$ in time proportional to the number of predecessors in D_I.

EXPERIMENTAL METHOD

Given the frequency values specified in the original CPCS–PM knowledge base {0,1,2,3,4,5}, we studied the mappings with associated probabilities shown in Table 1.

The second parameter studied was the maximum number of values allowed in variable domains. A binary-valued approximation of 4-ary diseases and IPS nodes was carried out as follows: for four-valued parent-child variable pair (d,x) and its two-valued counterpart ($d2$,$x2$), we map

1. P($x$absent| d=absent) to P($x2$=absent| $d2$=absent), and hence P($x2$=present| $d2$=absent) = 1 -P($x2$=absent| $d2$=present).
2. P($x2$=absent| $d2$=present) as 1 - 1/3{P(x=absent| d=mild) + P(x=absent| d=mod) + P(x=absent| d= severe)}.

These variations resulted in six sub networks derived from the original CPCS BN. We ran a suite of test cases on each of the six sub networks.

Test Cases: We generated test cases for the network by simulation in the QMR knowledge base. We generated 10 cases for each disease, resulting in 30 test cases. The terms in the test cases were mapped to the CPCS network. Because both are derived from the Internist-1 knowledge base, there was a good correspondence between the two terminologies. Findings not present in the CPCS BN were not included in the analysis. When we had set as evidence he findings from the test cases, we recorded the posterior probabilities for the 3 disease nodes after we did inference on the networks.

Table 3. The average posterior probability and 95% confidence interval for the true diagnoses and the misdiagnoses.

Network	Average Diagnosis probability	Average Misdiagnosis probability
standard n–ary	0.9458±0.0688	0.2357±0.0784
standard binary	0.9907±0.0120	0.2419±0.0723
categorical n–ary	0.7433±0.1439	0.0364±0.0246
categorical binary	0.8017±0.1417	0.0198±0.0122
curvilinear n–ary	0.7610±0.1419	0.0277±0.0134
curvilinear binary	0.8090±0.1367	0.0209±0.0093

The QMR simulation mode limited the number of test cases we were able to use because it generated cases with overlapping findings. We attempted to acquire cases from published clinico-pathological conferences but the limited domain of our selected sub network was a constraint.

RESULTS

Using multiple comparison [6] we found no statistically significant difference between the categorical or curvilinear mappings, but there was a significant difference between these mappings and the standard mapping, as shown in Table 3. The average probability for the correct diagnosis is higher in the networks with the standard mapping , but the probability assigned to the incorrect diagnoses (false-postives) is also higher. The curvilinear and categorical mappings show a much lower misdiagnosis rate than the standard mapping.

A two-sample t-test [6] of the binary and n–ary networks revealed no statistically significant difference for the standard (95% confidence interval -0.156, 0.117), categorical (95% confidence interval -0.135, 0.118), or curvilinear (95% confidence interval -0.137, 0.115) mappings.

The confidence intervals are approximate because we have assumed normality for results which are bounded by 0 and 1. An alternative method of analysis which may give more accurate intervals is the bootstrap sampling technique [12]. We did not have the resources to carry out bootstrap analysis for this paper.

DISCUSSION

The standard mapping yielded higher posterior probabilities for the correct and incorrect diagnoses compared to the other mappings. The significance of this finding depends on utility assignments when using this network for decision making. Perhaps one explanation for the relatively high misdiagnoses rate for the standard mapping is that it assigns high probability values to intermediate frequencies (2, 3) which are very common in the CPCS–PM, and therefore the CPCS–BN, and may result in greater weights given to findings which should be assigned lower probabilities.

It is, perhaps, surprising that the curvilinear and categorical mappings do so well compared to the standard mapping, given the extreme probability numbers used (for example, none between 0.1 and 0.9). This finding suggests that diagnostic performance in this belief network is not very sensitive to the exact probability numbers.

The statistically insignificant difference in performance between the n-ary and binary representations is very interesting. It suggests that the additional effort to develop 4-level instead of binary variables will not be justified by improved diagnosis. The number of probability numbers which need to be specified goes up exponentially with the domain size. For example, for each finding that can be caused by five (n) diseases, you need to specify six (n+1) probabilities for the binary case (Noisy-OR with a leak), compared to 48 (4-1)[1+n(4-1)] probabilities for the four-level case (Noisy-MAX). Hence, the saving in knowledge-engineering effort from using binary instead of 4-level variables is substantial.

These results should be considered as preliminary, for a number of reasons: The test cases are easy, in that they contain a full set of findings, and can be explained by a single disease. In future research, we plan to try harder cases (including phased introduction of findings related to their cost), a more complete network, other mappings, and other sub networks. If the findings hold up in future studies, they could be of substantial practical importance in guiding the development of belief networks with an appropriate balance of effort in knowledge engineering and diagnostic performance. At the very least, these findings should give reassurance to those expert physicians providing expertise to create belief networks who are concerned about the precision with which they can assess subjective probabilities.

ACKNOWLEDGMENTS

This work was supported by NSF Grant Project IRI-9120330, and by computing resources provided by the Stanford University CAMIS project, which is funded by grant number LM05305 from the National Library of Medicine of the National Institutes of Health. The authors thank R.Miller for providing us with access to the CPCS knowledge base, and to Lyn Dupré for her editorial input.

References

[1] Cooper, G. F. A diagnostic method that uses causal knowledge and linear programming in the application of Bayes' formula. *Comp Biomed Res,* 22:223 –237, 1986.

[2] Henrion, M. Practical issues in constructing a Bayes' belief network. In Levitt, T., Lemmer, J. F., and Kanal, L. N. (eds), *Uncertainty in Artificial Intelligence 3*, pages 132–139. North Holland, Amsterdam, 1988.

[3] Middleton, B. et al. Probabilistic diagnosis using a reformulation of the Internist-1/QMR knowledge base-II. Evaluation of diagnostic performance. *Meth Inf Med*, 30:256–67, 1991.

[4] Miller, R. A., Pople, H. E. J., and Myers, J. D. Internist-1: An experimental computer-based diagnostic consultant for general internal medicine. *N Eng J Med*, 307:468–476, 1982.

[5] Minsky, M. A Framework for representing knowledge. In Winston, P. H. (ed), *Psychology of Computer Vision*, pp. MIT Press, Cambridge, MA, 1975.

[6] Ott, R. L. *An Introduction to Statistical Methods and Data Analysis*. Wadsworth, Belmont, CA, 1993.

[7] Parker, R. C. and Miller, R. A. Using causal knowledge to create simulated patient cases: the CPCS project as an extension of Internist-1. *Proceedings of the Eleventh Annual Symposium on Computer Applications in Medical Care,* Los Alamitos, CA, pages 473–480. IEEE Computer Society Press, 1987.

[8] Pearl, J. *Probabilistic reasoning in intelligent systems*. Morgan Kaufman, San Mateo, Ca., 1988.

[9] Peng, Y. and Reggia, J. A. A probabilistic causal model for diagnostic problem solving - Part I: Integrating symbolic causal inference with numeric probabilistic inference. *IEEE Trans SMC*, SMC-17(2):146–162., 1987.

[10] Pradhan, M. et al. Knowledge engineering for large belief networks. *Uncertainty in Artificial Intelligence,* Seattle, Washington, pages 484–490. Morgan Kaufmann, 1994.

[11] Shwe, M. A. et al. Probabilistic diagnosis using a reformulation of the Internist-1/QMR knowledge base-I. The probabilistic model and inference algorithms. *Methods of Information in Medicine*, 30:241–55, 1991.

[12] Tibshirani, R. and Efron. B. Bootstrap methods for standard errors, confidence intervals, and other measures of statistical accuracy. *Stat Sci*, 1:54-77.

Probabilistic Constraint Satisfaction: Application to Radiosurgery

Russ B. Altman, MD, PhD and Rhea Tombropoulos, Section on Medical Informatics
Stanford University Medical Center, MSOB X-215, Stanford, CA 94305-5479
altman@camis.stanford.edu, rzt@camis.stanford.edu

ABSTRACT

Although quite successful in a variety of settings, standard optimization approaches can have drawbacks within medical applications. For example, they often provide a single solution which is difficult to explain, or which can not be incrementally modified using secondary "soft" constraints that are difficult to encode within the optimization. In order to address these issues, we have developed a probabilistic optimization technique that allows the user to enter prior probability distributions (Gaussian) for the parameters to be optimized as well as for the constraints on the parameters. Our technique combines the prior distributions with the constraints using Bayes' rule. The algorithm produces not only a set of parameter values, but variances on these values and covariances showing the correlations between parameters. We have applied this method to the problem of planning a radiosurgical ablation of brain tumors. The radiation plan should maximize dose to tumor, minimize dose to surrounding areas, and provide an even distribution of dosage across the tumor. It also should be explainable to and modifiable by the expert physicians based on external considerations. We have compared the results of our method with the standard linear programming approach.

INTRODUCTION

There are currently well-developed techniques for parameter estimation and optimization that are generally applicable over a wide range of science and engineering problems [5]. Unfortunately, the application of standard optimization methods within medical applications can be problematic. First, these methods do not typically provide any sort of confidence bounds in the parameter values chosen. Second, they give no insight into the possible interdependence of parameter values. Third, they often require an entirely new calculation if new information is provided dynamically. We approach optimization within a paradigm of probabilistic constraint satisfaction that solves these problems.

Constraint Satisfaction and Optimization

Constraint satisfaction is a problem solving paradigm in which legal values for a set of variables are sought, subject to constraints on both the possible values for each variable as well as the relationship between values of different variables [7]. A constraint satisfaction problem is formulated by defining 1) a set of variables whose values are sought, 2) the set of possible values (the domain) for each variable, 3) the relationships between variables (the constraints). When the parameters are continuous variables, then the problem of finding values that satisfy the constraints optimally is isomorphic to the problem of optimizing the variables so that some error function is minimized. We have described an algorithm for probabilistic constraint satisfaction that should, therefore, be useful for general optimization [1,2]. We represent the set of possible values for a variable as continuous parametric distributions over the range of possible labels. Initially, a variable distribution is described based on some prior knowledge of the range of possible labels (assumed to be Gaussian). The constraints between variables are probability distributions over functions that depend on the structural variables (described below). As constraints are introduced, they cause changes in the probability distribution for all the variables. The resulting probability distributions are the posterior probability distributions of the values for all variables.

Radiosurgery

Radiosurgery is a method for ablating brain tumors with high intensity radiation [3,4,6,8,9]. The main challenge in radiosurgery is to develop dosing schemes for which the dose to tumor is maximal and homogenous, while the dose to surrounding healthy tissue (especially tissues involved in critical functions or which are very sensitive) is minimal. With the advent of high performance robotic arms to position the xray source, it has become possible to plan radiosurgical procedures in which the xray beam impinges upon the tumor from multiple angles, so that healthy tissues receive low doses compared to the tumor. The problem of maximizing dose to the tumor and minimizing dose to healthy tissues becomes one of setting the strengths assigned to a set of xray beams impinging upon the tumor from different angles. The precise models for determining dose to a region [8] are too expensive to use for optimization of beam intensities, but the dose through a region, **S**, can be roughly estimated as the sum of the intensities of the beams which pass through the region (see Equation 11).

In general, the dose through tumor tissue should exceed some critical value, and the dose through normal tissue should be less than some safe value. The goal of an optimization program is to find values of the individual beam intensities that satisfy these constraints. Schweikard et al have reported a system which uses standard linear programming to solve this problem. It has been shown to perform well [8,9]. It is subject, however, to the pitfalls of standard optimization. It may not always converge, does not provide information about the range of intensity values compatible with the dosing goals, and provides no information about which part of the optimization is difficult. We have therefore attempted to replicate its performance using a system that maintains second order information about the parameter values, such as variance and covariance of beam intensities.

MATHEMATICAL FORMULATION

We represent an optimization problem as a vector of parameters (each parameter is a node in the constraint network). Each parameter has a prior probability distribution over the range of possible variable values. In our current implementation, we represent each distribution by its first two moments, the mean and variance. The mean values of each parameter are stored in a state vector, **x**. For a structural model with M parameters, the state vector is:

$$\mathbf{x} = \begin{bmatrix} x_1 & x_2 & x_3 & \cdot & \cdot & \cdot & x_M \end{bmatrix} \quad [1]$$

The second moment of the state vector is stored in a matrix. The diagonal elements of the matrix contain the variances of each parameter. The off-diagonal elements of the matrix contain the covariances between parameters.

$$\mathbf{C(x)} = \begin{bmatrix} \sigma_{x_1}^2 & \sigma_{x_1x_2} & \cdot & \sigma_{x_1x_M} \\ \cdot & \sigma_{x_2}^2 & & \cdot \\ \cdot & & \cdot & \cdot \\ \sigma_{x_Mx_1} & \cdot & \cdot & \sigma_{x_M}^2 \end{bmatrix} \quad [2]$$

If we have no information about the relationships between parameters, then the covariances are zero. As information about the relationship between parameters is gathered (as described below), the covariances may become non-zero.

Taken together, the mean vector, **x**, and the covariance matrix, **C(x)**, represent an uncertain estimate of the possible parameter values. In general, two parameters may have a complicated functional relationship. The covariance is simply a linearization of this relationship that specifies whether the values of the two parameters are correlated. Although a primitive summary of potentially complicated dependencies, the covariance is often sufficient (especially using iterative techniques to reduce estimation error) for capturing important parameter relationships.

Constraints involving the elements of the state vector, **x**, can be used to update the parameter estimates within **x** and **C(x)**. A constraint, **z**, is represented with two components; a deterministic function, **h(x)** that specifies how the value of the measurement depends on (and can be calculated from) the structural parameters in **x**, and a stochastic component, **v**, that specifies the uncertainty or tolerance in the information.

$$z = h(x) + v \quad [3]$$

In this work, **v** is assumed to be distributed normally with mean zero. We have found that inequality constraints (in which the equality of Eq. 3 becomes an inequality) can often be approximated with appropriate Gaussian distributions.

Given a new constraint, the parameter estimates can be updated using Bayesian measurement update formulae, as is used in the Kalman Filter [5]. These formula introduce non-zero covariances between all parameters that are involved in the constraint. New values for **x** and **C(x)** are calculated as follows:

$$x_{new} = x_{old} + K\left[z - h(x_{old})\right] \quad [4]$$

$$C(x_{new}) = C(x_{old}) - KHC(x_{old}) \quad [5]$$

where

$$K = C(x_{old})H^T[HC(x_{old})H^T + C(v)]^{-1} \quad [6]$$

and

$$H = \left.\frac{\partial h(x)}{\partial x}\right|_{x_{old}} \quad [7]$$

Simply put, the new estimate for **x** is based on the old estimate plus a weighted difference between the observed and predicted value of **z**. The weighting factor, **K**, is proportional to the ratio of the uncertainty in the current estimate and the uncertainty in the constraint.[1] If **h(x)** is nonlinear in **x**, then errors in the linearization of **h(x)** can be reduced by using a modified update formula [5].

These update formulae use the information in the covariance matrix to make concerted changes in parameter values. Thus, introducing a constraint that provides information about parameter x_i, will modify the value of variables which are highly correlated with x_i. However, if the relationship between parameters is nonlinear, then the covariances may not lead to precisely correct new values. We have described an iterative procedure to effectively minimize these errors [1].

With the measurement update equations, we can solve a constraint satisfaction formulation of optimization.

---

[1]Note that the term within the reciprocal is a first order estimate of the uncertainty in the measurement as predicted by the model, since the variance of z, $C(z) = C(h(x) + v) = C(h(x)) + C(v) \approx HC(x)H^T + C(v)$.

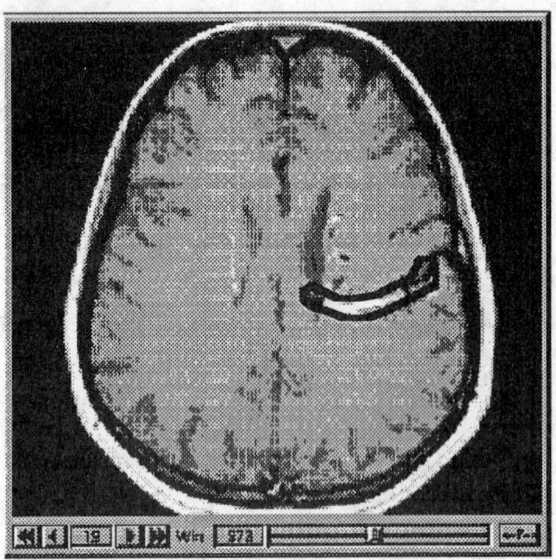

Figure 1. CT slice of tumor (middle right) used in testing.

A starting set of parameters is generated (based on previous experience or with a broad, uninformative prior distribution) and measurements are introduced (serially or in one large vector of values) to update the estimates of mean and variance. The final values of **x** and **C(x)** represent the posterior distribution of the parameter values that satisfy the constraints. We define the residual error for each constraint as follows:

$$E_i = \frac{h(x_{new}) - z_i}{\sqrt{\sigma^2_{v_i}}} \qquad [9]$$

where E_i is the error for an individual constraint, **z** is the measured value, $\mathbf{h}(\mathbf{x_{new}})$ is the predicted value based on the best estimate, and σ is the variance of $\mathbf{v_i}$.

APPLICATIONS TO RADIOSURGERY

For radiosurgery, the vector to be estimated, **x**, contains the values of the beam weights for *N* beams that impinge on the tumor mass:

$$x = \begin{bmatrix} w_1 & w_2 & w_3 & \dots & w_N \end{bmatrix} \qquad [10]$$

We generate one constraint for every volume element through tumor or sensitive tissue. If there are M such volume elements, then a constraint for the individual volume element through which a subset S of the N beams pass is represented as:

$$D_S = \sum_{i \in S} w_i + v \qquad [11]$$

D_S, is the target dose for the volume element (based on its status as tumor or normal). **v** is a random variable describing the tolerance we have for variation in the value of D_S. Given a starting value for the parameter vector, and all the constraints, we can calculate an improved estimate of the parameter values.

Example and Evaluation

We illustrate the performance of our method on a tumor that is shown in Figure 1. The irregularity of this tumor makes it a good test of the ability to refine the beam intensities. As a control, we applied the standard linear programming algorithm. For this tumor, there are only two types of tissues: normal and tumor. The linear programming technique finds a set of beam weights which produce a dose to all tumor tissues between 2000 and 2300 R (100 Rad = 1 Grey), while minimizing total dose to normal tissue. We translated these constraints into normal distributions; tumor tissues were constrained to have a mean dose of 2100 R with a variance of 1000 R^2.

The initial mean values for the beam weights were set to 150 R with a variance of 1600 R^2. The mean value is based on an estimate of how many beams travel through the tumor, and what the average dose to the entire tumor should be. The variance is chosen to allow a range of values, while minimizing the possibility that the program chooses a negative weight for a beam (a physical impossibility). The computational procedure was as follows:

1. Using the starting parameter estimates, all constraints were used to update the parameter estimate.
2. Any beam weights that were negative after step 1, were set to 0, and removed from the optimization.
3. The overall satisfaction of constraints is measured, using Equation 9. If there is no change in the result (within a user defined tolerance), then the algorithm halts.
4. If the residual errors are still large, the remaining beam weights were retained and used for another round of updating with the constraints (that is, loop to step 1).

Evaluation

In order to evaluate the internal consistency of our result, we analyzed the the distribution of errors for all constraints. The average error for all constraints is 1.57 SD. The error distribution assures us that the optimization was able to find a solution that is reasonable with respect to the provided constraints.

A more significant evaluation of our result entails a comparison with the "gold standard" of linear programming. There are two parameters with which we compared the methods: ability to deliver dose specifically to the tumor (that is, match the contour of the tumor precisely and minimize dosage to surrounding normal tissue), and ability to deliver tumor dose homogenously (that is, all tumor regions get approximately the same dosage). Figure 2 compares the ability of linear programming and probabilistic optimization to deliver adequate radiation to tumor cells. Figure 2AB shows for each of the two methods, the three-dimensional contour of volume elements that receive least 50% of the maximum

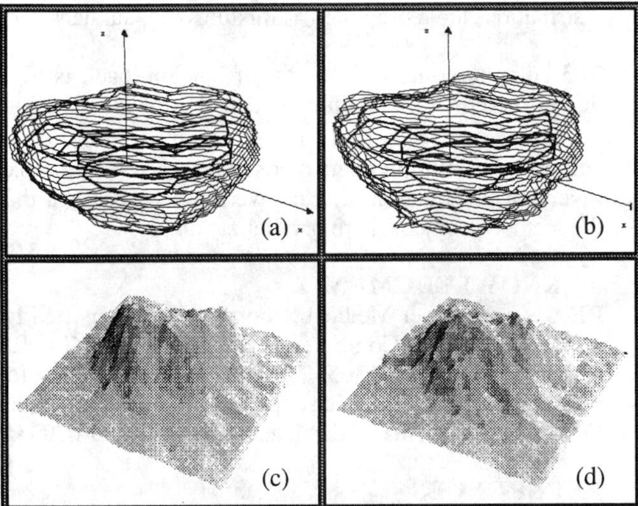

Figure 2. 2A and 2B show contours of volume elements receiving at least 50% of maximum dose. They each contain the contour of the tumor, as defined by an expert. 2C and 2D show the tumor dose on the slice of tumor shown in Fig 1. for each method. (2B/2D = our method).

dose delivered to any volume element. Superimposed upon these contours are the tumor contour defined manually be an expert physician. Ideally, all tumor volume elements will have nearly 100% maximum dosage, and the drop off would be precipitous. In practice, we examine the way in which the 50% contours match the manually segmented tumor boundary to get a feeling for the rate at which the tumor dose falls at the edges of the tumor. Figure 2CD demonstrates, for a single section through the tumor, how the incoming xray beams concentrate the dose within the tumor.

The homogeneity of dose distribution is illustrated by Figures 2 and 3. In the ideal, Figure 2CD would have a flat plateau in the area of tumor, and a steep drop off to zero for the surrounding area. Both linear programming and probabilistic optimization provide quite good approximations to a plateau. Figure 3 plots the volume of tumor exposed to increasingly greater percentages of the maximum dose. For example, it shows that for both results virtually the entire tumor (of volume 3800 mm^3) receives at least 80% of the maximal dose received by any tumor volume element, but that this ratio falls off rapidly so that only about half the volume elements (2000 mm^3) receive 90% or more of the maximal dose. Only about 15% of voxels receive 95% or more of the maximal dose. The integrated area of the curves in Figure 3 is a measure of the submaximal radiation or *efficiency*. For a perfect dose scheme, the integral should be 100. Both the linear programming and constraint satisfaction approaches produce efficiencies of 88%.

We conclude that the probabilistic optimization provides solutions that are compatible with linear programming

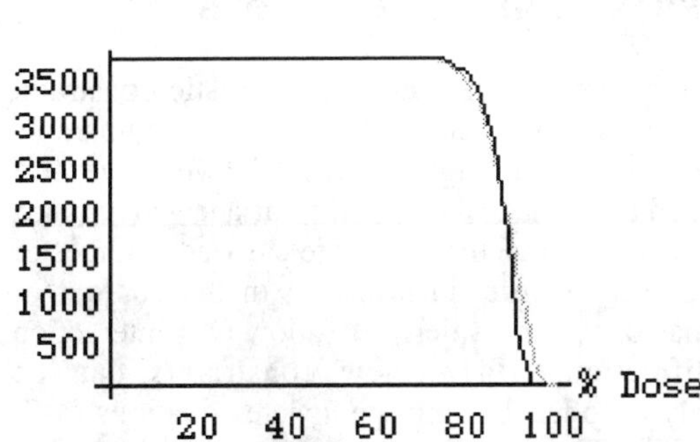

Figure 3. The number of tumor volume elements (mm^3) receiving a percent of the maximum dose (black is our method). The tumor volume is 3800 mm^3 and virtually all the tumor receives at least 80% of the maximum dose.

methods. We have now run other comparisons (not reported here) that produce similar agreement. The chief advantage of our method is the additional information provided by the probabilistic optimization. First, we have explicit confidence in the values for each beam strength. Figure 4 shows a plot of distribution of variances for all beams. These variances provide specific information that can be used to understand which beam values are critical to the dosage. For example, most of the beams have a variance between 10 and 40, indicating that these beams can be adjusted 3 to 7 units without significant effect on the final dose. Some beams, however, have variances up to 80 or more, which indicates significantly more flexibility for adjustment.

Secondly, the covariance matrix provides information about the correlated beam strengths. This allows us to identify key subsets of interacting beams (perhaps across multiple constraints, and not apparent by a scan of individual constraints). For example, Figure 5 plots the largest covariances within the final set of nonzero beams. This information suggests which clusters of beams (and the tumor regions they affect) are tightly linked.

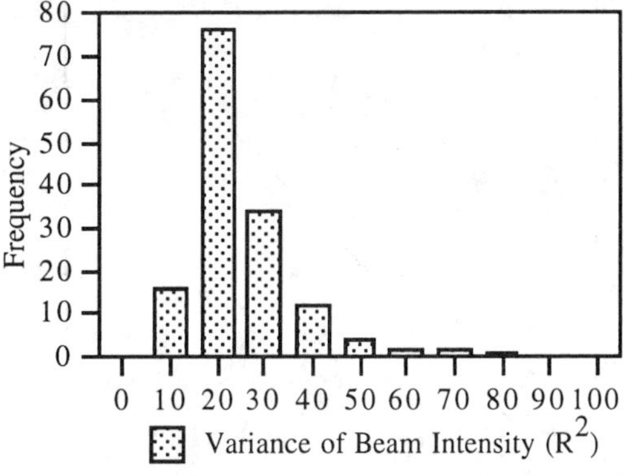

Figure 4. Histogram of the variance of beam intensities for 152 final nonzero beams. Most beams are defined tightly (with variance of 20 R^2), but some have more freedom to change values.

DISCUSSION AND CONCLUSIONS

These results demonstrate that a probabilistic constraint satisfaction formulation can produce answers comparable with linear programming. Although we have not demonstrated any practical use of the variance/covariance information, we believe that there are clear advantages of having the second order information in the context of semiautomated systems which will allow user interaction and modification. First, new constraints can be immediately introduced using the update equations (4-7) given above. The covariance information allows all beams to be updated in a concerted fashion. Second, information about variance of beam intensities can be used to immediately recognize which beams have a narrow therapeutic range, and which can be varied within a broader set of values.

This approach to parameter estimation has proven quite versatile in a number of domains, including the estimation of macromolecular structure, model driven CT image segmentation, and automated interpretation of MRI images of the cervical spine [1]. It is possible to solve a large variety of general optimization problems within this framework: the variables make up the state vector, and the constraints are the conditions that restrain the optimization function.

The use of two moments of a distribution can be limiting: there are clearly constraints on structure that may be multimodal or in some other way non-Gaussian. Also, we may want to represent non-normal posterior distributions for our variables. The introduction of higher moments adds computational complexity. However, because of their importance for some problems, we are currently investigating ways to relax the assumption of normality in the context of massively parallel computers. We have recently reported an extension in which arbitrary distributions are represented as mixtures of Gaussians [2].

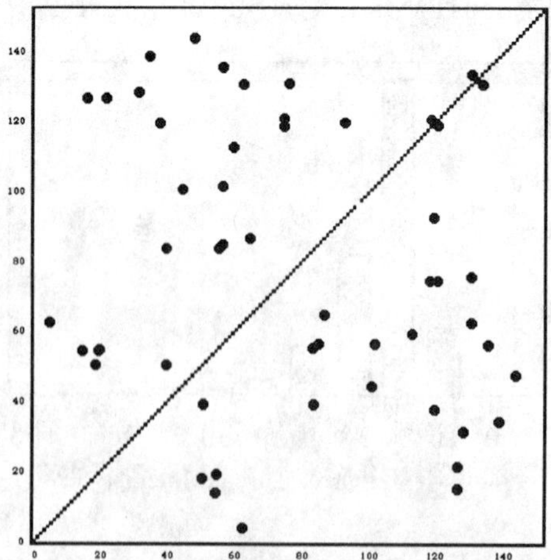

Figure 5. Covariance matrix (as defined in Eq. 2) showing largest covariances among 152 nonzero beams in the probabilistic solution.

The computational complexity of our approach is high due to the cost of maintaining second order information. There are matrix multiplications which are $O(N^3)$. In addition, for multiple-valued constraits, there is a matrix-inversion in Equation 6. However, we have shown that the method is amenable to parallelization [2].

ACKNOWLEDGMENTS

RBA is a Culpeper Medical Scholar, and is supported by NIH LM-05652. Computers provided by the CAMIS resource, NIH LM-05305. Thanks to J.F. Brinkley for useful comments. RZT is supported by the Sheik Enany Fund, Lorraine Ulshafer Fund, and NIH grant LM-07033.

REFERENCES

[1] Altman, R. B. *A probabilistic algorithm for calculating structure: Borrowing from simulated annealing.* Proceedings, Ninth Conference on Uncertainty in Artificial Intelligence, Washington, D.C., July 1993, Morgan Kaufmann Pub., San Mateo, CA pp. 23-31.

[2] Altman, R.B., Chen, C.C., Poland, W.B., Singh, J.P. *Probabilistic constraint satisfaction with non-gaussian constraint noise.* Proceedings, Tenth Conference on Uncertainty in Artificial Intelligence, Seattle, WA, August, 1994, Morgan Kaufmann Pub., San Mateo, CA, pp. 15-22.

[3] Betty, O.O., Munari, C., and Rosler, R. Stereotactic Radiosurgery with the Linear Accelerator: Treatment of Arteriovenous Malformations. Neurosurgery, 24(3): 311-321, 1989.

[4] Brahme, A. Optimization of stationary and moving beam radiation therapy techniques. Radiother. Oncol., 12:127-140, 1988.

[5] Gelb, A., *Applied Optimal Estimation.* 1984, Cambridge, Massachusetts: MIT Press.

[6] Larsson, B., et al. The High Energy Proton Beam as a Neurosurgical Tool. Nature, 182:1222-3, 1958.

[7] Mackworth, A.K. *Consistency in networks of relations.* Artificial Intelligence. 8, 99-118 (1977).

[8] Schweikard, A., Adler, J.R., and Latombe, J.C., Motion Planning in Stereotaxic Radiosurgery. Proc. IEEE Int. Conf. Robotics and Automation, Atlanta, CA, May 1993, 1909-1916. (Extended version to appear in IEEE Tr. Robotics and Automation.)

[9] Schweikard, A., Tombropoulos, R.Z., Adler, J.R., and Latombe, J.C., Treatment planning for a radiosurgical system with general kinematics. in press, Proc. IEEE Int. Conf. Robotics and Automation, 1994.

Formalizing & Implementing Practice Guidelines

Development and Evaluation of a Computer-Assisted Management Protocol (CAMP): Improved Compliance with Care Guidelines for Diabetes Mellitus

David F. Lobach, MD, PhD, MS, and W. Edward Hammond, PhD

Division of Medical Informatics, Department of Biomedical Engineering, and Department of Community and Family Medicine, Duke University, Durham, N.C.

ABSTRACT

Disease-specific standards for directing patient management are becoming increasingly important. These standards, however, are often not followed because they are not sufficiently integrated into the clinical care setting. In this study we describe the development and evaluation of a Computer-Assisted Management Protocol (CAMP) of care guidelines for diabetes mellitus. While other studies have shown improved compliance with rule-based reminders, the CAMP customizes disease-specific care guidelines to individual patients over time. We evaluated the effect of the CAMP on compliance with guidelines in a prospective, randomized controlled study. The study was performed at a family practice clinic where much of the patient record is maintained electronically on The Medical Record (TMR). The management protocol was developed from standards published by the American Diabetes Association. Fifty-eight providers were randomized to either receive or not receive the CAMP for diabetes. Compliance with standards was assessed by chart audits of all encounters with diabetic patients during the study interval. The following conclusion was made: the Computer-Assisted Management Protocol resulted in a statistically significant improvement in compliance with diabetes care standards.

INTRODUCTION

Limited financial resources and increasing emphasis on primary care in a managed care environment are driving medical care delivery to become more efficient and cost-effective without sacrificing quality. One major approach to achieving the goals of efficiency and quality is through the standardization of care for specific diseases [2,3,5,10]. Care standardization efforts have included development of care maps, critical pathways, and care guidelines [14]. While the standardization efforts are laudable, they often fail to have the desired effect because they are not sufficiently integrated into the clinical setting. Non-compliance with care standards can have both adverse medical and legal consequences [6]. While many factors contribute to this compliance failure, a primary cause is the limitation of the human care provider as an information processor [8]. Computerization of medical knowledge can be used to augment provider information processing. Several previous studies have shown that computer-generated, rule-based reminders can improve compliance with individual guidelines [4,8,9,11], but others have shown that reminders alone are insufficient to effect compliance [7,13]. No studies to date, however, have computerized an existing set of disease-specific care guidelines for use in the clinical setting. In this study we describe the development and evaluation of a Computer-Assisted Management Protocol (CAMP) for the continuing care of patients with diabetes mellitus. The CAMP provides a novel way to computerize domain-specific medical knowledge from disease-specific care guidelines and integrate this knowledge into the clinical setting. It allows customization of recommendations based on data in a patient's electronic medical record and evolution of these recommendations over time. Diabetes mellitus was selected for the prototypic CAMP for several reasons. Diabetes is a common disease affecting more than 5% of the adult population in the United States. Its diagnosis is quantitative and relatively unambiguous. Chronic management of diabetes requires monitoring of several laboratory parameters and serial physical examinations common to all patients. Care guidelines have been published by the American Diabetes Association (ADA) and are relatively well accepted as standards [1,5]. Lastly, encounters with diabetic patients are relatively time- and information-intensive leading to an increased need for efficient information processing. In this study we evaluated the impact of a CAMP for diabetes mellitus on provider compliance with guidelines in a primary care setting.

METHODS

Study Design

The effect of the CAMP on compliance with disease-specific guidelines was evaluated in a controlled, prospective, randomized study conducted from September 1993 through February 1994 at the Duke Family Medicine Center (DFMC). Retrospective data was obtained from the 6 months prior to the start of the study (March 1993 through August 1993) to determine baseline compliance levels. DFMC is a free-standing, full service primary care clinic and site of the Family Medicine Residency Program affiliated with Duke University Medical Center. The clinic had a total of 74,738 patient visits in fiscal year 1993. At the start of the study, the clinic employed 58 primary care providers and 6 specialists. The primary care providers included 25 faculty (21 physicians, two physician assistants, and two nurse practitioners), and 33 family medicine residents. All the primary care providers were randomly assigned to either receive or not receive the CAMP by standard randomization techniques. The randomization was not constrained by level of training since there is no evidence to suggest that training level alone affects compliance with care guidelines [13]. Providers in neither group were aware that they had been randomized in order to study the effect of the CAMP on their compliance with guidelines. At the start of the study, providers who were designated to receive the CAMP were sent a letter informing them that the CAMP developed from the practice consensus guidelines would be printed on the encounter forms for their diabetic patients. This letter also described how the CAMP functioned and solicited feedback about incorrect recommendations. Prior to the initiation of the study, a representative level of exposure to diabetic patients and diabetes care was defined. In order to consider a provider's compliance score a valid representation of their practice patterns for diabetes, the provider had to have contact with at least six unique diabetic patients and to have assessed diabetes care in at least 12 encounters during the study period. The CAMP was designed to integrate into the DFMC electronic medical record system, The Medical Record (TMR). TMR is a comprehensive electronic medical record system that supports a complete database of patient information [12]. TMR modules in operation during the study included demographic information, scheduling, accounting, problem lists, subjective and physical findings, encounter summary, medications, quality assurance, and laboratory orders/results.

Development of the Computer-Assisted Management Protocol

To diminish non-compliance with care standards due to provider disagreement with the standards themselves, consensus guidelines were developed among the providers at DFMC. The continuing care guidelines for diabetes published by the ADA were used as the initial template [1]. Faculty and resident consensus was obtained from the responses to two surveys and through discussions at practice management meetings. The consensus guidelines were completed three months prior to the initiation of the study, lessening the effect of recent exposure to care guidelines on provider practice patterns.

The consensus guidelines, summarized in Figure 1, were encoded in the existing Quality Assurance module of TMR. The the output from the program for the diabetes CAMP was printed on the first pageof an encounter form. Encounter forms at DFMC were

1. Foot examination every month in patients with diabetic neuropathy or history of lower limb ulcers
2. Annual complete physical examination
3. HgbA1c every 6 months
4. Annual urine protein determination
5. Annual cholesterol level
6. Annual ophthalmologic examination
7. Seasonal influenza vaccination (September-January)
8. Pneumococcal vaccination

Figure 1. *DFMC Care Guidelines for Diabetes Mellitus*

generated for each patient prior to the visit. These forms served as order/billing sheets, as well as summary lists for patient problems, medications, and health maintenance data. Initially the CAMP program identified all patients with diabetes listed as a problem in their electronic record who were scheduled to see a primary care provider. It then customized the guideline recommendations for the scheduled visit based on data in the electronic record. Laboratory and immunization data were historically available in TMR. CAMP providers could add data about the foot exam or physical exam in the feedback section of the CAMP (see below) to have this data also available to the CAMP. The patient's name, identification number, and CAMP were stored in a master file as a source list for encounters to be audited. The CAMP was then selectively printed only on the encounter forms of patients scheduled to see providers randomized to receive the CAMP.

A sample CAMP is shown in Figure 2. It lists the customized diabetes guideline recommendations and provides an area for written feedback/updating by the provider. The guideline feedback section also allowed the provider to indicate if the recommendation was offered but *declined* ("D") by the patient or *never* ("N") to be performed. When "never" was entered, a given guideline recommendation was permanently shut off for that patient. Feedback/updates from providers that were not automatically captured by TMR (e.g., a laboratory test performed at another facility) were manually entered into the patient's electronic record.

Data Collection and Analysis

Compliance with CAMP recommendations was determined by chart audit. Chart audits were selected as the "gold standard" for compliance since direct evaluation of the written documentation of the encounter was necessary to determine if diabetes care was assessed and if the recommendations were addressed during the encounter. Providers were considered compliant with a guideline if they performed the recommendation, commented that the

```
--------------------------------------------------------------------------------------------------------
CATEGORY       TEST            RECOMMENDED              LAST DONE        F/U DATE
--------------------------------------------------------------------------------------------------------
DIABETES       FOOT EXAM       AGE 18+ ONCE IN 1 MO                      *SUGGESTED*
               COMPLETE PE     AGE 18+ ONCE IN 1 YR                      *DUE NOW*
               HGBA1C          AGE 18+ ONCE IN 6 MO     9.1  09/10/92    *DUE NOW*
               URINE PROT      AGE 18+ ONCE IN 1 YR                      *DUE NOW*
               CHOLESTEROL     AGE 18+ ONCE IN 1 YR     257  09/10/92    DUE 09/10/93
               OPHTH EXAM      AGE 18+ ONCE IN 1 YR                      *DUE NOW*
               INFLUENZA       AGE 18+ ONCE IN 1 YR                      *DUE NOW*
               PNEUMOCOC       AGE 18+ ONCE                              *DUE NOW*
________________________________________________________________________________________________________
QUALITY ASSURANCE DATA COLLECTION
TEST                  PLACE           DATE           RESULT
FOOT EXAM  ______________________________________________________________  D______N______
COMPLETE PE____________________________________________________________  D______N______
HGBA1C  _________________________________________________________________  D______N______
URINALYSIS_______________________________________________________________  D______N______
OPHTH EXAM_______________________________________________________________  D______N______
INFLUENZA________________________________________________________________  D______N______
PNEUMOCOC  ______________________________________________________________  D______N______
```

Figure 2. *Sample Format for the Computer-Assisted Management Protocol for Diabetes Mellitus*

recommendation had been done in the past or was scheduled at a definite time in the future, or stated why a guideline was not being followed (e.g., financial limitations). Compliance was based solely on data derived from the paper chart. Diabetes was considered assessed if it was listed as a problem heading in the encounter note, if it was checked on the encounter form as a focus problem for the visit, or if it was dealt with in any two of the four sections of a progress note not specifically addressing diabetes. In order to standardize chart auditing, an audit protocol was used for every chart. Chart evaluations were recorded on an audit form generated from the encounter list in the master file described above. Data from these forms were entered into an electronic database (Paradox, Borland International, Inc., Scotts Valley, CA) for analysis. Comparison of patient demographic data between groups was done using a t-test for mean ages and Chi square tests for gender and race. Provider compliance scores were calculated as the number of required guidelines followed over the total number of required guidelines, and expressed as percent compliance. Comparison of compliance scores between the CAMP and No-CAMP groups was done with a two-tailed Wilcoxon rank sum test.

RESULTS

Derivation of Compliance Data

Initially, 497 patients were identified for possible inclusion in the study based on a listing of diabetes on their electronic problem list and on having at least one encounter during the study period with a provider enrolled in the study. Four hundred eighty-three (97%) of these charts were available for auditing after up to 5 chart requests were submitted for each chart. In 81 (17%) of the audited charts, the diagnosis of diabetes was incorrect. Most of these reflected errors in data entry, i.e. coding "family history of diabetes" (#250) as "diabetes" (#91) modified by "family history of." Forty-three (9%) of the charts were for patients who were not followed primarily at DFMC for diabetes. Every encounter in the remaining 359 charts (72%) that occurred during the study period with a study provider was assessed for compliance with guidelines. This resulted in 1265 encounters being audited. In 884 (70%) diabetes was addressed. In addition, for the 6 months prior the the start of the study, all encounters with study providers in which diabetes was a focus problem for the encounter were scored for compliance with guidelines. For the purposes of analysis, only compliance data from the encounters in which diabetes was a focus problem were used to derive provider compliance scores. Patients seen by CAMP versus No-CAMP providers did not differ significantly by age, race, or gender. The exposure to diabetic patients during the study is shown in Figure 3. The experience of the 58 providers is represented as a function of the number of diabetic patients seen versus the number of encounters in which diabetes was addressed. Based on the predefined criteria for minimum exposure to diabetic patient care, 16 providers of the CAMP group and 14 providers of the No-CAMP group qualified for further evaluation. The CAMP group consisted of 11 faculty members, 2 third-year residents, and 3 second-year residents. The No-CAMP group consisted of 9 faculty members, 3 third-year residents, and 2 second-year residents.

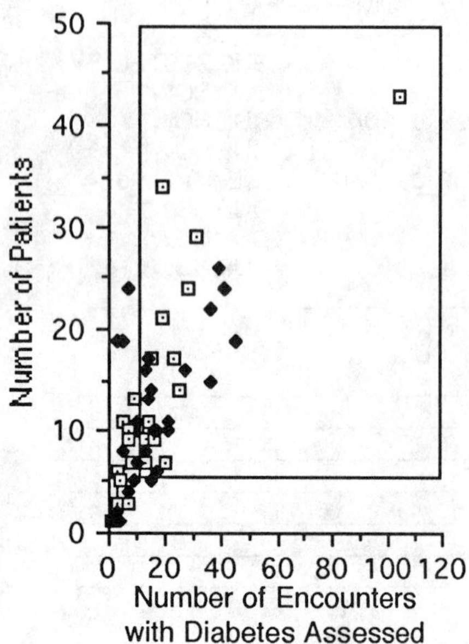

Figure 3. *Provider exposure to diabetes care. Diamonds represent CAMP providers. Squares represent No-CAMP providers.*

Comparison of Compliance Levels

Comparison of the compliance scores for qualified providers from both the CAMP and No-CAMP groups during the study is depicted in Figure 4. The providers receiving the diabetes CAMP had a

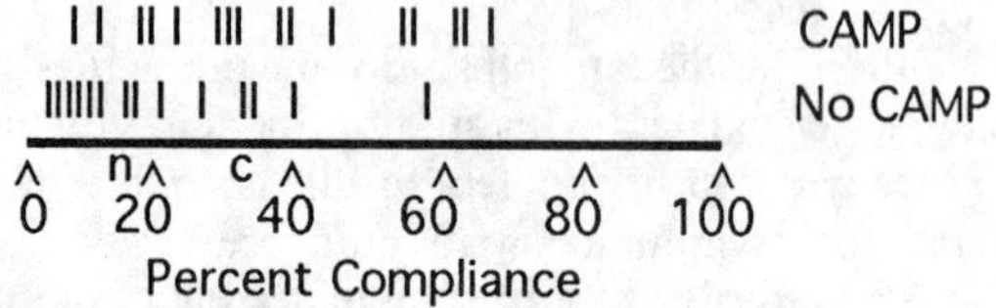

Figure 4. *Comparison of compliance levels between groups after introduction of the CAMP. Each "I" represents the compliance score for one provider.*

statistically significantly greater median level of compliance than the providers not receiving the CAMP (p=0.02) (32.0% versus 15.6%). Comparison of compliance scores between the same provider groups prior to the study were not statistically significantly different. The median baseline compliance levels during the 6 month prior to the implementation of the CAMP were 21.2% for the CAMP group and 18.0% for the No-CAMP group.

DISCUSSION

The significant difference in compliance levels between providers randomized to receive the diabetes CAMP and those who did not receive it demonstrates the effectiveness of the Computer-Assisted Management Protocol for improving compliance with diabetes care guidelines. The lack of difference between these two groups prior to the introduction of the CAMP underscores that the primary factor effecting the change in compliance was the CAMP.

A discussion of potential biases introduced into the study is warranted. The effect of not collecting encounter data from 3% of the patient charts initially identified could be a source of bias. However, this only slightly limited the total amount of data that could be collected, and there is no reason to suspect that compliance levels in the unevaluated charts were any different than those in the charts that were evaluated. Furthermore, the unavailable charts were relatively evenly distributed among the CAMP and No-CAMP providers. If this lack of chart availability suggests anything of significance, it is the limitation of a paper medical record as the primary repository for clinical data. The discovery that 17% of the study patients were incorrectly classified as diabetic reflects the cumulative errors in data entry by non-medical personnel and the lack of attention paid to updating and correcting patient problem lists by providers. While this finding should not bias the evaluation of provider compliance, it does underscore the need for greater accuracy in data entry and in data surveillance by providers. In order to drive medical knowledge modules, such as the diabetes CAMP, from data in the electronic patient record, the data must be accurate. The lack of difference in the demographics of the patients seen by the two study groups effectively eliminates the potential bias of patient age, gender, or race. The restriction of compliance data to only encounters dealing with diabetes was done to avoid requiring compliance with diabetes care guidelines during encounters in which the provider was focussed on other medical problems. This approach was felt to optimize a provider's opportunity to be compliant with the standards. The number of providers (55% of the CAMP group and 48% of the No-CAMP group) fulfilling the predefined requirements for exposure to diabetic patients was less than initially anticipated. These smaller numbers are due in part to the lack of availability of charts for auditing and the disqualification of some patients because they were wrongly labelled as diabetic or were primarily followed for diabetes at another facility. While the exposure criteria limited the sample size, these criteria were necessary to assure that the compliance score accurately reflected a provider's true practice pattern. Since the factors limiting the number of qualifying providers applied equally to both the CAMP and No-CAMP groups, there is no evidence to suggest introduction of bias at this level. Because providers in neither group were aware that their compliance with diabetes care guidelines was being studied, the Hawthorn effect was not considered to have had a significant impact on the study outcome.

The findings of this study have important ramifications for the delivery of health care in the United States. Computer-Assisted Management Protocols provide a mechanism to electronically represent medical knowledge and deliver this knowledge to the clinical setting. As the focus of the health care system shifts from a specialist-based, private payor system to a primary care-based, managed care environment, the primary care provider will be expected to see an increasing volume of patients and master an increasing breadth and depth of medical knowledge. No longer will domain experts (specialists) be the first level of care for most diseases. The development of care standards for specific diseases can assist the primary care provider in delivering high quality health care. Already, there has been an increasing effort to create such care standards. However, clinical standards are of little use unless they are available to providers in a timely, efficient way. As shown in this study, the CAMP as a computerized representation of medical knowledge is one effective tool by which practice guidelines can be integrated into the clinical setting. The CAMP also has a potentially important role in the evaluation of the care standards themselves. Many standards are assumed to favorably affect patient outcome but have never been proven to do so. By significantly increasing provider compliance with care standards, the use of CAMPs could allow direct evaluation of the efficacy of the standards in outcomes research.

In the future, it is anticipated that CAMPs similar to this prototypic diabetes CAMP will be developed. Further computerization of the patient record will also allow for real-time application of CAMPs during the actual clinical encounter. As shown in this study, now and in the future, CAMPs have great potential to improve compliance with care standards and ultimately enhance the quality and efficiency of health care delivery, by bringing care standards to the point of patient contact.

Acknowledgements

This work was supported in part by grant 1-T15-LM07071 from the National Library of Medicine. The authors wish to thank Ruby Grewal and Jim Collins for programming assistance, and Bill Wilkinson for advise concerning data analysis.

References

1. American Diabetes Association. Standards of medical care for patients with diabetes mellitus. *Diabetes Care* 1992; 15s: 10-13.
2. Ball JR. Practice guidelines and their role in quality assurance and cost effectiveness. *Quality Assurance in Healthcare* 1990; 2:31-36.
3. Burns LR, Denton M, Goldfein S, Warrick L, Morenz B, Sales B. The Use of continuous quality improvement methods in the development and dissemination of medical practice guidelines. *QRB* 1992; 434-439.
4. Barnett GO, Winickoff R, Dorsey JL, Morgan MM, Lurie RS. Quality assurance through automated monitoring and concurrent feedback using a computer-based medical information system. *Med Care* 1978; 16:962-970.
5. Clark CM, Kinney ED. Standards for the care of diabetes: Origins uses and implications for third-party payment. *Diabetes Care* 1992; 15s: 10-14.
6. Clark CM, Kinney ED. The potential role of diabetes guidelines in the reduction of medical injury and malpractice claims involving diabetes. *Diabetes Care* 1994; 17: 155-159.
7. Czaja R, McFall SL, Warnecke RB, Ford L, Kaluzny AD. Preferences of community physicians for cancer screening guidelines. *Ann Intern Med* 1994; 120: 602-608.
8. McDonald CJ. Protocol-based computer reminders, the quality of care and the non-perfectability of man. *N Engl J Med* 1976; 295:1351-1355.
9. McDonald CJ, Hui SL, Smith DM, Tierney WM, Cohen SJ, Weinberger M, McCabe GP. Reminders to physicians from an introspective computer medical record. *Ann Int Med* 1984; 100:130-138.
10. Murrey KO, Gottlieb LK, Schoenbaum SC. Implementing clinical guidelines: A quality managemnet approach to reminder systems. *QRB* 1992; 423-433.
11. Rosser WW, McDowell I, Newell C. Use of reminders for preventive procedures in family medicine. *Can Med Assoc J* 1991; 145:807-812.
12. Stead WW, Hammond WE. Computer-based medical records: the centerpiece of TMR. *M.D. Comput* 1988; 5:48-62.
13. Tape T, Campbell JR. Computerized medical records and preventative health care: success depends on many factors. *Am J Med* 1993; 94: 619-625.
14. Weingarten SR, Riedinger MS, Conner L, Lee TH, Hoffman I,Johnson B, Ellrodt AG. Practice guidelines and reminders to reduce duration of hospital stay for patients with chest pain. *Ann Intern Med* 1994; 120: 257-263

Comparison of Three Knowledge Representation Formalisms for Encoding the NCEP Cholesterol Guidelines

Justin Starren and Guochun Xie

Center for Medical Informatics
Columbia University College of Physicians and Surgeons
New York, New York 10032

Although many Knowledge Representation (KR) formalisms have been used to encode care guidelines, there are few direct comparisons among different formalisms. In order to compare their suitability for encoding care guidelines, three different KR formalisms were used to encode the National Cholesterol Education Panel (NCEP) guideline. PROLOG, a First Order Logic system, CLASSIC, a frame-based representation system, and CLIPS, a production rule system, were used in the comparison. All three representations allowed accurate encoding of the guideline. PROLOG produced the most compact representation, but proved the most difficult to debug. The lack of arbitrary disjunction in CLASSIC greatly increased the complexity of the encoding. Overall, the CLIPS representation was the most intuitive and easiest to use.

INTRODUCTION

There are now over 1000 different care guidelines, and more are added or changed almost monthly. Despite documented improvements in outcomes [1], guidelines have had limited penetration into general clinical practice. One reason for this is that no clinician can possibly remember all of the guidelines. Using computerized decision support systems to implement the guidelines has been suggested as a solution. Computerized medical logic has already been used to implement a number of care guidelines and guideline-like protocols. [2]

Several different knowledge representation (KR) formalisms have been used to encode care guideline knowledge. Although studies have compared different systems for the development of treatment recommendations [3], there has been little work directly comparing different schema for the representation of the same care guideline. In order to compare the suitability of different paradigms for representing a typical care guideline, we selected three of the KR systems at Columbia to encode the National Cholesterol Education Panel (NCEP) guideline:

- PROLOG: a First Order Logic based system
- CLASSIC: a frame-based representation system
- CLIPS: a production rule system.

The differences in ease of implementation and intuitiveness of representation will be discussed.

METHODS

The NCEP Expert Panel on Detection, Evaluation and Treatment of High Blood Cholesterol in Adults is now in its second version [4]. Like the first version, it presents its basic recommendations as block diagrams or tables. One of these is shown in Figure 1. An earlier version of the NCEP guidelines has been encoded by two other groups [5,6]. The NCEP guideline is one of the older and better known of the national care guidelines. The NCEP is quite specific about the thresholds and targets for dietary and drug therapy, but is less specific about the details. In particular, it does not state the exact sequence of drugs to be tried, or precisely when to determine that a particular trial of therapy is unsuccessful. Accordingly, only the unambiguous portions of the NCEP guideline was captured in the three KR representations.

Any extensions to the care guideline logic were limited to those which are clearly implicit in the guideline. For example, the guideline recommends testing cholesterol levels every 5 years. It also gives treatment recommendations based on cholesterol levels. This clearly implies that no treatment should be recommended based on a cholesterol level which is over 5 years old. Instead of using an out-of-date value, the system should stop and request that a new value be obtained. A similar expansion was required for each piece of data required by the careplan logic.

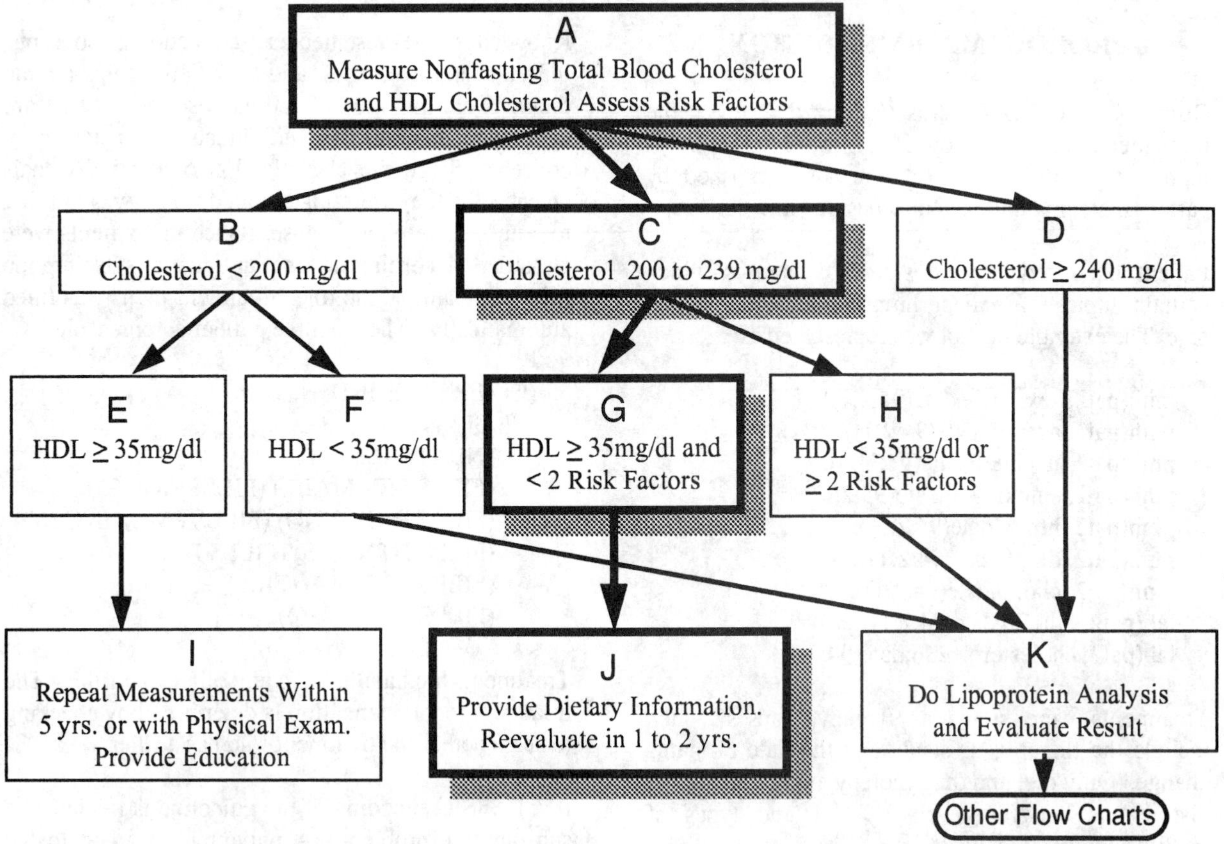

Figure 1. Part of the NCEP cholesterol guideline demonstrating initial evaluation of an uncomplicated patient. Letters were added for clarity. The highlighted path (A-C-G-J) will be used to show the differences between the representations. Also of significance is the fact that several decision paths diverge and then reconverge at box K.

The representation of time in computerized care guidelines has been the subject of considerable study. [5]. For the NCEP guideline, time considerations are limited largely to age of laboratory results and the duration of treatments. For that reason we selected a simple event-based time representation, rather than an interval based one.

For each implementation the patient data were encoded by hand in a form native to the representation. The specific representation syntaxes will be discussed under each of the systems. Data encoded included: patient identifier; laboratory results with times; risk factors; and, therapies with time of start. Correct implementation of the guideline (defined as the ability of each implementation to produce recommendations identical to ones generated manually from the published guideline) was considered a requirement for each implementation. Therefore, the accuracy of the systems was identical, by definition. The major criteria for comparison among the three representations was not the ability to correctly encode the guideline, but rather the difficulty in doing so.

A test set of patients was created for development purposes which were represented the eight different basic outcomes of the NCEP guideline. Additional patients were selected from the practice booklet developed by the NCEP. Since this booklet is based on the 1988 recommendations rather than on the new 1993 recommendations, the treatment recommendations were updated based on the new guideline. For this initial evaluation, no actual clinical cases were used. After initial development of each representation, these cases were used to test the system. In all cases, the initial implementations needed to be corrected to handle the practice cases. However, the representation varied significantly in the number of errors and the amount of effort required to correct them. For each of the implementations, an example patient is shown. The logic flow for this patient is highlighted as path A-C-G-J in Figure 1.

PROLOG IMPLEMENTATION

Quintas PROLOG was utilized for the implementation. Knowledge in PROLOG is represented as clauses. Inference is performed by pattern matching and resolution using Horn clauses.

Patient history data were stored as clauses which contain tuples of patient number, attribute, value, date. The example patient was represented as:

```
pmh(pat2, sex, male,date(94,2,1)).
pmh(pat2, age, 35,date(94,2,1)).
pmh(pat2, h_chd, 0,date(94,2,1)).
pmh(pat2, smoking, 0,date(94,2,1)).
pmh(pat2, htn, 1,date(94,2,1)).
pmh(pat2, dm, 0,date(94,2,1)).
pmh(pat2, chd, 0,date(94,2,1)).
lab(pat2, hdl, 70,date(94,2,1)).
lab(pat2, cholesterol, 236,date(94,2,1)).
```

Treatments were stored as therapy clauses which include the therapy, its status and the date of status change. Only diet and drug therapy are recorded. No distinctions between levels of diet and types of medication were included.

```
therapy(pat1,diet,on,date(92,1,1)).
```

A rule was written for each treatment outcome. Within the actual rules, information was accessed using CHECK_LAB and CHECK_PMH functions. The rule for the example patient is:

```
rule_j(PID) :-
  check_lab(PID, hdl, HDL,_),!,
  HDL >= 35,
  total_risk(PID, Risk),!,
  Risk < 2,
  check_lab(PID, cholesterol, C,_),
  C >= 200,
  C =< 239,
  print_rule_j.
```

Dates were represented using an internal PROLOG format. For time interval computations, this format is converted a second representation as a pair of integers corresponding to UNIX system time.

CLASSIC IMPLEMENTATION

CLASSIC is a frame-based description logic system. It is a special set of functions implemented in Lisp. Knowledge is represented as a collection of concepts, individuals, roles, rules, and the relationships among them. Concepts are defined as descriptions that are applied to individuals. Individuals are instances of concepts. Since the classification of the individuals occurred as they were instantiated, there was nothing to "run" in the typical sense. Once the patients were classified according to the automatic subsumption rules, the value of the role "treatment-plan" was filled automatically. The example patient is represented as:

```
(CL-CREATE-IND
  'PAT2
  '(AND PATIENT
     (FILLS SEX MALE) (FILLS AGE 35)
     (FILLS H-CHD NO) (FILLS SMOKING NO)
     (FILLS HTN YES) (FILLS DM NO)
     (FILLS CHD NO) (FILLS HDL 70)
     (FILLS CHOL 236)))
```

Treatments are handled like any other role filler. The treatment recommendation is determined by checking to see whether the treatment role has a filler.

In CLASSIC encoding of the guideline is treated as a subsumption problem. A patient is matched to the most specific subsuming concept, and the treatment recommendation determined on that basis. For example, in order for a patient to satisfy the criteria for box G it has to also satisfy box C, and therefore, box A. Thus, the concepts to classify the example patient to box J were.

```
(CL-DEFINE-CONCEPT  'OKLAB-PATIENT
  '(AND TESTED-PATIENT
      (FILLS TREATMENT-PLAN " ")))
(CL-DEFINE-CONCEPT
   'UNTREATED-PATIENT
   '(AND PATIENT
      (FILLS TREATMENT-PLAN " ")))
(CL-DEFINE-CONCEPT  'A-PATIENT
  '(AND UNTREATED-PATIENT
      OKLAB-PATIENT
      (FILLS CHD NO)))
(CL-DEFINE-CONCEPT  'C-PATIENT
  '(AND A-PATIENT
     (ALL CHOL
      (AND INTEGER
        (MIN 200) (MAX 239)))))
(CL-DEFINE-CONCEPT  'G-PATIENT
  '(AND C-PATIENT LOW-RISK-PATIENT
     (ALL HDL (AND INTEGER (MIN 35)))))
```

The handling of "or" relations in CLASSIC was complex, and required the creation of artificial branches and artificial roles. The representation of the path convergence for box K of Figure 1 is shown in Figure 2.

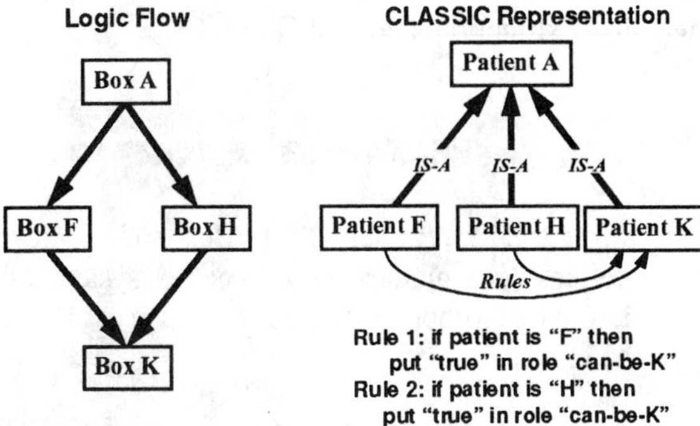

Figure 2. Representation of an "OR" convergence in CLASSIC.

CLIPS IMPLEMENTATION

CLIPS 6.1 is a forward chaining production rule system written in ANSI C by NASA. The knowledge in CLIPS is encoded in rules and functions. CLIPS also supports objects and individuals. Since it does not support automatic classification, we used templates for the creation of patient data structures. The CLIPS inference engine includes truth maintenance, dynamic rule addition and customizable conflict resolution strategies. However, these were not required.

Individual patients are stored as patterns of the type:

```
(patient-type(attribute1 VALUE1)
        (attribute2 VALUE2) ...)
```

This template was used for both history attributes such as "smoking" as well as numeric attributes such as "chol". Because CLIPS has a well developed default value system, it was used for the handling of missing history elements. Missing laboratory values are represented as -1. If the missing value is needed for a rule, the caregiver was prompted. The example patient was represented as:

```
(assert (uncalculated-patient
    (sex male) (name pat2) (age 35)
    (h-chd no) (smoking no)(dm no)
    (htn yes) (chd no) (hdl 70) (chol 236)))
```

For processing of the individual patients, the (uncalculated-patient (...)) data structure is converted to a (calculated-patient (...)) template which includes a numerically computed risk from the history attributes.

Unlike CLASSIC and PROLOG, CLIPS has no intrinsic time or date functions. In order to support date, a system call was executed to perform a UNIX date operation and store the date in a file. CLIPS then read the file and converted the value into a single integer. In a production implementation of this system, an external function could be written to provide date functions within CLIPS.

The rule based structure of CLIPS lent itself to a creation of explicitly defined states which were named based on their transitions among the boxes of the diagram (Figure 1). In addition, a "done" flag was added to force the logic to terminate when a treatment recommendation was generated. The final rule for the example patient was:

```
(defrule C2G2J "Rules to reach box J"
   ?f1 <- (calculated-patient (state c)
      (done no) (hdl ?hdl) (name ?name))
   (test (>= ?hdl 35))
  =>
   (printout t crlf "Patient " ?name
      " needs the following treatement:"crlf)
   (printout t ?treatment-j crlf)
   (modify ?f1 (done yes) (state j)))
```

Although the states were similar, in some ways, to the CLASSIC concepts, there was a fundamental difference. CLIPS allows states to be specified by rules with disjunctive conditions. Consequently, encoding path convergence in the guideline was straightforward.

DISCUSSION

PROLOG provided for the easiest construction of the patient database. In addition, it allowed for the storage of multiple sequential values for each patient and easy retrieval of the appropriate value. The inclusion of a human-readable date format was also quite convenient. The ability to specify arbitrary disjunctions allowed easy encoding of the convergence points in the guideline.

A well-known difficulty with PROLOG is with the control of backtracking. Because each lab result was a separate fact, it was possible for PROLOG backtrack from partial matches of current data into old data and, thereby, into incorrect conclusions. "Cuts" are a method in PROLOG for limiting such undesired backtracking. Unfortunately, the behavior of cuts is notoriously complex, and they were responsible for most of the errors encountered.

Although the automatic classification of CLASSIC seemed to be a natural representation for the block structure of the NCEP guideline, the difficulty of use overshadowed this. CLASSIC was by far, the hardest of the three systems to use, in large part because it required detailed instantiation of every possible outcome. There was no easy way to classify by exclusion. For example, every patient is either treated or untreated, (never both and never neither). Such a dichotomy was easy to encode in PROLOG and CLIPS, but both sides of the dichotomy had to be explicitly defined in CLASSIC. Fortunately, the ability to print the entire lineage of each individual greatly simplified the debugging.

Overall, CLIPS was the most useful of the three systems evaluated. The CLIPS approach, of states and rules, was the easiest to conceptualize. Patient attributes were easy to specify. No awkward manipulations were required to capture the logic. The only real disadvantage was the lack of built-in time and date functions. CLIPS and PROLOG required a similar number of program statements, while CLASSIC required almost three times as many.

Most important, all three representations proved adequate for encoding the guideline. Unlike the problems encountered by computerized diagnostic systems, care guidelines are specifically designed to be clear and unambiguous. Care guidelines for human use are often phrased in terms of "If symptom X, then give treatment Y." This type of explicit linkage between antecedents and consequents is ideally suited to both the rule structure of production-rule systems, as well and the Horn clause structure of PROLOG. There is no need to evaluate the relative merits of competing hypotheses. For a production-rule system, this means that there is no need for resolution of large conflict-sets. In addition, the NCEP guidelines is explicit that all information is either already available or it is requested. Therefore, there is no need to reason with incomplete data. Given all this, it is not suprising that, for this particular guideline, the resolution-based and the production-rule representations were a more natural fit to the problem. No hybrid representations were evaluated, and it is possible that one of these could prove superior to the systems tested here.

Acknowledgement

This work was funded in part by a National Library of Medicine Extramural Training Grant.

References

1. Grimshaw JM, Russell IT. Effect of clinical guidelines on medical practice: a systematic review of rigorous evaluations. Lancet 1993; 342:1317-22.

2. Johnston ME, Langton KB, Haynes RB, Mathieu A. Effects of Computer-based Clinical Decision Support Systems on Clinician Performance and Patient Outcome. Ann Intern Med 1994; 120:135-142.

3. Long WJ, Griffith JL, Selker HP, D'Agostino RB. A comparison of logistic regression to decision-tree induction in a medical domain. Comp. Biomed. Res. 1993; 26, 74-79.

4. Expert Panel. Summary of the Second Report of the National Cholesterol Education Program (NCEP) Expert Panel on the Detection, Evaluation, and Treatment of High Blood Cholesterol in Adults (Adult Treatment Panel II) JAMA 1993;269:3015-3023.

5. Rucker DW, Maron DJ, Shortliffe EH. Temporal representation of clinical algorithms using expert-system and database tools. Comput Biomed Res. 1990;23(3):222-39.

6. Weissfeld JL, Weissfeld LA, Holloway JJ, Bernard AM. A mathematical representation of the expert panel's guidelines for high blood cholesterol case-finding and treatment. Med Decis Making. 1990;10(2):135-46.

Towards Effective Implementation of a Pediatric Asthma Guideline: Integration of Decision Support and Clinical Workflow Support

Richard N. Shiffman, MD, MCIS
Center for Medical Informatics, Yale School of Medicine, New Haven, Conn. 06510

Successful local implementation of national guideline recommendations requires attention to factors that promote clinician compliance. Design of a computerized system is described that will implement recommendations from a recently published guideline for outpatient management of childhood asthma exacerbations. Logical analysis of the guideline shows that it is incomplete and contains several ambiguities that must be addressed before the guideline can be operationalized. Once the user-audience is defined guideline decision points are examined and a structured data entry system is devised. Support of clinicians' workflow is provided by an integrated capability for encounter documentation, dosage calculation, and prescription-writing. A pen-based, graphical interface represents an appropriate platform for implementation of the system because of its ease of use and portability.

A clinical practice guideline can only be considered to be effectively implemented if its knowledge content is faithfully transmitted to healthcare providers and its recommendations are incorporated into their clinical practices. National policies are unlikely to influence the practice of individual practitioners if they are merely published and allowed to diffuse [1]. Grimshaw and Russell reported that guidelines are most effective when they incorporate patient-specific information and provide decision support concurrent with decision making [2].

A goal of this project is to develop a replicable process by which clinical guideline knowledge can be extracted, verified, and incorporated into a system that will influence the behavior of physicians toward adherence to the guideline. Knowledge, published recently in a clinical practice guideline, is reused and recommendations are integrated into a system that facilitates physician work patterns.

BACKGROUND

Clinical practice guidelines are being produced by a wide array of organizations in an effort to reduce inappropriate variations in clinical practice and to reduce unnecessary costs [3]. These clinical policies frequently embody high quality knowledge that is intended for implementation by a broad range of users including healthcare practitioners, quality assurance bodies, third party payers, and governmental policy makers. Well-crafted guidelines contain knowledge that is evidence-based, representative of the best current thinking in a given domain, and sanctioned by the sponsoring organization.

Guideline knowledge, therefore, represents a valuable resource that can be reused for the development of new knowledge-based systems. Such knowledge sharing requires translation of guideline knowledge into a form that is usable by knowledge based systems [4]. We have previously found that logical analysis using decision table techniques facilitates this translation process and may enhance the knowledge by ensuring its completeness and logical consistency [5].

Shortliffe defined a decision support system as any computer program designed to help health professionals make clinical decisions [6]. Such a system may include tools for information management (i.e., for storing and retrieving clinical knowledge), tools for focusing attention (i.e., for reminding users about problems that might otherwise be overlooked) and tools for patient-specific consultation (i.e., for providing tailored diagnostic and treatment advice). Successful use of decision tools is dependent on their integration into routine data-management tasks [7].

Clinical workflow support includes activities embedded in the process of patient care that enhance that care without directly affecting decision making. Workflow support is a critical factor in the acceptance and use of all computer systems. Automation of any activity is unlikely to be successful unless it produces a net benefit to offset the costs associated with its implementation.

APPROACH

Selection of practice parameter

Guidelines are most frequently published as text-based narratives or as clinical algorithms. This work applies logical analysis techniques to a recently published guideline from the American Academy of Pediatrics for management of asthma in practitioners' offices [8]. The guideline knowledge is presented primarily in algorithm format with appended annotations. A clinical algorithm is a stepwise procedure for making decisions about the diagnosis and treatment of a clinical problem that is published in a graphic format [9]. It represents the logic of clinical decisions concisely and explicitly and focuses clinicians' attention on relevant issues by defining a world of restricted breadth and depth [10].

This guideline for office management of childhood asthma exacerbations was chosen for a number of reasons, including:

- Asthma is a major health problem in pediatrics. It affects 5-10% of children and accounts for almost 1/4 of school absences. The hospitalization rate and the death rate from childhood asthma are rising and there is considerable variation in treatment [8]. Early, appropriate management of asthmatic patients may significantly decrease morbidity and mortality.
- The asthma management guideline was published recently and therefore reflects current thinking of asthma experts in the pediatric community. Much of the knowledge in the guideline is evidence-based.
- The guideline has been sanctioned by the American Academy of Pediatrics. Additionally, the American Medical Association Specialty Society Practice Parameters Partnership reviewed the guideline and found that it conformed to AMA attributes.
- The complexity of the guideline knowledge content is intermediate, i.e., more complicated than a one-line recommendation—e.g., premenopausal women should have Pap smears every 3 years—yet less intricate than a guideline that specifies comprehensive management of chronic disease over many years. The short time-line of encounters governed by the asthma guideline simplifies its implementation and makes compliance assessable.

Overview of guideline content

The guideline is intended to apply to children over 5 years of age with signs of airway obstruction, wheezing, and/or persistent cough who present to an office setting. It includes several recommendations that "may vary from common practice" including use of peak expiratory flow rate (PEFR) measurements and pulse oximetry, altered frequency and dosage of ß-2 agonists, and increased use of corticosteroids. The algorithm proceeds through 7 decision boxes and 13 action boxes to a disposition of each patient either by transfer to a hospital setting or discharge home with appropriate medication and follow-up.

The asthma guideline was published both in flowchart form (with appended annotations) and in a table. The algorithmic representation more clearly expresses the recommended sequence of clinical activities while the table modularizes the guideline into 5 groups of related activities ("Initial Assessment and Emergency Management", "Initial Treatment", "Follow-up Treatment", "Additional Treatment or Transfer to ED or Direct Admission to Appropriate Hospital Unit", "Additional Treatment and/or Hospitalize"). One might expect that translation of a flowchart-based guideline to a set of rules would be straightforward but several unanticipated problems required remediation.

Assessment of guideline logical integrity

Before a practice guideline can be effectively operationalized, it should be demonstrated to be logically comprehensive and consistent [5, 8, 11]. This requires analysis and extraction of relevant clinical decision and action variables.

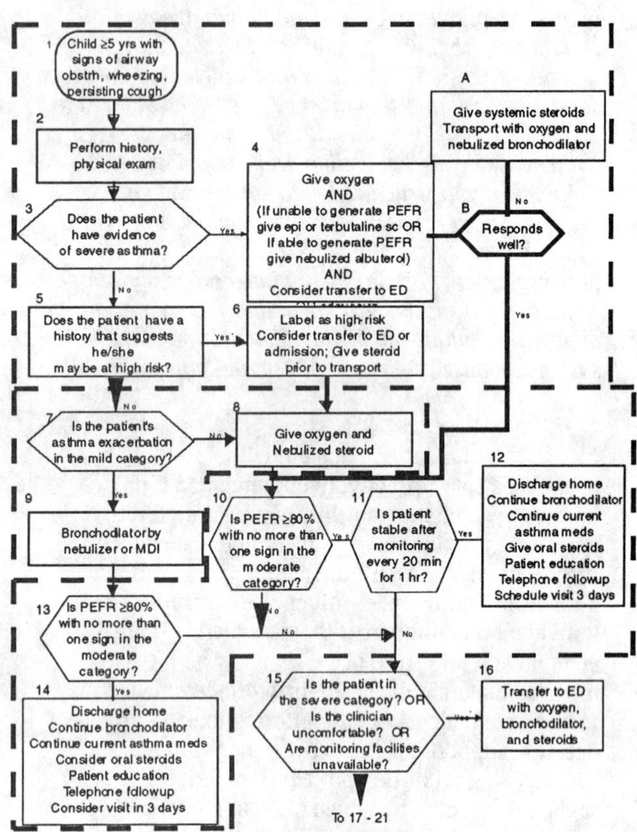

Figure 1. Flowchart display adapted from the published guideline for initial management of children with acute asthma in office settings. Three modules are indicated by dashed lines. Decision node and arcs added by the author are defined by heavy lines. (Reproduced by permission of *Pediatrics* Volume 93 page 123 ©1994)

The analysis is facilitated by modularization of the algorithm into cohesive and functionally independent blocks as shown in Figure 1. Such partitioning is an effective technique for simplification of complex decision problems [12, 13]. In this manner the number of variables pertinent to any single phase of the management sequence is limited, thereby decreasing the number of clinical rules that must be constructed. Also, activities within a single module occur contemporaneously so that temporal sequencing issues are ameliorated [14]. Only the sequencing relationships of whole modules needs to be considered.

In each module, an exhaustive set of possible values for each variable is determined and a Cartesian product defines all mathematically possible combinations of decision variables [5]. According to guideline recommendations, actions are appended to all combinations that are semantically possible to form rule sets. These rule sets are then subjected to decision table analysis to assess the guideline's logical integrity.

For this guideline, logical analysis identified several issues that required attention:

1. Incomplete logical expression. Despite its configuration as a flowchart, the guideline failed to explicitly indicate all the decision branches. As published, the algorithm incorporated 2 decisions within action box 4. The choice of subcutaneously injected vs. inhaled bronchodilators depends on "If the patient is able to generate a PEFR". The action box recommends that "If the patient responds well to the initial ...treatment" management should continue in box 10 although no linking arrow is included in the algorithm.

Likewise, action box 6 implies a linking arrow to box 8 that is not shown. It labels a group of patients as "High-Risk" but no subsequent decision box incorporates the high risk categorization in its decision making.

To remedy these problems, the algorithm was reformulated to indicate an additional decision box and its outcome actions. Linkage arrows were added to show the logical flow.

2. Ambiguous definition. Although this guideline is generally quite explicit with regard to test specification, medication dosing, and outcome measurements, it is logically compromised by several ambiguous definitions. Decision boxes 4 and 5 contain lists of parameters that respectively assess the severity of an attack and the risk status of the patient. They are each phrased: "Does the patient have...?" followed by a list of 7-9 parameters. There is no indication whether these assessments are combined by ANDs or ORs or "2 (or more) of the aboves".

In decision box #7 the user is asked to answer whether the asthma exacerbation is "in the mild category"? The published practice parameter includes a table from the National Asthma Education Program (NAEP) that characterizes 9 manifestations as mild, moderate, or severe, which presumably should be used for this determination. However, the guideline provides no criteria for interpretation of combinations of manifestations [15]. Is a patient with 6 manifestations in the mild category and 3 in the moderate category having a mild exacerbation? Examination of the original NAEP publication provides limited clarification: "(W)ithin each category, the presence of several parameters, but not necessarily all, indicate the general classification of the exacerbation".

To operationalize the guideline, precise definitions are necessary. Decision box 11 tests whether the patient is "stable after monitoring every 20 minutes for 1 hour", however stability is not explicitly defined. Also, the decision "If the patient responds well to the initial ... treatment" is considerably less rigorous than the later test (#10) "Is PEFR >80% with no more than one sign in the moderate category".

Finally, the published algorithm contains 2 ambiguities that are apparently due to typographical errors. Decision box 13 tests "PEFR >90%" whereas the equivalent section of the tabular representation tests for "PEFR >80%". Similarly, decision box 3 assesses PEFR "≥50%" for a finding of severe asthma whereas the tabular representation makes the more plausible test of "<50%".

After these logical deficiencies were corrected by consultation with local experts, decision table evaluation demonstrated that the guideline was logically complete and consistent. Input parameters were defined in the condition stub and potential outputs were specified in the action stub. Each column in the decision tables represents a rule that may be used to trigger pertinent decision support activities. The algorithm itself provides a view of the guideline pathway that facilitates decisions regarding workflow support.

Devise decision support that will facilitate adherence to guideline recommendations

Define the intended users. A specification regarding the intended audience for the application helps to determine the level and types of decision support required. Physicians and nurses have different needs, as do medical students and residents, and generalists and specialists. For example, medical students might find hypertext access to definition of terminology and a multimedia presentation of abnormal breath sounds in asthma to be pedagogically useful, while subspecialists probably would not. For this application, support was considered to be aimed at practicing, generalist pediatricians.

Examine the decision points in the guideline to determine potentially useful decision support information. Every decision in this guideline—except for the determination of risk level by consideration of historical factors—is based on an assessment of the patient's respiratory status. This uniformity facilitates design of a structured data entry system.

A graphical layout of all the clinical decision parameters and potential choices provides a useful reminder of the entire range of assessments that must be made at each decision point (Figure 2). Multiple factors are weighed (PEFR, respiratory rate, alertness, dyspnea, accessory muscle use, color, auscultatory findings, pulsus paradoxus, and evidence of extrapulmonary air) and an estimate of severity is formulated. Similarly, a list of criteria that determine high-risk situations (decision box #5) can be provided. McDonald, et al., have postulated that such reminders reduce oversights, i.e., they "improve the fidelity between a physician's actions and his intentions" [16].

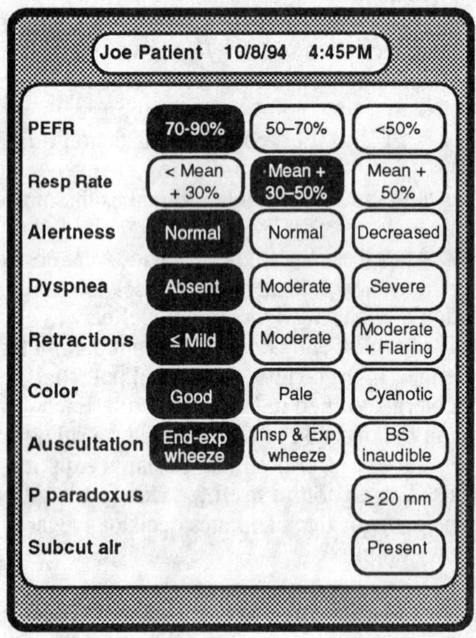

Figure 2. Input screen for assessment and documentation of asthma severity.

Entering the measured PEFR allows comparison with predicted values (which can be calculated from the patient's age and height). A clock function triggers reminders that reassessment is due.

Decision logic is used to trigger the appearance of alerts that indicate a variance from guideline recommendations. For example, printing discharge instructions for a patient who presents with moderate asthma that do not include a prescription for steroids prompts a reminder.

Additional decision support might include citations to relevant papers in the medical literature that support a given recommendation or indications of quality of evidence that support a particular recommendation.

Support workflow

Potential users were observed as they provided care for asthma exacerbations and surveyed regarding their needs. Perhaps the most valuable workflow support would come from automated documentation of interval clinical assessments. As each parameter is assessed at each decision point the program can maintain a record of the clinical evaluations. This information is useful for sequential comparisons of individual patient progress and can be a valuable source of data for retrospective evaluation of guideline adherence and effectiveness.

Examination of action boxes suggests additional areas for workflow support. This guideline recommends alternative dosages of bronchodilator based on the severity of the exacerbation. Medication dosages in pediatrics are adjusted based on the size of the child. The correct dosage for a given patient can be calculated based on weight and then automatically converted into a volume of bronchodilator solution to be dispensed into a nebulizer. Reminders of maximal dosages and frequency of repetition can be provided.

For patients who are discharged, materials can be printed including prescriptions for bronchodilators and steroids, patient education information, and follow-up instructions. For patients who fail to improve, software can provide the clinician with convenient phone listings for referral to emergency departments and ambulance services, and offer the possibility of electronic transmission of admission orders.

Interface and platform considerations

Implementation of this system would be facilitated by a platform that permits clinician mobility, is user-friendly, and is available at relatively low cost. The Newton PDA platform (Apple Computer Co., Cupertino, Calif.) provides an appealing graphical interface and intuitive pen-based input to help reduce physician reluctance to enter data.

Even with current technological restrictions these devices are capable of meeting the limited demands posed by this application. Most choices can be made by "tapping" gestures; for example, documentation of respiratory status can be performed by tapping on pertinent descriptor buttons (Figure 2) [17]. Text entry will be minimized since handwriting recognition capabilities remain limited. Wherever possible, known entries will be entered automatically, e.g., date and time. Choosing from drop-down menus (called "pickers") or slider "gauges" provides more accurate data input without introducing inefficiency.

DISCUSSION

Design of a system that brings about successful implementation of clinical practice guidelines recommendations is a challenge for medical informatics. Simply providing users with paper-based or on-line representations of published guidelines will likely produce less compliance than will integration of guideline information into the decision-making and documentation process. This paper describes the design of a system that deals with patient-specific information in real time and is intended to overcome the natural reluctance of many clinicians to use computer devices.

Furthermore, users must embrace and trust the guideline knowledge that is being implemented. Evidence-based, officially sanctioned guidelines provide a useful starting point; but this study re-emphasizes the fact that many current guidelines contain logical deficiencies that must be addressed and remedied [18].

If healthcare providers are to be expected to sacrifice some degree of professional autonomy to comply with guideline recommendations, some new benefit must accrue. Currently, for this asthma guideline and many others, data has not yet confirmed that compliance will improve patient outcomes. Therefore, to optimize user acceptance, the decision and workflow support that is provided must offset perceived disadvantages and inconveniences brought about by the new system.

The system described here will permit collection of data to facilitate outcome studies. Evaluation of the success of this project will require testing of hypotheses that use of this system does, in fact, promote compliance, change physician behavior, and improve patient outcomes.

References

1. Lomas J, Haynes RB. A taxonomy and critical review of tested strategies for the application of clinical practice recommendations: from "official" to "individual" clinical policy. Am J Prev Med 1987;4:77-94.
2. Grimshaw JM, Russell IT. Effect of clinical guidelines on medical practice: a systematic review of rigorous evaluations. Lancet 1993;342:1317–22.
3. Audet A-M, Greenfield S, Field M. Medical practice guidelines: Current activities and future directions. Ann Intern Med 1990;113:703-714.
4. Musen MA. Dimensions of knowledge sharing and reuse. Comput Biomed Research 1992;25:433–67.
5. Shiffman RN, Greenes RA. Improving clinical guidelines with logic and decision table techniques: application to hepatitis immunization recommendations. Med Decis Making 1994;14(3):145-54.
6. Shortliffe EH. Computer programs to support clinical decision making. JAMA 1987;258:61-66.
7. Shortliffe EH. Clinical decision-support systems. In: Shortliffe EH, Perreault LE, ed. Medical informatics: computer applications in health care. Reading, Mass: Addison-Wesley, 1990: 466-503.
8. American Academy of Pediatrics Provisional Committee on Quality Improvement. Practice parameter: office management of acute exacerbations of asthma. Pediatrics 1994;93(1):119-26.
9. Margolis CZ. Uses of clinical algorithms. JAMA 1983;249(5):627-632.
10. Abendroth TW, Greenes RA, Joyce EA. Investigations in the use of clinical algorithms to organize medical knowledge. In: Greenes RA, ed. Symposium on Computer Applications in Medical Care.Washington, DC: Computer Society Press, 1988: 90-95.
11. Field MJ, Lohr KL.Clinical practice guidelines: directions for a new program. Washington, D.C.:National Academy Press, 1990.
12. Hurley RB. Decision Tables in Software Engineering. New York: Van Nostrand Reinhold, 1983.
13. CODASYL. A Modern Appraisal of Decision Tables. New York: Association for Computing Machinery, 1982.
14. Rucker DW, Maron DJ, Shortliffe EH. Temporal representation of clinical algorithms using expert-system and database tools. Comput Biomed Research 1990;23:222-239.
15. National Asthma Education Program. Guidelines for the diagnosis and management of asthma. National Heart, Lung, and Blood Institute, National Institutes of Health, 1991.
16. McDonald C, Hui S, Smith D, et al. Reminders to physicians from an introspective computer medical record: a two year randomized trial. Ann Intern Med 1984;100:130-138.
17. McKeehan J, Rhodes N. Programming for the Newton: Software development with NewtonScript. Boston: AP Professional, 1994.
18. Shiffman RN. Clinical guidelines in medical practice. Journal of Medical Practice Management 1993;9:70-4.

Indexing Guidelines: Applications in Use of Pulmonary Artery Catheters and Pressure Ulcer Prevention

Robert A. Jenders, MD, MS; Greg Estey, EdM; Martha Martin, RN, MS; Glenys Hamilton, DNSc; Penny Ford-Carleton, RN, MS; B. Taylor Thompson, MD; Diane E. Oliver, MD; Randy Eccles, BS; G. Octo Barnett, MD; Rita D. Zielstorff, RN, MS; Joan B. Fitzmaurice, RN, PhD

Laboratory of Computer Science, Massachusetts General Hospital
Boston, Massachusetts

ABSTRACT

In a busy clinical environment, access to knowledge must be rapid and specific to the clinical query at hand. This requires indices which support easy navigation within a knowledge source. We have developed a computer-based tool for trouble-shooting pulmonary artery waveforms using a graphical index. Preliminary results of domain knowledge tests for a group of clinicians exposed to the system (N=33) show a mean improvement on a 30-point test of 5.33 (p<0.001) compared to a control group (N=19) improvement of 0.47 (p=0.61). Survey of the experimental group (N=25) showed 84% (p=0.001) found the system easy to use. We discuss lessons learned in indexing this domain area to computer-based indexing of guidelines for pressure ulcer prevention.

INTRODUCTION

Clinicians need to manage a large body of knowledge, using about two million pieces of information. Rather than storing such information randomly, experienced clinicians organize it into scripts structured around common clinical problems. They then use pattern matching to recognize and manage these problems in patients [1]. Adding to this complexity, clinical guidelines have been disseminated and used with some success to influence clinician behavior and to improve patient outcome [2]. Leading this effort recently has been the Agency for Health Care Policy and Research (AHCPR), with guidelines on several topics including pressure ulcer prevention [3].

In order to assist clinicians in the management of this information, some workers have developed computer-based access to patient care guidelines [4]. However, when multiple computer-based knowledge sources are made available, difficulty with interfaces and applying knowledge from different sources limits the utility of such systems [5].

With these challenges in mind, we have developed a computer-based system for providing problem-based access to knowledge used in troubleshooting pulmonary artery catheter waveforms. We chose this topic because knowledge among clinicians of the use of such catheters is variable despite their widespread use [6].

In this development we synthesized a knowledge base from a number of sources in the published literature and the opinions of local domain experts. We have studied prospectively the user satisfaction and impact on domain knowledge of an initial experimental group of users compared to a control group which did not use the system. In addition, based on this experience, we have begun to implement a computer-based system for access to the AHCPR guideline for pressure ulcer prevention.

PULMONARY ARTERY CATHETER SYSTEM DESIGN

The pulmonary artery catheter waveform troubleshooting system is implemented in the Toolbook authoring environment, running under the Windows operating system. This provides a robust graphical user interface coupled with the facility to develop prototype software rapidly. Though we might have used an expert system shell to organize and manage this expert knowledge, the relative simplicity of the rules governing the advice displayed by the system obviated this use.

The expert information [7] is organized hierarchically as depicted in Figure 1. At the upper level of the hierarchy, the user must choose one subtree of the hierarchy based on the anatomic location of the catheter: right atrium, pulmonary artery or pulmonary capillary wedge position. Once one of these large chunks of knowledge is chosen, the user then may access specific pieces of knowledge through the use of a graphical index. The user matches the catheter waveform of interest to one displayed by the system, selecting the one with the best match. Possible matches include topics such as damping, ringing and respiratory variation.

Level 0: *Anatomic site of the catheter tip*
- Right Atrium
- Pulmonary Artery
- Pulmonary Capillary Wedge

Level 1: *Problematic waveforms at a given catheter site*
- Catheter migration
- Damping
- Flat-line Pressure
- Irregular Rhythm
- Large Pulsations
- Normal Waveform
- Questionable Pressures
- Respiratory Variation
- Ringing

Level 2: *Description of Waveforms*
- Characteristics
- Causes
- Measurement
- Solutions

Figure 1. Hierarchy of knowledge of the pulmonary artery system. Each site at Level 0 is associated with each waveform of Level 1, each of which in turn is described by the four topics of Level 2.

The expert information pertinent to the selected waveform then becomes available to the user. This is organized in four categories: characteristics, causes, management and measurement. Each category then may be selected in turn to display information pertinent to identifying, isolating the cause of, improving and calibrating the problem with the catheter. A graphical design is used throughout, employing digitized waveform tracings, textual messages and digitized radiographs [7].

SYSTEM EVALUATION

The system was installed in a medical intensive care unit (ICU) which averaged three to five patients a day with pulmonary artery catheters in place. Another medical ICU was chosen as a control. The study group was the staff nurses of the ICUs and the resident physicians who rotated through these units each month. A total of 52 subjects agreed to participate in the initial study, including 33 in the experimental group (28 nurses and 5 physicians) and 19 in the control group (11 nurses and 8 physicians). All subjects provided written, informed consent.

The experimental group was those participants who worked in the ICU in which the system was installed. Each participant received an orientation to the system from one of the authors. The control group was those nurses and physicians working in a separate medical ICU which supported pulmonary artery catheters but in which the system was not installed. Data were collected over a period of ten months.

All participants completed a 30-question test of knowledge about pulmonary artery catheters before and after the study period. This instrument is based on a tool used to evaluate computer-based instruction systems as previously described [7]. In order to develop this test, the system designers created approximately 70 multiple choice, single-best-answer questions which could be answered by using the system. These questions were validated by administering the test to other local experts, and based on their responses and comments 30 of these questions were selected for the final version of the test.

In the case of the physicians who rotated through the units, these tests were completed before and after their exposure to the units. Although several physicians rotated through both control and experimental units during the study period, each was included in only one arm of the study, based on which unit was first in the rotation order.

In addition, 25 users in the experimental group completed questionnaires designed to evaluate satisfaction with various aspects of the system as previously described [7].

RESULTS OF EVALUATION

In the experimental group, the mean test score

before exposure to the system was 13.85 (out of a possible 30) and after exposure was 19.18 ($p<0.001$ by two-tailed analysis). This represents a 38.5% improvement in the mean score. By contrast, the mean test score of the control group was 16.74 before the study period and 17.21 afterwards ($p=0.61$ by two-tailed analysis), which is an improvement of only 2.8%.

Seventy-five percent (N=25) of the experimental group completed a survey of computing satisfaction. Eighty-four percent found the system was always or almost always easy to use ($p=0.001$ by one-tailed analysis). Ninety-six percent found the information provided by the system always or almost always accurate ($p<0.001$). The format was found to be acceptable always or almost all of the time by 76% of respondents ($p=0.007$).

APPLICATION TO PRESSURE ULCER PREVENTION

Cognizant of this experience of indexing a clinical guideline using a graphical interface to produce a positive change in clinician knowledge, we have begun to implement a computer-based index for the AHCPR guideline for the prediction and prevention of pressure ulcers in adults [3]. This area was chosen because of the significant prevalence of the problem [8] and the availability of a guideline written by a national organization. This successor system also uses a graphical interface to index guideline knowledge, but it relies principally on an interlinked hierarchy of important themes which we have termed the concept index.

As in the pulmonary artery catheter advice system, the pressure ulcer system is implemented in Toolbook in a Windows environment. However, because of the number and complexity of the rules governing expert advice on this topic, we use a commercial expert system shell, NEXPERT OBJECT, to manage and process a rule-based system. NEXPERT functions as an expert system server which communicates with the Toolbook client using a Windows Dynamic Link Library.

In this environment, we have structured the text of this guideline around a central concept index. Such an index combines the functionality of a glossary (containing simple definitions) with a table of contents (containing a hierarchy of concepts and their constituent subparts) and a hypertext document (containing multiple threads between topics). This extends the hierarchical structure of the pulmonary artery system by allowing navigation between topics without necessarily traversing to a common node located above both topics in the hierarchy. The concept index superficially resembles the main menu of many computer-based education programs but extends this notion by permitting more robust navigation than such programs.

To create this concept index, we manually reviewed the guideline document and divided this knowledge into "chunks" such as friction and shear, mobility and moisture exposure. Each concept has a simple definition, like that which would appear in a glossary, but it also contains hierarchically organized knowledge which provides a detailed description of the concept, its measurement (if appropriate), interventions used in treating patients and appropriate literature references.

These structured concepts are stored in a relational database. A system user can browse the database contents by using the concept index module, which queries the database to retrieve the information requested by a user. Also, the user may click on "hot words" in the text of a display to display a definition or additional information about an unfamiliar concept.

In addition, since the concept index identifies in a structured fashion the factors which affect patient outcome in pressure ulcer prevention, we have used the index to develop a data entry tool for recording details of the examination of the skin and comorbid risk factors for the development of pressure ulcers. In tandem, using the AHCPR guideline and other sources [9], we have developed a set of rules which characterize a patient's risk for developing pressure ulcers and which describe interventions which can treat such ulcers or help prevent their occurrence.

The system uses both patient data structured by the data entry tool and the knowledge base of expert rules to provide advice to the end user. Specifically, the Toolbook client communicates patient data to the NEXPERT server. The server in turn uses these data to fire rules in its knowledge base which determine the patient's risk for pressure ulcer and indicate interventions based on this determination. This assessment, along with appropriate explanatory text read from the concept index database, is communicated back to the Toolbook client and displayed to the user. Thus, the output of the system consists of an assessment of risk and advice for reducing that risk. As additional guideline material for treating already extant pressure ulcers becomes available from AHCPR, we are incorporating this knowledge into the expert system knowledge base.

Further, we are encouraged by the satisfaction of our study population with the pulmonary artery catheter system and its intensely graphical user interface. The pressure ulcer domain offers many similar possibilities for graphical indexing. We have assembled a number of digitized images, including skin lesions and skin care products, and in a prototype system we have used these to help index the knowledge contained in the concept index.

As with the pulmonary artery catheter system, we plan to evaluate the impact on clinician knowledge once the system has been installed in a care unit. We also plan to evaluate its effect on patient outcome in terms of the nosocomial development of pressure ulcers.

CONCLUSIONS

We have found that the use of a graphical index to guideline knowledge permits easy and rapid access to expert knowledge. A pulmonary artery catheter waveform troubleshooting system indexed in this fashion has been accepted and found easy to use by a study population of nurses and physicians. Use of this system produced an improvement in domain knowledge in an experimental population when compared to a control group. We have extended this experience in graphical indexing through the use of a concept index in developing a computer-based system for prevention of pressure ulcers. This system permits structured entry of patient characteristics which then are processed by an expert system shell to assess risk for pressure ulcer development and to provide advice regarding risk reduction and treatment of existing pressure ulcers.

ACKNOWLEDGEMENTS

Dr. Jenders was supported by National Library of Medicine training grant 1-T15-LM07092 during the course of this work. He is currently affiliated with the Department of Medicine and the Center for Medical Informatics of Columbia University.

The authors also acknowledge support from the UMLS project, contract number 1-LM-1-3538, from the Agency for Health Care Policy and Research, grant 5 R18 HS06575 and from the National Library of Medicine, grant 5 R01 LM05200. We further appreciate a grant from Hewlett-Packard administered through Harvard University.

REFERENCES

[1]. Wyatt J. Use and sources of medical knowledge. Lancet 1991; 338:1368-1372.

[2]. Woolf SH. Practice guidelines: a new reality in medicine. III. Impact on patient care. Arch Int Med 1993; 153(23):2646-2655.

[3]. Panel for the Prediction and Prevention of Pressure Ulcers in Adults. Pressure ulcers in adults: prediction and prevention. Clinical practice guideline, number 3. AHCPR Publication No 92-0047. Rockville, MD: Agency for Health Care Policy and Research, Public Health Service, U.S. Department of Health and Human Services. May, 1992.

[4]. Oliver DE, Estey G, Ford P, Burke SM, Teplick RS, Zielstorff RD, Barnett GO. Computer-based access to patient care guidelines. In Miller RA ed. Proceedings of the Fourteenth Annual Symposium on Computer Applications in Medical Care. New York: IEEE Press, 1990; pp. 398-402.

[5]. Osheroff JA, Bankowitz RA. Physicians' use of computer software in answering clinical questions. Bull Med Lib Assoc 1993; 81(1):11-19.

[6]. Iberti TJ, Fischer EP, Leibowitz AB, Panacek EA, Silverstein JH, Albertson TE. A multicenter study of physicians' knowledge of the pulmonary artery catheter. JAMA 1990; 264(22):2928-2932.

[7]. Zielstorff RD, Barnett GO, Fitzmaurice JB, Oliver DE, Ford-Carleton P, Thompson BT, Estey G, Eccles R, Martin M, Jenders R. Providing clinicians with problem-based access to knowledge: troubleshooting pulmonary artery catheter waveforms. In Safran C ed. Proceedings of the Seventeenth Symposium on Computer Applications in Medical Care. New York: McGraw-Hill, 1994;

351-355.

[8]. Smith DM, Winsemius DK, Besdine RW. Pressure sores in the elderly: can this outcome be improved? J Gen Int Med 1991; 6:81-93.

[9]. Maklebust J, Sieggreen M. Pressure ulcers. Guidelines for prevention and nursing management. West Dundee, IL: S-N Publications, 1991.

Linking Knowledge-Based Tools with the Computer-Based Patient Record

Coverage List: A Provider-Patient Database Supporting Advanced Hospital Information Services

Frederick L. Hiltz, Ph.D. and Jonathan M. Teich, M.D., Ph.D.,
Department of Information Systems, Brigham and Women's Hospital, Boston, MA

ABSTRACT

We have developed a provider-patient database system, known as Coverage List, which maintains the associations between house staff and inpatients in a teaching hospital. Coverage List automatically links each patient to the proper resident when the patient is admitted, and updates the linkage whenever the resident coverage changes due to night or weekend coverage, physician illness, changes in clinical rotations, and other factors. Using this association, decision-support applications that detect significant clinical events can transmit them directly to the responsible resident. Sign-out and patient-review systems, which collect information on all of a physician's patients, always know the patients for whom that physician is responsible. Nurses who need to contact a physician about a patient issue always know which physician is covering that patient.

Coverage List also manages schedule entry and display for physicians, or for any other staff members. A physician can enter individual schedule changes, sign out her service and her pager for the day, and page consultants automatically without going through an operator. These functions support clinical practice directly and enhance the value of other clinical programs.

INTRODUCTION

Many hospital information systems applications share a need to know which physician is responsible for a patient at any given moment. Examples include:

- Physician order entry — to determine the primary physician responsible for co-signing orders;
- Sign-out systems and results review — to guide the physician through a review of all of her patients;
- Clinical event monitoring — so that significant events detected for a patient can be transmitted immediately to the physician;
- Medical records processing — to assign responsibility for discharge orders and summaries;
- Quality improvement programs — to determine provider-related variation in workup, treatment, and outcome [1].

Reliable, up-to-date provider-patient matching supports these services and enhances their utility. For example, when a physician reviews results or enters orders for her patients, the information system steps through a current list of patients to guide her. The computer provides a printed summary of all patients to assist her on rounds, or a consolidated to-do list to help manage tasks for the day. At the end of the day, she can use the list to review patients' progress and write sign-out notes for the night call doctor. Once she has signed out to him, his patient list shows his own patients plus the patients he is covering for her. Surveillance programs scan for abnormal lab results, new positive cultures, and other clinical events. They alert the current provider to exceptional occurrences by radio page, E-mail, and screen displays in the patient care areas.

The utility of an accurate provider-patient list extends past the computer functions themselves. Nurses and other staff members who need to page a physician about a patient-related issue often find that they have called the wrong one on the first try. Their jobs are made easier if they can easily find the name of the current provider.

Determining the identity of the responsible physician is not always a straightforward process [2]. In any hospital, particularly a teaching hospital, clinical responsibility for a patient can change frequently. The identity of the accountable physician at any given moment is subject to overnight and weekend coverage schedules, coverage for illness, changes in clinical rotation, and several other factors. For this reason, manually-maintained patient lists are often inaccurate.

We have developed a database and its suite of programs, called Coverage List, for the Brigham Integrated Computing System (BICS) [3,4], a comprehensive information system supporting a 751-bed teaching hospital. This suite consists of two main parts: a rule-based processor that handles the assignment of each inpatient to a provider who has current responsibility, and a schedule manager for entry, edit, and display of providers' jobs. Coverage List provides tools for easy entry, management and dissemination of schedules. These tools assist both providers and departmental administrators with these tasks.

The purposes of Coverage List are:

- to identify which provider to contact for any inpatient at any moment;
- to provide patient coverage and schedule information to other application programs as well as to people;
- above all, to be fast, friendly, and valuable enough to motivate busy physicians to use it.

OPERATION

Positions

The program's central concept is the *position* — one shift of one job. *Rotation positions* (or *primary positions*), which typically cover the patient Monday through Friday daytime, are so called because house officers often occupy them in rotations lasting weeks to months. Some, however, are permanently filled by faculty members or other attending physicians. *On-call positions*, typically nighttime and weekends, are usually occupied by a different provider each day. A *schedule* is a set of assignments of providers to positions.

The program does not associate patients directly with providers. Instead, it assigns each patient to a position (Figure 1), whose occupant takes calls about the patient. This principle is the key to separating patient-related matters like admission, discharge, and transfer from provider-related matters of rotation, sign-out, and temporary coverage. Patient coverage is a set of assignments of patients to positions; the patient and the provider meet only at the position.

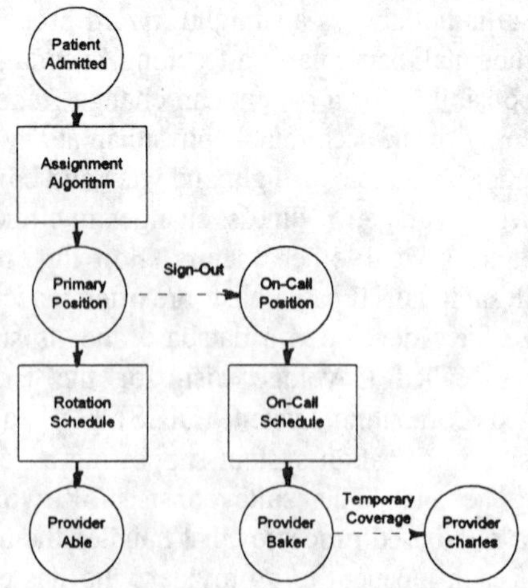

Figure 1. Assignment of patients using Coverage List.

A typical patient assignment in the cardiology service of the medicine department illustrates the concept: On admission the program assigns primary responsibility for a patient to the position "CCU Intern #2", according to the department's rules for assignment of new patients. During the day, calls go to Dr. Able, the scheduled occupant of that position. When Dr. Able signs out for the day (or at a predetermined time, if no sign-out occurs), Coverage List marks his position as signed out to the "CCU On Call Intern" position. The occupant of that position for tonight, Dr. Baker, now receives the calls and alerts. When Dr. Baker asks for a patient list or reviews her patients' current orders, she sees her own patients, plus all patients assigned to the positions that are signed out to her on-call position.

If Dr. Baker is called away from the hospital for personal illness or family emergency, she needs to ask her associate, Dr. Charles, to cover her assignments. She uses Coverage List's "Temporary Coverage" option to enter Dr. Charles' name into the database. From then on, the program diverts her patient list and her patient-related calls to him; optionally, she can forward all of her other radio pages as well. When a nurse asks who is covering this patient, Dr. Charles' name and pager number appear, followed by the names of Dr. Baker and Dr. Able with explanatory messages indicating the current chain of sign-outs. The name of the patient's attending physician, and any other clinicians concerned with the patient, are also displayed (Figure 2):

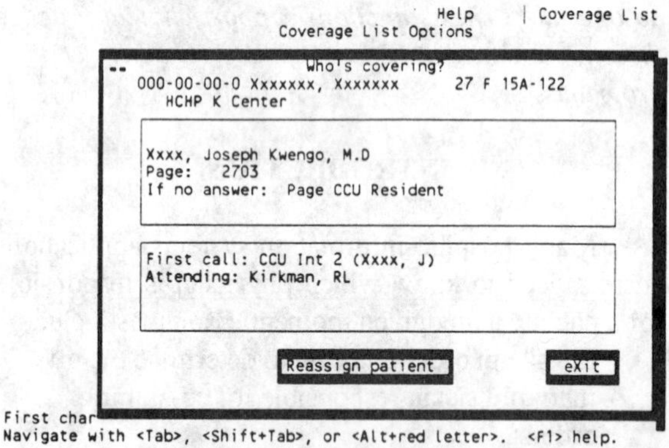

Figure 2. The "Who's covering this patient?" screen.

At the end of the month, the interns rotate to new services. Dr. Denton is now scheduled into the "CCU Intern #2" position, assuming primary responsibility for all of Dr. Able's former patients from this position.

DATABASE DESIGN

A small hierarchical database of seven parts supports the coverage list.

Department structure. This contains the names of the services and teams in each clinical department.

Providers. Linked to the BICS employee database, these records contain names, page numbers, and related information. They also indicate whether a provider is being temporarily covered by another due to illness, vacation or other cause.

Provider lists collect the names of providers into lists of faculty, attendings, residents, etc. in each department. Each position can be filled only by providers on certain lists associated with the position. This improves the speed and accuracy of entering schedules — only the first few letters of a name need be typed to identify a provider.

Positions. These attributes define a position (Figure 3):

- Its name.
- Its department, service, and team.
- Its type: rotation or on-call.
- Whether patients may be assigned to it for primary responsibility.
- Whether it appears on the hospital's consultants call list.
- Which actual patients are now assigned to it for primary responsibility.
- The provider lists that may be used to fill the position.
- Default sign-in and sign-out times for weekdays and for weekends.
- To what position it normally signs out.
- To what position it has actually signed out (if any), and when the sign-out is due to end.

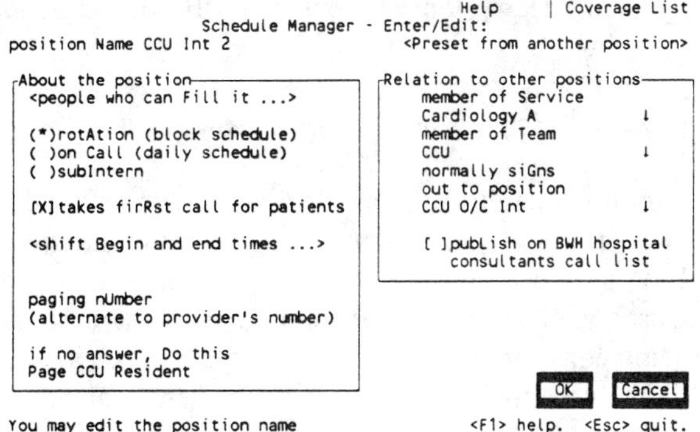

Figure 3. Screen describing a position.

Schedules are made from assignments that place one provider in one position (either rotation or on-call) from a starting date to an ending date. The universe of all assignments in Coverage List comprises a master schedule, far too large to examine or work on directly. Schedules are views of the master schedule. Each schedule contains a subset of positions and dates for easy viewing and editing. Multiple views of the same assignments are often used for convenience.

Patient responsibility. First call responsibility links each patient with exactly one position. Calls go to the last provider found in this sequence (See also figure 1):

1. The occupant of the primary position;
2. When this position is signed out, the occupant of the position to which signed out, iterated over a chain of sign-outs if necessary;
3. Whoever, if anyone, is temporarily covering for the provider found in 1) or 2), iterated over a chain of temporary coverage if necessary.

Inverted indexes. Outnumbering the base files 23 to 11, indexes provide rapid access to data in forms convenient for applications, for example, alphabetic lists of providers to fill a position.

FUNCTIONAL DESIGN

Schedule management

A schedule manager (usually a secretary or administrator) in each department administers the coverage list database, mostly by creating and modifying schedules. A table tool similar to a spreadsheet makes this task faster and easier than entering schedules on paper. The tool checks for conflicting assignments and distributes changes throughout the institution.

Schedule managers also maintain their departments' lists of providers, and they occasionally define new positions. Specific Coverage List functions perform these tasks.

User functions

Although the coverage list deals internally with positions and their occupants, it hides this concept from its users. Persons sign out to other persons, transfer patients to other persons, and cover for other persons.

The full-screen user interface (Figures 2, 3, and 4) is displayed with characters, not full graphics, but it works like Microsoft Windows™ to present the coverage list functions in a familiar environment.

Service sign-out is used by the primary physician at the end of the day to transfer responsibility for her patients to the on-call physician. As a fail-safe measure, if the departing doctor fails to use this function, Coverage List still assigns the patients to the on-call position at a designated time. As an incentive for physicians to use this function, the doctor can use this screen to change her radio page status to "out of hospital" without the need to call a telephone operator. She can also have the computer page the on-call doctor, so the two can meet to discuss patient issues. Additionally, the BICS Inpatient Sign-Out system [5], which is widely used to communicate patient status and data to the on-call provider, has a button to open this screen.

The primary physician can use the **Sign In** function to reactivate her pager and reclaim her patients when she returns to the hospital. Sign-in also occurs automatically at a designated time. If she does not do this explicitly, the program does it for her at the time she gave when signing out (Figure 4).

Physicians sign out about 1000 times per month and sign in about 20 times per month.

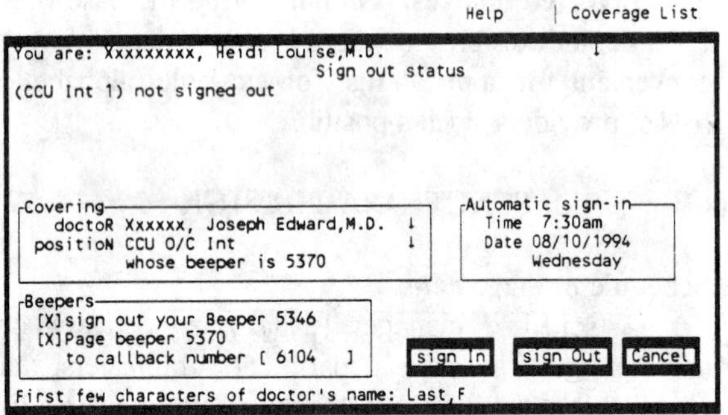

Figure 4. Service Sign-Out

View/Edit Patient List. The physician can view and print a list of those patients for whom he has first call responsibility and, when on call, those whom other providers have signed out to him. Team lists combine the patient lists of all providers on a care team, showing which physician is responsible for each patient. Patient rosters embellish the team list with admitting diagnoses and procedures from the computer, and notes added by members of the teams.

Sometimes, patients are reassigned arbitrarily to a different physician from the one determined by the department's rules. For example, a ward resident may determine that the intern who is supposed to receive a new patient has too many patients already, so the patient is assigned to another intern. "Add" and "Reassign" buttons on the Patient List screen allow Coverage List to keep track of these discretionary reassignments.

The **"Who's covering?"** function displays the physician responsible right now, her radio page number, whom to page if she does not answer, and the chain of sign-outs and temporary coverage back to the provider primarily assigned to the patient. Because of the popularity of this function, the name of the currently responsible physician now also appears at all times on the main patient-lookup screen. A "Who's on call?" screen shows names and page numbers of consultants and others on call right now, and offers to page them; this reduces the number of calls to the telephone operators.

View/Edit Your Schedule Assignments. Each physician can view or print his personal schedule, assembled from the universe of all schedule assignments. If a physician wishes to trade an on-call assignment with another physician, a parallel display box appears and shows the other physician's schedule. By marking one assignment in each physician's list and pressing a button, the assignments are changed in the database. The program warns of resulting conflicts and sends a confirming E-mail note to the parties involved and to the department's schedule manager.

Display Schedules. Anyone can display or print a department's schedules in a tabular format. One of the benefits of Coverage List is that a schedule change made at any workstation is immediately available at any other location in the hospital. This is in contrast to paper schedules, where a change would need to be made in every location where the paper schedule is posted.

PATIENT ASSIGNMENT ALGORITHMS

When a patient is admitted or transferred, departments assign the primary provider in many different ways: according to the patient's room, the team, the attending physician, the junior physician on the operating team, the resident on call tonight, and sometimes by combinations of these items. Some departments do not codify the process; the chief resident makes the assignments for each patient individually.

When a department establishes or changes its rules for assigning patients, a programmer encodes the rules in the M programming language and encapsulates the code into "methods" for inclusion in the database, either directly or by reference. The hospital admissions program sends admissions, transfers, and discharges to these patient-assignment "objects," which assign primary responsibility using the rules contained in the method. The patient appears on a physician's list without manual entry.

As noted, patients are sometimes assigned outside the rules for load-balancing and other needs. The

"Add" and "Reassign" buttons present on several screens adjust Coverage List's assignments as needed. About 8% of inpatients are reassigned this way during their stay.

USAGE

Clinicians' schedules and patient assignments are valuable to many other applications, from the critical (paging the right physician for a life-threatening lab result) to the mundane (determining who gets cafeteria vouchers for night call duty). A doctor can instruct the results-reporting system to step through her patient list or the team's patient list, reducing errors of omission. The BICS physician order entry system [6] optionally displays a physician's patient list, which not only allows quick access to any patient's orders but also provides an instant display of which patients need renewals or co-signatures, and which have pending alerts.

When signing out at the computer, physicians examine and edit patient summaries, guided by the same patient list, for the on-call physician's use [5,7]. Data suggests that these sign-out notes have reduced the increased risk of adverse events found in cross-covered patients [8]. The new BICS event-processing engine contains agents that monitor significant clinical events and send E-mail or radio pages to the appropriate covering physician [9].

Several other programs make use of Coverage List functions. During sign-out, the program sends changes in radio page status through a link to the hospital paging system. The new status tells any future caller not only that the doctor is signed out, but which doctor is now covering the service. Coverage List supplies the medical records department with a list of clinicians who worked with each patient, to assist the medical records staff in completing their records and chart analysis.

CONCLUSIONS

Usage of Coverage List is high: BICS users run programs from its menu an average of 300 times per day. Other applications call on its functions 400 times per day. Most of the hospital's clinical departments now use the schedule management functions. The ability of providers to modify their own schedules is popular with clinicians and administrators alike. Job schedules are valuable for non-providers as well. One department has completely replaced the in-house mailing of paper schedules with locally printed, up-to-date schedules from the computer.

We have found Coverage List to be a well-accepted and useful adjunct to the BICS system. It eases the job of secretaries who enter schedules, telephone operators who take calls for primary physicians and consultants, nurses and others who need to contact a patient's physician, and physicians who want to keep their patient lists up-to-date. The automatic patient list minimizes data entry by physicians, who need only enter exceptions to the program's assignment of primary responsibility for patients, thus lowering one barrier to acceptance of the HIS. Although work must be done by the programmer to construct the patient assignment algorithms for each department, programmer maintenance is low once these have been encoded.

References

[1]. G. Kuperman, B. James, J. Jacobsen, R. Gardner, "Continuous Quality Improvement Applied to Medical Care: Experiences at LDS Hospital," Med. Decis. Making **11**(4), 1991, pp. S60-65.

[2]. C. Kahn, "Computer-Aided Management of Residents' On-Call and Vacation Schedules," Am. J. Roentgenol. **154**(3), 1990, pp. 641-643.

[3]. H. Bleich, C. Safran, W. Slack, "Departmental and Laboratory Computing in Two Hospitals," MD Computing **6**, 1989, pp. 149-155.

[4]. J. Glaser, R. Beckley, P. Roberts, J. Marra, F. Hiltz, J. Hurley, "A Very Large PC LAN as the Basis for a Hospital Information System," J. Med. Syst. **15**, 1991, pp.133-137.

[5]. J. Teich, D. Potter, L. Petersen, T Brennan, "Sign-Out: a Continuous Integrated Inpatient Summary for Primary and Covering Physicians," Proc. AMIA Conference, 1994, p.93 (abstract).

[6]. J. Teich, C. Spurr, S. Flammini, J. Schmiz, R. Beckley, J. Hurley, M. Aranow, J. Glaser, "Response to a Trial of Physician-Based Inpatient Order Entry," Proc. SCAMC **17,** 1993, pp. 316-320.

[7]. R. Ram, B. Block, "Signing Out Patients for Off-Hours Coverage: Comparison of Manual and Computer-Aided Methods," Proc. SCAMC **16**, 1992, pp. 114-118.

[8]. L. Petersen, E. Orav, A. O'Neil, J. Teich, T. Brennan, "House Staff Adverse Event Self-Reporting Identifies Quality Problem, Then Documents Results of an Intervention," J. Gen. Int. Med., 1994, in press.

[9]. J. Glaser, J. Teich, G. Kuperman, "The Future of Clinical Information Systems: One Hospital's Perspective," Topics in Healthcare Info. Mgmt. *14* (1), 1993, pp.12-24.

A Comprehensive Computerized Patient Record with Automated Linkage to QMR

Charles R. Welford, M.D.
University of Illinois College of Medicine, Rockford, IL
President, Welford Medical Computing, Inc.

ABSTRACT

The author has developed comprehensive computerized charting software, Dr. Welford's Chart Notes Program, that interprets each portion of a patient record for the 4,653 QMR Findings and exports the identified Findings to a file that can be imported by QMR for immediate case analysis. The QMR Link utilizes a hierarchical Vocabulary System composed of approximately 20,000 terms and a "fuzzy logic" that identifies similar and implicit concepts as well as exact matches to QMR Findings. This system thereby makes it much quicker and easier to utilize QMR in evaluating a patient's illness.

INTRODUCTION

One of the most important capabilities of a computerized patient record is its ability to interface with other clinical software. Such interfacing is challenging because of differences in vocabularies among various programs.

QMR (Quick Medical Reference, Camdat Corporation) [1] is a program that generates a differential diagnosis after the user has entered a list of the patient's Findings (history elements, physical findings, and test results). Version 2.2 contains 4,653 different Findings.

Previous Work

Van Ginneken et. al. [2] mapped exact vocabulary matches in a structured computer-based patient record to a subset of QMR Findings that relate solely to auscultation of the heart. Shiffman et. al. [3] developed a speaker-independent natural language continuous speech recognition interface to 518 physical examination Findings in QMR. Kaplan [4] developed an interface to AI/Rheum that interactively responded to entry of the patient's chief complaints. Bouhaddou et al. [5] entered manually extracted items from patient records into Iliad for preauthorization of three surgical procedures. Feldman et. al. [6] evaluated free-text medical records of patients with ten diseases to identify core elements present in DXplain, QMR, and Iliad.

Dr. Welford's Chart Notes Program [7,8,9,10,11,12] is a comprehensive computerized patient record that allows the user to create both structured and free-text notes. It assists the user in recording a broad range of information about each patient, such as the patient's current and past history, physical examination, allergies, medications, diagnoses, and laboratory results, and incorporates a large number of other integrated features. Running on IBM-compatible DOS-based microcomputers, it is licensed to over 200 users throughout the United States and abroad. Using the program's accelerated text entry features, the average 323-word history and physical takes 149 ± 115 seconds to enter[13].

The author has developed QMR Link, a feature that interprets the information already stored in the patient record in Dr. Welford's Chart Notes Program and identifies virtually all of the QMR Findings described in the record. QMR Link exports the extracted information to a file that can then be imported by QMR (for Windows or DOS) for immediate case analysis.

METHODS

Vocabulary System

The program's hierarchical Vocabulary System recognizes over 13,000 elemental words and phrases and thousands of additional phrase patterns, including terms with single and multiple component meanings. Within each category, terms are organized in a tree-like structure with four layers of granularity. The user can extend this Program Vocabulary by adding both synonyms to existing terms and entirely new terms and classes of terms. The program also has a Vocabulary Updater that reconciles differences between the User-defined Vocabulary and Program Vocabulary when the Program Vocabulary is updated each quarter.

0195-4210/94/$5.00 © 1994 AMIA, Inc.

In creating QMR Link, the author added thousands of terms to the Vocabulary to enable the program to identify essentially all of the concepts implicit in the 4,653 QMR Findings. The Vocabulary includes common medical abbreviations, formal and informal medical terminology, eponyms, generic and brand names of medications, and a host of other medical and non-medical terms.

Parser

The program directs text to the QMR Link Parser sentence by sentence from the various portions of the patient record that have been selected by the user. The Parser examines the entire Vocabulary to assign concept numbers to each word and phrase in each sentence. It analyzes where clauses begin and end and applies various rules to determine where to distribute negation. It recognizes that "not just" and "not only" do not negate the item they precede, and similar subtleties of language.

After the sentence evaluation, the Parser identifies all of the QMR Findings that partially or completely match the concepts expressed in the sentence. It utilizes the hierarchical structure of the Vocabulary System to make inferences within classes. For example, a sentence stating that a patient is on phenobarbital triggers the QMR Finding regarding previous administration of a barbiturate, since phenobarbital belongs to the class of barbiturate drugs. The Parser also utilizes a "fuzzy logic" that allows it to identify more implicit information. For example, a sentence stating that a patient is producing sputum generates QMR Findings regarding cough, even though "cough" (a symptom) and "sputum" (a bodily substance) are not stored in the Vocabulary in the same category or class. The Parser links these together and thus "understands" that a patient producing sputum is implicitly having a cough.

The Parser adjusts the questions presented to the user based upon the user's previous responses. For example, a user who indicates that the patient has chest pain is asked more specific questions about the chest pain to determine which QMR Findings related to chest pain are present. If the user indicates that the patient lacks chest pain, the more specific chest pain questions are not generated. The Parser avoids posing questions that are mutually exclusive and thus could not be present in the patient simultaneously. The Parser also avoids asking the user the same question twice, further saving the user time.

The Parser adjusts some numeric quantities before evaluating their meaning. For example, a sentence stating that the leukocyte count is 15.2 is interpreted in the same manner as a sentence stating that the count is 15,200 and generates the QMR Finding, "WBC 14000 to 30000".

The Parser primarily recognizes Findings which are declared to be present in the patient, but it also acknowledges the absence of a number of Findings when they are declared not to be present.

Performance Analysis

Hardware. QMR Link performance was tested on an IBM 755C 486/DX4 notebook computer.
Software. QMR Link was tested using Dr. Welford's Chart Notes Program version 2.7B and QMR for DOS version 2.2. Statistical analysis was performed using SPSS for Windows Release 5.0.
Performance Tests. The author, a general internist, assembled the initial hospital admission notes from 25 of his patients who presented with uncertain diagnoses and were eventually diagnosed definitively. Five patients whose final diagnoses were not in the QMR database were then excluded. A wide variety of internal medicine cases were used, including common (acute myocardial infarction, deep vein thrombosis) and uncommon (leptospirosis, left atrial myxoma) diseases. The history, physical, and test results in each patient's admission note stored in Dr. Welford's Chart Notes Program were used, except that any definitive test result mentioned in the note was removed. The author manually entered Findings into QMR based on each note, recording the time elapsed, the number of Findings entered, and the rank and score within QMR of the patient's actual diagnosis after Case Analysis. The author then used QMR Link on the same notes, recording the same parameters. Cases in which QMR did not rank the correct diagnosis were given scores of 0.
Statistical analysis. Elapsed times, numbers of Findings generated, and QMR scores were

compared using two-tailed t-tests for paired samples. QMR ranks were analyzed using Wilcoxon matched-pairs signed-ranks test.

RESULTS

User Interface

The QMR Link User Interface is an integral part of the program's menu system. QMR Link Menu choices include Append file, Create file, Options, and Run QMR.

Options. The Options screen allows the user to specify which portions of the patient's record to evaluate for export to QMR. (Figure 1). The user

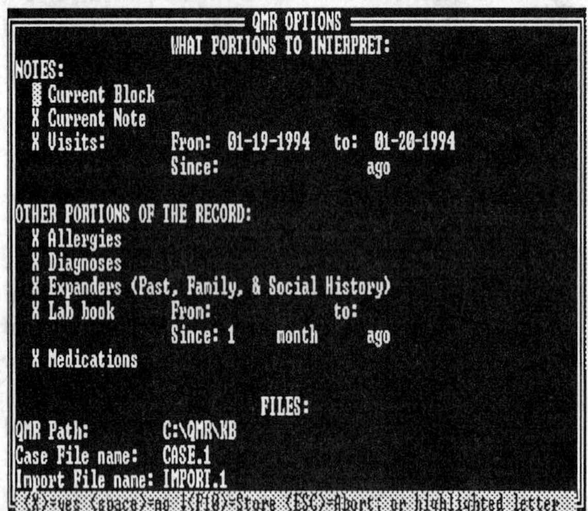

Figure 1. QMR Options

can specify a particular starting date for the patient's illness or an interval backward from today's date. The user can choose to export the Findings both directly to QMR and also to a "case file" that records the information in a different format that can be imported by other programs (such as a database program). The user can skip setting the Options and use the default or previously stored settings.

Next, the user generally chooses Create file, which activates the Parser to examine the portions of the patient record specified in the Options. As the Parser works, it presents two types of questions interactively to the user: Verifications and Clarifications.

Verifications. Verifications are questions that are generated when there is a virtually identical match between the text in the patient's record and a QMR Finding (Figure 2). The user is shown the Finding and asked to verify that this patient indeed has this Finding before sending it to the file. The user at this point can choose Yes to send the Finding, No to not send the Finding, Change to NOT Present to send the negation of the Finding , See Sentence to view the sentence upon which the question was based, and Abort to stop the QMR Link process altogether.

QMR LINK VERIFICATION

Lymph Node(s) Enlarged

Add this QMR Finding to file?

Yes, No, Change to NOT present, See sentence, or Abort?

Press <Y>,<N>,<C>,<A>,<S>, or <ESC>

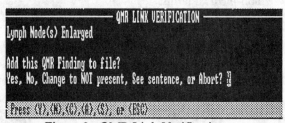

Figure 2. QMR Link Verification

Clarifications. Clarifications are questions that are generated when the Parser identifies a close but not identical match between the information contained in the patient record and one or more QMR Findings (Figure 3).

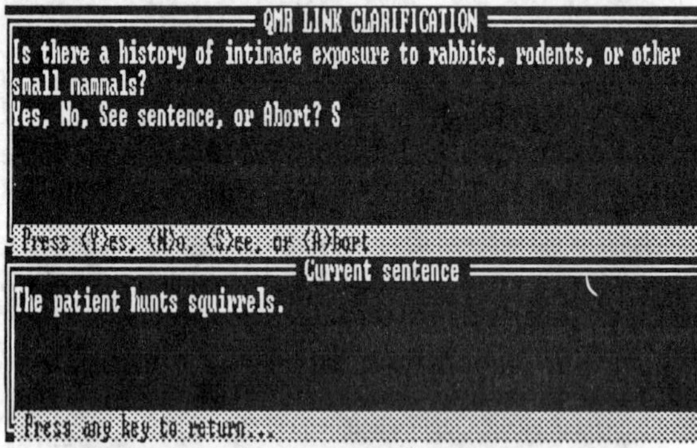

Figure 3. QMR Link Clarification

Clarifications are generated when the user's statements are inherently ambiguous, as well as when the user's statements are unambiguous but insufficiently specific to determine which QMR Findings are present in the patient. For example, if the user's statement indicates that the patient has diarrhea (without further modification), QMR Link asks Clarifications regarding whether the diarrhea is acute, chronic, profuse and watery, and intermittent, each of which is a separate QMR Finding. As with Verifications, the user can answer Yes, No, See Sentence, or Abort.

Running on an 80486 microprocessor, the program generates Clarifications and Verifications almost without pause, so that the user does not have to spend significant time waiting between questions for the next one to be generated.

The user can choose Append file to add more Findings to a QMR export file that had previously been created. The Run QMR menu choice causes the program to terminate but stay resident as it jumps to QMR. Upon leaving QMR, the user is returned to Dr. Welford's Chart Notes Program in the previous location.

QMR Use

Inside QMR for DOS, choosing Utility\Import imports the file created by QMR Link. The user can then choose Case\View to verify the accuracy of the Findings that were imported and edit the list further if necessary. Case\Analyze Case can then be activated in order to generate a differential diagnosis. In QMR for Windows, File\Open achieves all three of these steps. The user is spared the necessity of using the QMR Term Completer to enter those Findings already entered into the patient record, but can use the Term Completer to enter any additional Findings that were not stated in the patient record.

Performance Analysis

The 20 patient records had a mean length of 2992±705 characters. The author entered a mean of 17.8 Findings per case into the QMR Term Completer, in a mean of 337.7 seconds. QMR Link generated a mean of 43.4 Findings from the identical free text in a mean of 182.8 seconds. (Of this time, a mean of 30.7 seconds was taken by QMR Link to generate questions, and the remaining 152.1 seconds was the time required by the author to respond to these questions.) QMR Link thus generated Findings about 4.5 times faster than using the Term Completer manually. The rank and score of the correct diagnosis after Case Analysis were not significantly different using each method. (Tables 1 and 2).

In two cases, QMR did not present the correct diagnosis using either method. One was a patient with an atypical presentation of a left atrial myxoma. Another was a patient with a gastric ulcer who presented with prolonged exertional chest pain unrelieved by antacids. Both methods ranked acute myocardial infarction as the most likely diagnosis, which actually fit the patient's Findings better than the ultimate diagnosis. In a third patient with right colon angiodysplasia, QMR Link ranked this diagnosis #13 and manual entry did not rank the diagnosis at all. In a fourth patient with rheumatoid arthritis and a target diagnosis of hypervitaminosis D, manual entry ranked hypervitaminosis D as #6, whereas QMR Link correctly ranked rheumatoid arthritis as #1 but failed to rank hypervitaminosis D (and was counted as a failure to rank the target diagnosis).

	Findings	Time (secs)	Score correct diagnosis
QMR Link	**43.4±6.1 (S.D.)**	**182.8 ±53.2**	**144.6 ±99.1**
Manual entry	**17.8±4.7**	**337.7 ±67.5**	**149.7 ±101.0**
P	**<0.01**	**<0.01**	**0.682 (NS)**

Table 1: QMR Link vs. Manual Data Entry

	Among top 5	Below 5 on list	Not on list
QMR Link	65%	20%	15%
Manual entry	60%	25%	15%

Table 2: Rank location of correct diagnosis (P=0.477)

DISCUSSION

The full potential of a computerized patient record lies in its ability to extend the physician's ability to deliver high-quality care by providing tools that perform useful clinical functions. These tools often require interfacing the patient record with other clinical software, such as QMR.

QMR Link saves the user considerable time in utilizing QMR. By presenting virtually all of the relevant QMR Findings contained in the patient record as simple yes or no questions, the user can create a QMR case file much more quickly and completely than by using the QMR Term Completer. Thus, the user is not spending time typing statements into the Term Completer that were just entered into the patient record. Furthermore, the physician can enter the patient note as free text, and does not need the high degree of familiarity with QMR Findings necessary to correctly identify and enter the same Findings using the Term Completer.

The author is an experienced QMR user and types at 60 words/minute. Inexperienced QMR users or slower typists might take longer than 6 minutes to enter a case into QMR using the Term Completer. On the other hand, using QMR Link only requires that the user press the "Y", "N", or "C" keys in response to a series of questions, so that the time necessary to use QMR Link is not likely to exceed 3 minutes on a 3000-character note. Of course, users may spend additional time using other QMR features to refine the diagnosis once the case has been initially entered.

QMR Link has certain opportunities for further development. QMR Link evaluates laboratory results using only the units implicit in QMR's own Findings. For example, QMR has a set of Findings describing blood glucoses in mg/dl. If the user of Dr. Welford's Chart Notes Program refers to blood glucoses in some other system of units, QMR Link does not currently translate the number into the equivalent number of mg/dl before exporting the Finding. QMR Link does not parse for seven of the 4,653 QMR Findings. Although QMR Link is limited to interfacing with QMR's vocabulary, the same principles could be applied to mapping to other applications, such as the UMLS Metathesaurus. The performance analysis could be improved by using a larger number of randomly selected cases and a broad range of users.

The linkage between Dr. Welford's Chart Notes Program and QMR is an example of how free text can be successfully interpreted and transferred between two different programs to perform a very useful function that enhances the quality of patient care. Such applications make computerized patient records increasingly essential in providing outstanding health care.

ACKNOWLEDGMENTS

The author wishes to thank Ms. Andrea Welford for her invaluable assistance with this project, Ms. Andrea Doughty for statistical analysis, and all of the users who have contributed many suggestions in the program's development.

References

[1] Miller RA, Masarie FE: Quick Medical Reference (QMR): A Microcomputer-Based Diagnostic Decision-Support System for General Internal Medicine. Proc Annu Symp Comput Appl Med Care 1990;986-988.

[2] van Ginneken AM, Liem EB, Moorman PW: Integrating QMR with a Computer-Based Patient Record. Proc Annu Symp Comput Appl Med Care 1993;98-102.

[3] Shiffman S, Lane CD, Johnson KB, Fagan LM: The Integration of a Continuous-speech-recognition System with the QMR Diagnostic Program. Proc Annu Symp Comput Appl Med Care 1992;767-771.

[4] Kaplan RS: AI/Consult: A Prototype Directed History System Based Upon the AI/Rheum Knowledge Base. Proc Annu Symp Comput Appl Med Care 1991;639-643.

[5] Bouhaddou O, Frucci L, Cofrin K et al: Implementation of Practice Guidelines in a Clinical Setting using a Computerized Knowledge Base (Iliad). Proc Annu Symp Comput Appl Med Care 1993;258-262.

[6] Feldman MJ, Barnett GO, Morgan MM: The Sensitivity of Medical Diagnostic Decision-Support Knowledge Bases in Delineating Appropriate Terms to Document in the Medical Record. Proc Annu Symp Comput Appl Med Care 1991;258-262.

[7] Welford CR: Comprehensive Computerized Patient Record-Keeping Using Real-Time Natural Language Text Interpretation and Physician Quality Reminders. 1993 Spring Congress, AMIA. 1993;115.

[8] Berman AM: Dr. Welford's Chart Notes Program version 2.02. Med Software Rev 1992;1:5-6.

[9] Fox GN: Dr. Welford's Chart Notes Program, version 2.13 (4/92). J Fam Practice 1993;36:462.

[10] Burger M: Dr. Welford's Chart Notes Program. Arch Fam Med 1993;2:886-887.

[11] Kahn GS, Lynch T: Dr. Welford's Chart Notes. M.D. Computing 1994;11(2)100-106.

[12] Burger M: Four for Charts. Med Software Rev 1994;3(6):1-5.

[13] Welford CR: Comparison of Manual and Computerized Text Entry and Data Retrieval using Dr. Welford's Chart Notes Program. Submitted to CPRI 1992.

Construction of a Literature Database and its Use to Provide Probabilities for Decision-Analytic Models of Thrombolytic Therapy

John F. Murphy, M.D.,[1] Nilesh L. Jain, M.S.,[2,3] Calixto A. Romero, Jr., M.D.,[1] and Michael G. Kahn, M.D., Ph.D.[2]
[1]Cardiovascular Division; [2]Division of Medical Informatics; [3]Department of Computer Science; Washington University School of Medicine, St. Louis MO 63110

Probabilities for decision-analytic models are routinely obtained from the medical literature. This study describes development and use of a literature database to facilitate obtaining probabilities for decision-analytic models of thrombolytic therapy for acute myocardial infarction. Implementation demonstrates the concept of a literature database to be both feasible and effective. Specific difficulties encountered in the evaluation of continuous variables, the potential storage of actual probabilities, and the advantage for easy growth with the literature are discussed.

INTRODUCTION

The ability to develop a complete decision-analytic model and the merit that will be assigned to its recommendations rests heavily on the data used to provide probabilities for the model. Medical experts can be consulted to estimate the probabilities, but there are numerous pitfalls with this approach, including representativeness and the availability heuristic [1]. Probabilities for decision analysis are therefore usually obtained from the medical literature. However, extracting the required probabilities from the literature is a difficult and laborious task. No one source can appropriately include all the references required to attain the knowledge base necessary to develop the appropriate model and to furnish all the needed probabilities. A combination of electronic searches on MEDLINE and manual searches of bibliographies from papers and textbooks is necessary [2]. Once all the appropriate papers have been located, keeping track of all the clinical variables and the status of each variable in every paper quickly becomes unwieldy as the number of papers increases.

Precedent for a literature database to facilitate storage and retrieval of probabilities for decision-analytic models does not exist. Morris *et al.* have constructed a clinical trials database to support meta-analyses [3]. As discussed later it is a step forward but cannot serve an additional purpose of supporting decision analysis.

This study describes development of a literature database to provide appropriate clinical information on thrombolytic therapy for treatment of acute myocardial infarction. The database tabulates the papers so that papers pertaining to any clinical variable or outcome can easily be retrieved. The database is being used to provide information for decision-analytic models used to resolve current controversies in thrombolytic therapy for acute myocardial infarction. Several insights were gained from this process. The ability of the database to provide probabilities is directly dependent on the type of clinical variable to be evaluated in the decision-analytic model. Storage of actual probabilities would require assessment of each paper by database developers. The literature database is a way of organizing a specialized body of literature that allows physicians to master their paper collections with minimal effort. These issues and other specific advantages and disadvantages of the literature database are discussed.

LITERATURE DATABASE

There are over sixty clinical variables and outcomes that can influence the decision to administer thrombolytic therapy for acute myocardial infarction. Papers on thrombolytic therapy were assembled from MEDLINE in both broad searches and searches focused on individual variables. Manual searches of the bibliographies from these papers and from standard cardiology textbook bibliographies were used to increase the number of papers collected.

A database was then created with a data schema consisting of two tables. The first table stored information about every variable in every paper as a boolean value. Clinical variables included information on demographics, physical exam, myocardial infarction characteristics, medications, and outcomes. Papers that pertained directly to thrombolytic therapy and at least one variable were entered into this table. Citation information was recorded in separate text fields. The second table provided background papers for any

Author	GUSTO
Title	International randomized trial comparing four TL strategies for AMI
Year pubshed	1993
Journal	N Engl J Med
Citation	329:673-82

PATIENT CHARACTERISTICS

	Yes	No
Pt age	◉ Yes	○ No
Pt sex	◉ Yes	○ No
HTN	◉ Yes	○ No
Cholesterol	○ Yes	◉ No
diabetes	◉ Yes	○ No
other heart dis	○ Yes	◉ No
Prior MI	◉ Yes	○ No
Tobacco	◉ Yes	○ No
fibrinogen	○ Yes	◉ No
Prior CABG	◉ Yes	○ No
Prior PTCA	○ Yes	◉ No
Prior Cath	○ Yes	◉ No
Prior thromboly	◉ Yes	○ No
Recent surgery	◉ Yes	○ No
Peripheral vasc	○ Yes	◉ No
prior CHF	○ Yes	◉ No

	Yes	No
trauma	◉ Yes	○ No
CPR	○ Yes	◉ No
bleeding diathe	○ Yes	◉ No
GI GU bleeding	◉ Yes	○ No
intracranial tu	○ Yes	◉ No
Prior CVA	◉ Yes	○ No
prior CVA inclu	○ Yes	◉ No

PHYSICAL EXAM

	Yes	No
pulse rate	◉ Yes	○ No
weight	○ Yes	◉ No
blood pressure	◉ Yes	○ No
CHF Killip	○ Yes	◉ No
Mitral regurg	○ Yes	◉ No
cardiogenic sho	○ Yes	◉ No

Figure 1: View of one of the screens used for data entry. Shown at the top are the fields for the citation, and at the bottom is a partial list of the boolean clinical variables used for data entry.

given variable. These papers had supplemental medical knowledge to model the clinical situation and to represent the consequences of not giving thrombolytic therapy. These papers did not have any information about thrombolytic therapy, and hence were designated as background papers. These references were listed as citations and one text field for a one-word subject and were not further indexed. Actual probabilities were not stored in the database. The database was built using a commercial relational database, 4th Dimension (ACI US, Inc., Cupertino, CA).

Data entry was straightforward. Citation information of each paper was entered, then the presence of a clinical variable was recorded as the boolean value for that variable. The first data-entry screen is in Figure 1; it contains almost half of the boolean clinical variables stored for every paper and displays actual information from a clinical trial publication.

Papers were then retrieved by selecting any single variable or a combination of clinical variables, including basic citation information. For example, all papers with information on streptokinase, heparin, and mortality can be selected. The search for conditional probabilities can also easily be narrowed. For example, citations for papers which dealt with both location of infarct and post-thrombolytic ejection fraction can be retrieved; a manual search of the papers is then necessary to see if the ejection fraction outcomes are stratified by location of infarct.

DATABASE USE TO SUPPORT A DECISION-ANALYTIC MODEL

A total of 447 key publications have been collected and entered into the database thus far. There are 293 which directly pertain to thrombolytic therapy, and 154 which provide background information.

The database was then used to extract probabilities from the literature for decision-analytic models. The first decision-analytic model developed using the database sought to find the threshold of blood pressure above which thrombolytic therapy should be withheld because the risk of a hemorrhagic stroke and concomitant morbidity and mortality outweighed the benefit of decreased cardiac mortality. For all clinical events, the model required a probability of an event after thrombolytic therapy and the probability of the same event in patients not treated with thrombolytic therapy.

Papers were retrieved using the blood pressure, post-thrombolytic stroke, post-thrombolytic hemorrhage, and mortality variables. There were 9 background papers on hypertension and stroke. There were 107 papers which contained blood pressures. The blood pressures were all reported in very different fashions. One method was to report the mean of a population but not stratify the mortality [4]. Another method was to report ranges only, usually in the form of an upper boundary for exclusion criteria [5]. Some studies did some stratification with broad intervals and unspecified ranges for the first and last intervals [6]. No publications specifically addressed the question of what is the probability of a hemorrhagic stroke at a given specific blood pressure. The only way to combine these pressures to develop probabilities was to combine studies using exclusion criteria. For example, studies with patients with systolic blood pressures less than 200 mm Hg could be pooled and the needed probabilities extracted. The patient population and protocol used were not the same across studies, but the acute MI population entered into studies was relatively homogeneous with regard to risk factors for hemorrhagic stroke, such as female sex: roughly 80% of patients enrolled in virtually every study were male. A decision-analytic model evaluating patients with systolic blood pressure less than 200 mm Hg found they should receive thrombolytic therapy.

However, finding decision-analytic support for a recommendation to give thrombolytic therapy to this group as a whole will not provide adequate basis for the recommendation for the subgroup of patients with blood pressure between 190-200 mm Hg since their results are diluted by the entire population. The risk of hemorrhagic stroke stratified by blood pressure is required to answer the question about this narrow range of blood pressure, and the probabilities were not found in the literature. A sensitivity analysis will locate the threshold stroke rate at which the decision to give thrombolytic therapy changes, but the hemorrhagic stroke rate at a given blood pressure is essential because its comparison to the threshold is the basis for the recommended decision. Obtaining raw patient data from a clinical trial resolved this dilemma by providing the necessary stratification with the data, allowing attainment of the initial model goal of providing thrombolytic therapy recommendations for specific blood pressures [7].

DISCUSSION

The ability of the database to support decision-analytic models depends strikingly on the type of variable to be analyzed by the model. The medical literature, and hence this database, is generally well suited for probabilistic models involving ordinal or nominal variables, but a significant disadvantage is the inability to fully support decision-analytic models for continuous variables. This is readily apparent given the numerous ways in which an objective clinical finding, blood pressure, is reported in the literature. It can be presented as a demographic mean without outcome stratification by blood pressure, as a range with an upper limit given as an exclusion criterion, or with a minimal level of stratification but without a range. The various ways of reporting blood pressure are not a result of inattention to blood pressure in thrombolytic trials, but rather are part of a larger problem of reporting information on continuous variables. Even in trials for evaluation of the ability of a medication to lower blood pressure the blood pressures are not reported in a standardized way to facilitate the most accurate comparison [8]. This problem is easily extrapolated to other continuous clinical variables such as age, heart rate, respiratory rate, and weight.

One remedy to this problem is to use aggregate patient data to supplement the literature. This aggregate data can be in the form of an electronic medical record, the raw data from a clinical trial as was used in this study, a clinical data repository, or observational patient databases. The advantage of these sources is the ability to provide stratified data. These sources also provide conditional probabilities; several papers from a single trial do not have to be analyzed together to arrive at the conditional probabilities. The single source can ensure homogeneity of the patient population and a standard level of evidence, eliminating major steps requiring expert review. Probabilities are easier to retrieve, and no paper review is necessary. An electronic medical record would have the additional advantage of a robust amount of data on each subject whereas clinical trials often record only select clinical variables and outcomes. A second advantage of the electronic medical record would be the inclusion of all patients, not just those enrolled in trials where a statistically significant result is obtained; in short, publication bias would be eliminated [9]. Obtaining probabilities via a query instead of reviewing many papers would also save time.

Two additional steps could greatly expedite using the literature database to obtain probabilities. This first step is inclusion of study size; searches then could be limited to studies with a specific minimum number of patients. Second, the study design of each paper could be included as a set of boolean variables with the appropriate study design selected; the boolean format would in turn optimize searching. The decision-analytic modelers could then choose a level of evidence for their model, and then limit their search to only those papers with a study design which meets the required level of evidence.

The next step of actually storing probabilities and the fractions used to derive the probabilities would eliminate paper review by the decision-analyst and hence save a considerable amount of time. However, the paper review is not eliminated altogether but shifted to the literature database developers. Selecting papers to provide a probability requires identification of homogenous populations and a standard level of evidence to which each paper must adhere if its probabilities are to be included in the database. These are not small tasks. Identification of a homogeneous population requires homogeneous demographics, risk factors, medical illnesses, concomitant procedures and medications, and a uniform disease and disease stage. Identifying a standard level of evidence goes beyond study size and study design and includes all the quality assessment issues facing meta-analysis. Meta-analysis by definition seeks to combine quantitative data, and it is distinct from decision analysis in that it seeks to use published clinical trial data and arrive at a new standard of care [10]. Decision-analytic results aim at serving as a clinical guideline pending a clinical trial to establish a standard of care. The pitfalls in selecting publications and combining the results apply to both fields. The pitfalls are numerous and include specification of protocol, treatment assignment, selection bias, data-extraction bias, financial bias, statistical methods used, subgroup analysis, quality assessment and quality assessment methods, publication bias, economic impact, outcome definitions, confounding, and misclassification [11,12,13].

One proposal to address the obstacles to meta-analysis is to develop meta-analysis registers which will promote collaboration and provide a basis for methodologic research [14]. Another approach to these problems is the development of the aforementioned clinical trials database. Papers receive a quality score based on clinical protocol and experimental design [15]. Studies deemed to have sufficient quality are included in the list provided by the database which also stores study size, year of publication, agents used with doses, duration of therapy, additional therapy, and the percent of patients in whom therapy is effective. Modifications would be necessary to provide the quantified data necessary for decision analysis. First, all trial endpoints should be included and evaluated separately. Second, papers that include analysis of a different endpoint measured in the same patients should be included and incorporated to facilitate calculation of conditional probabilities. Third, database developers review papers focusing on protocol and design with little attention given to disparity among patients and outcomes. A more comprehensive review is necessary to furnish the probabilities needed for clinical decisions for specific patients. For its stated purposes of producing quick access to an updated list of clinical trials and selection of papers for meta-analysis, the clinical trials database should be lauded. The points raised here are meant to discuss its suitability for a different use, providing probabilities for decision-analytic models.

Once papers have been deemed worthy of use in calculating a probability, shortcomings in papers should be included by adjusting probabilities to account for them. An existing system which contains such corrective properties is THOMAS, a bayesian statistical expert system which takes a single paper, adjusts probabilities for statistical shortcomings, and when given prior probabilities and utilities packages the results into a clinical decision recommendation [16]. The incorporation of the entire above process in storing probabilities would transform the database into a knowledge base analogous to the creation of a disease profile in QMR, previously known as Internist-1 [17]. QMR investigators have attempted to standardize disease profile creation with a knowledge acquisition tool (QMR-KAT) to provide probabilities for diagnostic use [18]. QMR is an excellent educational and consultative resource, but selecting probabilities in this way may remove some of the probabilities essential to sensitivity analysis which validates all decision-analytic models. The probabilities are less likely to be excluded if the decision-analysts themselves review the papers. Conversely, including all published probabilities including those that are not applicable to the population considered and those that do not meet an essential standard of level of evidence will also give inaccurate probability ranges for sensitivity analyses. Hence there is a trade-off between reduced time for decision-analytic model development and careful selection of papers.

A separate objective of providing a source of background knowledge for decision-analytic model construction, distinct from finding probabilities to use in the model, is easily accomplished with a comprehensive literature database. Searching both tables of the database for references to a clinical variable will provide this information. Consequently, the literature database is an rich source of data for a single decision-analytic model, and it most appropriately serves as a source of data to evaluate comprehensively a medical intervention through decision analysis.

An important feature of the database is the ability to grow with minimal effort. As a new paper is published, it can be entered into the database as it is being read. Hence it adds only a few clicks of the mouse button to the usual "keeping up with the literature" physicians undertake. The number of variables to be considered also helps the researcher focus and read more critically and objectively without additional time spent reading. Aside from its purpose of providing probabilities, the database can be used by physicians to master their own journal collections.

In conclusion, the concept of a literature database to support decision analysis by providing background medical knowledge and probabilities is feasible, effective, and can grow with the literature. Decision-analytic evaluation of continuous clinical variables may require supplemental stratified data from another data source such as raw data from clinical trials. The storage of actual probabilities in the database would save time for model developers but would require extreme care to ensure accurate probability ranges for sensitivity analysis.

Acknowledgments

Dr. Murphy is a cardiology fellow supported by a training grant from the NHLBI. Dr. Kahn is supported in part by Grant #5-R29-LM05387 from the NLM.

References

[1] Dawson N, Arkes H. Systemic errors in medical decision making: Judgment limitations. J Gen Intern Med 1987; 2: 183-7.

[2] Dickersin K, Hewitt P, Mutch L, et al. Comparison of MEDLINE searching with a perinatal trials database. Controlled Clin Trials 1985; 6: 306-17.

[3] Morris RD, Lau J, Arena NJ, et al. A clinical trials database as a research tool in health care. Online J Curr Clin Trials 1992; Jul 17: Doc No 14.

[4] Topol EJ, Califf RM, George BS, et al. Coronary arterial thrombolysis with combined infusion of recombinant tissue-type plasminogen activator and urokinase in patients with acute myocardial infarction. Circulation 1988; 77: 1100-7.

[5] GUSTO Investigators. An international randomized trial comparing four thrombolytic strategies for acute myocardial infarction. N Engl J Med 1993; 329: 673-82.

[6] ISIS-2 Collaborative Group. Randomised trial of intravenous streptokinase, oral aspirin, both, or neither among 17,187 cases of suspected myocardial infarction: ISIS-2. Lancet 1988; 2(8607): 349-60.

[7] Murphy JF, Jain NL, Kahn MG, et al. The impact of hypertension on the risk of hemorrhagic stroke in thrombolytic therapy: An appraisal and hypothesis. 1994; Submitted for publication.

[8] Chalmers TC. Clinical trial quality needs to be improved to facilitate meta-analyses. Online J Curr Clin Trials 1993; Sep 11: Doc No 89.

[9] Levy G. Publication bias: Its implications for clinical pharmacology. Clin Pharm Ther 1992; 52: 115-9.

[10] Cook DJ, Guyatt GH, Laupacis A, et al. Rules of evidence and clinical recommendations on the use of antithrombotic evidence. Chest 1992; 102: 305S-11S.

[11] Sacks S, Berrier J, Reitman D, et al. Meta-analyses of randomized clinical trials. N Engl J Med 1987; 316: 450-5.

[12] Thompson SG, Pocock SJ. Can meta-analyses be trusted? Lancet 1991; 338: 1127-30.

[13] Spector TD, Thompson SG. The potential and limitations of meta-analysis. J Epidemiol Comm Health 1991; 45: 89-92.

[14] Dickersin K, Chalmers TC, Simes RJ, et al. Report from the panel on the case for registers for clinical trials. Controlled Clin Trials 1988; 9: 76-81.

[15] Chalmers TC, Smith, Jr. H, Blackburn B, et al. A method for assessing the quality of a randomized control trial. Controlled Clin Trials 1981; 2: 31-49.

[16] Lehmann HP, Shortliffe EH. THOMAS: Building Bayesian statistical expert systems to aid in clinical decision making. Comp Meth Prog Biomed 1991; 35: 251-60.

[17] Miller RA, Pople, Jr. HE, Myers JD. INTERNIST-1: An experimental computer-based diagnostic consultant for general internal medicine. N Engl J Med 1982; 307: 468-76.

[18] Giuse DA, Giuse NB, Bankowitz RA, et al. Heuristic determination of quantitative data for knowledge acquisition in medicine. Comp Biomed Res 1991; 24: 261-72.

Prompting Physicians For Cost-Effective Test Ordering in The Low Prevalence Conditions of Family Medicine

Robert M. Bernstein, Ph.D., M.D., C.M., C.C.F.P.
Gary R. Hollingworth, M.D., F.C.F.P.
William E. Wood, M.D., C.M., C.C.F.P.

Medical Informatics Research Group, Clinical Epidemiology Unit,
Department of Family Medicine, University of Ottawa

We have developed a computerized prompting system for test ordering which we feel will decrease the cost of investigations and at the same time promote an evidence based learning approach to test ordering. Prompting systems have been shown to be cost-effective but suffer from many disadvantages in the family practice setting. They tend to be difficult to modify by the user and contingent on an inflexible rule based structure. Many suggestions are ignored implying that they are not relevant. In family practice most conditions are of low prevalence. Prompting for test ordering where the pre-test likelihood of disease is small will result in a large number of false positives and many unnecessary repeat or confirmatory investigations and attendant anxiety unless the prompting system is specifically designed to be used in a low prevalence environment. PROMPTOR-FM (PRObabilistic Method of Prompting for Test ORdering in Family Medicine) was developed to overcome these perceived difficulties. It allows the physician to rapidly calculate the positive and negative predictive values of a test being considered based on the clinical index of suspicion. The physician is able to repeat the calculations and compare the results with previous calculations. By using PROMPTOR-FM repetitively, the clinician can learn to balance the risk of "missing" a rare but serious condition against the risk of falsely identifying disease with its downstream hazards and costs of further investigation. Prompting for test ordering is therefore uniquely tailored to each patient's situation.

I. INTRODUCTION

Governments are trying to control health care costs. The College of Family Physicians of Canada, and other professional organizations are developing practice guidelines and quality assurance programs. The success of these initiatives will depend on developing ways the practicing physician can initiate change in the course of his/her usual practice. An electronic record with integrated guidance is one such method.

We have developed a computerized prompting system for test ordering (PROMPTOR-FM - PRObabilistic Method of Prompting for Test ORdering in Family Medicine) which we feel will decrease the cost of physician test ordering and at the same time promote an evidence based learning approach to test ordering.

Prompting systems have been used and studied since the late 70's. They have been shown to be cost effective [1-4], however, they suffer from major disadvantages in the family practice setting. They are either poorly integrated with the process of usual care or they are rule based, inflexible, difficult to modify or update without programming, and result in many suggestions being ignored.[5] They do not distinguish situations of low prevalence of disease (as in much of family practice) from situations where the prior probability of disease is high, thereby potentially leading to inappropriately high test ordering. In addition, no learning seems to result from their use. (physicians revert back to old habits once the system is no longer available for prompting. [6]

Family practice is a low prevalence domain. The most common reason for visit in our clinic is hypertension which accounts for less than 5% of the visits. Many studies of the content of family or general practice confirm this frequency distribution of diagnoses [7]. Only 18 conditions have a visit frequency of over 1%. All the rest of primary care medicine has a visit frequency of less than one percent. Prompting for test ordering in these situations where the prior probability is low will result in a large number of false positives and many unnecessary repeat or confirmatory investigations unless care is taken to tailor the prompting system to the environment in which it is used.

Family and general practice residents are trained throughout most of medical school and much of residency by specialists in hospitals. Specialty medicine is high prevalence, and in hospital specialty wards the prevalence of the diseases in the domain of that specialty is high. Therefore trainees for general practice are taught and develop their attitudes and practices in conditions which do not mimic those which they will encounter after graduation in office based ambulatory primary care. Since the probability that a patient who presents to a cardiologist with chest pain has angina is high, and the probability of chest pain presenting in general practice being angina is low, therefore the approach to diagnostic testing must follow different paths.

II. OBJECTIVES OF PROMPTOR-FM

PROMPTOR-FM was developed to overcome the perceived difficulties with previous systems. The OBJECTIVES are: (a) to allow the physician to maintain his/her autonomy when ordering tests; (b) to allow the physician to become an active participant in the decision process when ordering tests, thus promoting active learning; (c) to allow the physician to understand the process of ordering tests in a low prevalence setting; (d) to promote an approach to test ordering based on the principles of evidence based learning;[8,9] and (e) to be a learning tool for trainees and a practical application of an evidence based curriculum.

There are 3 main reasons why tests should be ordered:

1. Case finding (suspicion of disease),
2. Screening for disease, and
3. Following or monitoring a known clinical condition.

PROMPTOR-FM is intended to be used for the first two. Its utility in case finding is clear, as it allows the physician to rapidly calculate the positive and negative predictive values of the test he/she is considering ordering based on his/her clinical index of suspicion. The physician is able to repeat the calculations and compare the results with previous calculations. The utility in screening is less obvious, since usually screening procedures appear to have been established by a consensus authority and are not usually questioned. However, many suggestions for screening in the Canadian Task Force [10-12] are discretionary and depend on the circumstances and risks of the individual patient. In these situations PROMPTOR-FM provides a guide to the usefulness of the screening procedure.

III. THEORETICAL PERSPECTIVE: PROMPTING IN LOW PREVALENCE CONDITIONS

The predictive value of a test is dependent on three variables: a) the sensitivity, b) the specificity and c) the pre-test likelihood, or prior probability of disease. For most practical situations sensitivity and specificity are fixed properties of a given test.[13] The pre-test likelihood however is a reflection of the clinician's judgment.

For example, the sensitivity of the mammogram for breast cancer is about 80 (i.e. the test will correctly detect 80% of individuals known to have breast cancer) and the specificity 90% (i.e. it will correctly identify 90% of those who do NOT have the disease)[14]. If a 50 year old woman presents with a small mobile painless breast lump we can make a judgment that although the presentation is atypical there is a certain probability of breast cancer and that probability may lead us to order a mammogram. We know that mammography is not totally reliable, so what confidence can we have in the result? The answer depends entirely on our judgment of the likelihood of cancer in this woman. If we had 100 patients JUST LIKE HER, we might suspect that 25% had breast cancer.[14] That clinical judgment is the pre-test likelihood. If these numbers are plugged into the PROMPTOR-FM program we will know that a positive test has a 73% probability of being correct and a negative test has a 93% probability of being correct. Both these estimates leaves us much more certain then the original 25:75, and give us reason to follow up a positive test, and some assurance that the benign nature of the exam is confirmed by a negative test.

However suppose this same woman had presented with a 3 cm fixed irregular mass and a family history of breast cancer in a first degree relative we might estimate that of 100 patients of her age, family history, physical findings etc. (i.e. JUST LIKE HER) 70% would have breast cancer. Would a mammogram help us to identify those? Putting these figures into PROMPTOR we discover that the positive predictive value is 95% and negative predictive value is 66%. We have confidence in a positive result, but a negative test is wrong 34% of the time. Since a positive result leads inevitably to biopsy and a negative test, having a significant risk of missing serious and life threatening pathology, will also lead to a biopsy, it calls into question whether we should order a mammogram in this setting at all.

What about screening a 40 year old woman who has read some of the latest articles in popular magazines and requests a mammogram, having no symptoms, signs or risks. Her prior probability of breast cancer is about 0.5% [15] and therefore a positive test is false 96% of the time. Of a thousand patients there would be 100 FALSE positives for only 4 true positives - clearly a waste of time and money, and worse if the false positives are followed up with more invasive and risky procedures. Screening at this age is not cost effective.

What is clear as the program is run repetitively is that the lower the prior probability of disease the less confidence we have in a positive result. In fact, even changing the sensitivity or specificity just to see what happens leads to little gain in clinical acumen unless we choose exceptionally good sensitivities or specificities. For a test with an excellent specificity the proportion of false positives falls making the test more useful in low prevalence or screening situations. A test with a 80% sensitivity, a 99% specificity used for a patient with a prior probability of just 5% yields a positive predictive value of 81%.

As the sensitivity rises we gain more confidence that we have not "missed" anyone. The clinician therefore can learn to balance the need to identify rare but serious conditions with the risk of false identification of disease and its downstream hazards and cost of further investigation. Each patient is unique and each situation is uniquely analysed. The investigations and be able to counsel the patient based on the facts of the case and the probabilities using a mathematical estimate of the consequences as a tool. The results of the calculations can be stored in the electronic record and/or printed for reference and patient education.

IV. DEVELOPMENT OF PROMPTOR-FM

A "BASIC" program which allows the user to determine the predictive value of a test based on the sensitivity, specificity and pre-test likelihood of disease was developed by Bernstein in 1989.[16] In addition, Hollingworth Wood and Bernstein developed a computerized electronic record for use in a family medicine musculo-skeletal clinic [17]. The two were then integrated.

The PROMPTOR-FM program is called by a "help" button at a point in the record when the physician is ordering diagnostic tests. Its use by the physician is intended to be discretionary although it can be made mandatory for teaching purposes. The program supplies the sensitivities and specificities of the common tests used in an orthopedic medicine clinic and allows the user to input others in the course of using the program.

Pre-test likelihood is always input by the physician as a reflection of his/her clinical judgment. The program asks the purpose of testing (case finding, screening or follow-up) and provides some guidance for each. Results of the calculations are displayed in a manner which "guides and teaches"[18] based on a 2 X 2 table. Suggestions are permissive. The physician can repeat the calculations with different clinical judgment and display the results of current and previous calculations for comparison.

V. EXAMPLE

In the example of the 40 year old woman above the program displays the prompting suggestion as follows:

DISEASE

TEST		Present	Absent	
	pos	4	100	104
	neg	1	895	896
		5	995	1000

For the mammogram	
with a sensitivity of	80 %
a specificity of	90 %
and a pre test likelihood of	.5 %
the POSITIVE predictive value is	3.9 %
the NEGATIVE predictive value is	99.9 %

This means that if your patient has a positive test this result will be true 3.9% of the time.

Of 1000 patients **just like yours**

you will find 4 **true** positive patients
to 100 **false** positives.

You will **miss 1** patient who has breast cancer.

DO YOU WANT TO DO THIS TEST?

VI. CONCLUSIONS

A. Low prevalence conditions call for different approaches to prompting for test ordering than when prevalence is high.

B. Prompting systems should guide and teach in the course of usual record keeping.

C. Cost effective test ordering depends on an understanding of the impact of the prior probability of disease on the predictive values of a test.

D. The most important variable in the calculation of the predictive values of a test is clinical judgment of the pre-test likelihood.

E. The downstream cost implications of inappropriate testing where the prior probability is low are enormous, both financial and in terms of the risk to patients from invasive follow up investigations or the unnecessary anxiety generated.

F. PROMPTOR-FM is a prompting tool which can provide the clinician with guidance to appropriate test ordering based on probability of disease, not just suggestions for testing based on diagnosis with a high probability of being ignored.

G. PROMPTOR-FM is designed to promote active learning in the process of guiding the clinician.

VII. REFERENCES

[1]. McDowell I, Newell C, Rosser WW. A Randomized Trial of Computerized Reminders for Blood Pressure Screening in Primary Care. Med. Care 1989;27:297-305.

[2]. McDowell I, Newell C, Rosser WW. Computerized Reminders To Encourage Cervical Screening in Family Practice. J.Fam. Pract. 1989 28:420-424.

[3].Tierney WM, McDonald CJ, Martin DK, et al: Computerized Display of Past Test Results, Effect on Outpatient Testing. Ann. Int. Med. 1987;107(4):569-574.

[4]. Tierney WM, McDonald CJ, Hui SL, et al: Computer Predictions of Abnormal Test Results, Effect on Outpatient Testing. JAMA, 1987;259(8):1194-1198.

[5]. McDonald CJ, Hui SL, Smith DM. et. al. Reminders to Physicians from an Introspective Computer Medical Record. A Two-Year Randomized Trial Ann. Intern. Med. 1984;100:130-138.

[6]. McDonald Clement J. Protocol-Based Computer Reminders, The Quality of Care and the Non-Perfectibility of Man. NEJM 1976;295(24):1351-1355.

[7]. Tailoring Family Medicine Residency Programs to Meet Community Needs, Department of Family Medicine, University of Ottawa, Can. Med. Assoc .J. 1984; 131:1205-1206

[8]. Elmslie, TJ. Integrating Research Findings into the Clinical Setting. in Tools for Primary Care Research Volume 6: Ways to Disseminate Research Findings and Have an Impact on Practice. Ed. Dunn E, Norton P, Stewart M, Tudiver F, and Bass M. Sage Publications 1994 in press.

[9]. Evidence Based Medicine Working Group. Evidence-Based Medicine: A New Approach to Teaching the Practice of Medicine. JAMA 1992; 268:2420-2425.

[10]. Canadian Task Force on the Periodic Health Examination: The Periodic Health Examination. Can. Med. Assoc. J. 1979;121:1193-1254

[11]. Canadian Task Force on the Periodic Health Examination: Periodic Health Examination Monograph: Report of the Task Force to the Conference of Deputy Ministers of Health (cat H39-3/1980E), Health Services and Promotion Branch, Dept. of National Health and Welfare, Ottawa, 1980.

[12]. Canadian Task Force on the Periodic Health Examination: The Periodic Health Examination: 1. Introduction. Can. Med. Assoc. J. 1989;141:205-207

[13]. Department of Clinical Epidemiology and Biostatistics, McMaster University. How to Read Clinical Journals: II. To Learn About a Diagnostic Test. Can. Med. Assoc. J. 1981;124:703-710

[14]. Diagnostic Strategies for Common Medical Problems. ed. Panzer RJ, Black ER, and Griner PF. American College of Physicians 1991.

[15]. Miller AB, Baines CJ, To T, Wall C. Canadian National Breast Screening Study: 1. Breast Cancer Detection and Death Rates Among Women Aged 40 to 49 Years. Can. Med. Assoc. J. 1992; 147:1459-1476

[16]. Bernstein, RM. A "Basic" Program: Determining the Predictive Value of Laboratory Tests.Canadian Family Physician, 38:1357-1360, June 1992.

[17]. G. Hollingworth, WE. Wood, R. Bernstein. A Self Entry Database for a Musculoskeletal Clinic in Family Medicine. Department of Family Medicine Research Inquiry and Opinion Conference Ottawa May 27, 1993.

[18]. Weed LL. Medical records that guide and teach. New. Engl. J. Med. 1968; 278(11):593-600

Evaluating the Impact of Decision Support Systems in Clinical Care

Development and Implementation of a Computer-Generated Reminder System for Diabetes Preventive Care

D.S.Nilasena[1,2], M.J.Lincoln[1,2], C.W.Turner[2,3], H.R.Warner[2], V.A.Foerster[1,2], J.W.Williamson[1,2], B.M.Stults[1]

Department of Medicine[1], Salt Lake Veterans Affairs Medical Center
Departments of Medical Informatics[2] and Psychology[3],
University of Utah, Salt Lake City, UT 84132

ABSTRACT

Diabetes mellitus is a chronic condition with several late complications that can be delayed or avoided through proper preventive health care. Although practice guidelines have been established to improve the preventive care in diabetics, dissemination of these guidelines among physicians and educational programs have been only moderately successful in changing physicians' practice patterns. Previous efforts, however, did not utilize computer-generated reminders. We developed a system of computer-generated reminders for diabetic preventive care. We completed an implementation of the system in the outpatient clinics of internal medicine residents at our institution. This paper describes the development and implementation of this system.

Our results showed that the system flagged an average of 13 items that deviated from diabetes guideline compliance, out of a possible 21 items per patient. The residents completed encounter forms used by the system for 37% of patients seen during a six month period. Physician users exhibited positive attitudes toward the use of guidelines which they judged improved quality at no additional cost of care. However, the complexity and length of the guideline encounter forms and the additional time demands proved to be significant obstacles to current routine use. Our experience will help to improve the system so that it is more usable and acceptable to physicians, especially in the future as health care increasingly makes use of electronic medical record systems.

INTRODUCTION

Diabetes mellitus (DM) is a chronic medical condition which is present in over 11 million persons in the U.S.[1] DM is directly responsible for over 140,000 deaths per year. The disease also contributes to several other causes of death, notably ischemic heart disease and cerebrovascular disease. DM is associated with numerous complications which cause significant morbidity and disability for diabetic patients, and ultimately can lead to their premature death. The medical treatment for DM and its complications is expensive. Treating late diabetic complications costs over $5 billion in hospital charges annually.[2] Although no cure currently exists for DM, experts believe that appropriate medical care can significantly reduce disease complications. Preventive interventions in DM can have substantial impact on health outcomes. [1]

Practice Guidelines for the Care of Diabetic Patients

The American Diabetes Association [ADA] has proposed guidelines for the care of diabetic patients. [3] Adherence to these guidelines could potentially reduce the complications of DM by a significant degree. [1] Thus, the successful implementation of these guidelines into medical practice could dramatically decrease the burden of suffering and the cost of health care for diabetic complications.

Despite the publication of DM practice guidelines and their dissemination to physicians, compliance with the recommended preventive care for DM patients has been low. [4,5] Although previous studies have shown that certain interventions can improve physician compliance with guidelines for diabetes care [6-8], the overall compliance level remained low for many elements of DM care. This low compliance following the dissemination of diabetes guidelines is similar to results from other guideline compliance studies, even those involving simple guidelines. [9] The complex decision-making logic required to apply diabetes guidelines in routine practice is likely to be an important reason for the observed low compliance rate.

The use of computer-generated reminders is one method that has been shown to be effective in improving physician compliance with practice guidelines for preventive care.[10-11] This method uses a computerized patient database and decision logic derived from selected practice guidelines to create reminders or prompts to physicians about recommended services for each patient. Computer-generated reminder systems have been successful in improving immunization rates, and screening rates

0195-4210/94/$5.00

for cancer, hypertension, and hypercholesterolemia [10,11]. The observed improvement in compliance is typically 10 to 20% more than that of control programs involving only education and monitoring. The key element of the computer-generated reminder intervention is the timely, individualized feedback that is given to the physician. At the present time, an evaluation of computer-generated reminder systems using diabetes care guidelines has not been reported.

This paper describes a stand-alone, computerized reminder system for seven interrelated DM preventive care guidelines. We evaluated the system's initial implementation with internal medicine residents in outpatient clinics. We also assessed the medical residents' attitudes about the system and about DM practice guidelines.

METHODS

Computerized Reminder System Development

1) Guideline selection and development: Individual guidelines for preventive care in DM were selected from those published by the ADA [3]. Additional guidelines were then identified from a review of available DM literature. The complications of DM can be divided into seven broad categories [3] :

macrovascular disease (coronary heart disease, peripheral vascular disease, and stroke)
nephropathy (chronic renal failure)
neuropathy (peripheral and/or autonomic)
retinopathy (severe vision loss or blindness)
foot disease (infections requiring foot amputation)
improper glycemic control (ketoacidosis (DKA) and hypoglycemia).
complications of pregnancy (congenital malformations and perinatal mortality)

The selected guidelines were organized into six categories corresponding to the above groupings of DM complications. Since our project was initially targeted at patients in internal medicine clinics, the pregnancy category was not directly addressed. The six guideline categories were:

- **Glycemic control**
- **Foot care**
- **Eye care**
- **Renal care**
- **Macrovascular care**
- **Neurologic care**

Each category was further divided into items performed at each visit and items performed annually or less frequently than every visit. The guidelines were then phrased concisely and assembled into flowcharts which presented the clinical decision logic and the necessary elements of care for each category.

A study group was organized which consisted of rural Utah physicians, physician assistants, and faculty members from the Department of Internal Medicine at the University of Utah. This group analyzed the flowcharts which were constructed from the guidelines selected originally. The study group made suggestions for changes in wording and content of the guidelines. The guidelines were also simplified and condensed in order to allow the easiest incorporation into the primary-care practice setting. These changes resulted in a set of revised guidelines and revised flowcharts for each of the six categories.

2) Encounter forms development: The clinical data needed to determine compliance with the revised guidelines and to drive the clinical decision logic were grouped into seven **encounter forms** to be used for data capture. Six of the forms, one for each of the six guideline categories, were designed to capture data from annual patient evaluations. The seventh encounter form was designed to collect data about care which should be performed at every visit. Most items on the encounter forms were simple Yes/No questions (for example: "Patient is currently on ADA diet"). The remaining questions had blank spaces for the written entry of numeric values such as laboratory test results ("Fasting blood glucose is ___"). The number of questions on a single form ranged from 5 to 15 and the seven forms together contained a total of 68 individual questions.

3) Computer algorithm and patient database development: The decision logic from the revised flowcharts and the data elements from the seven encounter forms were incorporated into a computer program written with Symantec C++ for the Macintosh. The program serves as an object-oriented longitudinal patient database for storing clinical information related to the revised DM guidelines. Data entry into the database is via a graphical user interface with dialog windows that are identical in structure and content to the seven encounter forms. This design is intended to facilitate data entry by a clinic clerk to whom completed encounter forms are returned by the physician. Baseline information about each patient (from manual chart review) and the responses to questions on any of the encounter forms are stored in the database for each patient, along with the date the information was recorded. Previous entries for an individual patient can be reviewed sequentially on the screen to verify the accuracy of the reminders generated by the program.

4) Health Maintenance report generation: The computer program uses the currently available data for a given patient to generate a printed paper **health maintenance (HM) report** for the patient's primary physician. This report includes demographic information, a summary of the patient's current DM preventive-health status, a schedule of upcoming or past due preventive-health activities for the patient, and clinical alerts about high-risk aspects of the patient's current profile. The report is intended to be placed on the front of the patient's chart so that the HM information will be available to the physician at the next clinic visit by the patient.

Implementation of the Reminder System

1) Recruitment of participants: All second and third years internal medicine residents at the University of Utah were oriented to the content of the developed guidelines, the encounter forms to be used, and the process of using the reminder system. Each of these residents sees patients in a weekly general internal medicine clinic at either University Hospital (UUMC) or the Veterans Affairs Medical Center (VAMC) in Salt Lake City. Thirty-five of the 36 residents agreed to participate in the pilot study which took place during the six months between October 1993 and April 1994.

2) Identification of diabetic patients: An attempt was made to identify all patients with DM at each of the sites who had a scheduled clinic visit within six months after the start of the project. The study included patients if they had been diagnosed with DM (Type I or II) and had been seen in one of the clinics or hospitals within one year prior to the initial data collection. Newly diagnosed patients and those receiving care at specialty clinics for diabetes were excluded. The main data sources used to identify DM patients were ICD-9 codes from hospital discharges and clinic billing lists, pharmacy records of diabetic medications, and laboratory data of patients with elevated blood glucose or hemoglobin A1c.

3) Putting the system into action: a cycle of feedback to the physician and capture of patient data: In this study, individualized feedback is given to each physician about preventive services that are recommended for each of their diabetic patients. This required a system of ongoing data collection about the services that the patient has received. The process is started by entering baseline patient data from a manual review of the patient's hospital and clinic charts into the computerized database. This information is used to generate an initial HM report about the patient with suggestions for preventive services that were overdue or planned. The report is placed in the patient's chart prior to the next clinic visit. At the time of this visit, the physician is given encounter forms to complete as appropriate for the patient. Following this, the physician returns the completed encounter forms for entry of data into the patient database. The new patient information is then used to generate a new HM report. This report would in turn guide the next preventive services that are provided to the patient, and the cycle would continue on from there.

4) Evaluation of the acceptability of the system: In order to assess the acceptability of the computer-generated reminder system by the physicians, a questionnaire was developed to determine physician attitudes to various aspects of the project. The usability of the encounter forms and the HM reports, the time required to incorporate the system into practice, and perceived obstacles to guideline compliance were addressed. Suggestions for system improvement were also solicited.

RESULTS

Implementation of the Reminder System

There were 221 patients initially identified with possible DM scheduled at the UUMC, of which 88 were scheduled more than once during the pilot study period. At the VAMC, there were 259 possible diabetic patients scheduled, of which only ten had more than one visit. Once the patients had been identified, an attempt was made 1) to locate and review their medical records, 2) to enter their DM related data into the computer database, 3) to generate an initial HM report, and 4) to place the report into their clinic charts prior to the scheduled visits.

Problems in the overall use of the system in this study included unavailable patient charts, canceled or rescheduled appointments, and failure to place the HM report in the patient's chart before a clinic visit. Because of these problems, only 49% of the initial diabetic patients identified were seen by a resident with the HM report available for review. This resulted in 93 patient visits at the UUMC and 141 visits at the VAMC available for evaluation.

The process of baseline chart review took an average of 15 to 20 minutes per chart to abstract the diabetes guideline related data. The time to enter the abstracted baseline data into the patient database was approximately ten minutes per patient. The generation of the initial and subsequent HM reports took an average of 30 seconds. Data entry from a completed encounter form into the patient's database required less than 45 seconds for an experienced data-entry person. The time necessary to complete a single encounter form by an uninterrupted physician was approximately 1.5 minutes.

The data from baseline chart review resulted in the identification of a substantial number of diabetes guideline items that needed attention by the physician to bring the patient's care into compliance. An average of 13.2 preventive care recommendations out of a possible 21, or 63%, were flagged for each chart. The categorization of items is shown in Table 1.

Table 1: Average Number of Preventive Care Recommendations Flagged per Patient following Baseline Chart Review

Category	UUMC	VAMC	Max.*
Eye Care	2.0	1.7	3
Foot Care	2.1	1.8	3
Glycemic Control	3.7	3.7	5
Macrovascular Care	1.6	1.7	3
Neurologic Care	1.7	1.8	2
Renal Care	2.1	1.5	4
Routine Visits	0.8	0.5	1
Total	13.9	12.5	21

* Max. = maximum possible flags for the category

Participation by the Resident Physicians

The number and type of encounter forms filled out and returned by the residents are shown in Table 2. The residents' participation declined after the first two months of the project, particularly at the VAMC clinics. The Routine Visit forms were completed more frequently at both sites (chi-square=18.3, $p<0.01$ for UUMC; chi-square=1.9, p=NS for VAMC), probably because this form was on the same sheet as the HM report. Overall, 37% of patients had one or more encounter forms completed and returned. On the average, there were 1.63 forms completed per patient visit. Specific reasons given for not always completing the encounter forms included lack of time during the clinic visit, lack of understanding of the use of the forms, lack of clarity about where to return forms, sub optimal organization of form content, and too many other existing paper forms to complete.

Table 2: Number of Completed Encounter Forms

Encounter Form Name	UUMC	VAMC
Eye Care	31 (33%)	16 (11%)
Foot Care	30 (32%)	19 (13%)
Glycemic Control	39 (42%)	19 (13%)
Macrovascular Care	30 (32%)	18 (13%)
Neurologic Care	30 (32%)	19 (13%)
Renal Care	31 (33%)	18 (13%)
Routine Visits	58 (62%)	24 (17%)
One or More Forms	60 (65%)	26 (18%)
Total Patients Identified	**93**	**141**

Acceptability of the System by the Residents

The acceptability questionnaire was completed by 33 of the 35 participating residents. The results revealed that at least 85% of the residents agreed that practice guidelines improved the quality of care and assisted physicians in providing care. Seventy percent did not believe that guidelines increased costs, and 70% did not think guidelines reduced the time it took to provide patient care.

While over half of the residents found the encounter form questions to be organized into useful groups appropriate for patient care, over 70% thought that the forms were difficult to use and did not reduce the time it took to provide care. The HM report was thought to be organized, accurate, and appropriate by over half of the residents. However, 74% did not think the report reduced time spent on patient care. Both the HM reports and the encounter forms were found by over 80% of residents to provide helpful reminders of aspects of DM care, and 35% believed this caused a change in their patient management.

The majority of residents believed that each of the categories of preventive care for DM had important effects on reducing long-term complications, and over 70% believed the glycemic control, foot care, and eye care had this effect. Over 75% of residents thought that each component of care (history, physical, lab, education, referrals) had an important impact on long-term outcome, with 88% finding patient education to be important.

Ninety percent of residents believed that the care they currently provided was in accordance with current recommendations, however, 77% also believed that their care would be improved by the use of practice guidelines. Over 80% thought that the guidelines used in this project were applicable to the diabetic patients they treat.

We found a number of differences between the UUMC and VAMC residents in their responses to the acceptability questionnaire. Although the small sample size did not allow these differences to reach statistical significance, there were six questions for which the VAMC and UUMC respondents differed by over 20%. For these six, the VAMC residents gave the encounter forms a less favorable rating. Compared to the UUMC group, the VAMC residents thought the encounter forms were more difficult to understand and use, made it more difficult to record patient care, increased the time it took for patient care, and were less appropriate for patient care than the UUMC residents. The VAMC residents also did not believe that attention to glycemic control, renal care, and neurologic care in diabetics had as strong an effect on long-term outcome as the UUMC group.

DISCUSSION

In this paper, we have described the development and implementation of a system of computer-generated reminders for diabetes preventive care. The system was effective in identifying and flagging an average of 13 diabetes guideline recommendations that required action by the physician to bring patient care into compliance. Once baseline data on a patient is entered, the system provided feedback about the current guideline compliance and generated a list of recommended preventive health services that were due. Typical visits required completing 2 of the 7 encounter forms, requiring less than 2 to 3 minutes. The forms could generate electronic medical records, actually reducing future documentation time.

The deficiencies in guideline compliance identified by the reminder system suggested a great potential for improved diabetic patient care with the use of the system. The seemingly low level of participation by the residents in this pilot study must be viewed within the context of intended system use. Since most of the diabetes guidelines are recommended at yearly intervals, the physician does not need to complete all seven encounter forms at every visit. If, for each diabetic patient, the physician completes eight to ten forms over a period of one year, the patient's care should be in compliance with the guidelines. Assuming the patient is seen four times a year, the residents in this study were participating at a level that could achieve compliance within one year. The complexity of the diabetes guidelines make it likely that certain services will be done by the physician often while others will be omitted in many patients. The reminder system that we have described can organize the preventive care guidelines for the physician to allow the delivery of timely and comprehensive diabetes preventive care.

Most residents believed that the guidelines: improve quality of care, have a beneficial effect on long-term outcomes, were appropriate for their own patients, and provided helpful reminders for many aspects of patient care. The residents did not respond positively to the organization of the forms or the extra time it took to complete them.

FUTURE DIRECTIONS

The findings of this study suggest a number of ways that this system can be improved. The use of encounter forms and HM reports in this study was problematic but in the future will not be needed as these guidelines become data-driven by electronic medical record systems. For the present, these paper forms should be reorganized and simplified to make them easier to understand and use. Getting specific input from the intended users will help to design forms that are more likely to be completed. More time should be spent giving a detailed orientation to clinicians on the mechanics of using the system and ways for them to incorporate it into their patient care routine. The training and support of clerical and nursing staff in the clinics would help in this regard. Also, direct entry of appropriate data by the patient, nurse, or clinic clerk could reduce the paperwork burden on the physician and increase acceptability of the system. Providing feedback to physicians about their relative performance in guideline compliance compared to their peers and their progress in achieving compliance could serve as an incentive to increase their use of the system. The ongoing development of an electronic medical record will greatly improve the utility of this system by making routinely collected patient data available to help drive the HM reminders. Once these changes are made, the system will become more readily used by clinicians, and the potential improvements in preventive care for diabetic patients can be realized.

REFERENCES

1. Anderson RM. The challenge of translating scientific knowledge into improved diabetes care in the 1990s. Diabetes Care; 1991; 14: 418-21.
2. Jacobs J; Sena M; Fox N. The cost of hospitalization for the late complications of diabetes in the United States. Diabet-Med; 1991; 8: S23-S29.
3. Clinical practice recommendations. American Diabetes Association 1990-1991. Diabetes-Care; 1991; 14 Suppl 2: 1-81
4. Harris ML. Testing for blood glucose by office-based physicians in the U.S. Diabetes Care; 1990; 13: 419-26.
5. Jacques CHM; Jones RL; Houts P; et. al. Reported practice behaviors for medical care of patients with diabetes mellitus by primary-care physicians in Pennsylvania. Diabetes Care; 1991; 14: 712-7.
6. CDC. Demonstration to improve care practices for diabetic patients in primary care centers - Florida. JAMA; 1987; 257: 1580-1.
7. Deeb LC; Pettijohn FP; Shirah JK; Freeman G. Interventions among primary-care practitioners to improve care for preventable complications of diabetes. Diabetes Care; 1988; 11: 275-80.
8. Maaze R; Deeb L; Palumbo PJ. Altering physicians' practice patterns - A nationwide educational experiment: Evaluation of the Clinical Education Program of the American Diabetes Association. Diabetes Care; 1986; 9: 420-5.
9. Lomas J; Enkin M; Anderson GM; et. al. Opinion leaders vs. audit and feedback to implement practice guidelines. JAMA; 1991; 265: 2202-7.
10. McDonald CJ; Hui SL; Smith DM; et. al. Reminders to physicians from an introspective computer medical record. A two year randomized trial. Ann Intern Med; 1984; 100: 130-8
11. Ornstein SM; Garr DR; Jenkins RG; et. al. Computer-generated physician and patient reminders. Tools to improve population adherence to selected preventive services. J Fam Pract; 1991; 32: 82-90

The authors would like to acknowledge Iona Thraen, Shelley Wood, and Charlene Weir for their assistance with this project, and Lee Min Lau for editorial suggestions.

This project was funded in part by the Special Fellowship in Ambulatory Care provided through the Department of Veteran's Affairs Medical Center in Salt Lake City.

A NEW KNOWLEDGE STRUCTURE FOR DRUG-DRUG INTERACTIONS

Gilad J. Kuperman, M.D., Ph.D.*, David W. Bates, M.D., M.Sc.*, Jonathan M. Teich, M.D., Ph.D.*
James R. Schneider, R.Ph**, Dina Cheiman, Pharm. D.**
Departments of Information Systems* and Pharmacy**, Brigham and Women's Hospital, Boston, MA.

ABSTRACT

We developed a program to automatically screen patients' medication profiles for pairs of interacting drugs. Since some drug-drug interactions are indicated by changes in physiological parameters (e.g., ciprofloxacin and theophylline leading to an elevation of theophylline levels), the program considered the patients' relevant laboratory parameters prior to generating the alerts. We developed an editor to facilitate maintenance of the knowledge base. We evaluated the program for 3 weeks in two satellite pharmacies. The program reported 160 alerts of which 5 resulted in a change in the patients' therapies (one per 500 patient-days of care). These five interactions were potentially very serious. An additional 3 alerts led to changes in medication administration times. Subjectively, the program is well received and continues to be in routine clinical use.

INTRODUCTION

Although drugs are an essential part of medical treatment, the use of medications often leads to undesired adverse events. Leape, et al.[1] noted that 3.7% of hospitalized patients had disabling injuries caused by medical treatments and the most commonly implicated treatment was medication use accounting for 19% of all injuries. Steel, et al.[2] noted that 9% of hospitalized patients incurred iatrogenic complications that were life-threatening or produced disability and medications accounted for 37% of the complications. Drug-related injuries are known as adverse drug events (ADEs). Examples of ADEs include allergic reactions, gastrointestinal bleeding, neurologic side effects, and metabolic abnormalities. The costs of ADEs are high: one study estimated the incremental costs associated with an ADE to be about $2000.[3]

Distinct from ADEs, several types of medication-related errors may occur during a hospital stay. A medication error is an error in the process of ordering or delivering a medication regardless of whether an injury occurred or whether the potential for injury was present.[4] Examples of medication errors include overdoses, underdoses, medications which are inappropriate given patient characteristics, orders for medications to which the patient is known to be allergic, and orders for interacting combinations of medications. Few medication errors actually result in ADEs and only a minority of ADEs are caused by medication errors. Bates, et al.[4] noted that 20% of 25 ADEs identified by chart review were caused by medication errors.

The goal of this project was to try to prevent medication errors and ADEs due to drug-drug interactions. Although the literature describes thousands of drug-drug interactions of varying severity,[5] previous studies have found that clinically important drug-drug interactions are relatively infrequent. Folli, et al.[6] found that out of 500 errors in 100,000 medication orders, only 9 were related to drug-drug interactions (overdoses and underdoses were much more common). The HELP system's drug alert monitor[7] finds only one important drug-drug interaction approximately every 500 patient-days. Medication orders that result in drug-lab interactions are twice as common. Out of 10,000 medication orders, Bates, et al.[4] found only one drug-drug interaction that caused an ADE. Even though serious drug-drug interactions are low frequency events, the resulting adverse events (while completely preventable!) may be devastating. The highly publicized death of Libby Zion a decade ago[8] was felt to be due partially to an interaction between meperidine and phenelzine. Indeed, this case caused a grand jury to suggest that computerized drug-drug interactions programs be considered for all level one hospitals in New York State. Additionally, malpractice suits resulting from drug-related injuries are difficult to defend[9] and although pharmacists often can detect medication orders that will result in an interaction, humans are fallible.[10]

We decided to implement an automated detection scheme because the data required to detect drug-drug interactions are present in our hospital information system,[11] because detecting such interactions is computationally relatively straightforward, and because of the potential importance of even a single such event.

METHODS

Setting: Brigham and Women's Hospital (BWH) is a 751-bed tertiary care hospital in Boston, Massachusetts. The Brigham Integrated Computer System (BICS) provides administrative, financial, and clinical computing services at the hospital.[11] A computerized pharmacy application is used by pharmacists to manage patients' medications. The BICS database contains a list of the medications that each patient is currently receiving.

Knowledge acquisition: We used empiric data on adverse events at BWH[4],[12] and surveyed the pharmacy literature to determine which drug-drug interactions may be life-threatening. Fifty-two serious interactions were identified. Eighteen of the pairs involved warfarin. Examples of other alerts are digoxin-quinidine (possible digoxin toxicity), antiotensin converting enzyme (ACE) inhibitors-potassium sparing diuretics (possible hyperkalemia), meperidine-monoamine oxidase (MAO) inhibitors (potentially fatal), and terfenidine-erythromycin (arrhythmia risk). The full list of interactions is available from the authors on request. For computational purposes, the data were stored in a database consisting of 3 fields: 1) drug A, 2) drug B, and 3) the message to be displayed if the patient is receiving both drugs. A knowledge base editor was created to facilitate knowledge base maintenance. For each interaction, the editor allows the drug names and the alerting message to be entered in a "slot-filling" approach. The editor also allows links to be created between the drug names and specific elements in the BWH drug database.

Linkage of drug names to BWH drug database: The BWH drug database consists of 9000 packages which, for management purposes, are collected into "rollup" groups (Figure 1). For example, all of the various erythromycin packages used in the hospital are contained in the erythromycin rollup group. The rollup categories were inadequate (i.e., too specific) for use in drug interactions. For example, MAO inhibitors (as in the meperidine-MAO inhibitor interaction) are contained in multiple rollup groups (e.g., phenelzine, tranylcypromine, etc.). We therefore created the concept of a "drug family" which is a collection of rollup groups (Figure 1) to be used in the drug interaction database. The drug interactions were therefore defined as interactions between pairs of drug families. Any individual patient's medication profile is defined in terms of drug packages however the associated drug families can be discerned by following the links shown in Figure 1.

Preliminary work and modification of knowledge structure: A program was written which reviewed all inpatients' computerized medication profiles and detected when patients were receiving pairs of interacting drugs. When the program was tested, it was found that many patients (60 per day) were generating alerts, yet there were few instances of clinical significance. A closer review of the interactions revealed why.

Twenty-eight (28) of the interactions were found to be mediated by alterations in measurable physiologic parameters such as potassium (K^+), prothrombin time (PT), urea nitrogen (BUN), creatinine, calcium, and various drug levels. For example, the life-threatening consequences of warfarin-related interactions involve an elevation of the PT which makes the patient more susceptible to hemorrhage and the simultaneous administration of potassium-sparing diuretics and potassium products may elevate the serum K^+ to dangerously high levels. Often, however, even when a patient is receiving both drugs in an interacting pair, the laboratory test which would be affected by the interaction remains normal, in which case an alert would not be necessary.

We therefore altered our knowledge structure to include the concept of a "relevant lab test" (Figure 2). The database structure of a drug interaction was extended to include a list of 0 or more relevant laboratory tests for each interaction. Each relevant laboratory test is described by 4 elements: 1) the name of the lab test, 2) a threshold value, 3) an inequality operator ("<" or ">") to

```
family           Hepatic Carbamazepine     Macrolid
                         Inhibitors         antibiotics
                              ↗        ↖        ↗             ↖
rollup          Isoniazid              Erythro          Clarithromycin
group
                    ↗        ↖        ↗        ↖              ↑
package      Isoniazid generic   Erythro   generic    Clarithromycin
```

Figure 1. Relationship between drug packages, rollup groups, and drug families in the BWH drug database.

Drug interaction data				Relevant laboratory tests			
Family A	Family B	Message		Labname	Threshold	Operator	Within
K-sparing diuretics	Potassium	Hyperkalemia	→	Potassium	4.7	>	4 days
Cyclosporine	Erythro	Renal Failure	→	BUN	25	>	3 days
			↳	Creatinine	2.5	>	3 days
Digoxin	Quinidine	Dig toxicity	→	Digoxin	2.0	>	5 days
Barbiturates	Warfarin	Warfarin less effective	→	Protime	13	<	3 days
etc.							

Figure 2. Knowledge structure for drug-drug-lab interactions.

indicate if "greater-than" or "less-than" the threshold is of concern, and 4) a "days-within" value indicating within how many days the test should have been performed.

The algorithm for alert detection was modified so that, even if both drugs were present in a patient's medication profile, the drug interaction alert would be suppressed if, for all of the "relevant labs" for that interaction 1) none of the last 3 test results were above or below (as indicated by the inequality operator) the threshold value, and 2) the laboratory test had been done within the "days-within" value.

For example, a patient receiving both potassium and potassium-sparing diuretics would only have the interaction reported if one of the three most recent serum potassium measurements was above 4.7 or if the serum potassium had not been measured in the last 3 days; a patient receiving both phenytoin and chloramphenicol would generate an alert only if any of the 3 most recent dilantin levels were above 20 or if no dilantin measurement has been performed within 4 days. Threshold values (i.e., K^+>4.7) were set so the alerts would be presented before the values became dangerous. The knowledge base editor was expanded so relevant labs could easily be defined.Since drug-drug interactions now often involve laboratory tests, we refer to these alerts as drug-drug-lab interactions, or DDLIs.

Program operation: The DDLI detection program runs daily at 7 a.m. All patients' medications are reviewed and the program generates reports which are reviewed later in the day by clinical pharmacists working in the hospital's four satellite pharmacies. The reports include relevant pharmacy, laboratory and demographic data (Figure 3). The pharmacists 1) review the alerts for significance, 2) collect further clinical information if necessary, and 3) contact a clinician if warranted. We decided to do background (batch mode) detection of interactions rather than real-time detection at the time of pharmacist data entry because a physician order entry project is under development[13] which soon will make programs relying on pharmacist entry of medication data obsolete.

Evaluation: For a 3-week period, data detailing the frequency and distribution of generated alerts were collected. We measured how often our modified knowledge structure suppressed an alert because a laboratory threshold value was not exceeded. We also kept data in two of the satellite pharmacies on 1) whether the patient's medications were changed as a result of the alert, and 2) how often additional data were required to establish the clinical significance of the alert.

```
=============== Drug-drug alerts -- 03/26/93, Alert # 6 ==================
Patient PATIENT, A in room 11D-72
MR #: 999-99-99-9 Age: 73   Sex: M
Patient on COUMADIN and BACTRIM.  Possible PROLONGED BLEEDING TIME
Patient had same alert recently on 03/23/93, 03/24/93, 03/25/93
  drug name                             dose        rt    sch       start date
WARFARIN SODIUM                         12.5 MG      PO    HS          03/23/93
TRIMETHOPRIM/SULFA                      160 MG       PO    BID         03/24/93
Relevant laboratory tests with age/sex specific normal values:
PT          37.3  03/25/93 10:20A  [nl:10 - 13]
PT          28.4  03/24/93  9:43A  [nl:10 - 13]
PT          26.4  03/23/93 10:37A  [nl:10 - 13]
```

Figure 3. Example of alert generated by DDLI detection program.

Table 1. Distribution of 160 drug-drug-lab interactions (DDLIs) captured over a 3 week period from two satellite pharmacies.

Interaction	%
ACE inhibitors and potassium	53%
Warfarin and other drugs	25%
Neuromuscular blockers and aminoglycosides	6%
Cyclosporin and erythromycin	6%
Phenytoin and other drugs	4%
Maalox and doxycycline	2%
Theophylline and other drugs	2%
Others	2%

RESULTS

The application has been in use since April 1993. The 3 week evaluation took place in June 1993. During the evaluation period, an average of 21.8 DDLI alerts per day were generated for the hospital as a whole. A further 38.3 alerts per day that might have been presented were suppressed because a relevant laboratory test did not exceed a threshold. Data were collected from two satellite pharmacies for 160 alerts. Table 1 shows the distribution of the alerts. Angiotensin converting enzyme (ACE) inhibitors/potassium and warfarin-related interactions accounted for 78% of the alerts.

Eight (5%) of the alerts were clinically significant. Five (3% of all interactions) led to a documented change in therapy (Table 2). This corresponds to a rate of about one clinically significant drug-drug interaction per 500 patient-days. Table 2 shows that the clinical circumstances surrounding the interactions requiring changes in therapy were potentially very serious (i.e., hyperkalemia, theophylline and digoxin toxicities, and excessive anticoagulation). Three interactions (2%) resulted in changes in medication administration times so that medications would not be administered concurrently (Maalox and doxycycline).

Pharmacists required additional data (e.g., medication administration times, other medication data, other laboratory data, etc.) to determine clinical significance in 18% of the alerts.

The program continues to be used routinely.

DISCUSSION

Although the DDLI detection program described here has a low specificity -- only 5% of interactions reported to BWH pharmacists led to immediate changes in medication therapy -- Table 2 shows that the program helped avert some potentially serious conditions. Gardner[7] reports that the physician compliance with the LDS Hospital drug alert detection system is near or at 100%, i.e., physicians nearly always change their prescriptions in response to alert messages. Several factors could account for the discrepancy between the two systems' performances including the differences in the knowledge bases and the fact that at LDS Hospital, pharmacists subjectively categorize alerts as "information-oriented" or "action-oriented" (the specificity figures apply only to the action-oriented alerts). It is interesting that the frequency of significant interactions found in this study was very similar to that found by Gardner (both about one per 500 patient-days).

Table 2. Interactions resulting in changes in medication therapy (with relevant laboratory results). Theoph = theophylline levels, PT = prothrombin time, K = potassium levels, Dig = Digoxin levels.

	Interaction found	Lab	Result	Action taken
1)	Ciprofloxacin-theophylline	Theoph	22.5	decrease theophylline
2)	Warfarin-trimethoprim/sulfa	PT	37.3	decrease warfarin
3)	ACE inhibitor-potassium	K	4.9	D/C potassium
4)	ACE inhibitor-potassium	K	5.4	add furosemide
5)	Digoxin-quinidine	Dig	2.2	change digoxin to every other day

Because a patient's medication profile continued to be scrutinized as long as the patient was in the hospital, it is unlikely that the screened-out alerts were clinically relevant (because an alert would have been generated if the laboratory value changed or if the test was not repeated shortly). A new medication started just prior to discharge, however, may have resulted in an adverse situation that would not have been discovered until after discharge. The scope of this project was limited to the inpatient setting.

The specificity of the BWH alerts could likely be increased if the threshold limits on the laboratory tests were changed. For example, BWH cardiologists like to keep the potassium values of cardiac patients "on the high side", i.e., close to 5. Many cardiac patients receiving ACE inhibitors and potassium thus generate DDLI alerts. These alerts could be squelched by increasing the potassium threshold value from 4.7 to, say, 5.0 or 5.1. However, the pharmacists are apprehensive about missing another patient's potassium that is creeping up. The pharmacists do not mind reviewing the small number of false positives that are generated and thus far have not asked for the threshold values to be changed. About 5-10 alerts per satellite per day are generated and review of the alerts is very quick (1-2 minutes) if additional data are not needed.

Another factor that may contribute to the low specificity is that in our study the BWH pharmacists only documented medication changes of which they were certain. It is possible that physicians, having been informed of a possible adverse situation may have changed the patient's medications at a later time, or otherwise modified their prescribing habits in response to the information, even though they did not respond immediately to the information.

Subjectively, the pharmacists feel the program provides them with worthwhile information and make time in their day to generate and review the alert report.

CONCLUSIONS

We developed a drug-drug interaction detection scheme that automatically reviews all BWH patients' medication profiles. We added the concept of a "relevant lab" for interactions mediated by changes in physiological parameters. We developed a knowledge base editor to manage rules and the linkages to the database. Over a 3 week period, 5 serious drug interactions (one per 500 patient-days of care) were detected that led to changes in patients' therapies. The program continues to be in routine clinical use.

REFERENCES

1. Leape LL, Brennan TA, Laird N, et al. The nature of adverse events in hospitalized patients. N Engl J Med 1991;324:377-384.
2. Steel K, Gertman P, Crescenzi C, Anderson J. Iatrogenic illness on a general medical service at a university hospital. N Engl J Med 1981;304:638-642.
3. Evans RS, Classen DC, Stevens LE, et al. Using a hospital information system to assess the effects of adverse drug events. Seventeenth Symposium for Computer Applications in Medical Care (SCAMC) 1993;17:161-165.
4. Bates DW, Boyle D, Vandervliet M, et al. Relationship between medication errors and adverse drug events. Clin Res 1993;41:526A.
5. Evaluation of drug interactions. American Pharmaceutical Association, Washington, D.C., 1990.
6. Folli HL, Poole RL, Benitz WE, Russo JC. Medication error prevention by pharmacists in two children's hospitals. Pediatrics 1987;79:718-722.
7. Gardner RM, Hulse RK, Larsen KG. Assessing the effectiveness of a computerized pharmacy system. Fifteenth Symposium for Computer Applications in Medical Care (SCAMC) 1990;15:668-672.
8. Asch DA, Parker RM. The Libby Zion Case: one step forward or two steps backward. N Engl J Med 1988;318(12):771-775.
9. National Association of Insurance Commissioners. Medical malpractice closed claims, 1975-1978. Brookfield, WI: National Association of Insurance Commissioners, 1980.
10. McDonald CJ. Protocol-based computerized reminders: the quality of care and the non-perfectibility of man. N Engl J Med 1976;295:1351-1355.
11. Safran C, Slack WV, Bleich HL. Role of computing in patient care in two hospitals. MD Comput 1989;6:141-148.
12. Bates DW, Leape LL, Petrycki S. Incidence and preventability of adverse drug events in hospitalized adults. J Gen Intern Med 1993;8:289-294.
13. Teich JM, Spurr CD, Flammini SJ, et al. Response to a trial of physician-based inpatient order entry. Seventeenth Symposium for Computer Applications in Medical Care (SCAMC) 1993;17:316-320.

Closing the Loop of Patient Care—A Clinical Trial of a Computerized Discharge Medication Program

Daniel Z. Sands, MD, MPH, Charles Safran, MD, MS

Center for Clinical Computing, Harvard Medical School and Beth Israel Hospital, Boston, MA

A frustrating time for hospitalized patients and their primary care providers is after discharge from the hospital, because of changes in patients' medications. We developed a computer program to improve the discharge process, by providing guidance to the physician writing the prescriptions, offering educational material to the patients, and providing electronic notification of medication changes to the primary care providers. During a one-year clinical evaluation of this system, in which use of the program was voluntary, 1000 patients were discharged through the program. House officers tended to use the program more often for patients who were older and in the hospital longer. Both house officers and primary care physicians found the program extremely useful, and the process took no longer than the manual method of creating discharge medication lists. Patients who were discharged using this program may have had better adherence to medication regimens. We conclude that computer-assisted compilation of a discharge medication list is a useful method for improving the discharge process.

In the 1990's, patients are hospitalized for ever-shortening lengths of time, and experience a greater intensity of activity in these hospitalizations than ever before. This trend is likely to continue, as health care reform and capitated payment further discourage the use of costly inpatient facilities. As a result, patients spend more time outside the hospital and primary care assumes increasing importance. This means that primary care physicians are busier than ever and are caring for increasingly ill patients outside the hospital, so that continuity of care from the inpatient to the outpatient setting becomes essential. At the same time, patients are expected to understand complicated lists of medications and instructions.

The effects are that ill patients are being sent home from the hospital not fully understanding changes in their medications, physicians and nurses cannot adequately educate patients about their medications, house officers are having difficulty developing an inclusive list of medications at the time of discharge, and primary care providers are spending large proportions of encounters trying to determine which medications their patients are supposed to be taking. Inadequate patient education about their medications leads to nonadherence to regimens[1] and contributes to adverse drug reactions[2]. Nonadherence is estimated to cost the United States $100 billion per year in health care costs and lost productivity[3].

We developed a computer program to respond to these problems, and investigated its efficacy through a clinical trial.

METHODS

Setting

The study was performed on the general medical service of Boston's Beth Israel Hospital, a 500-bed major teaching hospital of Harvard Medical School. For almost 20 years the hospital has had a heavily used integrated clinical information system, the CCC system [4]. For five years the general medical practice has used a part of the CCC system, the online medical record (OMR)[5], through which all aspects of outpatient primary care have been managed, including problems, medications, and notes. In addition to providing patient information, the system is heavily used for clinical decision support.

Problem Assessment

Patients' satisfaction with their education about medications at the time of discharge was assessed through a multi-hospital survey[6]. Interns, nurses, and primary care physicians were interviewed both singly and in small groups. Flow charts were constructed to outline the current process of sending a patient home from the hospital, focusing on medication-related issues. Problem areas were identified and solutions proposed.

System Development

A new process was outlined on a flow chart. The new process was able to take advantage of the information resources available on the CCC system, and implement our practice decision that the OMR medication list should be the current record of our patients' medications. The new system would be triggered by the house officer who had been caring for the patient in the hospital, and its use would be voluntary.

The system works as follows. Each medication that is ordered for the patient at the time of discharge is shown to the house officer for approval, discontinuation, or modification. To help with the decision making, the house officer can view the patient's OMR medication list or the online PDR while reviewing medications. Once the house officer has decided whether to approve, discontinue, or change the dosage of each of these inpatient drugs, the program checks the OMR medication list for drugs that may have been omitted and prompts the house officer to reevaluate these medications as well.

When the list is finalized, the program displays a list of all the medications the house officer is about to prescribe, sorted by therapeutic class. It also displays potential drug-drug interactions. On the basis of this information, the list can be edited.

Once approved, this list of medications is stored in the OMR as the patient's current medication list, which is then instantly available to outpatient providers who may be caring for the patient. The program then informs the house officer of any special blood tests that need to be ordered, according to the patient's specific medications.

The final discharge prescriptions and patient education monographs[7] are then printed on a laser printer, along with medication lists for both the paper chart and the patient. Finally, an electronic message is sent to the patient's primary care provider indicating which changes were made in the patient's medications.

Study Design

The study subjects were patients hospitalized for more than two days who were discharged from the medical service to their homes between Jan. 10, 1993, and Jan. 10, 1994. Eligible patients were those for whom more than two scheduled medications were ordered at the time of discharge. For patients hospitalized more than once, only the first eligible discharge was analyzed.

Nursing and secretarial staff on two floors in the hospital were taught to use new printers required for the intervention, and two other floors served as controls.

The discharge medication menu option was available to all house officers, but the actual discharge medication program was executed only if the patient being discharged was on an intervention floor. If the patient was located on a control floor, the program asked questions of the user about the number of prescriptions written and the time it took, but we did not allow online ordering of medications.

All medical interns were reminded about the program's existence by electronic mail monthly during the first three months of the study, and they were reminded again during house officer meetings early in the study and in the 11th month.

Data Collection

Details about program use were stored automatically. Comments from users were also collected. At the end of the study, the house officers, primary care physicians, and nurses were sent electronic questionnaires[8] inquiring about their use and satisfaction with the program.

Patient outcomes included the number of days until emergency readmission to the hospital, the patient's length of stay, and the number of medications the patient was given at the time of discharge. For patients who were readmitted within 30 days, readmissions attributable to medication errors were determined by the hospital's utilization review department (blinded to the study group of the patient).

Members of a random sample of English-speaking patients who were discharged during the first four months of the study from an intervention floor and from a control floor were contacted by telephone and asked about their satisfaction with their hospitalization, medication teaching in the hospital, and their adherence to discharge medication regimens. The questionnaire used the inquiries in an ongoing study[6], augmented with questions adapted from the Medical Outcomes Study[9].

Other data collected were patient demographic and insurance information, the number of procedures performed during the hospitalization, the number of inpatient medications at the time of discharge, whether the patient was followed in our hospital-based group practice, where the OMR is used for outpatient care, and whether the patient had an illness related to HIV infection (major diagnostic class of 25).

Statistical Analysis

Analysis was performed on an intention-to-treat basis. Fisher's exact test and two-tailed t-tests were performed on categorical and continuous variables, respectively. The same tests were also used to determine and adjust for the composition of each floor. Chi squared tests for trend were applied to program usage data. Secondary analyses were performed to identify the patients for whom the intervention was actually applied, and the effect of it. All analyses were performed using SAS[10].

RESULTS

Baseline Data

Three thousand nine hundred and sixty-four patients were discharged from the intervention floors and 2237 from the control floors during the study period. Two thousand one hundred and sixty-five patients met the entry criteria for inclusion in the analysis, 63 percent of whom were from the intervention floors. There were no differences between the intervention and control groups with respect to sex, ethnic group, age, proportion receiving outpatient care at Beth Israel, insurance status, HIV status, length of hospitalization, number of procedures, or number of inpatient medications.

User Data

Eighty-three percent of primary care providers responded to the survey with a median response time of 1 day. Almost 90 percent said that notification of medications at the time of discharge saved them time, and more than 90 percent felt that electronic notification was the most useful.

Seventy-one percent of house officers responded to the survey with a median response time of 2 days. Sixty-one percent of those said they had used the program, and 68 percent of the users felt it made deciding about medications easier. Seventy-seven percent felt that the program took no more time than the manual process, and 41 percent felt that it saved them time. More than half felt that their clerical work was easier, and more than 82 percent felt the program was usually helpful. All thought that it was worth the time and effort needed to use it.

Of the house officers who had not used it, 93 percent felt such an approach would be useful. Reasons for not using the program included not knowing it existed and not knowing how to use it.

Seventy-two percent of nurses responded to the survey with a median response time of nine days. Half had remembered receiving printouts from the program, 82 percent felt that it made their clerical work easier, and 30 percent were more comfortable teaching patients with this information. About half felt that the patient attained more knowledge because of this information.

Patient Data

There was no difference in length of stay, time to emergency readmission, or number of medications prescribed between the two groups. The amount of time spent doing the discharge medications was significantly lower in the intervention group (12 vs. 6 minutes, p=0.048); this was offset by slightly more medications (7.4 vs 6.3, p=0.052), so the number of minutes per medication was unchanged (1.3). One adverse drug event was determined to be contributing to early unplanned readmission, and this occurred in a patient from the control group.

The program was used for 38 percent of eligible patients during the study period. The proportion ranged from 42 to 69 percent during the first five months of the study (χ^2 for trend=0.02, p=0.88), and from 19 to 33 percent after the arrival of the new interns (χ^2 for trend=5.4, p=0.02; see Figure 1).

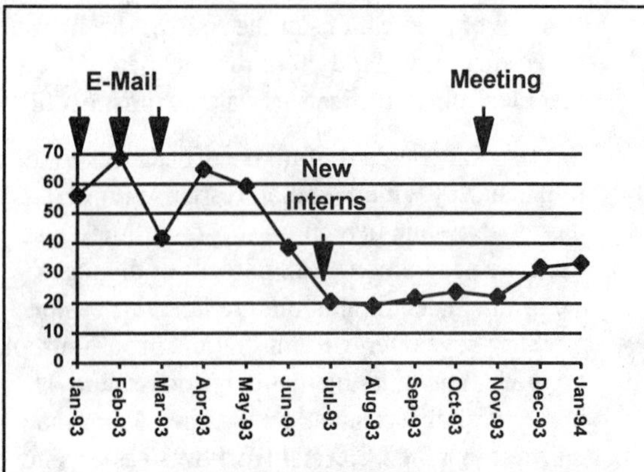

Figure 1 Percent usage of program by month

Patients for whom the program was used tended to be older and had longer hospitalizations. There was no difference in the number of procedures, HIV status, insurance status, number of medications in the hospital, or whether or not the patient was followed in our group practice.

Patient questionnaire results revealed no statistically significant differences between groups, but there was a tendency towards improved self-reported compliance in the patients who received the intervention (96 vs 87 percent, p=0.3).

CONCLUSIONS

We conclude that a computerized system to help interns develop a list of medications at the time a patient is discharged from the hospital, to print patient educational materials, and to communicate these changes to the primary care providers is helpful and felt to be worthwhile by house officers, primary care providers, and nurses. Patients receiving printed educational materials had better adherence to their medical regimens, although part of this might be explained by patient characteristics that we could not measure. The program was preferentially used for older patients with longer hospitalizations, probably because the house officers' perceived benefit of using the program was greater for more complex cases with greater potential for mistakes, drug-drug interactions, and inadequate medication teaching. We found no statistical differences in intervals to emergency readmissions or in rates of adverse drug events causing readmissions.

There are three possible explanations for the lack of statistically significant differences in patient outcomes. One is that the program had no real benefit. This seems unlikely given the face value of the system and the uniform direction of the results.

Another possibility is that the program was effective but that we did not have statistical power to show that it was, because of inadequate sample size and/or high variability of outcomes. This is quite possible given the small samples in the patient survey, the high variability of time to subsequent admissions, and the low frequency of adverse drug events that were thought to contribute to unplanned readmissions. We are currently trying to decrease the population heterogeneity by performing a matched analysis of the data.

The third possibility is that we did not measure the proper outcomes—measuring the impact of such a complicated intervention is difficult. We could have assessed patient knowledge by querying patients about specific features of their discharge medications, and we could have observed primary care visits to determine whether medication regimens were more accurate, or being followed more precisely, saving time during the visits. These measures may be included in future studies.

Sixty-one percent of the eligible house officers used the program for 38 percent of the eligible patients. Although this is quite good in a purely voluntary system, could we have increased it? It was clear that interns needed to be reminded about the system when it was first available, and e-mail and meetings certainly helped in that regard. It is interesting that use among the new interns increased without reminders or education, suggesting that the new interns found the program useful independent of reminders.

Perhaps the new interns should have been pursued as vigorously as the first group, or perhaps we should have petitioned the department of medicine to mandate that all interns use the system when sending patients home from the hospital. One of the difficulties we had was that the program was not universally available on all the floors on which the interns took care of patients. Perhaps a time-series or crossover trial would minimize this problem. Other factors that affect an intern's decsion to use the program include the amount of time saved, the encouragement of the nursing staff, the desire to provide good patient care, and the praise of the attending physicians.

Several issues arose after the system was installed. For example, once the nursing staff began to see the laser-printed patient education materials, they wanted to use the program earlier in their patients' hospitalization, so that they might teach patients several days before discharge. The interns were unwilling to take the time to plan their patients' discharge medications earlier, but we made the educational material available to nurses on demand at any time.

Another problem was that the interns felt we were printing too much. They wanted to be able to suppress the printing of educational materials (for patients in whom they felt such information would not be needed or would be detrimental to their care plan) or of specific prescriptions (in patients who already had certain medications at home), and we have decided to allow this.

The primary care physicians who received the most benefit from this program (and the ones who were surveyed) were those in our hospital-based group practice, where the OMR is used. Since many of our inpatients receive primary care in physicians' offices outside of the hospital, we are implementing a system that sends automatically (by fax) a list of medications to these practices at the time of discharge.

The last issue is that this program was not intended to assist in the care of patients not being discharged to their homes. For these discharges, printed prescriptions are no longer neccessary, but medication decisions remain important, and a large amount of clerical work is involved. We are enhancing the program to offer the creation of an inter-agency referral form, thereby providing incentives for the use of this system even for patients who are not sent home.

In view of user satisfaction and the apparent value of this program for patients sent home from the hospital, we are making it available to the whole medical service and later to the entire hospital. As the OMR becomes available to other specialties and to community-based providers, this discharge medication program will become increasingly useful.

References

[1]. Medication regimens: causes of noncompliance. Washington, DC: Office of the Inspector General, Department of Health and Human Services, June 1990:12-4.

[2]. Kessler DA. Communication with patients about their medications. New Engl J Med 1991;325:1650-2.

[3]. Noncompliance with medications: an economic tragedy with important implications for health care reform. The Task Force for Compliance, Baltimore, MD, 1993.

[4]. Bleich HL, Beckley RF, Horowitz GL, Jackson JD, et al. Clinical computing in a teaching hospital. N Engl J Med 1985;312:756-64.

[5]. Safran C, Rury C, Rind DM, Taylor WC. A computer-based outpatient medical record for a teaching hospital. MD Comput 1992;8:291-9.

[6]. Cleary PD, Edgman-Levitan S, Walker JD, Gerteis M, Delbanco TL. Using patient reports to improve medical care: a preliminary report from 10 hospitals. Quality Management in Health Care 1993;2:31-8.

[7]. NDDF. First Data Bank, The Hearst Corporation, San Bruno, CA.

[8].Bloom SM, White RJ, Beckley RF, WV Slack. Converse: a means to write, edit, administer, and summarize computer-based dialogue. Comput Biomed Res 1978;11:167-75.

[9]. DiMatteo MR, Hays RD. Adherence to cancer regimens: implications for treating the older patient. Oncology (supp) 1992;6:50-7.

[10]. PC SAS, Release 6.04. SAS Institute Inc., Cary, NC.

Warfarin 2.0 - a Computer Program for Warfarin Management. Design and Clinical Use.

Alvaro Margolis,M.D.(*), Francisco Flores,M.D.,Comp.-Anal.(*) , Mónica Kierszenbaum, M.D.(*), Zully Cavallo,M.D.(*), Bibiana Botti,M.D.(*), Enrique D'Ottone,M.D.(**), Norberto Tavella,M.D.(**) and Jorge Torres,M.D.(*)
Clínica Médica "C" (*) and Depto. de Cardiología (**),
Hospital de Clínicas, Montevideo, Uruguay.

ABSTRACT[1]

Warfarin 2.0 is a computer program that helps physicians optimize treatment of outpatients with warfarin. The main reason for its development was to achieve a good anticoagulation level, avoiding both undertreatment -- which causes thromboembolic complications -- and overtreatment -- which causes hemorrhagic complications. The program was also designed to help educate the anticoagulated patient, standardize warfarin management and audit results of what had been done. The philosophy of continuous quality improvement was applied. Warfarin 2.0 is in clinical operation in the University Hospital, Montevideo, Uruguay, and it has also been used since the end of 1993 in the Favaloro Foundation, Dept. of Hematology, Buenos Aires, Argentina. The results from the first 15 months of use in Montevideo showed an increase in the number of patients being followed (from 91 to 132) and the average number of visits per patient (from one visit every 10.6 weeks to one every 6.5 weeks): The frequency of visits has been in the internationally accepted ranges since the program was implemented. Better anticoagulation levels were achieved after an adjusting period. Unfortunately, the number of undertreated patients is still large, and a thorough analysis of the data is going to be undertaken to continue improving warfarin management.

INTRODUCTION

Uruguay is a small country of 3 million people located between Argentina and Brazil, bordered by the River Plate and the Atlantic Ocean. With a literacy rate of about 96% and life expectancy over 70 years, it also has a disease profile similar to developed countries, with a high prevalence of cardiovascular morbidity and mortality. The University Hospital (Hospital de Clínicas, Montevideo) is a tertiary care center with well-trained physicians and other health care providers, but with very scarce resources. Internists and Cardiologists are in charge of large numbers of anticoagulated patients, and attend to them when a thromboembolic or hemorrhagic complication occurs. Most of the complications are seen in ambulatory patients, and are often due to incorrect use of the drug or infrequent patient visits. Therefore, a computerized solution was proposed. The computer program was designed to emphasize patient education, standardization of treatment and audit of results.

Another important reason for the development of the program is the recent inclusion of non-rheumatic atrial fibrillation as a definite indication for anticoagulation [1]. However, these results were obtained in controlled clinical conditions, in academic institutions, with selected patients. The challenge is to translate these excellent results into routine clinical practice.

Several other computer programs that deal with oral anticoagulation have been developed [2,3,4,5,6,7,8]. However, their approach has been different from ours in several ways: all the British programs relied on empirical formulae to define dosage and date of next visit, and this approach does not allow the physician to understand the rationale for the decision. The same problem is encountered when using pharmacokinetic models or neural networks. In this paper we report on the design of a rule-based system that has been in clinical use for 15 months.

MATERIALS AND METHODS

Program design

One of us (AM) wrote a preliminary version of the program as a thesis project during Internal Medicine training [9]. From that first approach to the problem, the medical concepts and a general modular approach were established. The current version is written in CLIPPER, using DGE V.4 as a graphical library. The program is written for a 386 or higher IBM-PC compatible computer [10]. The system uses a parametric design, i.e., it can be modified by changing the files that the system uses for running. Among the modifiable modules are the main menu and the data entry modules for the first and subsequent visits. It has a normalized system of archiving data -- only positive data are archived, and these data are coded, which saves disk space (all the files with the current data use about 300 kb for all patients). However, the main advantage of using coded data is that information is retrievable for decision support.

The program was designed to be used by physicians, most of whom are not computer-literate,

[1] Correspondence to : A. Margolis, Dept. of Medical Informatics, University of Utah, Room AB193, SLC UT 84132 USA

0195-4210/94/$5.00

in a user-friendly and consistent way. The program also provides both technical and medical help on-line. The following modules are used (presented in the order most frequently used in clinical practice):

1) *Data entry for the first and subsequent visits.* On the first visit, demographic data, dates of use of anticoagulant, reason for anticoagulation, risk for embolic or hemorrhagic events (previous systemic embolism, gastroduodenal ulcer, alcoholism, etc), current medications and prothrombin time (PT) expressed in INR are recorded. The importance of reporting PT in INR (International Normalized Ratio) as a standardized expression of PT has been previously stressed [11]. INR is close to 1 in the normal population, and has a broad therapeutic range from 2 to 4.5, depending on the disease -- the upper limit has been decreased in recent years. In this article, the PT is always expressed as INR. On subsequent visits, a systematic review of complications, new medications and compliance with treatment are reviewed and entered. All these data are stored using a hierarchical coding system.

2) *An algorithm* uses the above data to suggest a dose and a date for follow up. Also, alerts are triggered in particular cases. The algorithm is the **core** of the program, but would be worthless if not used in the context of the whole system. The knowledge in the algorithm is based on the third Consensus Conference on Antithrombotic Therapy [12]. Nevertheless, since not every detail of antithrombotic therapy was considered by this conference, a detailed analysis of different possible problems was done. The variables considered included: presence of mechanical heart valves, age, last prothrombin time (PT), ratio of the last two PTs, time elapsed since warfarin was started, time elapsed since the current dose was administered, history of new drugs taken, history of bleeding, previous systemic embolism, diseases that can potentially cause bleeding, unstable PT values, alcoholism, extremely high warfarin dosage, ball valve prosthesis, use of an NSAID, distance to the clinic and non-compliance with treatment or scheduled visits. Consider a real case as an example:

- Twenty-five year old male patient.
- mechanical heart valves in the aortic and mitral areas for eight years.
- sinus rhythm.
- past history of duodenal ulcer and upper gastroduodenal bleeding two years ago. No recurrent bleeding thereafter.
- anticoagulated with warfarin for eight years.
- receiving warfarin, 5 mg 3 times a week, 7.5 mg 4 times a week, for the last three months.
- no new drugs , no problems reported.
- previous INR: 3.1 -- it was done 6 weeks ago.
- today's INR: 3.1.
- lives close by Montevideo.
- good compliance with treatment for the last 7 months.

The algorithm suggests:

- an INR goal of 2.5 to 3.5.
- since this goal has been met, no dose adjustment is recommended.
- recommendation of maximum interval until next visit of 6 weeks, because of stable anticoagulation levels, no new drugs added, no recent complications and the fact that the patient lives close to the Capital. If the patient had lived farther away, the recommendation would have been 8 weeks, which is the maximum allowed by the system's logic, according to the third Consensus Conference.

The following alerts are triggered:

- the patient has a condition that predisposes bleeding complications: duodenal ulcer.
- the patient has missed two or more appointments.

3) *A patient data retrieval system,* that helps the physician decide if the algorithm takes into account all the problems encountered with his/her patient. It includes the patient history, a graphical representation of the last 6 INR results and the average daily warfarin dosages, and the alerts and the rules used by the algorithm in this case. Referring to the previous example, some conditions were not considered: gender (the physician may insist on precautions to planning a pregnancy because of the teratogenic effects of warfarin), location and number of mechanical heart valves, and heart rhythm (none of these conditions were considered by the Consensus Conference, but they may affect the incidence of thromboembolic events), long term INR results (stability can also be determined using the graphical display of the last 6 INRs and dosages).

4) *Printouts:* after defining whether the suggestions should be modified or not, an instruction is printed for the patient, and a copy is included in his/her medical history. Also, on the first visit one page of general instructions about the use and potential problems of warfarin is given to the patient. If the patient has to go to the dentist, a printout is provided for the dentist explaining warfarin treatment in that situation.

5) *On-line medical help* is available throughout the program. It includes warfarin interactions with other drugs, what to do if the PT is high or the patient has had bleeding, risk of bleeding with warfarin, laboratory standardization of the PT, etc.

6) *Backup procedures and other tasks:* after seeing all the patients on a given day, a hard copy summary backup of all the visits is done, as well as a compulsory backup to diskette. A printout list of patients who have been rescheduled is given to the receptionist, and letters are sent to the patients who were scheduled but did not come.

7) There are two other important modules: one is *statistical software* for analysis; the other allows us

to *access the hierarchical vocabulary*, with a graphical interface that allows users to add new terms to the data dictionary.

Data analysis

Three periods are compared : 1) Pre-computer phase: nine months of prospectively collected data before the use of the software, from March to November 1992. 2) Computer phase 1 (implementation of the software): the first six months of use of the program, when modules were developed and incorporated, and the main changes to the software and the logic were undertaken. This period began in December 1992 and ended in May 1993. 3) Computer phase 2: the last nine months of use of the software. This last period started in June 1993 and ended in February 1994. Since the PT of the first visit was not impacted by the program, it was not included in the analysis in all three periods.

Patients were divided according to the therapeutic goal: 1) PT in INR = 2.0 to 3.0, for patients who do not have a mechanical heart valve. 2) A higher goal in patients with mechanical heart valves. This goal varied throughout the follow up: at the beginning (pre-computer phase and first three months of follow up with the computer) the goal was a INR = 3.0 to 4.5, with the ideal being as close as 3.0 as possible; we based this goal on the second Consensus Conference [13]. After the third Consensus Conference was published, we decided to adapt the goal to the one suggested by the third Conference (2.5 to 3.5). Therefore, we applied a more general goal (INR = 2.0 to 4.5) to compare all three periods for patients with mechanical heart valves, as suggested by Poller et al [4], for auditing purposes .

Statistical analysis: the results were converted to discrete values, dependent on whether the INR result at each visit was within a certain range or not. Chi-square analysis was then performed. Significance was set at the conventional 5% level. The Yates correction was used when comparing 2 by 2 tables.

RESULTS

There were 151 patients registered at the clinic in the two year period. Thirty-one of them (20%) had an INR goal of 2 to 3, and 120 (80%) had a higher therapeutic goal due to the presence of a mechanical heart valve.

Table 1 shows that there was a 45 % increase in the number of patients seen in Computer phase 2 compared to the Pre-computer phase and a 137% increase in the number of visits. This was due not only to the number of patients but also to the number of visits per patient. The percentage of missing values of PTs in INR was 1 % in the two year period, usually because they were not expressed in INR format.

Table 1 : Administrative data from the two-year follow up, beginning in March 1992 and ending in February 1994.

	Pre-comp. 9 months	Comp. 1 6 months	Comp. 2 9 months
# patients	91	107	132
# visits	336	386	796
Patients per visit	9.33	15.44	12.84
Interval between visits	10.6 weeks	7.2 weeks	6.5 weeks

Results for the two therapeutic goals are shown separately, since the populations were different and the knowledge base was not exactly the same for the two goals.

Higher goal (INR = 3.0-4.5 in the first year, 2.5-3.5 thereafter):

The characteristics of the population are as follows: the average age was 55 +/- 14 years. The dose of warfarin was in each phase 5.47 +/- 2.11, 5.15 +/- 1.93, 5.23 +/- 2.03 (range 1 to 13 mg per day).

The rate of INR results within the more general therapeutic goal suggested by Poller (2.0 - 4.5), for auditing purposes, is shown in Table 2. Even if there was a similar percentage within the general goal of 2.0-4.5 in all periods, there was an increase in the number of patients being overtreated (INR>4.5) during Computer phase 1, and a decrease in this number during Computer phase 2 compared to the two previous ones. While more patients were overtreated in Computer phase 1, fewer patients were undertreated compared to the other two periods.

Table 2 : Percentages of visits spent in various INR bands. Higher therapeutic goal.

	Pre-comp.	Comp. 1	Comp. 2
2.0 - 4.5	73.42 %	73.70 %	74.65 %
< 2.0	16.66 %	11.03 %	18.70 %
> 4.5	9.90 %	15.26 %	6.64 %
# of visits	222	308	647

The results of analyzing the different therapeutic ranges for the last 12 months, when a goal of 2.5-3.5 was established, are shown in Table 3. The number of patients in the therapeutic range +/- 0.5 (in this case, 2.0 to 4.0) significantly increased from 65.7% to 75.8% -- comparing March-May to December-February and considering the range 2.0 to

4.0, p=0.03. The number of patients being overtreated decreased to 2.8% for the last three months. This figure is significantly smaller than the pre-computer phase: 9.90%, p=0.0045 . The number of undertreated patients is more important than those overtreated, and has increased in the last period to values slightly greater than the pre-computer phase.

Table 3 : Percentages of visits spent in various INR bands during the period when the higher goal was 2.5 to 3.5. (March 1993- Feb. 1994)

	March-May	June-August	Sept. - Nov.	Dec. - Feb.
2.5-3.5	44.6 %	40.0 %	38.2 %	42.8 %
2.0-4.0	65.7 %	67.7 %	67.0 %	75.8 %
2.0-4.5	73.7 %	72.7 %	72.6 %	78.6 %
< 2.0	9.7 %	19.5 %	17.9 %	18.6 %
> 4.5	16.6 %	7.7 %	9.4 %	2.8 %
# of visits	175	220	212	215

Lower goal (2 - 3):

The characteristics of the population are the following: the age was 62 +/- 13 years. The dose was (in consecutive periods) 4.51 +/- 1.29, 3.90 +/- 1.21 and 4.02 +/- 1.49 (range 1 to 9 mg daily).

The ranges of anticoagulation for the three periods are shown in Table 4. The number of patients undertreated is important and has increased, but the range of patients under "broad range" (goal +/- 0.5, in this case 1.5 to 3.5) has also increased. The number of patients that were overtreated during Computer phase 1 is high, and there was also a greater dispersion of values during that time.

Table 4 : Percentages of visits spent in various INR bands. Lower therapeutic goal.

	Pre-comp.	Comp. 1	Comp. 2
2.0 - 3.0	48.4 %	43.6 %	44.8 %
1.5 - 3.5	77.4 %	72.7 %	81.6 %
< 1.5	3.2 %	9.0 %	13.6 %
> 4.5	0 %	5.5 %	2.4 %
# of visits	31	55	125

CONCLUSIONS

When Warfarin 2.0 was put into use in this population of patients, we knew it was going to be difficult to improve on the status quo, since many patients were on stable anticoagulation levels, and the whole population was within internationally accepted rates of success [4]. However, there was room for improvement with the computer program due to long periods between visits, the possibility of standardizing care, and the chance for better patient education and control. The group most likely to benefit were those patients who were newly started on warfarin and those who were non-compliant. The compulsory use of the INR, a standard measurement of PT, was another element that could improve anticoagulation with warfarin [14].

Warfarin 2.0 had the following impacts on the *processes* involved in patient care: 1) The frequency of visits increased, with an average visit per patient every 10.6 weeks in the first nine months and every 6.5 weeks in the last nine months. The frequency of visits is now within the recommended ranges [12]. 2) Seven to eleven minutes dedicated exclusively to anticoagulation, with a standard questionnaire, selective data retrieval, a standard management guideline and a printed instruction to the patient each visit.

The overall *results* regarding anticoagulation are promising in patients with a goal of 2.5 to 3.5 (80% of the patients). A large majority of them were in the therapeutic ranges most of the time, and showed steady improvement over the months. Still, there were a large number of visits with patients' INR results under 2, these results are being audited individually to clarify the reason. The results in the group of patients with a lower goal are acceptable, but there is room for improvement, particularly in the undertreated group. Case by case auditing will be done. The philosophy of continuous quality improvement was applied [15,16]. A goal was established, and a reduction in variability both in processes and outcomes was pursued. The cycle was then restarted as a part of a continuous improvement effort.

There were problem areas in the study as well: a number of patients were overtreated during the implementation phase -- Computer phase 1 --. The number was not as large as that reported in other series with the same goal [4]. Particular attention has to be paid to the first phase of implementation of a clinical information system, because the sum of the impact on the environment and problems with the system logic could be detrimental rather than beneficial.

We did not separate the overall change to the environment from the program logic while we were analyzing the impact of Warfarin 2.0 on the levels of anticoagulation. We were interested in dealing with warfarin management from a global perspective. Otherwise, it would have been a basic clinical experiment, not a practical development.

We are also aware that intermediate outcomes (in our case, amount of care provided and PT results) were not necessarily a reflection of end results (major bleeding, thromboembolism, death) [17]. There is a module in the program to trace patients who stopped attending the clinic. These patients may then have had a severe complication that would have gone undocumented otherwise. After this step, a thorough report and analysis will be done. Since the goal of anticoagulation ultimately depends on an equilibrium between risk of major bleeding and thromboembolic complications [18], this analysis would be helpful if the sample size is large enough. At this time, the size of the population would allow us to demonstrate substantial differences only, and preliminary data does not show this kind of result.

Warfarin 2.0 uses rules to represent knowledge. This strategy allows the clinician to understand the reasoning of the program. There are other strategies, some of them validated within clinical practice [2-5], and others still experimental to a greater or lesser degree [6-8]. It would be useful to identify the cases where each approach yields the best results, and combine them.

It will be important for our perception of transferability issues to observe the success and modifications that have to be made in the Favaloro Foundation in Buenos Aires. This site follows about 100 patients a week.

The development of a computerized decision support system is a complex task. Furthermore, its implementation is even more challenging. However, computers are excellent tools for providing real-time feedback to physicians. The complexity of the task should not undermine our efforts.

Acknowledgment

We would like to acknowledge the support provided by Quimica Ariston, Cardiology and Laboratory personnel, and Drs. Alfredo Alvarez Rocha and Juan Alonso. We are also indebted to Drs. Reed Gardner and Victoria Foerster for the revision of the manuscript.

References

[1] Singer DE. Randomized trials of warfarin for atrial fibrillation. N. Engl. J. Med. 1992; 327(20):1451-3.

[2] Wilson A, James AH. Computer assisted management of warfarin treatment. BMJ 1984;289:422-4.

[3] Ryan PJ, Gilbert M, Rose PE. Computer control of anticoagulant dose for therapeutic management. BMJ 1989;299:1207-9.

[4] Poller L, Wright D, Rowlands M. Prospective comparative study of computer programs used for management of warfarin. J Clin Pathol 1993;46:299-303.

[5] Hunt B. Development of a MUMPS-based anticoagulant management system. British Journal of biomedical Science 1993;50:117-124.

[6] Farrow L, Mungall D, Raskob G, Hull R. Predicting the daily prothrombin time response to warfarin. Ther drug monitor 1990;12(3):246-9.

[7] White RH, Mungall D. Outpatient Management of Warfarin Therapy: Comparison of Computer-Predicted Dosage Adjustment to Skilled Professional Care. Ther drug monitor 1991;13(1):46-50.

[8] Narayanan MN, Lucas SB. A Genetic Algorithm to Improve a Neural Network to Predict a Patient's Response to Warfarin. Meth Inform Med 1993;32:55-8.

[9] Margolis A. Anticoagulación crónica con warfarina. Un programa piloto. Monografía de postgrado, Marzo 1991. Escuela de Medicina, Montevideo.

[10] Margolis A, Flores F, Cavallo Z et al. Warfarin 2.0. Un programa de computación para el manejo de la anticoagulación crónica con warfarina. Revista Médica del Uruguay (in press).

[11] Hirsh J. Is the dose of warfarin prescribed by american physicians unnecessarily high? Arch Intern Med 1987;147:769-771.

[12] Dalen JE, Hirsh J (guest Editors). Third ACCP Consensus Conference on Antithrombotic Therapy. Chest 1992;102(4):303-549 (Supplement).

[13] Soffer A (Editor in Chief). Second ACCP Consensus Conference on Antithrombotic Therapy. Chest 1989;95(2):1-169 (Supplement).

[14] Bussey HI, Force RW, Bianco TM et al. Reliance on Prothrombin Time Ratios Causes Significant Errors in Anticoagulation Therapy. Arch Intern Med 1992;152:278-282.

[15] Laffel G, Blumenthal D. The Case for Using Industrial Quality Management Science in Health Care Organizations. JAMA 1989;262:2869-2873.

[16] Berwick DM. Continuous improvement as an ideal in Health Care. N Engl J Med 1989;320:53-6.

[17] Echt DS, Liebson PR, Mitchell LB et al. Mortality and Morbidity in Patients Receiving Encainide, Flecainide, or Placebo. The Cardiac Arrhythmia Supression Trial. N Engl J Med 1991;324:781-8.

[18] Rosendaal FR, Cannegieter SC, van der Meer FJM et al. A Method to Determine the Optimal Intensity of Oral Anticoagulant Therapy. Thrombosis and Haemostasis 1993;69(3): 236-239.

Support for Research & Imaging Neural Networks

Identification of Low Frequency Patterns in Backpropagation Neural Networks

Lucila Ohno-Machado, MD, MHA
Section on Medical Informatics, Stanford University School of Medicine
Stanford, CA 94305 machado@camis.stanford.edu

Although neural networks have been widely applied to medical problems in recent years, their applicability has been limited for a variety of reasons. One of these barriers has been the inability to discriminate rare classes of solutions (i.e., the identification of categories that are infrequent). In this article, I demonstrate that a system of hierarchical neural networks (HNN) can overcome the problem of recognizing low frequency patterns, and therefore can improve the prediction power of neural-network systems. HNN are designed according to a divide-and-conquer approach: Triage networks are able to discriminate supersets that contain the infrequent pattern, and these supersets are then used by Specialized networks, which discriminate the infrequent pattern from the other ones in the superset. The supersets that are discriminated by the Triage networks are based on pattern similarity. The application of multilayered neural networks in more than one step allows the prior probability of a given pattern to increase at each step, provided that the predictive power of the network at the previous level is high. The method has been applied to one artificial set and one real set of data. In the artificial set, the distribution of the patterns was known and no noise was present. In this experiment, the HNN provided better discrimination than a standard neural network for all classes. In a real data set of nine thousand patients who were suspected of having thyroid disorders, the HNN also provided higher sensitivity than its corresponding standard neural network (without a corresponding decay in specificity) given the same time constraints. I discuss the reasons why the sensitivity achieved by systems of divide-and-conquer hierarchical neural networks is superior to that of non-hierarchical neural network models, the conditions in which the algorithm should be applied, potential improvements, and current limitations.

NEURAL NETWORKS AND CLASSIFICATION

Neural networks, also known as connectionist systems, or parallel distributed processing models, are computer-based, self-adaptive models of artificial intelligence (AI) that were first developed in the sixties, but that reached great popularity only in the mid-eighties, after the development of the backpropagation algorithm by Rumelhart et al. [1]. Initially derived from neuroscientists' models of human neurons, neural networks now encompass a wide variety of systems (many of which have no intention to mimic the human brain). Classification, or pattern recognition, is one of the most common uses of neural networks in medicine, and is usually implemented as a supervised machine-learning method because the system needs a set of training cases to estimate its internal parameters, or weights. Typically, no rules or other traditional AI knowledge representation schemes are used in neural networks (with the exception of hybrid models). Figure 1 shows the basic components of a neural network. Input values are multiplied by weights that are adjusted iteratively every time a set of patterns is presented. The results of the multiplication are passed through an activation function in each "hidden" unit of the intermediate layer of nodes (in our figure, the activation function is the sigmoid). The activation values for the units of the "hidden" layer will then be multiplied by the weights of the second layer, and the results of these operations will subsequently pass through the activation function of the output layer, providing the final solution.

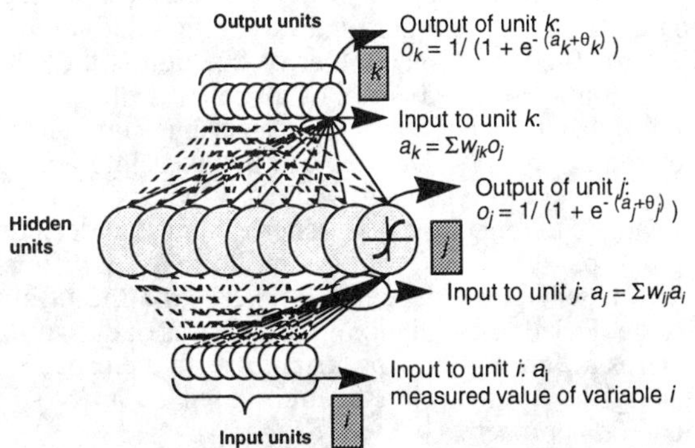

Figure 1. Basic components of a neural network

Usually, the output node that has the highest activation at the end of the training phase will indicate the predicted category. In a classification application, inputs are generally composed of the attributes of each instance in a data set, and outputs constitute classification categories. For example, a neural network that was designed to classify patients suspected of having thyroid disease, such as the one depicted in Figure 2, may have as inputs laboratory values, history data, and physical-examination items. The outputs are the classes *hypothyroidism*, *hyperthyroidism*, and so on. In medicine, neural networks have been used in many different applications, such as automated diagnosis of myocardial infarction [2], prediction of length of stay in intensive care units [3], decision support for assessing the adequacy of weaning patients from ventilators [4], prediction of the mechanism of action of new drugs [5], and radiology applications [6,7,8,9]. The backpropagation algorithm for supervised classification is the most frequent algorithm employed in medical applications of neural networks [10].

The backpropagation algorithm applies a steepest-descent (or hill-climbing) method to minimize an error function, and therefore it inherits steepest-descent's well-known problems: the existence of local minima, the possibility of having multiple solutions, and the difficulty of assuring that the solution found is optimal. Nevertheless, none of the limitations mentioned above has prevented backpropagation-based neural networks from being useful in a variety of real-world settings. However, researchers should fully understand the limitations of the backpropagation algorithm and its multiple variants to benefit maximally from its use.

0195-4210/94/$5.00

RECOGNITION OF RARE PATTERNS

Even though researchers in medical informatics are often looking for low frequency data or rare patterns, the latter are difficult to recognize in certain types of machine learning methods, including backpropagation-based neural networks. The difficulty is often due to the fact that the utility of a classification is not taken into account by the methods employed, and that the error that needs to be minimized is not weighted accordingly. The standard error function to be minimized in a backpropagation-based neural network is usually

$$E(w) = \frac{1}{2}\Sigma[\zeta_i - O_i]^2 \qquad \textbf{(1)}$$

where w is the weight matrix, ζ_i is the expected output for pattern i, and O_i is the output provided by the network [11]. The changes in weights in the backpropagation algorithm are proportional to the first derivative of the error function. Since the error function is the result of the sum of squared errors of all patterns, the patterns with higher frequency will have a stronger influence in the weight changes. Utilities can be taken into account in the process of changing weights if the error function is changed to reflect the researcher's interest in detecting a given pattern. In the latter case, however, a different network will have to be trained each time the utilities change. I tried to avoid mixing the process of classifying patterns according to their attributes with the process of making the optimal classification based on a decision-theoretic approach.

Machine-learning methods of classification provide inexpensive means to perform classification. Backpropagation-based neural networks are able to perform classification reliably, provided that the frequency of the relevant patterns is not low. With the increasing number of electronic clinical databases, and the increasing costs of manual processing, it is likely that machine-learning applications will be necessary to detect deviant procedures and unexpected outcomes. These patterns are infrequent, but their detection is important. Therefore, there is a need to enhance the predictive power of the machine learning methods, especially the detection of low frequency patterns, without a decrease in specificity.

Traditional classification methods, such as linear-discriminant analysis, also have difficulties in detecting infrequent patterns [12]. If the variability of the most frequent classes is high, then a rare class may be considered just another instance of the most frequent class, and no discrimination will be possible. On the other hand, if all classes are equally represented and they are separable (linearly separable, if the simplest form of neural networks — the perceptron — is used), then the neural network should be able to make the distinction. A large number of medical applications in which classification is desired have the goal of discriminating a pattern of low frequency (e.g., "thyroid disease", "bad prognosis") from a pattern with high frequency (e.g., "no disease", "good prognosis"). For example, if only a very small group of patients who have undergone by-pass surgery have prolonged lengths of stay in hospital, this category will hardly be recognized by most machine learning methods. These are, however, exactly the patterns that need to be studied and followed more closely. Another example is screening for certain diseases, which is considered beneficial even when the prevalence of the condition is low but the overall benefit of detecting a case justifies the costs (e.g, screening for congenital hypothyroidism, a disease that has a prevalence of 1/4,000) [13]. Unless neural network applications address the problem of discriminating low frequency patterns, their use in medical applications will not scale up to useful real-world applications. The issues of (a) considering the utility of a classification and (b) creating mechanisms to allow the discrimination of rare patterns must be addressed. In this article, I will focus on the latter.

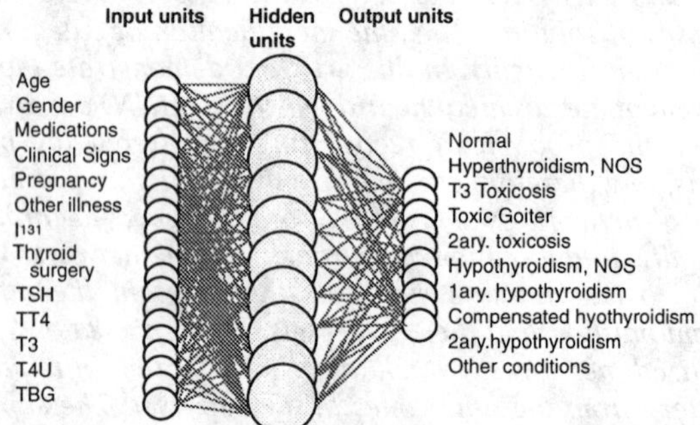

Figure 2. A generic neural network for thyroid diseases

HIERARCHIES OF NEURAL NETWORKS

The HNN is an architecture of neural networks in which the problem is divided and solved in more than one step. Figure 3 shows how a hierarchical system of neural networks should operate: the first classifier, or Triage Network, divides the data set in smaller subsets, which will then constitute the inputs for the Specialized networks.

DATABASE RECORDS

TRIAGE NETWORK

SPECIALIZED NETWORKS

Figure 3. Hierarchical neural network

Electronic data from medical records are entered in a Triage network. This network filter instances that should be further processed by Specialized networks.

The application of multilayered neural networks in more than one step allows the prior probability of a given pattern to increase at each step, provided that the predictive power of the network at the previous level is high (i.e., the area under the ROC curve is greater than 0.5). For example, suppose a researcher needs to discriminate four categories of patterns in a given data set. Among the patterns, there exists one that corresponds to only 1 percent of the patterns. The other categories have prior probabilities of 5, 44, and 50 percent. By applying a classifier that can reliably discriminate a set of two categories from the other patterns, and applying another classifier to the results of this pre-classification, the total number of patterns in the second step is decreased, and consequently the frequency of a given pattern increased. This increase in frequency allows a hierarchical neural network classifier to discriminate patterns faster, as I will demonstrate. The hierarchical model assumes that the first classifier is able to discriminate a superset of some categories, which includes the desired one, from the other ones. Since in any of these reliably constructed supersets the prior probability of a category in the set is higher than that of the initial sample, this process will yield higher posterior probabilities for the desired class than the one used by the classifier that attempts to make all distinctions in one single step.

Using Bayes rule, where X is a vector of attributes, and C_i is a category, we have:

$$P(C_1|X) = \frac{P(X|C_1)P(C_1)}{\Sigma P(X|C_i)P(C_i)} \quad (2)$$

In the two-category case, the equation becomes:

$$P(C_1|X) = \frac{P(X|C_1)P(C_1)}{P(X|C_1)P(C_1) + P(X|\neg C_1)P(\neg C_1)} \quad (3)$$

Assuming that $k_1 = P(X|C_1)$ and $k_2 = P(X|\neg C_1)$ are constants, and that $P(\neg C_1) = 1 - P(C_1)$, we can see in Eq.4 that whenever $P(C_1)$ is increased, the posterior probability $P(C_1|X)$ is also increased.

$$P(C_1|X) = \frac{k_1 P(C_1)}{(k_1 - k_2)P(C_1) + k_2} \quad (4)$$

Therefore, if the prior probability of a class is augmented in the training set and the sensitivity and specificity of the network remain unchanged, the posterior probability of the class is increased. In other words, if the Triage and the Specialized networks of the hierarchical system in Figure 3 each have the same number of weights as that of the generic system (and consequently the same potential for achieving the same sensitivity and specificity after training), they can perform better than the non-hierarchical system can.

This process confirms the intuition that if by any reason the prevalence of a pattern is increased, while everything else remains unchanged, the posterior probability of that pattern, given the same set of attributes, is increased. Therefore, if a Triage network is applied and is able to reliably discriminate a set that contains the desired pattern, an increase in the prior probability of that pattern will occur, also causing an increase in the posterior probability of that pattern in the corresponding Specialized network. The question remains whether Triage and Specialized networks with a smaller number of weights than that of the corresponding Generic network can also perform better than the non-hierarchical system. If the *total* number of free parameters (weights) in both systems is the same, the Triage and Specialized networks will certainly have *fewer weights* than the Generic network. The two following experiments were designed to answer this question.

EXAMPLE I: SORTING BINARY NUMBERS

In order to evaluate the power of HNN in classifying low frequency patterns, and to compare it to a standard neural network, I created an artificial data set using a known distribution. In the artificial data set, four categories (Category 0, Category 1, and so on) have to be discriminated. There were two attributes for each pattern, which constituted the binary representation of the number assigned to each of the classes ("00" was the pattern that corresponded to Category "0," "01" corresponded to Category "1," "10" corresponded to Category "2," and "11" corresponded to Category "3"). Each input unit corresponded to one digit of the binary number. All the units were binary. The inputs patterns, frequency of each type of pattern, and the expected output categories are shown in Table 1.

Table 1: Distribution of patterns for Example I

Pattern	Frequency	Output (Category)
00	44%	0
01	1%	1
10	5%	2
11	50%	3

I tested the hypothesis that the HNN could discriminate low frequency patterns earlier (i.e., requiring fewer training cycles) than a standard neural network could, provided that the systems had the same number of weights. Figure 4 shows how the hierarchical system of neural networks works. A standard feed-forward neural network that tries to classify the patterns in just one step was created for comparison. Classification in the HNN was done in a supervised manner in each step. The neural networks of the first-level (Triage networks) discriminate patterns 0 and 1 from patterns 2 and 3. The two networks for the second-level (Specialized networks), discriminate between patterns 0 and 1 and patterns 2 and 3, respectively. Note that the *total* number of weights in the HNN is the same as that of the standard neural network (i.e., the total number of parameters that needed to be estimated in each of the systems is controlled to be the same).

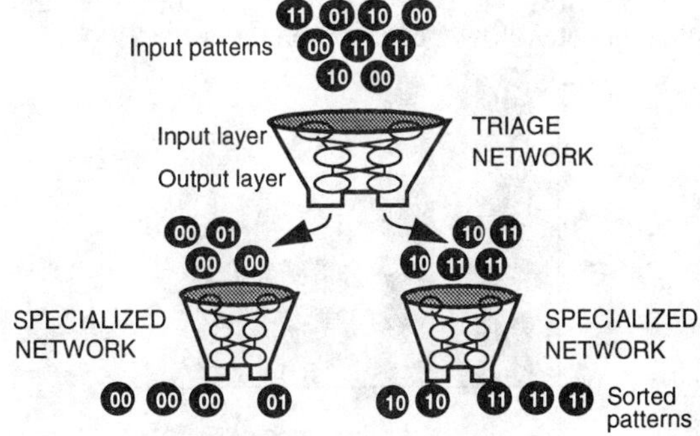

Figure 4. Sorting binary numbers

Table 2 displays the number of parameters to be estimated (weights), the number of training cycles (epochs), and the average time that each system took to converge to a perfect solution. A perfect solution was defined to be achieved when the activation of the correct output unit was at least twice that of the other output units. No noise was added to the data. Training was done by epochs. I performed 10 simulations for each system, starting with different initial weights. All networks were trained with a fixed learning rate of 0.01 and no momentum term. The overall time spent for making the perfect classification was significantly reduced ($p< 0.01$) with the use of HNN. I did not run Specialized networks in parallel, even though by doing so time could be reduced even more. It must also be taken into account that one epoch in the non-hierarchical network takes longer than one epoch in any of the networks in the hierarchical system, given the smaller number of weights in each of the networks of the latter, and the smaller number of patterns in the Specialized networks.

Table 2: Comparison of systems for Example I

System	Units	Weights	Epochs†	Time ‡
Standard NN	10	24	148,791	50 min 53 sec
Hierarchical NN	18	24	14,623	2 min 37 sec
Perceptron	6	8	11,119	2 min 00 sec
Hierarchical Perceptron	12	12	6,437	36 sec

† Average of 10 runs. Refers to the detection of pattern 1.
‡ Average time on an HP9000 workstation. Considers longest epoch in the hierarchical system.

Although the nature of the problem allows a simple perceptron (a one-layered neural network) to converge to a solution, my study focused on the behavior of the backpropagation algorithm for multilayered neural networks. The perceptron's performance on this problem (see Table 2) was extremely good, as expected, but it would not be as good in the case of a non-linearly separable problem, as we will see in Example II. A multilayered neural network that has enough hidden units can approximate any function [14], and its applicability is therefore much broader than that of a perceptron. Furthermore, a hierarchical system of perceptrons also proved to converge faster than a standard perceptron did in this example.

Figure 5 displays the number of epochs (in fact, the logarithm of the number of epochs, given the orders of magnitude involved) required for the standard neural network to learn patterns that have different frequencies in Example I. As we can see, the standard neural network requires an overwhelming number of training cycles to detect low frequency patterns.

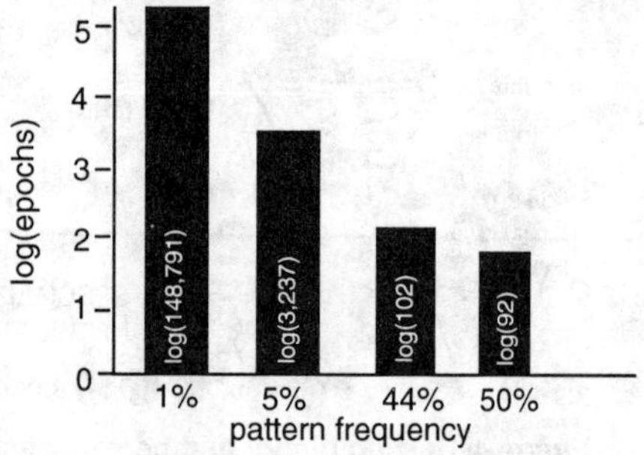

Figure 5. Number of epochs and pattern frequency

One might still argue that the pre-selection of subsets that were themselves linearly separable introduced a bias in favor of the hierarchical system. I also ran the same experiments dividing the subsets in a different way, such that patterns "00" and "11" would be separated from patterns "01" and "10" in the Triage network. This grouping would require that the Triage network would be able to solve a non-linearly separable problem first, and is by far the worst possible grouping: the Hamming distance between patterns in the same group is twice that of patterns in other groups. Furthermore, the proportions involved would require the Triage network to detect a subgroup that had a low frequency value itself (the patterns "01" and "10" constitute only six percent of the total number of patterns). The HNN exhibited a peculiar behavior: four of the ten networks converged to a solution after relatively few epochs (mean: 34,944), but the other six did not converge to a perfect solution even after $4x10^5$ epochs. This result indicates that the groupings should be done by similarity of features, rather than be based purely on pattern frequencies. Therefore, merging rare patterns that do not share similarities into a group simply to increase their frequency in the training set does not help. Patterns have to be similar for the Triage network to work.

Another experiment, in which the pattern distribution was changed to the one shown in Table 3, proved that the difficulties encountered by the Triage network were not related to the combined low frequency of the group "01" and "10", but to the fact that the similarities within the groups were low. None of the ten Triage networks built for this experiment converged to a perfect solution after $4x10^5$ epochs. Pattern similarity seems to be the key factor in determining the success of HNN.

Table 3: Another distribution of patterns for Example I

Pattern	Frequency	Output (Category)
00	1%	0
01	45%	1
10	5%	2
11	49%	3

Evaluation of a test set was not necessary in this artificial example because the categories were *defined* as being the decimal representation of the binary numbers. The systems would have exhibited the same performance on any test set composed of the same patterns, independent of their distribution. Overfitting was not a concern for exactly the same reason.

In order to determine whether (a) the difficulties that standard neural networks had to detect low-frequency patterns in the artificial data set would be reproduced in a real-world data sets, which often contain missing values and noise, and (b) the proposed solution would also be applicable in more complex problems, the following experiment was designed.

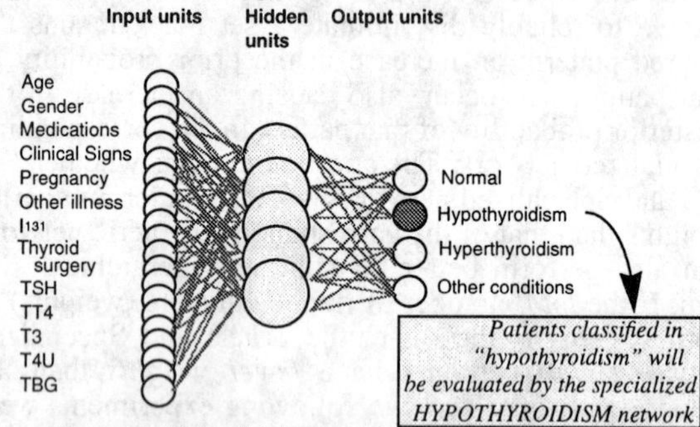

Figure 6. Thyroid diseases triage neural network

EXAMPLE II: THYROID DISEASES

I used a set of 9,172 patients suspected of having thyroid diseases, obtained from the data repository at University of California at Irvine [15]. The same data set was used by Quinlan to demonstrate the performance of decision trees in diagnosing hypothyroidism [16]. I used a subset of 4,586 patients to train the networks. A standard neural network discriminated ten different diagnoses. It consisted of 22 inputs, 10 hidden units, and 10 outputs. The standard neural network, or Generic network, was shown in Figure 2. In the HNN, the Triage network was dedicated to discriminate patterns of *hypothyroidism, hyperthyroidism, normality, and other thyroid conditions*. The rationale for establishing these groupings was based on the assumptions that (a) patients in each group shared similar attribute values, and (b) even if not all the specialized networks were able to refine the solution and obtain a final diagnosis, the partial diagnoses provided by the Triage network could be clinically useful. Figure 6 shows the Triage network. The Specialized network for hypothyroidism, shown in Figure 7, takes as inputs all patients that were classified in *hypothyroidism* in the Triage network and discriminate the patterns of *primary hypothyroidism, secondary hypothyroidism, compensated hypothyroidism, and hypothyroidism not otherwise specified.*

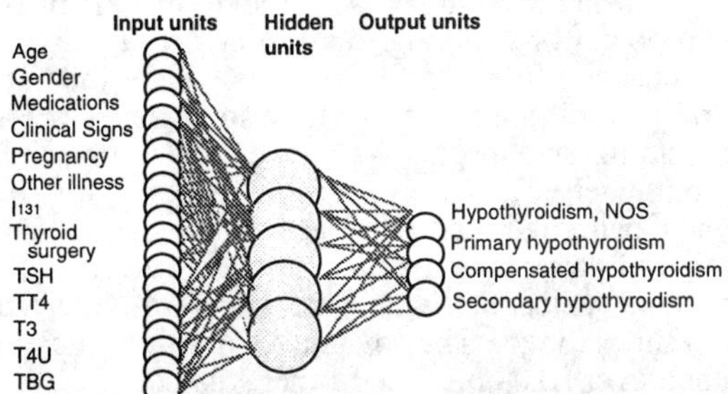

Figure 7. Hypothyroidism neural network

Table 4 shows the distribution of the output categories in the training set. Some patients had more than one diagnosis. Input attributes included age, gender, current medications, pregnancy status, previous thyroid surgery, presence of other illness, treatment with ^{131}I, clinical signs, and laboratory values for TSH, T_4, T_4U, T_3, and TBG. Missing values were imputed as their means (in the case of continuous variables) or their mode (in the case of categorical variables).

Table 4: Distribution of patterns for Example II

Output Category	Frequency	Percentage
normal	6771	72.52
Hyperthyroidism, NOS	193	2.07
Primary hyperthyroidism	21	2.25×10^{-3}
Toxic goiter	18	1.93×10^{-3}
Secondary hyperthyroidism	9	9.64×10^{-4}
Hypothyroidism, NOS	1	1.07×10^{-4}
Primary hypothyroidism	239	2.56
Compensated hypothyroidism	419	4.49
Secondary hypothyroidism	8	8.57×10^{-4}
Other conditions	1658	17.76

The networks were trained as long as the error rate in a test set of 4,586 patients was declining. When the error in the test set started to increase again, the stopping criterion was reached, and training was discontinued. The networks were not trained up to convergence to avoid overfitting [17]. Figure 8 illustrates the stopping criterion used on our networks. More details on an earlier implementation of HNN and the data set used for making the automated diagnosis of thyroid conditions can be found in [18]. Table 5 shows the time that the different systems took to reach the stopping criterion.

Table 5: Comparison of systems for Example II

System	Weights	Epochs	Time†
Standard NN	426	37,948	56 h 5 min 19 sec
Hierarchical NN	410	18,511	4 h 59 min 45 sec

† Time on an HP9000 workstation.

The time performance of hierarchical systems was clearly the best. The perceptron was not able to discriminate rare patterns even after 4×10^5 epochs, indicating that the problem was probably non-linearly separable.

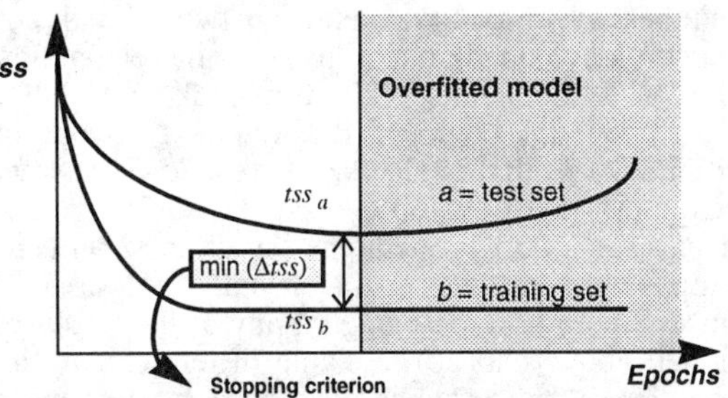

Figure 8. Avoiding overfitting in neural networks

Table 6 shows the sensitivities and specificities of the different systems after 90 minutes of training for the class *hypothyroidism*. Table 7 shows the equivalent numbers for the pattern *compensated hypothyroidism*. These numbers are based on the test set. Note that the increase in sensitivity obtained by using HNN is not coupled with a marked decrease in specificity. The superiority of the hierarchical system was clearly demonstrated in this complex problem. Not all possible subsets of variables were tried, but the results clearly confirm what was learned from the experiment using the artificial data set: HNN can learn rare patterns faster than their non-hierarchical counterparts, provided that the groupings are defined based on pattern similarity.

Table 6: Prediction of class *Hypothyroidism*

System	Sensitivity	Specificity	Epochs	Time†
Standard NN	49.25%	98.97%	650	90 min
Hierarchical NN	79.35%	98.82%	1,800	90 min

† Approximate time on an HP9000 workstation.

Table 7: Prediction of *Compensated Hypothyroidism*

System	Sensitivity	Specificity	Epochs	Time†
Standard NN	41.83%	98.45%	650	90 min
Hierarchical NN	65.87%	98.79%	3,800	90 min

† Approximate time on an HP9000 workstation.

DISCUSSION

Several authors have dealt with the decomposition of complex problems inside and outside the field of neural networks. The reasons for developing the hierarchical models of neural networks were in general very different from the ones presented in this article. Fukushima [19] developed the Neocognitron for eliminating the problem of space variations in the visual recognition of handwritten digits. The author was not specifically concerned with the frequencies of the patterns involved. He has also suggested that there were similarities between his architecture and the human visual cortex. Ballard [20] also developed a system of hierarchical neural networks for applications in machine vision, and he was particularly concerned with the problem that the backpropagation algorithm might not scale-up to complex networks. Hrycej [21] discussed modularization in neural networks. In his system, preprocessing of inputs was done in an unsupervised manner by a neural network, and the results of this factoring process were then imputed in the following networks. Frean was concerned with the problem of establishing the necessary number of units in a neural network, and consequently developed an algorithm for incremental addition of hidden units [22]. Romaniuk and Hall [23] developed the Divide and Conquer Network algorithm (DCN) that could also be related Frean's work. Hripcsak [24] developed a connectionist model for decision-support in medicine based on several backpropagation modules to incorporate real-valued and uncertain data. Even though many of the works mentioned above carried the name "Hierarchical Neural Networks", the systems developed by Jordan et al. [25] and Curry and Rumelhart [26] bear the most similarity to the one described in this article. Jordan proposed a system where many networks of experts would receive the system's inputs and compete for providing the best solution. A gating network decided among the experts' solutions. The system proposed in this article is different. Even though I propose a system were Specialized networks refine the partial solutions proposed by the Triage network, the decision on which network to use is done first, so not all experts need to be overburden with all data.

Curry and Rumelhart's work on the Mass Spectrometry Network (MSNet) is closely related to the one presented here. In that system, categories of chemical compounds are determined in a Top level network. The probability of belonging to a given group, allied to the original input attribute vector were then used by Specialized networks to refine the solution and get a final diagnosis. The authors were concerned with the fact that low frequency patterns would cause the performance of the network to decay, and they solved the problem of dealing with infrequent patterns by using a different strategy: they trained the network to recognize low frequency patterns by assigning a higher utility to these patterns. This procedure was done by modifying the learning algorithm, and processing the final output to reflect the consequent changes in posterior probabilities. My system, however, tried to disambiguate the process of diagnosing the categories from the process of using utilities while training to make an optimal decision based on a decision-theoretic approach. In my system, the diagnosis is based on the similarities between the patterns, and not on their relative utility. Once the diagnostic process is proven to be reliable and based mainly on the features presented by the inputs, the use of utilities and the decision on which category to choose should be straightforward. The selection of the best grouping at the Triage level may involve human participation, as in this study, or the clustering of examples by similarity-based algorithms, such as multidimensional scaling [27]. Rumelhart has also proposed the preprocessing of input patterns to eliminate the problem of low-frequency–pattern detection[1]. The preprocessing involves the replication of rare patterns up to the point where all categories have equal prior probabilities. A full investigation on the implications of this approach in terms of loss of specificity still needs to be done. As occurs in other systems, the rise in sensitivity of a classifier is tightly coupled with a decay in specificity. In screening large data bases, it is desirable that the rate of false-positives not be too high. Although I tried the replication method in the artificial data set — obtaining very good results with the standard neural network, as shown in Table 8 — application and evaluation of the method in the thyroid set is still under development. The problem of applying this strategy to the thyroid data set stems from the fact that the greater the number of patterns, the longer the time spent per epoch. In the training set, the network would have to handle approximately 67,710 instances per epoch if low frequency patterns were replicated to reach the same number of patterns of the most frequent category. The time spent per epoch would be therefore more than seven times longer. The advantages of this replication method over HNN must be further studied.

Table 8: Another system comparison for Example I

System	Weights	Epochs†	Time ‡
Standard NN	24	304.8	6 sec
Hierarchical NN	24	857.4	9 sec
Perceptron	8	124.4	2 sec

† Average of 10 runs. Refers to the detection of all patterns.
‡ Average time on an HP9000 workstation. Considers longest epoch in the hierarchical system.

Although I have demonstrated the superiority of HNN over standard neural networks, given specific time constraints, further enhancement of classification results could be achieved by implementing methods for pruning small weights and therefore reducing the number of free parameters allowed in the system [28]. Future work includes the study of misclassified cases to make sure that the gold-standard was correct and comparison with other statistical methods of pattern recognition. A principled way to establish the groupings at intermediate stages of the hierarchical systems needs to be developed. The adequacy of clustering methods for this purpose has to be tested. I am currently working on an implementation of HNN in the analysis of a large data set of HIV infected patients, in which investigation of these issues will be pursued. There are a number of medical applications other than the ones mentioned here that could benefit from HNN. As structured electronic medical records become more common, screening large data sets for unusual patterns may be greatly enhanced by the use of HNN. The unusual patterns detected by the neural networks can then be processed by a number of manual or computer-based decision-support applications. Database mining for knowledge discovery in large databases may also benefit from the power and simplicity of HNN.

1. Rumelhart DE. Personal communication, 1994.

CONCLUSION

The number of epochs required to train a neural network to detect patterns increases exponentially with the decrease in pattern frequency. To minimize this problem, a HNN can be used. Two examples, which used an artificial data set to classify binary numbers and a real-world complex data set of patients suspected of having thyroid disease, indicate that hierarchical systems of neural networks can overcome the problem of low frequency pattern detection in backpropagation neural networks if the selection of groupings at each step is based on pattern similarity. Many medical problems are amenable to such decomposition and should benefit from the use of HNN, especially if the detection of low frequency patterns is required. Furthermore, a rational choice of groupings may be useful for providing partial diagnoses and even for explanation purposes.

Acknowledgments

I thank Prof. David Rumelhart, Dr. Michael Walker, Prof. Mark Musen, Prof. Edward Shortliffe, Prof. Les Lenert, and Prof. Nils Nilsson for useful discussion in different stages and different aspects of the present work. I am solely responsible for any errors in the text. This work has been funded by the Conselho Nacional de Pesquisa (CNPq), Brazilian Ministry of Education. Computing facilities were provided by CAMIS, through grant LM05305 from the National Library of Medicine.

Reference

[1] Rumelhart DE; Hinton GE; Williams RJ. Learning internal representation by error propagation. In Rumelhart, D.E., and McClelland, J.L. (eds) *Parallel Distributed Processing*. MIT Press, Cambridge, 1986.

[2] Baxt WG. Use of an artificial neural network for the diagnosis of myocardial infarction. *Annals of Internal Medicine*, 1991, 115(11):843–8.

[3] Tu JV; Guerriere MR. Use of a neural network as a predictive instrument for length of stay in the intensive care unit following cardiac surgery. *Computers and Biomedical Research*, 1993, 26(3):220–9.

[4] Ashutosh K; Lee H; Mohan CK; Ranka S; Mehrotra K; Alexander C. Prediction criteria for successful weaning from respiratory support: statistical and connectionist analyses. *Critical Care Medicine*, 1992, 20(9):1295–301.

[5] Weinstein JN; Kohn KW; Grever MR; Viswanadhan VN; Rubinstein LV; Monks AP; Scudiero DA; Welch L; Koutsoukos AD; Chiausa AJ. Neural computing in cancer drug development: predicting mechanism of action. *Science*, 1992, 258(5081):447–51.

[6] Miller AS; Blott BH; Hames TK. Review of neural network applications in medical imaging and signal processing. *Medical and Biological Engineering and Computing*, 1992, 30(5):449–64.

[7] Scott JA; Palmer EL. Neural network analysis of ventilation-perfusion lung scans. *Radiology*, 1993, 186(3):661–4.

[8] Maclin PS; Dempsey J. Using an artificial neural network to diagnose hepatic masses. *Journal of Medical Systems*, 1992, 16(5):215–25.

[9] Wu Y; Giger ML; Doi K; Vyborny CJ; Schmidt RA; Metz CE. Artificial neural networks in mammography: Application to decision making in the diagnosis of breast cancer. *Radiology*, 1993, 187(1):81–7.

[10] Reggia JA. Neural computation in medicine. *Artificial Intelligence in Medicine*, 1993, 5(2):143–57.

[11] Hertz JA; Palmer RG; Krogh, AS. *Introduction to the Theory of Neural Computation*. Addison-Wesley, Redwood City, 1991.

[12] Gray NAB. Constraints on "learning machine" classification methods. *Analytical Chemistry*, 1976, 48(14):2265–8.

[13] U.S. Preventive Services Task Force. *Guide to clinical preventive services*. William and Wilkins, Baltimore, 1989.

[14] Hornik K; Stichcombe M; White H. Multilayered feedforward networks are universal approximators. *Neural Networks*, 1989, 2:359–66.

[15] Murphy PM; Aha DW. *UCI Repository of Machine Learning Databases* (on-line directory), University of California at Irvine, Department of Information and Computer Science, Irvine, CA, 1993.

[16] Quinlan JR Induction of decision trees. *Machine Learning*, 1986, 1, 81–106.

[17] Hecht-Nielsen, R. *Neurocomputing*, Addison-Wesley, Reading, 1990.

[18] Ohno-Machado L; Musen MA. Hierarchical neural networks for partial diagnosis in medicine. *Proceedings of the 1994 World Congress on Neural Networks*, San Diego, in press.

[19] Fukushima K. Neocognitron: A hierarchical neural network capable of visual pattern recognition. *Neural Networks*, 1988, 1:119–30.

[20] Ballard D. Modular learning in hierarchical neural networks. In Schwartz, E.L. (ed) *Computational Neuroscience*, Bradford, London, 1990.

[21] Hrycej T. *Modular Learning in Neural Networks*. John Wiley and Sons, New York, 1992.

[22] Frean M. The Upstart Algorithm: A method for constructing and training feedforward neural networks. *Neural Computation*, 1990, 2:198–209.

[23] Romaniuk SG; Hall LO. Divide and conquer neural networks. *Neural Networks*, 1993, 6(8): 1105–16.

[24] Hripcsak G. Using connectionist modules for decision support. *Methods of Information in Medicine*, 1990, 29:167–81.

[25] Jordan RA; Nowlan SJ; Hinton SJ. Adaptive mixtures of local experts. *Neural Computation*, 1991, 3:79–87.

[26] Curry B; Rumelhart DE. MSnet: A neural network that classifies mass spectra. *Tetrahedron Computer Methodology*, 1990, 3:213–37.

[27] Shepard RN. Multidimensional scaling, tree-fitting, and clustering. *Science*, 1980, 210:390–8.

[28] Weigend AS; Rumelhart DE; Huberman BA. Generalization by weight-elimination applied to currency exchange rate prediction. *1991 IEEE International Joint Conference on Neural Networks*, 3:2374–9.

Modeling Brain Adaptation to Focal Damage

Sharon Goodall*, James A. Reggia*+, and Sungzoon Cho°
Depts of Computer Science* & Neurology+, Univ. of Maryland College Park, MD 20742
° Dept of Computer Science & Engr., Pohang Inst of Science & Technology, Pohang, Kyungbook 790-784, Korea

Determining how feature maps in the cerebral cortex adapt to sudden, focal damage is important for gaining a deeper understanding of neurological illnesses such as stroke. In this paper we describe a neural model of the region of primary sensory cortex related to upper extremity proprioception, and show how the feature map there reorganizes following a simulated lesion. A perilesion zone with decreased activity appears and then gradually expands with time. These results differ from those seen with previous models of cortical lesions, and offer an alternative mechanism to the "ischemic penumbra" seen in certain types of stroke.

INTRODUCTION

As neural modeling technology has matured during the last several years there has been an increasing interest in adopting neural models to simulate disorders in neurology, neuropsychology, and psychiatry. For example, models of memory loss in dementia, epilepsy, aphasia, dyslexia, and schizophrenia have been studied to obtain a better understanding of the underlying pathophysiological processes. A recent review summarizes this rapidly growing area of research [8].

Many past computational models of the cerebral cortex have concentrated on map formation since this is a prevalent organizational structure in the mammalian brain[9]. A *cortical map* refers to a representation of the body surface or external world over the two-dimensional surface of the cerebral cortex. Cortical maps preserve a similarity relationship for input patterns, and can be divided into two classes. For *topographic* maps, similarity of input patterns is measured in terms of their geometric proximity; they occur, for example, in mammalian somatosensory cortex. For *feature* maps, the similarity measure can represent any functional correspondence of the input patterns. The well-known map of orientation-specificity in visual cortex provides an example. While computational models of topographic map formation have been studied previously [5, 7], there has been very little work on cortical lesioning with this class of maps. Feature maps, which generalize the concept of topographic maps, have also been modeled [4, 6, 9] but to date no cortical lesioning studies have been done with this type of map to our knowledge.

In this paper we describe the use of a neural model to simulate adaptation of the cerebral cortex to a sudden focal lesion such as occurs in stroke. Stroke is a major health problem in the United States: it has long been the third leading cause of death, and it carries an annual economic cost of over $13 billion [1, 3]. In spite of this and the complex, incompletely understood pathophysiological processes involved, very little past work has been done to develop a computational model of stroke. In fact, the one previous study that attempted to model a small cortical lesion was not successful in producing the spontaneous reorganization seen in experimental animal studies [5]. Only during the past year was a neural model of cortex that spontaneously reorganizes following an acute focal lesion first reported [2, 10]. When a small lesion was introduced into the cortical representation of the sensory surface of the hand, the model cortex reorganized so that the hand surface originally represented by the lesioned area spontaneously reappeared in adjacent cortical areas, as has been seen experimentally. Both of these studies applied lesions to topographic maps only.

Recently, we developed a model of cortical feature map formation based on proprioceptive input from a simulated upper extremity [4]. Proprioceptive cortex receives sensory information from muscles, tendons and joints enabling the nervous system to determine extremity position and movement. In this paper we focus on sensory information about muscle length and tension. In contrast to the maps used in previous lesioning studies of model cortex, this map is not a topographic rep-

0195–4210/94/$5.00 © 1994 AMIA, Inc.

resentation of skin surface but is a feature map of individual sensory features (e.g., individual muscle lengths and tensions). Surprisingly, the pattern of reorganization observed was quite different from that seen with previous lesion simulations of a topographic map [2, 10]. A region of decreased activity surrounding the lesion developed and then gradually expanded. In the following, we describe this result, offer an explanation for why it occurs, and describe how it may relate to recent empirical observations made in animal models of stroke.

METHODS

We briefly review our model of proprioceptive map formation [4], and then describe how it is lesioned.

Model Arm

Fig. 1 shows the structure of the neural model of the proprioceptive cortex. Inputs to the arm layer are calculated from a simulated model arm. This model arm is a great simplification of biological reality, and is intended as only a first effort for modeling feature map formation in the motor and somatosensory cortex [4]. It consists of upper and lower arm segments, connected at the elbow. It has only six generic muscles or muscle groups, each of which corresponds to multiple muscles in a real arm. We assume that there are four muscles that control the upper arm and two muscles that control the lower arm. Abductor and adductor muscles move the upper arm up and down through 180°, respectively, while flexor and extensor muscles move it forward and backward through 180°, respectively. The lower arm flexes and extends as much as 180° in a plane, controlled by lower arm flexor and extensor muscles. When the model arm is placed into a specific spatial position, it generates input signals to the cortex from the sensory neurons ("arm layer" in Fig. 1) that indicate individual muscle lengths and tensions. The biologically-oriented input to our model, based on muscle stretch and tension, distinguishes it from several previous robotically-oriented neural models of arm control where input is typically derived from a camera (e.g., [9]). Further details on the model arm can be found in [4].

Neural Computations

The model neural network has two separate layers of units (Fig. 1), an arm layer and a proprioceptive cortex layer. The arm layer consists of

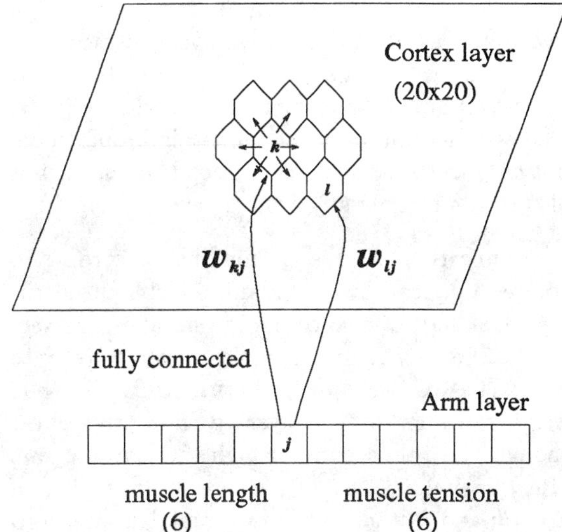

Figure 1: Structure of Neural Network Model

12 units which represent six muscle length and six muscle tension measures. A length unit becomes active when the corresponding muscle is stretched, while a tension unit becomes active when the corresponding muscle produces tension through active contraction. Each unit in the arm layer competitively distributes its activation to every unit in the cortex layer. The connection weights were trained starting from an initial random uniform distribution. The proprioceptive cortex layer consists of a grid of 20 × 20 units. Each unit represents a cortical column, and is connected to its six immediate neighboring units in a hexagonal tessellation. To remove edge effects, units on the edges of the cortical sheet are connected with units on the opposite edges forming a torus.

A competitive activation mechanism is used to control the spread of activation [4]. One distinct feature of a competitive activation mechanism is its ability to induce lateral inhibition among units, and thus to support map formation, without using explicit inhibitory connections. The activation level of unit k at time t, $a_k(t)$ is determined by

$$\frac{da_k(t)}{dt} = c_s a_k(t) + (max - a_k(t)) in_k(t) \quad (1)$$

where

$$in_k(t) = \sum_j c_p \frac{(a_k(t) + q) w_{kj}}{\sum_l (a_l(t) + q) w_{lj}} a_j(t). \quad (2)$$

Here $c_s < 0, c_p > 0, max > 0$ and $q > 0$ are constants. The weight of the connection from unit j to unit k is denoted by w_{kj}, which is assumed to be zero if there is no connection between the two units, as is the case with some intracortical connections. Weights are a function of time, but activation levels change much faster than weights. The output from unit j to unit k is proportional not only to the sender's activation level $a_j(t)$, but also to the receiver's activation level, $a_k(t)$.

Connection weights are modified according to competitive learning, a variant of Hebbian Learning that tends to change the incoming weight vectors of the output units (cortical layer units) into prototypes of the input patterns. Only the 4800 weights from the arm layer to the cortex layer change and this occurs through the learning rule $\Delta w_{kj} = \eta[a_j - w_{kj}]a_k^*$, where $a_k^* = a_k - \theta$ if $a_k > \theta$; and 0 otherwise (η is a small learning constant). The value θ is fixed throughout training.

Map Formation

A version of the neural model described above was trained as follows. Random input signals to the muscles were simulated as inputs to the model arm. These inputs specified positions of the model arm in 3-D space. From these model arm input values, arm layer muscle length and tension inputs were calculated. One thousand random input patterns, covering the input space, were presented to the network during training, after which further training did not produce qualitative changes in the trained weights. The neural model parameters were set empirically as follows. For cortical units, decay constant c_s and ceiling max in Eq. 1 were set to -4.0 and 5.0 respectively. Their q and output gain parameter c_p values in Eq. 2 were set to 0.001 and 0.9, respectively. For arm layer units, q and c_p values in Eq. 2 were set to 0.1 and 0.8, respectively. The learning rate η and θ value in the learning rule were empirically set to 0.1 and 0.32, respectively.

The trained network produced several results. Muscle length and tension maps formed during training. To examine the formation of muscle length and tension maps, the network was analyzed to determine which muscle length and tension input each cortical unit responded most strongly. Twelve input patterns were presented, each having only one muscle length or tension unit (arm unit) activated. Since the arm units represent the length and tension of the six muscles of the model arm, each test pattern corresponded to the unphysiological situation where either the length or tension of only one muscle is activated

```
B B - D D - C F - - - F F O O - F - O O
 E C C - D - B B F O O - - - O E B B - E
  E E C C F - - B F D D E B B - E E C C -
   D D - - F F O - - - D E E B C - D C C -
    F O O - B B O E E C C - - B C F D D - F
     F F O O B B - - E C C - - - - F F O O -
      - B - - E C C - D D - F F O O - F O O E
       E B B - E E C C D D - B F - O E - - - E
        E C C - - D - - F F O B B - D D E C C -
         - - - F F D O - - F O O - - - D E C B F
          F D O - F F O O B B - - E E C C - - B F
           F D O O - - - E E B C C D E - F F O O -
            - - - E E B C - E E C C D D - B F F O O
             E C C - E B C C D D - F F D O B B - - E
              E B C - - - - F D D O - F F O O B - D D
               D B B F - O O F F - O O B B - - E - C D
                - - B F F D O O - - - E E B - - E E C C
                 F O O - - D D E - B - E E - C C D D - F
                  F F O E - C - E E B C - D D C C D D - -
                   B B - E E C C - - - B F D D - F F - O -
```

Figure 2: Cortical units tuned to muscle length after training.

```
- - - - - - - F - - - F F - - - F - - -
 E - - - - - - - F - - - - - - E - - - E
  E E - - F - - - F - - E - - - E E - - -
   - - - - F F - - - - - E E - - - - - - -
    F - - - - - - E E - - - - - - F - - - F
     F F - - - - - - E - - - - - - F F - - -
      - - - - E - - - - - - F F - - - F - - E
       E - - - E E - - - - - - F - - E - - - E
        E - - - - - - - F F - - - - - - E - - -
         - - - F F - - - - F - - - - - - E - - F
          F - - - F F - - - - - - E E - - - - - F
           F - - - - - - E E - - - - - E - F F - - -
            - - - E E - - - E E - - - - - - F F - -
             E - - - E - - - - - - F F - - - - - - E
              E - - - - - - F - - - - F F - - - - - -
               - - - F - - - F F - - - - - - - E - - -
                - - - F F - - - - - - E E - - - E E - -
                 F - - - - - - E - - - E E - - - - - - F
                  F F - E - - - E E - - - - - - - - - - -
                   - - - E E - - - - - - F - - - F F - - -
```

Figure 3: Cortical units trained to upper arm extensor (E) and flexor (F) muscle lengths after training.

(this was *not* the case with the training patterns). A cortical unit is taken to be "maximally tuned" to an arm input unit if the activation corresponding to the input unit is largest and above a threshold of 0.5.

Fig. 2 shows the maximal tuning of cortical units to muscle length after training. The muscle lengths are labeled as follows: E for upper arm extensor, F for upper arm flexor, B for upper arm abductor, D for upper arm adductor, O for lower arm extensor and C for lower arm flexor (e.g., the unit in the upper left corner of the cortex is maximally tuned to the upper arm abductor (B) for muscle length). Cortex units marked "-" were found not to be tuned to the length of any muscle. Clusters of units responsive to the same muscle became more uniform in size after training. The size of the clusters ranged from 2 to 10 before training, but ranged from 3 to 4 after training, and their shape became more regular.

```
O E - - F - E E - F F - O E D D C F - -
O - C C - - - - B B B O O - D C C - - O
- B C C D D O - B C C D F - B - E D D -
B B E D D F O - E C D F F B B E E D F F
- E E - F F D - E - B F - D O E D F F -
O O - C C D D - - B B - - D - - C C - -
O - B C B - * * * * * * * * - B B C - -
F - B E - - * * * * * * * * - B E E D -
F - E E - - * * * * * * * * - O E D - F
- O O D C - * * * * * * * * - O D C C -
- O F C C - * * * * * * * * - - - B B -
- F F B E - * * * * * * * * - F F B E -
- B B E E - * * * * * * * * - F O E E -
C B O O O - * * * * * * * * - O O D - C
- D O O B B - - - - - - B B - O D D C C
D D F F B B E D D F F - B B - F F - - E
D - C C - E E D F F O O E C C F F - E E
- - C - - O O B C - O D D C C B B O O -
B - E D D F B B C - D D - - B B - O F B
B E E D F F - E E - F F - E E D - F F B
```

Figure 4: Muscle length tuning of cortex layer after lesion.

```
- O O - - - - - C C F F O - - - B E E D
- B - C C - - - E - F O B C C - - - D D
B B E C - - O E E D F B E C D O O - F F
B E E D - F O E D - - E E D - O O - F -
- E D - F F O - - - - - - - F F B C C -
O O - B F - - - - - - - - - - B E C - -
O - B B C - * * * * * * * * - E E D D -
- - E E - - * * * * * * * * - - D D F -
- - E O - - * * * * * * * * - - O F F -
D D O O - - * * * * * * * * - - B B C -
D F F B - - * * * * * * * * - - E E C D
- F B B F - * * * * * * * * - - E D D -
- C C D F - * * * * * * * * - - O O - -
E E E O - - * * * * * * * * - F F B B -
E D D O - - - - - - - - - - - F F B B E
- F F B - C C - - - C - B B C C - - - E
- F B B E C D B O D D - B E C D - C O -
- - B E E D D E E D F O E E D D C O O -
C - - - - F F B - F F O O - D F F B - C
C - O - - F B B C C - O - - - F B B E C
```

Figure 5: Muscle length tuning of cortex layer after further training.

Although difficult to see in Fig. 2, clusters of units tuned to antagonist muscles were usually pushed maximally apart from one another during training. Consider the clusters shown in Fig. 3, where only those units tuned in Fig. 2 to upper arm extensor (E) and flexor muscles (F) are displayed. After training, the clusters of "E"s and "F"s are generally pushed maximally apart, evenly spaced and more uniform in size. The network thus captures the mechanical constraint imposed by the model arm that two antagonist muscles cannot be stretched at the same time.

Lesioning the Model

For this study, an 8 by 8 contiguous patch of the cortex layer in the trained network was lesioned to simulate a sudden focal lesion such as occurs in stroke. For lesioned cortical units, the activation of the unit was fixed at 0.0. In addition, connections to lesioned cortical units were severed. The effect of the lesion on map formation was examined immediately following the lesion and after continually training the network with 4000 additional random patterns. A copy of the intact trained network before lesioning was also continually trained with the same 4000 random patterns to serve as a control. Little change was seen in the feature map with the control network.

RESULTS

Our study of simulated lesions in a proprioceptive cortical map has produced strikingly different results from those found with topographic maps [2, 5]. For example, Fig. 4 shows the muscle length map of the cortex layer immediately following the focal lesion. The lesion site is marked by "*"s. A perilesion zone of relatively inactive cortical elements ("-"s) appears. With time, as the map reorganizes in the context of continued proprioceptive input, the perilesion zone gradually expands, as is seen in Fig. 5 (after 4000 further random input stimuli). This perilesion zone is due to loss of intracortical excitatory connections from the lesioned region to surrounding elements, and it expands due to synaptic changes of the competitive learning process. There is also dramatic reorganization of the rest of the map, with 68% of the remaining elements changing the muscle group to which they are most sensitive (compare Figs. 4 and 5). However, the rearrangement may not be as complete as the figures suggest, since the maps show maximal tuning of cortical units. With further learning, the perilesion zone enlarges slightly and reorganization of the map continues.

Further evidence of the dynamics of the perilesion zone of inactivity is provided through an analysis of the mean activation level of cortical units averaged over all the test input patterns. We examined the mean activation level of cortical units at various distances from the lesion site. Before the lesion was introduced, the mean activation level of all regions was 0.18. Immediately after the lesion, the mean activation of the cortical units directly adjacent to the lesion site (distance d=1) dropped to 0.04 and additional training of the lesioned network produced a further drop to 0.01. Cortical units at distance d=2 from the lesion experienced a slight increase in mean activation immediately following the lesion(0.20); further training produced a drop in mean activation to 0.09. Cortical units at a distance d=3 experienced a significant jump in mean activation level to 0.32, which diminished somewhat with training (0.29), while those at distances greater than 3 experienced an increase after training (0.20 following the lesion, 0.27 after further training). For the cortical layer as a whole, the mean activation following the lesion was 0.21, even after training.

Most interesting are the results seen at a distance d=2 from the lesion site. These cortical units are responsive immediately following the lesion, suggesting that there is potential for preventing growth of the perilesion zone of impairment. However, after further training, they too become part of the inactive region, as evidenced by the decreased mean activation level for this zone after training. Immediately following the lesion, elements bordering the lesion channel a greater percentage of their output to cortical units at a distance d=2 from the lesion site. However, synaptic changes from further training reverse this effect, thereby extending the inactive perilesion zone.

CONCLUSIONS

A model of cortical map formation based on proprioceptive input from a simulated upper extremity was used to simulate brain adaptation to a sudden focal lesion such as transpires with stroke. A region of depressed activity surrounding the lesion site appeared immediately following introduction of a sudden focal lesion, and gradually increased in size with further training of the neural model. This result is strikingly different from that seen with model topographic maps [2, 10], and developing a better understanding of the different mechanisms involved is an important research priority. The inactive perilesion zone seen here is particularly interesting because it resembles the ischemic penumbra described in stroke, where neurons surrounding a brain infarction can be dysfunctional but not dead [3]. Our results suggest the hypothesis that in some situations part of the ischemic penumbra may be caused by a loss of lateral excitatory connections from the lesioned region, and this may worsen due to normal synaptic plasticity. This contrasts with the more generally held view that the dysfunctional lesion area is caused by borderline ischemia only.

This computational model of feature map adaptation to sudden focal damage is of interest to the modeling community as a whole as it demonstrates that current neural network models can be used effectively to study diseases. Neural models that simulate disorders compliment traditional methods for examining brain disorders. Lesion size and location can be controlled and uniformly varied over large numbers of hypothetical subjects. The simulations also permit detailed inspection of the mechanisms underlying brain disorders.

Acknowledgement: This work was supported by NINCDS awards NS 29414 and NS 16332.

References

[1]. AHA. *Stroke Facts*, AHA, Dallas, 1989.

[2]. Armentrout S, Reggia J and Weinrich M A. A Neural Model of Cortical Map Reorganization Following a Focal Lesion, *Artificial Intelligence in Medicine*, 1994, in press.

[3]. Caplan L. Stroke, Butterworth, 1993.

[4]. Cho S, and Reggia J. Map Formation in Proprioceptive Cortex. *Internat. J. of Neural Systems*, 1994, in press.

[5]. Grajski K, and Merzenich M. Hebb-Type Dynamics is Sufficient to Account for the Inverse Magnification Rule in Cortical Somatotopy, *Neural Computation*, 2, 1990, 71-84.

[6]. Miller K, Keller J, and Stryker M. Ocular Dominance Column Development, *Science*, 245, 1989, 605-615.

[7]. Pearson J, Finkel L, and Edelman G. Plasticity in the Organization of Adult Cerebral Cortical Maps: A Computer Simulation Based on Neuronal Group Selection, *J of Neuroscience*, 7(12), 1987, 4209-4223.

[8]. Reggia J. Neural Computation in Medicine, *Artif. Intell. in Med.*, 5, 1993, 143-157.

[9]. Ritter H, Martinetz T, and Schulten K. *Neural Computation and Self-Organizing Maps*, Addison-Wesley, 1992.

[10]. Sutton G, Reggia J, Armentrout S, and D'Autrechy C. Map Reorganization as a Competitive Process, *Neural Computation*, 6, 1994, 1-13.

Interpretation of Doppler Blood Flow Velocity Waveforms Using Neural Networks

Nazife Baykal[1], James A. Reggia [2], Nese Yalabik [3], Aydan Erkmen [4], M.Sinan Beksac [5]
Depts. of Computer Science[1,2] & Neurology[2], and Inst. for Adv. Comp. Studies[2]
A. V. Williams Bldg., University of Maryland, College Park, MD 20742 USA
Middle East Technical University [1,3,4], Hacettepe University School of Medicine [5],Ankara

Doppler umbilical artery blood flow velocity waveform measurement is used in perinatal surveillance for the evaluation of pregnancy status. There is an ongoing debate on the predictive value of doppler measurements concerning the critical effect of the selection of parameters for the evaluation of doppler output. In this paper, we describe how neural network methods can be used both to discover relevant classification features and subsequently to classify patients. Classification accuracy varied from 92-99% correct.

INTRODUCTION

A major goal of perinatal medicine is to reduce perinatal morbidity and mortality [2, 7, 9]. Various noninvasive technologies are used in fetal surveillance. Umbilical artery blood flow velocity waveform (henceforth "umbilical artery waveform") measurement is one of these methods that is widely used in clinical practice (see Figure 1). However, a serious debate has focussed on the predictive value of doppler studies. The most critical issue is the parameters used. Such parameters generally include the Pulsatility Index (PI), Resistance Index (RI), and A/B (Systolic Diastolic) Ratio [6, 8, 11]. The exact biological meanings of these parameters are not clear.

One of our motivations for studying this subject is to explore feasibility of an automated system for classifying umbilical artery waveforms. Another one is to explore the possibility of using neural network learning methods to discover and use classification features. In particular, we apply a way in which an unsupervised learning method can be used to discover key data features that can serve as input to a supervised pattern classification model.

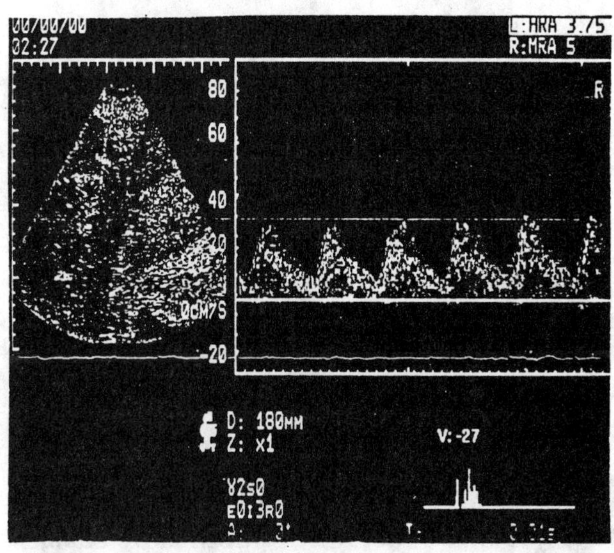

Figure 1: Example doppler waveform.

In this study, we used two different neural network methods for the development of an automated system for the analysis of umbilical artery waveforms. First, a modified Kohonen's self organizing feature map (SOFM) algorithm [5] is used for automatic feature extraction and clustering of the preprocessed doppler signal. Map features are then used as input to a back propagation training algorithm to classify an umbilical artery waveform as normal, abnormal or suspicious. The test results obtained by our model are compared directly with actual patient outcome (i.e., not

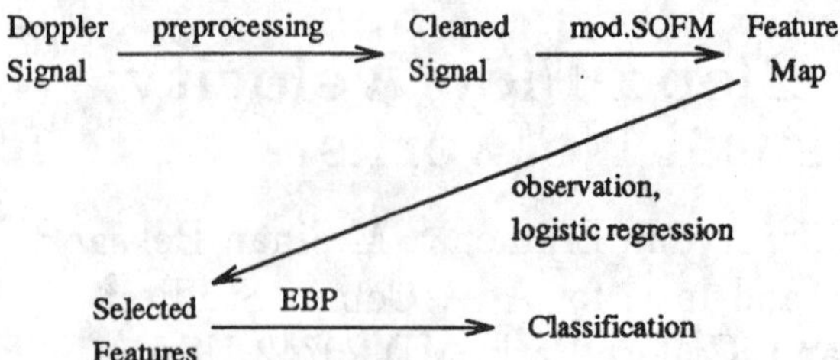

Figure 2: Procedure used in this study.

with physician classification of the waveform).

METHODS

The main steps in interpretation of doppler umbilical artery waveforms include preprocessing, map formation, feature extraction, feature selection and classification respectively (see Figure 2).

Preprocessing Waveforms

Umbilical artery waveforms are acquired by a 3.75 MHz duplex pulsed wave doppler probe during the data acquisition phase. Doppler images are then transferred from ultrasound to computer environments by means of a frame grabber. Averaging, thresholding edge detection, smoothing and image clearing are the main processes in the course of image analysis. For feature extraction, filtering algorithms are applied to digital waves in order to reduce noise which is inherent to doppler equipment and to the process of digitization of analog images. Averaging using a sliding window technique is first applied to umbilical artery waveforms within the thresholding process. Waveforms are further enhanced from the background by global thresholding. The edge of an umbilical artery waveform is detected by using Robert's Gradient operator [3]. Then, 4x4, 4x3, 3x4 & 3x3 masks are used to smooth and clear umbilical artery waveform signals to remove irrelevant details coming from the background of raw images and render waveforms more recognizable and crisp in form as seen in the Figure 3.

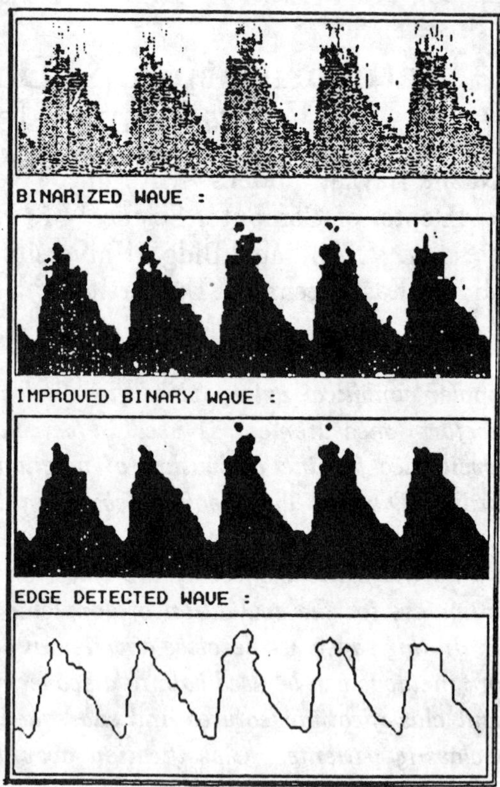

Figure 3: Preprocessing steps of BFVWs.

Map Formation with a Modified SOFM

Kohonen's SOFM is an unsupervised learning algorithm [5] that modifies the internal state of the neural network in order to model features found in the training data. No training response is prespecified for any training input. In this study, a modified SOFM is used for map formation and automatic feature extraction. Our algorithm is similar to SOFM except for a parameter ϕ in the learning rule:

$$w_i(t+1) = w_i(t) + \alpha(t)\phi(t)(x_i(t) - w_i(t)).$$

Excitation term ϕ(t) is defined to be

$\phi = (\gamma - \mu)/\gamma$ where;

γ = topological radius of neighborhood, and

μ = topologic distance from winner.

Input vectors to the SOFM are the preprocessed umbilical artery waveform signal patterns. This input space has dimension 300 which is the length of the processed signal.

Figure 4: Schematic illustration of map.

			S	S						
			S	S	N	N				
	S	S	S		N	N		N	N	N
	S	S	S		N	N		N	N	N
					N	N				
	A	A	A				A	A		
	A	A	A				A	A		
	A	A	A							

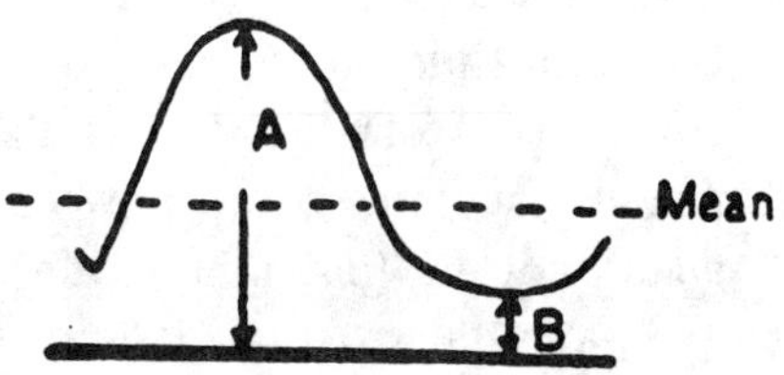

Figure 5: Widely used BFVW parameters.

The output of the system is an 11x11 array of processing units. Initially, all of the incoming connections to the output nodes are assigned small random weight values and the rate of weight tuning is 0.5. During learning a set of training umbilical artery waveform signals are shown to the network.

At the end of the training process we obtained six different clusters of umbilical artery waveforms as shown in Figure 4. The map elements are labeled as N (normal) S (suspicious) or A (abnormal) if the most of the waveforms mapped onto it have actual outcome normal, suspicious or abnormal respectively.

Feature Extraction

Various different indices have been used for quantitative assessment of umbilical artery waveforms. The most commonly used indices are the Pulsatility Index (PI), ABR (A/B ratio, Systolic/Diastolic ratio) and the Resistance Index (RI) [2, 9, 10, 8] defined as:

$$PI = (A - B)/Mean$$

$$ABR = A/B$$

$$RI = (A - B)/A$$

A, B and Mean are shown in Figure 5. From the automatic feature extraction and clustering phase and previous studies we observed that these indices are inadequate to evaluate umbilical artery waveforms [1]. For this reason, we extracted features from the normal, abnormal and suspicious clusters. We observed the general signal form and differences between waveforms from cluster to cluster and between pregnancy weeks. We identified features such as slope, fetal pulse rate, pulse width, peak values from FFT (fast Fourier transform) of the signals, A-B and pregnancy week that correlated with specific classes. Starting with 11 initial parameters, we used step-down logistic regression [4] to identify seven important and linearly independent features: A-B, ABR, FFT, slope, fetal pulse rate, pulse width and pregnancy week. Note that only one of the features discovered in this fashion (ABR) is among the three most widely used features described above.

Application of Error Back Propagation

The input vector represents the seven computed new parameters of umbilical artery waveforms. The network structure used in our experiments has one input, one hidden, and one output layer. The output layer has three nodes corresponding to classes normal, suspicious and abnormal.

We performed experiments on approximately 600 umbilical artery data sets having different gestational weeks belonging to 199 normal and high risk pregnancies. Patients are observed for their clinical conditions during the pregnancy period and they get an outcome grade between 0 and 5 for the worst and best case, respectively. Experimental data consists of multiple recordings from each of 56 abnormal (outcome grade less than 2.5), 88 suspicious (outcome grade between 2.5 and 3.8) and 55 normal (outcome grade between 3.9 and 5) patients' waveform. Clinically, data acquisition starts with the 14th gestational week and continues every four weeks. The data from weeks 14 to 40 were separated into seven groups. Clustering and feature extraction enable us to find out the common similarities within each gestational week group and then these groups are trained independently. Observed clinical conditions and outcome grade of the patient are used as the basis of classification criteria (i.e., not a direct physician classification of the waveform). Normal classification is assigned for outcome grade between 3.9 and 5 and pregnancy condition has one of the following a) normal pregnancy, normal outcome (ideal normal); b) normal but undesirable condition may exist; and c) normal, bad obstetrical history. Abnormal classification is assigned for outcome grade between 0 and 2.4 and if there are a) fetal problems; or b) perinatal and intrapartum problems and bad outcome. Pregnancy condition and outcome that do not belong to any of these classifications are labeled suspicious. According to these situations, computed features of the umbilical artery waveforms from patients having known outcome are choosen as the desired values of our error back propagation algorithm.

RESULTS

The basic result of this study is the reliable interpretation of umbilical artery waveforms for fetal well-being. Our simulation results are compared with the actual outcome and results are shown on the Table 1. Column GW records gestational weeks of data collecting for each group. TRAIN P# (TEST P#) is the number of training (test) patterns used for each group. Training cases were selected if they were good representations of their cluster (Figure 4); test cases were randomly selected (except training cases were excluded). Correct classification CORR is computed by

Table 1: Classification results.

GW	TRAIN P#	TEST P#	CORR.
14-15	20	40	92.50%
16-19	30	60	95.00%
20-23	40	60	96.67%
24-27	40	70	98.57%
28-31	40	60	98.33%
32-35	40	60	98.33%
36-40	30	50	96.00%

$$(100 * c)/t$$

where; c = the number of umbilical artery waveforms that are classified the same as actual outcome; and t = the total number of test samples of the same gestational week.

In our simulations, we used a different set of patients including normal and high risk pregnancies (number in each class varies between 6 to 27) for training and testing for each gestational weeks as shown in Table 1. Sensitivities and specificities for classification performance run between 83.33% to 100% for each group.

As seen from Table 1, at the beginning of the pregnancy less accurate results are obtained. The main reasons for this situation may be less training data; and the normal (ideal) form of the signal changes very much from patient to patient.

DISCUSSION

Blood flow velocity waveform measurements are widely used in perinatal surveillance [6, 8]. Different fetal blood vessels are used to evaluate fetal health. Umbilical artery waveform measurement is the most popular one in doppler studies. Good blood flow in the umbilical artery reflects good oxygenation of the fetus, and is of vital importance.

Various parameters are used for the interpretation of doppler waveforms. However, there are no clear cut criteria to evaluate doppler waveforms. This situation has motivated us to develop an automated system for the reliable evaluation of umbilical artery waveforms for perinatal surveillance. In the literature, Pulsatility Index (PI), Resistance Index (RI) and A/B ratio are the main parameters in clinical practice, although they are highly correlated with each other. The heterogeneity of doppler technology and probable interindividual variation of semi-automated determination of doppler parameters are also important issues in obtaining accurate results. Another critical issue is the representative meanings of doppler indices.

Based on the remarkable accuracy of our system predictions, we conclude that an automated system for classification of umbilical artery waveform is feasible and shows high correlation with outcome. Further, the unsupervised modified SOFM method proved to be a very powerful approach to discovering key features in a complex data. Our system may become an automated preliminary report and decision assistance. In addition, seven features of umbilical artery waveforms were discovered that had strong predictive power. These features deserve further study in a prospective fashion.

Acknowledgement: This study is conducted collaboratively with the Hacettepe University School of Medicine, Department of Obstetrics and Gynaecology. This work was supported by the Turkish Scientific and Technological Research Association (TUBITAK).

References

[1] Baykal N, Erkmen A, Yalabik N, Beksac S & Altintas I. Evaluation of Doppler Blood Velocity Waveform Indices for Perinatal Surveillance using BPT Algorithm,*2nd Turkish Sym. on AI and Artif. Neural Networks*, Istanbul, Turkey, 1993

[2] Farmakides G, Schulman H, Winter D, Oncey J, Guzman E. & Penny B. Perinatal Surveillance Using Non-Stress Testing and Doppler Velocimetry, *Obstet Gynecol.* 71:184-187, 1988.

[3] Gonzales RC & Wintz P. *Digital Image Processing*, 2nd Edition, Addision-Wesley, 1987.

[4] Hosmer D. & Lemeshow S. *Applied Logistic Regression*, Wiley, 1989.

[5] Kohonen T. *Self Organization and Associative Memory*, Springer Verlag, 1990.

[6] Ruissen C.V, Drongelen MMHP, Hoogland MJ, Jager W & Hoeks APG, Characteristic of The Umbilical Artery Velocity Waveform as a Function of Measurement Site, *Gynecol Obstet Invest* 30:212-216, 1990.

[7] Schulman H, Fleischer A, Stern W, Farmakides G, Jagani N & Blattner P, Umbilical Velocity Wave Ratios in Human Pregnancy, *Am J Obstet Gynecol* 148 985-990, 1984.

[8] Thompson RS, Trudinger BJ & Cook CM, Doppler Ultrasound Waveforms in The Fetal Umbilical Artery : Quantitative Analysis Technique, *Ultrasound in Med Biol* 11: 707-718, 1985.

[9] Trudinger BJ, Cook M, Gilles WB, Connelly A, & Thompson RS, Umbilical Artery Flow Velocity Waveforms in High Risk Pregnancy, *Lancet* 188-190, 1987.

[10] Trudinger BJ, Gilles WB, Cook CM, Bombardieri J, Collins L, Fetal Umbilical Artery Flow Velocity Waveforms and Placental Resistance: Clinical Significance,*Br J Obstet Gynecol* 92:23-30, 1985.

[11] Wladimiroff JW, vd.Wijngaard JAGW, Degani S, Noordam MJ,V.Eyck J & Tonge HM, Cerebral and Umbilical Arterial Blood Flow Velocity Waveforms in Normal and Growth-Retarded Fetuses, *Obstet Gynecol* 69:705-709, 1987.

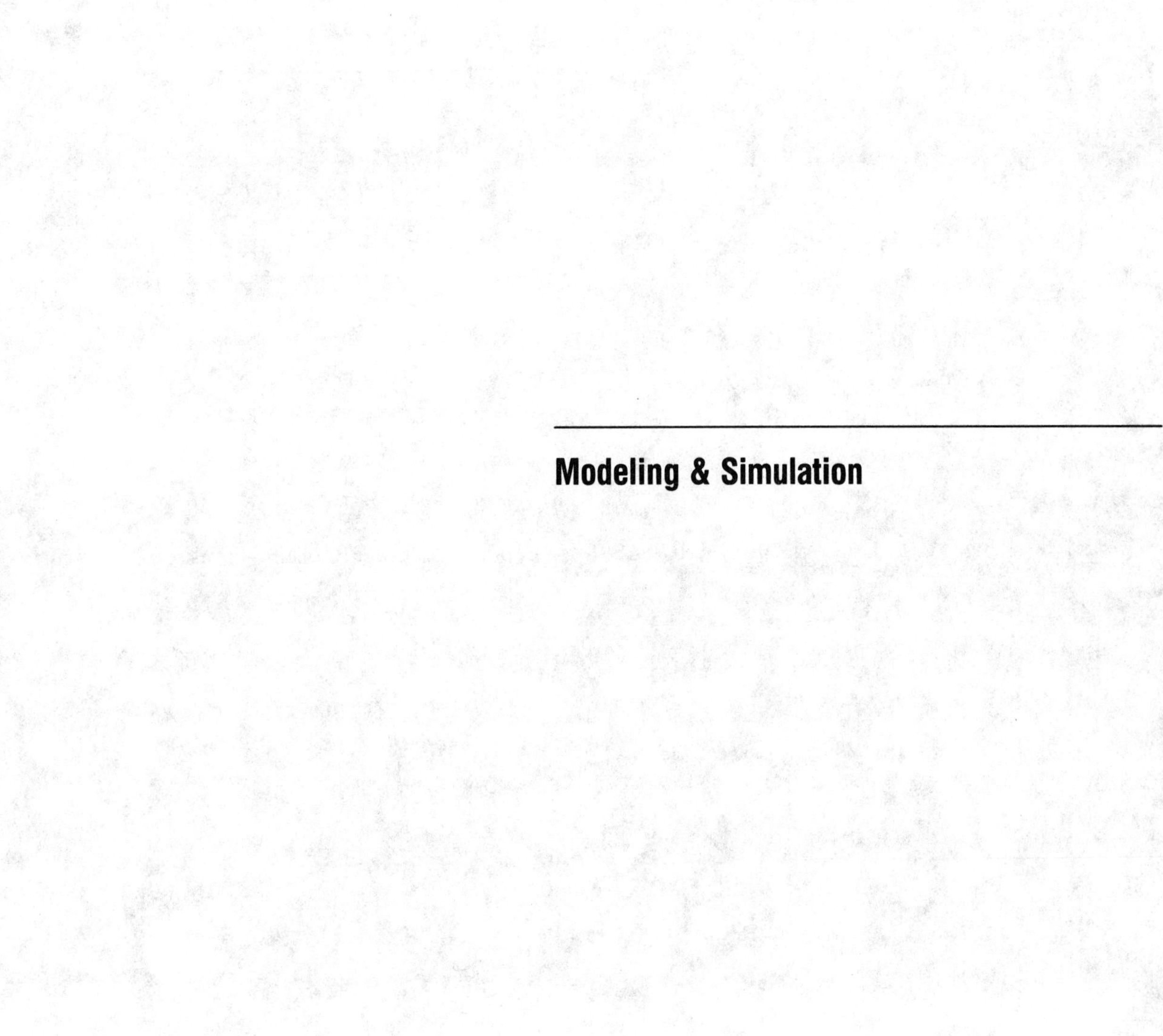

Modeling & Simulation

Modeling Cortical Spreading Depression

James A. Reggia* & David Montgomery+
Depts. of Computer Science*+ & Neurology*, and Inst. for Adv. Comp. Studies*
A. V. Williams Bldg., University of Maryland, College Park, MD 20742

Cortical spreading depression is a wave of electrical silence and biochemical changes that spreads across the cerebral cortex. Recently there has been a growing recognition that it may be an important pathophysiological event in a number of neurological disorders. In this paper, we describe a reaction-diffusion model of the extracellular potassium changes that are a central part of this process. Simulations with the model show that an appropriate stimulus evokes a moving wave of increased potassium with many similarities to that seen experimentally. The resultant model is a useful computational tool for future study of the effects of spreading depression on the cortex.

INTRODUCTION

Cortical spreading depression (CSD) is an expanding wave of temporarily suppressed electrical activity and biochemical disturbances that propagates across the cerebral cortex at a rate of about 2 - 5 mm/min (illustrated schematically in Fig. 1) [1, 3, 6, 10]. It can be initiated by topical application to the cortex of various chemicals (potassium, excitatory aminoacids, etc.), or mechanical/electrical stimuli. The exact physiological events involved in CSD are not completely understood, but the most generally accepted hypothesis is that the release of potassium ions (K^+), and possibly neurotransmitters such as glutamate, is the critical event. It is observed that as K^+ diffuses through the cortex, nearby regions first show a slow, small increase in extracellular K^+, followed by a dramatic rise once the K^+ level exceeds about 10 mM. The markedly elevated extracellular K^+ concentration depolarizes neurons and leads to suppression of their firing of action potentials.

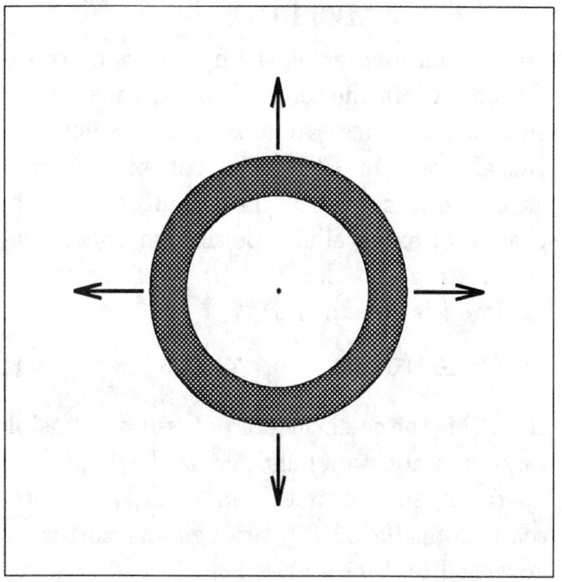

Figure 1: Annular wave of CSD (shaded) arising from a stimulus site (dot at center).

CSD has attracted attention recently due to suspicions that it may be an important pathophysiologic component of disorders such as migraine, cerebral ischemia and head trauma [5, 9, 16]. For example, it has been postulated that CSD may initiate migraine attacks and cause the associated aura [8]. In spite of this, there have been very few previous efforts to computationally or mathematically model CSD [1, 15, 17]. Because of the growing recognition of the clinical relevance of CSD, it is timely to develop a computational model that can be used to complement experimental work. Accordingly, we describe a model of the genesis and propagation of increased potassium during CSD and simulations that validate its behavior. The goal was to produce a model that was both robust to reasonable changes in parameters and computationally efficient when used with large, two-dimensional cortical regions. In the following, we first describe the mathematical model of CSD we have developed, and then present the results of numerical simulations with it. We conclude with a discussion contrasting our model with previous related work.

METHODS

Our model focuses on the dynamics of extracellular K^+ in the cerebral cortex since potassium disturbances are most likely the critical causal event in CSD. The cortex is viewed as a two-dimensional sheet and the rate of change of extracellular potassium concentration $K(x,y,t)$ at location (x,y) of the cortex at time t is governed by

$$\frac{\partial K}{\partial t} = D\nabla^2 K \ + \ f(K). \quad (1)$$

Here D is the coefficient of potassium diffusion (assumed constant) and ∇^2 is the Laplacian operator, so the first term of Eq. 1 represents diffusion of K^+ through the cortex as governed by Fick's Law [12].

The second term $f(K)$ in Eq. 1, which we take to be independent of cortical location and time, represents the local dynamics of extracellular potassium. These local dynamics must meet at least four requirements: homeostatic maintenance of resting extracellular potassium level $K_r > 0$ (approx. 3 mM in the cortex), a threshold $K_\theta > K_r$ beyond which elevated K triggers explosive subsequent growth in K, a ceiling $K_m > K_\theta$ above which K does not rise, and restoration to normal K levels that reflects post-wave intracellular resequestration of potassium. To capture these behaviors our model uses

$$f(K) = A(K - K_r)(K - K_\theta)(K - K_m)(K + 0.1) - rK \quad (2)$$

where $A < 0$ is a rate constant, and resequestration of potassium r is modeled as

$$\frac{\partial r}{\partial t} = B((K - K_r) - Cr) \quad (3)$$

where $0 < B << |A|$ and $C > 0$ are constants.

The quartic polynomial forming the first term in Eq. 2 satisfies the first three requirements outlined above. For example, if K is just above (below) K_r, then this polynomial is negative (positive), tending to return K to K_r (Eq. 1). The second term, $-rK$, provides for restoration of K to its resting value during the recovery phase. Eq. 3 represents the slow (B small) resequestration of potassium that rises in the face of increased K; as can be seen in Eq. 1 and 2, when r is elevated there is a tendency for K levels to fall. Our formal model expressed in Eqs. 1-3 is similar in form to, and in part inspired by, previous mathematical models of wave-like phenomena, such as calcium activation waves on the enclosing membranes of amphibian eggs [2, 7] and the FitzHugh-Nagumo model of action potentials in neurons [4, 11].

In the computer implementation of this model, both the spatial structure of the cerebral cortex and time are discretized. The cortex is represented as a two-dimensional array of elements, each of which represents a small volume of cortex (say 25 microns wide [13]). A hexagonal tessellation of the cortex is assumed, so each element has six immediately adjacent neighbor elements. Each cortical element i has its own extracellular potassium value K_i and resequestration value r_i governed by Eqs. 1-3. Initially, each element starts with $K_i = K_r$ and $r_i = 0$. This is a fixed point of the system (i.e., the model is initially in an equilibrium state) since with these values $\frac{\partial K_i}{\partial t} = 0$ and $\frac{\partial r_i}{\partial t} = 0$ for all elements i. The model's behavior is then studied numerically after perturbing it from this equilibrium state by simulating the external application of potassium to one or more elements j by raising the value K_j for those elements. In the simulation results described below, a time step of 0.25 is used, and a 100x100 element cortical region is modeled with opposite edges connected (forming a torus) to avoid edge effects. Parameter values used in the simulations reported here are D=0.75, A=-0.3, $K_r = 0.03$, $K_\theta = 0.2$, $K_m = 1.0$, B=0.0001, and C=10.0. These parameter values, determined empirically, produce a good waveform and the K values obtained can be viewed as one-hundredth of actual extracellular K^+ concentration in mM units.

RESULTS

The key result of our simulations is that a localized area of elevated potassium evokes a traveling wave of markedly elevated potassium that slowly propagates in an expanding annular region. For example, clamping the K value of a hexagonal cluster of seven elements to $K = 1.0$ for 1000 ticks leads to a potassium wave as depicted schematically in Figure 1. These simulations verify that the formal model represented by Eqs. 1-3, when simulated in a discrete fashion, can generate potassium waves. Further, when such waves, traveling in opposite directions, collide with one another, they obliterate each other, just as occurs experimentally. A wave is followed by a refractory period. Wave speed approximated 0.2 elements per simulated time unit. If one takes simulated cortical elements to be 25 microns wide and calibrates simulated wave duration (Fig. 2, adjustable by varying B) with experimentally measured wave duration, the model's wave speed corresponds to roughly 5 mm/min, near the upper range of wave speeds observed experimentally.

Figure 2 illustrates the nature of the propagating potassium wave. The horizontal axis represents time, and the vertical axis represents the extracellular potassium concentration K (solid line) and recovery variable r (dashed line) of a single cortical element as the potassium wave reaches it. As potassium diffuses into the element, there is an initial slow rise in K, followed by a sudden dramatic rise, a gradually decreasing plateau, and a more rapid fall as the wave passes beyond the element. These features are similar to those seen experimentally.

To examine the stimulus required to evoke the potassium wave, we ran over 250 simulations varying the intensity, duration and size

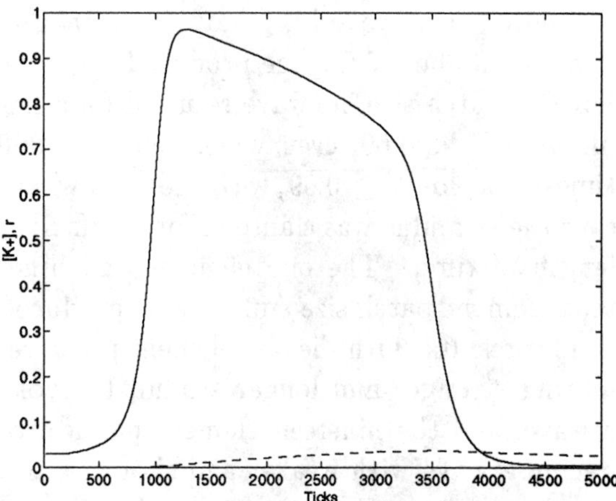

Figure 2: Extracellular potassium wave (solid line) and resequestration variable r (dashed line). Each "tick" is one iteration.

(1, 7, or 19 elements) of the hexagonal stimulus patch of elevated K. For all three stimulus sizes, a maximal stimulus ($K = K_m$) that persisted sufficiently long evoked a well-formed wave. For each patch size, however, there was a stimulus intensity $K < 1.0$ below which a maximal wave could not be evoked. As the patch size was increased, weaker and shorter duration stimuli were needed to elicit a maximal wave.

For example, to study the response to stimulus patches with seven elements, we varied the level of the clamped K from 0.0 to 1.0 and the duration of application of the stimulus from 100 to 5000 ticks (iterations). We ran approximately 100 simulations sampling points throughout the stimulus parameter space to get a general picture of the model's behavior, and then focused additional simulations on the interesting regions. In all of these simulations, one of two events occurred: either a strong sustained wave like that shown in Fig. 2 was evoked, with $K > 0.9$, or no wave resulted, and the potassium remained below 0.15 except in the immediate neighborhood of the stimulus. No intermediate strength waves were observed. The boundary between the two behaviors was quite sharp (line in Figure 3). All points on or above the line in Fig.

3 resulted in a wave like that shown in Fig. 2; all points below the line produced no wave. For this patch size, no wave resulted for stimuli with $K < 0.69$, even when held for 5000 timesteps. For $K \geq 0.69$, waves formed whenever the stimulus was clamped for a sufficient length of time. The one element and nineteen element patch size simulations produced similar results, with the one element patch requiring stronger and longer stimuli to evoke a wave, and the nineteen element patch producing a wave with weaker and shorter stimuli. Increases in the intensity or duration of the stimulus above the minimum threshold resulted in the wave being evoked sooner, but did not change the overall shape of the wave.

We also examined the total potassium added to the system and its relationship to the threshold for evoking a wave. The total potassium added was determined by subtracting, at each timestep, the K value that each stimulus element would have at the next time instant (from Eqs. 1 - 3) from the clamped K value, and summing this calculation for the duration of the stimulus. It was found that the lower the level of clamped K, the more total potassium had to be added to the system to evoke a wave.

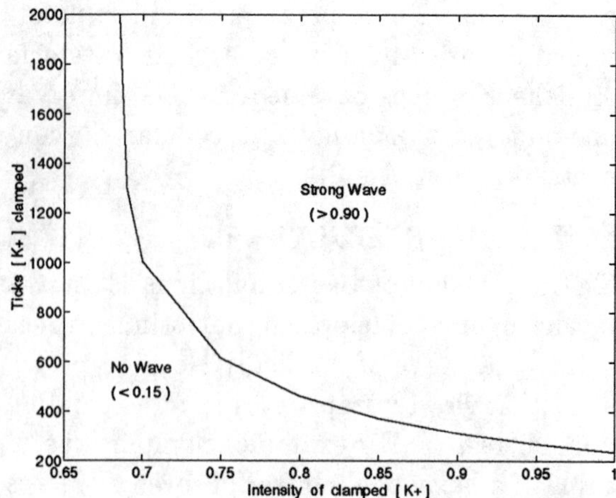

Figure 3: Threshold for evoking potassium wave in terms of intensity and duration of stimulus for a seven element hexagonal stimulus patch. Only stimuli on or above the line evoke a wave like that in Figure 2.

DISCUSSION

The growing interest in the clinical relevance of CSD has motivated us to develop a computational model of CSD so that its properties and effects can be studied theoretically. In this paper we have examined an important, presumably causative component of CSD, the spreading wave of dramatically increased extracellular potassium concentration. We showed that it can be simulated by a two-dimensional, reaction-diffusion system. As described above, numerical simulations based on the model confirm that it produces a propagating disturbance having several features similar to those seen experimentally.

Our model can be contrasted with three previous efforts to model various aspects of CSD. One previous cellular automata model represented the cortex as a two-dimensional spatial array of elements as we have done, but each element could be in only one of three discrete states (quiescent, depressed, or refractory) [15]. Elements changed state according to transition rules that did not explicitly represent physiological causative factors such as extracellular K^+ concentration. Our model differs in using a continuous-valued K^+ level at each element whose value is governed by two differential equations (Eqs. 1, 3).

Two other previous models of CSD used continuous representations of element states and reaction-diffusion equations as we have, but both considered only one-dimensional spatial distributions and used different local dynamics for extracellular K^+ (i.e., different formulas for $f(K)$). The earliest of these two models, attributed to A. L. Hodgkin, represented a wave of rising extracellular K^+ concentration but no restoration phase, and was apparently never simulated numerically [1]. The other one-dimensional model represented not only multiple intracellular and extracellular ionic changes, but also release of neurotransmitters and membrane potential [17].

This latter detailed model is more physiologically complete than the model we have developed, but produces a temporal waveform that is qualitatively less similar to experimental data than ours (Figure 2). Its complexity and computational expense would make it difficult to use in large, two-dimensional cortical simulations.

The model we have described in this paper will be used in future studies to learn more about CSD and its effects on cortical physiology. It will be extended to capture other presumably secondary biochemical changes of CSD, and will be combined with a computational model of cortical neural activity [13]. We intend to apply the validated model to study computationally various hypotheses about the role of CSD in neurological disorders such as stroke and migraine. Thus, from the perspective of modeling in general, our results support recent suggestions that computational models have an underutilized role to play in studying neurological disorders [14].

Acknowledgement: This work was supported by NINDS awards NS29414 and NS16332. We thank S. Goodall, J. Lohn, D. Perlis, and E. Ruppin for comments on a draft of this paper.

References

[1] Bureš J, Burešová O. & Křivánek J. *The Mechanism and Applications of Leão's Spreading Depression of Electroencephalographic Activity*, Academic Press, 1974.

[2] Cheer A. et al. Cortical Activity in Vertebrate Eggs, *J. Theor. Biol*, 124, 1987, 377-404.

[3] do Carmo R. (ed.) *Spreading Depression*, Springer-Verlag, 1992.

[4] FitzHugh R. Impulses and Physiological States in Theoretical Models of Nerve Membrane, *Biophys. J.*, 1, 1961, 445-466.

[5] Hansen A. Effect of Anoxia on Ion Distribution in the Brain, *Physiological Reviews*, 65, 1985, 101-148.

[6] Hansen A. & Lauritzen M. Spreading Depression of Leão, in Olesen J & Edvinisson L., eds., *Basic Mechanisms of Headache*, Elsevier, 1988, 99-107.

[7] Lane D, et al. Analysis of Wave Phenomena in a Morphogenetic Mechanochemical Model, *IMA J. Math. Appl. Med. Biol.*, 4, 1987, 309-331.

[8] Lauritzen M. Cortical Spreading Depression as a Migraine Mechanism, in *Spreading Depression*, R. do Carmo, ed., Springer-Verlag, 1992.

[9] Lauritzen M. et al. Persistent Oligemia of Rat Cerebral Cortex in the Wake of Spreading Depression, *Ann. Neurol.*, 12, 1982, 469-474.

[10] Leão A. Spreading Depression of Activity in the Cerebral Cortex, *J. Neurophysiol*, 7, 1944, 357-390.

[11] Nagumo J, et al. An Active Pulse Transmission Line Simulating Nerve Axon, *Proc. IRE*, 50, 1962, 2061-2071.

[12] Rashevsky N. *Mathematical Biophysics*, Dover, 1960, Chap. 1.

[13] Reggia J, D'Autrechy C, Sutton G. & Weinrich M. A Competitive Distribution Theory of Neocortical Dynamics, *Neural Computation*, 4, 1992, 287-317.

[14] Reggia J, Berndt R & D'Autrechy C. Connectionist Models in Neuropsychology, *Handbook of Neuropsychology*, Vol. 9, 1994, in press.

[15] Reshodko L. & Bureš. Computer Simulation of Reverberating Spreading Depression in a Network of Cell Automata, *Biol. Cybernetics*, 18, 1975, 181-189.

[16] Somjen J, Herreras O & Jing J. Spreading Depression and Neuron Damage, in do Carmo R (ed.), *Spreading Depression*, Springer-Verlag, 1992, 27-33.

[17] Tuckwell H. & Miura R., A Mathematical Model for Cortical Spreading Depression *Biophysical Journal*, 23, 1978, 257-276.

VentSim: A Simulation Model of Cardiopulmonary Physiology

Geoffrey W. Rutledge, M.D.
Section on Medical Informatics, Department of Medicine
Stanford University, Stanford, California 94305-5479
rutledge@camis.stanford.edu

ABSTRACT

VentSim is a quantitative model that predicts the effects of alternative ventilator settings on the cardiopulmonary physiology of critically ill patients. VentSim is an expanded version of the physiologic model in VentPlan, an application that provides ventilator-setting recommendations for patients in the intensive care unit.

VentSim includes a ventilator component, an airway component, and a circulation component. The ventilator component predicts the pressures and airflows that are generated by a volume-cycled, constant-flow ventilator. The airway component has anatomic and physiologic deadspace compartments, and two alveolar compartments that participate in gas exchange with two pulmonary blood-flow compartments in the circulatory component. The circulatory component also has a shunt compartment that allows a fraction of blood flow to bypass gas exchange in the lungs, and a tissue compartment that consumes oxygen and generates carbon dioxide.

The VentSim model is a set of linked first-order difference equations, with control variables that correspond to the ventilator settings, dependent variables that correspond to the physiologic state, and one independent variable, time. Because the model has no steady state solution, VentSim solves the equations by numeric integration, which is computation intensive.

Simulation results demonstrate that VentSim predicts the effects of a variety of physiologic abnormalities that cannot be represented in less complex models such as the VentPlan model.

For a ventilator-management application, the time-critical nature of ventilator-setting decisions limits the use of complex models. Advanced ventilator-management applications may include a mechanism to select patient-specific models that balance the trade-off of benefit of model detail and cost of computation delay.

MODELS FOR VENTILATOR MANAGEMENT

Numerous researchers have developed computer programs to assist the monitoring and treatment of patients in the intensive care unit (ICU) who receive treatment with a mechanical ventilator. These programs implement various methods, including protocols [13, 22], rule-based expert systems [7, 14, 18], causal probabilistic models (belief networks) [3], and mathematical models [19].

All programs that interpret patient data and make recommendations for the settings of a mechanical ventilator must rely on some model of patient response to the ventilator. Programs that incorporate mathematical models or belief networks may allow the user to examine the models and determine if the assumptions and simplifications these models make are valid for a specific patient. The user may also inspect the model predictions to verify that they match her expectations.

By contrast, protocols and rule-based expert systems implement symbolic models of patient responses that are opaque to the user. Users cannot inspect or test such embedded physiologic models, and may not be able to verify that the program's interpretation of a patient's physiology is valid.

VENTPLAN

VentPlan is a prototype ventilator management advisor (VMA) that explores the ability of a patient-specific mathematical model to guide the selection of optimal ventilator settings for ICU patients. VentPlan implements a classical three-compartment physiologic model to predict the effect of changes in ventilator settings [19].

VentPlan's mathematical model makes accurate predictions for postoperative patients whose abnormalities are well represented by a three-compartment model. For these patients, VentPlan's recommendations for changes to the ventilator settings were compared with the actual changes that were implemented by physicians. VentPlan's recommendations matched the sign of the actual changes in settings and correlated with their magnitude.

VentPlan's architecture allows it to take advantage of uncertain model predictions by computing the expected utility of the predicted effects of alternative ventilator settings. For patients with physiologic abnormalities not representable by a three-compartment physiologic model, VentPlan makes accurate predictions for small changes in ventilator settings, but not for large changes.

A clinically useful VMA should incorporate a model that is capable of representing the variety of physiologic abnormalities found in ICU patients.

VENTSIM

VentSim is a continuous time, continuous state simulation model that consists of a set of linked first-order differential equations that describe the circulation of oxygen and carbon-dioxide through compartments of the body.

VentSim expands the VentPlan model by including a detailed simulation model of a mechanical ventilator, and by increasing the number of circulation and airway compartments. The structures of VentSim and VentPlan are compared in Figure 1.

Ventilator component

VentSim's ventilator component simulates the constant mandated volume modes of a volume-cycled, constant-flow ventilator. The mechanical analog of the simulator is a rigid bellows with adjustable movement of a plunger during inspiration. In VentSim's default configuration, the plunger moves at constant velocity and compresses the desired tidal volume during the first part of the inspiration cycle. The simulator leaves a short inspiratory hold time after the plunger stops; during the inspiratory hold time, the bellows pressure equilibrates with the patient's airways.

During expiration, the ventilator pressure decreases to the value set for positive end-expiratory pressure, and outflow of air from the patient is limited by a variable outflow resistance (retard setting). Sample pressures and airflows during one cycle of ventilation of a simulated patient are shown in Figure 2.

Adjustable parameters of the ventilator component allow it to simulate most volume-cycled constant-flow ventilators. These adjustments include a maximum positive pressure, an inspiratory hold time, and an expiratory retard.

Differential equation modeling makes it straightforward to adapt the VentSim ventilator component to simulate any mechanical ventilator for which a complete description is available.

Airway component

VentSim's airway component has four compartments: a series anatomic deadspace, a parallel physiologic deadspace, and two alveolar compartments (Figure 1). Each compartment has an associated airway resistance

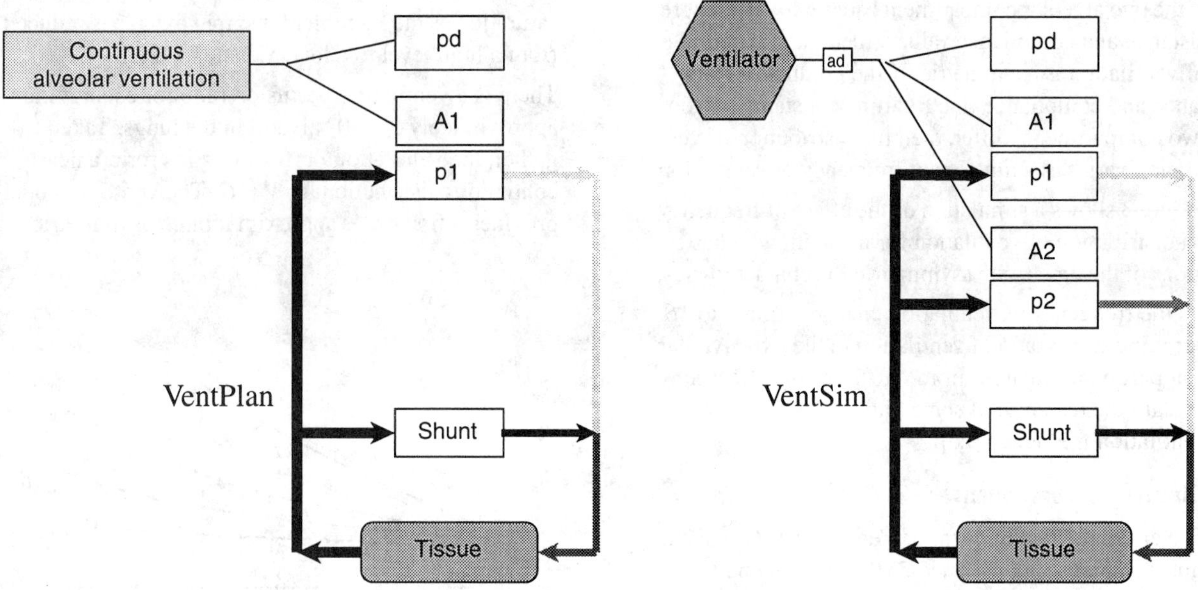

Figure 1. Comparison of VentPlan and VentSim model structures. Both models are sets of linked first-order differential equations. Blood carries oxygen and carbon dioxide in a circuit, as shown by arrows. VentPlan does not simulate the ventilator, but derives the total alveolar ventilation from the ventilator settings (the continuous alveolar ventilation assumption is indicated by the shaded rectangle). The compartments of VentPlan that correspond to the classic three-compartment model are (1) deadspace (pd), a compartment that receives ventilation but no blood flow, (2) a combined gas-exchange compartment with alveolar (A1) and pulmonary blood flow (p1) components, and (3) a compartment that corresponds to shunt. VentSim simulates a volume-controlled positive-pressure ventilator (indicated by a shaded hexagon) to compute airway pressures and airflows. The distribution of ventilation among the three ventilation compartments (pd, A1 and A2) depends on the resistance and compliance of each compartment, and varies with the frequency of ventilation. The VentSim model includes the components of the three-compartment model, plus a series anatomic deadspace (ad), and a second gas-exchange compartment (A2+p2). The presence of two gas-exchange compartments in VentSim allows it to predict the effects of asymmetric distribution of ventilation and perfusion.

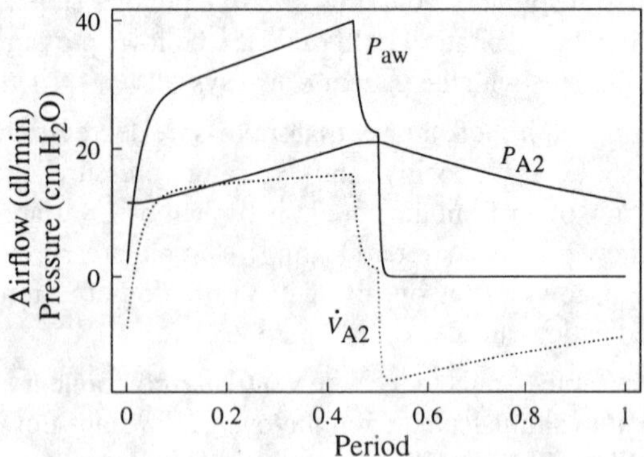

Figure 2. Sample ventilator simulation. The graph plots ventilator pressure at the mouth (P_{aw}), the pressure in one alveolar lung compartment (P_{A2}) and the airflow into one alveolar compartment ($\dot{V}_{A2}$) during one cycle of ventilation. Solid line, pressure; dotted line, airflow.

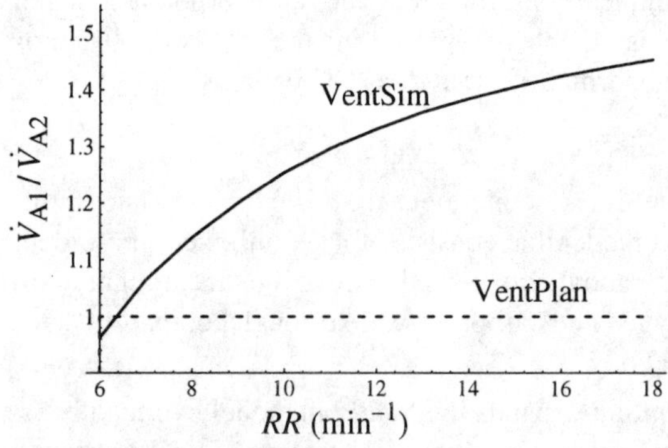

Figure 3. Simulation of the effect of asymmetric resistance-compliance (RC) on distribution of ventilation. The continuous line shows the ratio of ventilation in two alveolar compartments for a patient with asymmetric RC values. The dashed line shows the constant, symmetric ventilation of the single alveolar compartment of the VentPlan model. $\dot{V}_{A1}$, $\dot{V}_{A2}$, ventilation of the A1 and A2 alveolar compartments shown in Figure 1; RR, frequency of ventilation.

and a lung compliance. The airway component interacts with the ventilator component to predict the pressures, airflows, and volumes of ventilation at each point in the ventilator cycle. VentSim computes the tidal volumes for each airway compartment during the simulation, and, when all tidal volumes are unchanged during successive ventilator cycles, VentSim notes that the simulator has reached a cyclic steady state.

If the two alveolar compartments are set to different resistance and compliance values, then the distribution of ventilation is asymmetric. If the product of resistance and compliance (the RC time constants) of the two compartments differ, then the distribution of ventilation varies as a function of frequency of ventilation. Figure 3 shows a simulation of the effect of frequency on distribution of ventilation for a patient who has regions of the lungs with asymmetric RC characteristics. As the frequency of ventilation changes from 6 to 16 per minute, the ratio of ventilation in the two alveolar compartments changes from 1 to 1.4. This effect may explain the response of some patients to changes in ventilation frequency [26].

Circulation component

The circulation component of VentSim has two perfusion compartments (p1 and p2) that correspond to the two ventilation compartments (A1 and A2), in addition to shunt and tissue compartments (see Figure 1). The presence of a second perfused compartment that participates in gas exchange allows VentSim to represent asymmetric ventilation/perfusion distributions ($\dot{V}_A / Q$).

The ability to represent asymmetric $\dot{V}_A / Q$ is essential to describe accurately the effect of changes in inspired oxygen on the oxygen saturation. For example, in a simulation of a patient with severe asthma, the three-compartment model underestimates the fall in oxygen saturation as the fraction of inspired oxygen is reduced from a high level to a lower level (Figure 3).

There is a ventilation/perfusion ratio for each of the approximately 3 x 10^8 alveoli in the lungs. Taken together, the ventilation/perfusion ratios form a nearly continuous distribution for $\dot{V}_A / Q$. The VentSim model provides a first order approximation to asymmetric

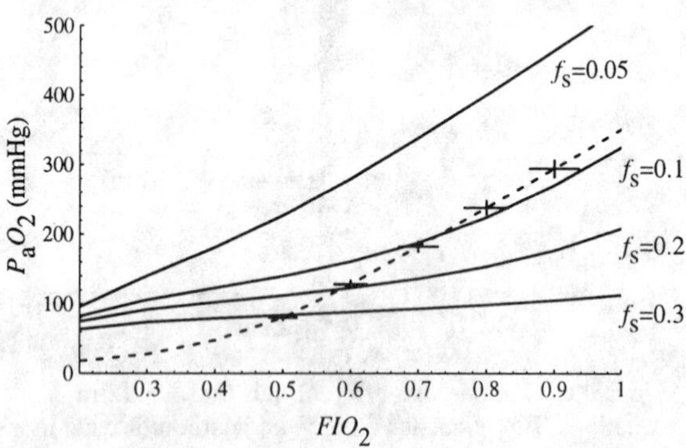

Figure 4. Effect of circulation compartments. The dashed line shows the VentSim model with parameters set to simulate a patient with a ventilation/perfusion mismatch (a moderate asymmetry in distribution of ventilation and perfusion, $\dot{V}_{A1} / Q_{p1} < \dot{V}_{A2} / Q_{p2}$). The continuous lines show the VentPlan model as the shunt fraction, f_s varies. Sampled data are shown as crosses on the dashed line. No value of f_s allows VentPlan to fit the data. (Variable names defined in legend to the Table.)

Table: VentSim and VentPlan variables

Model	Model parameters	Prediction variables	Control variables
VentPlan	$\dot{V}_{O_2}$, RQ, Q_T, f_s, V_{ds} HCO_2, Hb	P_aO_2, P_aCO_2, pH_a P_vO_2, P_vCO_2, pH_v, $\dot{V}_{A1}$	V_{Tset}, RR, FIO_2, $PEEP$
VentSim	$\dot{V}_{O_2}$, RQ, Q_T, f_s, f_{p1}, V_{ad} V_{pd}, R_{pd}, R_{A1}, R_{A2}, C_{A1} C_{A2}, C_{pd}, HCO_2, Hb	P_aO_2, P_aCO_2, pH_a, P_vO_2 $P_v\,CO_2$, pH_v, P_{aw}, V_{tidal} $\dot{V}_{A1}$, $\dot{V}_{A2}$, Q_{p1}, Q_{p2}, Q_s	V_{Tset}, RR, FIO_2, $PEEP$ P_{max}, $IEratio$

Variables: V, volume; $\dot{V}$, dV/dt; P, pressure; R, resistance; C, compliance; Q, blood flow; f: fraction; $\dot{V}_{A1}$, alveolar compartment ventilation; $\dot{V}_{O_2}$, metabolic rate; RQ, respiratory quotient; Q_T, cardiac output; f_s, shunt fraction; HCO_2, serum bicarbonate; Hb, hemoglobin concentration; V_{tidal}, delivered tidal volume; V_{Tset}, set tidal volume; RR, set rate of ventilation; FIO_2, set fraction of inspired oxygen; $PEEP$, set positive end-expiratory pressure; P_{max}, set maximum positive pressure; $IEratio$, set inspiratory/expiratory ratio. Subscripts: s, shunt; a, arterial; v, mixed venous; ds, total deadspace;, ad, anatomic deadspace; pd, physiologic deadspace; aw, airway; A1 and A2, ventilated alveolar compartments; p1 and p2, perfused pulmonary compartments.

V_A/Q by representing the distribution as $\{\dot{V}_{A1}/Q_{p1}, \dot{V}_{A2}/Q_{p2}\}$

IMPLEMENTATION

The author implemented the differential equations that describe VentSim as difference equations in a C program, then constructed a graphical user interface to study the behavior of the model. This interface allows a user to inspect model parameters, adjust ventilator settings, and observe the time-varying model predictions.

The VentSim model has 143 variables. A selection of the key model parameters, control variables, and prediction variables are shown in the Table.

Solution methods

The model equations are stiff—an airway component with very short time constants (due to low resistance and compliance of the anatomic deadspace) interacts with a circulation component that has much longer time constants. As a result, numeric integration of the full model is computation intensive. The initial implementation in C, on a desktop workstation (NeXT 68040/25Mhz), requires 53 seconds to simulate 20 minutes.

A second implementation reduced the computation delay by solving only for the steady state solutions to the model. The ventilator and airway components were first solved by numeric integration until a cycling steady state was achieved. Then, the circulation component was solved by searching for the roots of the equilibrium solutions [17], using values for the alveolar ventilation derived from the ventilator simulation. With this approach, VentSim now requires only 1.6 seconds to generate the steady-state solution to a change in ventilator settings.

The VentSim model is implemented as an external C routine that is separately compiled and linked to Mathematica, which provides symbolic and numeric manipulation methods in addition to graphical presentation tools [28].

DISCUSSION

Mathematical models are powerful tools for simulating the quantitative time-dependent behavior of complex, dynamic systems, such as the human cardiopulmonary system [5]. Quantitative models that focus on limited areas of physiology assist the study of individual physiologic concepts. For example, detailed models of the human airway led to insights on the distribution of airway resistance in normal and diseased lungs [26, 27], and to a better understanding of gas exchange in the respiratory system [24]. Detailed models of cardiovascular physiology allowed analysis of the effects of counterpulsation [1], of the effects of arterial grafts on cardiovascular function [10], and of the effects of therapeutic interventions on coronary sinus blood flow [20].

Models that include components from several areas of physiology allow the study of regulatory mechanisms and provide insight into the interactions among systems [2, 23]. An early and influential project in this area was a study by Guyton and colleagues of the behavior of a comprehensive model of renal and cardiovascular physiology, which led to new understanding of the mechanisms of blood pressure regulation [9].

Physiologic models also are useful to teach concepts to students of medicine and physiology. HUMAN is a comprehensive microcomputer-based model that allows students to perform a wide variety of physiologic experiments without performing animal or human experimentation [6]. Other examples of teaching models were developed in the areas of cardiovascular and respiratory physiology [12], anesthesia treatments [8, 16, 21], and ventilator management [4, 15].

An important problem in applying detailed simulation models to patients is that it is difficult to assess all patient-specific model parameters. For example, Wagner developed a 50-compartment model of lung ventilation and perfusion, but this model requires an inconvenient and expensive multiple inert gas study to determine patient-specific values for the model parameters [25]. The many parameters of Wagner's ventilation/perfusion model are underdetermined in all cases. In another study, Kaufman and colleagues demonstrated that, if only arterial blood gas data are available, the maximum number of perfusion compartments that are distinguishable is three [11].

An implementation of VentSim to assist in clinical care of ICU patients would require a method to determine patient-specific values of model parameters. This problem is addressed by the VentPlan architecture, which combines a belief network with a mathematical model. The belief network is a semi-quantitative model of the effect of disease states on the probability distributions of physiologic parameters; it computes conditional distributions for the parameters of the mathematical model. When the quantitative observations for a patient do not determine the value of all physiologic parameters, the model parameters are based on the prior distributions that are computed by the belief network [19].

The VentSim model includes a set of physiologic interactions that are sufficient to explain a variety of patient abnormalities, but it is by no means complete. For example, VentSim contains no representation of the phenomenon of hypoxic pulmonary vasoconstriction, and does not predict changes in cardiac output that may occur with increases in mean airway pressure. These, and other unmodeled physiologic effects, make it essential that any computer-based ventilator-advice system maintain a cautious estimate of the degree of model-prediction uncertainty.

The time-critical nature of decision making in the ICU limits the computation time that is available for evaluating complex models. Future ventilator-management applications may assess the tradeoff of benefit of model detail and cost of computation delay. This assessment would allow an application to select a model that is detailed enough to represent a patient's physiologic abnormalities and make accurate predictions, but not so complex that it delays treatment recommendations unnecessarily.

Acknowledgment

I thank Ross Shachter, Lewis Sheiner, and Lawrence Fagan for helpful discussions. George Thomsen developed the first VentPlan model and numerous model-solving techniques. Nora Sweeney and Maria Tovar provided valuable comments. I especially thank Edward Shortliffe for providing the environment for research in Medical Informatics at Stanford. This research was supported in part by Grant IRI-9108359 from the National Science Foundation and Grants LM-07033 and LM-04136 from the National Library of Medicine. Computing facilities were provided by the CAMIS Resource, LM-05305.

References

[1] Bai, J., Ying, K. and Jaron, D. Cardiovascular responses to external counterpulsation: A computer simulation. *Medical & Biological Engineering & Computing,* **30**(3):317–23, 1992.

[2] Barnea, O. and Sheffer, N. A computer model for analysis of fluid resuscitation. *Computers in Biology and Medicine,* **23**(6):443-54, 1993.

[3] Beinlich, I.A., Suermondt, H.J., Chavez, R.M. and Cooper, G.F. The ALARM monitoring system: A case study with two probabilistic inference techniques for belief networks. *Proceedings of the Second European Conference on Artificial Intelligence in Medicine,* London, UK, 1989, pp. 247–256.

[4] Boyle, J. RESPSYST: An interactive microcomputer program for education. *Physiologist,* **28**(5):452–3, 1985.

[5] Cellier, F.E. *Continuous System Modeling.* New York: Springer Verlag, 1991.

[6] Coleman, T.G. and Randall, J.E. HUMAN – A comprehensive physiological model. The Physiologist, **26**(1):15–21, 1983.

[7] Fagan, L.M., Kunz, J.C., Feigenbaum, E.A. and Osborn, J.J. Extensions to the rule-based formalism for a monitoring task. In Buchanan, B. and Shortliffe, E.H. (eds), *Rule-Based Expert Systems: The MYCIN Experiments of the Stanford Heuristic Programming Project.* Reading: Addison-Wesley, 1984, pp. 397–423.

[8] Gaba, D.M. and DeAnda, A. A comprehensive anesthesia simulation environment: Re-creating the operating room for research and training. *Anesthesiology,* **69**(3):387-94, 1988.

[9] Guyton, A.C., Coleman, T.G. and Granger, H.J. Circulation: Overall regulation. *Ann Rev Physiol,* **34**:13–46, 1983.

[10] Helal, M.A., Watts, K.C. and Marble, A.E. Hydrodynamic simulation of arterial networks which include compliant and rigid bypass grafts. *Journal of Biomechanics,* **27**(3):277–87, 1994.

[11] Kaufman, R.D., Patterson, R.W. and Lee, A.S. Derivation of VA/Q distribution from blood-gas tensions. *Br J Anaesth,* **59**(12):1599–609, 1987.

[12] Lefevre, J., Roucou, D., Lambert, K. and Maes, B. Simulation and computer-aided instructions in cardiovascular physiology. *Proceedings of the Conference on Computers in Cardiology,* Washington, D.C., 1988, p. 597.

[13] Menn, S.J., Barnett, G.O. and Schmechel, D. A computer program to assist in the care of acute respiratory failure. *JAMA,* **223**(4):308–312, 1973.

[14] Miller, P.L. Goal-directed critiquing by computer: Ventilator management. *Comput Biomed Res,* **18**(5):422-38, 1985.

[15] Petrini, M.F. Distribution of ventilation and perfusion: A teaching model. *Comput Biol Med,* **16**(6):431-44, 1986.

[16] Philip, J.H. Gas Man—an example of goal oriented computer-assisted teaching which results in learning. *Int J Clin Monit Comput,* **3**(3):165–73, 1986.

[17] Press, W.H., Flannery, B.P., Teulokolsky, S.A. and Vetterling, W.T. *Numerical Recipes in C: The Art of Scientific Programming.* Cambridge: Cambridge University Press, 1988.

[18] Rudowski, R., Bokliden, A., Carstensen, A., Gill, H., Ludwigs, U. and Matell, G. Multivariable optimization of mechanical ventilation. A linear programming approach. *Int J Clin Mon Comput,* **8**:107–115, 1991.

[19] Rutledge, G.W., Thomsen, G., Farr, B., Beinlich, I., Tovar, M.A., Sheiner, L. and Fagan, L.M. The design and implementation of a ventilator-management advisor. *Art Intell Med,* **5**:67–82, 1993.

[20] Schreiner, W. Computer simulation of the coronary circulation. *Simulation,* **59**(1):15–23, 1992.

[21] Schwid, H.A. A flight simulator for general anesthesia training. *Comput Biomed Res,* **20**(1):64-75, 1987.

[22] Sittig, D.F. *COMPAS: A Computerized Patient Advice System to Direct Ventilatory Care,* Doctoral dissertation, Dept. Medical Informatics, University of Utah, 1988.

[23] Sun, Y. and Chiaramida, S. Simulation of hemodynamics and regulatory mechanisms in the cardiovascular system based on a nonlinear and time-varying model. *Simulation,* **59**(1):28–36, 1992.

[24] Tomlinson, S.P., Lo, J. and Tilley, D.G. Time transient gas exchange in the respiratory system. *IEEE Engineering in Medicine and Biology Magazine,* **12**(3):64–70, 1993.

[25] Wagner, P.D., Smith, C.M., Davies, N.J., McEvoy, R.D. and Gale, G.E. Estimation of ventilation-perfusion inequality by inert gas elimination without arterial sampling. *J Appl Physiol,* **59**(2):376-83, 1985.

[26] Weibel, E.W. Lung morphometry and models in respiratory physiology. In Chiang, H.K. and Paiva, M. (ed), *Respriatory Physiology: An Analytical Approach.* New York: Marcel Dekker, 1989, pp. 1–56.

[27] Wiggs, B.R., Moreno, R., Hogg, J.C., Hilliam, C. and Pare, P.D. A model of the mechanics of airway narrowing. *J Appl Physiol,* **69**(3):849-60, 1990.

[28] Wolfram, S. *Mathematica: A System for Doing Mathematics by Computer.* Redwood City: Addison–Wesley, 1991.

From Chart Tracking to Workflow Management

Padmini Srinivasan
Gerard Vignes
Computer Science Department
(318) 231-5215
ps@cacs.usl.edu

Carol Venable
Anita Hazelwood
Toni Cade
Health Information Management
(318) 231-6629
cav0811@ucs.usl.edu

University of Southwestern Louisiana
Lafayette, LA 70504

Abstract

The current interest in system-wide integration appears to be based on the assumption that an organization, by digitizing information and accepting a common standard for the exchange of such information, will improve the accessibility of this information and automatically experience benefits resulting from its more productive use. We do not dispute this reasoning, but assert that an organization's capacity for effective change is proportional to the understanding of the current structure among its personnel. Our workflow manager is based on the use of a *Parameterized Petri Net* (PPN) model which can be configured to represent an arbitrarily detailed picture of an organization. The PPN model can be animated to observe the model organization in action, and the results of the animation analyzed. This simulation is a dynamic ongoing process which changes with the system and allows members of the organization to pose "what if" questions as a means of exploring opportunities for change.

We present, the "workflow management system" as the natural successor to the tracking program, incorporating modeling, scheduling, reactive planning, performance evaluation, and simulation. This workflow management system is more than adequate for meeting the needs of a paper chart tracking system, and, as the patient record is computerized, will serve as a planning and evaluation tool in converting the paper-based health information system into a computer-based system.

1 INTRODUCTION

Chart tracking, a basic function of the medical record department, is a legacy of the paper-based patient record, or *chart*. Although the task may be regarded as trivial, the benefits are by no means unimportant. In spite of the fact that most hospitals do tracking, charts occasionally disappear. Chart tracking programs exist which automate tracking tasks and allow the program's *operator* to keep tabs on active charts.

The research described in this paper is the result of work that was funded by LEQSF Grant Number 058-B.

We present, as the natural successor to the tracking program, a "workflow management system" which incorporates modeling, scheduling, reactive planning, performance evaluation, and simulation in a package . This workflow management system is more than adequate for meeting the needs of a paper chart tracking system, and, as the patient record is computerized, will serve as a planning and evaluation tool in converting the paper-based health information system into a computer-based system.

The current interest in system-wide integration seems to be based on the assumption that an organization, by accepting a standard for the exchange of information, will improve the accessibility of this information and experience benefits resulting from its more productive use. We do not dispute this reasoning, but instead the assert that a much greater benefit can be realized by focusing not on integration, but on the task of developing a realistic picture of the how the organization actually functions—not the obligatory company hierarchy diagram, but a mosaic of the interplay between technical and human resources within the organization.

For integration is change, and not change of some abstract, anonymous work process, but change of the way people work with one another, and the attitude with which they judge the costs and benefits of this cooperation. If enough people in an organization are convinced that change is not going to profit their own work, then they will either rebel against the policy, or, far worse, quietly appear to accept it but simply ignore it. It has been said that careless application of technology allows people to make more mistakes faster. As a corollary to this, we offer that enforcement of policies or protocols designed to promote integration will encourage *everyone* to make the *same* mistakes consistently, without hope of improvement except through revolution against the standards.

An organization's capacity for coping with change is proportional to the understanding of the current structure among its personnel. Organizations often embody years of evolution and accumulated tacit knowledge that is never made explicit and yet is vital. Modeling is an aid in the understanding of complex systems and problems. Modeling techniques can help to overcome human cognitive limitations and help with the management of change. Models of an organization serve to make tacit knowledge explicit, representing processes *and* people, viewed from various vantage points and related to one other in ways not restricted by the need to preserve a hierarchical structure.

Our workflow manager is based on the use of a PPN model which can be configured to represent an arbitrarily detailed picture of an organization. This model can be animated to observe the model organization in action, and the results of the animation analyzed—with far less time and effort than would be necessary for a similar study of the actual organization. This is not just a simulation which might be conducted once a year as an adjunct to the "time and motion" study. It is, rather, a dynamic ongoing process which changes with the system and allow members of the organization to pose "what if" questions as a means of exploring opportunities for change. It also offers the opportunity to evaluate the consequences of those changes by implementing them on a model of the actual system..

Section two of this paper describes an ordinary chart tracking program, and gives a listing of reports typically produced. Section three presents the *software architecture* for the workflow manager, with a breakdown of the functionality of its components. Section four presents the workflow model of a simplified health information system, and section five concludes the paper.

2 THE TRADITIONAL CHART TRACKING PROGRAM

The traditional chart tracking program is essentially an online card index, holding the current status of each chart entered into the system. It may or may not provide enhanced chart lookup and report generation features, but either way it is a relatively unintelligent aid to the human operator. As new status information about the completion of the chart is entered, the previous information may be overwritten, or perhaps saved as a log of *transactions*, i.e., changes made to the status of the chart as new information becomes available.

Aside from offering quick access to the status of a chart and a convenient report on the system's progress, there is no automated assistance to the human operator. No mechanism is provided to detect inconsistencies in the status of a chart, so when important events are not recorded—or are recorded incorrectly—the system is not aware of the error, and it is up to the operator to discover the problem and piece together the puzzle of what actually happened. Any intelligent, useful application of the information contained within the memory of the tracking program comes entirely from the human operator. As the number of charts in the system increases, the operator's ability to extract useful information and manage the system by "brute force" deteriorates.

The list below is compiled from various "wish lists," both published and from interviews, of desirable chart tracking reports. These reports serve as the basis for determining the functionality expected of an intelligent chart tracking system.

1. Medical Records Order List
2. Unavailable Medical Records List
3. Post-Dated Requests Summary

Figure 1: Workflow Management Software Architecture

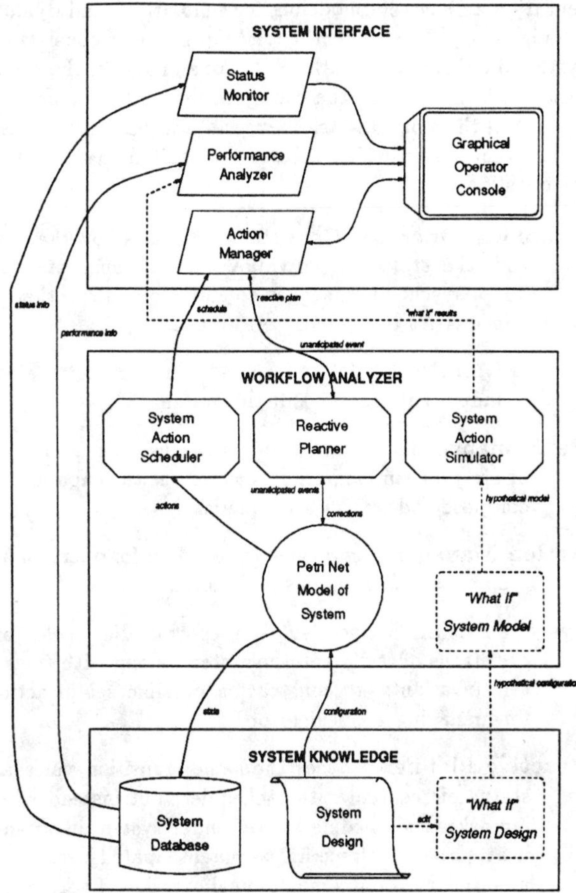

4. Down-Time Location List
5. Borrowers in Possession for Greater than 30 Days
6. Medical Record Department Activity
7. Restricted Medical Records Report
8. Delinquent Medical Records Report
9. Archived Medical Record Locations
10. Incomplete/Delinquent Letter Generation

3 SOFTWARE ARCHITECTURE OF A WORKFLOW MANAGEMENT SYSTEM

A diagram of the proposed workflow management system is shown in figure 1. The components of this architecture can be divided into three segments, system interface, workflow analyzer, and system knowledge. The *System Interface* allows the user to monitor the status of patient records, analyze the performance of the overall system, and manage the actions of the system. The *Workflow Analyzer* schedules normal system actions, drafts reaction plans to unanticipated events, and allows the user to pose "what if" situations and analyze the results. A Parameterized Petri Net

(PPN) [1] is used to animate and study a model of the system. Petri Net technology is used in knowledge representation and system modeling for simulations and dynamic management. The *System Knowledge* segment consists of a system database to store the status of all records, the system design which specifies the configuration of the model used to control the workflow analyzer, and alternative versions of the system design which the user has edited to pose "what if" questions.

Graphical Operator Console — displays for the operator the status of individual records, suggested and adopted schedules, suggested and adopted reaction plans, and metrics on system performance.

Status Monitor — determines and summarizes the status of individual records and the system.

Performance Analyzer — offers the user an assortment of pre-programmed reports as well as the capability to compose "ad hoc" status queries.

Action Manager — provides an interface for operator and system specified actions and alerts.

System Action Scheduler — uses transition rules and the status of records in the system, along with the system invariants, to construct a possible set of actions for managing medical records.

Reactive Planner — uses the same transition rules and status of records as the scheduler, but instead of being asked to schedule events under system invariants, it attempts to "force fit" an unanticipated event (e.g., unanticipated outcome, manual override of normal priorities ...) in the quickest and least obtrusive method available to it. The unscheduled event planner is the 911 service for the tracking system.

System Action Simulator — accepts a starting state for a hypothetical tracking system and proposes a schedule of actions for managing records. It animates this hypothetical system based on the conditions specified, and submits its results for performance evaluation.

Petri Net Model of System — represents the knowledge regarding the state and dynamic features of the information system, using multiple views to manage complexity in the representation. Section 4, an example workflow model, elaborates on this

System Database — stores the status of each record, and other related and necessary information.

System Design — provides the system with a set of inputs determining the PPN model for a particular system. These inputs include possible system actions along with their necessary and sufficient conditions.

"What If" System Design — is an operator-modified version of the system, used for representing and analyzing proposed changes to the actual system.

Figure 2: Workflow Model of a Health Information System

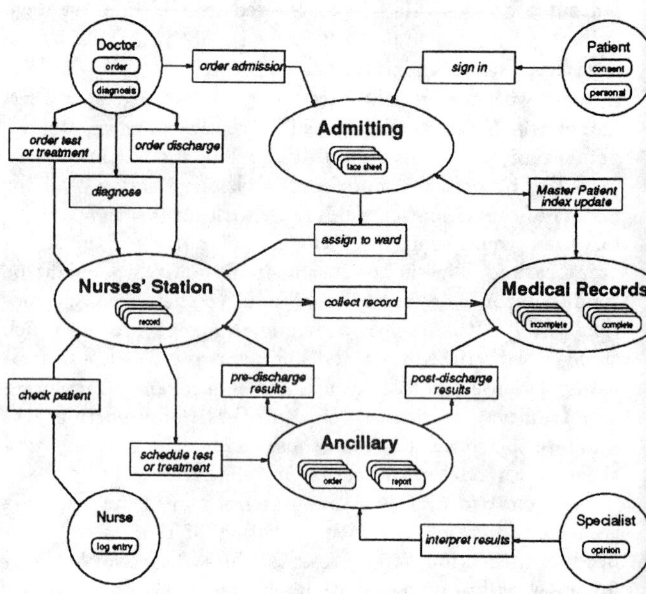

"What If" System Model — is the PPN model produced in response to the operator's "what if" design. It animates the model and makes results from the animation available for analysis.

4 WORKFLOW MODEL OF A SIMPLIFIED HEALTH INFORMATION SYSTEM

Figure 2 contains a simiplified view of the PPN for a hospital infomtion flow or chart movement. The oval and circular nodes are places, and represent department locations or personnel involved in the action. The rectangles are "transitions", and represent actions that can be applied to objects (records, information items) int the input "place" (from which an arc is directed to the transition) resulting in the objects being in the output "place" (to which an arc is directed from the transition) of the transition.

The theoretical underpinnings of this representation technique are discussed in [1]. Support of multiple views through parameterization is also discussed. Available PPN analysis methods allow the determination of useful properties of dynamic systems.

The medical records are "tokens" that move between places and are altered via transitions. The existence of a medical record in a place is necessary for transitions having that place as the input place to "fire" or operate upon that medical record. It is possible to associate time delays with a place or transition. Animations allow one to observe objects moving through transitions on the screen. An iconic and more intuitive interface is under development.

Simulating the system is equivalent to having the PPN model "run" (transitions fire) on an artificial set of medical records and events. The workflow analyzer can simultaneously "track" the status of the medical records by the state of the net, or its markings, stored in a database. Business process improvement planning is tantamount to altering the PPN model and carrying out a simulation-based performance analysis of the proposed system. The PPN representation of the system is the core of the workflow management software architecture. Prototype models for two healthcare institutions have been developed and demonstrated.

5 CONCLUSION

In this paper is presented a knowledge representation methodology and an associated software architecture that has been extensively and effectively used in manufacturing and command, control and communications applications. Considering the health information system as an information assembly and retrieval process and given the objective of cost reduction and rationalization in re-engineering this process, we propose this model based methodology for use in the healthcare institutions. Chart tracking is identified as an existing function in health information management that can be directly extended for performance evaluation. Existing chart tracking systems are not model-based; they are log-based. They incorporate database capabilities but not simulation, planning and predictive capabilities. The workflow manager discussed accomplishes model-based chart tracking and provides the fundamental modeling and simulation capabilities neded for evaluation of strategies in business process re-engineering/automation.

6 REFERENCES

[1] "Parameterized Petri Nets and Their Application to Planning and Coordination in Intelligent Systems," P. Srinivasan, D. Gracanin and K. Valavanis, *IEEE Transactions on Systems, Man and Cybernetics*, Vol. 23, No. 10, Oct. 1993

[2] "Health Care Computing in the 1990s," K. C. Cerny, *Thinkwork.*

[3] "Work Is a Closed-Loop Process," Peter J. Denning, *American Scientist*, Vol. 80, July-August 1992.

[4] "Infomation Flow Models for Two Healthcare Institutions" P. Srinivasan, V. Yekkirala, and K. Dahlgreen, *USL Technical Report 15-94.*

Optimal Location for a Helicopter in a Rural Trauma System: Prediction using Discrete-Event Computer Simulation

David E. Clark, David R. Hahn, Russell W. Hall, and Robert E. Quaker
Department of Surgery, Maine Medical Center, and Departments of Statistics and Computer Science, University of Southern Maine, Portland, Maine

A discrete-event computer simulation was developed using the C programming language to determine the optimal base location for a trauma system helicopter in Maine, a rural area with unevenly distributed population. Ambulance run reports from a one-year period provided input data on the times and places where major injuries occurred. Data from a statewide trauma registry were used to estimate the percentage of cases which would require trauma center care and the locations of functional trauma centers. Climatic data for this region were used to estimate the likelihood that a helicopter could not fly due to bad weather. The incidence of trauma events was modeled as a nonstationary Poisson process, and location of the events by an empirical distribution. For each simulated event, if the injuries were sufficiently severe, if weather permitted flying, if the occurrence were not within 20 miles of a center or outside the range of the helicopter, and if the helicopter were not already in service, then it was used for transportation. 35 simulated years were run for each of 4 proposed locations for the helicopter base. One of the geographically intermediate locations was shown to produce the most frequent utilization of the helicopter. Discrete-event simulation is a potentially useful tool in planning for emergency medical services systems. Further refinements and validation of predictions may lead to wider utilization.

INTRODUCTION

The optimal placement of emergency vehicles in a given geographic area is a problem in which the techniques of operations research can be usefully applied. Expensive resources must be distributed in such a way that the delivery of emergency services is sufficiently rapid for all possible locations within the area and as rapid as possible for as many events as possible, but with a minimum cost (generally by minimizing the number of vehicles).

If certain (potentially oversimplifying) assumptions are made, some such problems can be solved analytically [1,2,3]. A greater degree of flexibility in modeling a system can be obtained by simulation; this approach has been useful in the evaluation of urban and suburban ambulance locations and performance in Tucson, Arizona [4], Lee County, Alabama [5], and Shanghai, China [6]. However, a simulation model for Emergency Medical Services (EMS) planning in rural areas previously attempted in Maine and elsewhere was unsuccessful because of excessive complexity, failure to involve decision-makers in the modeling process, and other validation failures [7].

Statement of the Problem

In the course of planning for possible helicopter service as part of a trauma system in Maine, we wished to model the use of this expensive resource for transportation of acutely injured patients to designated trauma centers. Specifically, we attempted to predict the optimal location of a single dedicated helicopter within the state, given the probable location of trauma centers, in order to maximize its usefulness for this patient population. A solution is not obvious on inspection, since the majority of the population in Maine is in its southern part, but the largest area is in its central and northeastern parts (Figure 1).

The ideal function of the helicopter is to provide rapid transportation over medium distances from the scene of a serious injury (trauma) or a nearby small hospital to a major hospital with specialized capabilities in the management of severe injuries (a trauma center). In this state, such centers are planned in Portland, Lewiston, and Bangor. Injuries occurring close to these centers can be transported by ground ambulance at least as easily as by helicopter. Injuries occurring far from a helicopter base would take too long or require refueling stops and are therefore impractical for helicopter transport. Of course, only a small percentage of injuries will be serious enough for medical reasons to justify using the helicopter, and specific "launch criteria" must be developed to guide emergency medical

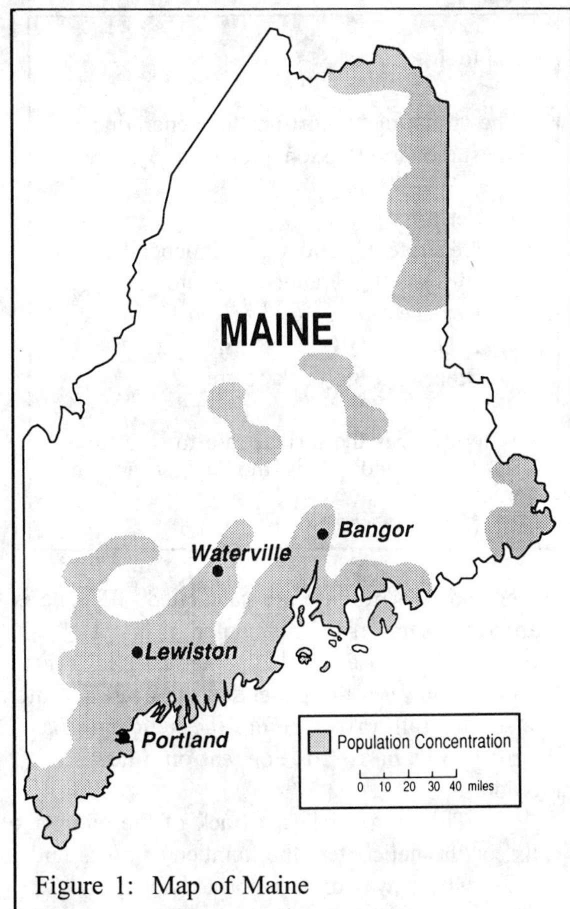

Figure 1: Map of Maine

personnel. Finally, at times a helicopter will be unable to fly because of weather, repairs, or concurrent demands.

Although most of the factors determining the availability and use of a helicopter are beyond human control, one factor which can be altered is the base location of the helicopter, which was the principal interest of our study. Each time it is used, there will be a short delay to get the crew on the helicopter, flight time from base to scene of injury, time spent at scene, flight time from scene to trauma center, time spent at the center, and time to fly back to base and prepare the helicopter and crew for another mission (Figure 2).

The critical times are from notification to arrival at the scene (since the helicopter carries paramedical personnel with higher training than local emergency medical technicians), and particularly the time from notification to arrival at the trauma center (where immediate surgical interventions can be undertaken).

MATERIALS AND METHODS

Computer programming was performed on a DEC computer system using the UNIX operating system. Programs were written in C, with subroutine calls to CSIM, a process-oriented simulation language based upon C [8]. The programs have subsequently been modifed for use with personal computers and DOS. Source code, with comments, is available upon request.

Input data, distributions, sources of randomness, and assumptions

The Maine office of EMS provided the time, date, and town location of all Maine EMS calls during 1991 classified by EMS personnel as "major trauma". The latitude and longitude of all Maine towns was also obtained [9] and entered into a computer file. Combining the location data from these two sources allowed us to plot the location of each incident and determine the frequency of incidents for each town. This empirical distribution was used for the model, which was therefore programmed to return town values randomly in the same frequency as they had occurred in 1991. Flying distances could be easily calculated from the latitude and longitude information.

Occurrence rates varied significantly for different times of day, seasons, and weekends versus weekdays. A nonstationary Poisson process seemed appropriate to model these arrival rates [6]. This resulted in the calculation of 192 average occurrence rates:

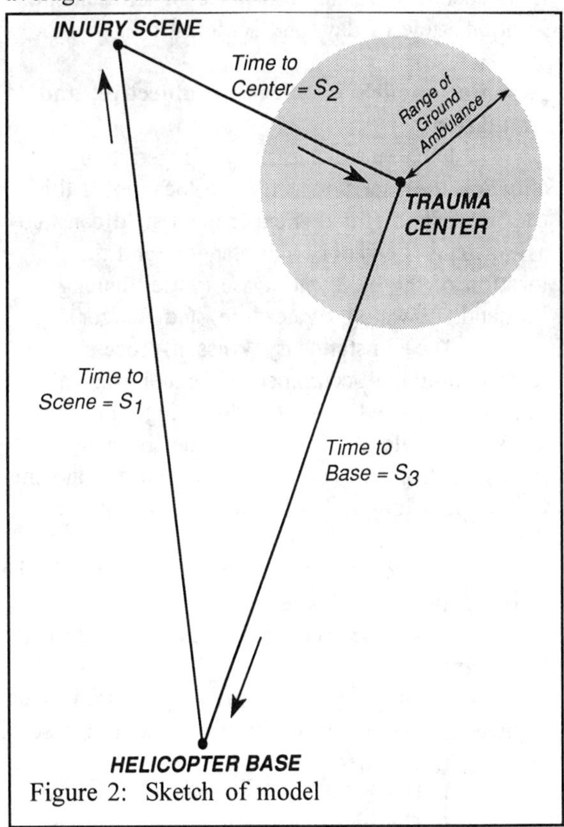

Figure 2: Sketch of model

For example, one rate was used for 6:00 A.M. to 7:00 A.M. for each winter weekend day (Friday, Saturday, or Sunday). A rough estimate of the percentage of "major trauma" calls which would be serious enough to justify the use of a helicopter was obtained, using trauma registry data [10] and based upon experience in other areas [11,12]. The present model assumes that the distributions of times and locations for these most serious injuries are the same as for all injuries classified by EMS as "major trauma".

Estimates of helicopter speed, range, and percentage of time unavailable for mechanical reasons (breakdowns, maintenance, etc.) were obtained from industry sources. Likewise, the time from notification to takeoff, time required at the scene of an accident, time for unloading the patient at a trauma center, and time for refueling and preparing the aircraft for another flight were estimated. In the absence of actual data on helicopter machine and crew performance, these are modeled as constants.

A rough estimate of percentage of time during which a helicopter would be unable to fly due to bad weather was made from data provided by the Northeast Regional Climate Center (Ithaca, N.Y.). We have also made the simplifying assumption that inability to fly because of weather is independent of the occurrence of an accident, location, time of day, and season.

Resulting model, justification, objective, and simulation

Each run of the simulation starts by allowing the user to specify the location of the trauma centers (for this experiment held constant as Portland, Lewiston, and Bangor) and the location of the helicopter base (varied among Portland, Lewiston, Waterville, and Bangor).

The nonstationary Poisson process representing the occurrence of "major trauma" events is initiated using the "thinning" algorithm shown in Table 1. The town is determined randomly from the empirical distribution, and the latitude and longitude of that town obtained as described above.

As each event (accident) is generated, the program determines whether:

1. The accident is serious enough to call helicopter.

2. The accident is not within 20 miles of a trauma center (ground ambulance will be faster).

3. Weather permits flying.

4. The helicopter is not already in use.

5. The helicopter is not being repaired.

If all the above are true, the distances from helicopter base to accident scene to each trauma center and back to base are calculated. If none is within the range of the helicopter, it is not activated; otherwise, the helicopter is used to get the patient and fly the patient to the nearest center. If a second call arrives before the helicopter has returned to its base, it is not sent on a new mission.

Table 1

The "thinning" algorithm for generating a nonstationary Poisson process [13]:

1. Set $t = t_{i-1}$
2. Generate U_1 and U_2 as independent uniform (0,1) random variates
3. Replace t by $t - (1 / \lambda^*) \ln U_1$
4. If $U_2 <= \lambda(t) / \lambda^*$, return $t_i = t$
   Otherwise, go back to step 2

Where $\lambda(t)$ is the arrival rate for the time interval t, and λ^* is the largest arrival rate.

The program keeps track of the number of calls for the helicopter, the number of times and reasons why it was or was not activated, and performance data for each event when it was activated. In addition to those reported here, performance measures included the mean and range of times from call to arrival at the scene of the accident, the mean and range of total times from the call until the patient arrives at the trauma center, and the percentage of the latter times under 60 minutes (the so-called "golden hour" thought to be a critical maximum in trauma management).

Each simulation run consists of one or more simulated years for a given helicopter base with random numbers taken from a single continuous stream. Each simulated year within a simulation run terminates at the end of the year. For this study, 35 years were simulated for each of the four possible helicopter base sites using four different non-overlapping random number streams. Data of interest were produced for each run and compared.

The chief objective, as described above, was to determine the optimal location for the helicopter base, as this is essentially the only factor which can be controlled. If all assumptions are correct, the number of missions flown is the statistic of importance, since it is further presumed that the seriously injured patients not transported by helicopter are at risk for complications or death as a result of the delay. Furthermore, to be financially viable, the helicopter should be given as many appropriate missions as possible in order to generate revenue, since its costs are largely fixed.

Verification of the program was achieved in several ways: Where possible, functions were written, compiled, and tested as separate entities. Functions were given values for which the results were known, and the known output values were then compared with those produced by the functions for correctness. Each section of code was checked by another member of the project team not involved in writing that section of code. The program was run for a simulated time period of 20 days and the results verified by hand. The effectiveness of the thinning algorithm was verified by obtaining the average number of trauma events for each time interval over 35 simulated years and comparing it (visually) with the input data.

RESULTS

Each simulated year was considered a terminating simulation (so that no "warmup period" was part of the model). A summary of the data is given in Table 2. The decision variable was the mean number of appropriate helicopter missions flown from each base, which ranged from 119 at Portland to 172 at Waterville.

Table 2

POSSIBLE LOCATIONS FOR HELICOPTER BASE

	Por	Lew	Wat	Ban
MISSIONS COMPLETED				
Mean	119.3	157.4	172.1	151.6
S.D.	8.9	12.6	11.9	12.5
TIME TO SCENE (hrs)				
Mean	0.64	0.59	0.56	0.67
TIME TO CENTER (hrs)				
Mean	1.49	1.44	1.42	1.57

Output analysis

From inspection of the results in Table 2, it appears that the most frequent usage of the helicopter occurred when it was based in Waterville. If its planned base in Portland is used as a standard, the mean difference of 52.8 missions is found to be significantly different by one-sided t-test (34 degrees of freedom, $p < .001$).

To select the best of k system configurations (in this case the best of 4 helicopter bases), a standard approach is that of Dudewicz and Dalal [14]: The random variable of interest (in this case the number of helicopter missions per year) is assumed to have a normal distribution for each configuration, but it is not necessary to assume that the variances for different configurations are equal. The problem is formulated such that we want the probability of selecting the best configuration to be greater than a specified value (in this case we choose 95%) provided that we do not care if a configuration is selected whose mean differs from the best configuration by less than a specified value d* (in this case we choose this "indifference amount" to be 10 helicopter missions per year).

Several runs of the simulations are done (at least 20 are recommended; we performed 35), and the sample standard deviations for each configuration are calculated (Table 2). The sample size required for each system i is given by

$$N_i = \max \left\{ n_0+1 \, , \, \left\lceil \frac{h_i^2 S_i^2 (n_0)}{(d^*)^2} \right\rceil \right\}$$

where n_0 is the number of runs in this sample, $S_i(n)$ is the sample standard deviation, and d* is the "indifference amount" described above; h_i is a tabulated value, which for $n = 35$, $k = 4$, and 95% confidence is approximately 3.02 [13]. The second statistic within the brackets evaluates to less than n_0+1 for all configurations. Thus, the number of runs is sufficient without further replications required for the Dudewicz/Dalal procedure, and we need only choose the configuration with the largest mean, namely basing the helicopter in Waterville.

CONCLUSIONS

Based upon the model described, we have concluded that of the four configurations tested, utilization of the helicopter for transportation of acutely injured patients will be most frequent if the helicopter is based in Waterville. There are, of course, numerous political and other considerations which would be more difficult to model, such as the possibility of patients transported across state lines, and the costs of maintaining the helicopter and its crew in different locations.

Possible extensions

More realism, at a cost of greater complexity, could be obtained by more detailed estimates of road travel times, either based upon historical data or road distances, and making allowance for the likely scenario of ground transport to a local hospital with subsequent interhospital transfer by air. In order to improve the model further, we would plan to incorporate weather data in the generation of trauma events to avoid the assumption of independence between the occurrence of an injury and the ability of the helicopter to fly. It may be possible to determine the geographic and time distribution only of the most serious injuries, and not simply to assume that they follow the same distribution of all "major trauma" events. Some of the constant times used could be modeled from estimates as triangular distributions or based upon data collected as the system is actually put into use. Although experimentation with a model may be time-consuming, the use of helicopters greatly increases the cost and risk of emergency transportation and it may be difficult to demonstrate a clear net benefit, particularly in areas of low population density [15]. Therefore, we believe the use of sufficiently detailed computer simulation holds considerable promise for helping decisions about helicopter utilization in rural trauma systems.

Acknowledgement

Although the authors are responsible for any errors in this manuscript, we are indebted to Dr. Muhammad El-Taha at the University of Southern Maine for instruction in simulation methodology and for a critical review of our work.

References

[1]. M.O. Ball, F.L. Lin. A reliability model applied to emergency service vehicle location. Operations Research 41:18-36, 1993

[2]. E.D. Hill III, J.L. Hill, L.M. Jacobs. Planning for emergency ambulance service systems. J Emerg Med 1:331-338, 1984

[3]. A.W. Neebe. A procedure for locating emergency-service facilities for all possible response distances. J Opl Res Soc 39:743-748, 1988

[4]. T.D. Valenzuela, J. Goldberg, K.T. Keeley, E.A. Criss. Computer modeling of emergency medical system performance. Ann Emerg Med 19:898-901, 1990

[5]. C.R. White, J.B. Best, C.K. Sage. Simulation of emergency medical service scheduling. Hosp Topics 70:34-37, 1992

[6]. Z. Zhu, M.A. McKnew, J. Lee. Modeling time-varied arrival rates: An application issue in queuing systems. Simulation 62:146-154, 1994

[7]. L.J. Schuman, H. Wolfe, M.J. Gunter. Ruralsim: The design and implementation of a rural EMS simulator. J Soc Health Syst 3:54-71, 1992

[8]. H.D. Schwetman. CSIM User's Guide, Revision 2. Austin, TX: Microelectronics and Computer Technology Corp., 1991

[9]. Maine Atlas and Gazetteer. Freeport, Maine: DeLorme Mapping Co., 1987

[10]. D.E. Clark. Development of a statewide trauma registry using multiple linked sources of data. Proc Annu Symp Comput Appl Med Care 17:654-658, 1993

[11]. A.R. Macione, D.E. Wilcox. Utilization prediction for helicopter emergency medical services. Ann Emerg Med 16:391-398, 1987

[12]. K.J. Rhee, R.E. Burney, J.R. Mackenzie, J. Flora. Predicting the utilization of helicopter emergency medical services: An approach based on need. Ann Emerg Med 13:916-923, 1984

[13]. A.M. Law, W.D. Kelton. Simulation Modeling and Analysis. New York: McGraw-Hill, 1991

[14]. E.J. Dudewicz, S.R. Dalal. Allocation of observations in ranking and selection with unequal variances. Sankhya B37:28-78, 1975, cited in [13]

[15]. J.P. Nicholl, N.R. Beeby, J.E. Brazier. A comparison of the costs and performance of an emergency helicopter and land ambulances in a rural area. Injury 25:145-153, 1994

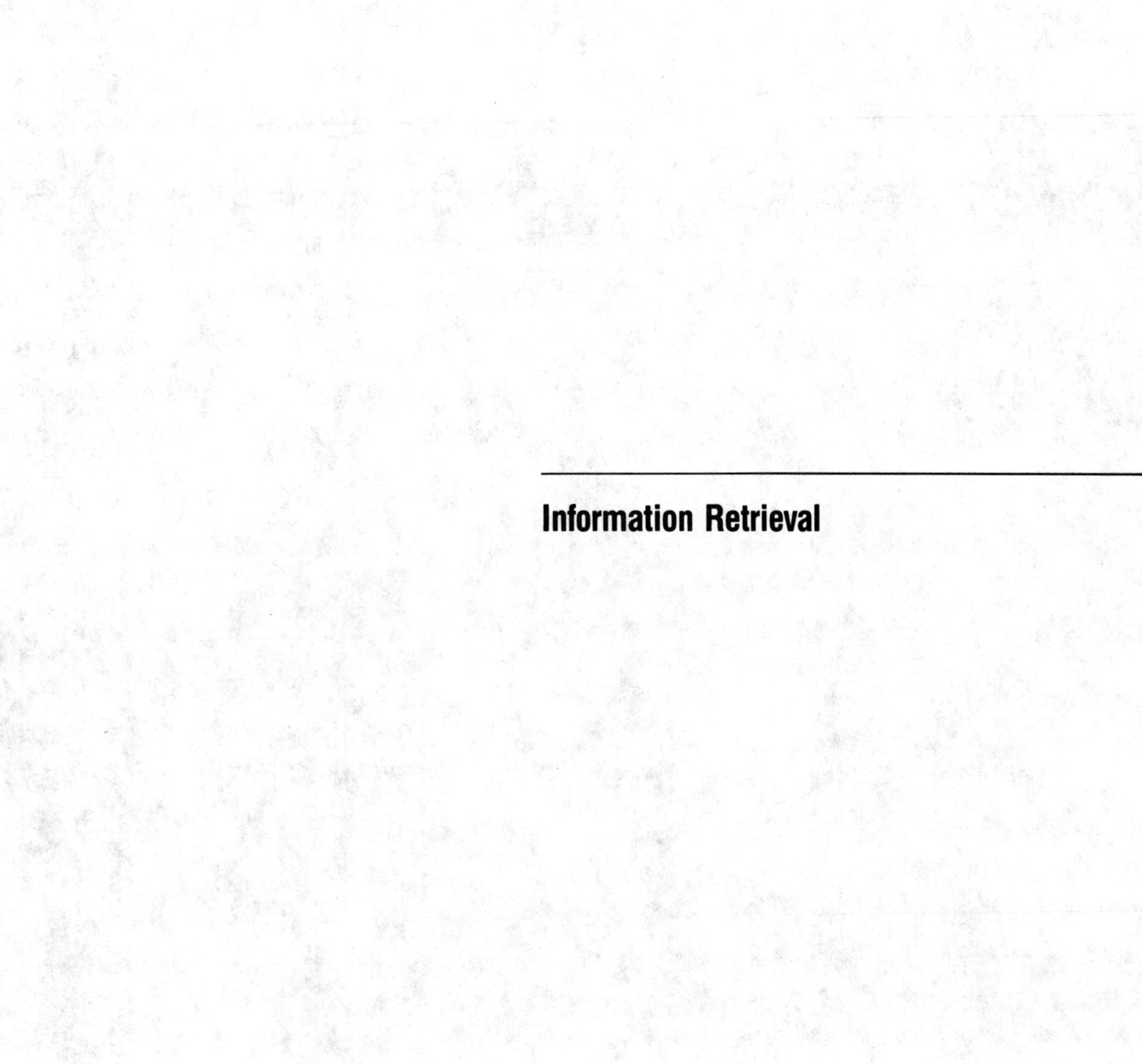

Information Retrieval

Towards New Measures of Information Retrieval Evaluation

William R. Hersh, M.D.
Diane L. Elliot, M.D.
David H. Hickam, M.D., M.P.H.
Stephanie L. Wolf
Oregon Health Sciences University, Portland, OR

Anna Molnar
Christine Leichtenstien
University of Ulm, Ulm, Germany

All of the methods currently used to assess information retrieval (IR) systems have limitations in their ability to measure how well users are able to acquire information. We utilized a new approach to assessing information obtained, based on a short-answer test given to senior medical students. Students took the ten-question test and then searched one of two IR systems on the five questions for which they were least certain of their answer Our results showed that pre-searching scores on the test were low but that searching yielded a high proportion of answers with both systems. These methods are able to measure information obtained, and will be used in subsequent studies to assess differences among IR systems.

INTRODUCTION

As information retrieval (IR) systems proliferate, it is necessary to assess their usefulness to clinicians. The most common approach for evaluating IR systems has been to measure usage frequency and/or user satisfaction. While usage frequency is easy to measure, it provides no insight into why the system was used or how successful the user was in finding information. Likewise, user satisfaction does not elucidate how users interact with IR systems and usually has not indicated user perceptions of the system's cost-effectiveness. Indeed, it has been shown that over a third of clinician users stopped using Grateful Med during a several-year period [1], and that usage dropped by two-thirds when access fees were imposed [2].

The next level of retrieval evaluation has been to measure users' success at retrieving relevant documents using indices such as recall and precision. While these indices provide a starting point at determining how much useful information is obtained from an IR system, they inherently are based on judgments of the relevance of documents to users' queries. Yet relevance is difficult to measure. Not only is interobserver agreement in relevance judgments low [3, 4, 5], but judgments of relevance are influenced by factors such as document order and expertise of the judge [6, 7].

Even if relevance judgments were valid, there are other problems with using recall and precision as measures of information retrieval [8]. There is the practical question about the definition of a retrieved document. We have seen users in previous studies who started out with a poor search, retrieving a large number of nonrelevant documents, but later refining the search to retrieve many relevant documents. In some cases, the poor search was just due to a typing error. Yet despite the ultimate success of the search, the recall and precision values were poor.

In the case of recall, the user's retrieval of more documents does not necessarily correlate with better searching success, as there is a great deal of redundancy in the medical literature. A related problem arises in the context of assessing differences between IR systems. In particular, how well do recall and precision actually represent "performance" of an IR system? Should the proportion of relevant documents obtained in the collection (recall) or search (precision) be the "gold standard" for performance? Knowing the quantity of relevant articles tells us nothing of the quality. It fails to indicate whether the information need that prompted the search was satisfied. Furthermore, when comparing two systems, while we may be able to show statistical significance between the results (with a t-test or some other appropriate statistical measure), we have no idea what constitutes a clinically significant difference.

To explore the feasibility of an alternative method to evaluate how well IR systems help users meet their information needs, we utilized an alternative approach, adapting methods previously used to evaluate a hypertext statistical textbook [9], a historical encyclopedia [10], and a series of biomedical factual databases [11]. The goal of adopting this approach was to assess how well users answered clinical questions with an IR system. The purpose of this study was to determine whether this method could measure information acquisition and thus be used as a method to determine the effectiveness of user interaction with the system.

0195-4210/94/$5.00 © 1994 AMIA, Inc.

METHODS

For this study we used two IR programs developed at Oregon Health Sciences University (OHSU). The first of these was SWORD, which features a natural language searching interface with relevance ranking. With SWORD, the user enters a free-text query and retrieved documents are ranked based on the "similarity" of their words to those in the query [12]. The second program was BOOLEAN, which utilizes a Boolean interface modeled after the Grateful Med system, where the words within each line are connected by logical OR, followed by the connection of each line with logical AND [5]. Both programs log every interaction with the user, including submitting a query, selecting a document to view, and browsing other documents. The database searched by both programs was an electronic version of the textbook, *Scientific American Medicine* [13], divided into over 6,600 "documents" based upon the hierarchical structure of the print version.

To measure information acquisition, we developed a ten-question short-answer test at the senior medical student level of difficulty (Table 1). The test questions were designed to have specific answers in the database, so that we had at least one document that provided the "answer" to each question. The test was given before and after searching, with the measurements of difference assessed by correctness of answers as well as changes in certainty of the answer.

All medical students from the senior class at Oregon Health Sciences University were sent a letter asking them to participate, of which 13 volunteered. Each student completed a brief questionnaire asking about prior computer experience, and we also obtained each student's class rank from the OHSU Dean's office. Both factors were used to stratify randomization of students.

The subjects spent a total of two hours in the experiment. After a brief introduction explaining the purpose of the experiment, they were given one-half hour to complete the ten-question test. At the completion of the test, they designated the five questions for which they had the least certainty about their answer. After a short break, they were oriented for 15 minutes to their computer and IR system, SWORD or BOOLEAN. Students then had up to 30 minutes to search for answers to the five questions for which they had greatest uncertainty about their original answers. They were required not only to answer each question, but also to give one or more document references that supported their answer.

The searching logs captured data about each query, including number of searches, total documents retrieved and viewed, and time taken. A *query* was defined as all of the interactions in attempting to find the answer to a question. A *search* was the entering of a search statement and retrieval of matching document titles. A document was considered *retrieved* if its title was in the list of document titles displayed after a search. A document was considered *viewed* if the user displayed the full text on the screen. For each user's query, we determined the number of searches, number of documents retrieved, and number of documents viewed. In addition to total number of searches, retrieved documents, and viewed documents for each query, we also calculated the number of each of these parameters required to reach an answer document.

The tests were scored independently by two members of the study team (WRH and SLW), whose interobserver agreement was good (kappa = 0.71). To assess information acquisition, a pre-test/post-test analysis was used. A McNemar's Test was performed for each test question, using data from those subjects who answered that question on the post-test.

RESULTS

A total of 13 subjects participated, six of whom used BOOLEAN and seven of whom used SWORD. There were no significant differences between the BOOLEAN and SWORD groups in computer experience or class rank. The average number correct on the initial ten-question test was 1.2, with no statistically significant difference between groups. The average number correct for the five questions searched upon was 4.1, again with no significant differences between groups (Table 2). Because there were no differences in general user characteristics or answers between the programs, the data were then pooled to determine information acquisition. Four of the ten questions showed a statistically significant difference in information found when using a searching program, while four others had a trend towards significance (Table 3).

Table 4 compares all of the questions in terms of searches done, documents retrieved, and documents viewed for each question, both in total as well as number required to retrieve an answer document. The majority of answer documents were found on the first search, within the top ten documents retrieved, and on the first document viewed.

Table 1: Ten questions for searching - answers in *italics*

1. A 60-year-old man from a poor socioeconomic environment is admitted with an acute illness characterized by mental disturbances, a sixth nerve palsy, and ataxia of gait. What specific emergency treatment is needed? *Thiamine.*
2. What percent of patients with Type II diabetes respond to oral hypoglycemic agents as their initial drug treatment? *60-70%.*
3. Mr. Rogers is seen in the Bend, OR Emergency Room. He states that he was bitten by a 'spider.' He is relatively certain that it was a black widow. What are the expected initial symptoms of the bite? *Muscular pain and rigidity.*
4. What organism is most commonly found in anaerobic osteomyelitis? *Bacteroides.*
5. You are seeing a diabetic man with severe gastropariesis. He has not improved on oral metoclopramide (Reglan) and was sent to you for additional treatment. What would you recommend? *Suppository form of metoclopramide.*
6. What electrocardiographic feature distinguishes Prinzmetal's angina from more typical angina pectoris? *ST elevation.*
7. Mrs. Towel, an 80-year-old woman on no medication, is seen for light-headedness and found to have a heart rate of 36 and third degree heart block. What is the most likely etiology of her heart block? *Lenegre's Disease* or *age-related changes in A-V conduction system.*
8. A strongly positive antibody test to which antigen is most typical of Mixed Connective Tissue Disease? *Anti-RNP antibody.*
9. What is the most common cause of sudden death among young athletes? *Hypertrophic cardiomyopathy.*
10. How is the organism which causes Rocky Mountain Spotted Fever transmitted? *Tick bite.*

Table 2: Test results for the study groups

	BOOLEAN	SWORD	Both
Number	6	7	13
Pre-Test Score (correct of 10)	1.8	1.6	1.7
Post-Test Score (correct of 5)	4.2	3.9	4.0

Table 3: Pre-Test/Post-Test results for each query

	Pre-Test		Post-Test		
Question	No. responses	% correct	No. responses	% correct	p
1	13	30.8	3	100	.08
2	13	23.1	6	83.3	.08
3	13	0	8	100	.005
4	13	23.1	9	100	.01
5	13	0	8	87.5	.008
6	13	0	12	100	.0005
7	13	0	4	25	.3
8	13	0	11	27.3	.08
9	13	15.4	1	100	.3
10	13	76.9	3	100	.08

We also performed a failure analysis of questions where the wrong answer was obtained, or where there was an unsuccessful retrieval or viewing (Table 5). Only four of the ten questions had any incorrect answers at all. The majority of these came from question 8, although almost all of those who got this question wrong retrieved the answer document, and over half viewed that document, indicating that perhaps it was a poorly worded question.

DISCUSSION

The purpose of this pilot study was to explore alternative methods of evaluating the performance of IR systems, based on ability to acquire information. Our results indicate that this approach is a viable alternative approach to measuring recall and precision, and may even be preferable, in that it indicates whether the searcher was able to use the system to find answers to questions. While this approach might not generalize to all uses of IR systems (i.e., the researcher who needed to find every relevant document on a topic), it appears to be appropriate for the specific questions that arise in the course of clinical practice [14].

One limitation of the study that was allowing subjects to choose only five questions to search. Not only did this make the statistical analysis more difficult, but it also made assessment of the adequacy of some questions difficult. In our next study, we will have users search on all questions in order to better assess the value of all questions searched by the IR system.

The next question is whether this approach will be able to allow comparison of different IR systems. To this end, we plan to compare two commercial MEDLINE systems that are used in the OHSU library, one of which features Boolean searching (*CD Plus*, CD Plus, Inc., New York, NY) and the other natural language searching (*Knowledge Finder*, Aries Systems, Inc., North Andover, MA) based upon clinical questions that were actually generated in the course of patient care during an information needs assessment study [15]. In this study, we will also compare these results with conventional recall-precision analysis.

ACKNOWLEDGEMENTS

This work was supported by Grant LM 05307 from the National Library of Medicine. The authors also thank Scientific American (New York, NY) for providing the text of *Scientific American Medicine* for this study.

REFERENCES

1. Marshall J. The continuation of end-user online searching by health professionals: Preliminary survey results. Abstracts of the Medical Library Association Annual Meeting. Detroit: Medical Library Association; 1990. Available from Medical Library Association.

2. Haynes RB, Ramsden MF, McKibbon KA, et al.: Online access to MEDLINE in clinical settings: Impact of user fees. Bulletin of the Medical Library Association. 1991; 79: 377-381.

3. Haynes RB, McKibbon KA, Walker CJ, et al.: Online access to MEDLINE in clinical settings. Annals of Internal Medicine. 1990; 112: 78-84.

4. Hersh WR, Hickam DH: A performance and failure analysis of SAPHIRE with a MEDLINE test collection. Journal of the American Medical Informatics Association. 1994; 1: 51-60.

5. Hersh WR, Hickam DH: A comparison of two methods for indexing and retrieval from a full-text medical database. Medical Decision Making. 1993; 13: 220-226.

6. Eisenberg M, Barry C: Order effects: a study of the possible influence of presentation order on user judgments of document relevance. Journal of the American Society for Information Science. 1988; 39: 293-300.

7. Schamber L, Eisenberg MB, Nilan MS: A re-examination of relevance: Toward a dynamic, situational definition. Information Processing and Management. 1990; 26: 755-776.

8. Hersh WR: Relevance and retrieval evaluation: perspectives from medicine. Journal of the American Society for Information Science. 1994; 45: 201-206.

9. Egan DE, Remde JR, Gomez LM, et al.: Formative design-evaluation of Superbook. ACM Transactions on Information Systems. 1989; 7: 30-57.

10. Mynatt BT, Leventhal LM, Instone K, et al.: Hypertext or book: which is better for answering questions? Proceedings of Computer-Human Interface 92. 1992: 19-25.

11. de Bliek R, Friedman CP, Wildemuth BM, et al.: Database access and problem solving in the basic sciences. Proceedings of the 17th Annual Symposium on Computers in Medical Care. 1993: 678-682.

12. Hersh WR, Hickam DH, Leone TJ: Word, concepts, or both: Optimal indexing units for automated information retrieval. Proceedings of the 16th Annual Symposium on Computers in Medical Care. 1992: 644-648.

13. Rubenstein R, Federman DD. "Scientific American Medicine." 1990 Scientific American. New York.

14. Gorman PN, Ash J, Helfand M, Beck JR: Assessment of information needs of primary care physicians. Proceedings of the Third Annual American Medical Informatics Association Spring Congress. 1992: 26.

15. Gorman P: Does the medical literature contain the evidence to answer the questions of primary care physicians? Preliminary findings of a study. Proceedings of the 17th Annual Symposium on Computers in Medical Care. 1993: 571-575.

Table 4: Searching results for all queries with both programs

Total searches done	
1	48
>1	17
Searches to find answer	
1st	51
After 1st	5
Not found	9
Total documents retrieved	
<=10	46
>10	19
Documents retrieved to find answer	
<=10	49
>10	7
Not found	9
Total documents viewed	
<=10	60
>10	5
Documents viewed to find answer*	
1	41
2-5	13
>6	5
Not found	6
Time per query (min.)	5.40

* There were three queries with answer documents viewed but not retrieved by searching due to answers being found by browsing through the database.

Table 5: Failure analysis

Query	Incorrect	Retrieved		Viewed	
		Yes	No	Yes	No
2	1	1	0	1	0
5	1	1	0	1	0
7	3	0	3	0	3
8	8	7	1	5	3
Total	13	9	4	7	6

Construction of a Medical Informatics Thesaurus

Nancy J. Ogg[*+], MaryEllen Sievert[*], Zong Rong Li[^], Joyce A. Mitchell[+]

[*]Dept. of Information Science, University of Missouri-Columbia
[+]Medical Informatics Group, University of Missouri-Columbia
[^]Medical Informatics Institute, Hubei Medical University, China

ABSTRACT

Medical Informatics needs a specific terminology that reflects the multi-disciplinary nature of the field and can rapidly change as the discipline evolves. Using the four primary methods of thesaurus construction, a group at the University of Missouri-Columbia is developing a thesaurus that meets these criteria and includes both user and literary warrant. The steps in construction include using existing thesauri, medical informatics literature, and the terminology of experts to produce a thesaurus arranged within a hierarchical structure.

INTRODUCTION

Medical Informatics is a constantly evolving, multi-disciplinary field which draws terminology from a variety of disciplines. When we tried to do original abstracting and indexing of medical informatics literature for the Medical Informatics Information Center at the University of Missouri-Columbia we realized a specific informatics thesaurus was needed. Several steps were taken to confirm that this need did exist and to identify its range.

First, we reviewed the history of the L Tree of MeSH[1] because it was the first vocabulary to include medical informatics terminology and is still used as a source of medical informatics terminology. We found that the current L Tree terms were not sufficient to cover the discipline because there were numerous major concepts not covered. An examination of the thesauri used in the contributing disciplines and of the medical informatics literature both confirmed our view and allowed us to develop a raw vocabulary of medical informatics terminology now in use. The resulting thesaurus will contain a manageable number of terms with an accompanying classification.

We believe that the medical informatics thesaurus we are developing more adequately covers the existing medical informatics discipline than anything currently does. It can also be quickly revised to include the rapidly evolving terminology of the discipline. The purpose of this paper is to present the steps we used to create this new thesaurus and to discuss our plans for further testing, refinement, and publication of that thesaurus.

METHODS

Our purpose in developing the thesaurus was to address both user and literary warrant in selecting terms for inclusion. User warrant means that the terms chosen for inclusion must be those which users in the field would use, while literary warrant means that the terms would be found in key documents in the literature of that discipline.

In order to achieve this goal, we looked at the four primary methods of thesaurus construction and used parts of each of them for our project. The four main methods of thesaurus construction, as identified by Lancaster[2], are to:

1. Generate the vocabulary empirically on the basis of indexing a representative set of documents;

2. Convert an existing vocabulary;

3. Extract the vocabulary from an existing, more general thesaurus or develop a specialized thesaurus within the framework of a general one;

4. Collect terms from diverse sources including glossaries, other publications, and from subject specialists.

The following discussion shows how we included facets of each of these approaches into our thesaurus construction.

Work on this project began in September 1992. A historical review of the MeSH L Tree was performed to ascertain the degree and nature of the changes made in the terminology in this source over the last thirty-three years.[3] A search of fifty titles from papers in the 1992 Symposium on Computer Applications in Medical Care (SCAMC) identified terms used in these titles that also appeared in the 1992 L Tree. Major concepts in the 1992 SCAMC for which no terms appeared in the L Tree were also identified. Examples of such concepts include Bayesian networks, knowledge bases and knowledge representation, heuristic approaches, electronic patient records, physician order entry, nursing systems and nursing informatics. These findings indicate that the L Tree would not suffice as a thesaurus for the medical informatics literature.

Because of the multi-disciplinary nature of the medical informatics field and the lack of a comprehensive thesaurus, seven thesauri from other fields were examined for relevant terminology for indexing medical informatics articles. The first step in the thesaurus construction was to compare the terminology in each of these thesauri to see which terms were used by all, some or only one of them. The thesauri used and the fields represented include:

Engineering field:

Engineering Information Thesaurus (EI)[4]
INSPEC Thesaurus[5]

Education/psychology field:

Thesaurus of ERIC Descriptors[6]
Thesaurus of Psychological Index Terms[7]

Medical field:

Medical Subject Headings (MeSH)[8]

Computer field:

Computer Select® Glossary of Terms[9]

Informatics field:

In-house list of indexing terms used at the Medical Informatics Information Center at the University of Missouri-Columbia.

Terms from each thesaurus were assigned a weight according to their importance in the informatics field. These weights were assigned to allow us to determine which terms were most significant to the literature. A term appearing in both the medical and the engineering terminology should be considered more important than a term carried only in the psychology terminology. Thesauri from the fields of engineering (EI and INSPEC) and medicine (MeSH) received a weight of two. The rest were assigned weights of one. The total weight for a particular term was determined by how many and which thesauri included the term.

The second step was to study the medical informatics literature to determine what terminology those who work in the field use. The literature examined came from journals and proceedings. The following journals were considered key medical informatics journals:

1. "Computer Applications in the Biosciences"

2. "Computers and Biomedical Research"

3. "Computers in Nursing"

4. "MD-Computing"

5. "Medical Informatics".

"JAMIA" was not in existence when this work was done, having published its first issue in January 1994. Also included were two major conference proceedings for the medical informatics field, SCAMC and MEDINFO.

From a total population of 1676 articles, 271 randomly selected abstracts were reviewed, a 30 percent sample. The entire sample was reviewed by two members of the project team to determine the key words used in the abstracts. As a further check, two senior members of the project team reviewed 30 percent of the sample again. A weight of one was given to each term selected by the first team and a weight of two to each term selected by the second team because the members of the second team have more expertise in determining which terms are significant. These weights were assigned so that, once the entire raw vocabulary had been assembled, decisions could be made on what terms to eliminate based on the number of occurrences of the term and the number of times it was selected by each reviewer.

The key terms from each abstract were then collected and entered into a database and the editing process began. The initial editing consisted of eliminating singular vs plural, lexical variants, and useless terms. The decision was made to prefer the plural over the singular form of terms with some exceptions for singular words that are considered a preferred over their plural form; for example, classification was preferred over classifications and terminology over terminologies. In determining the preferred term for lexical variants the noun was preferred over the verb form and either of these was preferred over the adjective form again with some exceptions for preferred usage. The literature and the weights that had been assigned throughout the development of the raw vocabulary assisted us in determining the preferred variant of a term. A number of terms were eliminated because they were useless terms; for example, megabytes or house officer care or interactive nature. These terms carried weights of one or two which meant they had only been chosen from one article by one or both of the members of team one and upon examination by the senior team members were determined to be meaningless terms for the vocabulary. Also, the term for an action was preferred to the term for the person performing the action; for example, education was preferred over educators and development over developers. We also eliminated any hyphenated terms in favor of the non-hyphenated terms as in computer-assisted instruction or CD-ROM. Phrases with extra unnecessary terms were eliminated in favor of the shortest version applicable. Examples of this include the exclusion of automatic indexing method and automatic indexing program in preference to automatic indexing and the exclusion of diagnostic decision support system and diagnostic decision support program in preference to diagnostic decision support. From an original 5759 terms these edits reduced the terms to 5462. Weights were added together when a term was combined with another to produce a total reviewer weight.

The third step consisted of a review of glossaries from experts in the field to see what terms they used in their texts. Blois[10], Covvey[11], Shortliffe[12] and Barnett[13] were used as experts for this section. The glossaries were reviewed to ascertain which terms were already included in the raw vocabulary. Terms not already included were added to the raw vocabulary. A weight of two was assigned to terms in the Barnett and Shortliffe glossaries because they are more recent publications. A weight of one was assigned to the Blois and Covvey terms. Therefore, a new term appearing in all four glossaries would carry a weight of six.

Finally, the terms identified in each of the first three steps were compared to one another to see which ones were present in which sources. For those terms that existed in both the literature and the thesauri, the weights for each source were included in the database. There were some terms found only in the thesauri. If the thesauri weight of these terms was four or above, they were included in the raw vocabulary list. The terms found only in the expert glossaries were added to the raw vocabulary as bolded entries so that they would stand out when terms were reviewed. They were reviewed for what sources they belonged to as well as their weight. This insured that they would not be eliminated simply because they had a low weight.

RESULTS

When all the terms had been identified, the process of refining the raw vocabulary began. The aim was to reduce the original 5462 terms to a manageable size which Batty defines as "as small as possible but includes everything with a good size being approximately 2000 terms."[14] First, we closely examined the terms with a literature weight of 1 or 2 because that weight meant the term was selected by only one or two reviewers and from only one article. There were 3368 terms in this category. We eliminated 1738 terms, or 52%, of them in this step which left 3724 terms in the vocabulary.

The next step in the refinement process was to create a group of categories and begin to create the hierarchical structure for the classification. The main concepts then were:

1. Business
2. Computer and Data Processing
3. Education
4. Engineering
5. Language/Library
6. Legal
7. Mathematics
8. Nursing
9. Dentistry
10. Veterinary Medicine

All terms were sorted into one of these categories. Terms that did not fit were placed in a separate category for further review. Many of the latter terms were eliminated from the vocabulary as unimportant. Examples of terms eliminated include crime, shared data, and system environment. The major categories were refined in the second step of this process to include:

1. Business
2. Computer and Data Processing with mathematics and engineering as sub-categories
3. Education
4. Health Care Informatics which includes the health category
5. Language/Library

The categories of legal, nursing, dentistry and veterinary medicine were absorbed into the other categories.

Once the terms were divided into categories, we began to establish a hierarchy of terms within each category. At this point, preferred terms were chosen for concepts which had several synonyms. Part of this final refinement was to decide how acronyms and geographic terms were to be handled. Not all acronyms were retained in the vocabulary. For those we did retain, it was decided to put the acronym in parentheses behind its spelled out version wherever it appeared in the thesaurus. Examples of this would be Computer Assisted Instruction (CAI) or Integrated Advanced Information Management Systems (IAIMS). For geographic names users of the thesaurus will be referred to the Z Tree of MeSH which contains a comprehensive listing of geographical place names.[15] Users will also be referred to the MeSH Subject Headings for specific medical terms as the purpose of this project was not to recreate the entire medical vocabulary but only to include terms that specifically addressed informatics and its related fields. The decision to handle acronyms, geographic names, and specific medical terms in this manner eliminated 1378 terms which gave us a total of 2315 terms remaining in the vocabulary.

When completed, our medical informatics thesaurus will contain a manageable number of terms, arranged within a hierarchical structure within the final five categories. The thesaurus will then be tested against the 1994 <u>SCAMC</u> titles to see if it contains the necessary terms to cover the concepts in the document. We also plan to test the document by sending it to experts in the field for their review, use and comments. Finally, we will publish the thesaurus in both a print and an electronic version.

DISCUSSION

The first formal work in the terminology of medical informatics was at NLM. They began to cover medical informatics terminology in a minimal way in their first L Tree developed in 1960. Major revisions to this L Tree in 1963, 1965, 1966, 1975, and 1987 have added new terms, eliminated terms and changed the hierarchical relationship of terms.

Rada and others[16] helped in this revision process in 1986 when they developed a medical informatics thesaurus. "It consisted of terms developed by an automatic merging of the thesaurus used by the "Association of Computing Machinery" and the Information Sciences component of the "Medical Subject Headings" from the National Library of Medicine (NLM). The terminology was then pruned by eliminating terms not related to those in the MEDINFO keyword list or not in the medical informatics literature." The terminology from this thesaurus was incorporated into NLM's 1987 version of the L Tree.

Currently Rada is working with the Committee for European Normalization (CEN) under the International Medical Informatics Association (IMIA). This work parallels our project. [17],[18] They have produced a new 200 word thesaurus.

Rada's terminology still leaves a wide area of informatics unrepresented since it is focused on the creation of a framework for standards development. The Rada et. al. work and this project also differ in methodology of thesaurus construction and size of the vocabulary.

Rada uses a computerized technique to extract possible terms. This method achieves literary warrant but makes little formal effort to ensure user warrant. He has published the list and requested comments from members of the informatics community. Our methods of construction were more extensive and varied and achieve both user and literary warrant. As shown, our approach uses literature review, thesauri review, review of expert glossaries, and comparisons of all sources for similarity to achieve both literary and user warrant for our terminology.

The small size of Rada's vocabulary (200) necessarily would force users to use broad terms for some concepts. With a larger thesaurus of 2000 or more terms the user is more likely to be able to achieve an acceptable level of specificity.

CONCLUSION

Our research first identified a need for a new medical informatics thesaurus. Then, using existing thesauri, medical informatics literature, and the terminology of experts in the field to identify appropriate concepts and terms, we are creating a new thesaurus to cover the discipline. Continued refinement will be accomplished by testing the thesaurus against the 1994 SCAMC titles and by asking experts in the field to use and review the thesaurus and give us feedback. The thesaurus will be published in both a print and an electronic format so that it is readily available for use by everyone in the field. We plan to support continuous revision of the thesaurus to keep it current with the ever expanding field of medical informatics.

References

1. Li Z, Ogg N, Sievert M, and Mitchell J. "On the Growth and Trimming of the L Trees of MeSH." Symposium on Computer Applications in Medical Care. 1993: 892.

2. Lancaster FW. Vocabulary Control for Information Retrieval. lst ed. Arlington, VA: Information Resources Press, 1972: 27.

3. Li Z, et al, 892.

4. Milstead JL. ed. Engineering Information Thesaurus. 1st ed. Hoboken, NJ: Engineering Information Inc, 1992.

5. Institution of Electrical Engineers. INSPEC Thesaurus. Old Woking, Surrey, Eng: Unwin Brothers Limited, 1991.

6. Houston JE. ed. Thesaurus of ERIC Descriptors. 12th ed. Phoenix, AZ: ORYX Press, 1990.

7. Walker A. Jr. ed. Thesaurus of Psychological Index Terms. 6th ed. Arlington, VA: American Psychological Association, 1991.

8. National Library of Medicine. Medical Subject Headings. Annotated Alphabetic List. Bethesda, MD: Medical Subject Headings Section, Library Operations, National Library of Medicine, 1992.

9. Lotus Development Corporation and Ziff Communications Company. Computer Select® Glossary of Terms. 5th ed. New York, NY: Ziff Communications Company, 1992.

10. Blois MS. Information and Medicine: The Nature of Medical Descriptions. Berkeley: University of California Press, 1984: 298 p.

11. Covvey HD, McAllister NH. Computers in the Practice of Medicine. Vol. I-Introduction to Computing Concepts. Reading, MA: Addison-Wesley, 1980: 266 p.

12. Shortliffe EH, Perreault LE, eds. Medical Informatics: Computer Applications in Health Care. Reading, MA: Addison-Wesley, 1990: 715 p.

13. Barnett GO. "Core Topics in Medical Informatics." Personal Correspondence, 1992.

14. Batty CD. Thesaurus Construction Workshop. 55th Annual Meeting of the American Society for Information Science (ASIS). Oct. 22, 1992; Pittsburgh, PA.

15. National Library of Medicine. Medical Subject Headings. Tree Structures. Bethesda, MD: Medical Subject Headings Section, Library Operations, National Library of Medicine, 1960-1992.

16. Rada R, Calhoun F, Mili E, Singer SJ, Blum B, and Orthnerr H. "A medical informatics thesaurus." MEDINFO '86. Washington, DC. Amsterdam: North-Holland, 1986: 1164-1172.

17. Rada R, Ghaoui C, Russell J, and Taylor M. "Approaches to the construction of a medical informatics glossary and thesaurus." Medical Informatics. 18(1). 1993: 69-78.

18. Rada R. "Vocabulary." SigBio. 14(1). Jan. 1994: 5-16.

Quantitative Comparison of Pre-explosions and Subheadings with Methodologic Search Terms in MEDLINE

NL Wilczynski, CJ Walker, KA McKibbon, RB Haynes
Health Information Research Unit,
Dept. of Clinical Epidemiology & Biostatistics,
McMaster University, HSC, Room 3H7,
1200 Main St W, Hamilton, Ont, Canada L8N 3Z5
(905)525-9140 x22311, FAX 905-546-0401, E-MAIL WILCZYN@McMASTER.CA

ABSTRACT

Objective: To compare the retrieval characteristics of subheadings with methodologic textwords and MeSH terms in MEDLINE for identifying sound clinical studies on the etiology, prognosis, diagnosis, prevention and treatment of disorders in general adult medicine.
Design: Analytic survey of the information retrieval properties of methodologic textwords, single methodologic MeSH terms, pre-explosions and subheadings selected to detect studies meeting basic methodologic criteria for direct clinical use in general adult medicine.
Measures: The sensitivity, specificity, and precision of search terms were determined by comparing the citations retrieved by the search strategies in MEDLINE with that of a manual review (the gold standard) of all articles in 10 internal and general medicine journals for 1986 and 1991.
Results: For treatment and diagnosis in 1991, and treatment, diagnosis, and etiology in 1986, pre-explosions yielded the highest sensitivity, with typical absolute increases exceeding 15%. For etiology and prognosis in 1991, and prognosis in 1986, textwords or MeSH terms yielded the highest sensitivity. In all cases the increase in sensitivity was coupled with a loss in specificity and precision.
Conclusions: Compared with searching with single methodologic textwords and subject headings, the detection of sound clinical studies on the diagnosis and treatment of disorders in general adult medicine was consistently enhanced by searching with pre-explosions, but at a price of decreased specificity and precision.

INTRODUCTION

It is important for clinical end users of MEDLINE to be able to retrieve articles that are both scientifically sound and directly relevant to clinical practice. MEDLINE, however, is a general purpose biomedical research literature database, with only a small proportion of articles reporting evidence that can be directly applied in clinical practice. A potential method for improving the detection of studies of high quality for clinical practice is the use of "methodologic search filters" [1]. A methodologic search filter is a search term or terms (such as 'random allocation' for sound studies of medical intervention) that select studies that are at the most advanced stages of testing for clinical application. The retrieval performance, however, of such terms on search recall and precision has not been fully tested. The purpose of this study was to test individual methodologic Medical Subject Headings (MeSH) terms and textwords in common use, and permutations and combinations of these MeSH terms and textwords for identifying studies meeting basic methodologic criteria on the etiology, prognosis, diagnosis, prevention and treatment of disorders in general adult medicine. In this paper, the information retrieval properties of subheadings are compared with textwords and MeSH terms. The retrieval properties of individual textwords and MeSH terms were reported previously [2]. Our results are of most interest to clinicians doing their own searches for clinically relevant and valid studies and for librarians involved in assisting clinicians to construct their own searches.

METHODS

The study compared the retrieval performance of methodologic search terms, pre-explosions, and subheadings in MEDLINE with a manual review of each article for each issue of 10 internal and general medicine journals for the 2 years 1986 and 1991. To evaluate MEDLINE strategies designed to retrieve studies meeting basic methodologic criteria for clinical practice, terms related to research design features were run as search strategies and treated as "diagnostic tests" for sound studies as determined by the manual review of the literature, treated as the "gold standard". Borrowing from the concepts of diagnostic test evaluation and library science, the sensitivity, specificity, and precision of MEDLINE searches were determined. The sensitivity of the MEDLINE search strategies was calculated as the proportion of correctly detected citations with relevant content and sound study methods among all relevant citations as defined by the manual review of the literature. This is equivalent to the library term 'recall'. Specificity was the proportion of irrelevant, unsound studies excluded by the search strategy. This differs from precision which is the proportion of all articles retrieved by a search strategy that are sound and relevant.

Manual Review of the Literature

For the years 1986 and 1991, 3 research assistants hand searched 10 journals, the same 10 in each year, for studies meeting methodologic criteria on the etiology, prognosis, diagnosis, prevention and treatment of human adult disease. The 10 journals searched were *American Journal of Medicine, Annals of Internal Medicine, Archives of Internal Medicine, BMJ (British Medical Journal* in 1986*), Circulation, Diabetes Care, Journal of Internal Medicine (Acta Medica Scandinavica* in 1986*), Journal of the American Medical Association, The Lancet,* and *New England Journal of Medicine*, including supplements. These journals were selected on the basis of impact factors and immediacy indexes [3], and to provide a broad range of publications, including both internal and general medical journals and both American and European authors.

Articles were classified for 'format', 'interest', 'purpose' and 'methodologic rigor'. 'Format' categories included 'original study', 'review', 'general article', 'conference report', 'decision analysis', and 'case report'. Articles with more than one format were classified for all that applied. An 'original study' was defined as any full text article in which the investigators had made first-hand observations. A 'review' was any full text article that was bannered review, had review in the title or in a section heading, or indicated in the text that the intention was to review or summarize the literature on a topic. A 'general article' was a general or philosophical discussion of a topic without original first-hand observation or a statement that the purpose was to review or appraise a body of knowledge, including unbannered news items, unbannered editorials, position and opinion papers, musings and psychosocial observations. A 'conference report' was defined as such by the journal but was reclassified by us as an original or review article when meeting those criteria. A 'decision analysis' was defined as the breaking down of the management of patients into component parts, defining routes of management and consequences of management based on alternatives, for the purpose of defining optimal methods of management. A 'case report' was defined as an original study involving less than 10 subjects. Items excluded from classification included bannered letters to the editor, book reviews, announcements, policy watch, editorials, commentaries, brief clinical observations, correspondence, news, obituaries, postgraduate and continuing education forums, and notices.

To be considered of 'interest' to the medical care of human adults the study had to be concerned with the understanding and management of clinical problems with clinical endpoints and recommendations for applications in human subjects, at least 50% of whom were ≥ 18 years of age at study entry. All format categories were classified for interest.

Articles classified as original studies, reviews, or case reports and of interest were classified for 'purpose'. Articles could have more than one purpose and were classified for all that applied. Articles were classified as 'etiology' when the content pertained directly to causation of a disease or condition; as 'prognosis' when the content pertained directly to the prediction of the clinical course or the natural history of a disease with the disease existing at the beginning of the study; as 'diagnosis' when the content pertained directly to the evaluation of a disease process, usually through comparing methods of arriving at a diagnosis; as 'treatment or prevention' when the content pertained directly to therapy, prevention or rehabilitation; and as 'something else' when the purpose of the study was something other than the above.

Studies in each purpose category were evaluated for 'methodologic rigor' and were assessed to determine if they met one key methodologic criterion specific to their purpose as shown in Table 1. These criteria were based on critical appraisal criteria for applied research [4] but were set at a minimal level in recognition that few published studies meet the full set of criteria for unbiased clinical evaluation.

Table 1. Key methodologic criteria by purpose of study

Purpose	Key methodologic criterion
Etiology	Formal control group: random or quasi-random allocation of participants to treatment and control groups; or the study was a non-randomized, concurrent control trial, a cohort analytic study with matching or statistical adjustment to create comparable groups, or a case-control study
Prognosis	A cohort of subjects all having the disease in question at baseline without the outcome of interest
Diagnosis	Provision of sufficient data to calculate the sensitivity and specificity of the test or likelihood ratios based on subjects who had all been tested on both the test and diagnostic standard
Treatment	Random or quasi-random allocation of participants to treatment and control groups
Review	Reproducible description of the methods for conducting the review

Inter-rater reliability was assessed for the classification of articles for format, interest, purpose and methods. In all cases the degree of agreement beyond chance was assessed by the kappa statistic and was greater than 0.80.

The sample size required to detect a 20% improvement in sensitivity for the comparison of one MEDLINE search strategy with another on the same topic was 73 methodologically sound studies in each of the purpose categories for each of the years 1986 and 1991 (type 1 error of 5%, one-sided, and a type 2 error rate of 20%).

Collecting Search Terms

To construct a comprehensive set of search terms, we began a list of methodologic subject headings and textwords and then sought input from clinicians and librarians in the United States and Canada through interviews of known searchers; requests on several electronic bulletin boards and in national publications, meetings and conferences; and requests to the National Library of Medicine and Canada Institute for Scientific and Technical Information. Individuals were asked what terms or phrases they used when searching for studies of etiology, prognosis, diagnosis, prevention and treatment and related review articles. Terms could be from MeSH, including publication types, check tags, pre-explosions (subheading pre-explosion groups together and retrieves subheadings that relate to the particular clinical category being studied; e.g. the subheading pre-explosion therapeutic use includes the subheadings administration & dosage, adverse effects, contraindication, and poisoning in addition to the subheading therapeutic use) and subheadings, or textwords denoting applied research methodology in titles and abstracts of articles. The list, excluding inaccurate terms, appears in the Appendix. Some of the terms and phrases were different for the 2 years as some of the corresponding terms changed definitions and some terms retrieved 0 citations for the 10 journals in 1986 and/or 1991.

DATA COLLECTION

Manual ratings of articles in the 10 journals for 1986 and 1991 were recorded on data collection forms, and the bibliographic information, including the 8-digit unique identifier, for the articles in those journals was captured from MEDLINE. Each journal title was searched in MEDLINE for 1986 and 1991 and the publication types 'editorial,' 'comment,' 'letter' and 'news' were eliminated from the search using the boolean 'AND NOT' operator.

The MeSH terms and textwords to be tested were searched in MEDLINE for 1986 and 1991 for the 10 journals. The unique identifiers were captured and then linked with the manual review data.

TESTING STRATEGIES

All methods terms were tested, both individually and in combination, and the sensitivity, specificity, and precision was calculated. For 1991 there were 27 etiology terms, 28 prognosis terms, 25 diagnosis terms, and 26 treatment terms. For 1986 there were 20 etiology terms, 22 prognosis terms, 25 diagnosis terms, and 20 treatment terms (see Appendix).

RESULTS

The results of the manual review of the journals was previously reported [2]. Briefly, the total number of original, review and case report articles in 1991 was 3495, and in 1986 was 3682. Less than half of the studies cited met basic criteria for scientific merit for clinical application.

For 1991, the sensitivity, specificity, and precision of the single best terms and subheadings are presented in Table 2. The corresponding figures for 1986 are presented in Table 3.

Table 2. Sensitivity, specificity and precision for single best terms and subheadings in 1991

Category	Search strategy	Sensitivity	Specificity	Precision
1991				
Etiology	Risk (tw) (best single term)	0.67	0.79	0.15
	Etiology& (px)	0.63	0.56	0.07
	Etiology (sh)	0.40	0.78	0.09
Prognosis	Exp Cohort Studies (best single term)	0.60	0.80	0.11
	Mortality (sh)	0.53	0.93	0.20
Diagnosis	Sensitivity (tw) (best single term)	0.57	0.97	0.33
	Diagnosis& (px)	0.80	0.77	0.09
	Diagnosis (sh)	0.59	0.88	0.13
	Diagnostic use (sh)	0.26	0.96	0.18
Treatment	Clinical Trial (pt) (best single term)	0.93	0.92	0.49
	Therapy& (px)	0.95	0.62	0.15
	Therapeutic Use& (px)	0.89	0.70	0.18
	Therapeutic Use (sh)	0.70	0.84	0.24
	Drug Therapy (sh)	0.63	0.84	0.23
	Prevention & Control (sh)	0.26	0.91	0.16
	Therapy (sh)	0.14	0.90	0.08

For sensitivity, pre-explosions out-performed methodologic textwords and MeSH terms in 5 out of 8 instances. For treatment in 1991 and 1986 the single terms yielding the highest sensitivity, 'Clinical Trial (pt)' (93%) and 'Random: (tw)' (82%), were out-performed by 'Therapy& (px)' (95% for 1991 and 91% for 1986). For diagnosis in 1991 and 1986 the term yielding the highest sensitivity 'Sensitivity (tw)' (57% in 1991 and 43% in 1986) was out-performed by 'Diagnosis& (px)' (80% in 1991 and 79% in 1986). For etiology in 1986 the best single term 'Risk (tw)' (61%) was out-performed by 'Etiology& (px)' (68%). In all cases, however, use of the pre-explosions resulted in a loss in specificity with a corresponding loss in precision. For example, the 2% gain in sensitivity achieved when searching with 'Therapy& (px)' rather than 'Clinical Trial (pt)' in 1991 was coupled with a drop in specificity from 92% to 62% and a drop in precision from 49% to 15%.

Table 3. Sensitivity, specificity and precision for single best term and subheadings in 1986

Category	Search strategy	Sensitivity	Specificity	Precision
		1986		
Etiology	Risk (tw) (best single term)	0.61	0.89	0.16
	Etiology& (px)	0.68	0.53	0.05
	Etiology (sh)	0.36	0.77	0.06
Prognosis	Prognos: (tw) (best single term)	0.56	0.97	0.29
	Mortality (sh)	0.44	0.95	0.18
Diagnosis	Sensitivity (tw) (best single term)	0.43	0.98	0.30
	Diagnosis& (px)	0.79	0.74	0.06
	Diagnosis (sh)	0.62	0.89	0.09
	Diagnostic use (sh)	0.16	0.96	0.10
Treatment	Random: (tw) (best single term)	0.82	0.95	0.53
	Therapy& (px)	0.91	0.62	0.13
	Therapeutic Use& (px)	0.83	0.64	0.13
	Drug Therapy (sh)	0.66	0.81	0.19
	Therapeutic Use (sh)	0.63	0.81	0.18
	Prevention & Control (sh)	0.16	0.94	0.12
	Therapy (sh)	0.13	0.90	0.07

DISCUSSION

Our findings show that in most instances, pre-explosions can achieve higher sensitivity for detecting sound clinical studies in MEDLINE than single methodologic textwords, subject headings, or subheadings but at the cost of lower specificity and precision. These results were not found for prognosis and were inconsistent for etiology, suggesting that improvements in indexing are needed here.

It is worth noting that we had a pre-screening step in the development of our search strategies. When searching for each journal title in MEDLINE the publication types 'editorial', 'comment', 'letter', and 'news' were excluded from the search using the boolean 'AND NOT' operator. This pre-screening step would have no effect on the sensitivity calculated for the combinations of terms as studies meeting the key methodologic criterion were defined by the manual review of the literature. This step would, however, result in improvements of specificity and precision. Thus, searchers would be advised to include this pre-screening step if maintaining similar levels of specificity and precision are of concern.

The search strategies presented here can aid searchers, particularly clinicians who are inexperienced in constructing complex searches, to retrieve studies that meet at least one major criterion for scientific merit for applied health care research while filtering out studies with weaker designs. Such filters are bound to retrieve 'false positive' articles and miss others that should be retrieved. Retrieved articles must be further evaluated by the user to determine their methodologic soundness and clinical applicability. 'False negative' articles can only be retrieved by hand searching journals or other labor-intensive means.

Other possible quality filters such as ordering journals by impact factors and citations exist but we do not know how these methods compare with our search filters. However, even among the best journals only a small proportion of articles met the quality criteria we used.

One limitation of this study was that only priority journals were included in the search. Also, only the abstracts and titles of citations could be searched for textword inclusion. However, one of the strengths of this study was the highly reproducible classification of articles in the manual hand searches which served as the gold standard.

For most research purposes, we recommend that the search term with the highest sensitivity be used in the MEDLINE search so that key articles will not be missed. In back file searches the most appropriate term may differ and the search should be modified appropriately. For clinical searches, higher precision may be desirable especially if there is redundance in the literature being retrieved.

Future research will have to address how these search terms perform when they are combined in all possible permutations and combinations of MeSH terms and textwords.

Appendix. Complete List of Search Terms

Notes: Terms with 0 citations retrieved in 1986 are marked with *; terms with 0 citations retrieved in 1991 are marked with †; terms with < 10% sensitivity in 1991 are marked with ‡; terms with < 10% sensitivity in 1986 are marked with §; truncation is noted by :; the & indicates a subheading pre-explosion.

Etiology

MeSH terms: exp case control studies§; case control studies*; retrospective studies‡§; exp cohort studies; cohort studies*; exp longitudinal studies; longitudinal studies‡§; follow-up studies§; prospective studies; cross-sectional studies‡§; exp causality*; causality*; risk factors*; exp risk; risk‡; logistic models*; odds ratio*; etiology& (px); etiology (sh);
Textwords: cohort§; risk; etiol: or aetiol:; odds and ratio:§; causation and causal:‡; relative and risk; case and control:; case and comparison‡§; case and referent*†.

Prognosis

MeSH terms: exp cohort studies; cohort studies*; exp longitudinal studies; longitudinal studies‡§; follow-up studies; prospective studies; prognosis; exp morbidity§; morbidity‡§; incidence*; exp mortality§; mortality‡§; cause of death*‡;infant mortality‡§; maternal mortality‡§; maternal mortality‡§; survival rate*; survival analysis*; mortality (sh);
Textwords: natural and history‡; prognos:; inception and cohort*‡; clinical and course§; predict:; outcome:; clinical and consequence:‡§; prognostic and factor:; morbidity‡§; course.

Diagnosis

MeSH terms: exp sensitivity and specificity§; sensitivity and specificity§; predictive value of tests§; ROC curve*‡; exp diagnostic errors‡§; diagnostic errors‡§; false positive reactions‡§; false negative reactions‡§; diagnosis, differential‡§;diagnosis& (px); diagnosis (sh); diagnostic use (sh);
Textwords: sensitivity; specificity; predictive and value:; post and test and probabilit:†§; post and test and likelihood†§; likelihood and ratio:‡§; false and rate‡§; false and positive‡; false and negative‡§; receiver and operat: and characteristic‡§; roc‡§; independent and comparison‡§; mask: and comparison*‡; blind: and comparison‡§; gold and standard‡§; pre and test and probability:*†; pre and test and likelihood*†; independent comparison*†.

Treatment

MeSH terms: exp research design; research design‡§; double-blind method; random allocation‡; exp clinical trials*‡; clinical trials‡; multicenter studies*‡; randomized controlled trials*‡; clinical trial (pt); exp multicenter studies*†; multicenter study (pt)*; randomized controlled trial (pt)*; comparative study; single-blind method*‡; placebos‡§; prevention & control (sh); therapy& (px); therapy (sh); drug therapy (sh); therapeutic use& (px); therapeutic use (sh);
Textwords: random:; placebo:; double and blind:; mask:‡§; single and blind:‡§; controlled and trial:.

ACKNOWLEDGEMENTS

The study was supported by the Ontario Ministry of Health and the National Library of Medicine (R01 LM04696-03).

References

[1]. Haynes RB, McKibbon KA, Fitzgerald D, Guyatt GH, Walker CJ, Sackett DL. How to keep up with the medical literature. V. Access by personal computer to the medical literature. Ann Intern Med 1986;105:810-6.

[2]. Wilczynski NL, Walker CJ, McKibbon KA, Haynes RB. Assessment of methodologic search filters in MEDLINE. Proc Annu Symp Comput Appl Med Care. 1994;17:601-5.

[3]. Science Citation Index. Vol. 16: Journal Citation Reports, 1984. Philadelphia, Institute for Scientific Information; 1985.

[4]. Sackett DL, Haynes RB, Guyatt GH, Tugwell P. Clinical epidemiology: a basic science for clinical medicine. Second Edition. Little, Brown and Company, Boston, 1991.

A Pre-search Estimation Algorithm for MEDLINE Strategies with Qualifiers

Rulane B. Merz *, Christopher Cimino, M.D. †
G. Octo Barnett, M.D., Dyan Ryan Blewett, John A. Gnassi, M.D.,
Robert Grundmeier and Laurie Hassan

Laboratory of Computer Science
Massachusetts General Hospital
Boston, Massachusetts

ABSTRACT

Inexperienced users of online medical databases often have difficulty formulating their queries. Systems designed to assist them usually do not estimate how effective the initial search strategy will be before performing an actual search. Consequently, the search may find an overwhelming number of citations, or retrieve nothing at all. We have developed an estimation algorithm to predict the outcome of a MEDLINE search. The portion of the algorithm described here estimates retrieval for strategies containing qualifiers. In test searches, the estimate reduced the trial-and-error of strategy formulation. However, the accuracy of the estimate fell short of expectations. Our results show that pre-search estimation for strategies with qualifiers cannot be performed effectively with only the occurrence data that is presently available. They further imply that automated search intermediaries can benefit from medical knowledge which expresses the relationships that exist between terms.

INTRODUCTION

In their brief summary of the history of databases, Neufeld and Cornog wrote that "databases can almost be said to have created the information industry as we now know it" [11]. Unfortunately, end-users often have difficulty retrieving the information they need. Walker *et al.* [15] studied technical failures of online searches of MEDLINE® , a biomedical database provided by the National Library of Medicine (NLM). They listed several causes of failure: the use of redundant terms or terms that are too general, strategies that are too restrictive, nothing in the database on the topic, and the use of terms that infrequently index a document. Kingsland *et al.* [7] noted that in April 1991, 28% of the searches conducted with the aid of a tool designed to facilitate the use of MEDLINE retrieved no citations; 60% of these were caused by users ANDing terms which were valid, but for which the intersection was null.

We developed QUESTAR (QUery ESTimation And Refinement) to help construct effective initial strategies by predicting the outcome of a search [9, 10]. QUESTAR uses data about the frequency with which terms occur in the database to determine how concepts are related, and thus how often they can be expected to appear together. It obtains the frequency data from the Metathesaurus (Meta), a knowledge source created by the National Library of Medicine's Unified Medical Language System® (UMLS) project [8, 13].

The version of QUESTAR discussed here was designed using Version 1.1 of Meta (Meta-1.1). Currently it is restricted to MEDLINE queries, since Meta-1.1 contained complete occurrence data only for MEDLINE's vocabulary of index terms (Medical Subject Headings, or MeSH).

Previous Work

A system which performs some pre-search estimation is "Animal Welfare Tome.SEARCHER" (AWTS), an intelligent system developed by TOME Associates of London UK [12]. AWTS aids inexperienced users who want to search Agricola, the online agricultural database of the United States Department of Agriculture's National Agricultural Library. It allows a query to be entered as free text, extracts the main concepts, and forms an initial search strategy. It is limited in scope to a single domain (animal welfare), and requires that a dictionary of terms and a classification hierarchy be built.

*now at Hughes Information Technology Company. Work performed while a student at Massachusetts Institute of Technology

† Albert Einstein College of Medicine

Chong developed a formula to estimate the percentage of relevant documents that a strategy would retrieve [1]. The formula depended on knowing two things. First, it required the user to prioritize the databases to be searched and the terms in the strategy according to their relevance to the query. Second, it depended on predetermined measures of how much each database and each term would reduce the number of relevant documents that would not be retrieved. These measures were *ad hoc* and did not necessarily reflect what would actually happen. The formula also assumed the independence of concepts in the strategy. Such an assumption has been shown to be unrealistic [5, 14].

Other estimation algorithms have been developed for clustered databases and probabilistic retrieval systems [3, 16, 17]. These algorithms are not directly applicable to keyword-based databases that depend on Boolean retrieval (*e.g.*, MEDLINE). In addition, some of the algorithms require an initial search to be performed so that the frequencies of the terms in the strategy can be determined.

METHODS AND PROCEDURES

QUESTAR's estimates are calculated from Meta's occurrence data for MEDLINE. The occurrence data are of three types. The number of citations which are indexed by a given MeSH heading is the total *frequency of occurrence* of the term in the file. Meta also contains a record of the number of times the term is marked as a MeSH main heading, indicating that it is a main concept in the document. The number of citations which are indexed by a given pair of MeSH main headings is the *frequency of co-occurrence* of the pair. Finally, a MeSH main heading can be combined with *qualifiers*, terms which narrow the focus of the concept described by the main heading. The number of citations indexed by a given main heading/qualifier combination is the frequency of occurrence of the combination.

QUESTAR had reasonable estimates for MeSH headings without co-occurrence data or qualifiers and for MeSH headings with co-occurrence data but without qualifiers [9, 10]. However, it must employ a different method to find the estimate when terms are attached to qualifiers; it must account for the effect a qualifier will have on the retrieval for a concept.

An example will help to explain the estimate for queries with qualifiers. Assume that QUESTAR is given the MeSH main heading/qualifier combinations "zidovudine/therapeutic use" (Z/tu), "AIDS/physiopathology" (A/pp), and "AIDS/drug therapy" (A/dt). The occurrence, co-occurrence and main heading/qualifier occurrence data are given in Tables 1, 2 and 3.

Table 1: Occurrence Data

MeSH main heading	Occurrence Frequency
Zidovudine (Z)	616
AIDS (A)	8291

Table 2: Co-occurrence Data

MeSH main heading pair	Co-occurrence Frequency
Z and A (ZA)	282

Because of the absence of co-occurrence data for pairs of MeSH main heading/qualifier combinations, QUESTAR must use a modified form of the equation given in [9] for queries without co-occurrence data. First, it computes the probability that a combination will appear in an article by dividing the frequency of occurrence of the combination by the total number of articles in the source when the frequency data were collected. It multiplies each of the occurrence probabilities together to obtain the probability that all of the combinations will appear in an article, thereby (falsely) assuming that the occurrences of the combinations are statistically independent. Finally, it multiplies the result by the total number of articles currently in the source to get the expected number of articles that will be retrieved.

For our example, the initial estimate is

$$Estimate = \frac{Z/tu}{T_1} * \frac{(A/pp + A/dt)}{T_1} * T_2 \quad (1)$$

where

T_1 = total number of citations in the source when the occurrence data were tabulated

T_2 = total number of citations currently in the source

Note that if more than one qualifier is attached to the main heading, the frequency of occurrence is the sum of the frequencies of occurrence of the individual main heading/qualifier combinations.

A correction factor is needed, however; the combinations are not independent. If co-occurrence data are available for the MeSH main headings, a correction factor called the *co-occurrence ratio* can be used [10].

$$Ratio = \frac{co\text{-}occurrence(term_1, term_2)}{occurrence(term_1) * occurrence(term_2)} * T_1 \quad (2)$$

The co-occurrence ratio measures the statistical dependence between terms without qualifiers. If it

Table 3: Combination Occurrence Data

MeSH main heading/qualifier	Occurrence Frequency
Zidovudine/therapeutic use (Z/tu)	358
AIDS/physiopathology (A/pp)	142
AIDS/drug therapy (A/dt)	629

is less than one, the two terms are negatively dependent; fewer citations are retrieved than would be expected if the terms were independent. If it is equal to one, the terms are independent, and if it is greater than one, the terms are positively dependent.

MEDLINE had 730,259 citations when the occurrence data in Meta-1.1 were compiled. Using this as the value for T_1, the co-occurrence ratio of the two main headings in our example is 40.3.

To use the co-occurrence ratio, QUESTAR sorts the main headings in ascending order by the magnitude of their ratios. Since the maximum number of articles that will be retrieved by a strategy is bounded by the smallest number of articles that will be retrieved by any pair of terms, QUESTAR begins its calculation of the estimate with the most-negatively/least-positively dependent pair (the pair with the smallest ratio). It multiplies the occurrence probabilities of the terms in the pair combined with their qualifiers to obtain the likelihood that the combinations will appear in the same article. It then multiplies the product by the co-occurrence ratio to correct for its assumption of independence.

Since our example has only two main headings, we simply multiply the estimate by the co-occurrence ratio.

$$Estimate = \frac{Z/tu}{T_1} * \frac{(A/pp + A/dt)}{T_1} * 40.3 * T_2 \quad (3)$$

The co-occurrence ratio is an insufficient measure of the dependencies present in a query with qualifiers. In experiments conducted with the ratio as the only correction for the assumption of independence, the estimate often failed to predict actual retrieval results. Closer inspection of documents retrieved by the queries in conjunction with discussions with physicians identified relationships that exist between qualifiers as an important cause of the discrepancy. A term qualified by "therapeutic use," for example, is more likely to co-occur with a term qualified by "drug therapy" than with a term qualified by "manpower." If more than one term in the query is attached to qualifiers, the dependencies between the qualifiers increase the error in the estimate.

In an effort to quantify the relationships between qualifiers, we computed the co-occurrence ratios for pairs of qualifiers. An online search of MEDLINE was performed to find the occurrence frequencies of the qualifiers and the co-occurrence frequencies of all possible qualifier pairs. The ratio of actual co-occurrence frequency vs. predicted co-occurrence frequency for each pair was then computed using Equation 2 and stored online.

QUESTAR incorporates the additional measure of dependence provided by the qualifier ratios. As previously mentioned, when a term is included in the estimate, the estimate is multiplied by the co-occurrence ratio of which the term is a part. The qualifiers attached to the terms in the co-occurrence ratio are then grouped into pairs consisting of one qualifier from each term. The least-dependent pair of qualifiers, or the pair with the smallest ratio, is found, and the estimate is multiplied by this ratio.

The qualifier ratios in the example are 1.5 and 9 for tu/pp and tu/dt, respectively. Since tu and pp are the least-dependent qualifiers, QUESTAR multiplies the estimate by 1.5. The final estimate is therefore

$$Estimate = \frac{358}{T_1} * \frac{771}{T_1} * 40.3 * 1.5 * T_2 \quad (4)$$

As of January 29, 1993, MEDLINE (1990-93) had 1,051,039 citations. Using this as the value for T_2, substituting in T_1's value and truncating produce a final answer of 32 citations. An actual search retrieved 119 citations.

RESULTS

We collected 24 MEDLINE search strategies containing qualifiers from physicians. QUESTAR computed estimates for these strategies and classified them as either too narrow, acceptable or too broad. The range of acceptable values was 15-30 citations; this was an *ad hoc* definition, based on the need to retrieve at least some useful information, an intuition as to how many citations a busy physician is willing to examine, and our philosophy that it is better to retrieve too much than too little. The estimates were compared with actual search results.

QUESTAR correctly classified 71% of the strategies. Thirteen of the strategies contained a single main heading with a qualifier; 69% of these were classified correctly. Inaccurate predictions may have been due to the sample size; the occurrence frequencies of MeSH main heading/qualifier combinations are small relative to the size of MEDLINE.

Five of the strategies contained multiple main headings, one of which was attached to a qualifier; 80% were classified correctly. However, the accuracy of QUESTAR's predictions was reduced when more than one qualifier was present, even when the estimate included a correction for the relationships

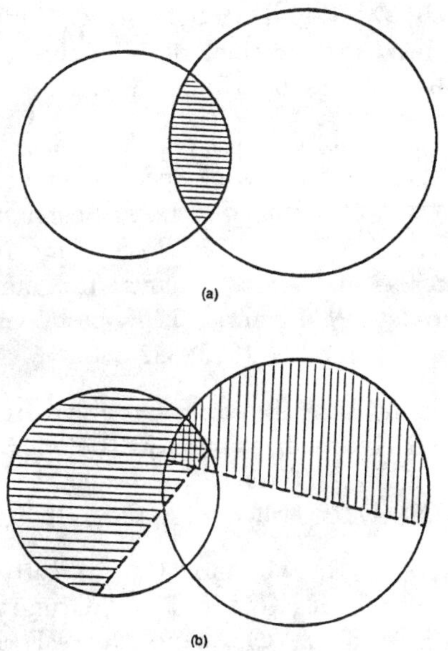

Figure 1: The effects of attaching qualifiers to MeSH main headings. (a) The lined area represents the intersection of two MeSH main headings. (b) The lined areas represent the fraction of the main headings which occur with a particular qualifier. The crosshatched area is the intersection of the MeSH main heading/qualifier combinations.

between qualifiers. Six of the 24 strategies contained more than one main heading/qualifier combination; QUESTAR classified 67% of them correctly.

Discussions with physicians provided an explanation for the drop in accuracy. Not only are qualifiers dependent on each other, but their presence changes the way concepts relate to each other (Fig. 1). For example, the drug "dipyridamole" is not the best medication to prescribe for treating "coronary disease." Adding the qualifier "therapeutic use" to "dipyridamole" and the qualifier "drug therapy" to "coronary disease" decreases the likelihood that the two terms will appear in the same document. Evidence for this conclusion is found in a study performed by Cimino *et al.* [2], which investigated the relationships implied by qualifiers.

DISCUSSION AND CONCLUSION

The estimation algorithm for strategies with qualifiers was not as accurate as we had been led to expect by our previous experiments using strategies without qualifiers. Some inaccuracies are inherent in the use of occurrence data to predict retrieval. Documents stored in MEDLINE reflect the research topics of interest to the medical community at a given time. With new discoveries and the rapid growth of knowledge, the content of the database shifts and changes. Acquired Immunodeficiency Syndrome (AIDS), for example, did not attract much attention until the 1980s, and the term was not added to the MeSH vocabulary until 1983. The occurrence data do not predict these changes, although they do show a history of changes which have already taken place and give some idea of the trends in the literature at the time the data were taken.

Inconsistencies in indexing are also reflected in the occurrence data. Citations on the same subject may be indexed differently, and some citations may be indexed erroneously. In a study of the consistency of MEDLINE's indexing, Funk and Reid [4] found that MeSH main headings, representing concepts that are highly important to the document, are indexed consistently 61.1% of the time. MeSH main headings with qualifiers are indexed consistently only 43.1% of the time. Other studies have shown that the MeSH terms selected vary with the indexer [6]. While QUESTAR knows how many documents have been indexed with a particular term, it cannot determine the accuracy of the indexing. This may lead to reduced or irrelevant retrieval in a search.

In addition to the inaccuracies introduced by the occurrence data, QUESTAR lacks knowledge of the relationship between qualified main headings. Its algorithm assumes that the interdependencies among qualifiers are uniform across MEDLINE; however, the actual relationships depend on the main headings to which the qualifiers are attached. Certain types of medical knowledge would have predictive value, but QUESTAR currently does not contain such knowledge.

Although advances in technology provide access to the information in MEDLINE with no incremental cost, a pre-search estimator can often benefit the user. A search may be time-intensive, especially on small systems with a slow, single-disk CD-ROM; ineffective strategies would create frustration and waste time. An end-user who needs up-to-date information from the definitive source must still perform an online search. Since the cost of an online search is affected by the search strategy and by how much information is retrieved, an algorithm that identifies badly-formulated strategies before a search will reduce the expense. Finally, it is important to avoid overwhelming the naive user with data or providing too little data to be of help. The ability to predict how many articles a strategy will retrieve allows the strategy to be improved before the search, increasing the likelihood that it will retrieve some articles of relevance to the user.

Future Work

QUESTAR already performs some query refinement based on its estimates in an effort to ensure that at least a few citations related to the user's query will be retrieved [10]. The next step would be to incorporate the ability to solicit feedback from the user. The user would not only designate which of the retrieved citations are most relevant to his or her query, but would also choose the most relevant index terms from those citations. QUESTAR could then reformulate the strategy with the chosen terms.

QUESTAR's lack of knowledge about the interactions between concepts introduces error into the estimates. It is not likely or reasonable to expect that complete occurrence data will be available for every possible kind of query. Medical knowledge is more robust and applies to many different kinds of questions. An important area of future work would be to encode the medical information that describes how concepts and qualifiers relate to one another.

Acknowledgments

The authors would like to express their thanks for the technical assistance of Ms. Cindy Schatz, Reference Librarian, Countway Medical Library, Harvard Medical School. This work was supported in part by NLM contract [N01-LM-8-3513] and in part by an educational grant from the Hewlett Packard Corporation. MEDLINE and the Metathesaurus are trademarks of the National Library of Medicine.

References

[1] Chong, H. F. L., *Recall Estimation for Information Retrieval Assistance*, MIT Department of Electrical Engineering and Computer Science, Bachelor's Thesis, 1986.

[2] Cimino, J. J., Mallon, L. J. and Barnett, G. O., "Automated Extraction of Medical Knowledge from Medline Citations", *Proc. of the 12th Annual SCAMC*, Greenes, R. A. (ed.), 1988; 180-184.

[3] Cooper, W. S., Gey, F. C. and Dabney, D. P., "Probabilistic Retrieval Based on Staged Logistic Regression", *Proc. of the 15th International Conference on Research and Development in Information Retrieval*, Belkin, N., Ingwersen, P. and Pejtersen, A. M. (eds.), June 1992; 198-209.

[4] Funk, M. E. and Reid, C. A., "Indexing Consistency in MEDLINE", *Bulletin of the Medical Library Association*, April 1983; 71:176-183.

[5] Harper, D. J. and van Rijsbergen, C. J., "An Evaluation of Feedback in Document Retrieval Using Co-occurrence Data", *J Doc*, September 1978; 34(3):189-216.

[6] Hersh, W. R. and Greenes, R. A., "Information Retrieval in Medicine: State of the Art", *M D Computing*, 1990; 7(5):302-311.

[7] Kingsland, L. C. III, Syed, E. J. and Lindberg, D. A. B., "Coach: An Expert Searcher Program to Assist Grateful Med Users Searching MEDLINE", *MEDINFO 92: Proc. of the 7th World Congress on Medical Informatics*, Lun, K. C., Degoulet, P., Piemme, T. E. and Rienhoff, O. (eds.), September 1992; 382-386.

[8] Lindberg, D. A. B. and Humphreys, B. L., "The UMLS Knowledge Sources: Tools for Building Better User Interfaces", *Proc. of the 14th Annual SCAMC*, Miller, R. A. (ed.), 1990; 121-125.

[9] Merz, R. B., Cimino, C., Barnett, G. O., Blewett, D. R., Gnassi, J. A., Grundmeier, R. and Hassan, L., "Q & A: A Query Formulation Assistant", *Proc. of the 16th Annual SCAMC*, Frisse, M. E. (ed.), 1992; 498-502.

[10] Merz, R. B., *A Pre-Search Estimation Algorithm to Improve Search Strategy Formulation for Medical Databases*, MIT Department of Electrical Engineering and Computer Science, Master's Thesis, 1993.

[11] Neufeld, M. L. and Cornog, M., "Database History: From Dinosaurs to Compact Discs", *JASIS*, July 1986; 37(4):183-190.

[12] "TOME.SEARCHER on Animal Welfare", TOME Associates Ltd., Report and User Guide, June 1990.

[13] "UMLS Metathesaurus", UMLS Fact Sheet, National Library of Medicine, Bethesda, MD, November 1992.

[14] van Rijsbergen, C. J., "A Theoretical Basis for the Use of Co-occurrence Data in Information Retrieval", *J Doc*, June 1977; 33(2):106-119.

[15] Walker, C. J., McKibbon, K. A., Ryan, N. C., Ramsden, M. F., Fitzgerald, D. and Haynes, R. B., "Methods for Assessing the Competence of Physicians' Use of MEDLINE with GRATEFUL MED", *Proc. of the 13th Annual SCAMC*, Kingsland, L. C. III (ed.), 1989; 441-444.

[16] Yu, C. T., Luk, W. S. and Siu, M. K., "On the Estimation of the Number of Desired Records with Respect to a Given Query", *ACM Trans. on Database Systems*, March 1978; 3(1):41-56.

[17] Yu, C. T., Meng, W. and Park, S., "A Framework for Effective Retrieval", *ACM Trans. on Database Systems*, June 1989; 14(2):147-167.

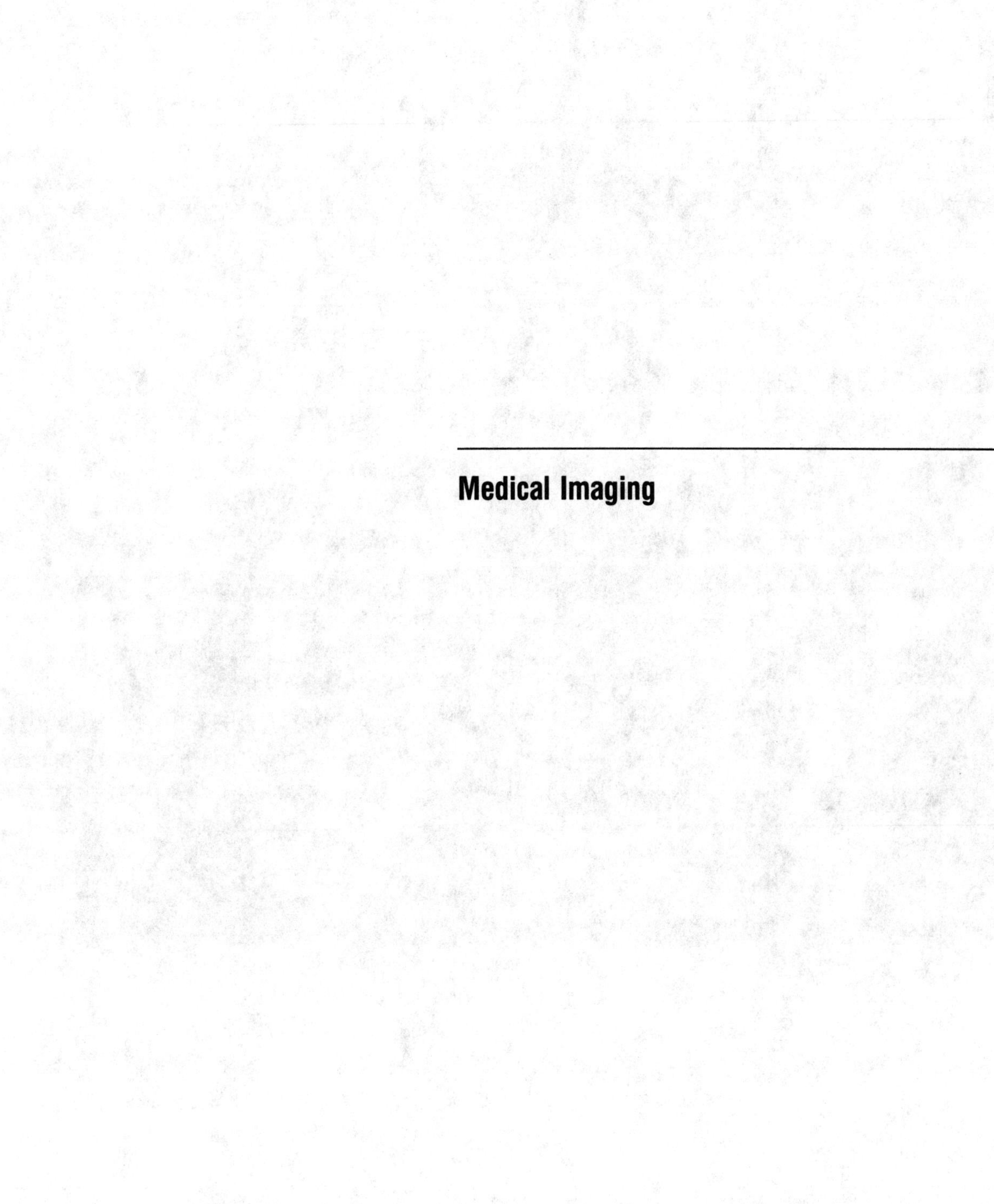

Medical Imaging

Preliminary Impacts of PACS Technology on Radiology Department Operations

Eliot Siegel, M.D., Chief, Radiology Service, Baltimore VA Medical Center
Austin Brown, Kenneth Leventhal & Company, Washington, D.C.

ABSTRACT

The potential benefits of digital imaging to clinical operations focuses on both quantitative and qualitative improvements. In the future it is postulated that it will totally replace analog imaging, creating the 'filmless' Radiology department. Although this could result in dramatic savings in film costs, realization of this scenario will require continued improvements in the performance and cost of component technologies, acceptance by the medical and legal communities of the reliability of the medium, and changes in the practice and process of radiology.

Baltimore VAMC has recently become one of the truly 'filmless' radiology departments through use of a leading commercial Picture Archiving and Communications System (PACS) and DHCP's Digital Imaging System. This document outlines the results of a preliminary assessment of PACS technology as it is installed at Baltimore, and its impact on operations.

INTRODUCTION

Archiving diagnostic radiology films and reports presents a significant challenge to hospitals and healthcare institutions. In a typical radiology department, archives hold all diagnostic patient images taken over the past several years. Older films -- those up to seven years old -- are usually kept elsewhere to satisfy legal requirements. Over the course of a year it is not uncommon to conduct 24,000 such examinations, requiring the unique identification and storage of upwards of a quarter million patient films.

Medical images are central to the careful diagnosis and successful treatment of patients. Retrieval and use of these films is one of the greatest logistical problems faced by hospitals. Because of the importance of these films and competition for them among different care providers within the institution, it is not unusual for radiology films to be missing. This results in tremendous frustration among clinical staff, and leads to highly paid clinicians searching for films both within and outside the Radiology department.

These and other problems associated with management of film archives routinely impede the timeliness of patient care. Not only do they present logistical hurdles, they can also impact the quality of patient care itself by requiring that studies be repeated -- needlessly irradiating the patient a second time -- or lack of consideration of prior medical history in formulating a diagnosis. In response to these challenges, Picture Archiving and Communication Systems (PACS) are being developed to expedite the retrieval and simultaneous use of medical images, providing functionality to scan, index, and compress data.

This study outlines the results of a preliminary assessment of this technology conducted at the Baltimore VAMC as part of VA's HOST program. This institution has installed a state-of-the-art digital imaging system using the DHCP Digital Imaging System and a commercial PACS system. New capabilities provided by these systems are being used to implement one of the first truly filmless radiology departments now on record.

Overview of PACS Technology

PACS evolved as clinicians sought ways to improve access to medical images. Consequently, the design of these systems emphasizes the use of networks and distributed processing to enable comprehensive access to images stored centrally. Other considerations that have helped shape development of the technology focus on new developments in radiological devices themselves. In the past decade, CT, MRI, and ultrasound scanners have all used advanced technology to improve the quality of medical images taken of soft tissues. All of these devices record images digitally, and account for roughly 20% of the volume of a typical hospital. X-rays, a technology dating from the turn of the century, continue to record images using analog techniques. These images must be concerted to a digital format before they can be used in a PACS. These systems have only become technically feasible due to

Study Question	Indicators
Digital Imaging improves patient care ...	... by increasing the availability of images ... by increasing the accessibility of images ... by enabling better diagnosis ... by enabling physicians to spend more time with patients
Improves Service Levels...	... by reducing processing time ... by reducing reading time
Facilitates BVAMC's Educational Role...	... by better enabling 'curbside consults'

Figure 1. Study Hypotheses

improvements of several component technologies over the past several years.

Among the most important performance characteristics of imaging systems is the resolution at which images are stored and displayed. Analog technologies record 8 - 12 bits per pixel, using a multi-tone gray scale to map images. In converting these to digital format, the image is divided into a matrix of pixels. The depth of data recorded for each pixel can vary from 12 to bits. The quality of an image is enhanced as the size of the matrix is increased, increasing the number of pixels, and hence, the resolution of the image. These two dimensions -- the size of the matrix and the number of bits per pixel -- define the diagnostic quality of images. Although there is no agreement as to what precision is needed to routinely ensure ease and accuracy of diagnosis, these criteria are generally used to rank the utility of PACS.

Note that these criteria apply only to analog images such as chest X-rays. CT, MRI, and ultrasound images are filmed and recorded digitally at 8 bits per pixel. However, these types of images make up less than 20% of the workload of a radiology department.

METHODOLOGY

Initial research developed an understanding of the technology and its use and acceptance in the commercial marketplace. This pointed to several macro-level impacts that could be expected from introduction of digital imaging. From this basis, interviews with radiology staff and physicians identified several specific hypotheses to be addressed in a comprehensive assessment of the technology. For each hypothesis outlined in Figure 1, both measurable and subjective indicators were agreed upon.

Over the course of the ten week project a structured task plan was used to coordinate activities that included interviews, shadowing physicians and staff, and formulating analyses that developed each of these perspectives.

FINDINGS

At the outset of the assessment it was agreed to measure the success of digital imaging technology by collecting data concerning several specific hypotheses.

Digital Imaging Improves Patient Care

... by increasing the availability of images

Evidence collected suggests that in a manual environment there is significant competition for patient films. The most immediate and credible measure of this competition is the 'hit rate' or the probability of finding a desired film. At BVAMC this was approximately 90%. This competition can also be gauged by the demand for images. The frequency of requests for archival images was 37 minutes during the course of an average workday.

Competition for films will be wholly eliminated by digital imaging. This will be the single most important contribution the technology makes in improving clinical practice.

... by increasing the accessibility of images

Whereas availability refers to the ability to locate films, accessibility addresses the issue of where they can be retrieved. In current practice images are routinely interpreted in a wide variety of locations close to the point of care. Light boxes are situated strategically throughout the clinics, inpatient wards, and ORS.

Once the PACS system is fully operational there will be 53 DHCP digital imaging terminals throughout the house, and an additional 20+ commercial terminals. This will not be a significant change from the status quo.

... by enabling better diagnosis

There are many dimensions to this issue, all relate to defining the improvements possible by use of the technology.

From a film quality perspective, digital imaging provides the same precision as analog techniques for typical computed radiology images. Some downsizing is required. However, the full implications of this reduction is not well understood from a clinical perspective, and the literature itself does not draw any definitive conclusions.

The second perspective is that of the timeliness of diagnosis. The most telling measure of this is the time required for an outpatient film to be carried back to radiology to be read. This delay in formal diagnosis will be eliminated through use of digital imaging technology. Another measure of this is the turnaround time for portable exams. The study conducted demonstrated that it took less than one hour to respond to a portable request, and an additional half hour before it was first read. This second component could be significantly reduced through use of digital imaging technology.

The last perspective is that of the tools available to clinicians in reviewing images. In a manual environment, the only tools commonly used were the hot box and the magnifying glass. In the computer environment these tools are much more sophisticated, and are augmented by others that have no counterpart in current practice.

In summary, digital imaging will promote accurate, timely diagnosis. Moreover, it will provide clinicians with new analytical tools that could lead to improvements in the practice of care.

... by enabling physicians to spend more time with patients

Physicians universally agree that full implementation of digital imaging will allow them to deliver more direct patient care. As evidence of this, every 37 minutes during the course of a weekday a physician presents at radiology looking for a film. The time in vested in each of these episodes directly detracts from providing care.

Digital Imaging Improves Service Levels

The second premise is that digital imaging will make significant improvements in the level of services provided by radiology.

... by reducing processing time

Use of phosphorus plate technology will not yield any improvements over current practice. In a manual regimen image processing takes on the order of 90 seconds. This will continue to be true using the phosphorus plate processor.

... by reducing reading time

The time invested in reading images is the product of a variety of factors, only a few of which will be influenced by use of digital imaging. Ongoing research is being conducted to determine the full impact of the technology.

Digital Imaging Facilitates BVAMC's Education Role

The third premise is that introduction of digital imaging will significantly enhance BVAMC's educational capabilities.

... by better enabling consults

In an operating environment based on use of films, consults are necessarily face-to-face. Consults are not rare, but the time required to leave the ward and go to radiology do make them relatively infrequent from a physician's perspective. Introduction of simultaneous review of images will enable a true interactive consultation from anywhere in the facility.

DISCUSSION

Adoption of computer technology has profound implications for operations. Improvements in computer support have a direct impact on the process and practice of care, which in turn begin to transform organizational roles and structure.

Impacts on Practice

Widespread adoption of digital imaging will engender practice improvements and innovations that could significantly improve patient care. A number of specific innovations can be expected.

Radiologists will play a larger role in clinical decision making. This will be manifest in the frequency of consultations. For the first time, digital imaging will make it possible for the full integration of Radiologists in the real-time interpretation of images. Manual systems do not permit this because of the logistical problems of finding films, and the requirement for physicians and Radiologists to meet and discuss images. As physicians become familiar with the system and its capabilities, it can be expected that on-line consultations over the phone in which images are simultaneously viewed from remote locations will increase.

The routine of reading films will incorporate use of tools provided by PACS technologies. Both commercial and DHCP systems offer diagnostic tools superior to those available in a manual operating environment. As Radiologists and others that make diagnoses become familiar with these tools, a new regimen for interpreting images may arise that routinely takes advantage of these capabilities.

The impact of these practice changes will be to enhance the role of Radiologists by making their skills more widely available and by making their diagnoses more comprehensive.

Impacts on Process

As production in radiology shifts from a film-based to an image-based process, procedures required to support production can be expected to change. For example, real-time interpretation and diagnosis could evolve. In a manual environment there is a significant delay between ordering a film and receiving a radiology report. Often the most significant delay is that between completing an exam and having a Radiologist make an interpretation.

The key cause of both these types of delays is that patient films must be physically carried from one location to the next. Digital imaging eliminates this by providing images instantaneously. This new capability will facilitate the evolution of real-time reading, where instead of interpreting images in batches, Radiologists may be able to keep up with production as it occurs. Real-time reading will no doubt require reassessment of basic support systems and procedures.

Another example is the elimination of most archive activities. Handling films as they are processed, routed, read, archived, and retrieved currently consumes a majority of the time and attention of radiology staff. Implementation of digital imaging would remove most of these requirements. Once processed, images will be wholly automated.

The value of these changes will be to reduce inherent complexity and thus streamline operations, reducing most measures of radiology turnaround time.

Impacts on Jobs

The reduction in process complexity enabled by digital imaging will necessarily change the roles -- the jobs -- of individuals employed in the Radiology Service. A number of specific changes can be anticipated.

Labor investments now made in archiving activities can be redeployed. As the department transitions to a filmless environment, it is envisioned that archived films will be converted to digital format when a patient presents for treatment. This will most likely be done by the Film Library staff. Consequently, the role of these individuals will shift from that of managing files to inputting images using a digital scanner.

Responsibilities for systems management can be added. Effective use of PACS will require the active participation of mangers or supervisors in managing the system and its data.

The impact of these changes will be to change the skill mix of the Radiology staff. Depending on the balance achieved, this could increase labor costs in the Service.

Impacts on Organization

The last dimension of operations that will be impacted by use of digital imaging is that of organizational structure. The premise is that as jobs evolve along new lines, the structure of the department will also change.

It is difficult to guess how this evolution will take place, but its general direction is clear -- to reorient radiology from a 'factory for films' to a more clinical focus. The rationale for this is that use of film erects barriers that distance radiology from direct patient care. These barriers include the availability and access of film and the manual production systems that have grown up around it. As digital imaging eliminates the use of film these barriers will fall. This will enable Radiologists, Radiographers -- and the services they provide -- to be better integrated in the mainstream of patient care activities.

In summary, use of digital imaging will create efficiencies in the practice of radiology and in the production processes that support it. Primary benefits will be the elimination of problems associated with film handling and management. Secondary benefits touching on jobs and organizational structure will not be realized without concomitant practice and process changes.

ACKNOWLEDGEMENTS

This work was funded by the Medical Information Resources Management Office, Department of Veterans Affairs as part of the HOST program.

References

[1] Hess, Thomas, "Rigid demands make image archiving the black hole of PACS development." *Digital Imaging,* Nov 1987.

[2] Inamura, Kiyonari, "Basic IMAC Concepts." *1990 IEEE Proceedings*, 1990.

[3] Demetriades, James, "Optical Storage Technology for MUMPS-based Systems." *MUG Quarterly,* Vol. XX, No. 1.

[4] Dayhoff, Ruth, "Providing Image Management and Communication Functionality as an Integral Part of an Existing HIS." *SPIE 1990,* 1990.

[5] Gomez, Enrique, "Online Archiving using Optical WORM for VA DHCP Systems." *MUG Quarterly*, Vol. XX, No. 1.

[6] Staff, "UCLA Research with Optical Disk Drives for Medical Imaging." *IMC Journal,* 1990.

[7] Cannavo, Michael, "Low-Risk Strategy for PACS calls for Modular Phase-In." *Diagnostic Imaging,* Oct. 1988.

[8] Cannavo, Michael, "Optical Disk Drives and Jukeboxes Transform Radiology Data Storage." *Diagnostic Imaging*, Oct. 1988.

[9] Cannavo, Michael, "Communications Still Weak Link in Implementation of PACS." *Diagnostic Imaging*, Jan. 1990.

The Role of Object Representation in the Design of the Intelligent Radiology Workstation

Katarzyna J. Macura, M.D., Ph.D.
Robert T. Macura, M.D., Ph.D.

Department of Radiology, Medical College of Georgia, Augusta, GA

The paper describes the design of the Intelligent Radiology Workstation (IRW) that is intended to handle heterogeneous radiologic data (text, image, video) and radiologic knowledge in such a way that it is easy to store, access, use, and repurpose. An object-based structure is used to combine the relational database, hybrid knowledge base, and hypermedia within a common framework. Functions such as data entry and retrieval, browsing, and intelligent processing of data are available in the single environment. IRW open architecture allows radiologic digital resources to be used for clinical practice, diagnosis support, education, and research.

INTRODUCTION

Efficient organization of the modern medical setting depends on computer support that offers fast and easy access to an information resource for decision making and teaching. The need for passive information resources as well as interactive decision support tools led to the research on development of intelligent computer workstations [1][2]. The major limitation of the current computerized information resources is that they are available only through isolated applications that are incompatible in terms of hardware, software, and user interface environments. There is a need for unified information access and standards, and for application independent frameworks for delivery of medical information. The information resources should be separated from the organizational structure for viewing and interacting with them [3]. But at the same time, they must be integrated to facilitate the exchange of data and knowledge.

The goal of our research is to implement the Intelligent Radiology Workstation (IRW). IRW is intended to handle heterogeneous medical data (text, image, video) and complex medical knowledge and to manage information so that it is easy to store, access, use, and repurpose. IRW should facilitate cross-disciplinary activity by providing uniform standards for the exchange of information. To meet these objectives, computer technologies that are usually treated in isolation must be integrated within a single environment. IRW must provide tools to store data (databases); apply knowledge to data (knowledge based systems); interrelate information from different sources using different media (hypermedia); and use knowledge and inference to make retrieval and use of information easy. The use of the object representation paradigm allows combination of the database, knowledge base, and hypermedia into a framework for viewing all these technologies as parts of the IRW. The only requirement is that the object-oriented structure refers to all the data and knowledge representations within the IRW modules. This paper presents work in progress. We describe the way we are using object representation to build a uniform platform for IRW.

INTELLIGENT RADIOLOGY WORKSTATION DESIGN

Radiologic Object Representation

The fundamental feature that will make the IRW responsive to the user is it provides the user with an abstract data and knowledge model that closely resembles the user's model of the real world. The basic structural unit of the IRW is an object. When thinking about medical problems, we often think in terms of objects: of diseases, of diagnostic methods, of treatments. Moreover, when we think of a particular disease or syndrome, we think of it as a whole; data such as signs and symptoms, laboratory values, diagnostic procedures, treatment and prognosis are associated with it. Each medical domain approaches the same diagnostic problem using different diagnostic and treatment methods, and different classification patterns and semantics. Thus, medical objects are composite objects. They will have as many profiles as there are subspecialties that deal with a given medical problem. Our goal is to design a radiologic profile for medical objects that represents the radiologic image model. The radiologic image model (Figure 1) consists of:

A. ***Image data objects***:

1. Acquisition data
2. Real image data: pixel value, sequence, measurements portraying anatomical relations and chemical or physical processes that are associated with the patient state
3. Image-related data objects: look-up-tables, regions of interest, file formats
4. Image access data: procedures for storage and retrieval operations (methods indicating the location

and the way to access physical data, how images are gathered within files, I/O operations and computer resources required to handle the image object, e.g. compression techniques).

B. *Non-image data objects*:

1. Domain-specific data objects: classifications, differential diagnosis, verbal descriptors for coding image content, image annotations for explanation/commentary
2. Clinically-related data objects: patient description, clinical history, indications for examinations

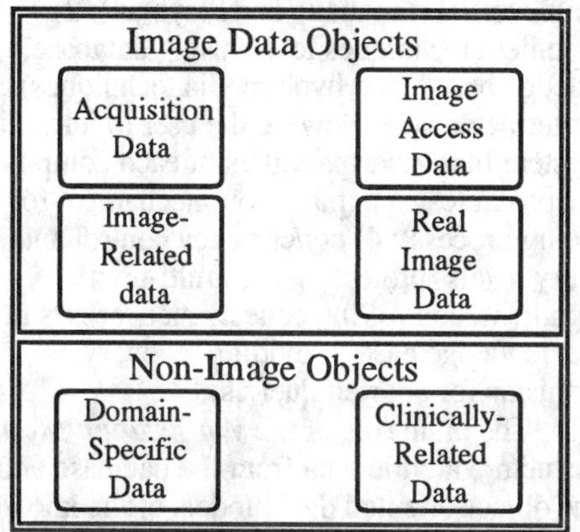

Figure 1. Structural Description of Radiologic Images

Database

The database forms the kernel of any information system. In the IRW environment, multiple databases will serve as sources of medical data, and the purpose of querying the system will not be predefined. IRW will manipulate independent data. The concept of data independence is simple; data should be stored in such a way that data is not specifically associated with any particular application. A relational database guarantees the independence of data. The basic data structure supported by the relational database is a table. Only one data item is allowed in any cell in a relational table (atomic data type). Objects in opposition to the atomic data type are structured data types. A relational database management system needs to be extended to allow creation of structured objects. A single object can possess several attributes (each is an atomic data type) as well as methods that manipulate the attributes. Objects are related by is-a-part-of links. Composite objects are defined as tree structures that are searched by recursively checking the relationship is-a-part-of until all objects making up a tree are identified.

Knowledge base

Knowledge-based systems separate the domain knowledge that is contained in the knowledge base from the general control knowledge that is mostly built into the inference engine. IRW knowledge base is a hybrid system that combines case-based reasoning (CBR) with rule-based technology. Each radiology subspecialty has its own rules and methods. Thus, there are multiple domain-oriented radiology knowledge bases in our system that are called the ***Case Bases.*** The descriptive knowledge is kept in object hierarchies and relations, while heuristic knowledge is stored in rules. In addition to organizing knowledge in inheritance hierarchies, objects are also linked to rules. Rules are linked to the attributes of objects using attached predicates. Attached predicates allow the invocation of rules from within objects. Thus, in addition to attributes and their values within the object, there is separate information that refers to attached rules. The objects in the Case Bases refer to cases. Groups of cases are arranged in a hierarchy in which higher level cases represent prototype cases - classes, and lower level cases represent factual cases - instances (Figure 2). The initial search involves prototype cases and then expands to search through the factual cases to find the closest match. In this approach, knowledge of the domain used to structure and index cases supplements the information included in the cases themselves.

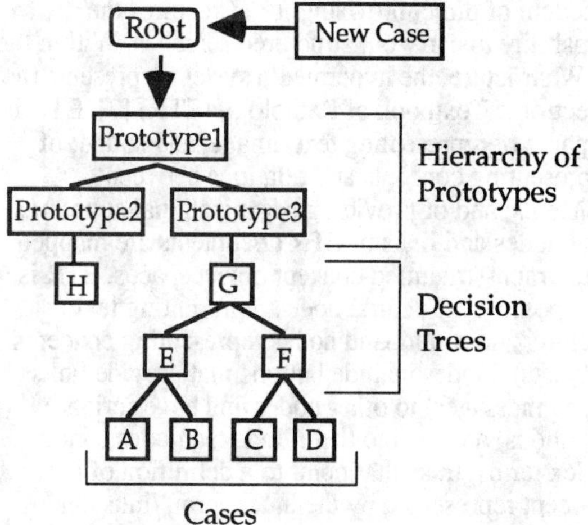

Figure 2. Case Hierarchy

For indexing purposes, we use a *hierarchical image description vocabulary* that is composed of basic observations and interpretations that form a continuum, in which higher level findings incorporate lower level findings [4]. Using this approach, the image details are coded using both basic observations such as the CT density of cerebral contents (e.g., appearance relative to brain tissue such as hyperdense, isodense, hypodense, CSF density, below CSF) and higher level findings that express interpretation of basic observations (calcified, blood, cyst, fat, etc.). The hierarchical ***Index*** communicates with the Controlled Vocabulary. The idea of using the finding-diagnosis continuum to describe medical images has been outlined by Greenes et al [5].

The structure of cases for a particular radiologic domain is kept in the domain-oriented Case Base, whereas the hierarchical Index is separate and is common to all the Case Bases in the knowledge base. Multiple radiologic Case Bases communicate with each other through the inference engine. The third component of the knowledge base is the Differential Diagnosis Manager (***DDM***) that is intended to use the Bayesian (probabilistic) network to compute the likelihood of diagnoses and generate lists of diagnostic hypotheses. Probabilistic networks have been applied successfully in the domain of pathological diagnosis [6].

Hypermedia

Hypermedia enhances the user interface in an important way. The ability to browse is generally the strongest reason for using hypermedia. Hypermedia can be browsed by following links, by searching the network for a particular string, keyword, or attribute value, or by navigating through a visual representation of the hypermedia network such as a map. The combination of hypermedia with a database and knowledge base needs to limit the freedom of direct browsing. IRW requires the capability to carry out structured searches. Within the IRW structure, the hypermedia system represents the Electronic Textbook of Radiology (ETR) [7]. ETR is capable of representing text, image, and sound; of representing concepts and relations between concepts; and of providing organizational structures. The nodes and links of ETR documents are mapped into graph-structured concept object spaces. ETR is composed of structural nodes representing text, picture, and sound, and nodes representing concepts (objects). Nodes include buttons that provide links (send messages) to other nodes and have scripts (methods) attached to them. Indexed nodes contain index terms, links that point to a definition of the concept represented by the index term, links that point to related terms or synonyms (links to the Controlled Vocabulary), and links that correspond to appropriate columns in relational tables that can be used to find documents that share a particular index term. The communication with the relational database provides a decomposition of the node (text document, image, sound file) into a set of index terms. A link to a particular column in the table is present if the corresponding index term describes the content of the document. This feature allows attachment of the radiologic thesaurus to the system and use of the Unified Medical Language System tools to map from the IRW vocabulary to another. ETR contains organizational and inferential links. Indexing links move the user from an indexed node to the corresponding index entry for that node. Is-a links indicate membership in a category, as in semantic networks. Has-a links describe the properties of nodes and are used to implement object-like capability. Rules are used to define links, implement predicate attachments on links, filter links, and execute actions.

Workstation Manager

Coupling a relational database with a knowledge base and hypermedia requires more than simply passing data through the import/export facilities of the cooperating systems. It requires an integration of systems and their behavior at each of several levels: 1) language level (syntax); 2) development techniques level (using database, knowledge based, and hypermedia techniques); 3) user interface level (allowing the user to interact with one system that has capabilities of each component and incorporates an explanation mechanism for the reasoning process); 4) concurrency control and recovery levels (protecting the multi-user environment, controlling concurrent accesses to the same knowledge base, providing recovery mechanisms for aborted queries).

The main role of the ***Workstation Manager*** is to structure atomic data from the database and to use the object-oriented data models of the knowledge base, and hypermedia, and link the relations expressed in the knowledge base and hypermedia to the relations expressed in the relational database (Figure 3).

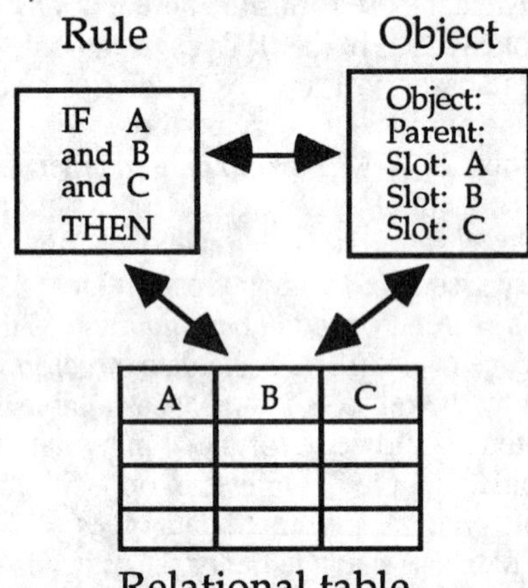

Figure 3. The relationship between logic, objects and the relational table

Mapping between objects and relations easily provides the inheritance feature, in which each relation can inherit attributes from its parent relation. The Workstation Manager recognizes the class objects represented in the knowledge base and hypermedia and brings records from the database to create instance objects. It needs to compose simple atomic items that are stored in the relation tables into the structured data items (objects). The Workstation Manager directs the search of the database, record by record, to return the next instance for the current object. The database system uses set-at-a-time retrieval compared with the record-at-a-time retrieval of hypermedia and the knowledge based system. Close integration between the knowledge based system, hypermedia and database requires an implementation of cursors on the database side that steps through a relational table one record at a time. These cursors provide access to necessary data stored in the database to be used by the Workstation Manager. Another function of the Workstation Manager is to apply knowledge to data through incorporated algorithms that identify and prioritize data according to chosen criteria. The Workstation Manager allows use of hypermedia in conjunction with a knowledge base through its indexing nodes and inference links. The Workstation Manager also assists in query formulation, as it permits the vocabularies of the user and the ***Controlled-Vocabulary*** of the system to converge prior to carrying out a search (Figure 4).

DISCUSSION

IRW is intended to support several goals: 1) Abstraction (the ability to have both decomposition and composition); 2) Modifiability (the ability to modify a part of the system without unexpected side effects in other parts); 3) Maintainability (the ability to make easy enhancements and adaptations); 4) Portability (the ability to have a system that is easily transferred from one computer system to another); 5) Reusability (the ability to reuse an existing code along with data and knowledge). The object-oriented system design promises to accomplish these goals.

Coupling existing computer technologies allows expert knowledge to be encoded in the same environment with a database and hypermedia system, so functions such as data entry, report generation, browsing, and intelligent processing of data are mixed together. The object-based metastructure allows integration of different computer technologies within one organizational framework. By developing hierarchies of objects (according to classification standards), we can describe medical problems in a more natural way than when using procedural approach. Inheritance creates possibilities for reusing the code. Domain-oriented class libraries can be flexibly used by different applications by assembling appropriate class objects drawn from the libraries. To access and assemble data for a specific application, the application must include the code that establishes the desired relationships among data. Although the application programs that access data stored within the relational database may evolve or change, this

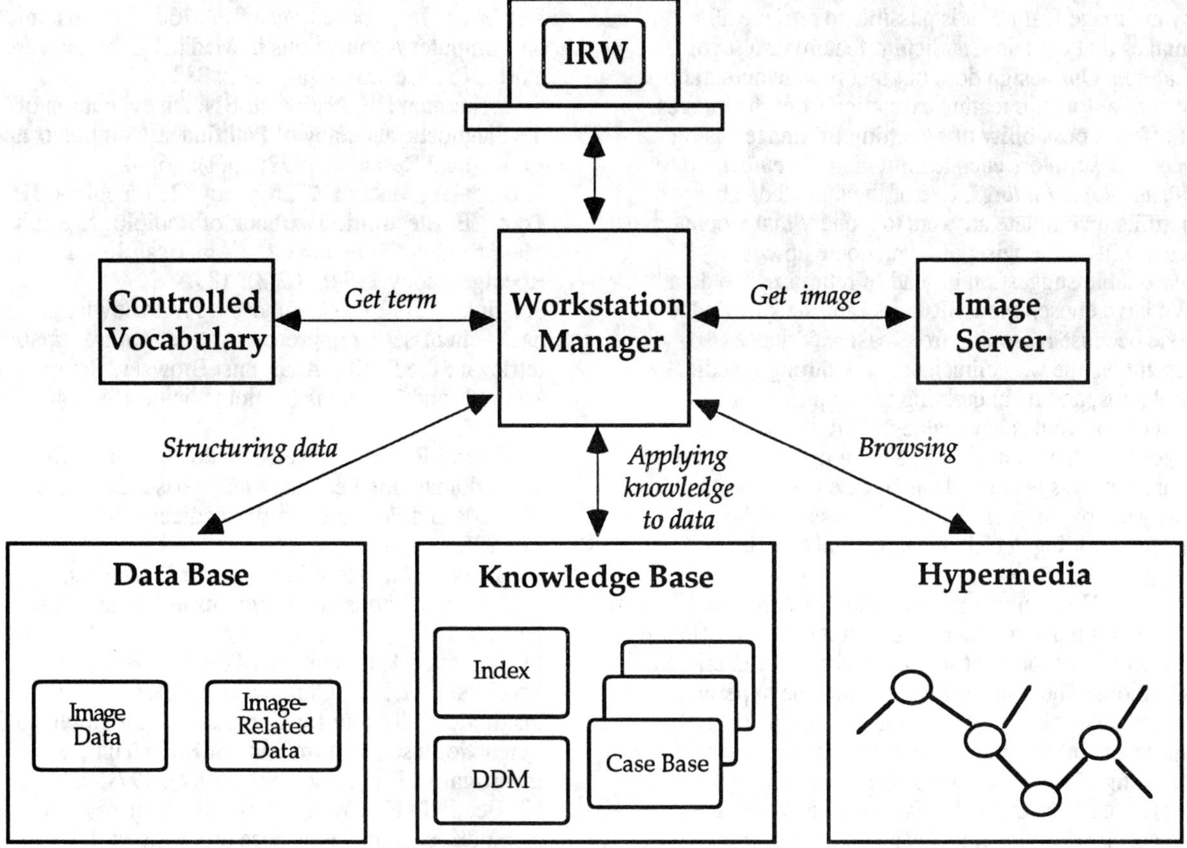

Figure 4. Intelligent Radiology Workstation Framework

possibility cannot affect the way the data is logically organized or physically stored. Most knowledge based systems have not incorporated database technology, which has resulted in systems in which knowledge is difficult to create, modify, merge, or export to other systems. Our design attempts to resolve this problem and avoid redundancy. The unified environment requires that an item of data be unique. Thus, although different applications refer to the same data, there is only one table that lists a particular data item and each data item is listed only once. Relational databases do not handle abstract data types and structured data items. The advantage of the extended relational database is that it structures atomic data and maintains the relational model, which gives data independence.

The extended relational model has been used to structure the *Digital Anatomist Browser* [8]. The use of multiple knowledge bases in conjunction with the relational database has been implemented in a feature dictionary, *MEDAS* [9].

Objects also provide a firm foundation for knowledge representation and inference. Integration of the relational database, knowledge base, and hypermedia permits the expression of complex queries and the use of content-based visual queries. For example, since each radiologic feature is identified by name in the knowledge base as well as by an image feature, it is possible to retrieve all images that contain a particular feature or a set of features. Our design does not incorporate automatic or semiautomatic feature extraction from the images. It offers a possibility of searching for images using verbal descriptors encoded into a *hierarchical index of radiologic findings*. Use of the knowledge base permits incomplete answers to a query that would have failed otherwise, or it can come up with a reasonable suggestion instead of returning "no data." We have chosen the CBR model for the knowledge base because reasoning from past experience resembles the way clinicians think through medical problems, and its underlying techniques refer to objects, attributes, and values. CBR also adds the algorithm that identifies the similarity between cases stored in the system and a new case that is being analyzed by the user. CBR techniques are especially useful in aiding decision making and teaching [10][11].

Hypermedia browsing tools interrelate information using various types of media and offer an excellent environment for quick assistance in clinical situations. The user may just browse the hypermedia system and select terms for subsequent queries. This approach ensures that the user understands the meaning of the terms and uses them in a way that the system also understands. Hypermedia is also a powerful educational tool. The concept of merging the browsing tool with the knowledge base to assist pathologists in the diagnosis of breast disease has been described by Heathfield et al [12].

Our system is currently in the implementation phase. The system is being written in the C++ on the Macintosh platform. Several steps remain to be completed before we can fully realize the contribution of the system design.

Reference

1. Swett HA, Fisher PR, Cohn AI, Miller PL, Mutalik PG. Expert system-controlled image display. Radiology 1989; 172(2): 487-493.
2. Giger ML, Doi K, MacMahon H, Nishikawa RM, Hoffmann KR, et al. An "intelligent" workstation for computer-aided diagnosis. Radiographics 1993; 13: 647-656.
3. Greenes RA. A "Building Block" Approach to Application Development for Education and Decision Support in Radiology: Implications for Integrated Clinical Information Systems Environments. Journal of Digital Imaging 1991; 4(4): 213-225.
4. Macura RT, Macura KJ, Morstad BD, Binet EF, Trueblood JH. Feature-Coded Image Database. In Boehme JM, Rowberg AH, Wolfman NT (Eds.): Computer Applications to Assist Radiology. Carlsbad, CA: Symposia Foundation, 1994; 313-318.
5. Greenes RA, McClure RC, Pattison-Gordon E, Sato L. The Findings-Diagnosis Continuum: Implications for Image Descriptions and Clinical Databases. In: Proceedings of the 16th Symposium on Computer Applications in Medical Care. New York, NY: McGraw-Hill, 1992; 383-387.
6. Heckerman DE, Nathwani BN. An evaluation of the diagnostic accuracy of Pathfinder. Computers and Biomedical Research 1992; 25(1): 56-74.
7. Binet EF, Macura RT, Macura KJ, Trueblood JH, Toro VE. Electronic Textbook of Radiology: Brain Mass Module. Supplement to American Journal of Roentgenology 1994; 162(3): 189.
8. Brinkley JF, Eno K, Sundsten JW. Knowledge-based client-server approach to structural information retrieval : the Digital Anatomist Browser. Computers Methods and Programs in Biomedicine 1993; 40: 131-145.
9. Nayemi-Rad F. A feature dictionary supporting a multi-domain medical knowledge base. Computer Methods and Programs in Biomedicine 1989; 30: 217-228.
10. Turner RM. Using Schemas for Diagnosis. Computer Methods and Programs in Biomedicine 1989; 30: 199-207.
11. Macura RT, Macura KJ, Toro VE, Binet EF, Trueblood JH, Ji K. Computerized Case-Based Instructional System for Computed Tomography and Magnetic Resonance Imaging of Brain Tumors. Investigative Radiology 1994; 29(4): 497-506.
12. Heatfield HA, Winstanley G, Kirkham N. A menu-driven knowledge base browsing tool. Medical Informatics 1990; 15(2): 151-159.

Dr. Browse, A Digital Image File Format Browser

Alan H. Rowberg and Thurman Gillespy, 3rd.
Department of Radiology
University of Washington
Seattle, WA

The emerging widespread adoption of the Digital Imaging Communications in Medicine (DICOM) standard will increase the demand for radiologic image transfer between radiologic image acquisition, archive, display and printing devices. Unfortunately, there are and will continue to be many devices that do not and will not support this standard, especially older radiologic equipment and devices from non-radiologic vendors. Determining the image file format characteristics of images from such equipment is often difficult, and done on an ad hoc basis. We have developed a software tool that assists users in determining the image file format parameters of unknown radiologic images.

BACKGROUND

Discussions of data formats in both the engineering and the radiology literature have included descriptions of formats which are proposed as standards [1-4] or formats used by specific software [5-7], and reviews of commonly available image formats [8-11]. More recently, the American College of Radiology and the National Electrical Manufacturers Association (ACR-NEMA) have developed and published the DICOM standard [12-17], which is being embraced by the majority of radiology equipment manufacturers for their new equipment. Unfortunately, little has been written about how to determine if a given digital image is in one of the common formats, in a format which can be easily decoded, or in a format so cryptic that decoding it will require a great deal of effort. The typical imaging scientist is motivated by specific problems, and applies techniques to a given unknown image until either that image format is adequately understood or the problem is viewed as not having a practically reachable solution. In the past there has been little impetus for anyone to explore the general process of image format determination in a logical manner.

METHODS

To determine the file format of unknown radiologic images, the following steps are suggested:

1. Obtain any *a priori* information.

In most circumstances one can get the image matrix size (horizontal and vertical image axis dimensions) and other information, such as pixel size, image location, patient name, and other demographics from the scanner. The filename itself may provide clues about the file format. While the name may contain an identifier such as an exam number, it may also contain information about the format, such as a TIFF file which has the extension .TIF or a Targa file with .TGA as its extension.

A photograph of the image made on the scanner will usually contain much of this information, in addition to showing the nature of the image and the anatomy involved.

2. Examine file sizes of related files.

In a situation where one has a group of related image files with little or no information about the file format, it is usually best to start with a list of a group of related files and compare their sizes. Image file sets from a CT exam without data compression may begin with a file of archive or patient identifiers. Next there may be one or more files of localizer images. Then there will be a series of image files, usually of equal length and all in the same format.

Changes in file length may be due to compression, changes in image size, or to different image types, such as localizer and axial images.

3. Is the file compressed?

Images which are already compressed will show little or no additional compression when processed by any standard compression program (e.g. StuffIt, PKZIP or UNIX compress). The headers of such image files are often not compressed, so some additional compression may be achieved. Unfortunately, images which are compressed can rarely be "decoded" without very specific information about the file format and method of compression. Fortunately, many imaging modalities allow images to be stored in both compressed and non-compressed formats, so the image might be obtained again, this time in a non-compressed format.

4. Estimate the header size.

The header size is estimated by multiplying the horizontal matrix size by the vertical matrix size and an estimate of the number of bytes per pixel. Often subtracting this number from the file size gives the exact length of the header for the image. Usually the entire header is in the file before the image and there is no trailer record after the image.

Header size = File size - (v * h * n)

where v = vertical image dimension, h = horizontal image dimension, and n = number of bytes per pixel (usually 1 or 2, but can be higher).

For many images, these steps alone will be sufficient for deriving enough information to display the image. Typically, an image display program can import and display the image after the information on matrix size, bytes per pixel, and size of header is entered into the program.

5. View the header with an ASCII editor.

Headers do not usually change in size from image to image (unless variable length fields such as comment fields are present.) The file can be examined with a hex/ASCII editor or file viewer and the location and nature of many fields may be obvious, since the contents of some fields (such as patient name) are known from the process of doing the scans and printing the images.

Often one will recognize a common image format like TIFF and others, especially if the image source is a peripheral device (not a scanner) such as a teleradiology system. TIFF files begin with either the two characters II or MM. A file which is based on the ACR-NEMA version 2 format will have the version name in ASCII in the file.

DR. BROWSE SOFTWARE TOOLS

The first tool is an ASCII browser. It will look for ASCII text in the file and display the text, in a manner simpler than any hex editor.

One mode gives a dense display of all text and another gives the address of each string, in hex and decimal.

The tool is able to drop 1 and 2 character words, which are usually extraneous characters, and words over 20 characters, which are most likely strings of a compressed image.

Header items which are ASCII are easy to locate and decode. Many are in ASCII, even for decimal/floating point values such as pixel size. Integer values are a little more difficult to find, but a data set with judicious variation of one value at a time will help. For instance, a series of slices with the slice number changing by one for each image will allow one to locate the slice number relatively easily.

Floating point values are usually conspicuous by a repetitive pattern every 4th byte. While the ieee floating point format is common, decoding other formats will require knowledge of which computer is used on the scanner.

Date formats also may follow a standard format, often 4 bytes for date/time, but may be in other formats.

The second tool is the Image Browser, which allows the user to examine any image file, regardless of the nature of the file, and get useful information, if not a viewable image.

The file is first displayed with an estimate of the image matrix size and header length based on the file size. This is chosen from a set of common matrix sizes, so as to minimize the number of characters left over, which are assigned to the header.

A default window width and window center are set, and they can be adjusted by the user. Alternatively, they can be calculated from the minimum and maximum values in the image and set so that the window will cover the range

$$WW = max - min + 1$$

$$WC = min + WW/2$$

where WW is the window width and WC is the window center.

The user can change WW and WC as desired. These may also be adjusted using alias names of Brightness and Contrast, but if the user invokes using the alias, the sign of changes in brightness is the opposite of WL. Contrast gets greater as WW gets smaller.

Then the user can change the image width and view the result. If the file is compressed, it will look very random. If it is uncompressed then the user can change the width, either by typing in a new value or using arrow keys to change it one pixel at a time. If the image is larger than the screen the user can pan within the image.

The user can then change the estimate of header size. Typically this is done first using the left arrow key to align the left edge of the image, then the UpArrow to skip one line at a time to align the top of the image. Finally, the bottom of the image can be adjusted to determine if there is a trailer or residual buffer after the image.

Thus the image area can be determined using an interaction with visual feedback, essentially a visual scroll.

The third tool calculates histograms of the image values. If the image format is not immediately apparent then one can do histograms on single bytes, pairs of bytes or triples. Peaks in these histograms will suggest first-order difference compression, or flag values which have special meaning in the format.

RESULTS

Dr. Browse was evaluated on nine unknown image sets, including the Elscint CT, GE CT Advantage, GE Windows Workstation, Hitachi CT, Picker CT, Picker MRI, Philips MRI, and two Fuji Computed Radiography formats. In all cases the alphabetic portions of the headers were located immediately, but it took some effort to conclusively identify some of the numeric items. Four of the formats were decoded essentially immediately, and two were decoded after just a few minutes of exploration. The remaining three were compressed formats, and were decoded only after several hours effort, although Dr. Browse revealed that they were compressed when it first displayed the images.

DISCUSSION

While many aspects of decoding an image format are much easier using these automated techniques, the power of the technique is particularly apparent when looking at an uncompressed image format with 2-byte pixels. Typically, the values are around 1000, so one byte is approximately 4 (4 times 256) and the next byte is a nearly random number. If one simply examines these bytes with a hexadecimal editor it is difficult to determine which low-order byte corresponds with which high-order byte. If the image starts on an even byte in the file instead of an odd byte, it may mimic the difference between low-byte first vs high-byte first formats (little endian vs. big endian). While the appearances of the files seen in a hexadecimal editor screen may be similar, the differences when viewed as images are dramatic.

If one is examining the bytes in the wrong order, either because the header length is off by one byte or because the byte order is wrong, the image may appear to be very noisy, having roughly an equal number of black and white values, with very little grayscale visible, yet show some evidence of the overall structure of the image, especially at high-contrast edges. If this is corrected inappropriately, the image will become recognizable but appear very similar to a first-order difference image. The vertical edges of the organs will be surrounded by black or white arcs, because of errors in whether the high order or low order byte are processed first. The user can rapidly change the byte order or change the header length by 1 byte, which will instantly correct the errors in the image.

Some programs offer some of the features of Dr. Browse, but with somewhat less convenience. Image, a public domain program produced at NIH, offers the ability to set horizontal and vertical image size, as well as header size, but is available only for the Macintosh computer. KBVision (Amerinex Artificial Intelligence Inc, Amherst, MA) is a commercial program with similar capabilities, but runs only on UNIX systems, such as Sun or Silicon Graphics.

CONCLUSIONS

While one can decode most image formats using a standard disk file utility program, the use of a specialized program, like Dr. Browse, makes the process much faster, simpler, and more reliable. Information on program availability is available from the AMIA forum on CompuServe (GO MEDSIG) or using Mosaic to read www.rad.washington.edu or by e-mail to rowberg@u.washington.edu.

References

1. Todd-Pokropek A, Cradduck TD, Deconinck F. A file format for the exchange of nuclear medicine image data: a specification of Interfile version 3.3. Nucl Med Commun 1992 Sep. 13(9). P 673-99.

2. Ando Y, Hashimoto S, Ohyama N, Inamura K. Current status of Image Save and Carry (IS&C) standardization. Comput Methods Programs Biomed 1992 May. 37(4). P 319-25.

3. Cradduck TD, Bailey DL, Hutton BF, deConninck F, Busemann-Sokole E, Bergmann H, Noelpp U. A standard protocol for the exchange of nuclear medicine image files. Nucl Med Commun 1989 Oct. 10(10). P 703-13.

4. Wicks DAG, Barker GJ, Plummer DL, Edited by: Lemke HU, Rhodes ML, Jaffe CC, Felix R. A general image file format. Computer Assisted Radiology. Proceedings of the International Symposium, CAR '91 pp. 471-6. 1991.

5. Noz ME, Maguire GQJr. QSH: a minima but highly portable image display and handling toolkit. Computer Methods and Programs in Biomedicine. vol.27, no.3. pp. 229-40. Nov.-Dec. 1988.

6. Young IR, Ling DHO, Bell DA, Edited by: Adlassnig KP, Grabner G, Bengtsson S, Hansen R. MIDAM-a generalised system for integrating medical images and patient records. Medical Informatics Europe 1991. Proceedings. pp. 174-8. 19-22 Aug. 1991.

7. Englmeier KH, Fink U, Hilbertz T. Visualization of multimodal image information in medicine. Proc Annu Symp Comput Appl Med Care. 1992. P 25-9.

8. Graef GL. Graphics formats. BYTE. vol.14, no.9. pp. 305-6, 308-10. Sept. 1989.

9. Maguire GQJr, Noz ME. Image formats: five years after the AAPM standard for digital image interchange. Med Phys. 1989 Sep-Oct. 16(5). P 818-23.

10. Wiltgen M, Gell G, Schneider GH. Some software requirements for a PACS: lessons from experiences in clinical routine. International Journal of Bio-Medical Computing. vol.28, no.1-2. pp. 61-70. May-June 1991.

11. Baumann P. Edited by: Abel D, Ooi BC. Database support for multidimensional discrete data. Advances in Spatial Databases. Third International Symposium, SSD '93 Proceedings. pp. 191-206. 1993.

12. Wang Y, Best DE, Hoffman JG, Horii SC, Lehr JL, Lodwick GS, Morse RR, Murphy LL, Nelson OL, Perry J. et al. ACR-NEMA digital imaging and communications standards: minimum requirements. Radiology. 1988 Feb. 166(2). P 529-32.

13. Seshadri SB, Khalsa S, Arenson RL, Brikman I, Davey MJ. An image archive with the ACR/NEMA message formats. Proceedings of the SPIE - Medical Imaging II. vol.914, pt.B. pp. 1409-15. 1988.

14. Horii SC, Hill DG, Blume HR, Best DE, Thompson B, Fuscoe C, Snavely D. An update on American College of Radiology-National Electrical Manufacturers Association standards activity. J Digit Imaging. 1990 Aug. 3(3). P 146-51.

15. Bidgood WDJr, Horii SC. Introduction to the ACR-NEMA DICOM standard. Radiographics. 1992 Mar. 12(2). P 345-55.

16. Best DE, Horii SC, Bennett W, Thomson B, Snavely D. Review of the American College of Radiology--National Electrical Manufacturers' Association standards activity. Comput Methods Programs Biomed. 1992 May. 37(4). P 305-9.

17. Horii SC, Bidgood WDJr. PACS mini refresher course. Network and ACR-NEMA protocols. Radiographics. 1992 May. 12(3). P 537-48.

Planning Diagnostic Imaging Work-up Strategies using Case-Based Reasoning

Charles E. Kahn, Jr., M.D.
Section of Information and Decision Sciences, Department of Radiology,
Medical College of Wisconsin, Milwaukee, Wisconsin

ISIS is a developmental decision support system that helps physicians select diagnostic imaging procedures. It uses case-based reasoning, an artificial-intelligence approach that emphasizes reasoning and planning from prior experience. The development, training, and evaluation of a prototype system were used to guide the development of ISIS. To realize a clinically useful system, particular emphasis has been placed on increasing the depth and breadth of case-based knowledge, enhancing the explanatory capabilities of the system, and refining the human-computer interfaces to include a critiquing approach.

INTRODUCTION

How does a physician plan a patient's diagnostic imaging work-up? The physician might consider similar patients and the radiological procedures that were performed in those cases. Using this knowledge, the physician would decide which imaging procedure to request.

Case-based reasoning (CBR) is an approach to computer-based cognition that involves reasoning from prior experiences: new problems are solved by recalling and adapting solutions that were used to solve old problems [1,2]. CBR systems can be particularly useful in domains where well-defined causal models or extensive statistical data are lacking.

The knowledge base, or "memory," of a CBR system consists of cases indexed by their pertinent features. The dynamic operation of a CBR system involves: (1) encoding new cases and storing them into memory, (2) activating (retrieving) cases from memory that are pertinent to the current situation, and (3) adapting the actions of retrieved cases to compute a course of action for the current situation.

ISIS (Intelligent Selection of Imaging Studies) is a case-based decision support tool being developed to help physicians select appropriate radiological procedures [3]. It provides computer-based expertise in the domain of diagnostic imaging procedures such as computed tomography (CT), ultrasound (US), and magnetic resonance imaging (MRI). ProtoISIS, a prototype case-based system, learned the use of ultrasonography and body CT from 200 actual, consecutive requests from imaging procedures, from which it achieved 84% accuracy in classifying new cases [3]. This report discusses the directions taken in the development of ISIS based on lessons learned from the clinical trial and evaluation of ProtoISIS [4].

PROTOTYPE SYSTEM

Exemplar-Based Learning

ProtoISIS is based on a CBR shell called Protos. Protos performs case-based classification: it learns to classify cases based on associations between categories and exemplary cases ("exemplars") [5,6]. Protos attempts to classify a new case by matching it to cases with similar features. We implemented CL-Protos, a version of Protos in the Common Lisp language [7], in Macintosh Common Lisp 2.0 on Macintosh IIsi and PowerBook 180 computers (Apple Computers, Cupertino, Calif.).

An "exemplar" is a case that particularly represents the specified category. Each exemplar in Protos consists of a name, a set of features and a classification. Each term known to the system may have an abbreviation and one or more synonyms. This information is supplemented by explanations that relate two or more terms. When a new case is presented, Protos gives the user the choice to pre-classify the case or to let Protos suggest a classification. If no suitable case is found, Protos asks the user to classify the case and to provide an explanation that relates the features of the case to the specified category.

Terms and Relations

In ProtoISIS, a case consists of a request for an imaging procedure. The order number is the case name, the clinical indications and questions to be answered are the features of the case, and the imaging study performed is the classification. Each semantically descriptive item — case name, feature, or category — is a "term"; terms can have synonyms, abbreviations, and relations to other terms.

To establish conceptual relationships between terms such as features and categories, ProtoISIS elicits explanations from the user. These relationships allow ProtoISIS to distinguish new cases from previously learned exemplars, and to link the case's features to its classification. Subsumption ("is a"), causal, functional, definitional, and part/whole relations can be defined.

For example, case PT070 has features FATTY-FOOD-INTOLERANCE and RIGHT-UPPER-QUADRANT-PAIN. The imaging-procedure category for this case is GALLBLADDER-ULTRASOUND; this term has the synonym US-GALLBLADDER and the abbreviation US-GB. In addition, ProtoISIS knows that GALLBLADDER-ULTRASOUND is a specialization of ULTRASOUND-PROCEDURE, which is in turn a specialization of IMAGING-PROCEDURE.

Because the original Protos system did not contain a verb to express the concept "detects" or "reveals," the verb VISUALIZES was substituted for ENABLES to relate imaging procedures and the conditions they reveal. Relations can be qualified by the terms ALWAYS, USUALLY, SOMETIMES, and OCCASIONALLY. For example, to the question "How is RIGHT-UPPER-QUADRANT-PAIN related to US-ABDOMEN?", one could answer: "US-ABDOMEN USUALLY VISUALIZES GALLSTONES" and "GALLSTONES SOMETIMES CAUSES RIGHT-UPPER-QUADRANT-PAIN."

These explanations allow ProtoISIS to create a semantic network that relates the cases, features, and imaging procedures (Figure 1). In addition, ProtoISIS creates "remindings" from the case's features to its imaging-procedure category, such as from RIGHT-UPPER-QUADRANT-PAIN to US-ABDOMEN, if it judges the feature's association with the category to be sufficiently strong. Strength is determined in

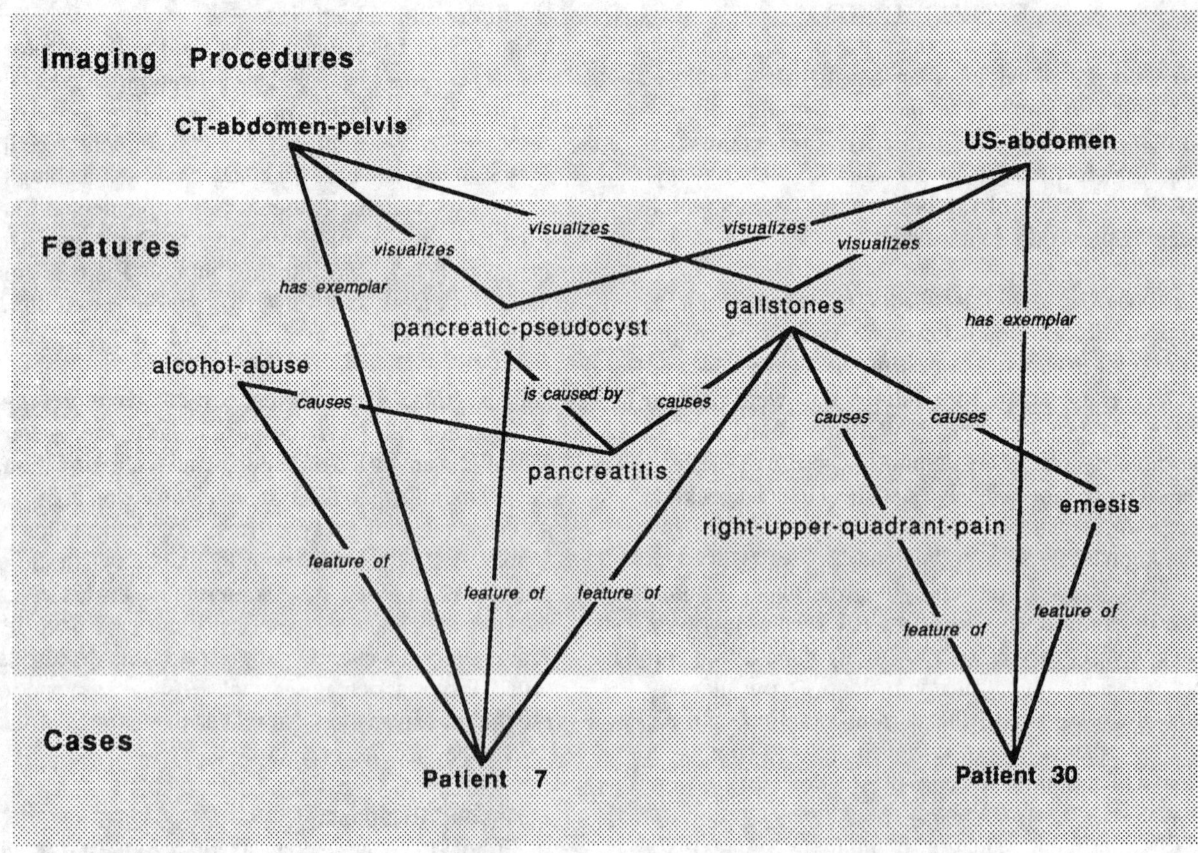

Figure 1. Semantic network of terms created by ProtoISIS.

part by the verbs (*e.g.*, CAUSES, DETECTS or DEFINITION IMPLIES) and the qualifiers (*e.g.*, ALWAYS, USUALLY) that express the relationships that lead from the feature to the category. These remindings allow ProtoISIS to associate features of new cases with relevant categories.

Performance of Prototype System

ProtoISIS was trained with 200 actual cases of body CT and ultrasound requests from one week of radiology department records. To test the system, 100 new, consecutive ultrasound and body CT cases, grouped into four sets of 25 cases each, were presented sequentially. After each case's identifier and clinical features were entered, the system attempted to assign the correct category to each case. If ProtoISIS was unable to assign a category or assigned an incorrect category to a case, we added that case and pertinent explanations into memory. ProtoISIS incorporated into its knowledge base all new terms — such as abbreviations, synonyms, and features — that were encountered in the test cases whether or not the case to which they belonged was itself added.

After training, ProtoISIS incorporated a total vocabulary of 527 terms: 200 case names, 28 imaging procedures, 37 abbreviations, 40 synonyms, and 222 features. Of the nine CT procedures, CT-ABDOMEN-PELVIS, CT-CHEST-ABDOMEN-PELVIS, and CT-CHEST had the most exemplars (33, 22, and 16, respectively). Among the 19 ultrasound procedures, US-KIDNEY, US-ABDOMEN, DOPPLER-ABDOMEN and US-HEAD had the most exemplars (29, 26, 14, and 11, respectively). All other imaging-procedure categories had six or fewer exemplars. Each exemplar consisted of one or more features: 66 exemplars (33%) had only one feature, another 77 (38%) had two features, and none had more than seven features. All but 13 (5.9%) of the 222 features had remindings to one or more imaging procedures. The great majority of features (76.4%) had remindings to only one imaging procedure; none had remindings to more than three imaging procedures.

In classifying imaging-procedure requests, ProtoISIS demonstrated satisfactory performance (Figure 2). Only three of the 100 test cases required new imaging-procedure categories: CT-ABDOMEN-DRAINAGE, CT-LIVER-BIOPSY, and US-AORTA. Overall, ProtoISIS correctly classified 72% of the imaging-procedure requests on the first attempt. Its performance improved as it gained experience: in the last two test series, it correctly classified 84% of the cases presented, compared with only 56% in the first series.

In many of the incorrectly classified cases, the correct imaging procedure received the second highest matching score. On average, 40% of cases included terms that had not been encountered previously; given the small number of training cases, the large vocabulary of medicine, and the variety of ways that a single medical concept can be expressed, this finding is not surprising.

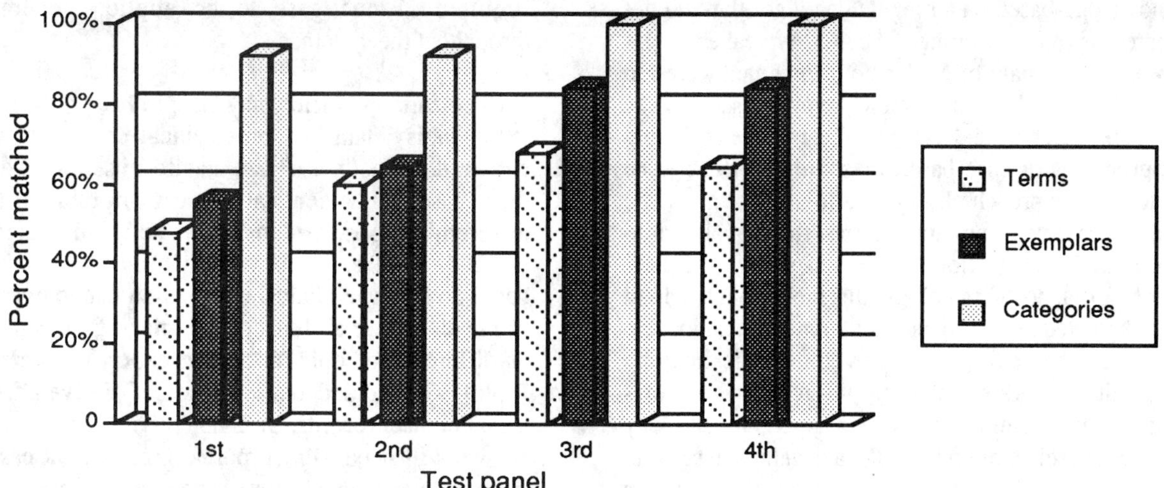

Figure 2. Performance of ProtoISIS. "Terms": cases that did not require additional terms or explanations. "Exemplars": cases that successfully matched an existing exemplar and were categorized correctly. "Categories": cases that did not require an additional category.

PRODUCTION SYSTEM

Case Structure and Reasoning
ISIS builds on the framework of ProtoISIS and incorporates two additional properties to overcome the prototype's deficiencies. First, ISIS distinguishes between known features (patient history) and those being queried (clinical questions). In addition to the procedure requested and the clinical information provided, each case includes information about the procedure actually performed, the imaging technique or protocol, and clinical questions to be asked of the referring physician. Second, ISIS treats imaging procedures as a elements of a plan, rather than as categories. ISIS can modify a plan's components instead of creating a unique category for each imaging protocol. This approach facilitates proper sequencing of imaging procedures and offers much richer interaction between computer and physician.

Interaction with Physicians
Although CL-Protos provides efficient and easily understandable interfaces, evaluation of their use in ProtoISIS found them unsuitable for physicians. In ISIS, the user interfaces limit the functionality of the system to those features needed by physicians. In addition, information being entered or presented must be clustered in ways that corresponds to typical clinical scenaria. Because most commercial radiology information systems are based on VT100-type 24-line, 80-column displays, integration with such systems requires special attention to the user interfaces to assure ease of use.

Some of the explanations generated by the Protos knowledge-based pattern matching algorithm did not represent valid reasoning. The most typical error was to present a chain of explanatory links that were too heavily dependent on the first exemplars seen by the system. Effort is underway to integrate the critiquing approach with case-based reasoning in ISIS. The critiquing approach allows ISIS to propose a revised or alternative plan and allows the physician to override its suggestions. In a consultative specialty such as diagnostic radiology, this mode of interaction and knowledge sharing is essential to the relationship between the radiologist (who knows the imaging procedures) and the referring physician (who knows the patient). Critiquing has been applied to radiology procedure selection in DxCON, a developmental rule-based system [8]. This approach allows more robust interaction between the physician and the decision support system.

DISCUSSION

As medical imaging technology has advanced, selecting appropriate diagnostic imaging procedures has become increasingly complex. Collaborative planning of imaging work-up strategies by radiologists and referring physicians has been limited by the large number of consultation requests. A computer-based "proxy" for the radiologist could help referring physicians select optimal diagnostic imaging procedures.

Existing decision support systems for radiological procedure selection include rule-based systems [8-10], hypertexts [11,12], and belief networks [13]. The development of ProtoISIS demonstrated that case-based reasoning can be applied successfully to the task of selecting diagnostic imaging procedures and that such a CBR system can be much simpler to construct and validate.

CBR systems offer other advantages. Knowledge acquisition (learning) for CBR systems is uncomplicated. Existing cases can be used to train the system; a causal model or deep understanding of the domain is not required. Also, human experts often have greater ease distilling their knowledge into examples rather than rules. CBR systems can explain their reasoning by referring to prior cases and generalizations of these cases. They can operate under incomplete knowledge and can adapt with experience; this flexibility is especially important in rapidly evolving domains such as medicine. CBR systems are computationally efficient and their network of relations between terms allows knowledge acquired in one case to be applied generally throughout the system.

Two potential problems may have to be addressed in ISIS: noisy data and prototypical cases. In the current domain, "noise" can manifest itself as two or more cases with identical clinical information but different proposed plans (*i.e.*, selected imaging procedures). Physicians may choose different plans based on identical clinical information due to overlap of the diagnostic abilities of the imaging procedures or difference of opinion among expert physicians. ProtoISIS included only "episodic" derived from actual clinical records. It is not yet clear whether or not we will need to incorporate prototypical cases; these are hypothetical cases that summarize published data or medical practice guidelines.

Case-based reasoning has been applied experimentally in medicine to diagnosis of hearing disorders [5,6,14], diagnosis of heart failure [15,16], and planning of radiation therapy protocols [17,18]. Although these systems have undergone some degree of validation, none is in routine clinical use. Once ISIS has been completely validated, it will integrated with our department's radiology information system, where it will provide interactive, on-line expertise to physicians at all times of the day, and be available to physicians in their work areas, such as clinics, inpatient wards, intensive-care units and the emergency department. Our radiology department performs more than 200,000 procedures annually, including about 36,000 imaging procedures. This setting will provide an excellent "production system" test, and will serve as a pilot project for "scaling up" the system to include all radiology procedures. ISIS offers an opportunity to study the role of case-based reasoning in day-to-day medical decision making, and has potential to significantly improve the quality and cost-effectiveness of medical care.

Acknowledgments

The author gratefully acknowledges support from the 1993 American Roentgen Ray Society Scholarship. CL-Protos, written by Daniel L. Dvorak, is based on the Protos system originally developed by Ray Bareiss and Bruce W. Porter at the University of Texas at Austin.

References

[1] Riesbeck C, Schank R. Inside Case-Based Reasoning. Hillsdale, NJ: Lawrence Erlbaum, 1989.

[2] Kolodner JL. An introduction to case-based reasoning. Artif Intel Rev 1992; 6:3-34.

[3] Kahn CE Jr, Anderson GM. Case-based reasoning and imaging procedure selection. Invest Radiol 1994; 29:643-647.

[4] Kahn CE Jr. Clinical trial and evaluation of a prototype case-based system for planning medical imaging work-up strategies. In: Aha DW, ed. Case-Based Reasoning: Papers from the 1994 Workshop. Menlo Park, CA: AAAI Press, 1994: 138-142.

[5] Bareiss ER, Porter BW, Wier CC. PROTOS: an exemplar-based learning apprentice. Int J Man-Machine Studies 1989; 29:549-561.

[6] Porter BW, Bareiss R, Holte RC. Concept learning and heuristic classification in weak-theory domains. Artif Intel 1990; 45:229-263.

[7] Dvorak D. CL-Protos User's Guide. Austin, TX: Artificial Intelligence Laboratory, Department of Computer Sciences, The University of Texas at Austin, 1989.

[8] Swett HA, Rothschild M, Weltin GG, Fisher PR, Miller PL. Optimizing radiologic workup: an artificial intelligence approach. J Digit Imaging 1989; 2:15-20.

[9] Kahn CE Jr, Messersmith RN, Jokich MD. PHOENIX: an expert system for selecting diagnostic imaging procedures. Invest Radiol 1987; 22:978-980.

[10] Kahn CE Jr. Validation, clinical trial, and evaluation of a radiology expert system. Methods Inf Med 1991; 30:268-274.

[11] Greenes RA, Tarabar DB, Krauss M, et al. Knowledge management as a decision support method: a diagnostic workup strategy application. Comput Biomed Res 1989; 22:113-135.

[12] Kahn CE Jr. A radiology hypertext system for education and clinical decision making. J Digit Imaging 1991; 4:207-212.

[13] Haddawy P, Kahn CE Jr, Butarbutar M. A Bayesian network model for radiological diagnosis and procedure selection: work-up of suspected gallbladder disease. Med Phys 1994; 21:1185-1192.

[14] Bareiss R. The experimental evaluation of a case-based learning apprentice. In: Hammond K, ed. Proceedings of a Workshop on Case-Based Reasoning. San Mateo, CA: Morgan Kaufmann, 1989: 162-167.

[15] Koton P. A medical reasoning program that improves with experience. Comput Methods Programs Biomed 1989; 30:177-184.

[16] Koton P. Evaluating case-based problem solving. In: Hammond K, ed. Proceedings of a Workshop on Case-Based Reasoning. San Mateo, CA: Morgan Kaufmann, 1989: 173-175.

[17] Berger J. ROENTGEN: case-based reasoning and radiation therapy planning. In: Proceedings of the 16th Annual Symposium on Computer Applications in Medical Care. New York: McGraw-Hill, 1992: 210-214.

[18] Berger J. Knowledge acquisition and design support in a medical domain. In: Leake DB, ed. Case-Based Reasoning: Papers from the 1993 Workshop. Menlo Park, CA: AAAI Press, 1993: 141-146.

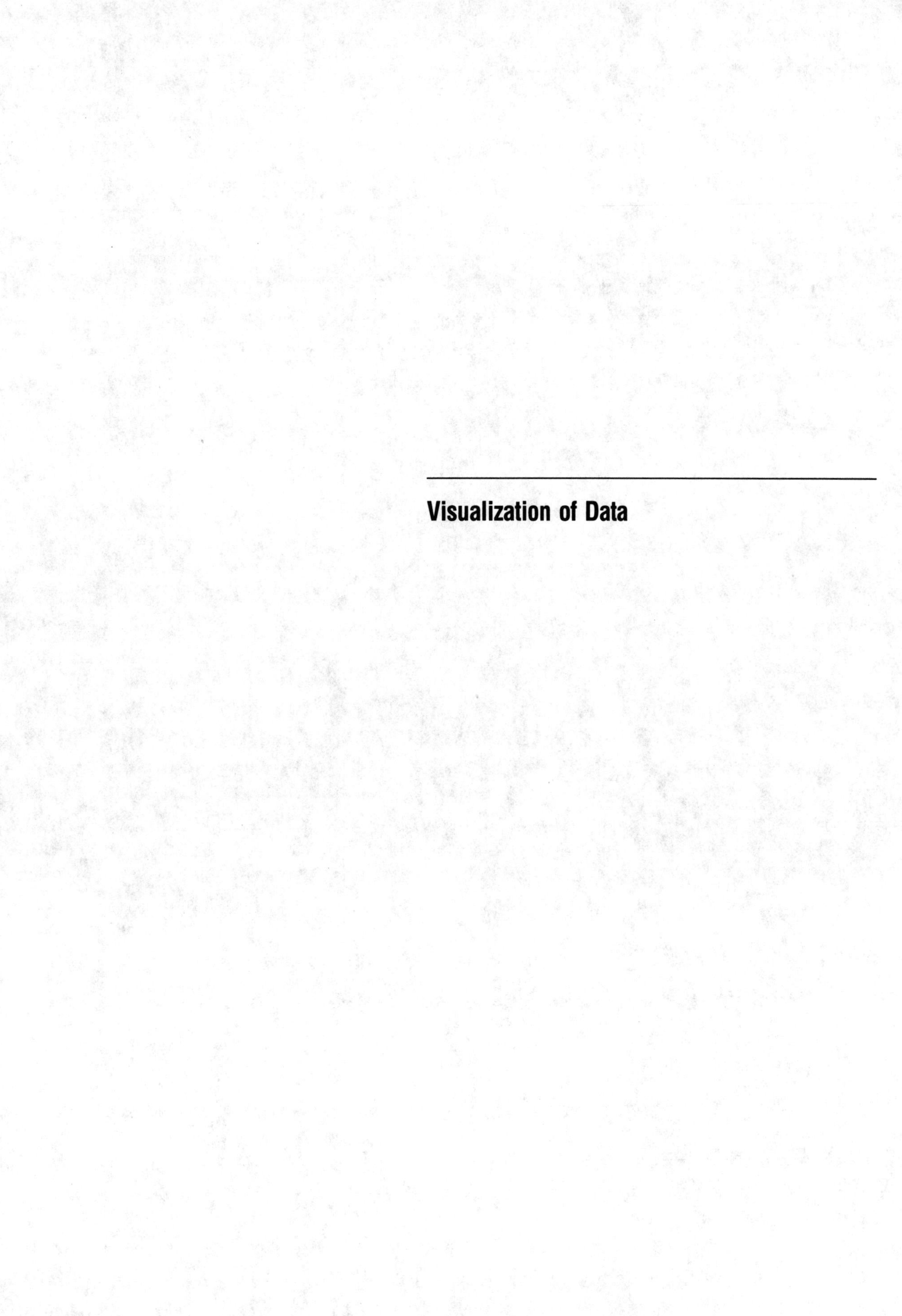

Visualization of Data

Monitor-Driven Data Visualization: SmartDisplay

James Fackler and Isaac Kohane, Children's Hospital and Harvard Medical School

Exhaustive display of all available clinical data, particular in data-rich environments like the intensive care unit, can easily overwhelm the ability of clinicians to comprehend the clinical status and evolution of their patients and may reduce their ability to detect pathological trends in a reliable and timely manner. SmartDisplay is a system we have designed that restricts the data sets displayed to time-lines of those parameters that are relevant to the patient context and to the particular care provider. The relevance criteria are provided by monitoring programs which may range in complexity from simple threshold alarms to full-fledged diagnostic engines. SmartDisplay can specify which parameters to display and the time intervals during which they should be displayed.

INTRODUCTION

In intensive care units, it is not unusual for a patient to be instrumented with a half-dozen probes generating over twenty signals sampled very frequently (between every few milliseconds to every minute). The same patient will also have fluid flux noted every hour or half hour. A number of clinical measurements and laboratory studies will be obtained every day or every few hours. Clinically significant physiological effects may occur over seconds (e.g. increased heart rate) to weeks (increased creatinine clearance). Knowledge of the data trends may provide the clinician with an opportunity to observe (even over multiple caregivers) such effects and therefore change therapy accordingly. A graphical summary of this data may permit rapid communication of these trends [1].

Most commercially available bedside critical-care monitors only provide two types of data display: a view of all signals monitored over the last 30 to 60 seconds and a summary view that allows the user to scroll (sometimes at varying levels of temporal resolution or granularity) through the last few hours to days worth of data. Such capabilities are often grossly inadequate to communicate effectively to the clinician what important events may have happened or are happening to the patient. To begin with, the data displayed on these monitors contains, at the most, 25% of the data which can be obtained on-line and in real-time [2]. Furthermore, a patient will be in the ICU for days or even weeks. Consequently, simply displaying a scrolling window over a two-week history of each measured parameter is likely to be unhelpful.

The nature of the data visualization requirements can be perhaps best considered in the context of the monitor responsibilities of an ICU nurse. Typically, he will be intermittently watching the monitors for evidence of current or impending cardiopulmonary pathology and therefore will be interested in only the last few minutes of monitored data (e.g. the heart rate as measured from the ECG). However, there are some parameters that are worth tracking over the entire period the patient was monitored. For instance, prior to administering a specified dose of a potentially toxic, renally-cleared antibiotic, knowledge of how much of the antibiotic was administered over the past week and at what level of serum creatinine would serve as a check to avoid erroneous dosing. The question this begs is: which parameters should be displayed and what period of time should each parameter display cover? This paper describes one methodology for answering this question and some examples of its use in critical-care data sets obtained at Children's Hospital.

The intuition that underlies the approach we have taken is that existing decision support programs that are capable of monitoring primary or "raw" bedside data provide important clues as to which parameters are relevant to display and when. Whether these monitoring programs implement simple boundary or threshold alarms or provide full-fledged differential diagnoses, the presumption is that they have been engineered to flag relevant data items or collections of data in a timely manner. Furthermore, even if the specifics of a hypothesized fault are incorrect, simply displaying the data that triggered the hypothesized fault may serve as a useful alert of a current or impending pathological trend or event. The central contribution of the research described here is in providing a language and an interpreter to translate the outputs of a wide range of monitoring programs into relevant data displays using off-the-shelf display technologies. We call this language and its interpreter SmartDisplay.

Related Work

Significant work has been accomplished in transforming numerical data into novel, concise visual metaphors that summarize large data sets (e.g. [1,3,4]. The investigations of Cousins and Kahn [5]. are closest to our own interests. They has been particularly influential in the design of the display layout or formatting components of the SmartDisplay language.

DESIGN ASSUMPTIONS

In the design of SmartDisplay we have made some simplifying assumptions about the format

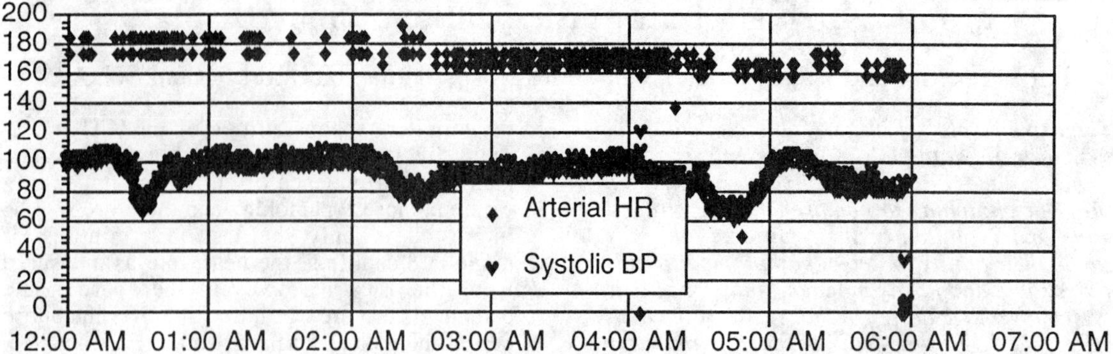

Figure 1: Six hour plot of heart rate and systolic blood pressure both measured via intra-arterial catheter.

of the data displayed. If these assumptions prove to be too limiting, we can revise them subsequently.

First, we assume that the clinician will be viewing clinical data trends on a rectangular screen of fixed area. Within the rectangular area are one or more horizontal lanes, vertically stacked, each with potentially independent temporal granularity or scale along the abscissa. Each horizontal lane or *time-line* can be independently labeled with a legend. One or more parameters can be plotted within each horizontal lane with the parameter value determining the position of a point or bar along the ordinate of a time-line.

Second, we assume that SmartDisplay will not control when a SmartDisplay specified set of time-lines (a *display set*) is executed. Nor does it control for what length of time the executed display set will remain on the screen before it is updated. These decisions are dependent on the particular class of monitoring programs that trigger the execution of a display and therefore require control logic that is outside the scope of SmartDisplay.

Third, we assume that display sets of interest will vary with the clinician (nurse, respiratory therapist, physician) observing the patient and the particular patient.

Finally, SmartDisplay should be able to support all the classes of monitoring programs listed below and be able to generate the displays described for each class.

Threshold/boundary alert

Display: If pH < 7.2 at time *t1* then display pH and pCO2 for a 24 hour interval prior to *t1*.

Single or Boolean combination of simple filters:

Display: Whenever: mean Heart Rate (HR) < 80 for at least 60 seconds and mean Systolic Blood Pressure (SBP) > 200 for at least 2 minutes then display Diastolic Blood Pressure (DBP) from the beginning of the interval of HR < 80 to the end of the interval of SBP > 200.

Automated abstraction engines

Programs such as Shahar's RÉSUMÉ [6] and Russ' TCS [7] automatically generate abstractions of primary data over time and parameter value. Display: For all abstracted intervals of increasing diastolic blood pressure, display heart rate during these same intervals.

Pattern-driven trend-detection engines

Some programs such as TrenDx [8] and DIAMON-1 [9] distinguish between competing knowledge-engineered archetypal patterns of parameter variation over time by comparing the degree to which primary data match or fit these archetypal patterns. Display: For the leading archetypal pattern engineered to detect falling blood pressure associated with manually-assisted ("hand-bagging") ventilation, display the heart rate during the interval from 2 minutes prior to the drop in blood pressure until the end of "hand bagging".

SPECIFICATIONS FOR THE SMARTDISPLAY LANGUAGE

We will motivate the specification for the SmartDisplay Language by working through an example monitoring task on patient data obtained from the Children's Hospital Multidisciplinary Intensive Care Unit. Figure 1 illustrates a graph of HR, SBP and DBP over a six hour period of a patient with Adult Respiratory Distress Syndrome.

SmartDisplay requires that for each relevant output or *trigger* of a monitoring program the following tuple or *display set* should be defined:

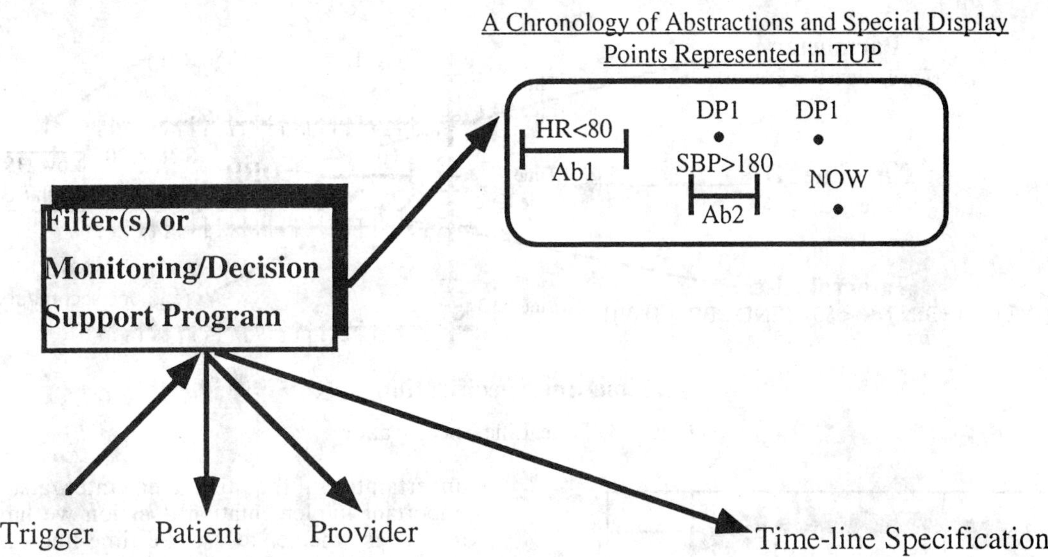

Figure 2: SmartDisplay Display Set Specification

{Provider, Patient, Chronology, Trigger, Time-Line Specification}

where *provider* specifies the class of provider for which the display set is appropriate, and *patient* the patient for which the display set is appropriate. *Trigger* provides a pointer to the output of a monitoring program that triggered the execution of this display set. For example, if the following pair of filters: mean Heart Rate (HR) < 80 for at least 60 seconds and mean Systolic Blood Pressure (SBP) > 200 for at least 2 minutes generated an alert in a monitoring program, the alert would constitute the trigger of the display set. *Chronology* specifies a set of partially ordered points and/or intervals and their temporal relationships. This partial order is expressed in the temporal representation language of the Temporal Utility Program (TUP) [10]. The intervals and points represented in the chronology are referenced in the Time Line Specification which controls what actually appears on the clinician's display screen. Chronologies must be generated by any monitoring program designed to communicate with the SmartDisplay interpreter. In the example we have used, the chronology would include the duration and relative order of the intervals of HR < 80 and SBP > 200. In addition to the points and intervals in the chronology the SmartDisplay interpreter also recognizes references in the Time-Line Specification to two privileged time points: NOW (the present, in real-time) and TimeTriggered (the time the trigger was issued by the monitoring program). Figure 2 illustrates the components of the display set tuple.

A time-line specification determines how a graphing program will display each parameter along the horizontal lanes or time-lines described above. Time-line specifications are lists of the following form:

{(TL-ID, parameter,label, scale,{interval list})}

where *TL-ID* uniquely identifies a horizontal lane or time-line on the fixed rectangular display. *Parameter* specifies which parameter is to be plotted, *label* specifies a textual annotation for the time line. Labels are most useful if they bear a direct relationship to the alert message of the trigger. The *interval list* describes those times during which the specified parameter should be displayed. The intervals in the interval list are specified with respect to the interval endpoints and other points of the TUP chronology generated by the triggering monitoring program. *Scale* is the suggested time-scale or temporal resolution for that time-line. It can be overridden by the SmartDisplay interpreter if it does not permit the display within the fixed width of the display area of parameter values during times covered by the interval list. Figure 3 diagrams an instance of a time-line specification for the pair of HR and SBP filters described above. Figure 4 diagrams the time-line generated by the example display set tuple.

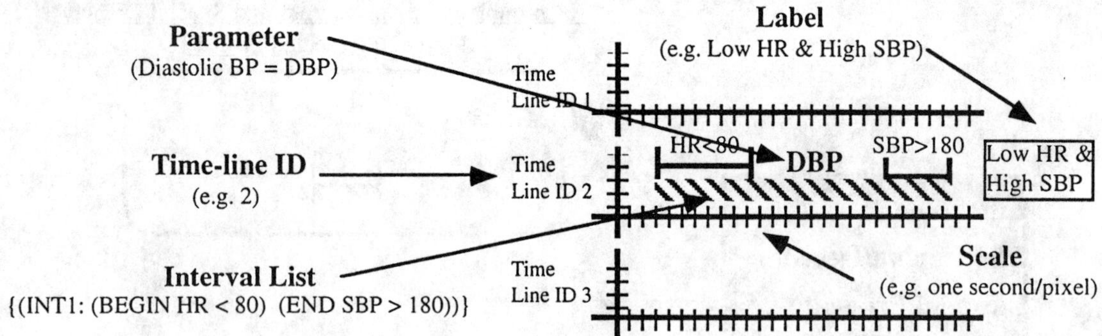

Figure 3: Time-Line Specification.

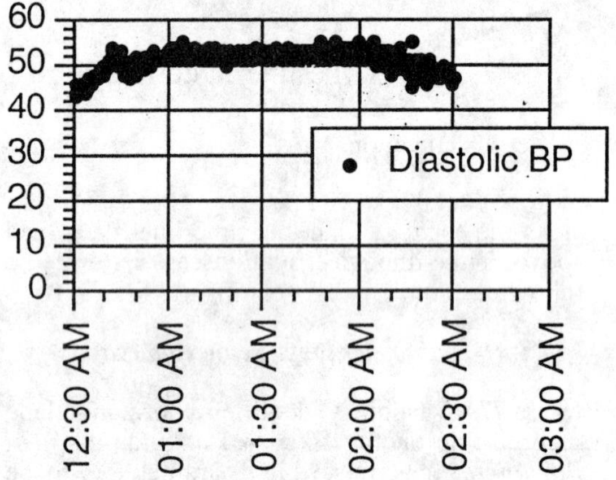

Figure 4: Result of Execution of Example Display Set.

Although the example we have used is contrived and quite simple, the SmartDisplay language enables the specification of a wide range of displays. Multiple parameters can be plotted across each time-line in multiple (disjoint or overlapping) intervals and temporal granularity can vary across time-lines. This would enable a knowledge engineer to write a display set that, when triggered, could show along one time-line the immediate hemodynamic effects of a drug and along another time-line the entire history of the intervals during which the patient received infusions of that drug.

IMPLEMENTATION STATUS

Earlier in the development of the display language we attempted hand-simulations of the operation of the SmartDisplay interpreter using TrenDx as the monitoring program [11]. These simulations led to the current definition of the SmartDisplay language. We are currently implementing the SmartDisplay interpreter. The program is currently able to plot displays whose chronologies only contain intervals with fixed endpoints. That is, there cannot be temporal uncertainty in the displayed intervals. One important implementation decision we have to resolve is whether to use the time-line display source code that Dr. Michael Kahn has kindly provided (from his earlier work on this subject [5]) or instead have the SmartDisplay interpreter generate graphing commands that are then executed by a commercial graphics package. Several graphing/plotting software packages available on personal computers now support some level of interprocess communications (e.g. OLE or AppleEvents). However, we have yet to determine if these packages can provide the SmartDisplay interpreter with sufficient control of the display through the available interprocess communications protocols.

CONCLUSION

We have described a language, SmartDisplay, that is intended to exploit the operation of a wide range of monitoring programs to focus the attention of clinicians onto a relevant subset of the available measured patient parameters by displaying them over specified intervals.

As it is currently defined, the SmartDisplay language has some significant limitations. First, it requires that a knowledge engineer select the relevant intervals and parameters and encode the display sets for each monitoring program intended to work with the SmartDisplay interpreter. Second, the language does not have any provision to direct the synthesis of a single display for each parameter when it is specified in multiple display sets (e.g. when two monitoring programs specify the display of heart rate).

Also, we have yet to answer several important questions. These include:

• Does SmartDisplay improve the rate at which clinicians accurately detect pathological processes? Is any change in performance related to the amount of data presented compared to commercial display systems?

• What are the control issues regarding the duration and update frequency of each display? How do these issues depend upon the nature of the monitoring programs?

Answers to these questions require testing SmartDisplay in conditions closely approximating clinical practice. In the short term however, we are working on completing the implementation of the SmartDisplay interpreter.

References

1. Tufte, E. R. *Envisioning Information*; Graphics Press: Cheshire, CT, 1990.

2. Fackler, J. C.; Kohane, I. S. Integration of sparse data from a clinical workstation with continuous data from bedside monitors. In: *Sixth Annual IEEE Symposium on Computer-Based Medical Systems.* Ann Arbor, Michigan: IEEE Computer Society Press, 1993:289-294.

3. Cole, W. G.; Stewart, J. G. Metaphor graphics to support integrated decision making with respiratory data. *International Journal of Clinical Monitoring and Computing* 1993, *10*, 91-100.

4. Wenkebach, U. Visualization of large datasets in intensive care. *Proceedings of Sixteenth Annual Symposium on Computer Applications in Medical Care.* 1992, 18-22.

5. Cousins, S. B.; Kahn, M. G. The visual display of temporal information. *Artificial Intelligence in Medicine* 1991, *3*, 341-357.

6. Shahar, Y.; Tu, S.; Musen, M. Knowledge acquisition for temporal abstraction mechanisms. *Knowledge Acquisition* 1992, *1*, 217-236.

7. Russ, T. A. Using hindsight in medical decision making. *Computer Methods and Programs in Biomedicine* 1990, *32*, 81-90.

8. Haimowitz, I. J.; Kohane, I. S. An Epistemology for Clinically Significant Trends. In: *National Conference on Artificial Intelligence.* Washington, D.C.: 1993:176-181.

9. Steimann, F.; Adlassnig, K. P. Clinical monitoring with fuzzy automata. *Fuzzy Sets and Systems* 1994, *61*, 37-43.

10. Kohane, I. S. Temporal reasoning in medical expert systems. In: *MEDINFO 86/Fifth World Congress on Medical Informatics.* R. Salomon, B. Blum and M. Jørgensens, Eds., Washington, D.C.: Elsevier Science Publishers, 1986:170-174.

11. Fackler, J.; Haimowitz, I. J.; Kohane, I. S. Knowledge-based Data Display Using TrenDx. In: Technical Report SS-94-01: *AAAI Spring Symposium: Interpreting Clinical Data.* Palo Alto: AAAI Press, 1994: 37-41.

Visualization and Analysis of Co-occurrence and Cross-tabulation data in Medical Research

Joseph I. Bormel, M.D., UCLA Center for Health Sciences
Linda R. Ferguson, Ph.D., UCLA Office of Academic Computing

ABSTRACT

Analyzing raw data can be prohibitively time consuming. A variety of graphical techniques have been developed to address this problem. Although graphical analysis can provide a simple yet comprehensive overview of a large dataset, often these techniques fail to capture the essence of data trends. In addition, the ability to easily query any component of the data subset frequently remains burdensome. In this paper, we present a general method to address these issues for cross-tabulation tables and provide examples of their use in medical research.

INTRODUCTION

Graphical display of information in medicine presents a variety of challenges[1]. For many applications, simple numerical tables of frequencies provides the first step in analyzing the patterns in the data set. Often, the next step in looking for patterns is summarizing all observations in a database along two axes to form a cross-tabulation or co-occurrence table. Frequently, these methods of viewing data fail to reveal important trends.

Recognizing significant patterns of disease progression in a large patient population over time is a task which demonstrates these difficulties. We recently studied a cohort of 410 patients from Cooperative Systematic Studies of Rheumatic Diseases (CSSRD) clinics[2]. These patients were entered from ten university-based rheumatology clinics in a prospective study within one year of onset of connective tissue disease (CTD). The purpose of the study was to gain a better understanding of progression or remission of undifferentiated connective tissue diseases (UCTD). Correlation between disease features at entry and subsequent remission were examined to identify features at entry that predict remission. These 410 patients were divided initially into 18 disease subgroups which over time redistributed into 25 disease subgroups. We identified disease progression via transition paths between disease subgroups, which show the number of patients who eventually develop another disease or enter remission versus those who remain in the same disease subgroup.

We developed a graphical exploratory method to find the important relationships in the data, as well as to facilitate more in-depth examination. First, we used a statistical program's procedure (SAS's proc freq, a frequency determining procedure) to produce a cross-tabulation table to show *Inital Diagnoses* and *Final Diagnoses*. This table showed the number of patients with each disease at entry into the study (initial diagnosis) and which disease category they were in at the last examination (final diagnosis). An example of such a table is shown in **table 1**. As described in this paper, we then developed a Visual Basic program to generate a graphical display of the data which supported further analysis on an interactive basis. This method is applicable to all forms of cross-tabulation tables, whether they arise from statistical packages as ours did, or relational database models of computerized patient records.

BACKGROUND

Exploratory Data Analysis (EDA) software facilitates unstructured, iterative visual exploration of relationships in complex datasets with the aid of multiple graphical displays linked to the data's information content. EDA methods can be essential in analyses of data sets because they can provide perspectives which would otherwise be obscured or completely hidden, especially when the data volume and variation contained is massive. EDA methods have been used in conjunction with statistical methods to build prediction models in medicine and psychiatry[3,4]. In addition to proving useful in enabling study of data from multiple perspectives and uncovering elusive data trends, it is also a powerful communications tool in the subsequent presentation of these findings.

To successfully view large amounts of clinical data, it is necessary to integrate a database management system, graphical

Table 1

TABLE OF Initial Diagnoses BY Final Diagnoses

Initial Diagnoses / *Frequency, Percent, Row Pct, Col Pct*	**Final Diagnoses**: Missing	Bad disease1	Bad disease2	Dead	Mild disease1	Remis-sion	...
Bad disease1 (Bad_dz1)	25 6.10 28.74 21.19	33 8.05 37.93 67.35	3 0.73 3.45 6.67	8 1.95 9.20 21.62	5 1.22 5.75 13.89	9 2.20 10.34 27.27	...
Mild disease1	27 6.59 31.40 22.88	4 0.98 4.65 8.16	10 2.44 11.63 22.22	3 0.73 3.49 8.11	24 5.85 27.91 66.67	7 1.71 8.14 21.21	...
Bad disease2	21 5.12 33.87 17.80	1 0.24 1.61 2.04	29 7.07 46.77 64.44	5 1.22 8.06 13.51	0 0.00 0.00 0.00	4 0.98 6.45 12.12	...
Mild disease2	13 ...	10 ...	1 ...	2 ...	4 ...	7 ...	... ...

display and statistical software. [5] We were not aware of any program that would integrate with the SAS system to perform the interactive graphical EDA techniques necessary. We therefore developed the Visual Basic program described in this paper.

METHODS

Our initial representation of our study population's disease course, shown in **table 1** was produced using the SAS PROC FREQ procedure. The table shows initial visit diagnosis by final visit diagnosis in an abbreviated fashion and using generalized labels (e.g. *Bad disease1* instead of the actual disease name). All possible courses a patient could take are represented by cells in this table. The full table included 18 categories of initial diseases (shown in the rows) and 25 categories of disease at the completion of the study (shown in the columns). In this sample table, the first cell containing 25 represents 25 patients with an initial diagnosis of 'Bad disease1' whose final diagnosis state was 'Missing'. Similarly, the next cell down containing 27 represents patients who initially had 'Mild disease1' whose final diagnosis was 'Missing'. This table did not convey a clear sense of our data due to the large number of cells, size disparity between adjacent rows and columns, sparseness and separation over multiple pages. Thus, it was difficult to identify the significant transition paths that link patients' initial and final diagnoses.

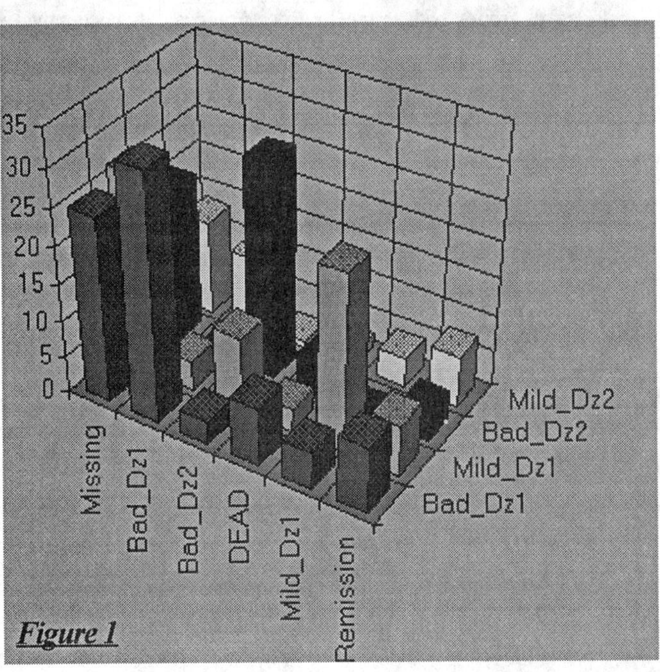

Figure 1

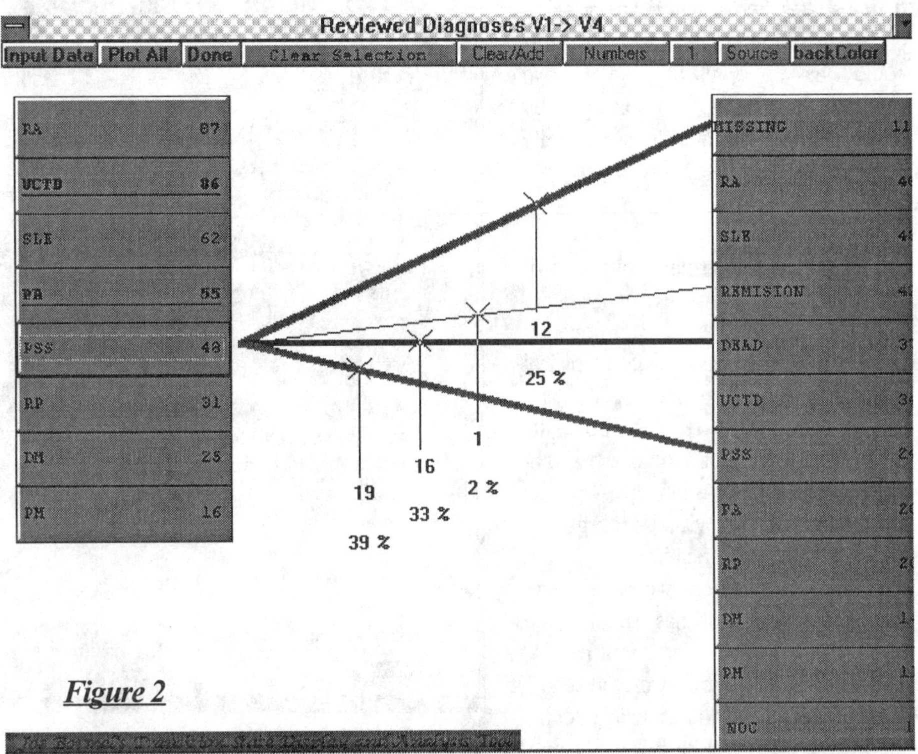

Figure 2

To facilitate interpretation, the next step was to convert the table into a graphical format. This can be done in many ways using a variety of graphing tools and techniques[6].

A graphical depiction of **table 1** using a three dimensional model (created with Microsoft Excel, in **figure 1**) was only a slight improvement. It did not communicate the flow of patients between subgroups. To overcome this, a pilot program was written to graphically represent the number of patients following each transition path. This tool was subsequently extended in Visual Basic to allow interactive query of patient subpopulations, by user subgroup selection and automatic generation of procedure code to statistically analyze those subgroups.

A sample display produced by this Visual Basic program is shown in **figure 2**. The initial disease selected in this case is PSS (Progressive Systemic Sclerosis)[7]. It was selected by pointing to the button containing the legend "PSS" with a mouse and selecting it with a mouse button press. This caused the distribution of these patients' disease courses to be displayed. For example, the top line, connecting PSS on the left to MISSING on the right, represents 12 patients, or 25% of all of the 48 patients initially diagnosed with the disease PSS. Any patient subgroup can be selected in this way, with the specific disease progression pattern instantly displayed. The interactive nature of this process combined with the clearing of data which is unrelated to the currently chosen subgroup helps to selectively focus the user 's attention.

Although this example demonstrates two categorical variables, each containing a diagnosis, the table could have represented any two categorical variables. For example, by selecting age group and disease severity variables, a display of this relationship would result.

Based on this visual exploration of the data, the correlates of patients' disease transitions were subsequently studied in the traditional statistical manner with chi square, logistic and categorical models. For example, the effect of age on likelihood of achieving a remission was studied[8]. The availability of this visual tool greatly facilitated the identification of relevant variables. In addition, we have found that this visual tool has enabled the results of complicated multivariate models to be summarized and presented more effectively to nontechnical people.

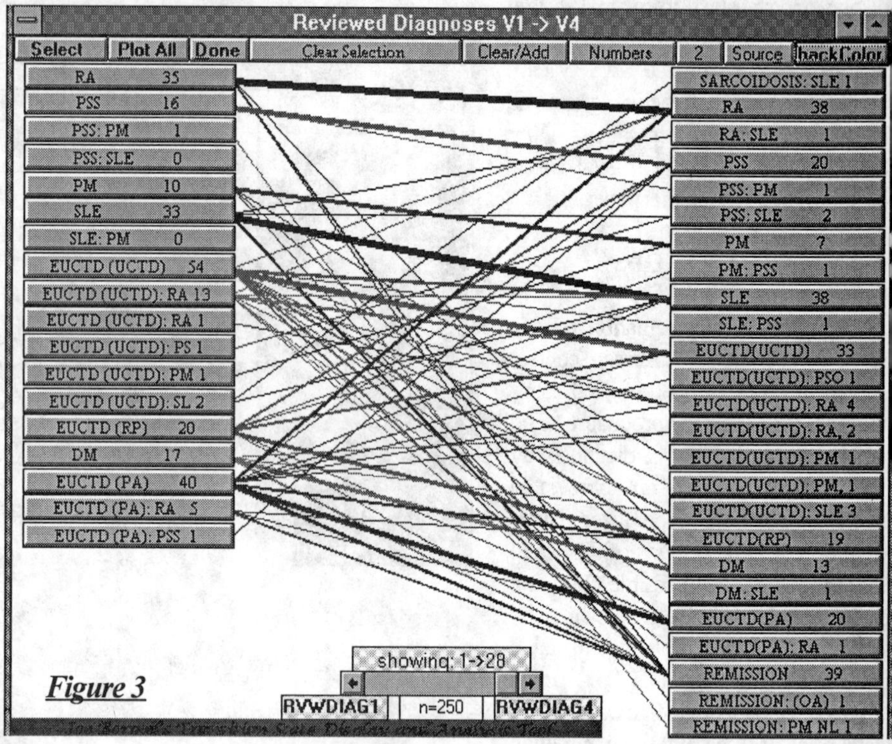

Figure 3

SYSTEM DESIGN

Implementing this method involved the use of two programming languages, Visual Basic and PERL[9]. Visual Basic is a commercial programming language sold by Microsoft Corporation. It is well suited to building graphical user interfaces and to quickly developing simple programs. There are many books and articles which describe programming in this language.

The second language, Perl, was developed by Larry Wall in 1986. It officially stands for Practical Extraction and Report Language and is ideal for extracting data from files and reformatting the data for other purposes. It is distributed with source code and is available at no charge. In the application described above, a Perl program translated the SAS PROC FREQ output into data more easily usable by the Visual Basic code.

In the course of developing the visualization engine and enhancing its interactive capabilities, it became clear that SAS's data subsetting and analysis capabilities and SAS's expressivity were fundamental components for powerful interactive analysis. For these reasons, we have been developing a generalized graphical front-end for data analysis which is specifically designed to facilitate analyses of disease transition in populations over time. The user can interactively select variables contained in an application's tables, and the Visual Basic program will graphically depict the relationships.

Using this approach, co-occurrence data containing large numbers of subsets can be quickly examined. For example, **figure 3** summarizes the disease course of the 250 non-missing patients in the earlier mentioned study. All transition paths, even those containing only one patient is shown. Thicker lines represent larger numbers of patients. Because of the density of information, this display is of limited use. However, some large patterns are evident. Also, on a color display, the display is slightly more useful.

To exclude subsets that occurred less frequently, a threshold can be adjusted to allow the user to focus on the larger groups. This signficantly reduces the cluttered appearance. The result is shown in **figure 4** which contains the same data as **figure 3**, but excludes all groups with less than 8 occurrences. By successively increasing this threshold, the interface allows you to decompose

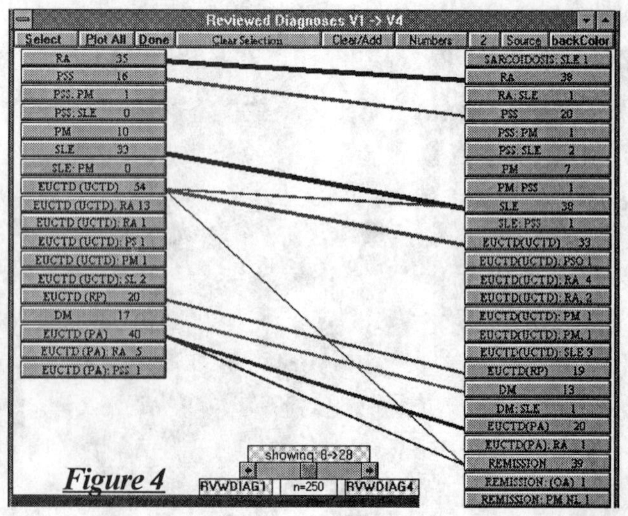

Figure 4

the data to its most coarse features. Similarly, the threshold can be incrementally decreased to reveal the full granularity.

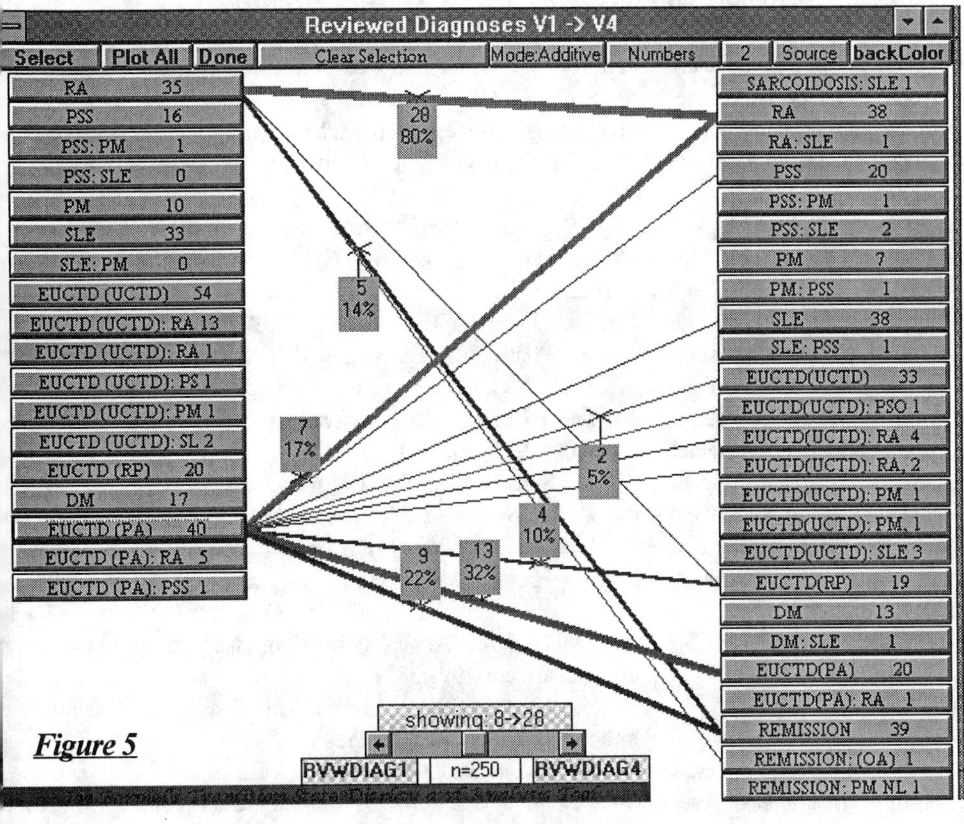

Figure 5

This technique also supports the direct visual comparison of multiple groups simultaneously. For example, the behavior of populations expected to have comparable distributions is shown in **figure 5**. Although it was anticipated that the Rheumatoid Arthritis (RA) <top left> and Early Undifferentiated Connective Tissue Disease/PolyArthritis (EUCTD(PA)) <bottom left> groups would have a similar distribution, it is visually apparent that the EUCTD(PA) group showed a considerably more variable course. Although the majority (80%) of the patients initially diagnosed with RA remained with RA as their final diagnosis, the EUCTD(PA) patients did not have nearly as predictable a course. By overlying data in this way, it is also possible to direct the computer to lump together groups that have similar characteristics for further analysis. This was implemented for SAS and is shown in **figure 6**. By visually selecting the subgroups of interest, a SAS program (procedure) is constructed by Visual Basic. A similar technique could have generated structured query language (SQL) code for a relational database. The size of the resultant group, in this case 35 patients, is shown in the title bar of the window where the procedure appears. You will also note that there is a button labeled "Show Selection" which will show just the selected transition paths. This subsetting can be built up interactively to include any combinations of subgroups, including groups not currently displayed.

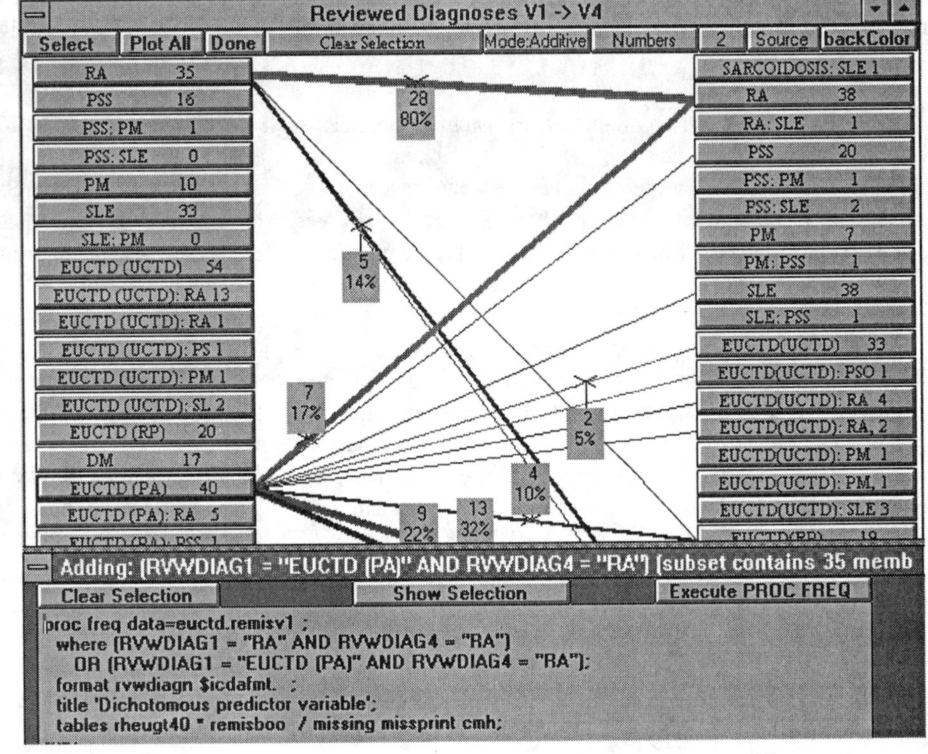

Figure 6

Finally, this tool has proven to be an effective way to communicate the contained relationships to others. We therefore added the ability to relocate displayed elements and dynamically connect the transition paths, to allow demonstration of another dimension of relationships such as groupings of related categories. Techniques like this, as well as the judicious use of color allow the user to selectively focus on the hilighted relationships, and to re-frame the view by changing the order or spatial relationships of elements. This is useful in identifying additional data relationships and for teaching purposes.

By using this tool, several patterns in our data became apparent. The remission rates for undifferentiated polyarthritis and rheumatoid arthritis were not different, although many of the undifferentiated polyarthritis patients had a milder disease course. These findings are shown in **figure 5**. The Visual Basic system, by writing the appropriate SAS program code, made it easier to find the correlates of disease course. Predictors of remission were determined by selecting subgroups from the visual display and conducting statistical tests for symptoms and laboratory values. The resulting predictors of remission included seronegativity, low sedimentation rate and low tender joint counts[8].

CONCLUSION

Significant improvements in quantitative data display result from visual representations achieved through graphical user interfaces. The use of custom graphics to visualize cross tabulation tables can augment existing tools such as statistics packages, speed interpretation of data, and facilitate presentation of complex analytical results. Prior techniques for data representation did not convert co-occurrence information into an interactive graphical display. Our system enabled us to graphically visualize important relationships in the data and facilitated in-depth examination of co-occurrence data.

We hope to extend this approach to automate analysis of independent variables. This will be done by facilitating menu selection of logical independent and dependent variables, generating dichotomized variables where indicated, and then summarizing these relationships through programmatically generated and dispatched statistical procedures and data steps.

Future substantive applications include analyses where a large number of discrete variables are associated with an outcome. Examples include sociological studies of occupational mobility, management studies of firm birth and attrition, or quality assurance studies of defect data. A variety of implementation paths are possible including development within the SAS System as a user-defined procedure (e.g., using SAS/TOOLKIT), as a SAS application (modeled after SAS/ASSIST which features pull-down menus with "point and click" options), or entirely in Visual Basic.

REFERENCES

1. Cole, W.G., *Integrality and Meaning: Essential and Orthogonal Dimensions of Graphical Data Display.* in Proceedings of the Seventeenth Annual SCAMC Convention. 1993. Washington, DC. McGraw Hill.

2. Alarcon G.S., et al. *Early Undifferentiated Connective Tissue Disease. I. Early Clinical Manifestation In A Large Cohort Of Patients With Undifferentiated Connective Tissue Diseases Compared With Cohorts Of Well Established Connective Tissue Disease.* Journal of Rheumatology, 1991 Sep, 18(9):1332-9.

3. Politser PE; Berwick KM; Murphy JM; Goldman PA; Weinstein MC. *Uncovering Psychiatric Test Information With Graphical Techniques Of Exploratory Data Analysis.* Psychiatry Research, 1991 Oct, 39(1):65-9.

4. Stinson CH; Horowitz MJ. *Psyclops: An Exploratory Graphical System For Clinical Research And Education.* Psychiatry, 1993 Nov, 56(4):375-89.

5. Herrmann FR; Safran C. *Exploring A Hospital-Wide Database: Integrating Statistical Functions With ClinQuery.* Proceedings of the Annual symposium on computer Applications in Medical Care, 1991:583-7.

6. Tufte, E.R., The Visual Display of Quantitative Information. 1983, Graphic Press.

7. Bulpitt K.J., Clements P.J., et al. *Early Undifferentiated Connective Tissue Disease: Iii. Outcome And Prognostic Indicators In Early Scleroderma (Systemic Sclerosis).* Annals of Internal Medicine, 1993 Apr 15, 118(8):602-9.

8. Bormel, JI, Clements P, Paulus, H, Ferguson, L. *Early Undifferentiated Connective Tissue Disease (Euctd) Study: Remissions In Patients Presenting With Polyarthritis.* American College of Rheumatology 57th Annual Scientific Meeting. 1993.

9. Wall, Larry and Randal L. Schwartz, Programming Perl, 1991 O'Reilly & Associates.

TRADEMARKS

ACKNOWLEDGMENTS

Dr. Bormel is currently a fellow supported by the National Library of Medicine (grant LM07092-01).

Thanks to Kevin Nechodom at the CSSRD in Salt Lake City, Utah, for unwavering support, encouragement, and constructive feedback. Thanks to Dr. Douglas S. Bell of the Design Systems Group at the Brigham and Womens Hospital, Boston, Massachusetts for the concept of threshold views which greatly improved the display capabilities. Thanks to the UCLA Division of Rheumatology and the CSSRD for the opportunity to develop this project, and to the Laboratory of Computer Science at MGH for assistance completing this paper.

Making the Relationships Visible: Testing Alternative Display Design Strategies for Teaching Principles of Hemodynamic Monitoring and Treatment

Judith A. Effken PhD, RN, CNA, Hartford Hospital, Hartford CT;
Nam-Gyoon Kim PhD, and Robert E. Shaw PhD, Center for the Ecological Study of Perception and Action, University of Connecticut.

A hemodynamic monitoring and control task was used to explore the utility of perceptually based displays to teach basic hemodynamic principles. The baseline display showed discrete values of key hemodynamic data elements. Alternative displays showed (a) anatomical relationships between those elements, and (b) causal constraints. Critical care nurses and student nurses used simulated "drugs" to correct simple hemodynamic disturbances using the three displays. Showing the anatomic constraints on pressure and flow improved treatment coordination by novices. Showing how etiological factors related to symptoms shortened the time required to reach a criterion level of performance and improved treatment coordination for both novices and experts.

INTRODUCTION

Over the past twenty years, sophisticated monitoring devices have become commonplace in critical care units and have proved beneficial in many ways. The new technology provides an observable window on what may be an otherwise unobservable state of the patient and allows clinicians to obtain rapid, frequent, repeated measures of physiological parameters so clinicians can detect potential problems before overt symptoms develop and titrate various drugs to maintain patient parameters within optimal ranges. But these innovations in critical care technology have also produced new problems [1]. Despite their many technological improvements, most monitoring devices still function as "single-sensor-single-indicator" devices [2]. That is, for each device used, a single variable is recorded. From the various data elements generated by independent sensors, clinicians must select and integrate those parameters relevant to the immediate situation. This results in sequential, piecemeal data gathering [3] that, in physiological monitoring tasks, precludes a more coherent understanding of the interrelationships of system functions and their underlying physiologic mechanisms [4].

Even though newer computer network-based monitoring systems are attempting to bring signals and alarms into a consistent format, they have not been able to solve what is essentially a multivariate analysis task for the clinician [5]. The clinician must still decide which information to use at a given time and how those variables relate. It is this task that educators teaching hemodynamic monitoring find most difficult for their students to learn.

The problem clinicians face can be understood as an example of the more general problem of perception. That is, how does an observer achieve the mapping of very many atomic elements into the perception of a chair, a sunny day, or an old friend? Similarly, how does the clinician as perceptual system achieve the mapping of very many atomic elements into a few categories of information? Given the equivalence of the clinical and perceptual problems, knowledge gained from the study of perception may be useful in creating displays that will be useful in teaching diagnosis and treatment.

One potentially useful concept is Gibson's characterization of information as higher-order invariants--patterns of persistence and change that structure the relevant medium in ways that are specific to the environmental facts they represent [6, 7]. For example, in vision, the source of information is the optic array which is structured by light reflecting off the various surfaces and substances that make up the environment. The transitions in the patterning of light are specific to the faces and facets of surfaces. Since this kind of structure is available to be perceived from the outset, it need not be added by the perceiver.

Additional support for this line of thinking comes from research on expertise. Studies of chess players [8, 9] have shown that experts rely heavily on their ability to detect familiar patterns. Clinicians too rely heavily on perception. Clinical experts easily detect the underlying structure of a previously experienced class of problems [10, 11]. Indeed, for experts, perception often precedes conception [10].

We have used Gibson's theory of direct perception to develop display designs that exploit perception by showing the inherent relationships between data elements. The purpose of this paper is to explore the utility of these displays as devices for teaching novices the complex relationships that underlie hemodyamic monitoring and treatment.

DESIGNING THE DISPLAYS

Traditionally, the inherent complexity of hemodynamic processes has seemed to demand one description for arterial hemodynamics, another for cardiac hemodynamics, etc. Overall descriptions are rarely seen. One exception is a well-known approach of Guyton [12], in which the major components of the hemodynamic system are treated as interconnected compartments in an effort to understand the more global relationships between pressures and flows. Guyton has developed a computer simulation which, in its most basic version, shows the intrinsic constraints on pressure. Arterial, venous, and atrial pressure and cardiac output are dependent variables, and fluid volume, contractility, and resistance are independent variables in the Guyton simulation.

The Guyton data were presented in three different visual formats: a traditional "strip-chart" display [5], an integrated balloon display, and an etiological potentials display. Drug controls are the same for all displays. Participants use six generic "drugs" to treat observed hemodynamic problems. Drugs act on the etiological factors--resistance, contractility, and volume. Participants select a drug and dose, then press a mouse button to give discrete "drug" doses.

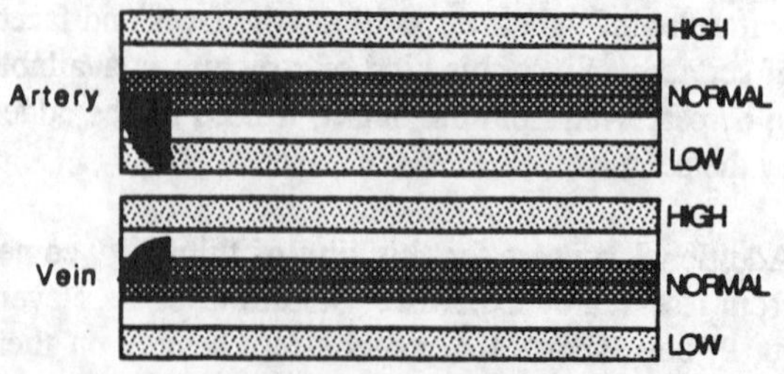

Figure 1. Arterial and venous pressures in TSD

In the traditional strip-chart display (TSD), arterial, venous, and atrial pressure, cardiac output, and resistance are shown as separate bar graphs (Figure 1). The vertical axis is color-coded for target range (green) and danger (red) regions. Values for each parameter are selected by sampling the Guyton simulation at one-second intervals.

The goal of the integrated balloon display (IBD) is to make visible the anatomical constraints on blood pressure and flow (Figure 2). By making the connectivity of the system visible, we hoped to teach participants to anticipate the effect of a change in one component, for example, a drop in right atrial pressure, on a subsequent change in another component, for example, cardiac output. The three pressures are shown as changes in the horizontal dimension of three ellipses (balloons). We have used the "balloon" image as a kinematic analog for the underlying dynamics of blood vessels, which have balloon-like characteristics [13]. The left ventricle is shown as a "bellows" to show the heart's forcing function on blood flow. Two parallel lines connect each compartment to the next. The connector between the arteries and capillary bed indicates changes in resistance by a change in the diameter of the distal end of the connection (a "funnel" metaphor). A bar graph shows overall system status (the mean of the standardized, absolute distances from normal for the four dependent variables).

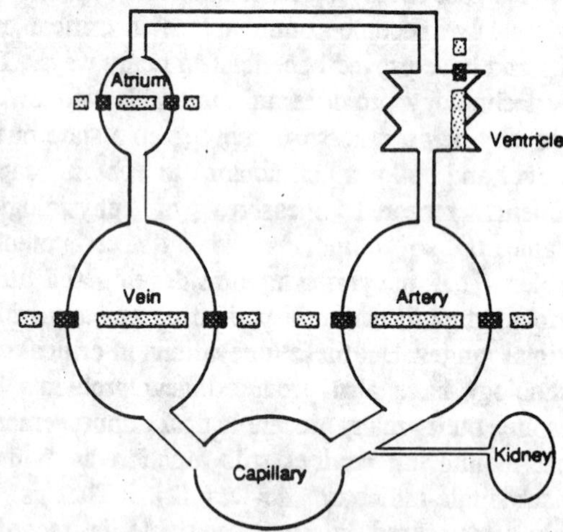

Figure 2. The integrated balloon display

Although the integrated balloon display shows how pressures and flows are constrained by their anatomical connections, it does not show how etiological factors in the model (fluid volume, resistance, and contractility) relate to changes in pressure and flow. Because the etiological components do not have a one-to-one relationship with pressure and flow, learning these relationships is not trivial. To make the relationships clear, a third (etiological potentials, or EPD) display was designed. In EPD, arterial, venous, and atrial pressure, and cardiac output are shown as vertices of a four-sided figure. When values are normal, the figure approximates a square and is located at the center of the window. The square can move in a two-dimensional (etiological) space defined by horizontal and vertical bars that cross at the center of the window. The vertical bar indicates contractility (heart strength); the horizontal axis shows resistance. Fluid changes are shown by an expanding or shrinking square.

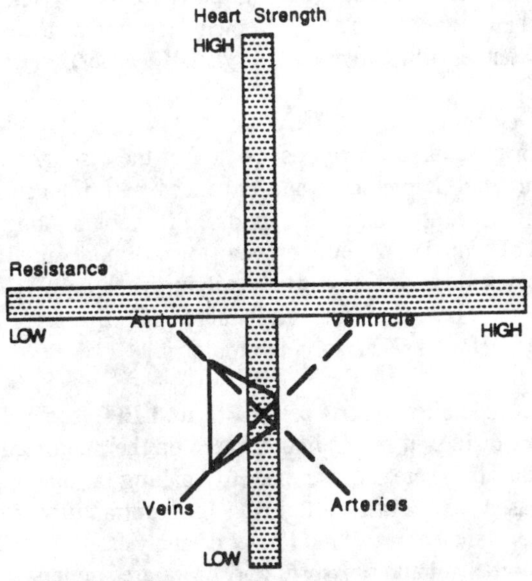

Figure 3. The etiological potentials display

In sum, the strip-chart display shows the values of three pressures and cardiac output as five separate graphs. Presumably, to coordinate treatment, the observer must already know, or must learn, how these discrete values relate. The integrated balloon display provides explicit information about how pressures and flow are connected anatomically. We assume that by seeing how anatomy constrains the values pressure and flow can take, the observer will be able to predict how a change in one will affect others. The etiological display attempts to make explicit how changes in etiological components relate to changes in pressure and flow.

The dynamic simulations were developed and presented on a Sun 4/260 workstation equipped with a 19 inch color monitor and Sun View graphics tools. Participants observed changes in pressure and flow that corresponded to certain disease states and corrected those states using the simulated drugs. To create a scenario ("illness"), the experimenter changes the value of any or all of the control parameters in the Guyton equations. In the experiment reported here, test scenarios were created in conjunction with clinical experts by varying three parameters (resistance, contractility, and fluid volume) to create "illnesses" such as high blood pressure, heart failure, or hypervolemia.

COMPARING THE DISPLAYS

We expected that learning to coordinate treatment quickly and accurately with the traditional strip-chart display (TSD) would be increasingly enhanced by the integrated balloon display (IBD) and the etiological potentials display (EPD) for all participants. However, because experienced critical care nurses are familiar with traditional displays, we expected that they would be able to use each display quite well. In contrast, we expected that student nurses would experience more difficulty learning to use the traditional strip-chart display (TSD) and show continued improvement with each succeeding enhancement (IBD and EPD).

Method

Participants. Six experienced critical care nurses currently enrolled as graduate students at the University of Connecticut School of Nursing served as the "expert" group. Critical care experience of this group ranged from 1-14 years with a mean of 6.17 years. The "novice" group was composed of six senior nursing students at the University of Connecticut.

Design and procedure. Three display types (TSD, IBD, and EPD) and three scenarios (low fluid, high resistance, and low contractility) were within-subjects variables in the mixed design. Participants were shown scenarios depicting common clinical problems and were asked to treat observed "illnesses" using the simulated "drugs."

Participants were given instructions that explained the purpose of the experiment, briefly explained hemodynamics, then described the three displays. The experimenter demonstrated changes participants might see the model undergo with each display. Participants then practiced using the drugs on each display (in a normal state) until comfortable with their use. In practice trials, participants were shown the same scenarios used in the test condition, but at different absolute values. Participants were required to solve each scenario with each display before beginning the experiment. In the test situation, each scenario was presented twice in each display condition. Presentation order of displays and scenarios was randomized.

Results

In addition to the number of practice trials required to solve each scenario using each of the displays, we recorded the number of scenarios solved in the test condition. Other performance measures, such as the time to initiate treatment, percentage of time in the target range, and number of drugs used have been reported elsewhere [14]. Finally, participants were asked to rank order the three displays for their usefulness as a teaching tool at three times during the experiment: after the initial instructions, after the practice trials, and at the end of the experiment.

Number of practice trials to criterion. The number of practice trials participants needed to solve each scenario once with each display ranged from one to six. A 2 (skill level) x 3 (display type) x 3 (scenario) ANOVA revealed, as predicted, a significant main effect of display type $F(2, 20) = 4.61$, $p < .05$. Participants required a mean of 1.63 trials to solve scenarios with TSD or IBD; but only 1.1 trials for EPD. In fact, for all but one subject (an expert), EPD resulted in one-trial learning. Experts required an average of 1.6 trials to solve each scenario with each display type; novices required an average of 1.4 trials. The ANOVA showed that this difference was not significant, $F < 1.0$.

Number of scenarios solved. In the test condition, experts performed very much as anticipated, solving 90% of the scenarios experienced with both TSD and IBD and 97% with EPD. As predicted, novices had more difficulty with TSD and improved significantly with each display enhancement. Novices solved 72% of the scenarios with TSD, 89% with IBD, and 100% with EPD (actually surpassing the experts). A 2 (skill level) x 3 (display type) x 3 (scenario) ANOVA showed that the display differences were significant, $F(2, 20) = 4.26$, $p < .03$. Skill level means (experts = 91.7% and novices = 87%) were ordered as predicted, but this difference was not significant, $F(1, 10) = 1.24$, $p > .10$.

Participant preferences. Participants were asked to rank order the three displays (a) for the purpose of instructing students about blood pressure and flow and (b) for the purpose of solving problems quickly. Experts consistently preferred the integrated balloon display as a teaching tool. Novices' opinions varied greatly and changed over time. Initially, three novices preferred IBD, two preferred EPD, and two preferred TSD. By the end of the experiment, five novices preferred IBD and two preferred TSD. EPD had become the second choice of five novices.

After trying each display, novices unanimously preferred EPD for solving problems. In contrast, experts' preferences varied. At the conclusion of the experiment, three preferred EPD, two preferred IBD, and one preferred TSD. Experts frequently related their preferences to their own learning style (e.g., whether or not they were a "visual" learner).

Discussion

In general, the results showed that the display types ordered as predicted and enhanced performance for novices more than for experts. IBD took as long as TSD to learn, but proved to be more useful--particularly for novices--in solving problems. EPD was easy to learn and more effective for all participants when solving problems.

Anecdotally, experts seemed to find EPD somewhat confusing. It seems likely, based on their comments, that they are accustomed to making a diagnosis based on preload, afterload, and contractility--with resistance at a different level of analysis. When the more available pressures and flows are immersed in the etiology space as an abstract object, experts may become rather disoriented. Even though problems can be solved simply by reducing the error in one of the three etiological dimensions (contractility, resistance, or fluid), some experts focused their attention on the changes in the shape of the "square."

When the context provided by the explicitly shown anatomical linkages in IBD was reduced to allow us to immerse pressure and flow measures into the etiology space, at least part of the semantics usually available to the expert was lost. Less familiar with that context, novices were not bothered by this loss. Consequently, they often performed as well as--or slightly better than--experts when using EPD.

IMPLICATIONS

Although we used a specific task domain (learning the fundamentals of hemodynamic monitoring and control) to test our approach to display design, our interest lies in identifying principles that can be generalized to the design of interfaces for a variety of educational--and practice--settings. Even in their current stage of development, the displays offer a useful alternative for enhancing hemodynamic monitoring training. Experts particularly liked having a tool they could use to play "What if?" by observing the effects of different drug combinations on pressure and flow. It is unlikely that any of the displays tested here will replace current critical care displays completely, in part because of the need to monitor accuracy of data produced by sensors. However, since the objective of the enhanced displays (IBD and EPD) is to show relationships, not specific values, it is hoped that what is learned with these displays will transfer to facilitate performance with more traditional displays.

The experiment reported here measured performance in a specific task. It did not attempt to ascertain exactly what subjects learned from each display (or from the experiment in general). Moreover, the extent to which what is learned with one display transfers to another remains an open question. Although the simulation we are using includes only the intrinsic constraints on hemodynamics, by using Guyton's more complex simulations, we can extend the displays to include other physiological constraints (baroreceptors, etc.) without changing the basic graphics. Our experimental task is admittedly simpler than hemodynamic monitoring in the "real world," so whether our results will generalize beyond this setting remains to be seen.

The results of the study suggest strongly that the learning and practice of complex diagnostic and treatment skills such as hemodynamic monitoring can be facilitated for experts, as well as for novices, when natural relationships or constraints are enhanced by a perceptually-based display. Showing the anatomic constraints on pressure and flow improved treatment coordination performance by novices. Showing how etiological factors related to symptoms shortened the time required to reach a criterion level of performance and improved performance for both novices and experts.

Acknowledgments

This research was partially supported by National Science Foundation grant #IRI8902755 and a grant from the Research Foundation at the University of Connecticut.

References

[1] Sinclair, V. (1988). High technology in critical care: Implications for nursing's role and practice. Focus on Critical Care, 15, 36-41.

[2] Goodstein, L. P. (1981). Discriminative display support for process operators. In J. Rasmussen & W. B. Rouse (Eds.), Human detection and diagnosis of system failures (pp. 433-449). New York: Plenum

[3] Woods, D. D., O'Brien, J. F., & Hanes, L. F. (1986). Human factors challenges in process control: The case of nuclear power plants. In G. Salvendy (Ed.), Handbook of Human Factors (pp. 1724-1770), New York: John Wiley & Sons.

[4] Shoemaker, W. (1992). Monitoring and management of acute circulatory problems: The expanded role of the physiologically oriented critical care nurse. American Journal of Critical Care, 1, 38-53.

[5] Deneault, L. G., Lewis, C. M., Debons, A., Stein, K. L., & Dewolf, A. M. (1990). An integrative display for patient monitoring. Proceedings of the Human Factors Society 34th Annual Meeting, (pp. 514-517). Santa Monica, CA: Human Factors Society.

[6] Gibson, J. J. (1966). The senses considered as perceptual systems. Boston: Houghtin-Mifflin.

[7] Gibson, J. J. (1979/1986). The ecological approach to visual perception. Hillsdale, NJ: Lawrence Erlbaum Associates.

[8] De Groot, A. D. (1965). Thought and choice in chess. The Hague: Mouton.

[9] Chase, W. G., & Simon, H. A. (1973). Perception in chess. Cognitive Psychology, 4, 55-81.

[10] Benner, P. (1984). From novice to expert: Excellence and power in clinical nursing practice. Menlo Park, CA: Addison-Wesley.

[11] Dreyfus, H. L., & Dreyfus, S. E. (1986). Mind over machine: The power of human intuition and expertise in the era of the computer. New York: The Free Press.

[12] Guyton, A. C. (1980). Arterial pressure and hypertension. Philadelphia: W. B. Saunders.

[13] Crane, H. D. (1973). Switching properties in bubbles, balloons, capillaries and alveoli. Biomechanics, 6, 411-422.

[14] Effken, J. A. (1993). Coordination of hemodynamic monitoring and treatment performance. Unpublished doctoral dissertation, University of Connecticut, Storrs, CT.

Managing and displaying different time granularities of clinical information

Carlo Combi (°), Francesco Pinciroli (°*), Giancarlo Musazzi, Cesare Ponti

° Dipartimento di Bioingegneria del Politecnico di Milano
* Centro di Teoria dei Sistemi del CNR, Milano

ABSTRACT

We approach the need of representing by powerful graphical user-interface the granularity of the temporal clinical information. In this work we present some contributions, to suitably display such temporal clinical information. The graphical representation relies on a temporal clinical data model able to manage data having different granularities.

1. INTRODUCTION

In the medical field, information has often a temporal dimension specified at different accuracy. Furthermore, temporal information can subtend the concept of instant or the concept of interval.
Let consider, for example, the following sentences:

1) "At 17:30 of July 18, 1992, the patient was hit by infarction"
2) "In 1989 the patient suffered from hypertension; hypertension lasted six months"
3) "Starting from June 15, 1989, the patient assumed diuretics for four months"
4) "In the visit of May 24, 1990, the physician measured a systolic blood pressure of 140 mmHg on the patient"
5) "From 17 hours to 19 of March 27, 1989, the patient suffered from abdominal pains"
6) "At 16:30 of October 26, 1990, the patient finished suffering from renal colics; they lasted five days"

Generally the above sentences consist in one atemporal proposition plus an expression specifying the temporal dimension. The atemporal proposition can concern various types of clinical information. The sentences set listed here above shows that clinical information has different sources. For example, it can derive straight from what the patient narrates, from what the physician wrote in preceding medical records, or it can be related to objective data collected during follow-up visits.
In the sentence 1) the instant is specified at the level of minutes, while in the sentence 4) the instant is specified by the unit of measure of days. In the sentence 2) the starting instant is given by the unit of measure of years, whereas months are used for the duration. In the sentence 3) days and months specify respectively the starting instant and the duration of the interval. The sentence 5) specifies, by the unit of measure of hours, the starting and the ending instants of the pathological event. Finally, the sentence 6) specifies by minutes the ending instant of the pathology, whereas it uses days for the duration. Although the physicians do not have any difficulty in performing a human processing of so different temporal specifications, such a variety makes very hard any computer processing.
Medical databases and medical expert systems literature report many contributions approaching the management of temporal clinical information [1, 2, 3, 4]. Recently a need has been emphasized: the **time management at different levels of granularity** [5, 6]. The granularity of a given temporal information is the level of abstraction at which the information is defined [7]. For database systems based on the calendar time, granularity is the unit of measure used for the time scale.
In systems allowing to store and to manage temporal clinical data, the users want displaying the clinical information effectively. A **suitable graphical representation tool** should be the proper answer [8]. The graphical representation should allow to clearly qualify and quantify the temporal dimension of clinical information. Furthermore, the representation should allow to take visually both qualitative and structured comparisons between clinical events themselves [9].
The effort described in this paper deals with defining a graphical representation of the temporal dimension of clinical data, given at different levels of granularity. The graphical representation relies on a temporal data model allowing to manage in a powerful way the temporal dimension of data to be stored in a database [1].

2. THE TEMPORAL CLINICAL DATA MODEL

The aims subtended to the proposed temporal clinical data model are multiple [1]:

- allow to express of the temporal dimension of the clinical information by different and mixed granularities;
- represent and manage the temporal dimension of clinical information in a homogeneous and unified way;
- allow to make operations on temporal dimensions of the clinical information and to establish relations between temporal clinical data;
- manage and model more types of clinical information, identified in the atemporal parts of the above sentences.

2.1. The temporal ontology

The model allows to represent the temporal clinical information by the concepts of *temporal assertion* and of *interval* [1].

Let be *temporal assertion* an assertion composed by a proposition and a temporal interval. Let be E a temporal assertion expressible by the tuple <E_p,E_i>: this tuple means that the proposition E_p is true in the interval E_i.

Let be *interval* a closed set of contiguous elementary instants, i.e., instants defined at the level of seconds, specified by the tuple:

<starting instant, duration, ending instant>

This tuple allows to specify the temporal dimension of all the mentioned sentences.

It is possible to define *instants* at various levels of granularity:

years: *<year>*
months: *<year, month>*
days: *<year, month, day>*
hours: *<year, month, day, hour>*
minutes: *<year, month, day, hour, minute>*
seconds: *<year, month, day, hour, minute, second>*

A *duration* can be specified by combining:

years	*months*	*days*	*hours*	*minutes*	*seconds*

Besides these numerical values, a duration can assume two particular values: *undef*, in case it is not possible to determine the duration itself; ε, for duration of one or more orders of magnitude lower than seconds. A couple of *elementary instants* allows to univocally represent both instants and durations. Let be *elementary instant* a temporal point, on the discrete time axis, expressed by the units of measure of seconds, that is the lowest considered in the model.

Two elementary instants identify the upper and lower bound of the set of time points, the instant can coincide with. For instance, the elementary instants, expressed as "6/15/89, 0 hours, 0 minutes, 0 seconds" and "6/15/89, 23 hours, 59 minutes, 59 seconds", univocally characterize the starting instant of the interval of the sentence 3), expressed as "6/15/89". In an analogous way, two distances between elementary instants identify the upper and lower bound of the set of time distances, the duration can coincide with.

2.2. The temporal clinical assertions

The data model defines many temporal clinical assertions. The choice performed in the data model for the atemporal part of the temporal clinical assertions consists in identifying suitable syntactic structures for the different types of clinical information. According to the predefined sentence structure, terminological freedom is given in describing the particular clinical information. The following attributes identify the syntactic structure of the atemporal part of the temporal assertion *diagnosis*:

- *Pathology*: it is the only mandatory part, to make the temporal assertion meaningful. It contains the specification of the pathology, the patient suffered from.
- *Localization*: it specifies the anatomic part, the pathology influenced.
- *Quantifier*: it specifies the strength of the pathology.
- *Specifier*: it enriches the description of the pathology by further details.

Likewise, the following attributes identify the syntactic structure of the atemporal part of the temporal assertion *therapy*:

- *Drug name*: it is the only mandatory part, to make the temporal assertion meaningful. It contains the specification of the drug taken by the patient.
- *Category*: it characterizes the therapy by terms as "Emergency", "Usual Posology", "Maintenance".
- *Quantity*: it specifies the drug quantity of each taking.
- *Unit of measure*: it specifies the unit of measure used to specify the taken drug quantity.
- *Frequency*: it specifies how many times the patient must take the drug in a certain period.

The temporal clinical assertions related to follow-up visits partially differ from those related to anamnestic information, because their atemporal part is usually less structured; it refers to quantitative data coming from measurements performed on the patient. The temporal dimension of all the data collected during a visit coincides usually with the follow-up date. In the model the entity *follow-up visit*, containing a set of temporal clinical assertions with the same temporal dimension given by the entity *interval*, from which the entity *follow-up visit* inherits.

The sentence 4) is an example of a temporal clinical assertion coming from data collected during a follow-up visit. In the same visit other

temporal assertion could be present, having the atemporal part as:
Diastolic blood pressure equal to 80 mmHg
or
Heart rate: 88 bpm

3. GRAPHICAL REPRESENTATION OF THE PATIENT CLINICAL HISTORY

During the displaying of the temporal clinical data stored for a certain patient, it is very useful the physician has at disposal a system able to represent, by suitable graphical notation, the temporal dimension of the clinical events belonging to the patient history. This way, the physician obtains a synoptic view of the clinical history of the patient.
The temporal dimension of the clinical events can have different granularities: temporal relations between events cannot always be stated with certainty. Anyway, the graphical representation of the clinical history must allow the physician to establish if some temporal relations between clinical events may exist. For example, if the events "acute myocardial infarction at 17:30, July 28th 92", "taking of acetyl-salicylic acid from August 13th 1992 for 10 months", and "abdominal pains for six months starting from August 1992" compose the clinical history of the patient, the displaying system, by a suitable graphical symbology, should allow the physician to immediately identify the temporal localization and the extension of the intervals related to the three clinical events. In this case, the physician should immediately establish that a) the myocardial infarction is before both the other events, b) the abdominal pains finished before the therapy finished, while c) the abdominal pains could be started before or after the taking of acetyl-salicylic acid started.
We considered various factors in designing the system for the displaying of the patient clinical history:

- representing the granularity of the intervals of the considered clinical events, in respect with the starting instant, the duration, and the ending instant;
- representing the temporal dimension, given by more intervals, of the full clinical history or of a partial history, using all the available space on the screen;
- representing a reference time axis, to give an absolute time location of the clinical events. Many different chronological reference marks should be displayed.

3.1. Design of the graphical symbology

The graphical symbology used to display the intervals allows the physician to easily understand the temporal localization of the considered clinical event. The representation highlights that a starting instant or a finishing instant of an interval can coincide with a generic elementary instant (expressed at the granularity of seconds) belonging to a set of elementary instants, which is related to the used granularity. Furthermore, the representation highlights that a duration of an interval can coincide with a distance between elementary instants, belonging to a set of time distances, which is related to the used granularity.
We introduced ad-hoc graphical symbols to display durations assuming one of the two special values ε or *undefined.* If the duration assumes the value ε, we use a square inside the rectangle representing the starting instant of the interval. Inside the square the character ε, if data concerns therapies or diagnoses, is displayed; in this case, obviously, the extension of the square is predefined and it is not significant of the duration of the interval. A rectangle extending to the upper (lower) bound of the time axis represents the duration assuming the value *undefined.* The label *"undef"* inside the rectangle further highlights this feature.
Fig. 1 depicts some of the graphical symbols used if the duration does not assume one of the two special values ε or *undefined.*
Some border-line situations have been considered: if the temporal extension of a clinical event is too small to be efficaciously on the screen, the horizontal dimension of the rectangle representing the clinical event is forced to be the same of the vertical dimension stated for each symbol.
Finally, suitable labels and colors related to the particular clinical event complete the graphical symbology. If the event is a diagnosis, the label contains the particular pathology occurred in the interval. If the event is a therapy, the label contains the particular drug name taken in the interval. If the event is a follow-up visit, the label contains the name of the physician performed the visit.

4. SYSTEM DESCRIPTION

We implemented and tested the user-interface able to graphically display the clinical history of the patient on a temporally oriented medical record for PTCA patients, which are undergoing to several follow-up visits. For these patients the narrative data have to be updated also during the follow-up period.

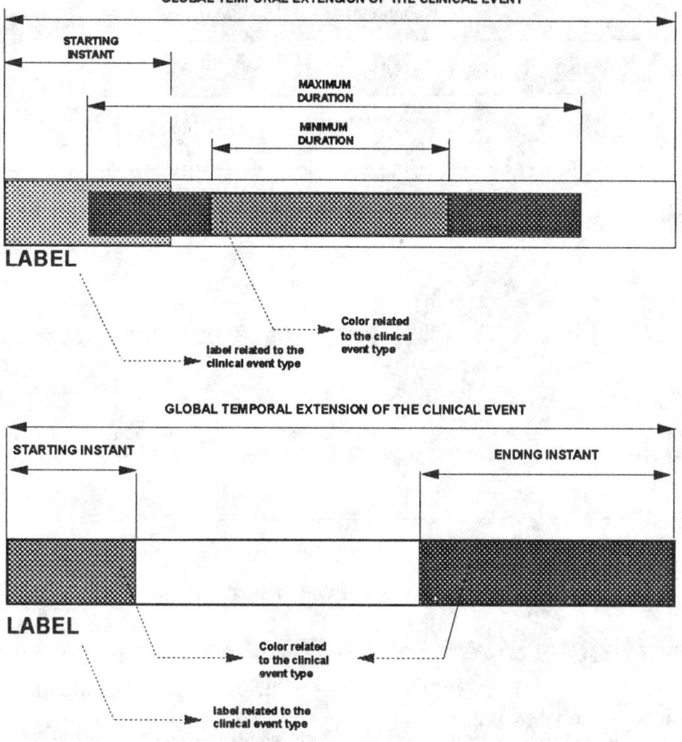

Fig. 1 Graphical symbology for the representation of the temporal dimension of diagnoses and therapies, if the duration does not assume particular values ε or *undefined.*

The figure highlights two capabilities to show a time interval; a further capability allows to show the ending instant and the duration of an interval. In the symbol at the top of the figure the duration is given in an independent way from the starting or the ending instant.

Historical data and follow-up data have to be managed in a global way, to monitor the status of the patient. We implemented the user-interface software on a Unix Sun SparcServer470; we developed the user-interface using OpenLook™ libraries with the C++ language. The clinical data are stored by the OODBMS ONTOS™.

4.1. The displaying system for the temporal clinical data

By the defined graphical symbols the physician can display the temporal dimension of all the clinical data of a patient. The physician can easily perform the displaying of suitable clinical sub-histories; he can add or remove temporal clinical events from the set of the represented ones. For each new selection of the clinical events to display, the bounds of the time axis on the screen are fixed so that the space on the screen is fully used; at the same time all the selected clinical events are completely displayed.

The reference marks on the time axis are stated in respect with the displayed temporal extension. The physician, however, can both move the bounds of the displayed time axis and choose the temporal distance between the reference marks. The physician can also enlarge the representation of the time axis. This way, the selected time axis is not completely displayed: the physician can display the parts of the selected time axis by a scrollbar. Finally, by vertical lines starting from each reference mark it is possible to identify more precisely the location of each represented interval in respect with the others and with the time axis.

The window *timepanel* allows in the Open Windows™ environment to display in a suitable window the clinical history of the patient. The fig. 2 shows an example of the window *timepanel*.

The window *timepanel* has the ID data of the considered patient as title. The window gives many options allowing the user to customize the displaying of the patient clinical history. The button labeled by "*Options*" allows to open a menu having three options labeled by "*Zoom Width*", "*Zoom Height*", and "*Redefine Extreme Instants*", respectively. Finally, on the window *timepanel* some buttons allow to dynamically control the bounds of the displayed time axis. The buttons labeled by ">" and "<", if selected, cause a shift of the lower bound and of the upper bound of the time axis. The button labeled by a time unit allows to choose the step for the shift.

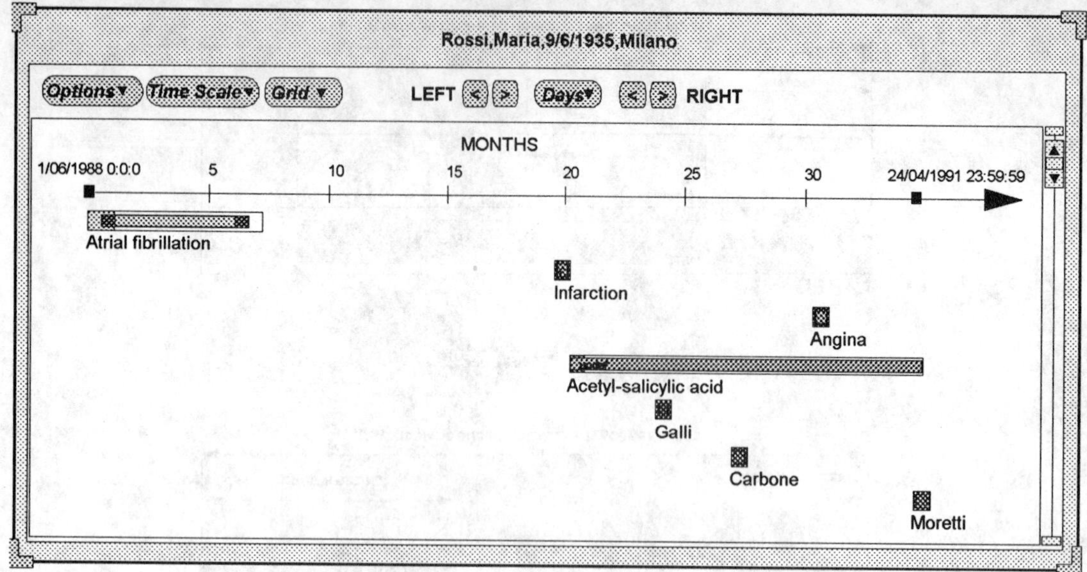

Fig. 2 An example of the window *timepanel*

5. CONCLUSIONS

The most relevant features of the work are:

- **Definition of a temporal clinical data model, to manage temporal clinical information given at levels of granularity**. The temporal clinical data model assumes the *interval* as fundamental concept; it relies for its computational properties on the concepts of *instant* and *duration*. The concept of *temporal assertion* has been introduced, to consider entirely information having a temporal dimension. Temporal clinical assertions have been proposed to manage data related to diagnoses, therapies and visits.
- **Design and implementation of a graphical user-interface able to represent the clinical history of the patient.** We designed and implemented a system able to represent the temporal dimension of the clinical events of the patient clearly and efficaciously. Clinical events with different time granularities compose the clinical history of a patient. We defined a suitable symbology, to manage some types of clinical information; the symbology allows to visually understand the different time granularities of the clinical events.

Acknowledgments

This research was partially funded by contributions from: MURST-40% funds "Informatica Medica" and "Bioingegneria del Sistema Cardiovascolare"; Department of Electronics and Informatics and Department of Bioengineering, Politecnico di Milano; C.T. S., Consiglio Nazionale delle Ricerche.

References

[1] Combi C. Time Management in Medical Records: Modelization, Implementation and Queries by Object-Oriented Techniques, Ph.D. thesis in Biomedical Engineering, in italian, 1993.

[2] Kahn M., Fagan L., Tu S. Extensions to the Time-Oriented Database Model to Support Temporal Reasoning in Medical Expert Systems, Methods of Information in Medicine, 30, 1991, pp.4-14.

[3] Larizza C., Moglia A. Stefanelli M. M-HTP: A system for monitorinig heart transplant patients, Artificial Intelligence in Medicine, 4, 1992, pp. 111-126.

[4] Das A.K., Tu S.W., Purcell G.P., Musen M.A., An Extended SQL for Temporal Data Management in Clinical Decision-Support Systems, SCAMC, 1993, pp 128-132.

[5] Pinciroli F., Combi C., Pozzi G. Object-orientated DBMS techniques for time-orientated medical record, Medical Informatics, 17, 4, Taylor & Francis, 1992, pp.231-241.

[6] Wiederhold G., Jajodia S., Litwin W. Integrating Temporal Data, in [10], pp. 564-579.

[7] Montanari A., Pernici B. Temporal Reasoning, in [10], pp. 534 - 562.

[8] Cousins S., Kahn M., Frisse M. The Display and Manipulation of Temporal Information, SCAMC, 1989, pp. 76-80.

[9] Chignell M.H., Singh G. Components of the Visual Computer: a Review of Relevant Tecnologies, the Visual Computer, September 1992, pp. 115-142.

[10] Tansel A.U., Clifford J., Gadia S., Jajodia S., Segev A., Snodgrass R. Temporal Databases: Theory, Design, and Implementation, The Benjamin/Cummings Publishing Company, Redwood City, CA, 1993

Section VII

Posters

Predictors of Nurse Adoption of a Computerized Information System as an Innovation

Carol A. Romano, National Institutes of Health, Bethesda, MD

This descriptive study focused on factors that influence the diffusion and adoption of an innovation after it is first introduced to members of a social system. The purposes of the study were 1) to explore a set of individual, technological, and organizational characteristics as predictors of hospital nurse adoption of a computerized information system (CIS) as an innovation, and 2) to investigate the effect of organizational position on innovation adoption. A computerized nursing information system for staffing, scheduling and productivity management was selected as the innovation.

INTRODUCTION

Computerized information systems are innovations used to support the management of clinical and administrative information. The exploration of factors that facilitate the adoption of innovations is needed so as to promote organizational and individual effectiveness in attempts to enhance quality and reduce costs. A review of the literature suggests that individual, technological, and organizational characteristics affect the diffusion and adoption of innovations. Prior studies, however, have not fully addressed a CIS as the innovation with nurses as the adoptors. In addition, the effect of organizational position has not been adequately explored.
[1,2].

METHODS / RESULTS

The sample included 193 staff nurses and 34 nurse managers in one large teaching research hospital. Instrumentation included use of the End User Computing Satisfaction Scale to measure adoption, the Index of Values Favorable Toward Change, the Distribution of Influence on Practice Scale and a questionnaire developed for this study. A self-report written survey method was used to test a set of 12 independent variables in relation to innovation adoption. Using multiple regression analysis, 43% of the variance in adoption was explained by 3 technology variable, 34% by 4 organizational variables, and 52% by all 12 predictors ($p < .0000$). A significantly lower level of adoption was found for managers compared to non-managers when either supervisor values ($F = 9.42$, $p < .05$), need ($F = 4.56$, $p < .05$), or peer values ($F= 4.68$, $p < .05$) was controlled ($df = 1.65$).

The results suggest that focus on the perceived advantages of an innovation, the perceived need, values held by peers regarding the innovation and use of communication mechanisms facilitate nurse adoption of a computerized information system as an innovation. A revised theoretical model for the study of innovation adoption was proposed based on the data analysis. The model asserts that a relationship exists among the categories of predictor variables and negates the hypothesized direct influence of adopter characteristics on adoption behavior. Implications for nursing include the need to focus strategies for planning, development and implementation of innovations on maximizing the significant predictors. Evaluation of the information management component of current nursing roles is also suggested.

REFERENCES

[1]. CA. Romano. Predictors of Nurse Adoption of a Computerized Information System as an Innovation
Diss Abstr, 1993; 54/04B:1893

[2]. CA. Romano. Diffusion of Technology Innovation. Adv Nurs Sci,1990;13:11-21

0195-4210/94/$5.00

Analysis of Three Coding Schemes: Can They Capture Nursing Care Plan Concepts?

Judith J. Warren, PhD, RN, James R. Campbell, MD, Mary K. Palandri, BSN, RN,
Robin A. Stoupa, BSN, RN
University of Nebraska Medical Center, Omaha NE

The purpose of this study was to determine the extent to which three major coding systems could capture the concepts used by nurses in the typical nursing care plan. Based on the results of a study conducted by the Codes Subcommittee of the CPRI Codes and Structure Work Group, the following coding schemes were studied: UMLS and SNOMED International. The NANDA Taxonomy was also included, as it is the major nursing coding system.

The CPRI study examined multidisciplinary progress notes. SNOMED International, followed by UMLS, was clearly the most comprehensive coding scheme from the schemes that were evaluated. However, most of nursing's documentation of the care process occurs in other types of formats, specifically the nursing care plan and flow sheets. This study collected discharge care plan summaries from patients: newborn, adult surgery and medicine, pediatric surgery, and adult oncology. The care plans were parsed into 372 different concepts.

The team used the same scoring methodology used by the CPRI research team: 0=no match, 1=conceptual match, and 2=exact match. The team met to review the parsed list to review the terms and whether the parsing was accurate. Each coded concept was reviewed by two researchers and the team reviewed all scoring decisions. Browsers developed for UMLS and SNOMED were used to look up the codes. NANDA was a manual look-up due to its brevity.

The average overall scores for nursing concepts were UMLS, 1.38, SNOMED, 0.85, and NANDA, 0.37. The percent of concepts coded was also calculated: UMLS 79%, SNOMED 55%, and NANDA 18%. Next each component of the care plan was analyzed: diagnosis, etiology, symptoms, outcome, treatment, and evaluation. The tables show the coding scores and percentages for each of the three systems.

UMLS does code nursing care plan with more granularity than SNOMED. UMLS incorporated the Iowa Nursing Intervention Classification (NIC) which is where UMLS outperformed SNOMED. The second area of increased coding ability occurred with etiologies. Many of the etiologies were of a psychosocial nature which are in UMLS but not SNOMED. NANDA continued to perform well in coding nursing diagnoses. UMLS coded more diagnoses due to the fact that some diagnoses were not listed in NANDA.

Lest this study be misunderstood, SNOMED was developed to capture medical concepts and is now moving into the domain of capturing patient-focused concepts. SNOMED has included an early list of NANDA diagnoses and may be including NIC. If these avenues are pursued, SNOMED may code nursing concepts in a more comprehensive manner and begin to match its ability to successfully code multidisciplinary data.

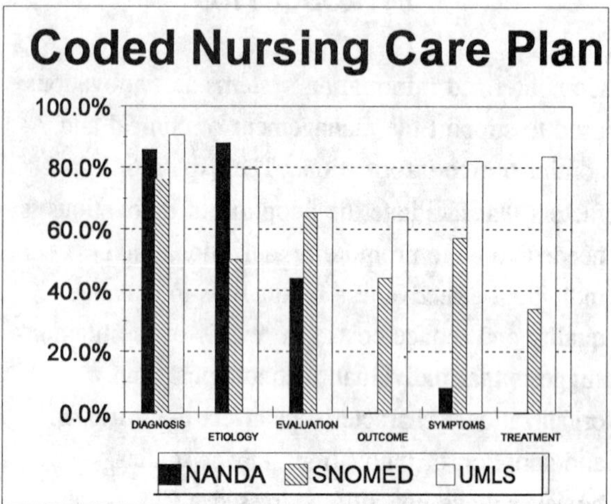

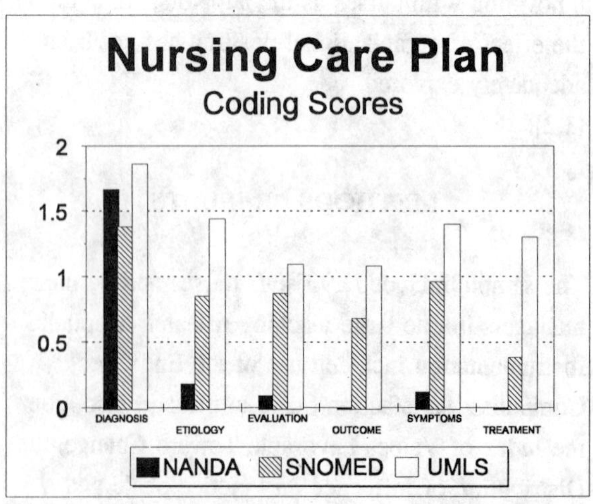

Nurse Manager's Use of Lotus 1-2-3 Template as Support for Decision Making for Nursing Hours, Staffing and Direct Nursing Costs per Day.

Richard D. Martorelli, M.B.A., C.P.A., Surgical Nursing, University of Pennsylvania Medical Center, Philadelphia, Pennsylvania.

Delivery of appropriate levels of resource utilization is the key to controlling costs in today's health care settings. Nurse Managers have a strategic and pivotal role in patient care delivery and health-care organizations, and have become more accountable for managing patient care, personnel and costs in the face of fluctuating patient activity. The most frequently used statistic for the measurement of nursing care and personnel staffing is Nursing Hours Per Patient Day (NHPPD). The purpose of the development of a PC-based spreadsheet was to provide the nurse managers with an easy-to-use, interactive tool from which changes in resource needs could be quickly determined from changes in patient volume and activity.

With increasing demands on hospitals to lower health care costs, and increasing needs to understand and manage expenses in a managed care environment, nurse managers have become more accountable for managing patient care and determining appropriate staffing requirements in the face of fluctuating patient activity. Mainframe programs exist that link volume/patient activity with payroll/scheduling programs, but these are expensive to implement and support. These systems also tend to be retrospective, and unable to help support decision making in a rapidly changing environment. The purpose of the development of a PC-based spreadsheet was to provide the nurse managers with an easy-to-use, interactive tool from which changes in resource needs could be quickly determined from changes in patient volume and activity.

At a university teaching hospital, where personnel management represents 80% of the Nursing Department's operating budget, a spreadsheet template, based in Lotus 1-2-3, was developed and customized for operation on 23,(100%), of the inpatient units. Traditionally, decisions made by nurse managers about staffing were done in a nonuniform method, mostly by relying on personal experience and clinical judgement. If any quantitative calculations were performed manually by the individual managers, this work could take up to an hour. The PC-based spreadsheet program requires minimal data input of daily patient census and staffing, and it calculates and displays the unit occupancy rate, the Direct Nursing Hours Per Patient Day (NHPPD), the direct nursing cost per patient day and the total direct nursing payroll per patient day. A comparison of the actual and budgeted patient activity and nursing costs is quantified and illustrated by graphic representation. Because of the software's capabilities, it is possible to obtain several iterations of patient staffing ratios in order to evaluate the one which best fits the budgetary constraints. Free text areas within the worksheet allow space for the nurse manager to enter unusual circumstances or special patient needs that may have affected the amount and cost of staffing. These notes can be stored and retrieved for later use in operational variance analysis. Because this PC-based commercial software program is easy to modify, changes in base-level assumptions, calculations or formatting can be accomplished with facility.

The nurse managers have used the spreadsheet on a daily basis for six months. As a result, the managers have 1) reduced the time for support of decision making from up to one hour to less than ten minutes; 2) applied consistent decision rules compatible with personnel resources; 3) increased flexibility in managing staffing assignments based on patient census and demand through the ability to easily identify resource changes required for different levels of activity. In addition, the storage of contemporaneous notes regarding resource use has enhanced the formal financial variance analysis process, by providing the manager with detailed information regarding peak activity periods that may not be obvious in monthly summary reports. Annual refinements of the basic spreadsheet, based on user comments, are planned, and development of an integrated summary report of period information is currently underway.

The Problem-Oriented Medical Synopsis: Coding, Indexing, and Classification Sub-Model

Frank W. Stitt MD, Departments of Epidemiology and Medicine
University of Miami School of Medicine, Miami, Florida

A clinical information system consists of four major components: the clinical database, decision support, data analysis (including outcomes), and the development system. We have created such a system using generally available database methodology. The system is documented using a conceptual model, a physical model, and sub-models for individual components. A key sub-model of the the clinical database, for record-keeping, has been defined for coding, indexing, and classification of the medical narrative typically encountered in medical records. We describe an approach to the development of the coding component that results in a hybrid system for recording information, locating indexed information, and summarizing it for analysis of outcomes. These are based on a primary term list—the problem glossary; SNOMed—the Systematized Nomenclature of Medicine (3rd. edition); and ICD-9-CM. The relationship with the UMLS is also discussed.

INTRODUCTION

We have developed a clinical database called the Problem-Oriented Medical Synopsis (POMS), based on work done over a twenty-year period. The conceptual schema of the system uses sub-models, and the record-keeping sub-model has been described elsewhere [1, 2]. Coding, indexing, and classification are critical components of clinical information systems, since a large part of the data in such systems consists of text, or narrative. Processing of "medical narrative" raises three fundamental issues. (i) How to **record** information: a standardized, preferred terminology is required, but such an instrument is not generally available for clinical problems; (ii) How to **locate** information selectively: this is done using a thesaurus of hierarchically organized nomenclature terms, such as SNOMed, the Systematized Nomenclature of Medicine; (iii) How to **summarize** information for analysis, using classification and aggregation. We have attempted to address this problem by combining the creation of domain-specific preferred terminologies with the modification of a classification system that is universal—ICD-9-CM, and a thesaurus of medical terms for indexing—SNOMed-III.

METHODS AND CONCLUSIONS

The preferred terminology we created is called the "problem glossary", and is strongly oriented towards general medicine and some of its subspecialties, such as infectious disease, oncology, and pediatrics.

A biaxial classification and a "tangled hierarchy" were used to form a semantic network: there are about 600 codes in each axis. **Axis 1** is a body organ-system classification, a hybrid anatomic-physiologic organization. **Axis 2** is a health care process classification: "process" is defined as *that which is done in the course of the management of a reason for encounter, problem, or disease identified by a provider in a health care setting.*

The problem glossary has been reviewed by expert groups across multiple domains, and is thought to be comprehensive and easy to use. The content of the glossary was also cross-checked against the 5,000 most frequently occurring terms in MEDLINE and Excerpta Medica literature databases (MeSH and MALIMET thesauri)—about 3,000 of these are clinical terms, after excluding drug names and procedures. Each term is indexed with as many SNOMed-III terms as are needed. The problem glossary terms have been compared with the UMLS Metathesaurus terms. It seemed from this comparison that primary clinical terms (symptoms, signs, and test findings)may be underrepresented in the UMLS, at present.

A hybrid coding, indexing, and classification system has been created for medical record keeping and analysis of outcomes. The **content** is comprehensive for the domain of internal medicine and its sub-specialties, especially for diagnostic statements.

The **titles** are clear and unambiguous, and are based upon sound lexical rules. The **keys** are numeric (based upon a 4-byte integer), and are thus highly efficient for use in databases. The terms can be used for statistical **aggregation,** since each term is indexed using ICD-9-CM.

References

1. Stitt FW. Clinical database management for medical records. In: Cote RA, Protti DJ, Scherrer , JR, ed., *Role of informatics in health data coding and classification systems.* Amsterdam: North-Holland, 1985:295-331. IFIPS/IMIA conference proceedings.
2. Stitt FW. The Problem-Oriented Medical Synopsis: a patient-centered clinical information system. In: Safran C, ed., Annu Symp Comput Appl Med Care. New York: McGraw-Hill, Inc, Health Professions Division, November 1993:88-92.

Positive efficiency findings using computer assisted ICD-encoding: 3,5 years of experience with the computerized patient record system PADS (Patient Archiving & Documentation System)

J.H. Hohnloser, University of Munich, Germany
H. Soltanian, University of Homburg-Saar, Germany

In daily routine there is a major discrepancy between what physicians do and what they document. From a medical information processing point of view amongst the more important functions physicians perform in their daily routine is the encoding of diagnoses using a standard vocabulary such as ICD-9. This paper presents evidence that through the use of the ICD-encoding module of a computerized patient record system (PADS, Patient Archiving and Documentation System) user compliance can be improved. "Bypassing" mechanisms can be partly reversed (up to 43 %), more coded diagnoses are documented (by 51 %) and those diagnoses documented are more complete (increase by 57 %).

INTRODUCTION

A computerized patient record system (PADS (Patient Archiving and Documentation System)) was developed at the University of Munich and used in ICU and CCU of one University of Munich medical hospital [1]. Amongst the systems' function is database management of automatic ICD-encoding.

This report we will focus on experiences the PADS ICD-encoding module and will present data to illustrate positive effects through system use.

MATERIAL AND METHODS

In our hospital before 1985 (phase I) no diagnoses were encoded. After 1985 (phase II) a German clinical modification of ICD-9 ("Lübecker Schlüssel") was used [2]. Doctors had to manually encode each diagnosis listed in the discharge summary. The discharge summary - amongst other sections - consists of diagnoses header, medical history and conclusion/summary. Diagnoses listed in the diagnosis header section of the discharge summary must be encoded using ICD-9. Frequently, those diagnosis were mentioned either in the medical history section or the conclusion/summary section.

After 1990 (phase III) diagnoses were encoded using the same ICD code but a semiautomatic computerized technique implemented as part of the computerized patient record system PADS was used instead of the manual encoding process.

In the analysis presented we compare the three phases: Pre ICD, Post ICD/Pre PADS and Post ICD/Post PADS. We analyzed the following parameters:

a) Total number of (free text) diagnoses in the discharge summary
b) Total number of ICD-encoded diagnoses in the discharge summary
c) Number of (free text) diagnoses in the medical history section
d) Number of (free text) diagnoses in the conclusion/summary section

The basis of this analysis for phase I and phase II were 200 traditional discharge summaries of ICU/CCU patients. This analysis was done manually. For phase III we analyzed 3153 admissions on ICU/CCU of 2792 patients between 1/90 and 6/93 with the help of a computer. In these patients 10414 ICD diagnoses were automatically encoded using PADS. Data were then jointly analyzed using PC based spreadsheet and statistics applications.

RESULTS

a) The mean number ($\pm$ SE) of free text diagnoses per admission for phases I, II and III respectively were 3.2 ± 0.73, 3.64 ± 0.33 and 3.34 ± 0.3, respectively (difference not significant).

b) The mean number of ICD-encoded diagnoses (0 in phase I) rose from 1.8 ± 0.31 (phase II) to 2.72 ± 0.24, a 51 % significant increase after installation of the computerized patient record system (see figure 1).

c.) The mean number of free text diagnoses in the medical history section rose from 0.5 ± 0.2 (phase I) over 0.92 ± 0.31 (phase II) to 1.0 ± 0.18 (phase III), a 84 % significant ($p < 0.001$) increase in free text diagnoses in the medical history section following the introduction of ICD-9 CM, which did was not reversed after the introduction of PADS.

d.) The mean number of free text diagnoses in the conclusion/summary section rose from 0 (phase I) over 0.81 ± 0.19 (phase II) and declined after installation of PADS to 0.45 ± 0.12, a 43 % significant ($p < 0.001$) reduction of diagnoses inappropriately escaping ICD-encoding.

e.) every single diagnosis encoded using the PADS ICD-encoder will allow only 100% encoding ("all or nothing" principle in phase III) as opposed to 46 % completeness in phase II thus assuring completeness of coding.

CONCLUSION

Our data indicate that

- only 50 % of all (free text) diagnoses are encoded manually using ICD-9 CM

documented data and even reverse "bypass" mechanisms developed by users to escape data coding.

LITERATURE

1. Hohnloser, J.H., Pürner, F. (1992) PADS (Patient Archiving and Documentation System): A computerized patient pecord with educational aspects. International Journal of Clinical Monitoring and Computing 9:71-84

2. Mansky T, Scriba PC, Fassl H, Friedrich HJ. [Diagnosis encoding: how and to what purpose? (editorial)]. Dtsch Med Wochenschr 1986;111(45):1707-8.

Transferring Knowledge From One System To Another

Charles W. Bishop, Ph.D, and Peter D. Ewing, M.D.,
Department of Medicine, School of Medicine and Biomedical Sciences,
University at Buffalo, State University of New York, Buffalo, NY

Although knowledge is contained in many systems, moving it from one system to another is not an easy task because each system is tailored in its own unique way and because knowledge configurations are usually copyrighted. To populate our FRAMEMED knowledge base we turned to the NLM Metathesaurus as a readily-available open source of knowledge. We were disappointed by the greatly variable granularity of the concepts and the lack of definitions that could be borrowed. Some reference books in electronic form seem attractive but reformatting will require excessive human intervention and copyright negotiation.

INTRODUCTION

Knowledge is ubiquitous and readily accessible. Moving it from one knowledge base to another without excessive human intervention is difficult because each knowledge base is organized along different lines. Additionally, most knowledge bases are copyrighted. FRAMEMED [1] has blocked out its organization for all medical knowledge but is faced with the problem of populating its knowledge base by importing reliable medical knowledge from whatever sources it can utilize.

METHODS / RESULTS

The National Library of Medicine's Metathesaurus [2] based on equating similar concepts from multiple systems was initially attractive. Difficulty soon arose because the various systems (eg, ICD, SNOMED) were not completely hierarchical (layers not distinctively coded) and had varying degrees of granularity, relating to the purpose for which these systems were created. Thus FRAMEMED found those lists to be of limited value in constructing its hierarchical lists (as well as identifying distinct concepts about which knowledge might be sought).

An additional difficulty in trying to utilize the Metathesaurus was the plethora of files (49). The 5 unit record files were most useful but each was as large as 30 megabytes and required copying to hard drive before it could be manipulated. Examination of records truncated to eliminate formatting characters and utilizing only 6 element abbreviations revealed a preponderance of chemical entries, most of which seemed of little immediate interest. Because of their origin in schemes devised for quite specialized purposes, many entries (eg, STR0001001 Inflammatory spondylopathies in diseases classified elsewhere) were unmatchable to the hierarchical concepts in the FRAMEMED knowledge base.

We were disappointed to find that many concepts in the Metathesaurus lacked definitions and that many of the definitions present were from Dorland's Medical Dictionary and hence copyrighted.

An encouraging development for knowledge transfer is appearance of some traditional reference books such as 'The Merck Manual' in electronic form. Their definitions, because they are very context-oriented, require extensive reediting before they might contribute to the FRAMEMED descriptive records. Much material in the Merck Manual could be invaluable for our relational records of diseases (eg, disease profiles) but cannot be immediately incorporated into our system because of differing phraseology for similar concepts.

In summary, the transfer of knowledge from one system to another is not easily accomplished at present because of diversity of system design (and terminology), and copyright prohibitions. Networking may be less successful in facilitating knowlege transfer than present optimists assert, mainly because of lack of standardization of terminology and formatting.

References.

[1] Bishop CW, Ewing PD. FRAMEMED, a prototypical medical knowledge base of unusual design. M.D. Computing, 1993,10:184-92

[2] UMLS Knowledge Sources. Unified Medical Language Sytem. U.S. Dept. of Health and Human Services, National Institutes of Health, National Library of Medicine, 4th Experimental Edition, April 1993, Bethesda, MD

Designing a Sub-Set of the UMLS Knowledge Base Applied to a Clinical Domain : Methods and Evaluation

A. Burgun[1], M.D., D. Delamarre[1], G. Botti[2], M.D., B. Lukacs[3], M.D, D. Mayeux[4], M.D., M. Bremond[5], M.D., F. Kohler[4], M.D., M. Fieschi[2], M.D., Ph.D., P. Le Beux[1], M.D., Ph.D.
1 Laboratoire d'Informatique Médicale, C.H.U., F-35033 Rennes, France. 2 Service de l'Information Médicale, C.H.U. la Timone, F-13385 Marseille , France. 3 Service Urologie, Hôpital Tenon F-75020 Paris, France. 4 Département d'Information Médicale, C.H.U., F-54035 Nancy, France. 5 Groupe Image, Ecole Nationale de la Santé Publique, F-94410 St Maurice, France

The UMLS is a complex collection of interconnected biomedical concepts derived from standard nomenclatures. Designing a specific subset of the UMLS knowledge base relevant to a medical domain is a prerequisite for the development of specialized applications based on UMLS. We have developed a method based on the selection of the appropriate terms in original nomenclatures and the capture of a set of UMLS terms that are linked to them in the network to a certain degree. We have experimented it as the foundation for a concept base applied to urology. Results depend on the exhaustiveness of the relationships between the Metal concepts. A preliminary analysis of the sub-base reveales that some adaptations of vocabulary and ontology are required for clinical applications.

INTRODUCTION

The UMLS is a vast repository of semantically categorized terms [1]. Designing a specific subset of the UMLS knowledge base relevant to a medical domain is a prerequisite for the development of specialized applications based on UMLS. We have developed a method to assist the researcher in that task.

METHODS / RESULTS

The method is based on the scanning of nomenclatures and the exploitation of the UMLS interconcept links . The first step consists in selecting the appropriate terms within some of the nomenclatures that have been incorporated in UMLS. During the second phase, the initial set of concepts is extended in order to build a consistent subset of the UMLS knowledge base. The process starts by locating in the Meta1 the concepts corresponding to the selected nomenclature codes. This operation enables one to integrate the information - stemming from any source of the UMLS - related to those concepts, and to free oneself from the structure of the original nomenclature in order to exploit the fulness of UMLS. Then the different kinds of links within the UMLS network are explored as follows : (1) addition of all the children -all i.e. at all levels- of the concepts (2) addition of all the parents (3) addition of the related concepts (4) addition of the parents of the related concepts. The programs run on UNIX platforms as C-Shell procedures that operate on the ASCII files of the CD-ROM UMLS Sources distribution.

That algorithm was applied to 47 initial concepts selected from MeSH and SNOMEDII in order to build a base of urology concepts. The final vocabulary includes 984 concepts, 1905 terms and 3030 interconcept relationships. The wealth of the resulting sub-base is a function of the exhaustiveness of the relationships within Meta1. That is the main limitation of our method. Noise is generated by the capture of terms from other medical domains. Among the 984 concepts of our urology sub-base, 681 (69%) were found to be relevant whether they were specific or not. The below figure shows how the selection of *Pyelonephritis* at the first step brings out *Arachnoïditis*.

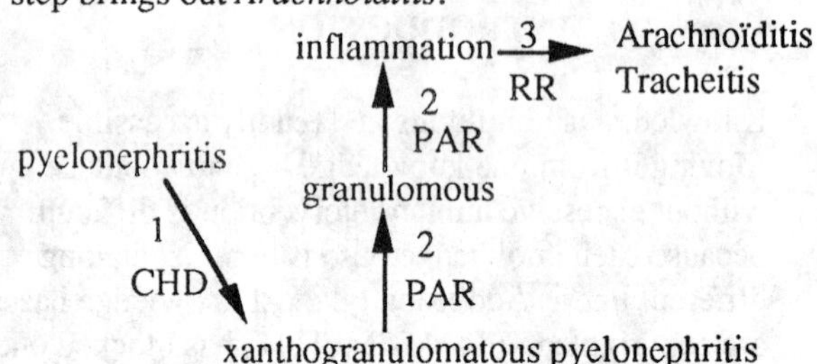

DISCUSSION

About the method : (1) The consistency of the sub-base is guaranteed since it represents the projection of the UMLS knowledge base on a specific domain. (2) It is well-adapted for the implementation of successive editions of the UMLS sources. (3) The sub-base is built up easily. (4) Further developments are required to reduce the noise.

About the resulting sub-base : (1) Because of the intended use of UMLS to facilitate information retrieval, the vocabulary may require some adaptations for clinical applications : clinical distinctions are missing -*Cryptorchism* and *Ectopic testis* are synonymous in Meta1. (2) Ontology may be adapted; for example a category *surgical approaches* is needed for the description of surgical procedures.

AKNOWLEDGEMENTS

The authors thank the N.L.M. for having provided the UMLS Knowledge Sources on CD-ROM.

Reference

[1]. Lindberg D.A.B., Humphreys B.L., Mc Cray A.T. The Unified Medical Language System, Methods of Information in Medicine, 1993; 32:281-91

Discern - An Integrated Prospective Decision Support System

Bob Johnson, Doug McNair, M.D., Ph.D., K. Kailasam, Rodger Reilly, Nancy Eklund, Glenn McCoy, Ed.D., and Patrick Jamieson, M.D.

We present a new integrated decision support tool, called Discern, for prospective case management within a comprehensive Healthcare Network Architecture (HNA). Discern is an event-driven, expert system tightly integrated into this architecture. It can perform a variety of actions including generating alerts, ordering tests, and entering results. Over 100 institutions use Discern to automate care processes. Discern was designed to meet the demanding requirements for effective decision support.

Introduction

Despite enormous investment in information technology, there is little evidence that hospital information systems (HIS) have improved healthcare productivity.
Decision support recognizes that intelligent management of patient information often requires more than simple data retrieval; this notion does not capture the concept of a dynamic care process, nor does it allow for active interventions. The HIS architecture at most institutions, however, is inadequate for the decision support tasks now demanded of them.

We started design on an integrated decision support tool, known as Discern, in 1988 and first deployed it in 1989. Discern, is a near real time, prospective, rule-based expert system fully integrated into the HIS system. The HIS components are tightly intrarelated in an architecture called the Healthcare Network Architecture (HNA).

Applications

A small sample of actual applications is shown in table one.

Sample Discern Applications
Allergy checking prior to contrast procedure
Ordering manual white blood cell differentials
Generating alerts in elderly patients on certain drugs
Pharmacy notification of pregnant patients
Billing for respiratory care procedures
Canceling tests that do not meet certain criteria
Ordering CSF culture if CSF white cells are increased
Warnings for dietary statuses that interfere with medications
Interpretation of iron studies
Notifying radiology of procedure cancellation
Adjust heparin dosage based on PTT
Notifying nursing of radiology procedure preparation
Checking for coagulation studies prior to surgery

Table One

Summarization of Complex Causal Diagnostic Hypotheses

William J. Long, PhD, MIT Lab for Computer Science, Cambridge, MA
Shapur Naimi, MD and M. G. Criscitiello, MD
New England Medical Center and Tufts Univ. School of Medicine, Boston, MA

The Heart Disease Program produces detailed causal diagnostic hypotheses for patients with cardiovascular diseases. This poster discusses our experience with summarizing these hypotheses for the physician. The basic approach is to merge the nodes of the structure indicating causal mechanism into the more important nodes. Analysis of the results shows that to generate effective summaries the identification of syndromes is very important, the definitions of the labels need to be carefully enforced, the causality of diseases should be supported by evidence and not just probability, and the sense of causal order must be carefully preserved.

1 INTRODUCTION

The use of detailed causal models for diagnosis enables the representation of many kinds of relationships allowing the diagnostic reasoner to make important distinctions not possible with simpler associations. However, more complex diagnoses may need explanation. We addressed this need for the Heart Disease Program (HDP)* in order to evaluate the program[1].

2 HEART DISEASE PROGRAM

Over the past ten years we have been developing the HDP to assist physicians in reasoning about the diagnosis and management of patients with cardiovascular disease[1]. The program uses the patient description and a causal physiologic model to generate detailed hypotheses for the differential diagnosis. A typical hypothesis is in figure 1.

The summarization procedure we developed merges nodes representing mechanism into the most closely associated important node and uses only the links needed to establish the structure of the diagnosis. Finally syndromes are recognized and combined into single nodes. The result of summarizing the hypothesis is in figure 2.

The summarization procedure did an effective job of shrinking the hypotheses and enabled effective evaluation. However, it was clear that the reviewer's objections were sometimes a result of inadequate exposition of the hypotheses in the summaries.

*The name has been changed from the Heart Failure Program to reflect the broader domain of application.

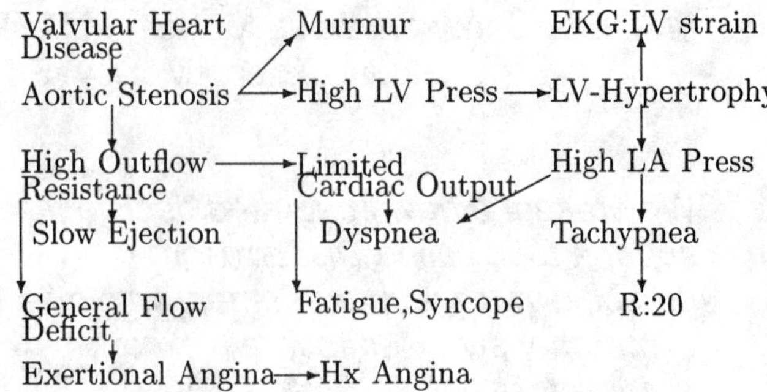

Figure 1: Fragment of a Hypothesis

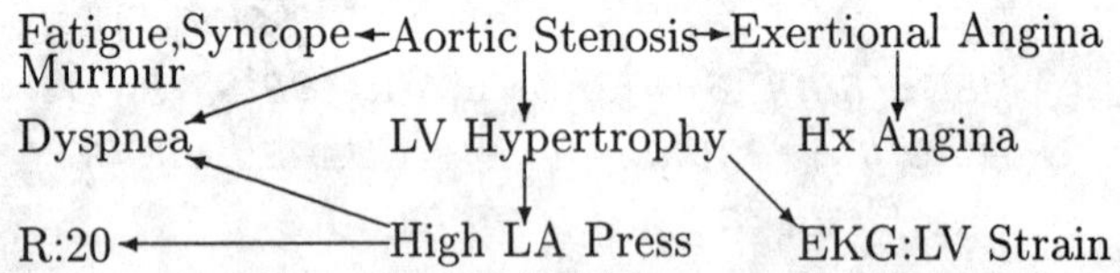

Figure 2: Summarization of Hypothesis Fragment

3 PRINCIPLES OF SUMMARIZATION

Our analysis of the summarization leads to some general principles. 1) The basic strategy of removing the mechanisms is correct. However, when only a part of the summary node causes an effect, the mechanisms are needed in a summary. 2) The sense of causality must be preserved in the summary, which may require additional knowledge. 3) The identification of syndromes is important and conveys more to the user than just the sum of the nodes. 4) Syndromes and node labels must be carefully defined to match the generally understood characteristics of acuteness, severity, or etiology. 5) A syndrome should not conceal other causes for part of the findings. 6) Unless there is evidence for a specific cause, secondary nodes or therapies should be linked to all possible causes. Nodes with a significant probability of being primary should be linked to none. 7) Mechanisms that establish a connection between nodes should remain in the summary.

References

[1] Long WJ, Naimi S, Criscitiello MG. Evaluation of a New Method for Cardiovascular Reasoning. Journal of the American Medical Informatics Association. 1994;1:127-141.

0195-4210/94/$5.00

Computerized Screening for Appropriate Dosing of Renally Eliminated Medications

Ramona Skinner, M.S., James Caldwell, Pharm.D., Paul Vitale, Pharm.D.,
Anne Arundel Medical Center, Annapolis, Maryland

A method of rapid screening for appropriateness of certain drug doses is described. The program extracts patient information from a hospital mainframe computer system, performs an estimation of creatinine clearance (CrCl), and prints a report of patients, drugs, doses, and CrCl for patients within a specified CrCl range.

INTRODUCTION

Proper dose adjustment of renally eliminated drugs offers clear benefit to patients and hospitals.[1] Patients benefit by reduction of morbidity and mortality secondary to dose-related adverse drug reactions (ADRs). For institutions, reduction of treatment cost and prolonged length-of-stay associated with ADRs is essential to quality improvement programs and financial survival. Secondary benefit includes direct reduction in drug cost in patients with reduced renal function.[2,3,4]

Based on the above, a need for an efficient method of screening patients requiring dose adjustments based on renal function was identified by the pharmacy department. The information systems and pharmacy departments worked together to develop an in-house program utilizing data from the active patient information files on the mainframe system.

METHODS/RESULTS

A monitored drug dictionary (MDD) was developed to allow creation and maintenance of a list of drugs to monitor. The MDD was designed to pull names and mnemonic bases directly from the pharmacy's main drug dictionary. Queries in the beginning of the program identify which location(s) to search (default ALL), a specific range of CrCl to include (default 10-50 ml/min), and a designation of where to print.

The pharmacy's location/name index is used to search for all patients currently on any of the drugs listed in the monitored drug dictionary. If identified as on a monitored drug, the patient's most recent serum creatinine is obtained from laboratory data. An estimated CrCl is calculated, using the method of Jelliffe, and used to determine if a patient is within the range of CrCl specified.[5] Information from patients thus identified is placed into a temporary file. The temporary file is sorted by location, room, and then bed. A final report is generated which includes: room, account number, age, drugs and doses/intervals from the MDD drugs, most recent Blood Urea Nitrogen (BUN) and serum creatinine with dates, and the calculated CrCl. Reports take approximately 3 minutes to compile and print.

Reports can be quickly scanned by a pharmacist to compare reported doses/intervals to standard dosage recommendations. More information is obtained as needed from the computer or the patient's chart. Physicians are then contacted when doses appear truly excessive.

This program provides an efficient means of identifying patients at risk for preventable dose-related ADRs. Patient care is enhanced while the institution enjoys cost avoidance and reduction. Reporting by location allows application of the program in the patient focused care arena. It illustrates maximal use of computerized information to directly improve patient care in health care institutions.

References

[1]. Matzke GR, Keane WF. Drug dosing in patients with impaired renal function. In: DiPiro JT, Talbert RL, Hayes PE, Yee GC, Posey ML, eds. Pharmacotherapy. A pathophysiologic approach. New York: Elsevier, 1989:589-98.

[2]. Peterson JP, Colucci VJ, Schiff SE. Using serum creatinine concentrations to screen for inappropriate dosage of renally eliminated drugs. *Am J Hosp Pharm* 1991;48:1962-4.

[3]. Johnson CT. Influencing dosing and selection of beta lactam antimicrobials in patients with reduced renal function. *Hosp Pharm* 1992;27:707,710-2,715-6.

[4]. Vlasses PH, Bastion WA, Behal R, Sirgo MA. Ceftazidime dosing in the elderly: Economic Implications. *Annals of* Pharmacotherapy 1993;27:967.

[5]. Jelliffe RW. Creatinine clearance: Bedside estimate. Ann Intern Med 79:604-605, 1973.

Pharmaco-informatics: More Precise Drug Therapy from "Multiple Model" (MM) Stochastic Adaptive Control Regimens: Evaluation with Simulated Vancomycin Therapy.

Roger W. Jelliffe, M.D., David Bayard, Ph.D., Alan Schumitzky, Ph.D., Mark Milman, Ph.D., and Michael Van Guilder, Ph.D.

Laboratory of Applied Pharmacokinetics, University of Southern California School of Medicine, CSC 134-B, 2250 Alcazar Street, Los Angeles, California 90033

ABSTRACT

MM stochastic control of dosage regimens permits essentially full use of information, either in a population pharmacokinetic model or a Bayesian updated MM parameter set, to achieve and maintain selected therapeutic goals with optimal precision. The regimens are visibly more precise than those developed using mean parameter values. Bayesian MM feedback has now also been implemented.

INTRODUCTION

In pharmaco-informatics, previous work showed the utility of NPEM population pharmacokinetic modeling, with discrete support points for the population joint probability density function. The points become multiple contending patient models to use to plan the initial MM dosage regimen for a new patient, and to update as feedback becomes available. We now describe a simulation of vancomycin therapy in which realistic errors are made in preparation and timing of doses, as well as in the measurement of serum levels.

METHODS

A 2 compartment population model of Vancomycin, previously developed using the NPEM2 program, had 28 support points, each of which had a value for each parameter, and its probability. Parameters were Vc, the apparent volume of the central (serum level) compartment, Kcp, the rate constant from central to peripheral compartment; Kpc, the reverse rate constant, and Kslope, the increment of elimination rate constant (Kel) for each unit of creatinine clearance (CCr). A nonrenal component, Kint, was fixed at 0.002043 hr^{-1}. A therapeutic goal of a stable serum vancomycin concentration of 15 ug/ml was chosen. Vancomycin was given by continuous IV in 3 infusion steps of 2 hrs each, followed by 3 steps of 6 hrs each, to achieve the goal of 15 ug/ml at the end of each infusion step.

The MM control strategy was evaluated by comparing it with conventional MAP Bayesian control, using a Monte Carlo simulation of a realistic clinical scenario containing errors in preparation (±10%) and timing (±12min) of the infusion steps, as well as serum assay error. Three days of therapy were simulated. Serum levels were "drawn" at 2, 4, and 8 hours into the regimen each day. Further, in a way that is never knowable clinically, the response of the simulated "true patient" (support point #15, chosen randomly), was also computed. The "true patient's" serum levels at 2, 4, and 8 hrs into the regimen were made available at the end of Day 1, and Bayesian updating was done. Therapy days 2 and 3 repeated the same scenario as Day 1.

RESULTS

The traditional MAP regimen, using mean population parameter values, was thus designed to achieve the goal of 15 ug/ml exactly. No consideration of therapeutic error was present. When that regimen was given to the 28 population support points, however, the serum level trajectories ranged from 9 to over 40 ug/ml, with 6 of the 28 trajectories (21%) being over 40 ug/ml.

In contrast, the MM regimen used all 28 support points of the Vancomycin population model instead of just the mean values, and computed the regimen to minimize the expected squared error in the achievement of the goal. The resulting 28 trajectories were much less variable, were better centered about the goal of 15 ug/ml, and ranged from 5 to 33 ug/ml.

The MM regimen thus delivered visibly greater precision than the traditional one. It used, for the first time, a real population pharmacokinetic model, that of Vancomycin. Further, the MM controller appeared to learn well from the feedback provided by the serum levels, and to control the simulated true patient well as it progressed from one feedback cycle to another. A user-friendly clinical version of the MM program is in development.

Acknowledgements

Supported by NIH grant LM 05401, and by the Stella Slutzky Kunin Research Fund.

A Hybrid Knowledge Based System for Therapy Adjustment in Gestational Diabetes

M.E.Hernando,MS, E.J.Gómez,PhD, R.Corcoy*,MD, F.del Pozo,PhD, M.T.Arredondo,PhD
Grupo de Bioingeniería y Telemedicina - GBT. ETSI Telecomunicación. Universidad Politécnica de Madrid. Spain
*Servicio de Endocrinología y Nutrición. Hospital Sant Pau. Universidad Autónoma de Barcelona. Spain

ABSTRACT

This poster describes a system to analyze self-monitoring data of gestational diabetic patients, for obtaining an assessment of their metabolic control with the final goal of supporting decision-making in therapy adjustment. The system is able to manage incomplete data and to make temporal reasoning under uncertainty, the two most important constraints when analyzing ambulatory monitoring data. Two different formalism have been used to represent and manage the knowledge: a dynamic Bayesian network and a production system based on rules. The outcomes provided by the whole system are: information on possible patient transgressions of the prescribed treatment and recommendations of treatment adjustments.

INTRODUCTION

Gestational diabetes affects 5% of pregnant women. This disease is manifested with high blood glucose concentrations and ketonuria. Complications can be avoided if normoglycaemia levels are achieved during pregnancy with a carefully planned diet and external insulin administration. Patient metabolism changes along time, and that motivates the need of continuous therapy modifications. Ambulatory monitoring in gestational diabetes implies patient self-monitoring measurements that are characterized by: 1) uncertainty in data reliability, and 2) frequent missing data.

The assessment of the metabolic patient state can be addressed using mathematical physiological models of glucose metabolism. The limitation of these approaches is that diet and insulin data, including timing, must be known to perform a feasible simulation. When ambulatory monitoring data are missed, it is not correct to assume data from the prescribed therapy, because patients do not strictly follow the prescribed diet and insulin therapy, and it is not feasible to request to them to record all their actions and modifications. To cope with these constraints, we propose a system that obtains the evolution of the patient metabolic state associated to a degree of uncertainty, according to the type, amount and reliability of monitoring data.

DESCRIPTION

Our approach is a hybrid knowledge based system that propose therapy adjustments by analyzing the patient ambulatory monitoring data. Two different formalism have been used to represent and manage the knowledge: dynamic Bayesian networks (DBN) and rules. Each of them is adequated to represent a different type of knowledge and to make a different type of reasoning, as described below.

First, a DBN is used to obtain the temporal evolution of the patient metabolic state from her monitoring data. This formalism can represent qualitative medical knowledge expressed as relations between causes and effects and their probabilities, and it also allows to make temporal reasoning under uncertainty of incomplete data. A DBN contains several dynamically chained subnetworks where temporal data can be entered. In our case, the basic structure is a network with 50 nodes that represents the metabolic situation for a day. The second step uses the production rule system to propose quantitative therapy modifications. The knowledge and data involved in this reasoning process are: the previously obtained patient metabolic state; the specific patient characteristics; the current therapy; and therapy modification criteria.

A prototype has been implemented in Ansi C on a Sun SparcStation. We have used the commercial software Hugin to develop the daily causal probabilistic network structure, a DBN software from Aalborg University, Denmark, to manage the dynamic structure and CLIPS 6.0 to implement the rule-based formalism.

A Digital EEG Laboratory - Distributed Systems for Data Acquisition and Clinical Support

Ernest C. Jacobs, Richard C. Burgess, Thomas F. Collura

Section of Neurological Computing and Engineering
Department of Neurology, Cleveland Clinic Foundation
9500 Euclid Avenue, Cleveland, Ohio

Recording electroencephalograms(EEG) and other neurophysiological signals traditionally involves dedicated analog amplifiers and multichannel stripchart pen-recorders. Modern instrumentation is now computer-based, providing analog-to-digital conversion and digital output using graphics CRTs and laser printers for display of waveforms. The emergence of digital systems provides a platform for integration of the various diagnostic instruments in a Clinical Neurophysiology Laboratory.

A typical analog instrument, such as an EEG machine, accomplishes data acquisition, signal processing, display, and archive functions all in a single, standalone unit. Using digital systems, it becomes practical to separate these functions into independent modules; for example, the EEG signal acquisition can be done at the bedside, with display of waveforms at a remote location at a later time. Furthermore, software-based systems can be dynamically reconfigured, so that a single digital system can perform the functions of several different analog instruments. Using standard computer networking, acquisition and waveform display systems can be distributed throughout the laboratory, in the operating rooms, at intensive care unit (ICU) beds, etc. Display systems can be located where most convenient for the physicians to analyze the waveforms, and can view data from any of the acquisition stations using a common user-interface. Waveform displays can be enhanced using computer signal processing and integration of textual annotations from a laboratory information system database. Paper output is drastically reduced, and can be centralized so that only a few printers are necessary for a large laboratory. Archive of digital data can likewise be centralized.

The Cleveland Clinic neurophysiology laboratory consists of 8 beds for 24-hour continuous EEG/video monitoring, 4 polysomnography beds for sleep evaluation, operating room and ICU monitoring, as well as performing more than 10,000 routine diagnostic studies per year. If traditional analog instrumentation were used, more than 50 miles of stripchart would be generated each day, at a cost of nearly $3 million / year for paper alone.

Analog systems have been replaced with a network (ethernet and TCP/IP) of 20 HP9000 series UNIX workstation-based acquisition and display systems for acquisition of neurophysiological waveforms and synchronized patient video recording. Three HP9000/835 UNIX time-sharing minicomputers provide operational and administrative support, including an extensive database management system for scheduling, reporting, archiving, and research queries; the database contains textual information for approximately 35,000 patient studies since 1989. Together, the real-time waveform data acquisition systems collect approximately 15 Mbytes of digitized waveform data per minute, 24 hours per day. These systems are used in assembly-line fashion to coordinate the activities of 10 physicians, 27 EEG technologists, 4 nurses, as well as secretaries and receptionists.

Custom application programs provide immediate access to data on any of the acquisition systems from any other system. Waveforms are reviewed at 5 screens per second (16 channels, 10 seconds), faster than the physician can turn pages using stripchart paper. Interesting segments of data can be identified and annotated, automatically by the computer or by a human reviewer. Advanced signal processing is integrated, including real-time montage reformatting, FFT, spike and seizure detection, cursor measurements, etc. Textual information from the clinical database can be incorporated. Interactive terminal sessions can be initiated with other information systems in the hospital, including the HIS, laboratory system, radiology reporting systems. Additionally, image processing software allows viewing radiological images (MRI, CT, PET) over the network.

0195–4210/94/$5.00

Classification of Red Blood Cell Images Using a Neural Network

Samavedam A. Krishna[1], MD; Joseph A. Orr[2], PhD; Dwayne R. Westenskow[2], PhD
[1]Department of Medical Informatics, [2]Department of Anesthesiology - Bioengineering Division
University of Utah, Salt Lake City, Utah

A back-propagation artificial neural network (ANN) has been used to classify images of red blood cells (RBC) based on morphological features. The sensitivity and specificity of the ANN for correctly classifying four categories of RBC have been obtained, at different levels of image noise and with increasing training of the ANN.

MATERIALS AND METHODS

Blood smears from four persons were photographed at 400x magnification; one person had normal cells (NC), one had microcytic hypochromic (MH) anemia, one had sickle cell (SC) anemia and one had hereditary spherocytosis (HS). The photomicrographs were transferred to computer media as 8-bit greyscale image files using a slide digitizer. The images were further manipulated using an image processing program, (NIH Image). Corrections were made for variation in background intensity of the images. Individual RBC were manually cropped from the photomicrograph images into separate files of 75 x 75 pixel size. From each RBC image, 5 values - the area, mean pixel density, standard deviation of pixel densities, integrated density and modal density - were obtained for pixels with greyscale values above the image noise threshold; two thresholds were used. These parameters were chosen for ease of acquisition and because they appeared to be independent descriptors of RBC morphology. Each set of 5 values constituted a pattern for presentation to the artificial neural network. At each threshold, 61 RBC were measured, with 14 NC, 16 MH, 13 SC and 18 HS cells, resulting in 61 patterns. For training the ANN, patterns at the same noise threshold were presented, as far as possible, in the order of one pattern per category following the other. As an important data pre-processing step prior to training and testing the ANN, all 61 values for each parameter were normalized to lie between -1 and +1.

Dartnet, a public-domain artificial NN simulation program, was used to classify the patterns. The ANN had 3 layers of neurons, with 5 neurons each in the input and hidden layers, and 4 in the output layer. Each input layer neuron received one of the 5 feature values in a pattern. Neuron outputs were passed on to all neurons of the next layer. For hidden and output layer neurons, outputs were calculated as logistic functions of summated inputs. Each of the 4 output layer neurons corresponded to one RBC diagnosis - determined by a high output value for one of the neurons and low values for the other three. The ANN was trained by modifying neuron interconnection weights by back-propation of error between actual ANN outputs and desired outputs for any training pattern. The ANN was trained and tested by cross-validation. One pattern of each category would be witheld during training and the ANN would be trained on the remaining 57 patterns of normalized values. After every 50 cycles of the training pattern set, the 4 test patterns would be presented to the ANN. Outputs in response to each of the 4 test patterns would be noted and the process continued till 2000 training cycles.

RESULTS

After all 61 patterns had been tested, the results were reorganized as true positive, false positive and false negative with respect to the true diagnoses for the test patterns. These results were then further compiled to generate the true positive rate (TPR) and false positive rate (FPR) for diagnosing each category of cells at each of the two thresholds. Using these values, the diagnostic performance of the ANN has been expressed in terms of sensitivity (= TPR) and specificity (= 1 - FPR) for diagnosis of each category of cells at each threshold.

The sensitivity and specificity for diagnosing the four categories of cells, at both thresholds (noise levels), stabilized after about 500 to 600 training cycles. In some cases, there was a marginal drop in sensitivity and/or specificity with increasing number of training cycles. At a threshold of 45 (greater noise), the best sensitivities were 0.64, 0.69, 0.77 and 0.94; the corresponding specificities were 0.96, 0.65, 0.98 and 1.0 respectively for NC, MH, SC and HS cells. At a threshold of 128 (lesser noise), the best sensitivities were 0.79, 0.69, 0.92 and 1.0; the corresponding specificities were 0.98, 0.93, 0.98 and 1.0 respectively for NC, MH, SC and HS cells.

CONCLUSION

Adequate to high sensitivity and specificity for identification of RBC images by an ANN using only a few image descriptors (5 parameters) can be achieved once regions of interest have been defined. The need for only a few training cycles is probably the result of pre-processing of data (by normalization); this contrasts with similar previous studies in which very large numbers of training iterations were used.

0195-4210/94/$5.00

Aspects of Risk Management Support for an Emergency Medicine Physician Workstation

Donald W. Rucker, M.D.[1], Richard S. Johannes, M.D., Scott W. Finley, M.D.[1], Stephen N. Kahane, M.D.
Clinical Information Advantages, Inc., Waltham, Massachusetts

Emergency departments are high risk sites for malpractice events. EMstation™ is an Emergency Medicine Physician Workstation that incorporates tools to reduce malpractice risk in near real time (at the time of documentation). Based on a Microsoft Windows 3.1 interface, physicians are led through color-coded templates addressing known failure modes in emergency medicine. Risk management opportunities available at the time of charting when the patient is often still in the department allowing real time risk reduction are explored.

CURRENT RISK MANAGEMENT EFFORTS

The emergency department is the third highest risk setting based on malpractice claims, following only obstetric and operating rooms. Studies of these suits have consistently shown that a small set of repetitive clinical errors (missed MI's, appendicitis, ectopic pregnancy, subarachnoid hemorrhage, meningitis, missed tendon lacerations, and retained foreign bodies within wounds) generates over 50% of dollars paid out to plaintiffs.

Currently manual audit such as chart review based on JCAHO criteria is a mainstay of risk management. These activities are generally based on handwritten or transcribed records. Current computerized efforts at risk management include clinical alerts, text string searches for high risk presentations, and electronically implemented documentation guidelines.

METHODS

EMstation 2.6 is a software and hardware package supporting both template based and free text dictation with an integrated database. It is written in Microsoft C with speech recognition by Dragon Dictate. EMstation represents over 40 person years of direct programming by a team of "C" programmers as well as a similar time spent by physicians designing templates. Templates support approximately 250 clinical scenarios. The core paradigm is the use of menu choices by voice or mouse. The templates are written in a programming language supporting Boolean logic to display text, calls to external databases or functions, and correct grammar for subject verb number agreement and complex noun phrases. At any point in generating the note, the physician can switch to free text.

INCORPORATING RISK MANAGEMENT

Risk management for high risk clinical presentations is incorporated directly into the templates rather than applied after the fact. The menus themselves highlight key symptoms, signs and lab examinations. Thus, in chest pain or related complaints, the physician is prompted for associated symptoms such as diaphoresis or palpitations (See Figure). Then he or she is asked about cardiac risk factors. Further on

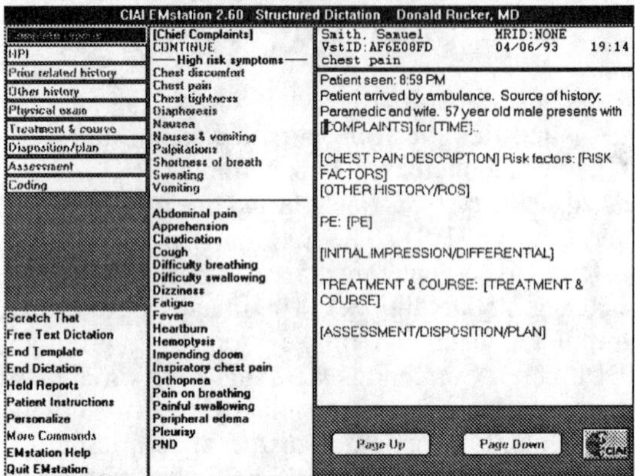

in the template, the EKG is prominently displayed as the leading diagnostic maneuver. All high risk items are displayed in red. Users can select additional items to the color red. Two specific risk management tools are incorporated. One is a package of customizable patient instructions available at any time. Secondly, an emergency medicine risk management syllabus is packaged as a hypertext browser.[1]. The integral database offers quality assurance and risk management review options as well. Database capture of notes is automatic.

CONCLUSION

Malpractice events are still relatively rare, so the next phase of research will likely have to focus on process measures rather than outcome measures. The EMstation architecture for graphic user interfaces, multiple modality data entry, mixed template and free text dictation, customization tools, syntax correction, an integral records database, and workflow support offers opportunities for both ease of use and risk management.

[1]. Henry, G. and N. Little, Managing Risk in Emergency Medicine, 1991, Ann Arbor: Medical Practice Management, Inc.

[1] Berenson Emergency Unit, Beth Israel Hospital and Harvard Medical School, Boston, MA
[1] NIH Clinical Center, Information Systems Department, Bethesda, MD

0195-4210/94/$5.00

Telemedicine in Support of Remote Medical Operations

David G. Gilbertson, MS, US Army Medical Department

This poster presents the United States Military Telemedicine project and how telemedicine is used to support United Nations medical operations in Croatia and Macedonia. A 40 bed inpatient facility in Croatia is using telemedicine to communicate with medical centers in Germany and the United States. Treatment stations in Macedonia have telemedicine connections to hospitals in Croatia, Germany, and the United States.

BACKGROUND

Telemedicine is used by the United States Military to enhance medical care at remote locations around the world. The Army Medical Research and Development Command and the Uniformed Services University of the Health Sciences (USUHS) have embarked on a prototype project to test the ability of telemedicine to enhance the capabilities of deployed military hospitals. The telemedicine project is uses off-the-shelf technology to transmit real-time video, data, and high resolution still-images. Croatia and Macedonia use high-speed satellite telephones to link to the global military telemedicine network.

MEDICAL APPLICATIONS

Telemedicine supports medical diagnosis, patient treatment, preventive medicine, video "soap notes", medical training (bilateral), patient documentation, supervision, and morale support for deployed medical personnel. The telemedicine project is designed to test the telemedicine technology and determine cost effective uses for this technology. The technological research issues are ease-of-use, reliability, and diagnostic quality of images. Medical researchers study the value of remote consultation, the ability to improve medical care, the value of video "soap notes", and the improvements in medical training. Operational issues include determining how telemedicine technology will be integrated with the routine health care delivery process.

TRAINING AND SUPPORT

The military recognized a need to train medical personnel on the technical and operational aspects of telemedicine. The USUHS designed telemedicine courses for medics and physicians. The medics course includes enhanced life saving training and training on how to use telemedicine consultation. Physicians are taught how to interact with the telemedicine equipment and how to use telemedicine to extend expert clinical knowledge to medics and physicians located in remote locations.

PRELIMINARY FINDINGS

The military is using telemedicine for several medical applications. Radiology and microbiology images are transmitted from Croatia to military hospitals in the United States. Final reports are electronically sent back to Croatia and Macedonia. Real-time patient diagnosis and treatment are accomplished using telemedicine. Medics and physicians are beginning to find a telemedicine "comfort zone". They are discovering how and when to use telemedicine. The project team is constantly improving the equipment, procedures, and system documentation.

CONCLUSION

Telemedicine will change the delivery of health care from the initial health care provider to the expert consultant. The current military implementation of telemedicine provides a fertile environment to study the impact of this technology. Advances made in the military telemedicine project will improve future humanitarian and military medical operations.

References

Goeringer, F. Hagmann, J. Fay, C.R.. Operation Primetime Project Plan, Army Medical Department Research and Development Command, 1994 January.

Sanders, J.H. and Tedesco F.J.. Telemedicine: bringing medical care to isolated communities. Journal of the Medical Association of Georgia, 1993 May, 82(5):237-41.

Hubble JP; Pahwa R; Michalek DK; Thomas C; Koller WC. Interactive video conferencing: a means of providing interim care to Parkinson's disease patients. Movement Disorders, 1993 Jul, 8(3):380-2.

Improving Outpatient Services - The Value of Information

JG Williams, JM Morgan, SC Greenway, WY Cheung
School of Postgraduate Studies in Medical and Health Care,
Maes-y-Gwernen Hall, Morriston Hospital, Swansea, SA6 6NL, UK

The quality of care delivered in outpatient clinics is influenced by many factors, not least the optimum management of time. This submission reports how the ability to analyse detailed patient data has enabled monitoring and improvement of the clinical service provided in a busy gastroenterological practice.

Clinical, administrative and demographic data have been collected on 2,000 consecutive patients referred to a specialist gastroenterology clinic in a busy general hospital in the UK. 15,000 items of clinical data have been recorded and analysed.

Analysis of outpatient visits by diagnosis has identified the five disorders which are most commonly referred, and the median number of follow-up visits each requires. Irritable bowel syndrome, gastro-oesophageal reflux and dyspeptic disorders tend to be seen only once. Ulcerative colitis and Crohn's disease tend to remain under follow-up long-term (median 4 and 6 visits respectively over 5 years).

Analysis of referral patterns of patients with irritable bowel syndrome has shown considerable variation in referring practice, both from primary and secondary care. A significant proportion are referred initially to other specialists, particularly surgeons and gynaecologists, with considerable variation as to whether tertiary referral occurs.

Discussion with primary care doctors (GPs), aided by agreed algorithms to guide initial management, has reduced the number of referrals, and enabled return back to the care of Gps many patients who would otherwise have remained under secondary care. This rationalisation of initial referral and shared care has led to an encouraging fall in the time patients spend waiting for an appointment (a widespread problem in the UK) from 9 to 2 months.

Not all patients, however, can be easily managed in primary care. Crohn's disease and ulcerative colitis are examples of chronic relapsing conditions, where the course is unpredictable. An analysis of the growth in demand for outpatient appointment time to follow up patients with these disorders has demonstrated that, if current trends continue, saturation of available appointment slots will occur within the next five years. This emphasises the need to transfer as many patients as possible back to the care of GPs.

To do this with confidence, a prediction of outcome is needed. We have monitored the disease activity of these disorders over time for all our patients, and demonstrated how this fluctuates. We are creating a detailed, coded knowledge base of clinical features, built upon the progress of real patients, so that we will in time be able to predict who is likely to do well, and can be discharged back to primary care with confidence.

Devolution of specialist care into the community is fashionable at present in the UK. The ability to identify which patients are seen, investigated briefly and discharged, has enabled prediction of the likely impact of open access services, and the creation of clinical guidelines for referral. For example, patients with gastro-oesophageal reflux or dyspepsia comprise a third of total referrals for an out-patient opinion, but only half of these are considered by the specialist to require endoscopy. Guidelines and monitoring are needed to ensure that patients are not inappropriately endoscoped via an open access service.

The length of time patients spend in their first consultation ranges from 10 to 30 minutes (median 19 min). The consultation takes an average of six minutes longer if a rigid sigmoidoscopy is performed. Patients with functional disorders (such as irritable bowel syndrome and non-ulcer dyspepsia) take five minutes longer than those with organic disease. This information enables more rational allocation of consultation times according to presenting complaint.

These data have been captured using a generic Clinical Information System (GeneCIS), which is currently under development at the School of Postgraduate Studies in Swansea. The generic concept aims to ensure that information is patient focused, rather than merely provider or carer based. Relevant data can be collected on all aspects of a patient's transit through care (during any period of illness), and progress can be monitored over time. GeneCIS is intended to support the broad spectrum of clinical care, and is currently in use in gastroenterology, urology and elderly care.

A Quantitative Method for Identifying Specific Educational Needs Among CD Plus Medline Searchers: A Pilot Study

Cheryl Chisnell, M.A., Kathel Dunn, M.S.L.S., Dean F. Sittig, Ph.D.
The Informatics Center, Vanderbilt University, Nashville, Tennessee

The Eskind Biomedical Library of Vanderbilt University recently provided remote access to MEDLINE using CD Plus' OVID software. Remote users had previous experience searching MEDLINE with other systems (in particular, Grateful Med, SilverPlatter, and Notis,) but not with the CD Plus interface. Our concern was that prior experience with a system would inhibit searchers from using CD Plus' system features correctly.

This study was developed to provide a quantitative method for measuring the educational needs of remote searchers based on the use of specific features of the CD Plus system. Data generated by this study will be used to develop targeted educational programs and materials.

Transaction logs generated by remote CD Plus users over a two week period were analyzed. Discrete system features, such as the use of textword or MeSH term searching, were counted. Since typical search sessions involve more than the use of a single feature, system features were also considered in combination. Librarians experienced with CD Plus generated rules, based on the use of system features, defining "bad searches." For example, a rule might be developed to isolate textword searches that failed to use limits, subheadings, boolean operators, or MeSH terms properly. For example,

Line #	Search Statement
1	retinoid.tw.
2	review.tw.
3	1 and 2

The first search term, *retinoid*, has an equivalent MeSH term but it was not used. Experience suggests that MeSH terms, when available, should be used first, though not exclusively, in the search process. A second problem is the lack of use of the "limit" feature. *Review* is searched as a textword instead of making use of MEDLINE check tags supported through the "limit" feature of CD Plus. The result of the misuse of features in this case is the oversight of several key articles.

Rules were developed and applied to the transaction logs to determine the significance of each type of searching. Analysis of the data indicates that remote users misuse CD Plus in several significant ways. Author only or textword only searches are more the norm than the exception. In addition, searchers browse through too much information without applying appropriate limits. Search precision can be increased by combining terms or using limits such as "English." Figure 1 represents initial results when several rules were applied to the transaction logs.

Initial results of this study indicate that the methodology developed can be successfully used to determine search habits and develop educational materials. The method could also be used to evaluate the effectiveness of educational program and materials instituted.

This work was supported in part by grants R29 LM05284 and G08 LM05443 from the National Library of Medicine.

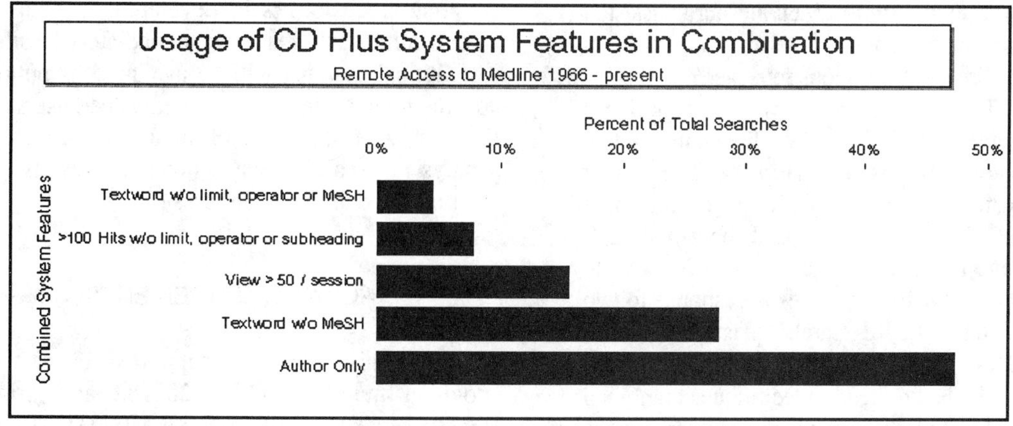

Figure 1

Using the Metathesaurus™ for Bibliographic Retrieval: A Pre-Implementation Study

Denise P. Radow, MSLS, Maryanne Blake, MSLS*, Ellen Howard, MLS, Cynthia Jones+, Linda Milgrom, MSLS*, Maren Ostergard+, Erika Shaffer+
*National Network of Libraries of Medicine Pacific Northwest Region, SB-55
Health Sciences Library and Information Center, SB-55
University of Washington, Seattle, WA 98195
+Graduate Student, School of Library and Information Science, Univ. of Washington

The Health Sciences Library and Information Center was awarded a contract from the National Library of Medicine to apply the Metathesaurus™, one of the Unified Medical Language System (UMLS) Knowledge Sources, to the University of Washington's online search interface, Willow. The overall plan is to make the Metathesaurus accessible both as a key index for MEDLINE searchers and as a terminology and concept resource to health information analysts. This poster describes a study which evaluated the use and utility of the Coach Metathesaurus Browser for MEDLINE search construction. Results of the pilot evaluation were incorporated into the implementation design.

These questions guided the design of this study: 1. What do searchers experience and report when using the Metathesaurus to construct MEDLINE searches? 2. Which features of the Metathesaurus browser do searchers consider useful for MEDLINE searching? 3. How do searches constructed using the University of Washington (UW) system compare with Metathesaurus-assisted searches, in selection of terms and also in number of relevant citations retrieved?

Ten clinicians with experience searching MEDLINE on the University system participated in this evaluation. The group included four physicians, three nurses and three dentists. Each searcher used both the UW system and the Coach Metathesaurus Browser to construct MEDLINE searches in response to two NLM "Gold Standard Search" questions.

In this study, qualitative and quantitative data collection techniques combined to capture a holistic, user-oriented view of the online search process. Using a "think-aloud" protocol, study participants' thoughts and reactions were audiotaped as they used the UW search interface and the Metathesaurus browser. Search activities were observed and tallied. Searchers also answered twelve scripted questions about the online tools. Each searcher's Metathesaurus searches were measured against his or her UW interface constructions, and both retrieval sets were compared to the "Gold Standard" retrieval set for each question.

Study participants reported satisfaction with the ability of the Metathesaurus to "map" their queries to appropriate controlled vocabulary, an improvement over the alphabetic MeSH browse list available on Willow. Other well-liked features included the concept definitions, MEDLINE postings information, and concept co-occurrence postings. The complexity of the Metathesaurus browser made it difficult for most study participants to evaluate it fully after one brief session. This repeated comment influenced the interface design process for implementation of the Metathesaurus at UW: a streamlined tool is in development, with the most important features immediately visible. Additional features will be available as buttons off the main screen, for more advanced users.

A full report of qualitative findings, analysis of search constructions and results will be presented at the poster session.

ACKNOWLEDGEMENTS

This project is supported in part by contract number 467-MZ-201782 and grants GO8-LM05620 and 1-F38-LM00031-01, all from the National Library of Medicine.

Increasing Access to Clinical Information on Hospital Wards

Cathy H. Eames M.S.L.S., Michele S. Klein, M.S.L.S.
Medical Library, Children's Hospital of Michigan, Detroit, Michigan

Medical library information resources can make a positive contribution to the clinical information needs of health care professionals. To increase availability of knowledge-based information and transfer information to its point of use, a CD-ROM resource library was networked and interfaced with the existing hospital information system at Children's Hospital of Michigan in Detroit, Michigan. Clinicians in 21 patient care areas now have access to the patient record, full-text pediatric journal information and the Micromedex CCIS database at one location.

INTRODUCTION

Children's Hospital of Michigan (CHM) is a 260 bed pediatric hospital that is part of the Detroit Medical Center (DMC) in Detroit, Michigan. The CHM experience of linking and relating the library to institution-wide computer networks can be traced back to 1987 [1]. At that time, screens were developed for requesting a LATCH (Literature Attached to the Chart) and for requesting patient education materials from the hospital-wide patient information system. These were given a procedure code so that they could be requested in the same manner as an x-ray or laboratory test. Two preformatted message screens were also developed, one for an article or book request, and one for a literature search or information request.

In 1992 an Information Systems Grant was funded through the National Library of Medicine to increase access to knowledge-based information in the patient care areas of the hospital. A multi-disciplinary Medical Information Systems Committee consisting of librarians, physicians, nurses, pharmacists, and information systems personnel advised the project's coordinators. This committee is still involved with the project's progress. A preliminary needs assessment of in-house and outside attending staff solicited input to determine the areas of greatest information need. This assessment supported previous studies in the literature reporting that clinicians wanted journal and drug related information which was physically close, either in their office or on the unit [2,3].

METHODS / RESULTS

To increase availability of information resources, full-text health science information in CD-ROM format has been linked to the CHM patient information system and provided to users at point of need on the wards. A fiber optic backbone was installed to the patient care floors and an Ethernet LAN configuration was used to add twenty-one microcomputers at nursing stations, in clinical conference rooms, the physicians' lounge, the Poison Control Center, the Drug Information Center and the nursing administration offices. The LAN was then connected, by means of an existing DMC FDDI campus ring, to a Tricord 40/50C file server with a CD-ROM tower at the DMC Campus Data Center. This was the link to full-text information. Another link was made by means of T1 lines to the DMC Troy Data Center where the computer containing the hospital information system was housed. Microsoft Windows and terminal emulation software were installed on each of the 21 PCs. Both the CD-ROM information and the patient information were brought together on the desktop PC with a Windows interface. This PC functions as both an order-entry and a clinical information workstation.

Doctors, nurses, allied-health personnel, and students now have access to the Micromedex CCIS and the CMC Research, Inc's library of pediatric journals and Yearbook series. Clinicians in patient care areas can now look at a patient's record, order a test, find information on a disease or drug and order a literature search or patient education materials, all at the same location.

Reference

[1]. MS. Klein. Adapting IAIMS to a hospital level. Bull Med Libr Assoc 1989;77:357-365.

[2]. SH. Woolf, et al. The medical information needs of internists and pediatricians at an academic medical center. Bull Med Libr Assoc 1989;77:372-80.

[3]. SP. Curley, et al. Physicians' use of medical knowledge resources: preliminary theoretical framework and findings. Med Decis Making 1990;10:231-41.

An SDI Program for Distributing Funding Opportunities using Electronic Mail

Paul M. Keenan M.S., Carol H. Montgomery, Ph.D.
Medical College of Pennsylvania and Hahnemann University

ABSTRACT

As the competition for funding increases, the need to make researchers aware of all available funding is becoming more acute. The solution presented here is a Selective Dissemination of Information (SDI) service which electronically mails funding information that matches a researcher's keywords. The keywords are part of extensive faculty profiles that make up a Faculty Expertise database. The funding information comes from the Sponsored Programs Information Network (SPIN) database. The software enables researchers to learn about appropriate funding opportunities without spending time actively searching for them.

INTRODUCTION

Over the past ten years there has been a concerted effort by both the federal government and commercial vendors to make funding information available in electronic forms. However, the information accessible to an individual researcher is often dispersed across several different systems, making it difficult to obtain a complete view of the available opportunities. The commercial comprehensive databases developed to date are often difficult for an inexperienced user to search.

In particular, young medical researchers and investigators entering new fields need help in identifying suitable funding sources. The solution presented here is to provide a Selective Dissemination of Information (SDI) service to make researchers aware of a broad spectrum of relevant funding opportunities. It is similar to the SDI system at the Yale School of Medicine for *Current Contents*.[1]

COMPONENTS OF THE SYSTEM

The SDI system matches keywords in a comprehensive Faculty Expertise Database with indexing terms from the SPIN database. The Expertise Database is available online and serves many other purposes, including informing faculty about each others' work and capabilities.

The Faculty Expertise Database was initially developed by collecting faculty information for the national BEST*North America database of expertise, as well as certain information of local interest only. In return for participation in BEST, the University received a file of its own faculty's records. These records were then loaded into a MUMPS (M) database designed by the project staff using a combination of M and M/SQL, a fourth generation relational database management system. The system platform is a MicroVAX 3100.

SPIN was selected because it is comprehensive, microcomputer-based, runs on a local area network, and uses a standard xbase format which could be manipulated with several types of PC database software. In our evaluation *SPIN* was found to have excellent coverage of new program announcements, and with a bi-weekly subscription has proven to be almost as timely as an online service. If necessary, library staff can also connect to the publisher's online service to retrieve the most recent program announcements.

In general, the SDI system has been received enthusiastically by researchers. Because it has been active only a few months, it is not yet possible to determine whether the system is having an impact upon the number or type of grant applications submitted by the researchers. This will be measured after a sufficient period of time has passed.

Acknowledgements

This project was supported by NIH Grant LM05373 from the National Library of Medicine. The assistance of Margaret G. Fallis has contributed immeasurably to its success.

References

1. Paton, John A. et al. "Online Bibliographic Information: Integration into an Emerging IAIMS Environment." in *Proceedings of the Sixteenth Annual Symposium on Computer Application in Medical Care.* McGraw-Hill, Inc., 1992, 605-609.

Structured Text Representations and Relevance Judgments: An Exploratory Study

Padmini Srinivasan

School of Library & Information Science
University of Iowa
Iowa City, Iowa, USA -52242
padmini-srinivasan@uiowa.edu

This paper presents results of an exploratory study on using a structured text and query model for analyzing relevance judgments made by users on retrieved texts [1] The structured model moves beyond keyword based text representation and retrieval. In particular it allows texts and queries to be represented by concepts embedded within the structural framework of complex objects. These objects preserves important text-based links between the selected concepts. The current study reveals a tendency for user judged relevance potential to decrease as the structure-based similarity between query and text decreases. This indicates that the structure-based retrieval model has the potential to conduct more precise retrieval than keyword based models. This supports our overall research goal of developing and investigating the structured retrieval model.

INTRODUCTION

The study is part of ongoing research on structure-based text retrieval wherein both texts and queries may be represented using complex objects. In the 1993 SCAMC session we presented the details of this model and its motivation [1] We have also discussed associated retrieval strategies and a prototype implementation in other work [4]. Here we focus on the ability of the model to explain (and therefore possibly predict) relevance judgments made by users.

METHODOLOGY & CONCLUSIONS

The analysis was conducted on a subset of the dataset used by Hersh et al. [3]. For each of 12 queries a maximum of 20 relevant and 20 non relevant texts were analyzed resulting in a total of 174 analyzed texts. In particular we focused on those queries where the majority of non relevant articles had the query concepts but not in central roles.

Four distinct steps were followed: 1) Extract structured representations from queries. 2) Extract structured representations from retrieved abstracts. 3) Compare query and text structures and describe the relationship between the two. 4) Compare query-text relationships (obtained in the previous step) to relevance judgments made by users.

The data analysis indicates that there is a tendency for relevance to decrease as the relationship between the query and text weakens. The analysis of these query-text relationships involves conceptual comparisons within a structured framework. To conclude, the tentative conclusions made here provides further support for continued development and investigation of the underlying structure-based text retrieval model. Our next step is to perform similar analysis on larger sets of queries and texts.

REFERENCES

[1] Hankom, L. L. and Srinivasan, P. Quality Retrieval of the Empirical Literature: A Structured Approach. *Proceedings of the SCAMC,* 1994.

[2] Haynes, R., McKibbon, K., Walker, C., Ryan, N., Fitzgerald, D., Ramsey, M. Online Access to MEDLINE in Clinical Settings. *Ann Intern. Med.* (1990), 112: pp. 78-84.

[3] Hersh, William R. Hickam, D. H., Haynes, B., McKibbon, K. A. A Performance and Failure Analysis of SAPHIRE with a MEDLINE Test Collection. *JAMIA* 1, 1 (1994), pp. 51-60.

[4] Rama, D. V. and Srinivasan, P. An Investigation of Content Representation using Text Grammars. *ACM Transactions on Information Systems*, January 1993

---

[1]The author is very grateful to William R. Hersh, MD for sharing the MEDLINE dataset which originated in an earlier study by Haynes & colleagues [2] and also for sharing the error analysis data generated in [3].

0195-4210/94/$5.00 © 1994 AMIA, Inc.

Trends in Students' Knowledge, Opinions, and Behaviors Concerning Dental Informatics and Computer Applications

W. Paul Lang, D.D.S., M.P.H., Thomas G. Green, Ph.D., and Jed J. Jacobson, D.D.S., M.S., M.P.H.

School of Dentistry, University of Michigan, Ann Arbor, Michigan 48109-1078

INTRODUCTION

No long term evaluations of dental students' knowledge, opinions, and behaviors regarding dental informatics and computer applications have been completed. A 1988 survey found junior dental students to be most knowledgeable about generic applications like word processing and least knowledgeable about dental applications [1]. A 1990 survey of first and fourth year dental students found both groups had little knowledge and experience with computers and informatics applications, but held favorable opinions about these issues [2]. Given the paucity of previous research, the goal of this investigation was to evaluate changes over time in knowledge, opinions, and behaviors of dental students concerning dental informatics and computers.

METHODS

A 74-item questionnaire was constructed to assess students' knowledge, opinions, and behaviors. Eighteen items having a three point scale (Agree, Undecided, Disagree; collapsed range: 0-18) were used to measure knowledge. Opinions were measured using 13 questions (Cronbach's alpha = 0.81) with a five-point Likert scale (Strongly Agree to Strongly Disagree; range: 13-65). Behaviors were assessed with 28 questions that measured the extent of experience with computers and informatics applications. A five point scale ranging from no experience to extensive experience was used (Range: 28-140). Demographic information was collected including age, gender, personal and parental ownership of computers, and numbers of formal computer courses completed. First (N=95) and fourth year (N = 91) students completed the survey in 1990. First (N=97) and fourth year (N=91) students completed the survey in 1993. The 1990 first year and 1993 fourth year students were the same group. Response rates ranged from 99 to 100%.

RESULTS

First Year Students (D1s). In 1993, 43.8% of D1s owned computers compared to 17.9% in 1990. No difference was observed in the numbers of computer courses completed. Knowledge scores were not different between groups, but 1993 D1s had a significantly lower opinion score about these issues than 1990 D1s (44.8 versus 52.2, $p<0.001$). The 1993 D1s reported more experience with computers than the 1990 D1s. Total experience scores were 47.4 versus 41.9 ($p<0.001$).
Fourth Year Students (D4s). There was no difference in computer ownership between groups. The 1993 D4s had completed more computer courses than the 1990 D4s (2.3 versus 0.9; $p<0.001$). There were significant differences in knowledge scores between groups with 1993 D4s answering about twice as many questions correctly ($P<0.001$). There were no differences in opinion scores. The 1993 D4s reported more experience with computers than the 1990 D4s. Total experience scores were 55.9 versus 41.3 ($p<0.001$).
First Year, now Fourth Year Students. There was no statistically significant increase in computer ownership during dental school. Students reported an average increase of one course. Mean knowledge scores of these students increased between 1990 and 1993 (8.0 to 14.1; $p<0.001$). Opinion scores did not change significantly. The group's mean experience score increased from 41.7 to 55.8 ($p<0.0001$).
Gender Differences. In 1990, 58.6% of D1 females reported completing ≥ 1 computer courses compared to 76.8% of males ($p<0.01$). Mean knowledge scores were significantly different with females having a mean score of 5.0 compared to 9.5 for males ($p<0.001$). There were no statistically significant differences in opinion scores or total computing experiences. In 1993, a difference in completed computer courses remained between the genders. Knowledge and experience scores had increased for both groups and were about equal. Opinion scores had not changed.

DISCUSSION

Students currently entering dental education are more likely to own a computer and to have experience with computers and computer applications. Interestingly, opinions of current new students were lower suggesting less enthusiasm for computing or more understanding of its limitations. D4s in 1993 displayed more knowledge and experience than 1990 D4s, and these increases may reflect the introduction of a required information management course in the fourth year. The 1990 D4s received little education on informatics or computing. Knowledge and experience increases are evidenced in the comparison of 1990 D1 scores with their own 1993 scores as D4s. Results suggest that at least knowledge differences between genders are addressed in dental school. In summary, students come more prepared and their computing and informatics knowledge and experiences are increased during their dental education.

REFERENCES

[1]. Feldman CA: Junior dental student survey of computers in dentistry, *J Dent Educ*, 53 (1989) 55.

[2]. Lang WP, Green TG, and Jacobson JJ: Students' knowledge, opinions, and behaviors concerning dental informatics and computer applications, *J Dent Educ*, 56 (1992) 195-9.

Preparatory Information

Carol L. Ireson, R. N., M.S.N., Cathie L. Velotta, R. N., M.S.N.
Department of Nursing, University of Kentucky Hospital
Lexington, Kentucky

Research has demonstrated the effect of preparatory information in reducing patient's negative responses to stressful experiences. Information about diagnostic procedures is unavailable to the clinicians due to rapidly changing technology and lack of exposure to the diagnostic experience. Therefore the purpose of this project was to disseminate procedure related sensory to the clinician to patients through the use of mainframe terminals and printers.

INTRODUCTION

Concrete, objective information has been demonstrated to have a positive effect on the patient's response to stressful diagnostic and treatment related experiences. Knowledge about this process has been developing since the early 1970's when Jean Johnson published her seminal work on the effect of accurate expectations on reactions to noxious medical exams [1,2]. Despite this knowledge, nurses do not consistently use this method in preparing patients for stressful health-related events. One explanation is that nurses are not actually present during most procedures and therefore do not have access to concrete information about what the patient experiences.

METHODS

In an effort to assist nurses to use the research related to the effect of using concrete, objective information, a project has been undertaken at the University of Kentucky Hospital. This project involve s Nursing, Information Management and the diagnostic departments. An instrument was developed to elicit procedure-related sensory information from all clinical diagnostic and treatment departments. individuals performing the procedures were asked to include a description of the procedure room including lighting, temperature, and general appearance; concrete objective descriptions about the sensations that patients experienced during and after the procedures; the length of the procedure; and the length of time required for interpretation of the results.

These concrete, objective descriptions written in terms that patients could understand were entered into the hospital information system mainframe. Access to the on-line information is available via terminals located at every hospital nursing station, nursing charting room, diagnostic department and clinic workstation. An index listing all of the procedures allows registered nurses and other clinicians to select the information needed for a specific patient. Nurses can use the information for verbal explanations or can give the patient a screen print copy.

An added benefit for the nurse having such detailed information is the ability to more appropriately schedule events in the patient's day.

References

[1]. J. Johnson. Effects of accurate expectations and behavioral instructions on reactions during a noxious medical examination. J. Pers. Soc. Psychol. 29:710-718.

[2]. N. Christman., K. Kirchoff., M. Oakley. Concrete Objective Information. IN: G. Bulechek. Nursing interventions: essentials nursing treatments. W. B. Saunders, Philadelphia, 1992.

0195-4210/94/$5.00

CC-IMED: The California Consortium for Informatics in Medical Education and Development

Anthony R. Kwak, Ed.D and Nikola Jurisic, Ph.D., University of California, Los Angeles
Parvati Dev, Ph.D., Stanford University
Helene M. Hoffman, Ph.D. and Anne Irwin, M.D., University of California, San Diego

The California Consortium for Informatics in Medical Education and Development (CC-IMED) began in late 1990 with an inaugural meeting of representatives from the medical schools in California. The representatives were individuals identified by the academic deans from each participating school as having major responsibilities related to computer-based instruction.

MISSION AND ORGANIZATION

From its inception, CC-IMED's focus has been on sharing, cooperation, collaboration, face-to-face meetings and open communications among its members. The stated mission of the consortium is "to provide a forum to promote the development, evaluation, dissemination, and utilization of technology-based medical education".

The organizational structure of CC-IMED has remained informal and small, limiting membership to the eight medical schools in California. Each school has one to two representatives who meet on an average of two to three times per year. There is no separate budget for the consortium and no membership fees. Travel, meeting, communications and project-related costs are assumed by the member institutions. There are no organizational officers, board of directors, or staff personnel. Responsibility for hosting, organizing and presiding over meetings or carrying out projects are shared among all members.

ACTIVITIES

Consortium activities and interests have included software evaluation, visual databases, resource sharing, curriculum databases, computer and informatics literacy, networking, multimedia computing, and faculty development.

An early consortium project was the development of a computer literacy assessment instrument which has been administered to incoming first-year medical students in California since the fall of 1991. The results of these surveys have assisted member schools in developing plans for computer-based instructional programs and facilities. Other surveys to assess students' medical informatics competencies and their use of computers in the curriculum are being developed for students at the end of their second and fourth years.

In 1992, the consortium published a *Curriculum Software Inventory* which describes the "successful" use of computer-based programs in the medical school curriculum. In addition to descriptive information about a program, each entry contains information on how a program is actually used in an institution, by what faculty and students, and why it has been judged as "successful". Multiple entries for a specific program provide data for comparing how a program is used in different institutions. Thus far, the inventory is providing valuable insights into the varying ways computer-based instruction in contributing to medical education.

Other consortium activities have resulted in a grant from Apple Computer Corporation which provided member schools with educational software development equipment and helped to establish a consortium internet server with additional assistance from Upjohn; established a special agreement for the sharing of consortium member developed *DxR* cases with the DxR Development Group; agreed to share patient cases developed for *Short Rounds*, a patient case multimedia presentation program develop by Stanford University, a consortium member.

CONCLUSION

The mission of the CC-IMED is a very broad and general one which reflects the rather diverse interests and needs of its members. As a consortia, it has evolved into a unique and open environment that has fostered cooperation, collaboration and innovation on many fronts. To date, it has provided its members with benefits far beyond their initial expectations and has resulted in accomplishments that could have been achieved only through inter-institutional sharing.

OA-Rehab: Designing a Personalized Exercise Program for People with Osteoarthritis

John C. Reid, Ph.D., Marian A. Minor, Ph.D., Joyce A. Mitchell, Ph.D., Timothy B. Patrick, Ph.D., Joyce Z. Griffin, Ph.D., James C. Cutts, III, Matthew Morrow, M.D., and Nancy Thompson
School of Medicine, University of Missouri, Columbia, MO

We describe the design of a multi-media performance support system (PSS) based on the documented benefits of a personalized exercise program for people with arthritis, on the known value of self-efficacy and stages of change, and on principles of learning theory. The poster will show examples of incorporating motivational and cognitive principles into a PSS.

INTRODUCTION

Although regular exercise is an effective therapy for rehabilitation of persons with osteoarthritis (OA) [1], people with OA may not exercise for three reasons. First, primary care physicians seldom recommend therapeutic exercises for people with OA [2], second, booklets about exercise may not be tailored to individuals' impairments [3], and third, people may have difficulty maintaining exercise without increasing their self-efficacy [4], or without having the intervention tailored to their stage of change [5].

Effective multi-media presentations should incorporate principles of instructional design [6]. These include using advance organizers, involving the reader by using pre- or post questions, enhancing storage and retrieval through reminders, prompts, and summaries, meaningful presentations, and increasing interest and attentiveness through personalization [7]. Our intelligent PSS includes advising, teaching, doing, and reference functions by combining an intuitive interface with an expert system and a database.

METHOD

We selected a PC platform based on availability of software, expense, flexibility, and local expertise. Since our audience were to be older adults with limited if any computer expertise and possible visual handicaps, we decided to use a large, touch screen, and eliminate keyboard and mouse input. The interface design was arrived at by examining other systems, by seeking advice from experts, and by group brainstorming sessions where we identified three main content ideas to repeatedly present to the user. We designed a supportive, social environment based on the demonstrated research effectiveness of Bandura's Social Learning theory, and from the literature on the value of social support in exercise maintenance. The program asks the client to perform tests for range of motion and strength, helps the client assign priorities to areas of improvement, and produces written instruction and an exercise videotape. The poster will illustrate examples of incorporating tests and assessments into a multi-media PSS.

References

[1]. MA. Minor, JE. Hewett, RR. Webel, SK. Anderson, DR. Kay. Efficacy of physical conditioning exercise in patients with rheumatoid arthritis and osteoarthritis. Arthritis Rheum 1989;32:1396-1405.

[2]. PA. Dexter. Joint exercises in elderly persons with symptomatic osteoarthritis of the hip or knee. Arthritis Care Res 1992; 5:36-41.

[3]. MA. Minor, JE. Hewett, RR. Webel, TE. Dreisinger, DR. Kay. Exercise tolerance and disease related measures in patients with rheumatoid arthritis and osteoarthritis. J Rheumatol 1988; 15:905-911.

[4]. BH. Marcus, VC. Selby, RS. Niaaura, JS. Rossi. Self-efficacy and the stages of exercise behavior change. Res Q Exerc Sport 1992; 63:60-66.

[5]. JO. Prochaska, CC. DiClemente, JC. Norcross. In search of how people change. Am Psychol 1992; 47: 1102-1114.

[6]. RM. Gagné, LJ. Briggs, W. Wager. Principles of instructional design. 3rd ed. New York: Holt, Rinehart & Winston, 1988.

[7]. JC. Reid, CM. Kardash, RD. Robinson, R. Scholes. Comprehension in patient literature: The importance of text and reader characteristics. Health Communication 1994;6: in press.

GIFIC
A Graphical Interface For Intensive Care

Michael F. Lesser, M.D.
LMI of Brevard, Inc.
Holmes Regional Medical Center

GIFIC (Graphical Interface for Intensive Care) applies a new graphical language paradigm to intensive care unit information. By using this new graphical paradigm. coupled to simple rule based decision making tools, a complete display of intensive care unit patient information can be placed on a single screen. This includes such diverse items as lab work, cultures, patient devices, input and output and imaging studies. This article represents the initial time/accuracy, and training time studies based on this technology. Preliminary data suggests that significant time savings, without loss of accuracy of assessment can be obtained with as little as 8 hours of training.

INTRODUCTION

When completing tasks in complex, dynamic domains observers must consider the relationships among many variables (integrated tasks) as well as the values of individual variables (focused tasks)[1]. This is precisely what physicians do in evaluating the complex illnesses typically seen in an intensive care unit when they review signs and symptoms, laboratory information, and results of specialized diagnostic studies. Recently a new graphical language paradigm has been applied to information in the intensive care unit producing a robust display of patient information. This display design is the first to provide an evaluable summary of a complex database of patient information, while at the same time, providing access to specific data points within the database, thus accomplishing proximity capatability[1] for both high proximity and low proximity tasks without the typical performance trade-offs between integrated and focused tasks[1]. This paper details the results of the first time/accuracy comparative study using this display technology.

METHODS / RESULTS

A double blind study was performed assessing a physicians ability to complete patient assessments under timed conditions using a typical chart and flowsheet vs a single piece of paper displaying the GIFIC printout. Assessment sheets were independently scored on a scale of 1 to 10, 10 being perfect accuracy.

All patients were picked at random by the nurse manager in the CCU and were unknown to all reviewing physicians. No patient examination was allowed, however the "Chart" physician did have access to all patient progress notes, histories and physicals, etc. The "GIFIC" physician had access to a single sheet of paper (the GIFIC printout).

The results of the first study are shown in Table I. Although the accuracy grades were not statistically different (paired T test, $p = 0.13$), the time differential was of high statistical significance ($p < 0.001$).

Table I

Pt #	GIFIC		Chart & Flowsheet	
	Min:Sec	Score	Min:Sec	Score
1	4:55	5	15:25	8
2	3:38	9	6:40	9
3	5:05	9	9:15	9
4	4:03	9	8:45	9
5	3:20	7	5:55	9
6	2:30	9	7:18	8
7	4:35	9	9:55	8
8	4:53	8	9:45	9
9	5:45	7	10:15	9
10	6:30	8	15:13	9
M	**4:33**	**8.0**	**9:50**	**8.7**

REFERENCES

1. Bennett, K.B., and Flach, J.M., Graphical Displays: Implications for Divided Attention, Focused Attention, and Problem Solving. Human Factors, 34(5), 513-533, 1992

Toward an EMRS: Object-Oriented Models of the Clinical Domain

Paulina S. Sockolow, M.B.A., David R. Petzko, M.S., C. Martin Harris, M.D., M.B.A.

University of Pennsylvania Health System
Office of Information Systems and Technology,
Philadelphia, PA 19104

As healthcare organizations plan to meet the increasingly complex information requirements of new patient care delivery systems, they must develop strategies for evolving their current health information systems toward an EMRS. One approach is to augment commercial systems with timely and valuable clinical decision support. This would communicate recommended standards of practice to physicians, and contribute to on-going efforts to improve the quality of patient care.

To test this approach, we developed a prototype clinical decision support system. Components of this prototype include objects which model the medical entities found in the real world and domain models of patient interactions with a health care system. The domain models are operational views of health care delivery, and provide an organizational framework for the information gathered during a patient's interaction with the health care system. Because these domain models maintain the context for the data gathered during a clinician/ patient interaction, they form the basis of our EMRS investigations.

The domain models show the interrelationships of a patient and the health care system. They are similar to conceptual models developed by other investigators [1]. Both include concepts such as patient, location, order, diagnostic procedure, etc. The conceptual models are intended to bridge the gap between the physical data model (the data organization within the database management system) and the logical data model (the application's view of the data) while isolating the domain experts from the data organization. Because we are using object-oriented methods, we can develop a single unified domain model which is directly representable in the underlying technology being used in our EMRS investigations. This single unified domain model is also equivalent to both the physical model (in the object-oriented database), and the logical model in the decision support application. Since there is a single unified domain model, system developers can work with domain experts using the expert's language. This results in applications that more accurately reflect the domain under consideration.

To develop our models, we formed reasonable statements of clinical care, taking into account both patient and clinician viewpoints. Our goal was to create statements that were as general as possible while at the same time specific enough to capture the important concepts associated with clinical care. The statements of clinical care were reviewed by clinicians from different areas for completeness. We performed an initial analysis of the statements using several object-oriented analysis and design methods including Object Behavior Analysis and Class/Responsibility/Collaboration (CRC) techniques [2] [3].

Once all objects in these statements were identified, we examined their attributes and relationships in order to identify similarities. These similarities can help identify abstract objects not immediately recognizable during preliminary analysis. We then developed a graphical representation using a notation suitable for illustrating objects, attributes and relationships [4]. We also implemented these objects in Smalltalk [5] in order to investigate how they might interact in and be useful for EMRS development. Our next step will be to verify these models and investigate several approaches to object persistence.

References

1. Johnson, S., *et al.*, *Conceptual Data Model for a Central Patient Database*. Proc Annu Symp Comput Appl Med Care, 1992. **15**: p. 381-385.
2. Rubin, K.S. and A. Goldberg, *Object Behavior Analysis*. 1993, ParcPlace Systems, Inc.
3. Wirfs-Brock, R., B. Wilkerson, and L. Wiener, *Designing Object-Oriented Software*. 1990, Prentice Hall.
4. *Object-Oriented Analysis and Design*. 1991, Semaphore Training.
5. *ParcPlace Systems, Inc.* 999 E. Arques Ave. Sunnyvale, CA 94086.

Providing Access to Healthcare Information Resources using Internet Gopher Technology as a Part of a State-Wide Medical Information Network

Elizabeth E. McColligan[1],M.S., M.P.H., Robert L. Samuell III[2],M.S., Warren T. Jones[2],Ph.D., William A. Moon[3],M.S., Susan Z. Pretnar[3],MBA and Merida L. Johns[1,2],Ph.D.

[1]Health Information Management, [2]Department of Computer and Information Sciences University of Alabama at Birmingham, [3]BlueCross BlueShield of Alabama Birmingham, AL

An Internet healthcare information resources Gopher server is described as a part of a state-wide medical information network. The development of the server and its design and operation are presented. The potential impact of this technology on the healthcare delivery process and issues associated with the use of public domain information resources are discussed.

INTRODUCTION

This poster describes the development of a healthcare information resources Gopher which provides access to healthcare information resources publicly available on the Internet. This application is a part of a larger on-going BlueCross BlueShield of Alabama project to develop a comprehensive state-wide electronic healthcare medical information system for use by the physician community in the State of Alabama.

The goal of this project was to identify potential healthcare information resources and to provide a facility for easy-to-use, friendly access to these resources. The underlying assumption of this effort was that timely access to accurate and up-to-date information will improve the healthcare delivery process. Not only will medical decision-making be enhanced, but patterns of practice can be improved and better patient education provided.

DEVELOPMENT PROCESS

The Internet is a world-wide network of computer networks connected by common protocols and gateways [1]. It is estimated that the Internet is comprised of over two million computer hosts serving over fifteen million users. It is a vast collection of information resources which can be accessed via a variety of communication services. The facilities for browsing and locating information on the Internet have been primitive in the past. A service called the Internet Gopher originated three years ago at the Computer and Information Services Department of the University of Minnesota and is commonly called 'the user interface to the Internet.' It was designed to provide quick and easy access to the information resources of the Internet, particularly for the casual computer user [2].

The Healthcare Information Resources Gopher Project has involved developing and deploying a Gopher server which provides physicians and healthcare practitioners with easy-to-use, friendly access to healthcare information resources on the Internet. While the focus was on healthcare information resources, other information resources were also made available (e.g. a collection of desk references).

The process of developing this application included the following tasks: tool selection; resource identification; menu design; server customization; client selection; user training; and project evaluation. Menu design and implementation was based upon a conceptual model of the information needs of the tasks comprising the healthcare delivery process. Information resources were matched to these tasks based upon the information needs of the task. Client software packages including several Windows-based Gopher and World-Wide Web browsers (e.g. MOSAIC) were provided. User training consisted of two one-day, hands-on seminars for physicians and healthcare practitioners and provided a general overview of Internet resources, services, and tools with examples drawn from the healthcare domain. While the formal project evaluation has not been completed, a preliminary subjective evaluation has been done and was quite favorable.

IMPACT

The Healthcare Information Resources Gopher Project extends the model of facilitating information access in a hospital setting to the ambulatory care setting, especially to those physicians in rural communities. The Internet is a valuable information resource for community physicians who are isolated from relevant information stores and are basically information "poor". Clinical information systems of the future will automatically link electronic medical literature relevant to a patient's diagnosis and a particular therapy [3]. Duke University Medical Center researchers have prototyped such a system. Internet Gopher technology was used to link medical resources with automated patient care plans [4]. This work is related to ongoing research in the area of information filtering being done by the group for Studies in Information Filtering of Electronic Resources at UAB, of which the work reported in this paper is one aspect.

ISSUES

Utilizing public information resources to support the healthcare delivery process presents a number of challenges, such as: control over Internet resources, network operational delays, client connection/software availability, access to subscription or fee-based services, information quality, and menu navigation.

Acknowledgements

Work on this project was funded by a grant from BlueCross BlueShield of Alabama.

References

[1] Hahn, Haley and Rick Stout, The Internet Complete Reference, Osbourne 1994.

[2] Wiggins, Rich, " The University of Minnesota's Internet Gopher System: A Tool for Accessing Network-Based Electronic Information", The Computer Systems Review, Vol. 4, No. 2, 1993, pp. 4-66.

[3] Shortliffe, E.H., L.E. Perrault, G. Wiederhold, L.M. Fagan (eds), Medical Informatics, Computer Applications in Health Care. Reading, Massachusetts: Addison-Wesley Publishing Co. 1990.

[4] Hales, Joseph W., Richard C. Low and Kevin T. Fitzpatrick, "Using the Internet Gopher Protocol to Link a Computerized Patient Record and Distributed Electronic Resources", Proceedings of the 17th Annual SCAMC, 1993, pp. 621- 625.

Emulating Cognitive Diagnostic Skills Without Clinical Experience: A Report of Medical Students Using Quick Medical Reference and Iliad in the Diagnosis of Difficult Clinical Cases.

Marvin E. Gozum, M.D.
Chief, Section of Medical Informatics, Division of Internal Medicine, Department of Medicine.
Jefferson Medical College, Philadelphia.

Diagnosing complex internal medicine cases has traditionally been the domain and hallmark of clinical expertise. However, the creation of a differential diagnosis list using abstracted case information can be seen as a database query function and has been emulated by software such as QMR and Iliad. To test this premise, twenty two sophomore medical students were taught how to abstract clinical data, and use QMR and Iliad to diagnose complex clinical cases from the New England Journal of Medicine. Half of the students were able to provide correct diagnoses within a list of ten. These preliminary results supports a notion that clinical diagnosis may be a skill independent of clinical experience.

INTRODUCTION.

The solution to complex clinical cases has been considered the result of years of clinical training. One clinical skill is developing an appropriate differential diagnoses, a process which may be seen as a database query. To test this premise, individuals with minimal clinical experience were asked to diagnose complex cases using software to provide expertise. [1]

METHODS/RESULTS:

Over ten, 1.5 hour, weekly sessions, 22 sophomore medical students were taught the concepts underlying the construction, philosophy and use of Quick Medical Reference (QMR) and Iliad [2]. The instructor had sophomores read the presentation of a difficult case from clinico-pathologic conferences (CPCs), taken from the New England Journal of Medicine. The medical students were told to select, at their discretion, all findings that needed analysis by a physician. The instructor offered no input into the validity of the student's selections. The student's expertise with computers varied, so students were formed into 6 groups, to minimize technical difficulties . Five complex cases were analyzed by students; these same cases were also analyzed by the instructor using Iliad and QMR. At the end of each five 1.5 hour laboratory sessions, the results of students and the instructor were compared with case discussants of the CPCs. The object of the exercise was to have the students arrive at the CPC diagnosis within the first ten diagnoses listed by Iliad or QMR as demonstrated by the instructor. The definition of "correct diagnosis" was strictly defined by being within the first ten diagnosis in a list. Further, associated diseases and diagnoses that were mentioned in the CPC but were not the concluding diagnosis were not considered as part of the correct diagnosis.

RESULTS.

Students were able to generate lists that contained a all possible diagnoses from the CPC. However, accuracy for the principle diagnosis varied greatly . Using Iliad, the instructor could only arrive at the diagnosis of the CPCs in 3/5 cases. Comparing instructor performance to the students, *one* group was consistently able to arrive at similar diagnosis, 5/5, within the top ten differential diagnosis presented by Iliad. In this group, it was one individual who was responsible for this performance. Of the five remaining groups, two groups were able to achieve the diagnosis within the top ten in 3/5 cases. Two groups were able to provide a diagnosis within the top ten, compared to the instructor in 2/5 cases. One group could not provide a diagnosis within the top ten in all cases. The same cases were analyzed using QMR. Of 6 CPCs, QMR arrived at the diagnosis in 5/6 cases, all within the first ten diagnosis listed using the "case" mode. These results suggest that diagnosis may be a skill independent of clinical knowledge. However, the inability of the students to narrow the differential diagnosis allude to the importance of clinical skill.

References:
1. Miller, R. Medical diagnostic decision support systems - past, present and future: A threaded bibliography and commentary. JAMIA 1994;1;8.
2. Lincoln MJ, Turner C, Hesse B, Miller R. A comparison of clustered knowledge structures in Iliad and in Quick Medical Reference. Proceedings the 12th Annual Symposium of Computer Applications in Medical Care, 1988. p.131-6.

A Tcl/Tk Based Graphical Interface to Medical and Administrative Information

Charles Webster[1] MD, MSIE, MSIS, Andrew Pople[2], Roseanne Silva[3], MSIN, Xiaofeng Wang[4], MS, Sean McLinden[1], MD

[1]Dept. of Health Information Sciences, Duquesne University
[2]Carnegie Group Inc., [3]Fiserv Inc., [4]Shadyside Hospital, Pittsburgh PA

FELIX is an front-end application processor, with an open systems back-end, that provides a uniform and intuitive interface to clinical and administrative information. It consists of an information browser, three clinical applications, and three management applications. FELIX was developed in a community hospital environment, but has conceptual and technical roots in medical informatics and the Internet.

INTRODUCTION

FELIX (FELIX Enables Limitless Information Exploration) provides a generic graphical interface for browsing medical and administrative information. It relies on a large number of industry standards such as TCP/IP, X11R5, SQL, Postscript and SGML. In particular, the interface was developed using a high-level X-windows graphical scripting language called Tcl/Tk [1] (which is currently also being ported to Windows and Macintosh platforms). We used real patient information and based our targeted applications on analysis of patient care processes at a local urban community referral hospital. We intended FELIX to be a vision of what is possible, a prototype to force us to confront the necessary integration of disparate technologies, and an inducement for clinicians and administrators to press for open systems file formats, programmatic interfaces and network protocols.

FELIX applications, are manipulatable from within a common, but customizable, information browser. The three clinical applications are a clinical document viewer that uses SGML formatted files to generate Tcl/Tk scripts which are then executed, a digital image and audio transcription system (used in radiographic scenarios), and a hypertext facility for viewing pathology images while linking phrases in text to objects in images. The three administrative applications are a real-time resource monitor that is dynamically updated from bar code readers on a network (used in this case to represent the amount of time that patients, tracked by "wanding" them into rooms, have spent in their current locations), a quality control and trend analyzer that allows retrospective display of activities such as weekly radiology procedures by ordering physician, and a visually intuitive resource scheduler that intelligently represents possible and impossible resource combinations (physician, nurse, room, and equipment).

FELIX would not have been possible without Tcl (tool command language), an application independent, embeddable interpreted command language, and TK, an X11 tool kit and widgets based on Tcl. The combination provides a high-level graphical scripting language that can be easily extended by writing C programs that become new Tcl commands. Applications created with Tcl/Tk can allow a user to dynamically modify their interface while working from within it. Many of the capabilities that support FELIX functions are extensions to Tcl created either by us (in the case of digital audio) or by members of the Tcl/Tk community and made available over the Internet (in the case of the photo and hypertext widgets and extensions to provide additional access to the UNIX environment).

Some of the ideas we explored included a double layer of menus that was retrieved from a database and configured by the user in order to obtain customized views of database content. Each retrieved "document" is actually an executable Tcl/Tk script that is generated from an SGML file or from the contents of a database. This allowed us to embed useful behavior while retaining flexibility, such as embedding buttons that turn into digital signatures or text widgets that adjust their size to the number of lines contained.

While FELIX relied on industry standard formats, application programming interfaces, and network protocols, none of the potential data sources were accessible, except by manually down-loading and translating data from proprietary hospital and departmental information systems. However, FELIX was built to demonstrate to hospital clinicians and administrators what they could have on their desktops if they invested in the required network infrastructure, and made sure that future information systems, and modifications of extant information systems, complied with open system standards. As a result, the hospital invested in an optical fiber backbone, began to subject departmental systems to open systems requirements, and pressed the vendor of the main hospital-wide clinical information system to make its data more accessible.

Reference

[1]. J. Ousterhout. Tcl and the Tk Tool kit. Addison Wesley, Reading, MA, 1994.

Medication History Display and Evaluation

Kathleen Daye, M.D.; Deborah Lashman, MSPH; John Pandiani, Ph.D,
Vermont Department of Mental Health/Mental Retardation

The centerpiece of the poster will be the Vermont Medication Graphics Project, currently being developed at the Vermont State Hospital with support from the Robert Wood Johnson Foundation.

The primary purpose of Project Medgraph is to improve the quality of medical care by presenting medication history in a graphic format. This allows prescribing physicians to make decisions on changes in the patient's medication regimen which are fully informed by past history, facilitating the development of the optimum medication regimen.

The evolution of medication administration record keeping from the pre-computer era to the future will be dramatically illustrated. A large photo of our hospital, with its classic nineteenth century architecture, will suggest the past, where medication administration records were handwritten and summarized, sometimes incompletely on lists. Narratives in which attempts are made to correlate medication with patients' symptoms are also shown, and contrasted to the same information displayed graphically. This highlights the problem of the inaccessibility of the large amount of complex information, which we needed to solve, in order to make medication prescription as rigorously scientific as it should be.

With Project Medgraph we commissioned the development of software to create graphs to organize and display medication records. The graphs consist of a series of timelines, each displaying in bold colors the different medications of a certain category which an individual patient received. The graphs show the dose as a percent of the usual daily dose, rather than in milligrams. Thus, one can tell at a glance, by the height of the columns, whether the dose is relatively high or low at a given point. Target symptoms are also graphed simultaneously, demonstrating medication effectiveness. These features make our graphs potentially useful to a much broader audience, including reviewers and the patients themselves.

For prescribing physicians, the graphs put the "big picture' in focus, which is so important when evaluating a medication regimen that spans years and involves multiple medications with significant cumulative toxicity. They can reveal clinical information about side effects that can be recognized clearly only in retrospect. For example, the graph below shows that multiple adverse events were strongly associated with a course of Nardil. This gives a more accurate picture of why this drug is now contra-indicated for this patient than we would have if we merely listed it as an "allergy".

Finally, the poster will depict the future evolution of the system, under a large photo of the earth as seen from outer space, suggesting the immense potential applicability of increased information accessibility through computerization. It will show the clinical graphs that could become available as soon as it becomes standard practice to record medication administration and clinical response directly into a computer database and our prototype software is upgraded to a state-of-the-art system.

The poster will also include imaginative spin-offs of the central concept of presenting medication administration graphically. For example, a computer display might give warning that the cumulative dose is in the range where there is increased risk of drug dependency or permanent harm such as the development of tardive dyskinesia. Spatial representations of huge volumes of data might reveal the causes of rare and deadly medication reactions.

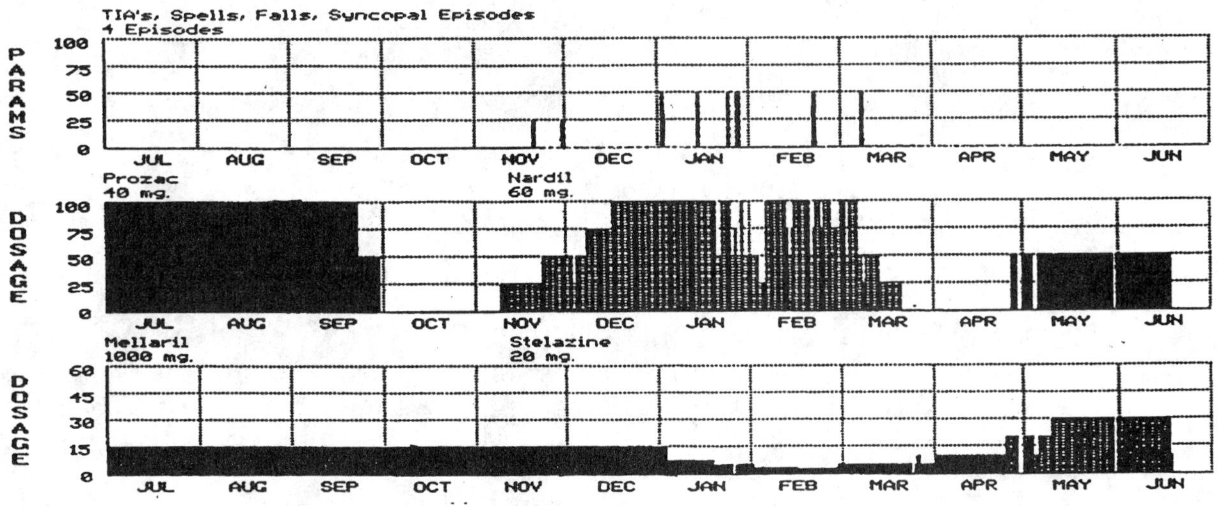

User Requirements for the Computerized Patient Record: Physician Opinions

Wally R. Smith, M.D., Raymond Zastrow, M.D.
Medical College of Virginia, Richmond Virginia, Falls Medical Group-Northwest, Milwaukee, Wisconsin.

Little has been written regarding physicians' user requirements for the computerized patient record (CPR). We questioned whether physicians uncomfortable with using computers and/or not favoring national adoption of the CPR desired different features than those reasonably comfortable with the CPR.

We mailed a two-page questionnaire to 248 physicians comprising the active membership of the Milwaukee County Medical Society. Sixty urban and suburban physicians (24.2%) responded. We asked them to rank how important each of 21 potential user requirements of a CPR was to them (most important=5 to least important=1). We also asked them to rank on a scale of 1 to 5 whether they favored the adoption of the CPR (FAV), whether they thought using computers was difficult (DIF), and whether they felt comfortable interacting with computers (COMF). We defined a CPR discomfort score (INDEX) = (Reverse of FAV) + DIF + COMF. We then compared ranks of physicians with less discomfort with the CPR (below median INDEX) vs. those of physicians with more discomfort.

Overall, 36 of the 60 physicians favored the adoption of the CPR (strongly agreed or agreed), 18 did not favor adoption (were neutral, disagreed, or strongly disagreed), and seven had no opinion. The top five most desired user requirements of the 60 physicians were legibility (LEG), a problem list and medications (PROBMED), a lifetime medical record (LIFETIME), easy transmission of information to consultants (CONSULT), and abstractability for research (RES). LEG, PROBMED, LIFETIME, CONSULT, LAB were the most desirable among 32 physicians with median or higher than median discomfort INDEX scores. LEG, PROBMED, RES, access to information from multiple locations (ACCMULT), CONSULT ranked highest among the 28 physicians with lower than median discomfort INDEX scores. Of interest, only the 11 physicians who found computers most difficult to use did not rank PROBMED in their top five most desired features, whereas all others ranked it second most important. Older physicians ranked access to laboratory data (LAB) in their top five most desired requirements, whereas younger physicians ranked ACCMULT, but not LAB, in their top five.

We conclude that legibility and having a problem list and medications almost uniformly rank as the most desirable user requirements of the CPR from physicians, and that level of discomfort with the CPR and/or age only slightly influences which features are most desired CPR requirements.

0195–4210/94/$5.00 © 1994 AMIA, Inc.

MODULAR INTEGRATED TRANSPLANT INFORMATION SYSTEM (MITIS)

L.P. Dang, Oklahoma Transplantation Institute; Steve Ireland, Oklahoma Transplantation Institute; Nazih Zuhdi, M.D., Oklahoma Transplantation Institute

In the continuing attempt to answer the question: "What can we do to improve the care and outcome of our organ transplant patients?" MITIS was developed. The Modular Integrated Transplant Information System (MITIS) is a client / server based information system which provides the Oklahoma Transplantation Institute staff with an online systemic view of transplant related patient data for essential clinical and research support.

Technical:

The Modular Integrated Transplant Information System operates on a Local Area Network under the Novell Netware 3.12 operating system. It functions as a part of the hospital wide FDDI backbone. This backbone extends throughout the hospital allowing MITIS to interact with other hospital systems.

Fundamentals:

The foundation of MITIS is a normalized collection of Structured Query Language (SQL) tables. These tables contain expansive transplantation information created with the concept of keeping the informaiton as consistent as possible across all organs; parsing the information only when deemed specific to each organ. Our goal is to view patient data on a systemic longitudinal view rather than as 'snapshots'.

Modules:

From the fundamental tables of the relational database system extends specialized fully interactive modules to further enhance the system. These modules interact at various levels providing the enduser a user friendly interface. These modules are clinical, research, statistical, graphics, finance, and teaching.

The most important module of MITIS is the clinical module. This module's main function is to provide up-to-date information on patients for the transplant medical staff. The second most significant module is the research module. This module can be used to create sub-populations for analyses. Prediction of drug mechanism and treatment viability can be evaluated. Neural networks can be implemented to create decision based models.

The remaining modules play a critical role in support of the clinical and research module. The statistical module provides basic statistical functions such as minimums, maximums, sums, averages, standard deviation and standard error. Further statistics include life tables, Kaplan-Meyer product limits, and T-tests for evaluation of significance. The graphics module provides graphical representation of a set or sets of data queried by the user. It can provide survival curves and longitudinal representation of various factors. Additional features will provide on-line access to transplant based images (X-rays, CT scans, etc.). The finance module will permit administrative personnel to summarize and report on costs, benefits and discrepancies.

The teaching module is the last but possibly the most important for development. It will provide transplant surgeons and residents the opportunity to evaluate case based scenarios and to implement reasoning for improved clinical practice in organ transplantation for tomorrow. The modules are developed to work concurrently as well as individually. The graphics module uses data from the statistical module to derive survival curves. The teaching module may use findings from the research module to enhance the case based scenarios. The graphics module will graphically represent longitudinal laboratory values for the transplant coordinator via the clinical module.

Conclusion:

As of March 31 1994, there were 34,493 patients in the United States waiting for transplants (number of patients registrations on the national waiting list)[1]. The number of transplant candidates far outweighs the number of organ donations. We must therefore promote organ donation and concurrently value each opportunity given for organ transplantation. Baptist Medical Center of Oklahoma realizes and believes in these beliefs, and will further develop the Modular Integrated Transplant Information System (MITIS). This will in turn provide us with the tools to improve transplant patient care and quality of life.

References

[1] UNOS Update, Vol 10, Issue 4, April 1994

Impact of Computerized Physician Order Entry on Physician Time

David W. Bates, MD, MSc (1), Deborah L. Boyle, BA (2), Jonathan M. Teich, MD, PhD (3)
Center for Applied Medical Information Systems Research (1,3)
Division of General Medicine and Primary Care, Department of Medicine (1,2)
Brigham and Women's Hospital and Harvard Medical School

ABSTRACT

We examined the effect of computerized physician order entry on housestaff time use patterns, using time motion techniques. For both medical and surgical house officers, writing orders on the computer took about twice as long (p<0.001), or 44 minutes for medical and 73 minutes for surgical house officers. Medical house officers recovered about half this time because some administrative tasks--e.g. looking for charts--were made easier. Within types of orders, sets of stereotyped orders took much less time with order entry, but one-time orders took longer. We have since developed strategies to make it easier to enter one-time orders.

INTRODUCTION

Computerized physician order entry, in which all orders are written directly on a hospital information system by physicians, has enormous potential for improving care, because it allows structuring of orders, and offers the opportunity to give providers feedback at the time they make decisions.[1] Nonetheless, experiences with order-entry to date have been mixed; a major problem has been that such systems take providers longer than pen and paper.[1,2]

We have recently implemented a physician order entry system at Brigham and Women's Hospital. To evaluate the effect of order entry on medical and surgical housestaff time, we undertook a study with the following goals: 1) to measure the time spent before and after order entry in ordering; 2) to evaluate specific types of ordering to determine whether they were differentially affected; 3) to measure time spent in activities which might be simplified using order entry.

METHODS

We studied medical interns, and first and second-year surgical residents, as they write most orders in our hospital. We refer to the period before implementation of order entry as Phase 1, which included 22 medical interns and 7 surgical house officers, and to the period after as Phase 2, including 28 medical and 5 surgical house officers. In Phase 1, a trained observer followed medical interns; each physician was observed continuously between 8 am and 5 pm. The physician's activity was recorded every thirty seconds. In Phase 2 medical data collection, and in both phases for surgeons, we used random reminder pagers to measure time use.

RESULTS

When time spent ordering was compared between Phase 1 and Phase 2, the percent for medical interns increased from 5.3% to 10.5% ($p<0.001$), representing 44 additional minutes per day, while for surgical house officers the corresponding figures were an increase from 6.4% to 15.5% ($p<0.001$), 73 minutes per day. However, the medical interns (but not the surgeons) recovered some time because of decreased time to perform activities expected to take less time after order entry: 9.4% to 6.1% ($p<0.001$), 27 minutes per day.

Daily and one-time orders accounted for the majority of this change, increasing almost threefold in percent total time (2.2% before, vs. 7.2% after order entry). However, sets of orders took less total time after order entry (1.7% vs 3.1%).

DISCUSSION

While physician order entry has tremendous potential for reducing costs and improving quality,[1] the first requirement is that it be fast enough to be usable. Computer order entry takes physicians about twice as long as paper ordering, and adds more time for surgeons than for medical interns, although it is faster for orders which are written in groups, and some time is recovered because of reduced time needed to perform other activities. We are currently implementing strategies to reduce the time required to write one-time orders.

1. Tierney WM, Miller ME, Overhage JM, McDonald CJ. Physician inpatient order writing on microcomputer workstations. JAMA 1993; 269:379-383.

2. Massaro TA. Introducing physician order entry at a major academic medical center. Acad Med 1993; 68:20-25.

Screen and Pathway Standards for Interfacing

Joel Buchanan, MD
University of Wisconsin Hospital and Clinics

INTRODUCTION

Clinical computing system architects face many challenges. Designers may integrate departmental systems across an enterprise or may provide interfaces between systems [1]. Replacement of existing departmental systems with a fully integrated institutional system is expensive. In addition, departments are frequently reluctant to sacrifice specialized functions. Finally, hospitals and other enterprises can install "off the shelf" systems faster than they can create their own integrated systems. Therefore, hospitals usually interface systems to some degree.

DATABASE VS.PATHWAY INTERFACE

Database interfaces can link departmental databases (e.g., lab, radiology, transcription) to a common clinical database (the *clinical repository).* This arrangement allows a common user interface to the clinical data in the repository. A single database, however, may not be capable of storing and retrieving all the varied types of clinical data (e.g., numerical tables, text, images). Therefore, the clinical repository frequently consists of more than a single database type. Because screen consistency is important to users [2], these heterogenous databases must be interfaced at the *pathway level.*

PATHWAY STANDARDS

A pathway is a set of menus, screens and links that appear united to the user. An interface at the pathway level requires rapid response between heterogeneous elements of the pathway. Also, the various pathway screens should offer consistency.

THE WISCR IMPLEMENTATION

At the University of Wisconsin we have created a clinician's pathway. This pathway is used heavily (more that 16,000 times per month). Lab, radiology reports, surgical pathology reports, clinic notes, admission notes, and operative notes are stored in the clinical repository, which was created with the SMS Lifetime Clinical Record software along with Inquire, by Info Data. Electronic mail service is provided with EMC2/TAO by Fischer. Electronic reference material is provided with the Computerized Clinical Information System by Micromedex.

The clinicians at the University of Wisconsin access this pathway across heterogeneous terminal and workstation platforms. We have optimized the uniformity between workstation platforms and between software packages. Uniformity for function keys such as *help, previous screen, scroll up, and scroll down* was achievable, because vendors have followed SAA CUA standards [3].

References

[1]. H. Bleich., W Slack. Designing a Hospital Information System: A Comparison of Interfaced and Integrated Systems. M.D. Computing., Vol. 9, No. 5, 1992.

[2] Guidelines for Designing User Interface Software. The Mitre Corporation., National Technical Information Service., 1986. (ESD-TR-86-278, ADA 177 198)

[3] W. Galitz. User-Interface Screen Design. QED Publishing Group., Wellesley, AM, 1993.

Quick Report for Psychiatric Emergency Rooms

Robert S. Kennedy, M.A.
Department Of Psychiatry
Albert Einstein College Of Medicine, Bronx, New York

ABSTRACT

Translating and pre-digesting the volumes of data from a psychiatric emergency room database into a simple, easy-to-review "quick report" offers a different approach to a rapid review of patient information. Clinicians from psychiatric emergency rooms in New York City were asked to describe the minimal amount of information they would wish to review from previous clinical visits. The smallest report was then constructed to offer the most information.

INTRODUCTION

Working in a Psychiatric Emergency Room places demands on staff to triage a patient with as much information as possible as quickly as possible. There is frequently a need for fast decisions. Traditionally, the clerk checks to see if the patient has had a previous visit and then he or she calls the medical record room to send the chart. This process can be time consuming and can delay appropriate treatment. This can be particularly crucial if the patient is a behavior problem, agitated or delirious.

BACKGROUND

One solution being explored at some of the Albert Einstein College of Medicine, New York, Psychiatric Emergency Rooms is the "quick report." Three of the Psychiatric ER's have a common database based on a scanned medical record[1]. The database contains information about each emergency room visit including such items as patient demographics, presenting symptoms, diagnosis, medications given, disposition etc. Having such a database makes it easy to look up information on a patient with prior visits and display it on screen or print out a clinical summary. Clinicians have requested a "just the facts" report with minimal but crucial information rather than a narrative type of summary report .

METHOD

The clinicians were asked what minimal crucial information would be most helpful from the database to assist them in reviewing information about a patient who presents at the ER and who has had previous visits. The items that the clinicians requested were reviewed and compiled into a "Quick Report". This report is available instantaneously via a printout or on screen from the database.

Initially, if you ask clinicians what information they <u>want</u> from a database, they usually respond "everything". Obviously, this would produce pages of data that would be difficult to read, especially if you wanted specific information in a hurry. Asking again, what information they <u>need</u> produced different results that opened a debate about necessary versus unnecessary information. After some discussions, a minimal data set was agreed upon.

The goal of creating this report was to list the most amount of important data (as deemed by the clinicians) in the least amount of space. Creating a small one-to-three line report seemed to be the most desirable type of print out that the clinical staff requested.

An interesting feature of this database is that information is stored in as little space as possible to keep storage demands at a minimum. The database generates information "on the fly", for example, a positive finding for a particular symptom will be recorded as a single digit then translated into a word or phrase as it is called to the screen or to a printed report. It is this speed and flexibility that can make a report such as this more powerful as a clinical assistant. Another interesting feature built into the emergency room database is the concept of an ALERT field. There are six ALERTS - serious medical illness, drug allergy/serious adverse reactions, history of criminal behavior, history of violent/assaultive behavior, history of serious suicidal behavior and history of giving false medical information. These alerts are important clinical "flags" that are incorporated into this report.

REFERENCES

[1] Salamon, I., Kennedy, R.S., A Clinical Information System for Psychiatric Emergency Rooms. <u>Hospital and Community Psychiatry</u>, , 43: 397-399, 1992

Relational Database Design: Evaluation of the Recognition, Isolation and Treatment of Hospitalized Patients with Tuberculosis

Edward N. Robinson, Jr. MD [1,2,4]
David Beard Ph.D. [3]

[1] Duke-UNC Training Program in Medical Informatics
[2] Department of Medicine
[3] Department of Radiology
University of North Carolina School of Medicine
Chapel Hill, NC 27594
and
[4] The Internal Medicine Training Program
Moses H. Cone Memorial Hospital
Greensboro, NC 27401-1020

Abstract

Hospitals have been charged with the the evaluation of their abilities to identify, diagnose, isolate and treat individuals with active tuberculosis. This evaluation can be facilitated by a properly designed relational database. Using Entity Relationship diagrams, a relational data model, and the process of normalization, a database was designed that will contain the information gathered in prospective surveillance of tuberculosis in a community hospital. Although the authors' intent is to implement the design using a personal computer and a commercially available relational database management tool (Microsoft Access), the design is independent of the management tool and can be applied to other systems.

Introduction

The decades long decline of infections due to Mycobacterium tuberculosis ended in 1984 [1]. As greater numbers of individuals with active pulmonary tuberculosis are admitted to health care facilities, the risk of transmission of tuberculosis to health care providers or other patients increases [2]. In recognition of this risk, a federal agency (OSHA) mandated the internal and periodic evaluation of how medical facilities identify, diagnose, isolate and treat those with active tuberculosis [3].

This is no simple task. Surveillance involves the collection of information about patients, physicians, admissions to hospitals and room assignments, the ordering, collection and results of mycobacterial cultures from a variety of sources, and the prescribing and administration of antituberculous medication.

Database Design Overview

An ER Diagram [4,5] was drawn representing the entities and relationships between entities involved in hospital tuberculosis control. The diagram was converted to a relational data model yielding tables designed to store information about physicians, patients, radiographs, prescribed antibiotics, room assignments, microbiologic cultures and physician encounters. Each relation was examined for multivalued, partial and transitive dependencies. A data dictionary containing attribute names and descriptions was compiled.

The database design is being implemented in a database management tool, Microsoft Access, and will be used in prospective quality assessment.

[1] Ellner et al. J Infect Dis 1993;168:537-51.

[2] Beekmann SE, Osterholm MT and Henderson DK. Infect Control Hosp Epidemiol 1993;14:228-232.

[3] Centers for Disease Control and Prevention. "Draft guidelines for preventing the transmission of tuberculosis in health-care facilities" Federal Register 1993;58:52810-54.

[4] Elmasri R, Navathe SB. Fundamentals of Database Systems. The Benjamin/Cummings Publishing Company, Inc. Redwood City, CA. 1989.

[5] McFadden FR, Hoffer JA. Database Management. The Benjamin/Cummings Publishing Company, Inc. Redwood City, CA. 1991.

An ACCESS-based Academic Attending Physician and Resident Rotation Evaluation Database

Tomás D. Valdivia, M.D., Beth A. Hartquist, M.D., Department of Internal Medicine, St. Paul Ramsey Medical Center, University of Minnesota

A database of residents' evaluations of their Internal Medicine (IM) rotations and attending physicians (APs) was created using ACCESS (Microsoft). The IM attendings and the corresponding inpatient or outpatient rotations from three academic settings (county hospital, VA, and University) are ranked by 130 different residents. For APs, reports show rotation specific, year average and, for comparison, all-AP aggregate values. For rotations, reports provide estimates of workload, didactic teaching, and overall desirability. Free text comments may be provided for all evaluations.

INTRODUCTION

Due to flagging interest in some primary care specialties and increasing pressures to alter the balance of subspecialist and primary care physicians, resident training programs are subject to unprecedented scrutiny and unanticipated down-sizing. In response, well-established, traditional IM residency programs now have "night float" teams and offer a greater number of ambulatory rotations. The resultant rapid change has created a need for tools to provide careful analyses of overall rotations and AP effectiveness.

DESCRIPTION

Interface: The system interface was developed using ACCESS's partial object-oriented, event-driven, visual programming paradigm that is also found in other Microsoft programming products (e.g., Visual Basic). Due to the busy schedule and moderate computer literacy of the intended users, the interface was designed to maximize ease of use and efficient data entry. Users are asked to mouse click radio buttons to indicate values on a Likert scale and perform a minimal amount of free text entry. Total evaluation data entry time varies depending on the user's computer skills, comfort, and the extent of their comments, but is approximately 5±2 minutes.

Data Elements: Information gathered from resident evaluators falls into two categories. First, the resident evaluates their ward or ambulatory rotation AP. The APs are rated on twelve attributes, each assigned a value by the resident based on a modified Likert scale: fund of knowledge, clinical judgment, overall professionalism, enthusiasm, teaching effectiveness, support of housestaff, involvement with students, punctuality, ability to allow the service sufficient autonomy, willingness to teach and appropriateness of rounding schedule. Amount of didactic teaching per week, number of salient clinical references and comments regarding the AP's strengths and weakness are also solicited.

The rotations are rated by the residents on the magnitude of clinical workload; adequacy of clinical knowledge resources (e.g., institutional and departmental libraries, on-line search tools, and Chief Resident files); overall effectiveness of concomitant conferences including grand rounds, and morbidity/mortality conferences; and, more generally, adequacy of facility support including ancillary services, on-call facilities, parking and meals.

Reports: A report summarizing AP performance on each of the twelve factors named above, with comparison values vis-à-vis that AP's previous months' values, and an aggregate of fellow APs' performance is provided to each individual AP. The residency coordinator uses aggregate AP performance summaries to carry out cross-hospital and cross-AP analyses. To underscore the importance of these evaluations, one of the three academic sites uses the aggregate reports in an equation to apportion incentive compensation.

Similar aggregate reports are employed by the clinical residency coordinator to help monitor hospital and rotation effectiveness.

System Usage: Although not required, user participation in the evaluation process is strongly encouraged by the Chief Residents at the each of the three University Affiliated hospitals. Despite the voluntary nature of participation, user involvement each month is approximately 80%.

System Requirements: The current system was developed in Microsoft ACCESS, version 1.1. It will run on any computer supporting Microsoft Windows version 3.1; an i486-66 or faster microprocessor and mouse or similar input device should be used.

0195-4210/94/$5.00

Converting Clinical Data into Information: Mapping Operational Hospital Data into a Time-Oriented Clinical Repository

Charles Rogerson, Ph.D.[1], Vinay Sabharwal[2], William W. Woo[1], John Foy, M.D.[3]

[1]Systems Architecture Group, TDS Healthcare Systems Corporation, San Jose CA,
[2]VS Associates, Fremont CA, [3]TDS Healthcare Systems Corporation, Atlanta GA
Email: crogerson@tds-hsc.com

ABSTRACT

The growing demand within healthcare enterprises for distributed, ad hoc query access to operational data integrated from multiple heterogenous data sources can be met through time-oriented clinical repositories stored in SQL-based relational databases using client-server architecture. Correctly mapping, transforming and loading operational data from proprietary non-relational data structures into relational schemas in an automated way when such data structures may change over time is a complex problem that has not been generally solved. We present a general solution based on data modeling, schema transformation and configurable mapping dictionaries. Large quantities of data from the operational patient care information systems at a cancer research hospital have been successfully mapped and loaded into relational databases to support clinical research, CQI, outcomes studies, decision support and other population-oriented analysis. Today's healthcare environment, with constantly changing regulatory and reimbursement requirements and rapidly evolving delivery systems, places unprecedented pressures for information on the clinical and financial leadership of the healthcare enterprise (HCE). Personnel at many levels of the HCE must be able to access and analyze the data now residing in multiple systems and data sources with ease and flexibility. Most clinical data still resides in *paper chart form* as unstructured text and typically is also maintained in multiple electronic stores and ancillary systems. To allow for *ad hoc* access to the data for a large patient population requires a methodology for Information Mapping that supports the transformation of diverse data from multiple data sources into a time-oriented clinical information repository. The Information Mapping methodology is used for defining the source and target systems as well as the mapping between the multiple data stores. It begins with the creation of source and target conceptual schemas and results in the population of the meta-data dictionaries. The initial conceptual source schema represents the initial scope of source data and the first cut of the source groups. It is important to note that the source data model is not a true, normalized data model. Rather, it is simply a collection of various bundles of data assembled into a collection of logical groups. The target conceptual schema represents the data that will be stored in the repository as a relational database. It clearly prescribes what must be captured and/or derived from the source systems. The target schema presently contains 21 tables and a total of 239 columns. The tables include Patient, Address History, Episode, Order, Physician, Diagnosis History, Pharmacy Charting, and Result, among others.These conceptual schemas are then embellished into logical schemas. The source and target logical schemas are the two key components upon which the information mapping is based.Once the source logical schema is completed two major tasks can begin. First the source schema will be used to map the data elements to the source logical groups. All the meta-data is captured into a separate data repository that catelogues all the relevant information. Once the target logical schema has been completed and validated, it must be defined in the meta-data repository.Once the source data elements (logical groups) along with the target (tables, columns) and the source and target schemas have been entered in the RML dictionaries, the last, but most important step is the information mapping itself. The mapping defines the data source and transformation for each field of a specific target schema. This mapping definition is also entered into the meta-data repository. The information mapping step relies on the accuracy of the data definitions of the source and target schemas and therefore is highly sensitive to changes in either the meta-data of each element or the source or target schemas. Very often modifications will be necessary in one or more of the logical schemas or the logical grouping; this will also affect the information mapping. It is recommended that a uniform procedure be instituted to regulate and synchronize such changes.

0195-4210/94/$5.00 © 1994 AMIA, Inc.

Building a Cooperative Institutional Model of IAIMS at the Yale - New Haven Medical Center

Perry L. Miller[1], John A. Paton[1], Nancy K. Roderer[1], C. Carl Jaffe[1], Jeffrey I. Clyman[1]
Mark A. Shifman[1], Joseph E. Sullivan[2], Marc Newman[2], Mark Tepping[2], Walter J. Hierholzer[1,2]
[1]Yale University School of Medicine and [2]Yale - New Haven Hospital, New Haven, CT

The poster describes the cooperative institutional structure which underlies the IAIMS activities at Yale - New Haven Medical Center. Whereas some institutions implement IAIMS via some form of centralized structuring of major computing units, for many institutions this approach may not be viable and a more cooperative model will be required. The poster describes the process through which our IAIMS project evolved, and outlines certain principles underlying such an approach.

The successful realization of an Integrated Advanced Information Management System (IAIMS) within a medical center demands vision, coordinated planning, and an integrated implementation of that vision at many levels [1,2]. One question that arises concerns the nature of the organizational structure required to support such a process. Does a medical center need a centralized structuring of its major computing and information units under the direction of a single Chief Information Officer? Or can an effective IAIMS project be carried out via a more distributed, cooperative model of responsibility [3], providing that the overall vision is firmly established?

There are several examples of medical centers which have adopted some form of centralized structuring of responsibility to support an IAIMS effort [e.g., 4,5]. At the same time, there are other institutions where a unified structuring of computing activities would be difficult to achieve. For example:

1. At many academic medical centers, the medical school and its associated hospital are separate corporate organizations. At such a center, even in the most centralized model, there would have to be a separate centralized computing structure within each organization.
2. At many medical centers, a major driving force towards IAIMS may come from within an academic unit of Medical Informatics. The individuals within such a unit, while committed to the IAIMS process, may not be interested in taking on the computing service responsibilities for the entire medical center. Nevertheless, such an academic unit may be able to provide much of the initial vision and a great deal of energy to help the different components of the institution carry out IAIMS successfully.

At the Yale - New Haven Medical Center (YNHMC), both of these conditions apply. The Yale School of Medicine is a separate organization from Yale - New Haven Hospital, although the two organizations work collaboratively on many different levels. In addition, a great deal of the initial vision that led YNHMC to embrace the IAIMS concept has come from what is now the Center for Medical Informatics. Over time, many other institutional units have come to share this vision. As a result, the current IAIMS project involves the cooperation of a number of different components within the medical center.

This poster describes the cooperative model of IAIMS that has evolved at YNHMC. As we describe, once the IAIMS model was adopted as an institutional goal, a broad range of related activities followed quite naturally. In the process, institutional computing ties between organizations within the medical center have been greatly strengthened at several levels, including the strategic level of planning and oversight and the operational level of system implementation.

Acknowledgement This work was supported in part by NIH grant G08 LM05366 from the NLM.

References

[1]. Lindberg DAB: The IAIMS opportunity: The NLM view. Bull Med Libr Assoc 76:224-225, 1988.
[2]. Matheson NW, Cooper JAD: Academic information in the health sciences center: Roles for the library and information management. J Med Educ 57:1, 1982.
[3]. Spackman KA, Elert JD, Beck JR: The CIO and the medical informaticist: Alliance for progress. Proceedings of SCAMC-17, 1993, pp. 525-8.
[4]. Stead WW, Borden R, McNulty P, Sittig DF: Building an information management infrastructure in the 90s: The Vanderbilt experiment. Proceedings of SCAMC-17, 1993, pp. 534-8.
[5]. Roderer NK, Clayton PD: IAIMS at Columbia-Presbyterian Medical Center: Accomplishments and challenges. Bull Med Lib Assoc 80:253-62, 1992.

A Surgical Services Management System - Toward Improved Communications and Operational Efficiency

Authors: DP Strum, MD; LG Vargas, PhD; JH May, PhD; JS Palmer, BS; HB Gunnerson, MD; WD Watkins, MD

Affiliation: Department of Anesthesiology and the Katz Graduate School of Business, University of Pittsburgh, 15213

INTRODUCTION

Today all health centers are subjected to severe financial, social, academic, political, and organizational pressures resulting from increased demands on services and limitations in health care resources. We estimate that surgical services expenditures in the United States will reach $170 billion in the very near future[1,2]. It seems clear that any inefficiency in the process of patient care involving surgical services could be extremely costly to individual hospitals and the nation as a whole. Likewise, the potential savings for hospitals that are not operating efficiently is enormous. Results of a preliminary study of surgical services indicate that significant increases in overall efficiency are possible at our institution.

To reduce costs and increase operating room utilization, we developed a real time communications and patient tracking system to provide a data driven method of work process management focused on patients and health care providers. A Situational Information Management System (SIMS) was developed collaboratively by the department of anesthesiology and the Artificial Intelligence in Management Laboratory of the Katz Graduate School of Business. The project objectives included academic fulfillment, improved business efficiency and cost effectiveness, improved staff morale, increased patient satisfaction, and statistical analysis of trends in utilization of surgical services. SIMS was conceived as a communications system but features automated patient and staff tracking using bar codes, utilization statistics, patient transaction receipts, and reactive and predictive scheduling.

METHODS

SIMS is an electronic bulletin board analogous to the monitors at air terminals and is capable of tracking patients from pre-surgical admission to post-surgical disposition. It is a distributed database with more than 40 fields of data functioning on a local area computer network. User interviews were conducted to determine which custom information should be displayed at each geographical location including admitting, same day surgery, holding area, operating suites, post-anesthesia recovery area, and the intensive care unit. At each location, displays were designed that mimicked lists and worksheets currently in use by health care providers at those locations.

Two types of data are displayed at each location: patient-specific data (patient demographics) copied from location to location with few changes, and site-specific data (local worksheets) edited and maintained locally. Each location has read and edit access to the local data it owns and maintains. The same location has read, but not edit privileges to similar data in other geographic locations. As patients are processed through surgical services, data ownership and editing privileges for the patient-specific data move with the patient. Ownership and edit privileges for site-specific data are retained locally. In each location, data are entered by health care providers directly caring for patients, but are available for viewing by health care providers across the surgical services network.

A peer to peer local area network was employed with read and edit privileges defined for each remote location. A distributed database was chosen with data stored locally and shared with remote sites through a coordinating server so that SIMS would be modular and robust (malfunctions are site specific while peer locations remain unaffected). We used a mouse-driven, click and drag software design in order to produce user-friendly software.

RESULTS

SIMS was written in LISP on Apple Macintosh (System 7.1). Object-oriented programming enables rapid prototyping allowing us to demonstrate our software and information displays to physicians, administrators, nurses, and ancillary personnel involved in the clinical care of patients. The prototype is used for knowledge acquisition and assists in the process of cultural change including how information management systems function in the health care environment. Utilization statistics from SIMS are used to do predictive scheduling and will assist in developing cost-based accounting systems for surgical services.

REFERENCES

1. Moore FD: Surgical streams in the flow of health care financing. Ann Surg 201:132-41, 1985.

2. Statistical Abstract of the United States, 1993.

Guardian: An Experimental System for Intelligent ICU Monitoring

Barbara Hayes-Roth, Serdar Uckun, Jan Eric Larsson, John Drakopoulos
Knowledge Systems Laboratory, Computer Science Dept., Stanford University

David Gaba, Juliana Barr, Jane Chien
Dept. of Anesthesiology, Stanford University
Palo Alto Dept. of Veterans Affairs Medical Center

We are developing an intelligent agent for patient monitoring named Guardian. It is applied to the post-operative monitoring and therapy management of cardiac surgery patients. Even though Guardian is an experimental system so far, we anticipate that in the short term it will be integrated with existing ICU information systems and critically evaluated on simulated patient cases. In evaluating the system, we aim to demonstrate that human-machine cooperation in information overload situations can improve the work environment of clinicians, improve health care delivery, and ultimately reduce health-care costs.

THE GUARDIAN SYSTEM

The Guardian [1] architecture is organized in two levels. The top level supports *cognitive* behaviors such as condition monitoring, fault detection, diagnosis, planning, and explanation. The lower level is the *physical* level, and it is responsible for a variety of behaviors regarding perception and action in the external environment such as data acquisition, perception of messages from clinicians, closed-loop control actions, and actions to communicate with clinicians. The physical level sends perceived information and feedback from action execution to the cognitive level, while the cognitive level sends control plans to the physical level. The two levels operate concurrently.

Each of Guardian's two architectural levels are based on an underlying "dynamic control model" of their own operations. At the cognitive level, the model is implemented as the BB1 blackboard control architecture [2]. At the physical level, the model is implemented in a simpler, but analogous form.

The knowledge representation in Guardian is based on a shared ontology for *intelligent monitoring and control (IMC)*. The IMC ontology defines the basic types of domain objects (concepts) and relations of interest (link types) to the tasks typically performed by Guardian and other possible IMC agents.

The current Guardian knowledge base focuses on the postoperative ICU care of patients who have undergone cardiopulmonary bypass. It is organized under six organ systems (cardiovascular, pulmonary, renal, hematological, neurological, and metabolic/endocrine). The knowledge base contains information on about 70 diseases and complications, 120 parameters, 200 signs and symptoms, and 100 treatment actions and plans. We continually revise and update the existing knowledge base in parallel with the development of Guardian's cognitive and physical skills.

REASONING COMPONENTS

At the physical level, Guardian has three major reasoning components. *Focus* performs a data reduction task while *tFPR* and the *Sign Evaluator* methods perform data abstraction tasks. At the cognitive level, Guardian currently possesses two diagnostic methods, (*MFM* and *PCT*), an integrated method for diagnosis and therapy management, (*ReAct*), and a protocol-based treatment method, (*SPIN*).

DISCUSSION

We are now embarking on a new phase of evaluation in which we will evaluate Guardian on a broader range of scenarios involving difficult problems such as multiple critical events, cognitive overload, and known cognitive "traps." In this study, we will compare Guardian's performance in critical situations with the performance of human experts under the same circumstances using an advanced simulator. We aim to identify whether an intelligent agent can be designed and fine-tuned to perform adequately in situations where the cognitive skills of human experts are seriously taxed. We hypothesize that human-machine cooperation under information overload situations can improve the work environment of clinicians, improve health care delivery, and ultimately reduce health-care costs.

This project is sponsored by NASA contract NAG 2-581 under ARPA Order 6822 and a grant from the Whitaker Foundation administered by NSF.

References

[1] B. Hayes-Roth et al. Guardian: A prototype intelligent agent for intensive-care monitoring. Artificial Intelligence in Medicine, 4:165–185, 1992.

[2] B. Hayes-Roth. A blackboard architecture for control. Artificial Intelligence, 26:251–321, 1985.

REAL-TIME EXPERT SYSTEM FOR ADVISING ANESTHESIOLOGISTS IN THE CARDIAC OPERATING ROOM

Aleksandar Timcenko, Ph.D. and David L. Reich, MD
Department of Anesthesiology, Mt. Sinai Medical Center, NY, NY 10029

Abstract *This paper describes the initial work towards building a distributed real-time expert system for advising anesthesiologists in the cardiac operating room. The goal of this project is to build a vigilant system that contains knowledge relevant to the practice of cardiac anesthesiology. The system is being designed to use this knowledge in conjunction with continuous automated patient data acquisition in order to provide clinically useful differential diagnoses and treatment recommendations in real time.*

1 INTRODUCTION

This report describes a prototype system that has been developed at The Mount Sinai Medical Center. This system attempts to go one important step further than existing systems [1,2,3] towards generating treatment recommendations in real time based upon on-line measurements, pharmacokinetic models and the patient's medical history. The goal of this project is to build a system that contains a reasonable amount of knowledge relevant for the practice of anesthesiology and to utilize this knowledge in conjunction with measurements of patient's state, knowledge of patient's medical history and pharmacokinetic models, providing responsive and useful information in real time. The system will be evaluated on case files generated from the CompuRecord (ARI, Pittsburgh, PA), of which approximately 20,000 are already available. The features of the system are:

- *Accuracy.*
- *Explanation.* The system needs to clearly present its "train of thought" and be able to respond to "what-if" questions
- *Responsiveness.* The system is designed to provide timely recommendations for treatment.
- *Truth maintenance.* The system maintains a network of interdependencies between differential diagnoses and computes their belief measures.

2 SOFTWARE ARCHITECTURE

The main software modules that comprise the expert system are (see Figure 1):

1. The **Rule Base** and the **Dictionary**. This module contains the algorithmic knowledge in the form of OPS-5 rules and lists of relevant information on diseases, drugs and procedures in form of hash tables.
2. **Knowledge Processing Module**, embedded within the LISP environment with OPS-5 interpreter
3. The **Pharmacokinetic Module** that contains simulation models of drug concentrations
4. **Data Acquisition** and **Signal Conditioning** modules that prepare measurement data and data trends for processing in the **Knowledge Processing Module**
5. **Concentrator Module** that serves as a "blackboard" for funneling data to other modules
6. (Optional) **Report Generation** module that prepares the output in the form of correct English sentences.
7. The **Hypertext GUI** that presents the system's advises in the form of hierarchical hypertext structure (see Figure 2)

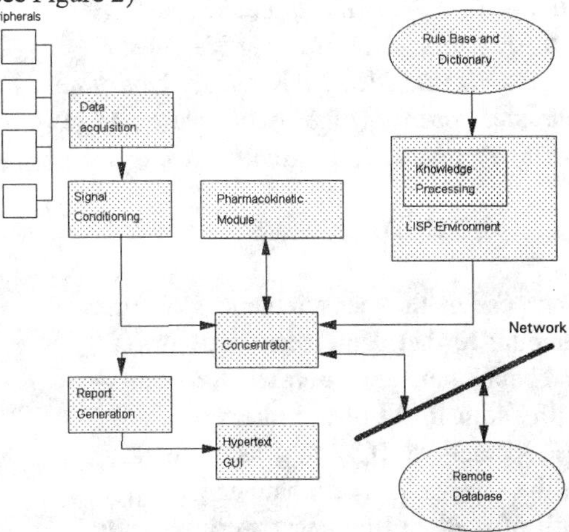

Figure 1. Main software modules of the expert system

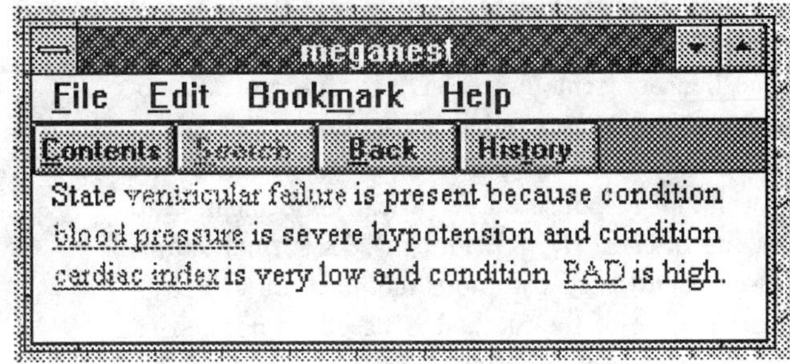

Figure 3. System's output in the hypertext form. Underlined clues are pointers to additional information.

REFERENCES

[1] Groth, T, Hakman, M., Hedlund, A., and Zaar, B., KBSIM/FLUIDTHERAPY: a system for optimized design of fluid resuscitation in trauma. *Comput. Methods Programs Biomed.*, 34(2-3):163-173, 1991.

[2] Schecke, T., Langen. M., Popp, H. J., Rau, G., Kasmacher, H., and Kalff, G., Knowledge-based decision support for patient monitoring in cardioanesthesia. *Int. J. Clin. Monit. Comput.*, 9(1):1-11, 1992.

[3] Sukuvaara, T., Koski, E. M., Makivirta, A., and Kari, A., A knowledge-based alarm system for monitoring cardiac operated patients -- technical construction and evaluation, *Int. J. Clin. Monit. Comput.*, 10(2):117-126, 1993.

Optimized Method Of Estimation Of Critical Flicker Frequency (CFF)

Vladimir A. Feshchenko, Ph.D., Ruth A.Reinsel, Ph.D., Robert A. Veselis, M.D.,
Department of Anesthesiology and Critical Care Medicine, Memorial Sloan-Kettering Cancer Center New York, NY 10021

The threshold frequency for perception of a flickering light (CFF) is an indicator of arousal of the cerebral cortex, and widely used both for clinical and research purposes [1]. The measurement is often based on the method of limits (MOL), presenting a flickering stimulus of steadily increasing or decreasing frequency. This method is not free from biases [2]. The method of constant stimuli (MCS) is more precise but may take more time, so the state of the subject cannot be considered as invariable [2]. We describe a time-saving, computer-controlled method based on MCS modified with feedback from previous responses.

METHOD/RESULTS

The main purpose of the measurement is obtaining the curve similar to that depicted in fig.1 or its derivative. The advantage of our MCS method consists in the adjustment of the interval of frequencies representing [f_{min}; f_{max}] as close as possible to the interval of real changes [f_L; f_H]. Light stimuli of random frequency were presented within a range bracketing the estimated CFF, and the subject pressed a button if the stimulus was perceived as flickering. Testing was continued until at least 10 stimuli (in practice, often many more) had been presented at each 1 Hz interval. Two values were compared as estimates of CFF: the frequency of an extremum of first derivative of this sigmoidal response curve (Fpeak) and mean value of the interval [f_L; f_H] (Fmean). 35 normal subjects have been tested using our method. Initial verification of the method is based on comparison with results obtained by MOL in a subset of 15 subjects on two different days. A device measuring CFF by MOL (Lafayette Instr. Co., Indiana) was modified to be computer driven via the counter-timer board. Special software has been developed by one of us (VF).

Stimuli were presented within a mean range of 6 Hz within which CFF was estimated. Fpeak and Fmean were highly correlated ($r=0.98$; $p<.0001$) and differed by only 0.20 ± 1.66 Hz (mean + std.dev.). Therefore we selected Fpeak as our estimate of the critical flicker frequency. For the full set of subjects (N=35) CFF estimated by Fpeak was 36.5 ± 4.8 Hz. For these subjects, CFF measured on 2 different days was not significantly different. Comparing Fpeak computed by our method to CFF measured by MOL (measured on 15 subjects), the two estimates of CFF differed by less than 0.1 Hz ($t= 0.062$, ns). Our technique took on average 6.2 min, comparable with the time required for MOL, but provided on average 147 trials for estimation of the probability distribution of CFF versus 20 trials in MOL, affording a two-fold increase in the reliability of CFF estimation.

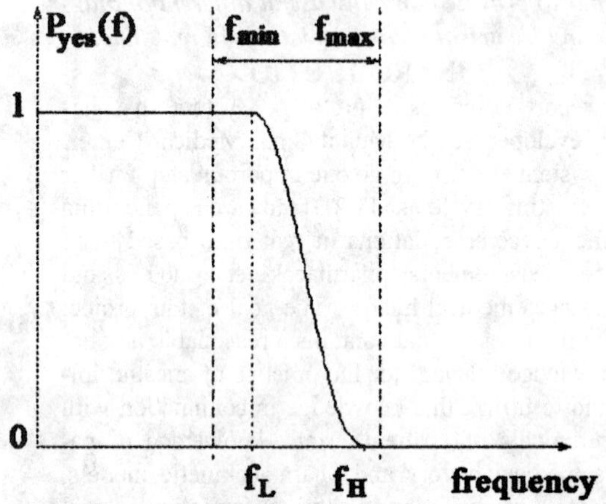

Figure 1. Heuristic dependence of the probability of perception of the light stimulus as "flickering" on the frequency of flicker.

We report a method to estimate CFF which includes desirable features of MCS, but is more rapidly performed. This is possible because we adjust the stimuli presented based on the subject's previous responses. Thus, most data are gathered around the actual estimate of CFF. Our method correlates well with the standard MOL. This method can be further optimized from the viewpoint of statistical precision and minimum time of measurement by reducing the number of stimuli presented to no more than 10 per bin so that measurement will take approximately 3 minutes. A further advantage of this technique is that the data are amenable to analysis by signal detection theory, yielding an estimate of response bias as well as of perceptual threshold.

References

[1]. I. Hindmarch. Information Processing, CFF Threshold and Benzodiazepines. Br J Clin Pharmac, 1980, 10:189-209.

[2]. B. Aufdembrinke. The Measurement of CFF. Pharmacopsychiatria 1982, 15 (Suppl.1): 5-8.

0195-4210/94/$5.00 © 1994 AMIA, Inc.

A Model-Based Simulator for Testing Rule-Based Decision Support Systems for Mechanical Ventilation of ARDS Patients

R. Matthew Sailors, B.E., Thomas D. East, Ph.D.*
Departments of Bioengineering, Medical Informatics*, and Anesthesiology*
University of Utah and Pulmonary Division LDS Hospital, Salt Lake City, Utah

A model-based simulator was developed for testing rule-based decision support systems that manages ventilator therapy of patients with the Adult Respiratory Distress Syndrome (ARDS). The simulator is based on a multi-compartment model of the human body and mathematical models of the gas exchange abnormalities associated with ARDS. Initial testing of this system indicates that model-based simulators are a viable tool for testing rule-based expert systems used in health-care.

INTRODUCTION

During the past decade, researchers at LDS Hospital have developed a series of computerized decision support systems for managing the mechanical ventilation of patients with ARDS. These protocols, as they are called, are data and time driven, rule-based expert systems which suggest changes in mechanical ventilator therapy based on current and past respiratory therapy and laboratory data. These protocols run within and directly access the integrated patient database of LDS Hospital's HELP system [1, 2]. The complexity of the protocol system makes the testing of the underlying logic and its exact implementation difficult and confusing. In the past, the only way to test the computerized protocols was to manually enter all of the necessary data into the computer in real-time. This is neither an elegant nor efficient means of testing. The objective of this work was to develop a new type of tool for testing rule-based expert systems: a model-based simulator of the human body. Model based simulators are able to dynamically adjust to the suggestions and requests of a rule-based expert system and are therefore an improvement over previous testing methods.

METHODS / RESULTS

The simulator is based on a multi-compartment model of the human body. The various compartments represent various physiologically distinct body tissues, such as arterial and venous blood pools, musculoskeletal system, central nervous system, and the three compartments of the Riley-Cournand lung. [3] The gas exchange abnormalities associated with ARDS were modeled using mathematical models describing the time-course changes sizes of the shunt fraction and dead space compartments of the Riley-Cournand lung. Gas exchange was also corrected for Positive End Expiratory Pressure (PEEP), cardiac output, and pH. [3, 4] It is important to understand the simulator compresses time to speed up the testing process. Time compression is achieved by starting the simulation's clock at a point in the past and then processing the model's equations rapidly enough that the simulator's clock moves faster than real clocks. This is a change from previous testing methods which were limited by the normal passage of time.

Since February 1, 1994, the simulator has been tested for more than 2000 simulated hours. The simulator's modeled physiologic responses were similar to those of ARDS patients treated in LDS Hospital's intensive care unit. During this period, fifteen individual patients were simulated and more than 900 instructions generated. The simulator dynamically changed the disease process model and made protocol-suggested therapy adjustments. Initial tests of the simulator uncovered two small programming syntax errors in portions of the protocols which deal with clinically rare conditions. These errors were quickly and easily corrected before they could cause any problems in the clinical use of the protocols.

Model-based simulators are an untapped, important, and useful addition to the toolbox of anyone who develops and tests expert systems used in health care .

References

1. Kuperman GJ, Gardner RM, Pryor TA, ed. HELP: A dynamic hospital information system. New York: Springer-Verlag, 1991:
2. Thomsen GE, et al. Clinical performance of a rule-based decision support system for mechanical ventilation of ARDS patients. Proceedings of SCAMC, 1993. Washington, D.C.
3. Riley RL, Cournand A. 'Ideal' alveolar air and the analysis of ventilation-perfusion relationships in the lungs. J Applied Physiology 1:825-847, 1949.
4. Dickinson CJ. A computer model of human respiration. Baltimore: University Park Press, 1977.

0195-4210/94/$5.00 © 1994 AMIA, Inc.

User Evaluation: PA Catheter Waveforms Troubleshooting System

R.D. Zielstorff, RN, MS; G. Estey, EdM; J.B. Fitzmaurice, RN, PhD;
M. Martin, RN, MS; G.O. Barnett, MD
Massachusetts General Hospital
Boston, MA

This paper reports on a user satisfaction survey of a system for consultation and education in troubleshooting pulmonary artery catheter waveforms. The twelve-item End-User Computing Satisfaction Questionnaire was used to assess users' ratings in four areas. On a scale of 1-5 (with 1 the lowest), the ratings were: Content, 3.5; Accuracy, 4.5; Format, 4.2; Ease of Use, 4.4, and Timeliness, 4.1. Comparison with ratings in a survey that included a variety of applications and settings is provided.

INTRODUCTION

The object of this evaluation is a microcomputer-based system for providing access to synthesized knowledge regarding characteristics, causes and management of PA catheter waveforms. Designed for physicians and nurses who practice in intensive care settings, the system contains content on approximately forty commonly and uncommonly encountered PA waveforms. Graphics and images are used extensively to explicate the knowledge [1].

METHODS/RESULTS

After ten months of use on a 19-bed cardiac intensive care unit, users of the system were surveyed to assess their satisfaction with the system. The instrument used was a short survey developed by Doll and Torkzadeh [2]. This twelve-item instrument uses a Likert-type scale to assess users' perceptions of five system components: Content, Accuracy, Format, Ease of Use, and Timeliness.

The questionnaire was distributed to users who met the following criteria: they used the system more than one time, they used it for a total of at least 8 minutes, and they viewed at least 20 screens. Of the 58 people who had logged onto the system during the experimental period, 30 users (52%) met the criteria.

Twenty-five out of thirty subjects returned the questionnaire, a response rate of 76%. On a scale of 1-5, the mean scores for the five dimensions of user satisfaction were: Content, 3.5; Accuracy, 4.5; Format, 4.2; Ease of Use, 4.4, and Timeliness, 4.1. The non-parametric Sign Test was used to see whether there was a significant number of mean ratings of 4 or more on each of the five components. Content is the only dimension that failed the test.

The average total score for the End User Satisfaction survey was 48.3, with a standard deviation of 8.56. This is very similar to the population statistics reported by Doll & Torkzadeh, where the average total score for a range of applications in several types of industries was 49.09, and the standard deviation was 8.30. The average total score of 48.3 for the PA Waveform Troubleshooting System falls in approximately the 40th percentile of total scores for all applications surveyed in the Doll & Torkzadeh study.

Although the experiment itself has been completed, the system is still in use on the experimental unit, and its use has expanded to other units within the hospital where knowledge of PA catheter waveforms is necessary in patient care.

References

[1] Zielstorff RD, Barnett GO, Fitzmaurice JB, Oliver DE, Ford-Carleton P, Thompson BT, Estey G, Eccles R, Martin M, Jenders R. Providing Clinicians with Problem-Based Access to Knowledge: Troubleshooting Pulmonary Artery Catheter Waveforms. In: Safran CS (ed). Proceedings of the Seventeenth Annual Symposium on Computer Applications in Medical Care. New York: McGraw Hill, 1993, pp. 351-355.

[2] Doll WJ, and Torkzadeh G. The Measurement of End-User Computing Satisfaction. MIS Quarterly, 1988, 12:259-274.

======================

Funded by Grant 5 R18 HS06575, AHCPR, PHS, USDHHS; Grant 1 T15 LM07092 and Grant 5 R01 LM05200, NLM, NIH, PHS, USDHHS; and by an educational grant from Hewlett Packard Corporation

The Representation of Time in Clinical Patient Simulations

Jihad Obeid, M.D., Bryan P. Bergeron, M.D.,
Luke Sato, M.D., and Ronald L. Rouse

Decision Systems Group of Harvard Medical School and M.I.T.
Brigham and Women's Hospital
75 Francis Street, Boston, Massachusetts 02115

Simulated clinical scenarios are generally compressed in time to enhance educational effectiveness and to minimize testing time. Designers should consider how to best control potential sources of distortion in the perception of time and how to best communicate the passage of time to the user.

INTRODUCTION

Clinical scenarios that would normally take days or weeks to unfold can be simulated in minutes, thereby allowing the user to experience several clinical cases in a single session. Despite the universality of time compression in patient simulations, there appears to be little effort in the way of standardizing how time is represented in either the underlying design or to the user.

Patient case simulations often rely on a variety of time progression techniques. For example, time may begin in step with real time and then jump to some point in the future or time may be compressed uniformly from start to finish. Further, the degree and nature of time compression may change from one event to the next.

Conventional simulation paradigms generally approach time as either a continuous, discrete, or mixed continuous/discrete entity. Regardless of how the passage of time is simulated, the user should somehow be made aware of its current value and rate of passage. Our experience with multimedia simulations indicates that there is need to continually display the simulated time, which provides a working context and a sense of urgency that can be advantageous, e.g., in a critical care simulation.

The commonest indicators of simulated time are analog/digital clocks and bar/slider displays. The optimal type of display is a function of the simulation design and the purpose of the simulation, e.g., testing or education. Bar and slider displays can be configured to provide a richer and more intuitive indication of time than can analog/digital clock displays. For example, bar and slider displays can simultaneously provide cues on the time remaining, time since the start of a simulation, and the relative progression of time in the simulation (e.g., what percentage of time is remaining). In addition, since bar and slider displays be calibrated in real or arbitrary time units, in either linear or non-linear markings, they can be used to provide an indication of intentional time distortions.

Although there will always be individual differences in the perception simulated time, a number of factors that influence this perception can be controlled. For example, perceived time is a function of the complexity of a patient case simulation and by the amount of activity required of the user. The more demanded of the user, in terms of navigation, parameter input, and mental processing, the faster both simulated and real times appear to pass. With this is mind, simulation designers can influence the perception of time by controlling simulation complexity, the difficulty of the simulated patient case, and the complexity of the user interface.

DISCUSSION

The simulation and representation of time in patient case simulations has been largely ignored. Given that there are differences in how simulated time progresses, the representation of simulated time is a potential source of user confusion that is compounded by the distortions due to individual differences in time perception. Clearly, the user must be given clues as to how simulated time can be expected to progress, and how their interactions and events within the simulation will affect the passage of time.

ACKNOWLEDGMENTS

This publication was supported in part by grants R29 LM04715-05 and LM07092 from the National Library of Medicine, by the Health Sciences and Technology Division of the Massachusetts Institute of Technology and Harvard Medical School, by the Office of Educational Development of Harvard Medical School, and by the American Board of Family Practice.

A Computer Simulation of the Hypothalamic-Pituitary-Adrenal Axis

Joseph Gonzalez-Heydrich M.D.[1], Ronald J. Steingard M.D.[1], Isaac Kohane M.D., Ph.D.[2]
Psychopharmacology Clinic, Departments of Psychiatry [1] and Division of Endocrinology, Department of Medicine [2], Children's Hospital, Boston

This paper describes the construction of a computer model that simulates the hypothalamic-pituitary-adrenal axis (HPA axis) regulation of cortisol production. It is presented to illustrate the process of physiological modeling using standard "off the shelf" technologies. The model simulates components of the HPA axis involved in the continuous secretion and elimination of cortisol, adrenocorticotropin (ACTH), and corticotropin releasing hormone (CRH). The physiological relations of these component pieces were modeled based on the current knowledge of their functioning. Rate constants, half lives, and receptor affinities were assigned values derived from the experimental literature. At its current level of development the model is able to accurately simulate the timing, magnitude and decay of the ACTH and cortisol concentration peaks resulting from the ovine-CRH stimulation test in normal and hypercortisolemic patients. The model will be used to predict the effects of lesions in different components of the HPA axis on the time course of cortisol and ACTH levels. We plan to use the model to explore the experimental conditions required to distinguish mechanisms underlying various disorders of the HPA axis, particularly depression. Efforts are currently underway to validate the model for a large variety of normal and pathological perturbations of the HPA axis.

INTRODUCTION:

The HPA regulation of cortisol is accomplished through a complex network of interacting components. Despite increasingly detailed knowledge about each of these <u>components</u>, it remains difficult to predict from this information how the <u>network</u> will perform. One possible approach to understanding network functioning is to build a simulation that allows us to model, quantitatively, the functioning of these components within the context of the network [1].

METHODS / RESULTS

Extend, (Imagine That, Inc. San Jose, Ca.) a simulation development tool was used to build the simulations on a macintosh computer. The granularity of mechanistic detail modeled was chosen to simulate the time course of ACTH and cortisol plasma levels observed during a standard test of HPA functioning, the Ovine-CRH stimulation test (oCRH stim. test). The following are the differential equations used:

Cortisol module: Eq. (1)

$$d[cortisol]/dt = k_1*[ACTH] + k_2 - k_3*[cortisol]$$

ACTH module: Eq. (2)

$$d[ACTH]/dt = k_4*[CRH]+k_5 - k_6*[ACTH] - (k_4*[CRH]+k_5)*I_{max}*[cortisol]/(K_d+[cortisol])$$

CRH module: Eq. (3)

$$d[CRH]/dt = \text{pulse function}, f(t) + k_7 - k_8[CRH]$$

Where [X] is concentration of X. k_n is a rate constant. I_{max} is the saturation level of inhibition. K_d is the dissociation constant for the glococorticoid II receptor (only inhibition at the level of the pituitary by cortisol was modeled [2]). The constants were estimated from published oCRH stim. tests in normal controls.

The results of the simulations were compared to published results of the oCRH stim. test in normal controls and patients with acute and chronic hypercortisolemia[3]. The program was able to successfully simulate 1) the plasma half lives of cortisol and ACTH and 2) the magnitude and timing of their peaks in response to an oCRH stimulation test in normal individuals and patients with hypercortisolemia .

This paper discusses the implementation with "off the shelf" software, of simulations that closely follow clinical and experimental observations. To proceed in further building this tool, we plan to generate a range of models and selecting the *minimal* or *optimal* model by applying formal criteria [1]. Fitting the constants of this model to actual patient's diagnostic tests should allow the estimation of otherwise inaccessible physiologic parameters and serve as guides to further basic and clinical research.

REFERENCES

[1] Carson, C. Cobelli and L. Finklestein. <u>The Mathematical Modeling of Metabolic and Endocrine Systems.</u> John Wiley and Sons. New York. 1983.
[2] Dayanithi and F. A. Antoni. Rapid as well as Delayed Inhibitory Effects of Glucocorticoid Hormones on Pituitary Adrenocorticotropic Hormone Release are Mediated by Type II Glucocorticoid Receptors and Require Newly Synthesized Messenger Ribonucleic Acid as well as Protein. <u>Endocrinology</u> 1989;125:308-13.
[3] B. Martin and S. Reichlin. <u>Clinical Neuroendocrinology.</u> F. A. Davis. Philadelphia. 1987.

0195-4210/94/$5.00 © 1994 AMIA, Inc.

Elders' Attitudes and Behavior Regarding ComputerLink*

Patricia Flatley Brennan, RN, PhD, FAAN, and Kathleen Smyth, PhD
Case Western Reserve University , Cleveland, Ohio

ComputerLink is a set of telecommunications modules designed to provide information, decision making assistance, and communication support to caregivers of persons with Alzheimer's disease. Over 19 months, each of the 47 AD caregivers had 12 consecutive months of access. There were a total of 3875 accesses to the AD caregivers' ComputerLink. Attitudes toward ComputerLink were assessed. Subjective and objective measures of use also were captured. ComputerLink users held generally positive attitudes towards the use of the computer network and tended to under-report the number of times they accessed the system.

INTRODUCTION

ComputerLink is a set of telecommunications modules designed to provide information, decision making assistance, and communication support to caregivers of persons with Alzheimer's disease (AD). Examination of attitudes towards ComputerLink aids in discerning motivation for use. However, use of ComputerLink may vary depending on whether it is measured by subjective or objective means. This paper examines elders' attitudes towards ComputerLink use, and explores differences in subjective and objective appraisals of use.

Instruments and Measures

Attitudes toward ComputerLink were assessed in a self-administered 20-item investigator-developed instrument. Based on other reports of users' reactions to using computers, subjects were prompted with single-word adjectives and asked to indicate in a likert-format the extent to which the adjective expressed how they had felt while using ComputerLink.

A passive monitoring system recorded each individual's use and noted screen sequences. Subjective appraisal of use was assessed by a single-item question that asked subjects' to estimate how often they had used ComputerLink during the previous year.

Attitudes towards ComputerLink

Thirty-five subjects completed the Adjectives Reactions to ComputerLink form. Listed below are the adjectives grouped by whether the adjective term connotes a positive or negative attitude toward ComputerLink, and the percent of persons reporting that use of ComputerLink engendered this attitude *Quite a Bit* or *Extremely*.

Positive	*Quite a Bit /Extremely*
Interested	75%
Excited	29%
Strong	18%
Inspired	32%
Enthusistic	52%
Proud	33%
Alert	31%
Determined	33%
Attentive	41%
Active	29%

Negative	*Quite a Bit /Extremely*
Distressed	39%
Upset	32%
Guilty	30%
Hostile	15%
Irritable	35%
Ashamed	15%
Nervous	33%
Scared	23%
Jittery	26%
Afraid	26%

Most subjects held favorable attitudes towards ComputerLink. ComputerLink engendered attitudes of "Interested" and "Enthusiastic" for over 50% of the respondents. Generally fewer than one-third experienced any negative feelings about ComputerLink; the most commonly expressed negative feelings were "Distressed", "Upset", "Irritable" or "Nervous"; these were identified by fewer than ten respondents each. Cross tabulations of each individual attitude revealed tight scatter around the median for postive-positive and negative-negative comparisons, and broad scatter for positive-negative comparisons.

Subjective and Objective Measures of Use

Number of Subject	***Subjective* Number of Logons**	***Objective* Mean (sd) Count of Logons**	***Objective* Range of Logon Counts**
10	8 or less	19 (14.1)	3-54
13	Monthly	60.6 (55.61)	7-170
16	Weekly	79 (66.26)	9-275
7	Once a Day	147 (80.9)	31-234
1	>Once a Day	590	590

These data demonstrate that most individuals underestimated their use of ComputerLink; individuals who believed they used the ComputerLink daily were the only ones who, on self-report, over-estimated their actual behavior. Most persons thought they had accessed ComputerLink once a week. Weekly logons for a calendar year would result in a count of 52 logons. The discrepancy between 52 and 80 may be explained by a early participation behavior in which individuals accessed ComputerLink frequently during the early weeks of the experiment, and then stabilized to a pattern of access every seven days.

*Support for this project came from a grant from the NIA, AG 8617, Patricia Flatley Brennan, PI. Some ideas resulted from discussion with Faye Payton-Cobb, PhD student, Weatherhead School of Management.

Section VIII

Electronic Posters

MODELING A COMPUTE ASSISTED INSTRUCTION FOR ABDOMINAL SURGICAL PATIENTS

Fendy H. Huang, RN, MSN Candidate & Mary A. Curran, RN, Ph.D.
Dept. of Adult Health Nursing, UNC-Charlotte, Charlotte, NC

INTRODUCTION

Patient education is a key component of health care. Nurses teach to improve the patient's level of understanding, knowledge, attitudes, and skills. This knowledge enhances the self-care abilities of the clients and promotes their health.

As a self-directed learning strategy, Computer Assisted Instruction (CAI) transfers the responsibility for the patient's education from the nurse to the patient. Therefore, a self-care focus is maintained and supported.

Research has investigated the use of CAI in patient teaching. A survey of this literature suggests that CAI impacts on patient education in the following ways:

1. CAI can be utilized, whenever the learner is ready or available to learn.
2. CAI provides instruction in a manner that can be viewed as infinitely patient, consistent, and tireless.
3. CAI allows privacy to overcome learning barriers due to embarrassing or sensitive content.
4. CAI enables the learner to proceed at his/her own pace and permits review of any sections which are not fully understood.
5. An interactive CAI program provides immediate feedback and specific reinforcement that is critical to effective and efficient learning.
6. CAI integrates graphics, sound, animation, and color to make the user interface friendly, entertaining, and well accepted.
7. CAI enables learner control and ensures the learner's active participation to enhance the learning process.
8. CAI helps ensure that standardized instruction is presented to every patient.
9. CAI can effectively supplement the time of health professionals, and therefore decrease personnel costs (1,2,3).

There are commercial CAI programs for patient teaching that focus on Diabetes and Renal disease. Little development has been done for general surgical patients who represent a large population served by health care providers (4). Preoperative teaching has been discussed in the literature since 1970. Teaching enhances the patient's understanding of postoperative regimens, decreases anxiety and postoperative complications, and promotes rapid recovery. Lindeman and Van Aernam (5) found structured preoperative teaching increased the adult surgical patient's ability to cough and deep breathe. CAI fits well into formulating a structured teaching tool for the pre-op patient. Surgical patients were, therefore, chosen as the target population to standardize pre-op teaching materials and improve post-op status.

PROJECT METHODOLOGY

The CAI program was developed under a Microsoft Windows® environment using Asymetrix Toolbook® 1.53, an object-oriented hypermedia program. The program includes a runtime version which allows for ease in transport.

The format is an interactive tutorial of sequential instructional content accessible in a non-linear manner. Using Gagne's nine events of instruction as a framework (6), contents relating to pre- and post-op activities (lab tests, consent forms, exercise, infection prevention, diet, and medication considerations) are presented. Patients choose the area of interest or skip areas that they already know. Use of color, graphics, and animation attracts the learners' attention.

Content is based on accepted health care practice. Evaluation and recommendations by nursing experts, instructional specialists, and patients further strengthened the program.

REFERENCES

[1]. Cartwright, M. (1988). Why not computers in patient education? Australian Journal of Advanced nursing, 5(4), 28-30.
[2]. Kahn, G. (1993). Computer-based patient education: A progress report. MD Computing, 10, 93-99.
[3]. Sinclair, V. (1985). The computer as partner in health care instruction. Computers in Nursing, 3, 212-216.
[4]. American Hospital Association (1994). AHA hospital statistics 1993-1994 Edition. Chicago: AHA.
[5]. Lindeman, C. & Van Aernam, B. (1971). Nursing intervention with the presurgical patient-the effects of structured and unstructured pre-op teaching. Nursing Research, 20, 319-332.
[6]. Gagne, R., Wager, W., & Rojan, A. (1984). Planning and authoring computer-assisted instruction lessons. In DF Walker & R Hess (Eds.), Instructional software: principles and perspectives for design and use. Belmont, CA: Wadsworth. (pp.57-67)

School Nurse's Assistant Expert Screening System

Duncan Belser, Allen R. Wenner, M.D., Matthew Ferrante, M.B.A.
Primetime Medical Software, West Columbia, SC 29169

Abstract

The School Nurse's Assistant is designed to aid the School Nurse by providing a diagnostic discovery tool that also educates the student through the use of multimedia. Response initiated questions focus on the most pertinent student risk factors: lifestyle choices such as alcohol, drugs, and sexual activity. Because the questions are patient driven, the student stays interested as only relevant questions are presented. The School Nurse's Assistant provides the school nurse with increased sociographic information, and delivers cost-effective information to high risk segments of the student population. The potential for successful intervention is dramatic.

Engineered to satisfy the needs of the secondary school systems of the United States for checking the social activities of high school students, The Nurse's Assistant uses techniques of artificial intelligence for medical screening and complements them with a multimedia presentation designed to catch the interest of the students. Specifically, the computer aids the nurse by asking a series of background questions that would ordinarily require much of the nurse's time. The Nurse's Assistant then creates a complete report of the student's problems and their symptoms.

The questions, which first appear harmless and general, progress based upon the student's responses. For example, while at the same time the student sees a seductive picture of a member of the opposite sex, a question of their encounters with a sexually transmitted disease is posed. "Have you or any sexual partner ever had *Granuloma Inguinale*?" the screen reads. The choices listed are "Yes," "No," "Maybe," "I Don't Know, "Pass," and "Show Me." If the student responds "Show Me," then the seductive picture becomes a detailed medical photograph of genitalia infected with the Venereal Disease. The question is asked again. However, the student who has not encountered such a disease can select "No" and move on. Another example of the artificial intelligence expert system employed in The Nurse's Assistant would be if the student indicated that he or a close friend consumed alcohol regularly. The program would then initiate appropriate sequencing to determine the extent of alcohol consumption and administer standardized alcoholism diagnostic tests if warranted. Thus, the students who do not have problems will not be questioned or receive information about symptoms while troubled students, on the other hand, will see detailed medical photographs designed to educate them for future encounters.

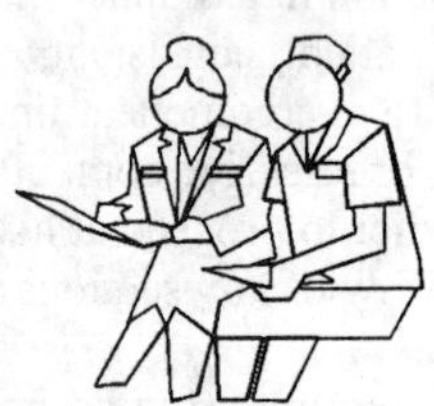

Studies have shown that adolescent student responses are likely to be honest since the questions are being asked by an impersonal machine rather than an adult (and remember, in the mind of a troubled adolescent, adults are the enemy).

For the nurse, this software can be used to operate more efficiently because it allows the computer to conduct the initial interview while the nurse can be attending another student. It also allows the detection of high-risk behaviors at an early stage, allowing for effective intervention. The main focus of this program is to shift the time of the school nurse away from routine questioning. By delegating this task to the computer, the school nurse will be able to spend more time for further education and counseling: these higher value activities are what will allow the school nurse to become more proactive in guiding student lifestyles.

Homeless Patients: Designing a Database for Nursing Documentation

M. A. Curran, RN, PhD*, K.E. Curran, DBA**, W.K. Cody, RN, PhD*
College of Nursing* & College of Business** UNC-Charlotte, Charlotte, NC

ABSTRACT

Care of the homeless in small out-patient clinic settings presents unique challenges in health care documentation. The transitory and infrequent episodic nature of client contact, as well as the inherent inefficiencies of the traditional paper chart, tend to minimize the collection of useful data for analyzing trends and patterns to identify and meet evolving health care needs.

INTRODUCTION

Meeting the health care needs of the growing homeless population is providing nursing with unique data collection and documentation challenges. These challenges are unique because of the typical transitory nature of the episodic encounters with homeless clients. This limited contact decreases accessibility to historical and current data and impedes the health care provider's ability to do more than meet immediate health care needs[1].

Further difficulties arise because of inherent inefficiencies in traditional paper systems of documentation. Manual documentation is labor intensive, results in decreased productivity, and often impedes the capture, storage and retrieval of information [2].

The lack of instant, or on-line, accessibility to patient information can create uncertainties in caring for any patient. This lack of available data seems especially prevalent with the homeless. Multiple psychosocial, as well as pathophysiologic problems are frequent findings [3].

Recognition of these problems has lead to development of a nursing documentation database that can be used in nursing-focused clinics that provide care to homeless populations. Client data from these sites can be collected, merged, and analyzed to identify population patterns. Identification of these patterns provides the opportunity to develop nursing interventions that could focus on health promoting, in addition to episodic, patient care.

PROJECT METHODOLOGY

The patient record was developed under a Microsoft Windows@ environment using Microsoft Access@, a relational database program. The relational structure was required because of the many-to-many or complex data relationships [4]. Access was used because of its intuitive interface, query language, ease of modification, stand-alone capability, and convenience.

The record began as computerization of existing documentation. However, it was quickly recognized that an exact paper to computer conversion was inappropriate. The system was redesigned based on a nursing model developed to address the health needs of homeless families [5]. this structure provided a more comprehensive interface that could focus on current and future health care needs.

Development was done by prototyping with multiple iterations based on user feedback [6]. This method involved the users and provided them with ownership and vested interest in the success of the system. In addition, real time usage increased the system's functionality.

The system currently provides a mechanism for rapid, but thorough documentation. Data entry can be initiated by the client and completed by the nurse.

Current efforts are underway to implement the system at other nursing-based homeless shelters. It is believed that this dissemination could result in a larger data source for analysis of health care trends in homeless populations.

References

[1] Institute of Medicine Homelessness, health, and human needs, Washington, DC: National Academy Press, 1988.
[2] Raygor, AJ. A study of the paper chart and its potential for computerization.. Computers in Nursing 1994, 12(1), pp. 23-28.
[3] Wright, JD, & Weber, E. Homelessness and health. New York: McGraw-Hill, 1988.
[4] Sheperd, JC. Database management: Theory and application. Boston: Richard D. Irwin, Inc., 1990.
[5] Berne, AS, Dato, C, Mason, DJ, & Rafferty, M. A nursing model for addressing the health needs of homeless families. Image, 1990, 22(1), pp. 8-13.
[6] Wetherbe, JC. Systems analysis and design. (4th ed.). New York: West Publishing Co., 1992.

NURSETALK: The Latest Addition to the Information Highway

K. Alden, RN, J. Dellinger, RN, A. Glasgow, RN, S. McCulley-Hall, RN, F. Huang, RN, L. Leatherwood, RN, N. Parce, RN, M. Pfaff, RN, D. Queen, RN, N. Richard, RN, L. Todd, RN, and H. Trahan, RN, MSN Candidates, UNC-Charlotte

ABSTRACT

NURSETALK is an electronic bulletin board system (BBS) developed to provide information and meet the communication needs of three different nursing organizations in North Carolina. It was designed and conceptualized from a user perspective to promote functionality and acceptance.

INTRODUCTION

In these times of cost containment, limited resources and rapid change, nurses are seeking effective methods to communicate ideas, share resources, and disseminate information relevant to the profession. Even with differing specialty foci, some issues and information are relevant to all practitioners.

BBSs offer an alternative to traditional communication methods and exemplify another way for nurses to utilize the power of the personal computer. The implementation of many BBSs has not, however, resulted in consistent usage by members of the targeted population.

These systems tend to be initiated by a single individual who perceives a need and implements his/her response to that perception. Many times this individual perspective, regardless of rationality, limits the acceptance of the system by the group [1].

To change this pattern of poor usage, decisions about content and structure need to be based on a user perspective. Because most nurses have limited experience with personal computers, the program also needs to provide a clear and intuitive environment for use.

PROJECT METHODOLOGY

NURSETALK is a BBS used primarily by nurses across North Carolina. It is a creative and cost effective application of computer technology to encourage and expedite communication within and between members of three organizations: the North Carolina Consortium of Sigma Theta Tau Chapters (the Consortium), the North Carolina Nurses Association (NCNA) and the North Carolina League for Nursing (NCNLN).

The original system was developed for the Consortium. However, economic and manpower problems forced the BBS to be unavailable for over a year. Members of the Consortium and the newly formed Council on Nursing Informatics of the NCNA requested reimplementation of the BBS. Rather than reinstate the existing system, a decision was made to start the development process from the beginning.

Development decisions were referred to a group of twelve nursing graduate students with minimal computer experience. This design group contained members from the three organizations. Their initial design and content decisions included structures for organizational information, an events calendar, forums, and shareware download facilities. Their purpose for the BBS was to provide information and enhance communication. Forums would allow users to participate in discussions or to ask pertinent questions of their colleagues [2.3].

Data and information were collected for inclusion in the BBS. Shareware selection was done through a group process and using compiled software rating scores. Forum topic selection occurred through group consensus after a review of nursing and lay literature on current issues.

The design and implementation of NURSETALK utilized group process and input. The result is a system that is based on a user's perspective and, hopefully, a user's needs. Whether to retrieve information, dialogue with one another about ideas, or access shareware, NURSETALK is a viable BBS for nurses of North Carolina.

References

[1] Dean, JW, & Sharfaman, MP. The relationship between procedural rationality and political behavior in strategic decision making. Decision Sciences Journal, 1993, 24(6), pp. 1069-1083.

[2] Brennan, PF. Computerlink: Electronic support for the home caregiver. Advanced Nursing Science, 1991, 13(4), pp. 14-27.

[3] Billings, DM. Computer conferencing: The "nurse" in the electronic school district. Computers in Nursing. 1991, 9(6), pp. 215-218.

The Emergency Psychiatry Nursing Assessment Report Framework: A Computer Program to Assist in Preparing Reports

Barry A. Tanner, Richard C. Marcolini, Eileen Howell, Jesse Bateau, and Irva Faber-Bermudez
Detroit Receiving Hospital and Wayne State University Medical School
Detroit, MI 48201

Abstract

EP Nurse is designed to guide the nurse through the interview and reporting process, and to produce a complete or nearly complete report of the nursing evaluation in emergency psychiatry. EP Nurse allows the nurse to produce a report in five to 10 minutes, accepting keyboard input for free-form text, and mouse clicks for selecting from lists of choices. Input includes identifying information, presenting complaints, substance use history, medical history and vitals, psychiatric medications, treatment history, history of mental illness, last hospitalization, family history of mental illness, nursing diagnosis, and nursing intervention. Written and on-line help and training were included to facilitate learning. The program includes an editor, based on HighEdit, which allows the nurse to review and modify the report prior to printing, and supports various fonts. Optionally, the nurse may save the report in ASCII format and load it into another word processor before editing or printing. We believe that EP Nurse reduces both errors of omission and errors of commission, and improves documentation in the medical record.

EP Nurse is intended to be used by licensed nurses familiar with the nursing assessment in emergency psychiatry. It is suitable for adult patients. EP Nurse requires MS Windows and nearly a megabyte of disk space for the program, runtime module, and help file.

A Computer Assisted Psychiatric Nursing Review: Modeling Nursing/Computer Analyst Collaboration

Karen DuBois, RNC, MSN, Nursing Information Systems Consultant/Computer Assisted Instruction Specialist, Penzance Professional Nursing and Health Career Development Center at The Presbyterian Hospital in the City of New York

Jeffrey Zucker, M.A., Programmer Analyst, Department of Nursing Education and Standards at The Presbyterian Hospital in the City of New York

Darlene Galashaw, RNC, MSN, Nursing Care Clinician at The Presbyterian Hospital in the City of New York

Transforming information in a changing health care environment is directly related to the collaboration of health care professionals and programmer analysts. Separate languages are spoken in the health care field and computer technology. These languages must be merged in an effort to translate health care content into appropriate electronic formats.

The process of collaboration between nurse content experts and a programmer analyst led to the development of a software program that has multiple uses for nursing. The final product was originally intended as a review course for psychiatric nurses taking the ANA certification exam. Many discussions with the programmer analyst enabled the nurse content experts to expand the objectives of this program to include clinical validation of psychiatric nursing skills, continuing education and/or orientation purposes.

The content experts were involved in teaching psychiatric nurses a two day lecture series in preparation for the ANA psychiatric mental health certification exam. In addition they oriented new nurses to the clinical setting and provided continuing education. The repetition of content in these areas prompted them to consult with a programmer analyst regarding the development of a computer assisted instruction course.

The content experts and programmer together developed a series of requirements for the program based on the computer platform, the targeted audience and the nature of the content. Since the materials were aimed at both in-hospital and home use, the program needed to be available in stand-alone and in networked environments. Further, the lack of graphics capabilities at many nursing computer stations mandated a text-only program. The targeted audience included nurses with little or no computer experience so the program needed to be simple, have easily available help information, and allow users to exit and return to the program at will. In addition, the team thought that the software needed to be flexible enough to adapt new information as it became available.

Taking these requirements into consideration, the programmer developed an authoring tool using C++ language. The tool does not require large amounts of disk space or memory and runs on any DOS computer, either networked or stand-alone. Aimed at the nurse with little computer experience, the software requires the user to be familiar with only six keys on the keyboard; and presents keystroke help and a description of the user's current location in the program on every screen. The tool accepts data in ASCII format so that information, questions, and scenarios may be changed and updated by anyone with simple word processing skills.

In addition to these platform and audience questions, the content presented special considerations: the development team perceived a need to have the software contain a representation of the ongoing evolving nature of the relationship between psychiatric nurses and their patients. The special nature of the psychiatric nursing relationship was partially preserved by a series of patient scenarios. Each topic area focuses on a specific (although fictional) patient. Users are presented with a scenario about the patient, asked some questions, then presented with further details in another scenario that includes changes in the patient status. Some topic areas include as many as six or more scenario changes so users are able to answer questions about several stages in the patient's progress. At any time the user may review the scenarios to use all of the information to answer the current question.

0195-4210/94/$5.00

An Innovative Approach to Gathering Functional Requirements

Karen Knecht, BSN, RN
Industry Specialist
Insource Management Group, Inc.

Frank Kopankiewitz
Systems Integrator
Insource Management Group, Inc.

Defining the functional requirements of the key clinical care providers is an important, foundational design activity for the development and design of clinical systems. A significant aspect of defining functional requirements is understanding the process of patient care delivery. Clinical information is an input as well as an output of patient care delivery. However, patient care delivery is not a single process but complex series of processes and activities involving many disciplines and departments. The ability to successfully automate the patient clinical information will be dependent on having a clear understanding of how patient care is delivered.

A key methodology in illustrating and describing patient care delivery is Process Mapping. It is a graphic illustration of how work gets done, who does the work, what information is required, and how that information is transformed. It describes the important linkages, hand-offs, and interactions that occur throughout patient care delivery Process Mapping takes a large, complex process and breaks it into smaller, more understandable components. This methodology reflects the cross organizational, cross functional work that is carried out through multiple settings within the health care organization.

A key tool developed to support the generation and documentation of process maps is ProMap. ProMap is a Windows based tool that utilizes a database software to generate reporting and graphic representations of the process. The interaction between the Process Mapping using ProMap will be demonstrated through real working models.

References:

Ball, M. and Collen, M., **Aspects of the Computer-Based Patient Record.** Springer-Verlag, New York. 1992.

Barry, C.T., Gibbons, L.K. *Information Systems Technology: Barriers and Challenges to Implementation.* **Journal of Nursing Administration.** 20(2). 40-42.

Bolens, M., Borst, F. Scherrer, J. *Organizing the Clinical Data in the Medical record.* **M.D. Computing.** 9(3). 149-155.

Bunschoten, B., *22 Years of Lessons Learned.* **Health Data Management.** June 1993. 24-27.
Gabrieli, E. *Standardization of Patient Care Documentation, Part 1.* **Journal of Clinical Computing.** 19(3-4). 39-105.

Gabrieli, E. *Standards for Electronic Medical record.* **Journal of Clinical Computing.** 20(1). 21-32.

Korpman, R., *Patient Care Automation: The Future is Now. Part 3. The Five Rules of Automation.* **Nursing Economics,** 8(5). 345-349.

Korpman, R., *Patient Care Automation: The Future is Now. Part 2. The Current Paper System- Can It Be Made To Work?.* **Nursing Economics,** 8(4). 263-267.

Lincoln, T., Essin, D., and Ware, W., *The Electronic Medical Record: A Challenge for Computer Science to Develop Clinically and Socially Relevant Computer Systems to Coordinate Information for Patient Care and*

Analysis. **The Information Society Journal.** 9(2).

National Conference on the Paperless Medical Record - Obstacles and Opportunities - December 8, 1992. Dallas, Texas.

Pferd, J. and Fuller, A., *User-Led Approach to Information Systems Investments.* **Society of Petroleum Engineers.** 1992. 83-92.

Reiser, S., *The Clinical Record in Medicine. Part 2: Reforming Content and Purpose.* **Annals of Internal Medicine.** 114(11). 980-1005.

Steen, E. and Dick, R., eds., **The Computer-Based Patient Record: An Essential Technology for Health Care.** National Academy Press. Washington, D.C. 1991.

Weed, L., *Medical Records that Guide and Teach.* **M.D. Computing.** 10(2). 100-114.

Getting Around in a Large Nomenclature File: Browsing SNOMED International

J. Craig Klimczak, D.V.M., Allen W. Hahn, D.V.M., Ph.D.,
MaryEllen Sievert, Ph.D. and Joyce A. Mitchell, Ph.D.

Medical Informatics Group and Veterinary Teaching Hospital
School of Medicine and College of Veterinary Medicine
University of Missouri, Columbia, MO 65211

We have developed a means whereby we can easily browse a very large (≈ 30 MB) file of a nomenclature vocabulary. "SNOMED International - A Vocabulary of Human and Veterinary Medicine" is such a file and has been proposed to serve as the basis for controlled vocabularies. The College of American Pathologists developed the nomenclature and the American Veterinary Medical Association has adopted it as a coding and interchange system for diagnoses, problems, procedures, etc. The nomenclature is also being brought into the Universal Medical Language System (UMLS) project of the National Library of Medicine.

SNOMED International has 12 modules and contains over 120,000 medical terms. This implementation is an appropriate step toward a comprehensive consistent codified nomenclature suitable for computer information interchange. However, because of its size, the system, in its distributed form, is difficult to use (printed form), necessitating numerous "page flips" and other delaying tactics when searching for a specific term. The text files furnished with the machine readable form of SNOMED are in Standard Data Format (SDF) with no handler for display and searching. It is left to the user to provide any form of usable display of the data.

We have developed a "Viewer" for these large files using a commercial information publishing tool - Folio Views from the Folio Corp., Provo, UT. We wrote a program in Turbo Pascal (Borland International, Scotts Valley, CA) to place the various SDF files from the distribution CD-ROM into a format suitable for inclusion into Folio Views. Included in the display format are synonyms, SNOMED codes, ICD-9 codes and connections to other modules of SNOMED (i.e. morphology, topography, etc.). Each of the separate items is presented in a different color to make for easy identification.

The viewer allows easy searching for codes and/or terms of interest to the user via the "Query" option in Folio Views. Hypertext links applied to the secondary hierarchies allow the user to become acquainted with the multiple hierarchies provided by SNOMED. Other links could be provided in various other formats limited only by the needs and imagination of the users.

The browser/viewer which we demonstrate, can run under DOS, MS Windows and Macintosh operating systems. Each platform can access the same file on the network with the platform dependent viewer so that only one data file need be available for network users. With the search facility, we are able to easily find profession specific terms (i.e., veterinary, nursing, etc.) and to just as easily cycle through all the occurrences of a particular word, phrase or clause. Color coding allows the user to easily note if the selection is a preferred term or a synonym.

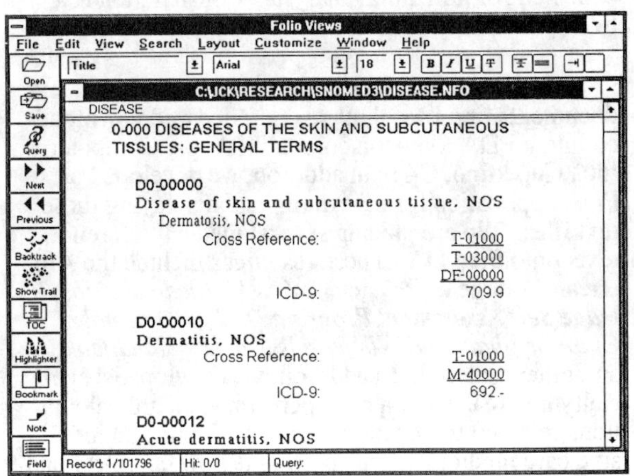

Figure 1 is a clip from the page display of the viewer.

We are using the system to develop a controlled vocabulary for our new electronic medical record currently under development and to assist in coding of diagnoses, problems, procedures, pharmaceuticals, etc. for importation and use.

This work was supported by a National Library of Medicine Training Grant, LM -07089 from the National Library of Medicine of the National Institutes of Health, Bethesda, MD.

The Constellation Project: Access to Medical Reference Information Using Personal Digital Assistants*

Steven E. Labkoff, MD[1], Sandeep Shah, MS(CS)[2], YongJoon Lee, BS[1], and Robert A. Greenes, MD, PhD[1]

[1]Decision Systems Group, Brigham and Women's Hospital, Harvard Medical School, Boston, Massachusetts
[2]K2 Consultants, Inc., Nashua, New Hampshire

The information needs of health care workers include access to not only clinical data, but educational resources, decision aids, and other professional and practice information. It has been shown that most of these information needs are not easily met by currently available material [1,2]. Analysis of access to CD ROM-based medical information has been analyzed by Osheroff et al [3]. This study illustrated only 62% of clinicians' questions could be resolved with this type of reference tool. New developments in personal digital assistant (PDA) technology make it possible to provide reference material and other information to clinicians where and when needed.

CONSTELLATION PROJECT

The Constellation Project is developing and evaluating the use of PDA-based information retrieval tools in two large Harvard-affiliated hospitals. PDA use is monitored by a program that records an audit trail of all transactions. This audit trail is later collected for utilization analysis. Constellation is a two-phased project as described below:

Phase I

We developed a program to convert content text documents into files that are compiled and downloaded into a PDA (Newton computer, Apple Computer, Inc., Cupertino, CA). In addition, we developed a PDA application for navigating and displaying these text files. We are placing several medical reference texts onto the PDA. These resources include the American College of Physician's (ACP) *Medical Knowledge Self Assessment Program IX*, *ACP Journal Club*, *Brigham and Women's Resident's Handbook*, and other material. In addition, we developed a specialty medical calculator to perform standard calculations relevant to general internal medicine and intensive care medicine. This portion is now complete and is the subject of the demonstration.

Evaluation of PDA use of these tools and content will be carried out during project deployment in the second half of 1994. Subjects will be medical residents at the Brigham and Women's Hospital and the Massachusetts General Hospital. A questionnaire (both electronic and paper) will be administered throughout the trial period as well as an analysis of the audit trail. The goal of this evaluation will be to assess how the PDA and its content will affect the ways house officers use reference information.

Phase II

Phase II of Constellation will create a link to the Brigham and Women's Hospital Clinical Information System with participation of the Information Systems department. This link will create a two-way dialogue between PDAs and IS servers. Uses of this link will include client-server requests for clinical data, educational material, resident sign-out procedures, and order entry via a wireless connection. Phase II feasibility studies are ongoing with implementation projected for late 1995 or early 1996.

DISCUSSION

Paper-based resources are useful for reference but are inconvenient to carry around the hospital or into the examination room. PDA technology places large textbooks on a small, light-weight memory card (about the size of a credit card). With potential wireless connectivity, PDAs will also be able to access non-local information. Our goal is to study the interactions between PDAs and medical house staff in two institutions. We hope to learn how access to this new information paradigm will affect the work-habits of the participants. We do not believe that it will ultimately be practical to store libraries of educational material on the portable devices themselves. Toward that end, as wireless communication facilities become more robust, we will adapt PDAs for use in client-server environments to access both education and decision support resources as well as clinical data.

REFERENCES

[1] Covell DG, Uman GC, Manning PR. Information needs in office practice: are they being met? Annals of Internal Medicine. 1985;103:596-9.

[2] Osheroff JA. Forsythe DE, et al. Physicians' information needs: analysis of questions posed during clinical teaching. Annals of Internal Medicine. 114(7):576-81, 1991 Apr. 1.

[3] Osheroff JA, Bankowitz RA. Physicians' use of computer software in answering clinical questions. Bulletin of the Medical Library Association. 81(1):11-19, 1993 Jan.

*Supported in part by grant LM07037 from the National Library of Medicine.

A Medical Information Resource Server: One Stop Shopping on the Internet

John Angelo Gnassi, MD, Joseph I. Bormel, MD, Dyan Ryan Blewett, MS,
Richard J. Kim, G. Octo Barnett, MD
Laboratory of Computer Science, Massachusetts General Hospital, Boston

THE PROBLEM OF RESOURCE ACCESS

For more than a decade now many medical information resources have been available to the researcher, practitioner, and student. Nevertheless use has generally been less than envisioned. We suggest that access has been impeded by a lack of standardization in the methods of resource access. If busy users have to learn different vocabularies, different styles and details of querying a resource, and different output formats, then they are discouraged from exploration and discovery, and may fail to recognize the applicability or utility of extant medical resources. Yet another deterrent, caused by lack of integration, is the frequently imposed requirement to interrupt current work to use an information resource.

With ever-increasing geographic spread and use of the Internet to provide high-speed connections to all kinds of information sources, various standards for browsing and interactive querying have emerged. The widespread distribution and rapid acceptance of the University of Minnesota Gopher protocol, its simple nature, modest system requirements, and the free availability of clients for diverse platforms have made it a reasonable standard to target for delivery of resources in general. We will demonstrate how it is useful for medical resources in particular.

THE PROMISE OF FAST, EASY ACCESS

We have developed, and are expanding and evaluating, a Gopher server that can respond quickly to queries to provide biomedical term definitions, medical care guidelines, disease characterization summaries, review article citations and abstracts, and cancer evaluation and treatment reviews. All the information comes from currently available electronic medical information resources: AHCPR Guidelines, DXplain, PDQ, UMLS Metathesaurus, and MEDLINE.

With this approach we hope to satisfy the need for truly unimpeded access to a few useful medical resources. Users can access, at least in part, much of the information directly from standard clients, such as Gopher or Mosaic. Developers can use the simple Gopher protocol to embed query ability into their applications. We have implemented this in our developing Student and Clinicians' Workstations, and the Decision Systems Group at Brigham and Women's Hospital has incorporated the ability to query our server in a demonstration radiology system.

ACCESS OVERVIEW

The usual method of interaction with the server is to first match a user's text string to the National Library of Medicine's (NLM) Unified Medical Language System (UMLS) Metathesaurus (Meta). This is a very large thesaurus of terms from many medical vocabularies; the UMLS also provides semantic relationships between terms. The server returns concepts that are matched and also identifies resources which could provide further information about those concepts. Additions to our local copy of Meta allow uniform use of other resources pointers.

The interaction is iterative: the user may select an offered resource and query our server again. By a variety of techniques, involving both queries to local databases and further queries over the Internet to remote resources, the information is captured and returned to the user, still using the Gopher protocol. Thus users can enjoy a uniform interface to access disparate resources, and developers can benefit from a common and simple programming interface to provide this capability from within their own applications.

REFERENCES AND ACKNOWLEDGMENTS

[1]. Humphreys BL, Lindberg DAB, *The Unified Medical Language System Project: a Distributed Experiment in Improving Access to Biomedical Information*, MEDINFO 92 Proceedings, 1992, pp. 1496-500.

[2]. Cimino C, Barnett GO, *Standardizing Access to Computer-Based Medical Resources*, 14th SCAMC Proceedings, 1990, pp. 33-7.

This work was supported in parts by the NLM (N01-LM-1-3538) and Hewlett Packard. Drs. Gnassi's and Bormel's fellowships are also funded by the NLM (1-TM15-LM07092).

AHCPR, DXplain, PDQ, MEDLINE, and Metathesaurus are trademarked.

Test Advisor: A pen-based computer program for Bayesian decision-making in the clinical setting

Mark H. Ebell, M.D.
Wayne State University, Dept. of Family Medicine, 4201 St. Antoine UHC-4J, Detroit, MI 48201

Bayesian decision-making is a potentially powerful tool for physicians. However, it requires calculation, and access to detailed information about pre-test probability of disease and test characteristics which may not be readily available.

A pen-based computer program (Test Advisor) has been written for the Microsoft Windows environment which helps physicians apply Bayesian decision-making to the care of their patients. It uses patient-specific data to help physicians select the best test for a patient's medical problem.

The computer program was written in Visual Basic Professional for Windows v. 3.0. This is a visual programming language with built-in support for database access, graphics, and pen input. The program stores information about pre-test probabilities, test characteristics, and the interface itself in a relational database. This information can be updated or changed by the user. In fact, because information about the interface is stored in the database, entirely new patient problems and their associated data can be entered by the end-user.

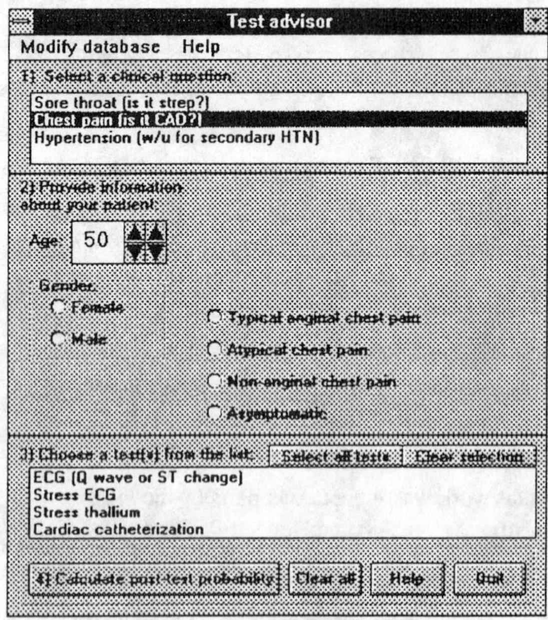

Figure 1. User interface

The basic interface is shown in Figure 1. The user begins by selecting the patient problem from the pull down list at the top of the screen. After a problem is selected, the mid-section of the interface is drawn based on the patient characteristics needed to calculate the pre-test probability. In the example of "Chest pain - is it CAD?", the program requests information about the patient's age, gender, and the type of chest pain they are experiencing.

At the bottom of the screen a list of possible tests is shown. The user can select one or more tests. When they press the <Calculate post-test probability> button, a bar graph is shown which helps them choose the test (Figure 2). The graph, while simple, provides the user with a great deal of information. For each test, the left edge represents the post-test probability for a negative test; the transition between colors at the middle of the bar the pre-test probability; and the right edge the post-test probability for a positive test. Cost is also shown to the left of each bar.

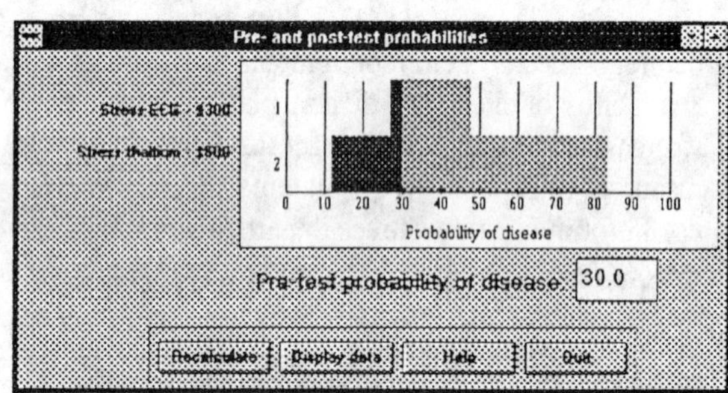

Figure 2. Output, showing cost, pre-test probability, and post-test probability for positive (right edge) and negative (left edge) tests.

Future work will involve expanding the number of problems addressed by the software, and rewriting it for other computer platforms. Currently these efforts are focused on the WinPad environment, an extension of the Microsoft Windows operating system designed for handheld, pen-based computers. Similar to the Apple Newton, these personal digital assistants (PDA's) will be especially useful for highly mobile professionals such as nurses, physicians, and mid-level providers.

0195-4210/94/$5.00 © 1994 AMIA, Inc.

The Ambulatory Care Information System -- Augmenting DHCP with PC Workstations and a Local Area Network

Steven H. Rappaport, M.D.
UCLA - San Fernando Valley Program, VA Medical Center Sepulveda CA

The Ambulatory Care Information System (ACIS) is a computer environment serving the clinical, administrative and educational information needs of the Primary Ambulatory Care and Education (PACE) clinics at the Sepulveda VA Medical Center. ACIS has been designed to help: (1) improve patient satisfaction with the ambulatory care encounter, (2) improve quality of care, (3) enhance provider education, and (4) promote the efficient utilization of ambulatory care services. In the past two years, ACIS has grown to encompass approximately 180 IBM compatible personal computers (PC's) linked by a local area network (Microsoft LAN Manager). The PC's share data residing on network file servers and are able to exchange data automatically with the VA Hospital Information System (DHCP). PC's are located in examining rooms, attending and pharmacist offices, clerical, administrative and patient education areas and nursing stations. Via wireless pen-based laptop PC's (AST GRID Convertible, Solectek wireless ethenet) housestaff browse patient records in examining rooms while documenting encounters in the presence of attending physicians in conference areas. ACIS has been in operation since October 1992 and currently assists in processing more than 250 patient visits each day.

ACIS offers a mixture of locally developed (using Toolbook by Asymetrix and Visual Basic by Microsoft) and commercial software applications. Clerical staff use ACIS for assistance in checking patients in and out of the clinic and in recording the activities that occur during visits. ACIS automates many of the interactions clerks routinely perform with the hospital mainframe and, via the graphical capabilities of PC workstations, is able to simplify data entry tasks. As patients check-in, ACIS automatically retrieves clinical data from DHCP and from local file servers, organizing these data into an encounter form customized to each patient visit. Clinicians and nurses use ACIS to view and add to a patient's problem list, prior progress notes, medication and laboratory profiles, allergy and immunization data, previous vital signs and selected recent orders. The system offers advice, based on locally and nationally developed practice guidelines, regarding what issues should be addressed in evaluating certain patient complaints and diagnoses. It also offers interactive disposition suggestions, home care instructions and test ordering options to nurses as they respond to phone calls from patients. Administrative staff use ACIS in analyzing provider practice patterns and in reviewing progress note quality for total quality improvement tasks. The commercial applications available through ACIS include on-line medical reference materials, patient education handouts and literature searching tools, expert differential diagnostic and decision support programs and directories of patient services and education classes.

ACIS helps increase patient satisfaction by promoting more efficient clinic operation and resource utilization. ACIS tracks the amount of time patients spend with providers and support staff and how much time is spent waiting. This facilitates an orderly passage of patients through the clinic and prevents patients from being forgotten. The system also identifies patients who have not had a visit with their primary care provider within a set time interval or patients who may benefit from services they are not receiving such as a geriatrics evaluation.

ACIS promotes the delivery of quality care and enhances provider education by offering rapid access to information. The customized encounter form and the electronic medical record capabilities of ACIS offer clinicians a more complete understanding of their patients, leading to more informed treatment decisions. Given easy access to medical textbooks and journals, providers may more frequently review medical literature and learn from clinical encounters. The problem specific prompts offered by ACIS additionally provide passive education as to what issues are important to address in evaluating and following patient problems.

By integrating the database capabilities of DHCP with the functionality of PC based clinical workstations and the adaptability of local area networks, ACIS has produced important benefits in the care of patients in the ambulatory care arena.

0195-4210/94/$5.00 © 1994 AMIA, Inc.

On-line Decision Support for Emergency Trauma Management

John R. Clarke, M.D.[1] Bonnie L. Webber, Ph.D.[2] Abigail Gertner[2]
Jonathan Kaye[2] Ron Rymon, Ph.D.[2]
[1] Dept. of Surgery, Medical College of Pennsylvania, Philadelphia PA 19129
[2] Dept. of Computer & Information Science, Univ of Pennsylvania
Philadelphia PA 19104-6389

The overall goal of the TraumAID project is to improve the delivery of quality trauma care during the *initial definitive phase* of patient management. To this end, we are applying artificial intelligence techniques such as rule-based reasoning, planning, and plan inference. The current system, TraumAID 2.0, consists of (1) an electronic version of the standard *trauma flow sheet* implemented in HyperCard, that allows information to be entered by a dedicated member of the trauma team called a "scribe nurse" during trauma resuscitation; (2) a *rule-based reasoner* able to draw diagnostic conclusions from patient findings and test results, and identify what management goals they imply; (3) a *planner* that takes the set of currently relevant goals and identifies what (partially-ordered) sequence of actions is most appropriate under the circumstances; and (4) two complementary modes of information presentation – a *graphic display* of TraumAID's recommended management plan that can be shown on a monitor positioned in the trauma bay, and a critiquing interface (TraumaTIQ) that uses the goals and plans computed by TraumAID 2.0 to interpret physician orders and comment on them when appropriate. Because both interfaces can present information at a time and place where it could make a difference to the quality and/or cost of patient care, both implement the ideal of *real-time quality assurance*.

Papers describing TraumAID have previously appeared in the literature [1, 2, 3, 4, 5, 7]. TraumAID 2.0 has been validated retrospectively, and its management plans found significantly preferable to actual care [1]. The system is about to be field-tested in the Emergency Center at the Medical College of Pennsylvania (MCP). The system to be field-tested links our HyperCard interface asynchronously to the core system executing in Macintosh Common Lisp on a Quadra 700. The development version, implemented in Lucid Common Lisp within X-Windows on a SPARCserver 690MP, interacts with the developer through a simple Tk/Tcl interface.

With respect to our proposed demonstration, we will use segments from videotapes of trauma resuscitations to convey the environment and activities of a trauma team in an Emergency Center, and demonstrate TraumAID's support for data entry during patient management, its capabilities for reasoning and multiple-goal plan formation, and both its graphic and critiquing approaches to real-time information delivery. Such videotapes have been used for educational purposes at the MCP Emergency Center for several years [6].

Acknowledgements

This work has been supported in part by Army Research Organization under grant DAAL03-89-C0031PRI, National Library of Medicine under grant R01 LM05217-01 and Agency for Health Care Policy and Research under grant R01 HS06740-01.

References

[1] Clarke, J.R., Rymon, R., Webber, B., Hayward, C., Santora, T., Wagner, D. and Ruffin, A. The Importance of Planning in the Provision of Medical Care. *Medical Decision Making* 13(4), October-December 1993, p. 383 (abstract).

[2] Clarke, J.R., Webber, B., Niv, M., Rymon, R., Gertner, A. and Kaye, J. The Care of Injured Patients: An architecture of Medical Knowledge. *Der Chirurg* (Special issue on surgical decision-making), to appear April 1994.

[3] Gertner, A. Real-time critiquing of integrated diagnosis/therapy plans. *Proc. AAAI Workshop on Expert Critiquing Systems*, Washington D.C., August 1993.

[4] Gertner, A. Ongoing Critiquing During Trauma Management. *Proc. AAAI Spring Symposium on Artificial Intelligence in Medicine: Interpreting Clinical Data*, Stanford CA, March 1994.

[5] Rymon, R., Webber, B. L. and Clarke, J. R., Progressive Horizon Planning – Planning Exploratory-Corrective Behavior. *IEEE Transactions on Systems, Man, and Cybernetics* 23(6). Special issue on Planning, Scheduling and Control, November 1993.

[6] Santora TA, Trooskin SZ, Blank CA, Clarke JR, Schinco MA, Trauma video tapes: impact on quality assurance and resident education. *J Trauma*, 1994 (in press).

[7] Webber, B., Rymon, R. and Clarke, J.R. Flexible Support for Trauma Management through Goal-directed Reasoning and Planning. *Artificial Intelligence in Medicine* 4(2), April 1992, pp. 145-163.

Integrated Ambulatory Care Resource Scheduling in Oncology

Farideh Majidi, M.S., John P. Enterline, M.S., Gloria Stuart
Michael Herman, Ph.D., Linda Langsdale, Lisa Lattal Ogorzalek, M.H.A, J.D.
The Johns Hopkins Oncology Center, Baltimore, Maryland 21287

In a modern managed-care environment, the scheduling of ambulatory care activities must be viewed as a series of closely related activities rather than a group of unique and independent events. These activities must be sequenced in a logical manner, and linked with a variety of information on other clinical, operational, and administrative activities. This article focuses on such an integrated scheduling system which supports the ambulatory care services at the Johns Hopkins Oncology Center.

INTRODUCTION

One of the many ancillary support applications developed around the OCIS decision-support data structure is an OPD scheduling and resource management system [1]. In fact, the OPD system is itself a operational decision-support system which uses data from other clinical and ancillary systems in the Oncology Center. Rarely does a patient in Oncology have a single event scheduled on a single day which does not relate to a variety of other information (Figure 1). Approximately 70,000 patient visits are scheduled and coordinated through this system annually. A great many of these visits involve multiple related appointments on the same day. In general, a scheduled event has close relations with other scheduled events, outcomes of clinical tests, clinical progress, available resources, clinical protocol requirements, and even events scheduled on other visits.

The ambulatory care component of the Oncology Center consists of four physically and logically unique clinics: Medical Oncology, Pediatric Oncology, Radiation Oncology, and a Medical Oncology consultation clinic. The ability to communicate and share data in real time is essential in this distributed environment. Patients frequently have appointments in multiple Oncology clinics during the same Oncology visit. Each of these clinics has a core of scheduling requirements which are identical, combined with an assortment of requirements which are unique to the clinic.

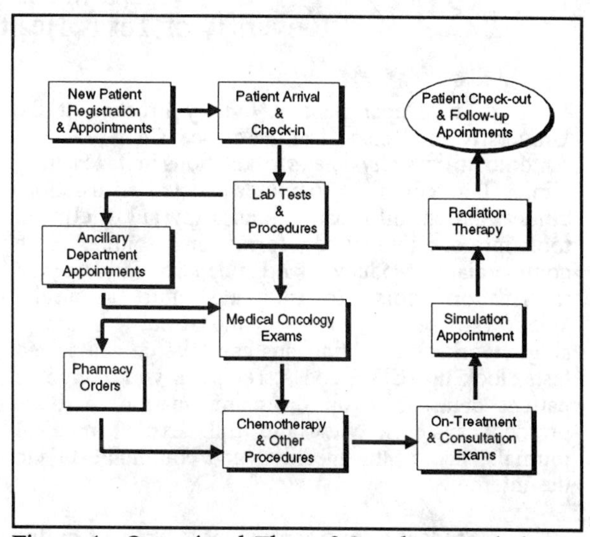

Figure 1. Operational Flow of Oncology Ambulatory Care Services.

The operational flow and management of outpatient services within Oncology are defined and conducted through this system. Patients, care providers, and ancillary support personnel know what to expect, and when it is expected. Resources are used to the greatest extent possible. All procedure and charge data are automatically collected in a complete, accurate, and timely manner. Additionally, this system provides a means of communication with other ancillary and clinical resources which are essential in the effective and efficient treatment of ambulatory patients. Such areas include the pharmacy system, blood product systems, inpatient services, laboratory systems, research systems, and other clinic systems. The computerized system which supports these resource scheduling activities is presented on-line in this demonstration.

REFERENCES

1. Enterline, J.P., Majidi, F.M., Ogorzalek, L.L., Stuart G.J. Patient-Centered Ambulatory Care Scheduling. Healthcare Information Management. Vol. 7, No. 3, pp. 33-38, Summer 1993.

Integrated Physician Workstation for Use in a Family Practice Teaching Clinic

James D. Legler, MD

Department of Family Practice
University of Texas Health Science Center, San Antonio

The Department of Family Practice at the University of Texas Health Science Center at San Antonio utilizes physician workstations in its teaching clinics that combine computer-assisted instruction, clinical patient information, and a myriad of clinical tools into one integrated information resource. Both commercial products and department-designed information tools are integrated into a single, Windows-based physician workstation. From a single workstation, clinicians can take computerized tests, look up ICD-9 codes, review a wide range of patient data, look up drug information, activate protocol systems, view the full text of medical journals, access the medline, and communicate via the internet.

Student testing consists of a series of online multiple-choice exams that both evaluate and educate third-year clerkship students as they rotate through our clinics. The exams cover 24 of the most common problems seen in primary care. Each exam consists of ten questions randomly picked by the computer from a battery of test questions developed for each topic area. After each exam, the students are shown their grades. They are then given the opportunity to review the questions again with the correct answers identified. A short explanation of each answer is provided. Students may repeat the tests as many times as required until a passing grade is obtained in each topic area.

Workstation connection to the teaching hospital's Novell network allows access to a wide range of clinical information on our patients. Laboratory data, radiology reports, discharge summaries, specialty consultation results, cardiac catheterization reports, and outpatient medication summaries are available on the patients seen in our clinics.

Diagnostic coding is performed via access to Code-Link(r), a commercial program that contains all known ICD-9 codes. For simpler searches, the workstation incorporates a database engine that searches for the 1500 most common codes used in our clinic.

The workstation incorporates Electronic Drug Reference(r) by Clinical Reference Systems to serve as an online source of drug information. Information about drug indications, contraindications, doses, interactions, and dosage forms is readily available. In addition, the program prints out a patient information sheet for each drug.

The workstation incorporates a series of protocol systems developed within our department that provide clinicians with a wide range of decision-support services. Among these protocol systems, PEDIATRICIAN is a program that generates a series of recommendations for well-children care based upon the child's age. Included is a listing of the history, physical, lab, immunizations, anticipatory guidance, development, vitamins, and follow-up for each standard screening age. Another protocol system, OBSTETRICIAN, generates a series of recommendations for each week of prenatal care.

On-line text retrieval is achieved by use of DiskPassage(r) to access a series of CD-ROM resources. At present, the CD-ROM library includes information stored from selected issues of Pediatrics, Pediatrics Infectious Disease Journal, Pediatrics in Review, The "Red Book" on pediatric infectious diseases, New England Journal of Medicine, and American Family Physician.

Modem communication with our health sciences library is achieved via TermPlus(r), a Windows-based communication program. From the library, clinicians can access medline information via the CD-ROM-based Plusnet(r) system. Communication with the library also allows access to campus mail, to our campus-wide information system, and to the burgeoning resources of the internet.

The First Two Years: Volume 1 of the Series:
Family Health Education on CD-I and CD-ROM

Antonino Abbolito, MD* and Marco Criscione, MD**
*Ospedale di Frascati (Roma) & ETAS-RCS (Milano)
**Dipartimento di Pediatria Università di L'Aquila

CD-I seems to be one of the less expensive and more attractive systems to perform Health Education's activities at consumer level. The costless hardware and the possibility of a full interactivity, together with the low end-cost of the programs, give to this new media good chances to became, on the incoming years, one of the most popular source of entraitenement and educational programs.

On the other end, once the contents of the program have been defined and images aquired is very easy to transfer everything on a different support, that is the CD-ROM, certainly more expensive, considering that a computer is required, but at the moment more diffused all over the world.

Family Health Education is a Series of programs on CD-I and CD-ROM that are going to be realised to give parents most of the informations thay need to help kids to grow up healthy.

The first two years is the number 1 of this series and is a multimedia publication that covers child development during the first two years of his or her life.

The first two years of a baby's lyfe are very important because most of the problems he or she could have in the future, if recognised, can be prevented or cured on time.

The contents of the CD-I is organised on a chronologic basis, following the major milestones in child development: hearing, seeing and psycho-neurological acquisition. Every development phase is covered by different thematic aspects: normal behaviour, the child's environment and common parental errors and misconceptions.

Particular attention has been given to the stimulation of child development and to the identification of physical and phsycological signs of discomfort and alarm ("when to consult a doctor").

Part of the publication is dedicated to the correct feeding of the infant and to the identification of his feeding needs and disturbances.

The informations are presented with images (still frame and full motion) graphics and animations. Text cards and spoken text are used to explain details on the topic discussed.

The program will be available in three languages, Italian, English and French. Spanish is also under consideration.

SIN-FM: (A Short Indexed Nomenclature of Family Medicine)

Gary Viner, M.D. C.C.F.P.
Robert M. Bernstein, Ph.D., M.D.,C.M., C.C.F.P.
Gary R. Hollingworth, M.D., F.C.F.P
Medical Informatics Research Group, Clinical Epidemiology Unit,
Department of Family Medicine, University of Ottawa

INTRODUCTION

We have developed a short indexed nomenclature of diagnoses, health problems, and reasons for encounter for use in family practice electronic records. It is in the "WK1" format and can be incorporated in electronic medical records. This defined vocabulary we believe provides some distinct advantages over other vocabularies currently in use.

In family and general practice a nomenclature must cover the breadth of illness, uncertain and ill defined diagnoses, symptoms and reasons for encounter. Current classifications cannot semantically represent these areas precisely. Family physicians cannot use mortality classifications for point of service data entry. ICD-9 and ICHPPC[1] require extensive training to be used effectively whilst ICPC[2] is not specific enough to be used to follow patients.

At a certain point a nomenclature is just large enough to minimize error. If it is too large then different terms may be chosen for the same entity; if too restricted appropriate terms may not exist for some entities, resulting in inaccurate data entry and subsequent inaccurate retrieval.

OBJECTIVES

To be usable at the point of service the vocabulary must be MONOAXIAL, requiring selection of just one term to represent a diagnosis or reason for encounter. It must enable the physician to find terms fast enough so that using the defined vocabulary is inherently preferable to writing free text in the chart. It must strike a balance between comprehensives and usability. It must be small enough so that a provider of care can walk through the hierarchical structure to locate an appropriate term and yet robust enough so that most clinical terms are present and can be found by a simple search algorithm, and for those that are not, another accurate term can be selected via the hierarchy.

The vocabulary must be easy to learn and therefore we have based SIN-FM on ICPC which has been validated for consistency in many international settings. Naive users can learn to use it as a classification without computer aided searching in less than half an hour. With the computer to act as a search instrument and the 10 fold expansion of terms in SIN-FM the new user needs only to know how to use his/her own search software. The need for knowledge of the underlying classification is minimized.

The structure of SIN-FM was designed so that terms are easy to find, thereby minimizing background error in coding (signal to noise). SIN-FM is a clinical nomenclature. Arcane terms which cannot be applied to patients, and terms such as "other diseases of the skin not elsewhere classified" cannot be part of a clinical nomenclature. ALL users have to know what else IS classified in order to interpret such a term.

STRUCTURE OF SIN-FM

ICPC with 3 digit ICD-10 mapped to it[3] was combined with a synonym dictionary and our own local vocabulary (based on ICHPPC). Each ICPC body system chapter was arranged hierarchically in sections of symptoms and complaints, non-specific disorders, infectious/ inflammatory disorders, neoplasms, trauma, and congenital disorders. Terms were then edited to make clinical sense. ICPC main headings and other common or clinically relevant conditions were identified as index terms. Each term (where possible) was identified by body site so that e.g. all symptoms and disorders of the shoulder can sort together. There is consistency from chapter to chapter with respect to the headings, hierarchy and coding scheme. Coding is derivable from the position in the hierarchy.

REFERENCES

1. ICHPPC-2 Defined: International Classification of Health Problems in Primary Care Oxford University Press, Oxford 1983.

2. ICPC: International Classification of Primary Care. ed. Lamberts H, and Wood M. Oxford University Press, Oxford 1987.

3. Obtained with gratitude from Dr. Maurice Wood.

0195-4210/94/$5.00 © 1994 AMIA, Inc.

ISIS: A Computer-Aided Education Program For Hypertensive Patients

CONSOLI Silla, MD
Unité Médico-Psychologique ◇ Centre de Prevention Cardio-Vasculaire
Hopital Broussais ◇ Paris - France

BEN SAID Mohamed, MD,
Service d'Informatique Médicale ◇ Hopital La Pitié-Salpétrière ◇ Paris - France

JEAN Jocelyne, RN
Service d'Hypertension ◇ Hopital Broussais ◇ Paris - France

Hypertension represents a major risk factor and plays a major role in the aggravation of the overall risk of premature cardio-vascular diseases [1, 2]. Unfortunately, statistical findings, reveal a failure among patients, to comply with the therapy [3] and make the health education of hypertensive patients even more necessary. A patient education computer program called ISIS[1 2] aimed to be a complementary method to the habitual educational techniques by bringing into patient education the pleasantness of the multimedia. It was developped on a color MacIntosh, using MacPaint, PixelPaint, MacroMind Director and MacRecorder. It runs on MacIntosh II and higher and requires 8 megabytes of RAM, a coprocessor and a color monitor of 13". It takes a 32 megabytes of disk space and is organized into 30 MacroMind Director files or movies. Macros use a high level language (Lingo) to control the navigation between files as well as the patient performance. The movies are made of sequential animations of "theatre stages" or computer screens. Up to 20 objects or "cast-members" fill the "stage" at one time. A spreadsheet facilitates the visualization of the "casts-members" arrangement into columns and provides additional channels to control the transition aspect and speed, the sound and the macros. Building simple animations is "trivial".
The clinical information is primarly represented with icons, developed using the guideline design in [4] [5].
ISIS alternates relaxing interludes with educational messages. The patient may navigate through the educational part by selecting one of the six modules: arterial pressure physiology, epidemiology, heart physiology, athersoclerosis, risk factors, drug therapy. The patient may also take the time and navigate through an imaginary trip in the ancient egyptian world. A randomized evaluation study showed the substantial benefit of using ISIS in patient education, particularly among patients whose initial health knowledge was low and the patients whose hypertension was known for more than 6 months. ISIS is actually used by hospitalized hypertensive patients and nurse students.

References

[1] Eugene Braunwald. *Heart Disease - a Textbook of Cardiovascular Medicine.* W.B. Saunders Company, Hartcourt Brace Jovanovich, Inc. the Curtis Center Independence Square West, Philadelphia, PA 19106, 1992.

[2] G. Plouin, F.P.and Chatelier, J.Y. Pagny, and T. Lang. Hypertension arterielle (epidemiologie, hemodynamique et physiopathologie, strategie de l'exploration et de la prise en charge. *Encycl. Med. Chir. (Paris, France), Coeur-Vaisseaux, 11302 A19, 9-1986, 12 P.*, pages 1–12, 1986.

[3] S.M. Consoli and M.E. Safar. Predictive value of the patient's psychological profile and type of patient-practitioner relationship in compliance with antihypertensive treatment. *Arch Mal Coeur*, 81 (Suppl HTA):145–150, 1988.

[4] A. Marcus. Graphic design for electronic documents and user interfaces. *ACM Press Eds*, pages 60–63, 1992.

[5] 0. Yukio. Pictogram design. *Kashiwashobo Eds*, pages 90–92, 1987.

[1] ISIS: Initiation Sanitaire Informatisée et Scénarisée
[2] ISIS is also a personage from the ancient Egypt

0195-4210/94/$5.00 © 1994 AMIA, Inc.

ScriptWriter™
A Relational Database to Manage Outpatient Medical Treatment

T. Bradley Tanner, MD (Tanner@ConnectInc.Com)
Clinical Tools, Inc., 5105 Bayard Street, Pittsburgh, PA 15232

ABSTRACT

ScriptWriter™ is database software designed to replicate the process of a physician writing a prescription. The software also includes standard demographic and progress note information; however the focus of the software is on automating the process of writing prescriptions. The software is especially adept at creating patient medication lists, generating medication histories and keeping track of medication expiration dates. Other strengths include its ability to organize patient assignments and assist in the generation of progress notes. The application is network capable and fully graphical. A psychiatric outpatient clinic is currently using the software. Practitioners in non-psychiatric settings can also benefit from the software.

DESCRIPTION

ScriptWriter™ is a database application written to simplify the process of treating outpatients. A physician using the software would access a patient's information from a list of patients assigned to him or her. The physician would then enter prescriptions on-line, using an interface similar to a blank prescription. The physician can retrieve previous medication trials to evaluate past treatment or list medications that will expire soon. A listing of prescriptions could be generated for reference by the patient, family, or caregiver.

The physician can also create progress notes that will automatically include standard demographic information (required for the presciption) and the previously entered medication information. The progress note system is relatively unstructured and supports free text input. Users can list patients for a given clinician and patient assignments to clinic staff. A nearby laser-printer prints all prescriptions, documentation and reports.

Implementation and Environment

An outpatient psychiatric clinic including 16 clinicians and 700 patients currently uses the software. ScriptWriter client software runs on 486 PCs running Windows for Workgroups™. These computers access the database file stored on a Windows NT™ server using both NetBIOS and TCP/IP protocols.

Scriptwriter requires a 486 PC and the Windows™ graphical interface. The software runs in both stand-alone and networked environments such as Windows for Workgroups, Netware™, or Windows NT. If desired, the client software can access a full SQL based database.

ScriptWriter uses a Microsoft Access™ client application to access the database. ScriptWriter includes the run-time libraries; there is no need to purchase Microsoft Access to run the software.

Confidentiality

The software protects confidentiality using user passwords that expire every 60 days. The database keeps track of all sign-on events, requests for access to patient information, and data entry. The site administrator can thus use the database to determine if authorized users are making improper data requests or entries.

CONCLUSIONS

The author has developed a simple database application to computerize the essentials of outpatient treatment, especially the prescribing of medications. The software provides a secure and straightforward assistant to providers of outpatient treatment.

Normal Human Structure: Comprehensive Courseware for Gross, Microscopic and Radiologic Anatomy

Richard Rathe, MD; Lynn Romrell, PhD; Kyle Rarey, PhD; Tom Hollinger, PhD; Linda Lanier, MD
University of Florida; College of Medicine; Gainesville, FL

INTRODUCTION

A firm understanding of normal human structure is essential to the practice of medicine and the other health professions. Much of this content is covered early in medical school, often during the first semester. At the University of Florida we have combined Gross Anatomy, Microscopic Anatomy, Embryology, Cell Biology, Radiologic Anatomy, and parts of Physical Diagnosis into a unified "Normal Human Structure" block curriculum. Students are required to cover more material in less time than ever before. They must also assimilate a huge volume of visual and spatial information for which traditional media have been less than adequate. To overcome these deficiencies we have developed interactive instructional programs for gross, microscopic and radiologic anatomy.

METHODS

Over the past three years our facility has produced more than twelve thousand teaching images. These were captured from a variety of sources including 35mm slides, plain xray film, video equipped microscopes, and direct videography. We selected the laserdisc as our archival and delivery media because this technology handles thousands of high quality images and full motion with ease. Our image archive currently contains the following:

- Several complete cadaveric dissections
- A cross-sectional anatomy collection
- A surface anatomy collection
- A complete histologic slide collection
- Electron micrographs of major tissues
- Normal radiographs, MRI, and CT
- Full motion fluoroscopy of major joints
- Fluoroscopy of major internal organs
- Abnormal radiographs for comparison

We used the HyperCard programming system to build interactive teaching modules based on these images. Our approach has been direct and pragmatic—concentrating on student efficiency and effectiveness. The programs share a simple user interface and support multiple learning styles. Common design elements include:

- Overall outline structure
- Linear, tutorial modes
- Quick look up, reference modes
- Self evaluation modes
- Visual indexes and browsers
- Hypertext cross-links

RESULTS

Microscopic Anatomy—This program is in its fifth year of use and has been well accepted by students and faculty. Having rapid access to images of every important histologic structure has allowed our students to efficiently preview before laboratory sessions. The program also contains a 1500 question quiz bank that is popular for review before exams.

Radiologic Anatomy—In its third year of use, this program allows students to review several hundred anatomic structures as they appear in all major imaging modalities. Students navigate by structure, image, or organ system. A visual quiz bank allows students to test their knowledge at any time.

Video Dissector—A complete guide to dissection is at the core of this, our newest program. Students are able to read about and **see** each step they need to perform. Unlike the actual cadaver, the program can be rewound to any point in the dissection for review. Students may also use the extensive practical exam module to gain confidence with what they have learned.

0195-4210/94/$5.00

Instant Medical History

Allen R. Wenner, M.D., Matthew Ferrante, M.B.A, Duncan Belser
Primetime Medical Software, West Columbia, SC 29169

Abstract

We introduce a knowledge-based patient driven screening expert system used in an outpatient family practice for 10,000 *consecutive visits. The nurse hands the patient a laptop computer. Using knowledge-based questioning, subjective complaints are collected directly from the patient. The questions are response driven. Simultaneous analysis of the pattern of answering also determines the direction of the questioning. If indicated by the patient's answers, standardized published self-rating and self-assessment scales from the medical literature are administered totally unseen by the patient. The patient's complaints are succinctly presented to the physician as he enters the exam room. The physician can usually glance at the positive answers and graphically depicted scales and arrive at a working clinical impression in a few seconds before he begins his interview. Both he and the patient are totally focused on the problem at hand. Limitless potential for enhancing physician productivity is evoked.*

Sir William Osler once said, "Talk to a patient long enough and he will tell you what is wrong with him." Ninety percent of diagnoses are made on the basis of the subjective history, five percent are made on the basis of the physical examination, and five percent are made on the basis of laboratory and X-ray studies. today's time-conscious medical practice, few physicians can ask every question that they would like to ask every patient. The standard of care requires that a complete history be gathered and documented on all patients.

Instant Medical History is a patient-driven computerized medical history expert system. It is designed for use while the patient is waiting to see the physician. The nurse or receptionist selects a symptom or any or all organ systems for review. The questions that follow are those the physician would normally ask in a live patient interview. Instant Medical History has extensive branching technology that uses the patient's responses to each question to initiate additional questions that become more specific. For example, in the "URI and Sinus" if the patient indicates that he has a fever, then he is asked several questions about the fever and each of these are followed up. These answers are translated into medical terminology to become the starting point for the physician who can usually glance at the output of medical terminology and have a correct diagnosis in mind. The physician has time to get that extra bit of information he needs to make a confident diagnosis -- before he even sees the patient!

For a routine office visit, Instant Medical History reviews the pertinent organ system or group of organ systems indicated by the nurse. When the patient indicates a complaint, the program will ask a set of secondary questions about the illness. Totally unseen by the patient are standardized self-rating scales and psychological tests embedded in the program. These tests are automatically administered if the patient answers positively to trigger questions or the pattern of answers is outside the parameters set in the system utilities. These tests are scored and the results are printed in numeric and graphical form for the physician. For instance, in the Review of Systems section "Health Habits," a patient who drinks alcohol will automatically be administered the CAGE Questionnaire. If he answers positively to any of the CAGE (Cut down, Annoyed, feel Guilty, Eye opener) questions, then a MAST, Michigan Alcohol Screening Test, is also administered. Because that title does not appear on the screen, the patients believe that these are simply the next questions in a series and that everyone gets the same questions. Thus, the patient is not embarrassed by being pre-labeled an alcoholic. The physician has obtained sensitive information about the patient's problem that both the patient and the doctor might feel uncomfortable discussing. Since the answers came directly from the patient, the patient is inclined to be more receptive to the physician's diagnosis of alcoholism.

Instant Medical History makes the office encounter less stressful for the patient so the doctor can concentrate on the most important task at hand, treatment.

0195-4210/94/$5.00

Use of Video to Communicate Possibilities for Integrated Information Management

Ann J. Olsen, M.B.A., M.A.
Informatics Center
Vanderbilt University Medical Center
Nashville, TN 37232-8340

As part of our information management planning process, Vanderbilt University Medical Center is using videos to capture, communicate, and obtain feed-back on end-user visions. In the spring of 1993, members of our Education, Patient Care, Research, and Administrative Domain Committees wrote scenarios to describe how they each might be working in five to ten years [1]. In December 1993, we completed a 10-minute video based on one of the Education Domain's scenarios. The video combines, through skillful editing, brief clips of interactions with existing applications and new screens prototyped with Microsoft Visual Basic to create illusions of new operational systems.

The video illustrates the following possibilities:

- Voice interaction with the computer.
- Integration of voice and electronic messages.
- Integration of individual calendars with the patient database and clinic appointments.
- Personalized information filtering.
- Continual updating of literature searches.
- Wide-spread network access to educational resources.
- Using educational modules to support direct patient care.
- Using a patient database to support clinical teaching.
- Enhanced faculty/student communication.
- Advance, off-site preparation for rounds with sharable electronic charts.
- Distance learning.
- Integrating evaluation with computer-based instruction.
- Automated resource scheduling.
- Sharable image resources to support teaching and research.
- Using telemedicine to provide specialist support of primary care providers.

This video has been invaluable in stimulating individuals and groups to think creatively about how information technologies might assist them. It has also been helpful to show groups such as our Medical Center Advisory Board what kinds of things we want to accomplish and to generate support for our new directions with information technology.

Videos offer an alternative to building prototypes or real world demonstration systems to communicate functional possibilities. A video can be used to demonstrate a wide variety of functions easily and quickly. The video format also supports the iterative process of identifying desirable function. As visions are shared through a video, flaws are identified and new ideas surface. New paradigms begin to emerge. A vision video can be updated to let the process start again. Videos also provide an alternative to technology fairs; they can reach broad audiences and present a clear vision.

In October 1994, we will complete a second video which will focus on patient care. This poster session will demonstrate both videos, show the screen prototypes, and provide information about the process used to create the videos (script writing, prototyping, voice overs, editing) and the resources required.

Reference

[1] Olsen AJ, Baker WL, Sittig DF, Stead WW: A Planning Process for a Fast Track to IAIMS. Proc 17th Symp Computing Appl Med Care, ed. Safran C, McGraw-Hill 1994: 544-548.

Acknowledgement

Video production was supported in part by National Library of Medicine Grant GO8 LM05443, awarded by the National Institutes of Health, Department of Health and Human Services.

Converting Interactive Laserdisc to Interactive Digital Video: A Demonstration Using the University of Washington Human Brain Animations

Chiang S. Jao, Ph.D., Daniel B. Hier, M.D. and Steven U. Brint, M.D.
Department of Neurology, University of Illinois, Chicago, IL 60612-7330

ABSTRACT

Interactive laserdisc is a powerful medium for the communication of subjects that involve 3D animation, rotations, or translations. This technology has been used to produce multimedia programs with full-motion animated video and CD-quality stereo soundtracks. The primary advantage of laserdisc technology over conventional videotape is the ability to randomly access and display video sequences or still video frames quickly. Furthermore, unlike videotapes, laserdiscs do not need to be rewound. Although computer-driven interactive laserdisc is a powerful multimedia teaching tool, there are disadvantages to this technique. First, a device driver must be installed on the computer to drive the laserdisc. Installation of these device drivers may be difficult and complex. Second, in the absence of a device driver or a computer interface on the laserdisc player, random access to the desired video sequence may be difficult or cumbersome. Third, video output from the laserdisc player cannot be displayed on the computer monitor unless a specialized video overlay card is installed in the host computer. These video overlay cards add expense and require additional specialized drivers. Fourth, it may be prohibitively expensive to create more than one or two training stations that consist of a computer, a computer monitor, a video monitor, and a laserdisc player. Fifth, some laserdisc programs lack audio tracks. Mixing in narration to laserdiscs lacking audio may be cumbersome. Finally, laserdisc-based educational programs require users to handle delicate videodiscs and run the risk of inexperienced users damaging the discs.

To address some of these disadvantages, we decided to build an educational brain anatomy program by converting laserdisc to digital video. We purchased a series of computer-generated brain animations from the University of Washington on laserdisc. These are an excellent set of brain animations that reveal anatomic relationships between multiple brain structures including the ventricles, the basal ganglia, hippocampus, and thalamus. Laserdisc is an ideal medium for conversion of these animations to digital video. We used the Intel Indeo Video technology (under the Microsoft Video-for-Windows environment) to capture sections of the laserdisc animations as audio-video-interleave (AVI) files. Cinepak CODEC compression technology offers more favorable data rates on AVI files. We collected more than 100 AVI files from the laserdisc. We then interleaved narration in the form of recorded audio waveforms (WAV) with the AVI files since no narration was on the original laserdisc.

Our driver program is implemented in KnowledgePro for Windows® (KPWIN), an expert system shell with hypermedia capabilities. KPWIN allows the system to communicate with external multimedia devices via MCI (Media Control Interface) commands. KPWIN calls external DLL (Dynamic Link Library) functions in Windows to issue these command strings. KPWIN implements a backward-chaining heuristic mechanism with IF-THEN statements. The hypermedia capability of the KPWIN allows the use of text, graphics, hypertext, and hypergraphics to link a functional execution. KPWIN supports a contextual indexing method to speed up data retrieval from external database files.

We designed a topic-oriented host window with button-driven control to play audiovisual files. Each button is associated with a list of subtopics related to the selected major topic. Every subtopic invokes the play of an audiovisual file on the host computer. A control panel allows the user to fast forward ahead or to freeze any video frame for extended viewing. The play of interleaved stereo soundtrack offers a narration for the displayed brain animation. By converting laserdisc to digital video, the program offers the advantages of the laserdisc technology but avoids the need of the laserdisc player during the operation of the program. The expert system technology and data indexing methods provide a powerful interface to the brain animations. We have developed an interactive multimedia-based animation program to teach medical students about the key brain components. The Brain Animation project gives the user a convenient tool to access computer-generated brain animations without requiring the use of a laserdisc player or VCR.

0195-4210/94/$5.00 © 1994 AMIA, Inc.

A "Listener/Viewer" for Phonocardiograms

Allen W. Hahn, D.V.M, Ph.D., Michael J. Knowles, M.S., and J. Craig Klimczak, D.V.M.
Medical Informatics Group and Veterinary Teaching Hospital, University of Missouri, Columbia, MO 65211

In 1987, Bergeron and Greenes[1] presented a program called HeartLab which allowed users to listen to prerecorded heart sounds in order to build their clinical skills. Inspired by some of the innovations from HeartLab, we present a Macintosh program which allows previously and simultaneously recorded heart sounds and single lead electrocardiogram (phonocardiogram) to be viewed on the screen and played back through the audio output circuitry of any Macintosh computer running System Software Version 7.1. The system currently uses data acquired with a commercially available hardware/software system from BIOPAC Systems, Inc. (Goleta, CA). The software system is AcqKnowledge™ Version 3.0. Other forms of acquisition could also be used as long as the file standards are followed.

The data acquired from the analog signal (AcqKnowledge) files are stored in a BIOPAC proprietary format, but with the aid of BIOPAC Systems, we transformed these files into standard AIFF files for playback of the sounds. The viewer reads the original acquired data and presents it to the user in a "strip-chart" window (see Figure 1). The viewer allows the user to scale the data at varying degrees of resolution in terms of amplitude and time. The amplitude can be increased or decreased to fit the user's needs, as can the time base which can be contracted or expanded at will. Standard scroll bars allow the user to scroll through the entire waveforms.

The system was written using THINK C for the Macintosh and the THINK Class Library, an object-oriented application framework package that defines a generic Macintosh application (Symantec Corp., Cupertino, CA).

In order to keep the size of the data files manageable we sampled the analog data at 2 KHz. A simple low-pass filter is connected to the sound output port when the heart sounds are played back in order to filter out switching transients and their accompanying noise. A high-quality stereo headset are speaker is attached to the filter output in order to listen to the sounds.

The digital phonocardiogram files can be transmitted over any digital network connection and stored along with other patient data. The sonic data can thus be used to document patient encounters, be sent for consultation, and analyzed with various forms of sound spectral analytic tools. In addition, respiratory or gastrointestinal sounds could also be captured for storage and transmission.

Using an object-oriented development approach facilitates future extensions and modifications of the program. In addition, the OOP approach allows much easier code reusability for other type of graphic applications.

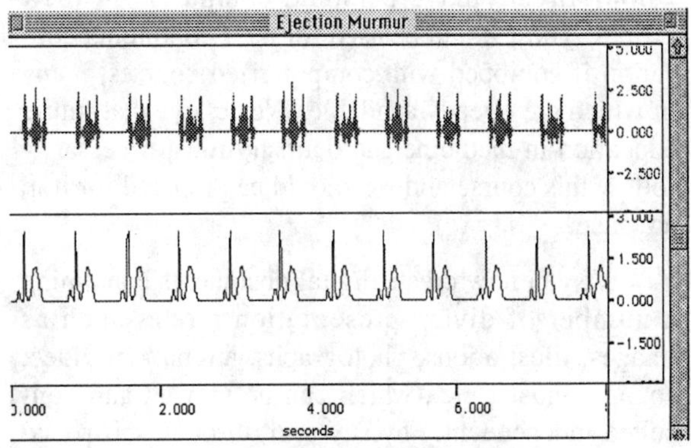

Figure 1

A copy of the strip chart display presented to the users. The sounds are the upper channel and the ECG is the lower channel. Each wave form can be vertically scaled independently and they may be time scaled concurrently. This particular sound is a systolic ejection murmur commonly heard in pulmonic or aortic stenosis.

1. Bergeron, B.P. and R. A. Greenes: "HeartLab and EKGLab:Skill-Building Simulations in Cardiology." Demonstration Digest- Proc.,11th Annual SCAMC. Nov. 1-4, 1987. pp 29-30.

Supported in part by a National Library of Medicine Training Grant LM-07089 and by the Gilbreath-McLorn Veterinary Research Fund.

Internet contacts: hahn@vth.vetmed.missouri.edu (AWH), VOX999@aol.com (MJK) and craig@vth.vetmed.missouri.edu (JCK)

Interactive-Multimedia Teaching of Medical Sciences in the 21st Century: The Temporo-Mandibular Joint.

Arto Demirjian D.D.S,.M.Sc.D., Professor of Anatomy
Benoit David B.D.I., Instructional Designer, Multimedia Specialist
Faculty of Dentistry, University of Montreal, Montreal, Canada

The technological revolution which has occurred over the last ten years in the field of computer sciences leads one to wonder about the future roles of teachers and students. In the light of this rapid change, one must also consider what the basic sciences curriculum in medicine and dentistry of the future will be; conventional course format or a different format? Should we consider replacing conventional laboratories with electronic presentations? Should we be scanning our documents (x-rays, texts, slides, etc....) for our files? Shouldn't we be placing computers in our university clinics? Let us not forget health professionals in private practice, many of whom already have personal computers in their offices. These could be used for their continuing education if equipped with computerized courses, many of which are already available. We believe that future education in medicine and dentistry must necessarily follow this course and we should be prepared for it in advance.

We can now create digital documents containing a number of divers presentation modes such as images, illustrations, photographs, animation, video, sounds, music, etc., which can be viewed and consulted independently by any user, through self-paced interactive structures "playable" on personal computers.

In the last five years, progress in information technology and the globalization of the industry has touched every corner of the world. This technological revolution has influenced all aspects of our daily lives, and the field of education has certainly not managed to escape this current. University level education in all domains has been particularly affected by this change. We believe that we have arrived at a point of no return and must continue in this direction in the 21st century. Are changes in medical and dental schools' curricula following this trend with enough force?

In order to prove the necessity of preparing such multimedia documents for the future generation, we prepared an interactive multimedia courseware on the Temporo-Mandibular Joint. The courseware is on CD-ROM, multilingual (English/French) and for both platforms (Mac and PC/Compatible). We chose the TMJ because of its clinical implications and the difficulties in diagnosing its syndromes. We also wanted to introduce the student to basic sciences' components of the joint and to show on the computer screen, all the latest imaging technologies in this domain.

The design of the instruction consists of a tutorial presenting the following chapters: Introduction, Osteology, Soft Tissues, Physiology, Pathology, Imaging and a self-assessment module in which the student can test his/her knowledge by going through several multiple choice and short answer questionnaires based on the textual content of the tutorial, as well as visual material, i.e. anatomical dissection material and several X-Ray images.

Besides the facility of access to dissecting room material and osteological specimens, the instruction is supported by animations & digital video clips as well as audio material, like the different physiological and pathological noises of the joint during the movements of the jaw. Medical illustrations are also included to present anatomical structures from the skin surface to the joint level, layer by layer, exposing structures in-between.

Aiming toward future implementation of computed-assisted instruction as a standard learning and teaching tool, this self-paced courseware was provided with monitoring options to provide each student with information about his/her progress, and giving them additional and useful help to reach the instructional objectives, thus mastering the subject-matter, with several user controlled options.

This monitoring is initiated by the user personalizing its usage of the courseware with a user name and a password. The users' activities are then monitored and recorded for later use and reference: which sections are accessed (which ones have not yet been seen). The user controlled options consists of the opportunity to take notes while using the courseware, which can be retrieved or printed at a later time. Bookmarks can be inserted and results from the different questionnaires are retrievable to evaluate the student's progress. The software can also list sections of the courseware where questions have been missed.

All pertinent information is stored in external files that we are using to conduct research in the field of educational technology, in regards to user's navigational patterns and usage of provided options.

0195–4210/94/$5.00 © 1994 AMIA, Inc.

Multi-format, multi-platform multimedia: *The Anatomy Project*

Thomas R. Gest[1] & Alan VanBiervliet[2]
Office of Educational Development & Department of Anatomy[1]
Department of Physical Medicine & Rehabilitation[2]
University of Arkansas for Medical Sciences
Little Rock, Arkansas 72205

The Anatomy Project is a series of instructional programs for health science education that use multimedia technologies to combine anatomical and clinical content in an artful manner. The titles of this series are available in a wide variety of formats, including videodisc, videotape, and CD-ROM. In videodisc format, *The Anatomy Project* is a proposed series of twenty-six videodisc titles comprising a comprehensive presentation of clinically-oriented human anatomy. Currently, eight titles of the twenty-six volume series are available: Introduction to Anatomy, The Eye, The Hand, The Heart, The Respiratory Tract, Neuroanatomy 1, Neuroanatomy 2 and Neuroanatomy 3. Each title is a double-sided videodisc (CAV) presenting the information in a variety of ways. Each side of each videodisc contains approximately twenty to twenty-five minutes of video tutorial, organized into three or four chapters of information per side. There is a glossary of terms on each side of each videodisc, and textual summaries of information for each chapter are also presented. Each chapter also presents an atlas and interactive questions with video tutorial remediation of incorrect answers.

The videodiscs of *The Anatomy Project* series can be used with a broad variety of hardware platforms. The information on each videodisc may be accessed at Level I (videodisc player only, no computer) via remote control or barcode workbook (using a barcode-equipped videodisc player). The videodiscs can also be used at Level II (using a program dump from videodisc to a Pioneer LDV6000 series or LDV8000 player, no computer). In Level II use, the program dump from the videodisc to the player has the effect of transforming the remote control unit into a "super remote", which accesses menus of information on the videodisc and enables the user to navigate through the information using these menus. Level III use involves computer control of the videodisc player, and there is a wide range of Level III options for use of *The Anatomy Project* videodiscs. Level III computer software is available for use on Macintosh computers using a two-screen system (computer monitor and videodisc monitor are separate), DOS computers using two screens, and Windows systems using either one or two screens.

The titles of *The Anatomy Project* series are also available on VHS videotape format. This allows delivery of the educational material using low-cost, available videotape players. The content of each title is covered in from five to eight videotapes, which provides the user more rapid access to selected topics.

The systems described above for *The Anatomy Project* use a videodisc or videotape player as the primary tool for delivery of the information. The newest delivery format for the titles of *The Anatomy Project* series is CD-ROM. The CD-ROM versions of *The Anatomy Project* titles are delivered using a multimedia computer system comprising CPU, monitor, CD-ROM drive and speakers. Navigation through the information in the digital adaptation of *The Anatomy Project* series is similar to the Level III Macintosh control software. For each title, there are seven or eight chapter tutorials, each of which presents between four to eight minutes of audio, still images and motion video. Textual summaries of tutorial information are also available. The high quality digital movie-based tutorials are one of the features that distinguishes *The Anatomy Project* from other CBI programs for human anatomy. There is a glossary of terms that provides for easy searching for words. An interactive atlas for each chapter presents labeled still images. By clicking on any labeled structure, the user can access tutorial or textual information about that structure. Interactive questions provide tutorial remediation of incorrect answers. The screen layout and user interface of the CD-ROM versions of *The Anatomy Project* were adapted and modified from the Level III Macintosh videodisc control software in order to accommodate the combination of still and motion video images, text, and navigation controls on the same screen.

0195-4210/94/$5.00 © 1994 AMIA, Inc.

Integration of Pen-based Computer Technology in Clinical Settings

Richard D. Acuff; Lawrence M. Fagan, Ph.D., M.D.; Thomas C. Rindfleisch;
Robert W. Carlson, M.D.; *Stanford University School of Medicine*
Mark S. Tuttle; David D. Sherertz; *Lexical Technology, Inc.*

In this demonstration, we will show how a set of existing or emerging technologies, particularly pen-based, mobile devices, could be applied to facilitate clinical tasks, including information access at the point of care.

Although clinical work is highly information intensive, few care providers are using computers in the clinical setting. A major reason for this has been the mismatch between the mobile clinician and the fixed computer workstation. Clipboard sized computers controlled via a pen-like stylus are making it possible to bring computers to clinicians. Making the computers a useful tool for the clinicians is the next challenge.

Integrating computerized tools into the highly evolved, time-critical pattern of the clinical environment is much more difficult than computing on the desktop. When sitting at a desk working with a computer, the user is generally focused on the computer, working on a task that is entirely embedded in the computer. In this setting, people seem to be tolerant of delays, complicated user interfaces, and large, noisy hardware devices such as keyboards and CRTs. In contrast, the clinician is focused on a task which is mostly external to the computer. In fact, the clinician would prefer to view the computer as a tool, just like a stethoscope or hammer, which are quick to hand, simple to use, effective, and out of the way when not being used.

This gives rise to several characteristics that are likely to be important in software systems that achieve broad clinical success. First, the system must be *responsive.* With thirty or more patients a day, every second counts. Of course, fast hardware is important, but careful software design plays as important a role. Good algorithms and careful coding are the first step. In client-server systems, delays can often be avoided by caching data from the server and pre-fetching potentially relevant data when the system is otherwise idle.

The system should be *flexible* to the user's needs. Physicians are often interrupt-driven and would be very unhappy if unable to switch patients in mid-exam. The system should allow the user to move freely between tasks (patient A, patient B, e-mail, schedule, phone, etc.), preserving the context of the idle tasks. This means no so-called system modal dialogs that lock-out the user from doing anything else until some task is complete. This characteristic is also important when responsiveness is less than ideal. There's nothing more frustrating than wanting to send e-mail while the computer is busy copying a file and has locked you out.

Any clinical system must be *simple to use.* Physicians already have enough to keep track of without adding complicated computer interfaces. Simple does not mean that the system should have its hands tied behind its back, however. By taking a small set of core concepts, such as a few pen gestures, buttons, and dialogs, and using them consistently it should be possible to build interfaces that convey data clearly, are self-prompting (i.e. it is clear to the user what actions are available), and provide the user with a complete set of relevant actions.

The various components of a clinical software system must be highly *integrated.* By having modules that talk to each other, a lot of work can be saved. At the most basic level, this means copying patient names to prescription forms. In a more advanced form, it could mean presenting the results of decision-support agents within the context of the medical record.

In considering these issues, we have developed a simple scenario-based mock-up to illustrate how interactions with an advanced clinical system could appear from the clinician's perspective. The mock-up is organized around a the longitudinal care of an oncology patient, and the clinicians caring for him. We show how electronic mail, filtered for urgency and delivered via a wireless network, can substitute for urgent but routine communications. We demonstrate a mechanism for recording medical findings that balances the inherently complex space of discourse of medical progress notes against the need for a simple user interface and capturing structured information. We show how medical reference knowledge sources can be seemlessly and efficiently accessed from the problem-list of the medical record, with data from the medical record being used to facilitate searching literature. Finally, we show how a decision support agent, in this case one that matches clinical trials with potentially eligible patients, can be used to support clinical care.

0195-4210/94/$5.00

Transforming Information for Computer-Aided Instruction: Using a Socratic Dialogue Method to Teach Gross Anatomy

Constantinou P., Daane S., Dev P.
Department of Anatomy and SUMMIT, Stanford University

ABSTRACT

Traditional teaching of anatomy can be a difficult process of rote memorization. Computers allow information presentation to be much more dynamic, and interactive; the same information can be presented in multiple organizations. Using this idea, we have implemented a new pedagogy for computer-assisted instruction in *The Anatomy Lesson*, an interactive digital teacher which uses a "Socratic Dialogue" metaphor, as well as a textbook-like approach, to facilitate conceptual learning in anatomy.

SOCRATIC TEACHING METHOD

Socrates taught using confrontational questioning: his effectiveness as a teacher lay in making students realize what they did not know. In using the "Socratic Dialogue" metaphor, we have addressed problems associated with student-computer interaction and data organization. Unlike passive textbook learning, Socratic questioning helps the student realize what she does not understand. The computer then provides the student with an easy way to search huge quantities of related information, from which she can understand the significance of both the question and answer. The Socratic metaphor also gives the software designer a method of organizing abundant information into a manageable format.

SOCRATIC DIALOGUE DATA ORGANIZATION

To create a "Socratic Dialogue" method for teaching anatomy, we organized anatomical data into a hierarchy of three types (Fig. 1):

1) At the lowest level are a series of "interactive labeled images" of anatomical dissections. Similar in purpose to an anatomy atlas, the user can click on any structure and to see its outline, name, and a sentence description. The user can access structures on these interactive images through an alphabetic index of the entire body.

2) At the intermediate level are a series of "cards," which roughly correspond to sub-sections of an anatomy textbook chapter. Each card contains an "icon" image, descriptive text of one or two paragraphs, and a multiple choice question. The goal of the "cards" is to present one or two key anatomical concepts. The user can access individual "cards" or sub-chapters through the Table of Contents.

3) The third and highest level is the "Socratic lesson," of which there are approximately 30 for each body region. An example is: "How does the gut change from a simple cylinder to an elongated, coiled structure?" Each Socratic lesson contains links to several "primitives" from the deeper two levels in the hierarchy. As the user navigates through "cards" and interactive images of a Socratic lesson, she is presented with complete information on individual anatomical structures, as well as building-block concepts through which she may understand the broader picture in terms of clinically relevant anatomy.

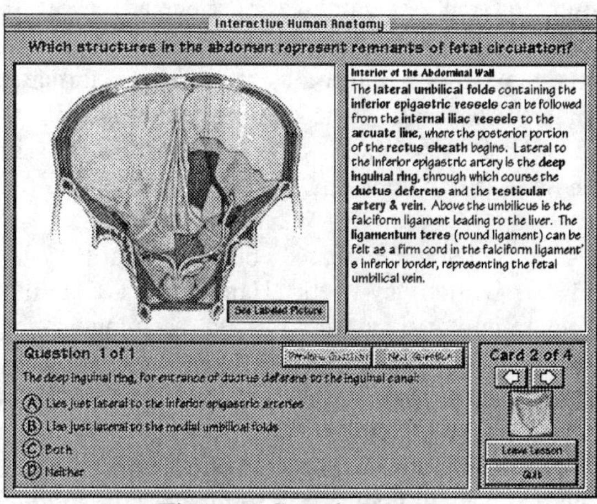

Figure 1. Sample Lesson

AUTHORING ENVIRONMENT

The Anatomy Lesson uses an authoring shell, in which all media, text, and questions are specified in an external text document which is loaded into memory at run-time. This data is authoring in a formation similar to that of a lecture. Thus, content revisions can be performed without any reprogramming, and work on the program can easily be distributed between a number of specialists. The Anatomy Lesson makes liberal use of animations to convey concepts, such as rotation of the gut or formation of the heart, which in the past have been difficult for students to understand from a textbook.

CONCLUSION

We have implemented a novel pedagogy for computer-assisted instruction in anatomy. Using an interactive "Socratic Dialogue" metaphor, we have addressed issues in student-computer interaction and in data organization.

The Anatomy Lesson was created with SuperCard on Apple Macintosh Computers, for the Freshman Anatomy course at Stanford University Medical School.

On-line Continuing Medical Education Employing A Graphical User Interface Bulletin Board System: The Children's Hospital DATALINE

Thomas J. Selva, M.D.
Assistant Professor, Dept. of Child Health
University of Missouri-Columbia Hospital and Clinics, The Children's Hospital
Chief System Operator: The Children's Hospital DATALINE BBS

On-line information access systems have long been in existence for the seasoned computer user, and indeed now are becoming rather common place in the arena of the home user. However, until recently information systems dedicated solely for the use of medical professionals lacked an interface that makes user interaction intuitive. Coupled with the complexities of setting up the appropriate communications hardware, accessing information systems can be somewhat bewildering for the practicing physician who has only a passing knowledge of computers.

Using a computer based bulletin board system (BBS) written by Seth Hamilton of Hamilton Telegraphics, we have established a communications and education system that makes user interaction intuitive and completely mouse driven. The BBS package allows full 256 color Super VGA graphics to be transmitted over standard phone lines at speeds rivaling standard color ANSI graphics. In addition, images compressed with the JPEG standard can be transmitted to the end user and displayed on the user's terminal screen with no interaction by the user (i.e. the user need not download the file, de-archive the image, and then display the image on the terminal screen). Image dithering is performed automatically to accommodate for each user system's graphics capabilities.

Electronic mail can be transmitted with full file attachments. Again, the system assumes the novice user and displays dialog windows requesting user input as the message entry process progresses. Mail can be downloaded to a text file or directly to the user's printer with no user interaction save for pushing a button on the terminal screen.

Using these two modalities, image display and message processing, a continuing medical education program has been established. A case summary is displayed in a scrolling text window with prompts for the user to examine images pertaining to the case at hand. Images can consist of radiographs, micrographs, or photographs. During the case presentation as well, questions are asked of the user. Answers to these questions are entered in a message window that is addressed only to the system operator. Open discussion of each case is available to the user through a message base designated as public.

Under the auspices of the American College of Continuing Medical Education, user's are required to submit specific information to fulfill registration requirements for each CME course. This information is obtained on-line from the user via "templates" which are dialog windows completely configurable by the system operator using a simple scripting language. Information from this registration "template" is combined with the user's personal information database and stored as a text file. At the end of each case cycle, this text file is forwarded via electronic mail to the Continuing Medical Education office at the University of Missouri-Columbia where certificates of completion are prepared.

Standard ANSI graphics are available for non-DOS users. At this time a terminal software package for DOS is available at no charge that will allow full use of color SVGA graphics. Client software for the Windows and Macintosh platforms is in progress. ANSI users can download each case in a self-extracting archive and view the case and images off-line. Case browsing software for the Windows platform is under development.

Using a toll free access line we have developed a sophisticated, yet simple system to allow physicians of all subspecialties and other medical professionals to hone their clinical skills without decreasing their in office practice time and without investing in expensive hardware.

0195-4210/94/$5.00 © 1994 AMIA, Inc.

Clinical Assessment - A Computer-Based Aid to Assessing the Clinical Problem Solving Ability of Medical Students

GO Barnett, DA Link, MJ Feldman, MA Coleman, KT Famiglietti, RJ Kim, WF Raila, P McArdle

Harvard Medical School, Massachusetts General Hospital, Boston, MA

Clinical Assessment, a computer-based program designed to assess the clinical problem-solving skills of medical students, has been developed by the MGH Laboratory of Computer Science and the Harvard Medical School Pediatric faculty. This objective method of evaluating student performance can supplement the traditional grading method used by the course director of a clinical clerkship.

The Clinical Assessment program employs a graphical user interface with mouse and keyboard input to provide a number of stages in which the student gathers information about a simulated patient's condition and formulates diagnostic hypotheses. The case begins with a limited amount of clinical information about the presenting symptoms of a patient with a classic pediatric problem. The student is instructed that since the setting for each case is the Emergency Room, the workup for the simulated patient needs to be focused and not exhaustive. The student enters an initial list of diagnoses which should be considered given the set of findings presented. Each diagnostic entry is analyzed using an interactive text recognition algorithm. The program may present possible word or concept lists if the student entry is not understood as entered. The student then chooses up to ten information items (symptoms, signs, etc.) from the History and Physical Exam menus with the instructions to select items which are useful in determining the diagnosis and the severity of the patient's illness. Immediate "results" are given for each item; some are text responses while others are multimedia responses in the form of images or sounds. The student enters a revised diagnostic impression and is then allowed to select information items from a Laboratory menu as well as the History and Physical Exam items until ready to make a final diagnosis. After entering the final diagnosis, the student identifies those information items selected during the workup which are believed to be the most useful in establishing the diagnosis and in estimating the severity of the disease. In the program's final stage, the student is presented a Therapy menu and orders treatment items pertinent for the simulated case and selects a disposition for the patient. Instructions specific to each stage of the program are provided on each frame. Students can enter a comment easily at any point in the interaction by clicking a button and writing the comment to a screen overlay note pad. Comments are then stored for author review.

In the present method of use, the student receives no immediate evaluation analysis from the program; instead, his/her performance is evaluated by the computer and made available as a case analysis report for a faculty member to review with the student. The scoring algorithm, a complex process which continues to be reviewed and modified, attempts to analyze several different components of clinical problem solving. These components include: diagnostic impressions at various points in the workup, selection of the most appropriate information to clarify the differential diagnosis while considering the risk/cost of each item, interpretation of the images and sounds presented as well as textual descriptions of findings, and justification of the final diagnosis from the information gathered. Less weight accrues to scoring for selection of appropriate therapy.

The Clinical Assessment program is now installed in several Pediatric Clerkship sites for student use and evaluation. The current version presents an annotated sample case and four examination cases to each student. Current cases are drawn from two categories: cough and fever, and abdominal pain. Cases under development include newborn respiratory distress, rashes, and anemia. An administrative system allows course administrators to register students, assign passwords and receive usage reports as well as individual case analysis reports. After pilot testing, the program will be used for grading in the core Pediatric clerkship, constituting about 10% of the final grade.

Supported in part by a grant from Hewlett Packard.

HOME HEALTH CARE CLASSIFICATION (HHCC) SYSTEM

By
Virginia K. Saba EdD, RN, FAAN, FACMI
Alan E. Zuckerman, M.D.
Georgetown University Medical Center
Washington, DC

ABSTRACT

The Home Health Care Classification (HHCC) System is a system designed to predict home health care needs and resource use for the Medicare population. The HHCC System translates clinical nursing parameters, medical parameters, ans socio-demographic data into a clinical case-mix classification for home health patients according to their expected care needs and utilization of home health resources.

The HHCC System is based on a conceptual framework using the nursing process to access patient information in a holistic manner. The Saba Taxonomies -- four sets of nursing of nursing parameters categorized by 20 home health components -- are used to not only assess, but also to code and classify care. They include: (1) 145 nursing diagnoses, (2) three expected outcomes, (3) 160 nursing interventions, and (4) four types of intervention actions. The patient is also assessed using 20 medical diagnoses and/or surgical procedure groups, and 10 socio-demographic data elements.

The HHCC System predicts: (a) **care needs** in terms of home health components and their respective nursing diagnoses and interventions; and **resource use** in terms of nursing and all provider visits (nursing, physical therapy, occupational therapy, speech therapy, medical social work, and home health aide). The medical assessment parameters and socio-demographic data elements are correlated with clinical nursing parameters.

The HHCC System is also designed to record the clinical care process for an entire episode of home health care by extending the clinical assessment parameters into critical care maps. It can be used to determine the cost of care, but also provide a prospective payment method for reimbursement.

The HHCC System is being used to run on a microcomputer using a portable notebook to facilitate ease of use for data collection. The HHCC System prototype is also available to run on the Apple Newton Notepad.

Creating and Evaluating the Department of Veterans Affairs Electronic Medical Record and National Clinical Lexicon

Michael J. Lincoln MD (1,2,5), Charlene Weir Ph.D. (1), Gordon Moreshead (3), Robert Kolodner MD (4), and John Williamson MD (5)
(1) The Salt Lake City VA Information Systems Center, (2) University of Utah Department of Medical Informatics, and (3) Director, Salt Lake City VA Information Systems Center, (4) Director, VA Medical Information Resources Management Office, (5) Salt Lake City VA Medical Center

The Decentralized Hospital Computer Program (DHCP) is a clinical information system now installed in 171 Veterans Affairs Medical Centers (VAMCs), 357 outpatient clinics, 163 nursing homes and domiciliary facilities, and dozens of private hospitals. DHCP forms the basis of Finland's national health care computer system. Few systems featuring DHCP's integrated, comprehensive suite of clinical, laboratory, and administrative functions have been successfully implemented in such a broad range of medical practice settings. Thus, DHCP may represent the most successful electronic medical record now in use. This poster is designed to inform medical informaticians who work with electronic records on three important DHCP developments: the new, electronic medical record and its graphical user interface, formative clinical evaluations of this system, and national VA standards for messaging and vocabulary.

The new, graphical clinician interface to the VA electronic medical record is called Order Entry/Results Reporting version 3.0 (OE 3). OE 3 can connect with existing DHCP databases and application programs, including Problem List, Progress Notes, Discharge Summary, Consultations, an expert system, Forum electronic Mail, and Clinical Notifications. The clinical functionality of OE 3 was specified by a national selection of VA clinicians who served on an Expert Panel (EP) empowered by the VA Clinical Applications Requirements Group. Therefore, OE 3 represents a nationally representative, working (not theoretical) synthesis of currently achievable electronic medical records functionality. The client graphical user interface for the OE 3 software is written in Microsoft's Visual Basic for Windows and interfaces to a server running the Massachusetts General Hospital Utility Multi-Programming System (MUMPS). OE 3 runs on a variety of easily and economically scalable hardware platforms, including PC-compatible clients interfaced to Digital Equipment Corporation Alpha reduced instruction set microcomputer servers.

Because inadequate evaluation has been an important explanation for the failure of many past medical informatics systems, the OE 3 software has undergone extensive formative evaluations. The presenters will report on a national series of usability tests of OE 3. In these tests, the subjects were VA clinicians who were tasked to use intermediate prototypes of OE 3 software to accomplish a suite of representative clinical tasks. Persons visiting the poster will be able to participate in "mini-usability tests", where they will review and run several generations of VA usability testing protocols in sequential versions of the VA OE 3 prototype. Written material summarizing the results of the OE 3 usability testing will be provided on the poster and as participant handouts.

Finally, the poster will summarize recent VA advances in adopting national standards for data representation. The summary will cover the design of the HL-7 messaging module in OE 3, and the OE 3 data structures which relate to the national VA Clinical Lexicon. This national Lexicon is based on the UML Metathesaurus. The Lexicon is an integral part of OE 3 and is now being released to VA hospitals to support the VA's Problem List component. The on-line component of the poster session will allow walk-up users to test the VA Clinical Lexicon's functionality.

The VA Computerized Patient Record - A First Look

Curtis L. Anderson, M.S. and Kevin C. Meldrum, M.S.
Information Systems Center, Department of Veterans Affairs, Salt Lake City, Utah

In support of its in-house DHCP Physician Order Entry/Results Reporting application, the VA is developing the first edition of a Computerized Patient Record. The system will feature a physician-oriented interface with real time, expert system-based order checking, a controlled vocabulary, a longitudinal repository of patient data, HL7 messaging support, a clinical reminder and warning system, and full integration with existing VA applications including lab, pharmacy, A/D/T, radiology, dietetics, surgery, vitals, allergy tracking, discharge summary, problem list, progress notes, consults, and on-line physician order entry.

The Department of Veterans Affairs (VA) is developing its first edition of a Computerized Patient Record (CPR). The VA approach is highlighted by a physician-oriented, graphical user interface to their in-house Decentralized Hospital Computing Program (DHCP) patient care modules. The VA's CPR is being developed around the concept that improved patient care and cost reduction could be achieved by providing a synthesized view of patient data across a variety of information sources and direct, on-line physician Order Entry and Results Reporting (OE/RR) [1].

In addition to gathering, synthesizing, and displaying patient results and treatments, the VA's CPR directly supports physician order entry through editable order sets, user-defined defaults, provider-specific patient lists, and real time, expert system-based order checking.

Emphasis was placed on developing a system which VA physicians would use. The VA CPR provides a graphical environment where physicians can examine results, review problems, observe active medications, and place orders all on the same screen. It also allows them to cut and paste results, treatments, problems, and other data into a progress note, reducing the need to enter the same information repetitively.

VA physicians using the CPR are greeted with a list of patients currently under their care and an accompanying list of clinically relevant alerts. Upon selecting a patient, the automated patient chart opens to the cover sheet. The cover sheet is a one page summary of the patient's current information. It typically includes problems, allergies, active medications, recent laboratory results, next of kin, clinical warnings and notifications, and a summary of past hospital and clinic visits. The user can select any item on the cover sheet for an expanded view of related information.

In the VA CPR, the physician user is in control. From the cover sheet, VA physicians can choose to move through the CPR to fit their needs. Among other things, the user can review and graph lab results over a specific period of time, enter or review a progress note, place and sign orders electronically, or add a problem to the patient's problem list. The system also allows for access to tools such as an on-line clinical calculator. Expansion of the on-line tool list to include literature searches, treatment protocols, drug references, and access to CD-ROM libraries is possible.

Underlying support for the VA's CPR comes in the form of a patient-oriented repository of clinical data, a VA-wide controlled vocabulary termed the "clinical lexicon", and standardized, HL7-content compliant communication between DHCP applications.

The VA CPR will be installed in more than 170 VA medical centers and clinics. Practicing VA clinicians provided functionality and usability guidance throughout the development process.

Reference

[1]. Sittig DF, Stead WW. Computer-based physician order entry: the state of the art. J Am Med Informatics Assoc. 1994;1:108-123.

INQUERY: Inference Net Retrieval of Encounter Notes in an Automated Medical Record

David B. Aronow, MD, MPH
Harvard Community Health Plan
Jay M. Ponte, BS
University of Massachusetts in Amherst

Harvard Community Health Plan (HCHP) is a large HMO, which has benefited from computerized medical records since its founding 25 years ago. The Automated Medical Record System (AMRS) of HCHP is a derivative of COSTAR IV and contains essentially the complete medical record more than 300,000 current members.

The data within AMRS is a strategic resource for both clinical and utilization management. The coded portions are used extensively. However, with the exception of resource-intensive manual chart review for quality measurement and research, the text portions of the AMRS resource are inaccessible and virtually ignored. HCHP has searched for ways to unlock this data and build into production systems the capacity to access, manipulate, extract and abstract text clinical data.

INQUERY is an advanced information retrieval system using an inference net model developed by the Information Retrieval Laboratory of Computer Science Dept. of the University of Massachusetts in Amherst. In order to better focus research in applied problem solving and to facilitate transfer to industry of technologies developed, the Computer Science Dept. established the National the Center for Intelligent Information Retrieval (CIIR), an NSF supported State-Industry-University consortium. HCHP has joined CIIR as a means of developing state-of-the-art tools for exploiting text data resources.

Asthma is the most common serious childhood illness and the greatest consumer of inpatient resources in children. Several quality improvement projects have been undertaken at HCHP concerning asthma care, one of which concerned the frequency and circumstances surrounding exacerbations. This study has a manual chart review component, part of which requires trained coders to identify AMRS encounter notes in which exacerbations are documented.

The question HCHP posed at CIIR was: **to what extent can an automated information retrieval system replace manual chart review of medical record encounter notes in support of quality measurement?** Specifically, can how well can INQUERY identify these 5% of all encounters of pediatric asthmatics which concern acute exacerbations.

This table-top demonstration will present the current release of the INQUERY engine accessed through both Windows and Macintosh interfaces, searching complete, sanitized AMRS records of HCHP members.

Features to be demonstrated include preprocessing of data files, SGML tagging, natural language query formulation, Boolean query formulation, AMRS encounter note retrieval, relevance feedback, query refinement, Phrase Finder automated query expansion system, interpretation of ranked document output, and recent results of experiments in classification of AMRS encounter notes. Hands on use of INQUERY will be encouraged.

Automated Medication System - Benefits For Nursing

D. Hurley

The Royal Alexandra Hospitals (RAH) is a 1,252 bed plus 160 bassinet, City of Edmonton and University of Alberta affiliated active treatment teaching center. It provides a wide range of general, specialized and tertiary care services to patients referred from central and northern Alberta, adjoining provinces and territories. Approximately 46,000 patients are admitted annually. The processing of medication orders plus the administration and documentation requirements consume a large portion of nursing time. Since 1988 the RAH's forty nursing units have been reaping the benefits of an automated medication system, which is part of an integrated hospital information system on two sites. A collaborative multi-disiplinary approach was utilized to develop a customized system for approximately 2,000 nurses, student nurses, nursing assistants, and unit clerks.

This presentation will provide an overview of the medication system beginning with the order entry process. There are numerous safety checks such as duplicate order and unverified order alerts. Also, the system is streamlined to accommodate nursings' diverse specialties.

The selection of each nurse's patient assignment will be discussed as well as the medication worksheets resulting from this selection process. Medication logging will be reviewed and will include the automatic narcotic tracking. The capability to log all medications for assigned patients has proven to be a definite time saver. The medication administration record is stored entirely in the system and is not part of the paper chart. A summary will be given of the numerous reports that are invaluable to nursing, with special emphasis on quality assurance. Additional availability of medication information such as the IV manual and Pediatric Drug Calculator will be addressed. An on-line demonstration of the system will be presented concurrently with the oral presentation.

Information Integration in a Decision Support System

D. L. Hudson*, M. E. Cohen#, P. C. Deedwania*&
*University of California, #San Francisco, California State University, Fresno,
&Veterans Affairs Medical Center, Fresno

Electronic medical records pose a challenge because of the complex types of data which are included. Decision support systems must be able to deal effectively with these data types. In the expert system demonstrated here, a diversity of data types are included. These data are processed by three different methods. However, the different methods of processing are transparent to the user. An overall rule-based interface integrates the different methods into one comprehensive system.

INTRODUCTION

Medical decision support systems fall into several categories: knowledge-based systems in which information is represented as rules, frames, or some other symbolic structure [1], data-derived systems such as neural networks and pattern classification [2], and modeling approaches in which mathematical techniques are used to develop approximate models of biological systems [3]. In all these approaches, the wide variety of data types which are present in medical records must be handled. In our approach, these methods are combined into one decision support system [4]. The handling of different data types by different models is transparent to the user of the system.

SYSTEM STRUCTURE

Data Types

Data types include crisp data, fuzzy data, temporal data, and numerical representation of chaotic analysis. Some data items which appear to be crisp, for example, test results, are more accurately represented as fuzzy numbers which indicate the degree of precision of the test. Four types of temporal data are considered: change in value from previous value, change in value relative to a specified time interval, duration data, and sequence data. A measure developed by the authors which determines the degree of variability in time series data is also included.

Knowledge-Based System

The knowledge-based portion of the system utilizes approximate reasoning techniques which allows weighting of antecedents and partial presence of symptoms. The rule base is used as the interface which invokes the neural network model or time series analysis if certain rules are substantiated.

Neural Network Model

The neural network model is a three-level feed-forward model based on a non-statistical learning supervised learning algorithm developed by the authors [4]. Input data can be of any ordered form, including binary, categoric, integer, or continuous. The network can categorize data into two or more classes, and also produces a degree of membership for each class.

Time Series Analysis

Time series data, such as electrocardiograms, are important measurements for many diagnoses. An ECG may have an overall interpretation which can be used in the rule-based component, or categorized to be used in the neural network component. However, other analyses may also prove useful. In the application shown, a measure of variability for 24-hour Holter tapes is used.

Application

The combination of these techniques is illustration in a decision support system for the diagnosis and treatment of heart disease, including the use of a rule base, a supplementary neural network model of exercise testing data (ETT), and a time series analysis for Holter data.

CONCLUSION

The hybrid system described here has been shown to be a useful decision tool in cardiology. The general structure is readily adaptable to applications in other areas of medicine, and has already been used in prognosis of outcome in carcinoma of the lung and melanoma.

Reference

[1].A. Kandel, G. Langholtz. *Hybrid Architectures for Intelligent Systems*. CRC Press, 1992.

[2].R.Sabbatini. Applications of connectionist systems in biomedicine. *MEDINFO*, 418-425, 1992.

[3].J. Michalis. Use of quantitative ECG-analysis for early detection and prediction of coronary heart disease. *Med. Informatics*. 10:207-214, 1985.

[4].D. Hudson, M. Cohen. A nonlinear neural network combined with symbolic processing. *Nonlinear Theory and Applications*. 937-940, 1993.

The PA Catheter Waveforms Troubleshooting System: A Demonstration of Simple Graphical Knowledge Access for Clinical Care

Greg Estey, EdM; Penny Ford-Carleton RN, MS; B. Taylor Thompson, MD; Robert A. Jenders, MD, MS; Diane E. Oliver, MD; Randy Eccles; Martha Martin, RN, MS; Rita Zielstorff, RN, MS; Joan B. Fitzmaurice, RN, PhD; G. Octo Barnett, MD
Massachusetts General Hospital, Boston MA 02114

The Pulmonary Artery Catheter Waveforms Troubleshooting System is a resource for on-site decision support and education now in use on several care units at Massachusetts General Hospital. The system provides access to clinically applicable information about specific pulmonary artery catheter waveform abnormalities, including characteristics, causes, interventions and measurement techniques. The method of access to information in the system is through waveform selection screens that depict prototypical waveform problems. Supplementary material is presented in structured tutorials and a glossary that is integrated with the troubleshooting screens using hypertext links. The presentation will highlight a number of lessons from our experiences with the development of this system and its introduction and use on care units. The principal points are:

a. The importance of knowledge resources that can be used by caregivers at the time when they need the knowledge. We developed this system to test our hypothesis that providing clinically applicable information resources on care units can be a powerful method of clinical education, particularly in areas of specialty expertise. The value of such a system to the experienced specialist may be less than that for the relative novice. We have found that the utilization of the system has increased when it has been made available in patient care areas where multiple staff are engaged in cross-training.

b. The importance of a user interface that requires virtually no training. Clinicians do not have time to spare for learning about complex user interface features. We set as a design goal that the user interface for this knowledge resource should be simple enough that it would be immediately clear to the first-time user how to proceed. We achieved this goal by:

- modelling the user interface design on a simplified model of problem-solving in the domain of PA catheter waveforms troubleshooting
- intensive use of graphical methods of presentation
- strict hierarchical organization of content
- repeated early evaluations of paper mock-ups and working prototypes with clinicians from the intended user populations

c. The primacy of credible content. For a knowledge resource to be seen to be worth using, the knowledge it conveys must be authoritative, current and consistent with local standards of practice. The resource must be comprehensive within a well-defined domain, so that caregivers can easily understand its scope. To meet these requirements, our project was pursued as a collaboration with clinical content experts who wrote, edited, and revised text, specified illustrations and evaluated early system designs. Obtaining expert collaboration entailed accommodating an extended consensus-building process. The large investment in content development and validation has yielded a system that has been able to move directly from research to adoption for use in critical care orientation programs run by the MGH Department of Nursing.

d. The importance of clinical opinion leaders on the units. Enthusiastic support from the clinical opinion leaders on the unit has proven to be a key determinant in the successful installation of this system. The leaders usually include the nurse manager, the medical director and especially those involved in consultation and staff training. Fully engaging these busy individuals requires providing clear models for system use. In the presentation we will walk through the system using written case scenarios we make available in order to provide additional structure in introducing the system in teaching.

This work has been supported in part by grants from the Agency for Health Care Policy Research (HS06575) and the National Library of Medicine (LM05200), and by an educational grant from Hewlett Packard Corporation.

The Mental Status Expert (MSE): An Expert System for Scoring and Interpreting the Mental Status Examination

Daniel B. Hier, M.D., Chiang S. Jao, Ph.D. and Steven U. Brint, M.D.
Department of Neurology, University of Illinois, Chicago, IL 60612-7330

ABSTRACT

The mental status examination is the most difficult and time-consuming portion of the neurological examination. A complete mental status examination requires the examiner to assess alertness, memory, language, praxis, gnosis, attention, and visual-spatial functions. Findings of the mental status need to be interpreted in terms of severity of deficits, nature of the deficits, likely etiology, and likely area of corresponding brain injury. The performance of an accurate, complete, and detailed mental status examination is a daunting task for the medical student or resident in training. Traditional mental status examinations show considerable inter-examiner variability for items administered and for interpretation of abnormalities. Even in academic settings, mental status examinations have little educational content.

We have developed an expert system to assist neurologists and other physicians in the scoring, interpretation, and reporting of the mental status examination. Our goal was to build an expert system with following desirable characteristics: (1) Encourage the use of a standardized protocol of mental status examination and minimize examiner's variability in the tests administered; (2) Score the patient's performance according to pre-determined normative data; (3) Use production rules to determine the presence of mental status deficits so as to minimize examiner's bias in the diagnosis of deficits; (4) Generate an attractive and legible consultation in text and graphics to convey findings; (5) Provide the user access to a stored knowledge-base of interpretative information that would enhance the educational content of the consultation; (6) Store patient findings in a database to allow future retrieval as well as analysis of aggregate data.

We designed a standardized mental status examination that sampled the following aspects of higher cortical functions: Alertness and Concentration (orientation, level of alertness, spell WORLD backwards); Language (naming, repetition, comprehension); Left Parietal Function (right-left discrimination, finger gnosis, calculating, writing, motor praxis); Right Parietal Function (dressing, drawing, neglect, extinction); Occipital Lobe Function (color naming, reading); Memory (recall); Frontal Lobe Function (verbal fluency, oral praxis, executive functioning). The standardized mental status examination was printed and then administered manually by examiners.

We designed a hypermedia-based expert system for patient registration and report writing. The system is implemented in KnowledgePro for Windows® (KPWIN). KPWIN is a rule-based expert system shell with object-oriented programming and hypermedia capabilities. The former capabilities reduced the complexity of program design and the latter ones allowed us to build an intuitive user interface with a minimum of screen clutter.

The Mental Status Expert (MSE) allows the user to input information in ten areas: Patient Demographics, Patient History, Basic Neurological Examination, Alertness/Orientation, Language, Left Parietal Lobe Function, Right Parietal Lobe Function, Frontal Lobe Function, Occipital Lobe Function, Memory, and Miscellaneous Functions. A button bar at the bottom of each screen allows the user to page forward/backward, quit, print the consultation, store findings in the database, or access an on-line reference library. The on-line reference library adopts a portion of text from *Topics in Behavioral Neurology* (Hier DB, Gorelick PB, Shindler AG; Butterworths Publishers, 1987). The MSE displays a paragraph of explanatory text about each chosen mental status deficit that can either be viewed on the screen or printed to be appended to the consultation. The MSE uses production rules (1) to decide the severity of deficits displayed in a bar chart; (2) to create a deficit summary to list all deficits currently diagnosed; (3) to retrieve explanatory text about any deficits diagnosed. The user may then append any further interpretative text he/she wishes to add. Patient findings are stored in a database file. This provides a permanent searchable record of the consultation for either review purposes or statistical analysis.

0195-4210/94/$5.00

DECISION TOOL -- A Graphical User Interface for Generic Markov Models

Brian D. Kan, M.D.[1], Harvey L. Levy, M.D.[2], John B. Wong, M.D.[1], Stephen G. Pauker, M.D.[1]
[1]Division of Clinical Decision Making, New England Medical Center
[2]Newborn Screening Program, Massachusetts Department of Public Health, Boston MA

INTRODUCTION

Markov modeling has become increasingly popular for medical decision analysis because it captures the interaction of events over time[1]. Unfortunately, Markov models are difficult to construct and debug, creating a barrier to their use in supporting patient care and health policy decision making. The availability of a generic Markov model to use as a template to frame a set of similar medical problems would simplify the use of such models in medical decision making and would enable users to capture the dynamics of a group of related medical problems without constructing a *de novo* model and without requiring the end user to become an expert in constructing decision models.

Much of the available software for medical decision making uses a command line or menu driven interface and is designed for decision tree construction [2, 3]. Because analysts who wish to use these generic templates may not be expert computer users, a graphical user interface would facilitate Markov model generation and decrease errors. Restricting the editing capabilities would prevent users from introducing errors to an existing tree by inappropriate modification. To test these hypotheses, a generic Markov decision tree and interface has been constructed to evaluate the cost-effectiveness of a variety of screening tests for newborns.

DESCRIPTION

We developed DECISION TOOL using Visual Basic 3.0 for Microsoft Windows, which allows integration of spreadsheet and graph components, Windows API (application programming interface) calls, as well as relational database commands. The decision tree was constructed using DECISION MAKER 7.0. DECISION TOOL consists of a main window, an editing window, and a results window. A translator is provided for converting between a tree in DECISION MAKER format and a tree in DECISION TOOL's relational database format, which is compatible with the Microsoft Access relational database. This allows database storage of both decision tree information and results of the analysis. Decision trees constructed using SMLTREE are also compatible with DECISION TOOL.

The main window contains both menu and tool bar access to all of the program's functions, including file management functions, DECISION MAKER calls, data editing, and simulation results. This window includes a spreadsheet which allows viewing of those parts of the decision tree which can be edited. DECISION TOOL calls DECISION MAKER to run a simulation.

Selected information in the model can be edited. Tree node names may be changed; comments can be added. Most variables can be changed in value, or can be changed to lookup a value in an indexed table, or to use an arbitrary expression or function. Variables represented by functions or tables can be graphed to facilitate the elicitation of subjective values from the user.

We developed a Markov cost-effectiveness model for neonatal screening which considers age at detection, severity of chronic illness, presence of an acute illness, compliance with therapy, and presence of another chronic illness using 63 states of health. The model contains 790 bindings, 169 nodes and 317 variables. Physicians not familiar with Markov modeling were able to instantiate the model and perform sensitivity analyses which examined neonatal screening for phenylketonuria, sickle cell anemia, and cystic fibrosis.

CONCLUSION

The ability to design a generic template model and provide a graphical user interface should facilitate the use of Markov models by users who are not decision analysts. We have developed such a generic Markov model for neonatal screening and have applied it to policy decisions facing a department of public health.

Acknowledgments This work was supported in part by State of Massachusetts Grant MCJ 258101 and NLM Grant LM07092.

REFERENCES

[1] Sonnenberg, F.A. Beck JR, Markov Models in Medical Decision Making: A Practical Guide, Medical Decision Making. 13(4), 1993:322-38.
[2]Sonnenberg, FA, Pauker SG, Decision Maker: An Advanced Personal Computer Tool for Clinical Decision Analysis, Proceedings of the Eleventh Annual Symposium on Computer Applications in Medical Care, Washington, D.C. IEEE Computer Society, 1987.
[3]Hollenberg, J, SMLTREE: The all Purpose Decision Tree Builder. Boston: Pratt Medical Group, 1985.

Interactive Data Analysis, Modeling, and Simulation: Available Now On a Desktop Near You

James L. Daly, MS, J. A. Fernandez-Pol, M. D., and James W. Fletcher, M.D.
St. Louis VA Medical Center, St. Louis, MO and St. Louis University Health Sciences Center

This electronic poster will illustrate the use of two powerful "off-the-shelf" tools for the transformation of data into information in a medical center setting. We have used these tools for clinical, research, and educational applications and have found them very useful not only for extending the mathematical capabilities of the individual user, but also for improving communications among users from diverse disciplines. Two important features shared by both programs are ease of use and effective information presentation and display. These features allow the user to concentrate on the formulation of the problem, leaving the tedious part of the problem solution for the computer.

The first program, ***Mathematica®****, is a "system for doing mathematics by computer."* ***Mathematica®*** *supports users with a wide range of mathematical sophistication in the solution of problems which have been formulated in "standard" mathematical format. The second program,* ***ithink™****, is used to create simulations of processes and to facilitate "what-if" analysis by presenting process variables in graphical or tabular form. The unique feature of* ***ithink™*** *is that the simulation builder /user specifies the relationships between process elements while the application supplies the "mathematics" to carry out the simulation. We have found* ***ithink™*** *to be a powerful tool not only for testing the predictions of completed models but also for the process of developing the models themselves. This is especially true in modeling processes which require input from several disciplines, where developers can see the results of their contributions in interactive "runs" of the process simulation.*

The insights gained from the collection and analysis of data associated with a given phase or stage of a process frequently lead to questions which may suggest a reformulation of the basic model. If the reformulation requires much "higher math", the development cycle is often extended due to the need for additional "expertise". In much the same way that "word processing" and "spreadsheets" amplified the capabilities of the end user to develop their subject-matter expertise, these programs extend the capability to create and validate mathematical models to the end-user.

APPLICATIONS

Modeling and Simulation

These applications, developed in **ithink™**, were formulated with input from subject matter "experts" who developed the simulations in an interactive manner.

Ambulatory Care Clinic Service: The relationships between patients served and various clinic parameters were studied, with results presented in graphical form.

Tracer Kinetics: The effects of physical decay and biological elimination are simulated in a manner which allows students to see the effects of varying model parameters.

Spread of Disease: The differential equations used to specify a model for the spread of AIDS were used to build a "compartment" model in which the mathematics required for the simulation were automatically produced.

Disk Storage Utilization for Data Archiving: In this simulation, the effects of various archiving strategies were studied with projections for disk storage requirements presented in both graphical and tabular form.

Computation and Analysis

Mathematica® was used to analyze data imported from the medical center hospital information system and to present the information in both hard-copy and animated displays.

Presentation of Bed Usage Data: Bed utilization data by service on a daily basis was analyzed for a two year period for trends and patterns.

Clinical Decision Making: Electronic notebooks for teaching basic decision making were developed and used for teaching Bayesian decision strategies.

Clinical Information Processing: Notebooks were developed to process "count" data from nuclear medicine studies, performing appropriate corrections and presenting results in graphical format.

Section IX

Theater-Style Demonstrations

The Regenstrief Medical Record System - Experience with MD Order Entry and Community-wide Extensions

Authors: Clement J. McDonald M.D., William M. Tierney M.D., J. Marc Overhage M.D. Ph.D., Douglas K. Martin, M.D., Brenda Smith, R.N., Cheryll Wodniak, R.N., Lonnie Blevins, Jill Warvel, Jeff Warvel, Jim Meeks-Johnson, Larry Lemmon, Tull Glazener.

Abstract:

The Regenstrief Medical Record System (RMRS) encompasses three hospitals on the Indiana University Medical Center campus, all of their clinics, and thirty off-campus clinic sites. It captures data for about 60,000 hospitalizations and 600,000 outpatient encounters per year. At present, over 800,000 patients and nearly 100,000,000 separate observations are carried by RMRS.

We have been deliberately opportunistic in the capture of clinical data. We capture laboratory and medication information from three different laboratory and pharmacy systems; vital signs and nursing observations from automated bedside machines (Vital Net) on one inpatient service; full text admission, discharge and visit notes, and surgical pathology, radiology, and nuclear medicine reports from three different dictation systems; EKG tracings and diagnoses from EKG carts; and registration and transfer information from three different ADT systems. We use HL7 as our principal message standard for linking these systems. We also capture a varying amount of fully coded patient information from patient- and clinic - specific encounter forms, and we code and record the diagnostic impressions from all diagnostic studies.

The medical records room tracks charts, enters case abstract information, and tracks chart completion through the system. When discharge dictations and operative notes are transcribed, the system notes that fact and alerts the physician to the need to electronically sign the report. As patients are admitted, the computer sends notice to the attending physician.

Researchers and managers can retrieve patients from the medical records system, based on the value of coded and numeric results, in seconds to minutes (depending upon the query). Raw text data can also be searched but the process is much slower.

At Wishard, where the system has been installed the longest, the computer contains everything but the provider's handwritten notes. Medicine service physicians enter all of their orders (inpatient and outpatient) directly into the computer order entry system. Surgery physicians enter all inpatient orders. The order entry system provides problem oriented order prompting; access to medical text book information; pocket rounds reports; warnings about allergies, drug and diagnosis interactions; and reminders about blocking conditions, consequent orders, and preventive care, triggered by rule-based guidelines.

The computer scans all laboratory results and vital signs as they are entered, looking for critically abnormal values. Any such results are transmitted directly to the physician via a pager with a 4x20 character LCD display.

In the homeless clinics the computer maintains the entire patient record and generates patient education sheets related to the patient's problem.

We have extended the system to thirteen mental health clinics, four HMO offices, ten community-based clinics, a number of homeless care sites, and two elderly care facilities located between one and eight miles from Wishard Hospital. Currently we are upgrading and expanding these links. We will add lines to the emergency rooms of two more hospitals (Methodist and Community East) and convert to Ethernet links over cable TV lines. We are developing interfaces to community pharmacy systems so physicians can obtain complete drug profiles on their patients and determine whether patients are complying with their medication orders.

We will demonstrate all components of this system.

Patient Care Applications on Internet

Octo Barnett, Edward Shortliffe, Henry Chueh, Judy Piggins, Robert Greenes, James Cimino, Mark Musen, Paul Clayton, Betsy Humphreys, Lawrence Kingsland III, PRC Rodgers

Harvard Medical School, Stanford, Columbia, National Library of Medicine

Introduction: Promise and Potential of National Networking

Knowledge Access in Clinical Workstation:

The Clinical Workstation (CWS) is an integrated computer-based workstation for recording and retrieving patient-based clinical information and accessing network-based clinical knowledge resources. Fundamental to the CWS strategy is a client-server architecture which makes use of multiple servers for different services. The demonstration will illustrate how an Oracle relational database at the Massachusetts General Hospital (MGH) is utilized as the server for the electronic medical record, while the National Library of Medicine (NLM) MEDLINE server in Bethesda and the Lab of Computer Science (LCS) DXplain server at MGH act as knowledge servers. By using a controlled clinical vocabulary, the CWS is able to use documentation entered by the clinician as the entry point to the knowledge resource servers. The NLM Metathesaurus is used to map the CWS clinical vocabulary (an extended version of COSTAR's vocabulary) to alternative source vocabularies (Mesh, DXplain) through a client-server API. While the knowledge servers are disparate in location and implementation, the clinician accesses the information transparently through a single interface.

Collaborative Infrastructure Tools to Develop Medical Information System Applications: the NLM/HPCC Collaboratory Project

Medical information systems to support the complex clinical problem-solving, patient-management, and continuing-education needs of health care professionals are necessarily complex. These systems must integrate a variety of services, including those providing clinical data and image access, education and decision support, and communication. Such services are currently available largely on disparate, often incompatible systems. A major challenge for medical informatics is how to decrease the redundant development of software components while simultaneously assuring compatibility among elements so as to facilitate integration both within institutions and among like-minded organizations.

Our Collaboratory Project is a joint effort involving medical informatics groups at Harvard, Columbia, and Stanford Universities, supported by the HPCC initiative of NLM. The goal is to develop a shared set of Internet tools and methods for building information systems from network-based component objects. Our system demonstration will show some of the shared tools that we are developing (for example, browsers for exploring and testing our network-based vocabulary server, and tools for shared access to clinical data and structured guidelines) plus a prototype clinical workstation application that is based on client-server access to such shared components.

Access to NLM databases through the Internet

The National Library of Medicine (NLM) is making increasing use of the Internet to broaden the distribution of its existing databases; to build new multimedia services that exploit the Mosaic client software and World Wide Web; and to make a range of system development tools, including the UMLS Knowledge Sources, more accessible and useful to the informatics community. In a demonstration that includes access to clinically interesting information services available on the Internet, NLM staff will illustrate how the UMLS Knowledge Sources can be employed to assist users in identifying and searching information sources relevant to particular health care or research questions.

The Virtual Hospital: Creating and Organizing a Ubiquitous Health Sciences Organization on the Internet

Michael P. D'Alessandro M.D.[1,2], Jeffrey R. Galvin M.D.[1], William E. Erkonen M.D.[1], David L. Lacey M.D.[1], David S. Curry M.S.L.S [3], Edwin A. Holtum M.S. [3], Donna M. Santer M.D.[4]

[1] Electric Differential Multimedia Laboratory, Department of Radiology, University of Iowa College of Medicine, Iowa City, IA, [2] Department of Radiology, Children's Hospital and Harvard Medical School, Boston, MA, [3] Hardin Library for the Health Sciences, University of Iowa, Iowa City, IA, [4] Division of General Pediatrics, Children's Hospital and Harvard Medical School, Boston, MA

Introduction

A physical organization is defined by its physical plant, the people who work within it, the knowledge they contain and the services they offer. A ubiquitous organization is a digital representation of the information and services of a physical organization that is made available to anyone at any time in any place. Creating a ubiquitous organization amplifies the attributes of the physical organization by extending its power and reach. Now, instead of people having to come to the physical organization for information and services, the ubiquitous organization comes to them whenever they need it.

Ubiquitous organizations can be created for physical organizations such as governments, libraries, schools, universities, and hospitals. We have created a ubiquitous organization which we call the Virtual Hospital which is a digital representation of the University of Iowa Health Sciences Colleges, Library, and Hospitals and Clinics. The Virtual Hospital contains digital representations of key medical center services which are continuously available at a distance, thereby serving as an efficient medical center extension.

Discussion

The Virtual Hospital therefore serves as a digital health sciences library for Iowa and the world. It contains information of use to patients and health sciences practitioners. The information contained within the Virtual Hospital may be used by health sciences practitioners at the time of patient contact to aid patient care or it may be used as continuing education material at a time and place that is convenient for the practitioner. It is now well recognized that our concept of education is changing. Universities need to focus on building life long learners, and must teach their students how to learn. In order to maintain their skills throughout a lifetime of practice, the health sciences practitioner must always be "in training." This continuum of training requires a continuum of information and this will be the function of the Virtual Hospital, providing an electronic umbilical to the practitioner throughout their career. By lowering the threshold for obtaining high quality medical information by putting information at their fingertips, health sciences practitioners may practice "just in time learning," which is the acquisition and review of information at the time it is needed, just before or during a patient encounter, when it will have the greatest impact on patient care and thereby improve the quality of medical care rendered unto patients.

Patient information in the Virtual Hospital includes "The Iowa Health Book" - a compilation of patient education and preventive medicine information, a Health Care Providers Directory for the University of Iowa Hospitals and Clinics (UIHC) to help patients choose a health care provider, and Post-Visit Follow-up and Home Care Instructions. Information in the Virtual Hospital for Health Sciences Students and Practitioners includes multimedia textbooks, teaching files, patient simulations, and diagnostic algorithms, access to the UIHC Informm patient information database, access to MEDLINE and other electronic resources at the Hardin Health Sciences Library, and Continuing Education materials including grand rounds, conferences and lectures.

The Virtual Hospital is constructed upon 4 computer software, hardware and communication standards which are all in the public domain: (1) The World Wide Web (WWW), a hypermedia client/server database technology, is used to organize the Virtual Hospital, (2) Wide Area Information Servers (WAIS), a client/server indexing and searching tool, is used to index the content within the Virtual Hospital, (3) The Internet, the data superhighway of today, is used to transmit the content of the Virtual Hospital to its users, (4) Mosaic, a client for the WWW and WAIS which is available for all popular personal computers and workstations, is used to display the information contained in the Virtual Hospital.

Connecting to the Virtual Hospital

Once connected to the Internet with a Mosaic client, set your Uniform Resource Locator (URL) to: http://vh.radiology.uiowa.edu/. If you do not have Mosaic, but you do have a communications program that can emulate a VT-100 terminal you may connect using the telnet command to log into the host "lemans.radiology.uiowa.edu" and then when prompted with "login:" type "lynx" and you will be on the Virtual Hospital Home Page.

Reference

[1]. Galvin JR, D'Alessandro MP, Erkonen WE, Knutson TA, Lacey DL. The Virtual Hospital: A New Paradigm for Lifelong Learning in Radiology. Radiographics 1994; 14:875-879.

This work is supported by grants from the National Library of Medicine, Apple Computer Inc., the University of Iowa Hospitals and Clinics and the University of Iowa College of Medicine.

Teaching Visual Thinking in Radiology

Robert T. Macura, MD, Ph.D., Katarzyna J. Macura, MD, Ph.D.

Department of Radiology, Medical College of Georgia, Augusta, GA

We have implemented a tutoring system, ***Radiology Puzzler****, for teaching visual recognition of intracranial lesions on radiological images. The system is designed to support the learning of radiological patterns through graphical case retrieval. Using radiologic feature samplers, the user may define brain lesion characteristics and use visual query when searching for reference cases. A rule-based module generates a hierarchical list of diagnostic hypotheses and provides a feed-back to the user. Relevant cases that match the sampler's index are retrieved from the case library for comparison with the case in question.*

INTRODUCTION

Recent discoveries in cognitive psychology emphasize the importance and influence of visualization on thinking [1]. Images are easily remembered and give more information than words. It has been hypothesized that in a visual domain such as radiology, perceptual learning, the outcome of which is a differential diagnosis set with associated probabilities, occurs earlier in the course of learning than the cognitive learning that depends on products of the perceptual process [2]. Learning an extensive reference set is thus a necessary prerequisite for radiological diagnosis [3].

The ***Radiology Puzzler*** is a computerized tutoring system that is designed to emphasize visual thinking in radiology education [4]. The system is intended to help first year residents develop visual fluency, enhance visual memorization, and improve indexing of mental images used in radiological diagnosis. The system provides a teaching environment that combines text, image, video and audio, and intends to mimic a real one-to-one teaching environment. The user learns radiology visual language by making a visual pattern matching with interactive feed-back.

SYSTEM ARCHITECTURE

The ***Radiology Puzzler*** consists of five modules:

Case Library (CL) - is a database of radiologic cases. A case consists of images, with diagnosis and radiologic finding indexes, and captions. CL provides cases for both testing and reference purposes.

Visual Concept Library (VCL) - is a pictionary of radiological findings (set of samplers linked to the images in the CL) with voice annotations.

Tutor Knowledge Base (TKB)- is a rule-based module that identifies deficiencies in the user's knowledge, selects strategies to present that knowledge to the user, controls dialog sequences in the *Dialog Window*, and generates differential diagnoses.

Explanation Library (EL)- is a library of video clips and teaching images that are presented to the user in the interactive mode.

User Data File (UDF) - is a database that holds information about the user's performance during the tutoring session.

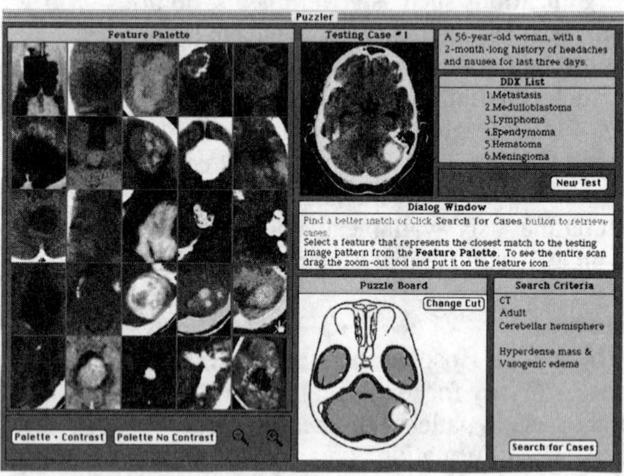

Figure 1. ***Radiology Puzzler*** screen

References

1. Kosslyn SM, Koenig O. *Wet Mind: The New Cognitive Neuroscience*. New York, NY: The Free Press; 1992.

2. Lesgold A, Rubinson H, Feltovich P, Glaser R, Klopfer D, Wang Yen. Expertise in a Complex Skill: Diagnosing X-Ray Pictures. In Chi M T H, Glaser R, Farr M J , eds. *The Nature of Expertise*. Hillsdale, NJ: Lawrence Erlbaum Associates, Publishers; 1988: 311-342.

3. Pizer SM, ter Haar Romeny BM. Fundamental Properties of Medical Image Perception. *J Digital Imaging* 1991; 4(4): 213-225.

4. Macura RT, Macura KJ, Trueblood JH, Binet EF. Radiology Puzzler: Artificial Intelligence-Based Game. Supplement to *Radiology* 1993; 189(P): 445-446.

ComuniCare™: Case Management & Clinical Decision Support Systems

Jay C. Taylor, Director, Medical Utilization Systems, Aetna Health Businesses
William T. McGivney, PhD, VP Clinical Evaluation & Research, Aetna Health Businesses
Arthur J. Steinberg, MD, VP Health Services, Aetna Health Businesses

COMUNICARE STRATEGY

Aetna Health Businesses (AHB) is migrating it's Utilization Management programs from a precertification transaction review process to a comprehensive case management strategy. This strategy will continue to position Aetna as a premier managed care insurance company in the 1990's.

To support the transition and delivery of this strategic offering, AHB is developing a new Comprehensive Case Management system with a family of integrated clinical decision support tools. These integrated systems provide full case management capabilities for the entire spectrum of care for a member/patient across all AHB health insurance products and customers. Knowledge base systems capture clinical information and provide service recommendations to AHB case managers. The clinical information, supporting guideline/policy, system recommendation and decision is stored in the case management system for local and central reporting.

COMUNICARE DEMONSTRATIONS

The system demonstration includes the following:

. How information and knowledge engineering analysis tools and methodologies were used to design ComuniCare™.

. Considerations for planning the rollout of a new distributed computing environment and national communications network.

. Demonstration of the MedQuery™ clinical decision support system, an integrated set of artificial intelligence and high performance document retrieval tools for clinical protocols and guidelines. Color human anatomy images are also provided.

. Demonstration of the comprehensive case management system, MedCase™, (e.g., precertifications, admissions, reviews, reevaluations, discharge planning, etc.).

ComuniCare™ provides complete audit capability for AHB's managed care business and provides flexibility in local medical management and reporting. This allows evaluation of clinical practice patterns with service quality and cost measures for operational, management and customer reporting.

UM BUSINESS BENEFITS

. Allows AHB to improve customer and provider relations: systems have been designed to support programs that are focused on the improvement of customer and provider relations (e.g., enhancing local reporting, reducing provider call backs, etc.).

. Decreases administrative costs and streamlines workflow: the service based workflow is supported and facilitated by integrated systems resulting in significant productivity improvements and operational cost savings.

. Facilitates quality and consistent decision making: policy and clinical guidelines are authored centrally, distributed electronically and used locally, ensuring consistency in service policy implementation and decision making across AHB networks nationwide. Changes to clinical policy are distributed nationwide overnight.

. Provides service flexibility: the distributed computing architecture provides flexibility in delivering functionality and information at local sites. National management and reporting is also supported by a central UM database.

. Provides opportunity for the delivery of ComuniCare functions to physicians' offices.

* ComuniCare, MedCase and MedQuery are trademarks of Aetna Life Insurance Company

0195-4210/94/$5.00

Integrated Clinical Workstations for Image and Text Data Capture, Display, and Teleconsultation

Ruth Dayhoff MD, Peter M. Kuzmak, Garrett Kirin
Washington Information Systems Center
Dept. of Veterans Affairs
8403 Colesville Rd, Suite 200
Silver Spring MD 20910
(301) 427-3700
E-mail: DAYHOFF@FORUM.VA.GOV

ABSTRACT

The Department of Veterans Affairs (VA) DHCP Imaging System digitally records clinically significant diagnostic images selected by medical specialists in a variety of hospital departments, including radiology, cardiology, gastroenterology, pathology, dermatology, hematology, surgery, podiatry, dental clinic, and emergency room. These images, which include true color and gray scale images, scanned documents, and electrocardiogram waveforms, are stored on network file servers and displayed on workstations located throughout a medical center. All images are managed by the VA's hospital information system (HIS), allowing integrated displays of text and image data from all medical specialties. Two VA medical centers currently have DHCP Imaging Systems installed, and other installations are underway.

VISUAL CHART DISPLAY SOFTWARE

The goal of the VA's DHCP Imaging System is to provide image and text data in an integrated manner that facilitates the clinician's making of patient care decisions in a timely and accurate way. This system is oriented toward providing the treating physician with a complete view of patient data, at the same time allowing consulting physicians to have access to the full range of data.

Clinicians use workstations to view screens of "thumbnail" images for all studies or procedures performed on a selected patient. This display option allows the user to interactively indicate radiology exams or individual images to be displayed in greater resolution. Radiology images grouped by examination are displayed first as thumbnail images, for further selection of full images for full resolution viewing. This software will be demonstrated.

HIGH RESOLUTION RADIOLOGY VIEWING STATION

A new capability of the DHCP Integrated Imaging System is support for a diagnostic quality high-resolution megapixel DOME display adapter (Md2K/EISA) and an Image Systems portrait-mode monitor (M21PMAX). The hardware will support a 1728 x 2304 16-bit gray scale image, for example a 14" x 17" chest digital xray. This state-of-the-art display technology is completely integrated with the DHCP Imaging System and provides support for teleradiology. The various capabilities of the display, including window/leveling, zooming, panning, and magnifying, will be demonstrated.

TELECONSULTATION

All VA medical centers and other VA facilities are connected by a wide area packet-switched network. The VA's electronic mail software has been modified to allow inclusion of binary data such as images in addition to the traditional text data. Medical reports can also be included in mail messages, and patient data can be transferred from the hospital information system at one medical center to another. Testing of the use of multimedia electronic mail for medical teleconsultation is currently underway at two sites. Multimedia mail consultation software will be demonstrated.

SUMMARY

The V.A. has emphasized integration in developing its hospital information system and in integrating text and image data. We believe there is a critical mass where systems work together to provide many more benefits than non-integrated systems.

PROTÉGÉ-II: A Suite of Tools for Development of Intelligent Systems from Reusable Components

Mark A. Musen, M.D., Ph.D., Henrik Eriksson, Ph.D., John H. Gennari, Ph.D., Samson W. Tu, M.S., and Angel R. Puerta, Ph.D.

Section on Medical Informatics, Stanford University School of Medicine, Stanford, CA 94305-5479 USA

PROTÉGÉ-II comprises a set of tools that developers use to build intelligent software systems. One tool, called MAÎTRE, allows developers to browse through and edit domain models (ontologies). Another tool, called DASH, takes as its input a domain ontology, and generatres as its output a graphical knowledge-acquisition tool that application experts can use to enter the detailed content knowledge necessary to define new applications. Other tools in the PROTÉGÉ-II collection allow developers to define the problem-solving methods that automate application tasks by making selections from a library of reusable problem-solving–method building blocks. PROTÉGÉ-II has been used to create knowledge-acquisition tools and the associated knowledge bases for a number of applications, including the decision-support components of the T-HELPER computer-based patient record system.

There are multiple dimensions of knowledge sharing and reuse [1]. Although much work to date has concentrated on development of standardized syntaxes for knowledge representation, the development of large-scale intelligent systems requires attention not only to representation of propositions about the world being modeled, but also to the control knowledge that allows complex problem-solving to take place.

For the past several years, our research group has been building a development environment, known as PROTÉGÉ-II, that permits developers to reuse knowledge in multiple ways [1]. Unlike PROTÉGÉ-I [2], which assumed that the performance system that interprets a knowledge base is based on a fixed problem solver (namely, a domain-independent version of the ONCOCIN expert system), our new architecture produces custom-tailored problem solvers based on the method configurations defined by PROTÉGÉ-II users. In particular, PROTÉGÉ-II supports libraries of reusable *problem-solving methods* that define, in domain-independent terms, the manner in which domain knowledge may be used to solve application tasks. Developers may select from a library of well-known problem-solving methods such as *episodic skeletal-plan refinement* [3], and configure those methods to create running application programs.

To build a knowledge-based system, a system builder uses the MAÎTRE tool to develop the domain ontology and either selects from the library the method that most closely fits the requirements of the application task, or constructs a composite method from the available methods and mechanisms. The system builder then uses the DASH tool to generate a graphical knowledge-acquisition tool based on the ontology. Domain specialists can then use this custom-tailored knowledge-acquisition tool to create a knowledge base.

PROTÉGÉ-II offers a new approach to the construction of intelligent systems—namely, the use of reusable building blocks that are at various levels of abstraction. PROTÉGÉ-II has been used to create a number of clinical applications, including the decision-support modules of the T-HELPER computer-based patient record system [4]. PROTÉGÉ-II demonstrates that the process of engineering and maintaining complex software systems can be enhanced through the use of libraries of appropriate components. The automated generation of domain-specific knowledge-acquisition tools should allow health-care workers to have a direct role in the creation and maintenance of a variety of clinical software applications.

Acknowledgments

This work has been supported, in part, by NLM grants LM05157 and LM05305, and by gifts from Digital Equipment Corporation and from the Computer-Based Assessment Project of the American Board of Family Practice. Dr. Musen is recipient of NSF Young Investigator Award IRI-9257578.

References

[1]. M.A. Musen. Dimensions of knowledge sharing and reuse. *Computers and Biomedical Research* **25**: 435–467, 1992.

[2]. M.A. Musen. Automated support for building and extending expert models. *Machine Learning* **4**:349–377, 1989.

[3]. S.W. Tu, Y. Shahar, J. Dawes, J. Winkels, A.R. Puerta, and M.A. Musen. A problem-solving model for episodic skeletal-plan refinement. *Knowledge Acquisition* **4**:197–216, 1992.

[4]. M.A. Musen, R.W. Carlson, L.M. Fagan, S.C. Deresinski, and E.H. Shortliffe. T-HELPER: Automated support for community-based clinical research. In *Proceedings of the Sixteenth Annual Symposium on Computer Applications in Medical Care*. Baltimore, MD, pp. 719–723, 1992.

Induction of Medical Expert System Rules based on Rough Sets and Resampling Methods

Shusaku Tsumoto and Hiroshi Tanaka
Department of Informational Medicine
Medical Research Institute,Tokyo Medical and Dental University
1-5-45 Yushima, Bunkyo-ku Tokyo 113 Japan
TEL: +81-3-3813-6111 (6159) FAX: +81-3-5684-3618
E-mail:{tsumoto, tanaka}@tmd.ac.jp

Abstract

Automated knowledge acquisition is an important research issue in improving the efficiency of medical expert systems. Rules for medical expert systems consists of two parts: one is a proposition part, which represent a if-then rule, and the other is probabilistic measures, which represents reliability of that rule. Therefore, acquisition of both knowledge is very important for application of machine learning methods to medical domains. Extending concepts of rough set theory to probabilistic domain, we introduce a new approach to knowledge acquisition, which induces probabilistic rules based on rough set theory(PRIMEROSE) and develop a program that extracts rules for an expert system from clinical database, using this method. The results show that the derived rules almost correspond to those of medical experts.

INTRODUCTION

One of the most important problems in rule induction methods is how to estimate the reliability of the induced results, which is a semantic part of knowledge to be induced from finite training samples. In order to estimate errors of induced results, resampling methods, such as cross-validation, the bootstrap method, have been introduced. However, while cross-validation method obtains better results in some domains, the bootstrap method calculates better estimation in other domains, and it is very difficult how to choose one of the two methods. In order to reduce these disadvantages further, we introduce the combination of repeated cross-validation method with the bootstrap method, both of which are studied as non-parametric error estimation methods or statistical model estimation ones in the community of statistics. The results show that this combination estimates the accuracy of the induced results correctly.

The paper is organized as follows: in section 2, we mention about probabilistic rules. Section 3 presents our new method, PRIMEROSE for induction of RHINOS-type rules. Section 4 gives experimental results. Finally, in section 5, we mention about Ziarko's related work, Variable Precision Rough Set Model.

RHINOS2 PROBABILISTIC RULES

Our approach is firstly motivated by automatic rule generation for RHINOS [5].RHINOS is an expert system which diagnoses the causes of headache or facial pain from manifestations. For the limitation of the space, in the following, we only discuss about the acquisition of inclusive rules,which are used for differential diagnosis. For further information,refer to [5].

Inclusive rule consists of several rules,which we call positive rules. The premises of positive rules are composed of a set of manifestations specific to a disease to be included for the candidates of disease diagnoses. If a patient satisfy one set of the manifestation of a inclusive rule, we suspect the corresponding disease with some probability. These rules are derived by asking the following questions in relation to each disease to the medical experts:*1.a set of manifestations by which we strongly suspect a corresponding disease. 2.the probability that a patient has the disease with this set of manifestations:SI(Satisfactory Index) 3.the ratio of the number the patients who satisfy the set of manifestations to that of all the patients having this disease:CI(Covering Index) 4.If sum of the derived CI(tCI) is equal to 1.0 then end. If not, goto 5. 5.For the patients suffering from this disease who do not satisfy all the collected set of manifestations,*

Due to difficulties with international mail delivery, this paper did not arrive in time to be placed in the proper order in the Proceedings. We apologize to the authors.

0195-4210/94/$5.00

goto 1. An inclusive rule is described by the set of manifestations, and its satisfactory index. Note that SI and CI are given experimentally by medical experts. For example, let us consider an example of inclusive rules. Let us show an example of an inclusive rule of common migraine(CI=0.75) as follows:

If
history:paroxysmal, jolt headache:yes,
nature: throbbing or persistent,
prodrome:no, intermittent symptom:no,
persistent time: more than 6 hours, and
location: not eye,
Then we suspect common migraine (SI=0.9, CI=0.75).

Then SI=0.9 denotes that we can diagnose common migraine with the probability 0.9 when a patient satisfies the premise of this rule. And CI=0.75 suggests that this rule only covers 75 % of total samples which belong to a class of common migraine.

Formally, we can represent each positive rule as a tuple: $\langle d, R_i, SI_i(, CI_i)\rangle$, where d denotes its conclusion, and R_i denotes its premise. The inclusive rule is described as: $\langle\{\langle d, R_1, SI_1(, CI_1)\rangle, \cdots, \langle d, R_k, SI_k(, CI_k)\rangle\}, tCI\rangle$. where total CI(tCI) is defined as the sum of CI of each rule with the same conclusion:$\sum_i CI_i$.

ROUGH SETS AND PRIMEROSE

Rough set theory is developed and rigorously formulated by Pawlak[9]. This theory can be used to acquire certain sets of attributes which would contribute to class classification and can also evaluate how precisely these attributes are able to classify data.

For the limitation of space, we mention only how to extend the original rough set model to probabilistic domain, which we call PRIMEROSE(Probabilistic Rule Induction Method based on ROugh Sets). And we denote a set which supports an equivalence relation R_i by $[x]_{R_i}$ and we call it an *indiscernible set.* For example, if an equivalence relation R is supported by a set {1,2,3}, then $[x]_R$ is equal to {1,2,3} ($[x]_R = \{1, 2, 3\}$).

Definition of Probabilistic Rules

We extend the definition of consistent rules to probabilistic domain. For this purpose, we use the definition of inclusive rules which Matsumura et.al [5] introduce for the development of a medical expert system, RHINOS(Rule-based Headache and facial pain INformation Organizing System). This inclusive rule is formulated in terms of rough set theory as follows:

Definition 1 (Probabilistic Rules) *Let R_i be an equivalence relation and D denotes a set whose elements belong to one class and which is a subset of U. A probabilistic rule of D is defined as a tuple, $< D, R_i, SI(R_i, D), CI(R_i, D) >$ where R_i, SI, and CI are defined as follows.*

R_i is a conditional part of a class D and defined as:

$$R_i \quad s.t. \quad [x]_{R_i} \bigcap D \neq \phi$$

SI and CI are defined as:

$$SI(R_i,D) = \frac{card\ \{([x]_{R_i} \bigcap D) \bigcup ([x]^c_{R_i} \bigcap D^c)\}}{card\ \{[x]_{R_i} \bigcup [x]^c_{R_i}\}}$$

$$CI(R_i,D) = \frac{card\ \{([x]_{R_i} \bigcap D) \bigcup ([x]^c_{R_i} \bigcap D^c)\}}{card\ \{D \bigcup D^c\}}$$

where D^c or $[x]^c_{R_i}$ consists of unobserved future cases of a class D or those which satisfies R_i,respectively. □

In the above definition, ***unobserved future cases*** means all possible future cases. So we consider an infinite size of cases, which is called *total population* in the community of statistics.

And SI(Satisfactory Index) denotes the probability that a patient has the disease with this set of manifestations, and CI(Covering Index) denotes the ratio of the number the patients who satisfy the set of manifestations to that of all the patients having this disease. Note that SI(R_i,D) is equivalent to the accuracy of R_i.

A total rule of D is given by $R = \bigvee_i R_i$, and then total CI(tCI) and total SI(tCI) is defined as: tCI(R,D) = CI($\bigvee_i R_i$,D), and tCI(R,D) = SI($\bigvee_i R_i$,D) respectively.

Since the above formulae include unobserved cases, we are forced to estimate these measures from the training samples. For this purpose, we introduction cross-validation and the Bootstrap method to generate "pseudo-unobserved" cases from these samples as shown in the next subsection.

Cross-Validation and the Bootstrap

Cross-validation method for error estimation is performed as following: first, the whole training samples $\mathcal{L}$ are split into V blocks: $\{\mathcal{L}_1, \mathcal{L}_2, \cdots, \mathcal{L}_V\}$. Second, repeat for V times the procedure in which we induce rules from the training samples $\mathcal{L} - \mathcal{L}_i (i = 1, \cdots, V)$ and examine the error rate err_i of the rules using $\mathcal{L}_i$ as test samples. Finally, we derive the whole error rate err by averaging err_i over i, that is, $err = \sum_{i=1}^{V} err_i/V$ (this method is called V-fold cross-validation). Therefore we can use this method for estimation of CI and SI by replacing the calculation of err by that of CI and SI, and by regarding test samples as unobserved cases.

On the other hand, the Bootstrap methods is executed as follows: first, we create empirical probabilistic distribution(F_n) from the original training samples. Second, we use the Monte-Carlo methods and randomly take the training samples by using F_n. Third, rules are induced by using new training samples. Finally, these results are tested by the original training samples and statistical measures, such as error rate are calculated. We iterate these four steps for finite times. Empirically, it is shown that about 200 times repetition is sufficient for estimation.

Interestingly, Efron[3] shows that estimators by 2-fold cross-validation are asymptotically equal to predictive estimators for completely new pattern of data, and that Bootstrap estimators are asymptotically equal to maximum likelihood estimators and are a little overfitting to training samples. Hence, we can use the former estimators as the lower bound of SI and CI, and the latter as the upper bound of SI and CI.

Furthermore, in order to reduce the high variance of estimators by cross-validation, we introduce repeated cross-validation method,which is firstly introduced by Walker[12]. In this method, cross-validation methods are executed repeatedly(safely, 100 times), and estimates are averaged over all the trials. In summary, since our strategy is to avoid the overestimation and the high variabilities, we adopt combination of repeated 2-fold cross-validation and the Bootstrap method in this paper.

Cluster-based Reduction of Knowledge

Reduction technique removes dependent variables from rules. This dependence is originated from algebraic dependence, that is , if $f(a_1, a_2, \cdots, a_n, a_{n+1}) = f(a_1, a_2, \cdots, a_n) = 0$ then a_{n+1} is dependent on $a_1, a_2, \cdots, a_n$. Hence, intuitionally, if the removal of one variable does not change the former consistent classification, we can remove this variable. In PRIMEROSE, we extend the concept of reduction to probabilistic domain: we delete an attribute when the deletion does not make apparent SI change. For example, if one rule support one class with some probability and other classes with some probabilities, we minimize its conditionals by the cluster-based reduction: that is, if the removal of one attribute does not change the above probabilities, we can remove this attribute.

This process means that we fix the probabilistic nature of the induced rules and is very effective when databases include inconsistent samples. This method is very similar to VPRS model introduced by Ziarko[13].

On the other hand, in the original Pawlak's models inconsistent parts is ignored and only reduction of the consistent parts is executed. For precise information, please refer to [9, 13, 11].

Algorithm for PRIMEROSE

Algorithms for rule induction can be derived by embedding rough set theory concept into the algorithms discussed in Section 2. An algorithm for induction of inclusive rules is described as follows:

1)Using all attributes, calculate all equivalent relation $\{R_i\}$ which covers all of the training samples, that is, calculate $\{R_i | \bigcup [x]_{R_i} = U\}$.
2)For each class D_j, collect all the equivalent relation R_i such that $[x]_{R_i} \cap D_j \neq \phi$. For each combination, calculate its possible region.
3)Calculate SI(R_i,D_j).
4)Apply probabilistic reduction of knowledge to each relation R_i until SI is changed(Minimize the components of each relation). If several candidates of minimization are derived, connect each with disjunction.
5)Collect all the rules, perform the cross-validation method and the bootstrap method to estimate utCI for each D_j.

EXPERIMENTAL RESULTS

We apply PRIMEROSE to headache(RHINOS's domain), meningitis, and cerebrovascular diseases, whose precise information are given in Table 2 and 3. These data are incomplete, and include many inconsistencies.

The experiments are performed by the following three procedures. First, we randomly splits these samples into pseudo-training samples and pseudo-test samples. Second, by using the pseudo-training samples, PRIMEROSE induces rules and the statistical measures. Third, the induced results are tested by the pseudo-test samples. We perform these procedures for 100 times and average each accuracy and the estimators for accuracy over 100

Table 1: Information of Database

Domain	Samples	Classes	Attributes
headache	121	10	20
meningitis	99	3	25
CVD	137	6	27

Table 2: Experimental Results (Comparison)

Domain	Method	Accuracy
headache	CART	62.8%
	AQ15	61.2%
	PRIMEROSE	74.4%
meningitis	CART	60.6%
	AQ15	67.7%
	PRIMEROSE	74.7%
CVD	CART	65.7%
	AQ15	73.0%
	PRIMEROSE	81.7%

trials. We compare PRIMEROSE with AQ15[6] and CART[1].

Experimental results are shown in Table 2 and 3. In Table 3, the first column shows estimators tested by the pseudo-test samples, as shown above. The second and third column denotes cross-validation estimator and the bootstrap estimator, respectively.

These results suggest that PRIMEROSE performs a little better than the other two methods and that the estimation of accuracy performs very well.

RELATED WORKS

Comparison with AQ15

AQ is an inductive learning method based on incremental STAR algorithm developed by Michalski [6]. This algorithm selects one seed from positive examples and starts from one "selector"(attribute). It adds selectors incrementally until the "complexes" (conjunction of attributes) explain only positive examples. Since many complexes can satisfy these positive examples, according to a flexible extra-logical criterion,AQ finds the most preferred one.

It would be surprising that the complexes supported only by positive examples corresponds to the positive region. That is, the rules induced by

Table 3: Experimental Results (Estimation)

Domain	Test	CV	BS
headache	74.4%	58.7%	91.6%
meningitis	74.7%	59.6%	88.3%
CVD	81.7%	70.1%	87.5%

AQ is equivalent to consistent rules introduced by Pawlak[9]. However, as shown in [9], the ordinary rule induction by rough set theory is different from AQ in strategy;Pawlak's method starts from description by total attributes, and then performs reduction to get minimal reducts,that is, rules are derived in a top-down manner. On the contrary, AQ induces in a bottom-up manner. While these approaches are different in strategies, they are often equivalent because of logical consistency, and this difference suggests that when we need the large number of attributes to describe rules, induction based on rough set theory is faster.

One of the important problem of the AQ method is that it does not work well in probabilistic domain [6]. This problem is also explained by matroid theory: inconsistent data do not satisfy the condition of independence, so we cannot derive a basis of matroid in probabilistic domain using the proposed definition, which is the same problem as the Pawlak's method,as discussed in Section 4. Hence it is necessary to change the definition of independence to solve those problems.

As discussed earlier,in PRIMEROSE, we adopt cluster membership as the condition of independence, instead of using class membership. Restricting the probabilistic nature, we can use almost the same algorithm as class-consistency based reduction. Then we estimate the probabilistic nature of the derived rules using some resampling plans, such as cross-validation method in this paper. This is one kind of solution to the above problems, and the similar approach can also solve the disadvantage of AQ.

Comparison with CART and ID3

Induction of decision trees, such as CART[1] and ID3[10] is another inductive learning method based on the ordering of variables using information entropy measure or other similar measures. This method splits training samples into smaller ones in a top-down manner until it cannot split the samples, and then prunes the overfitting leaves.

There are many discussions about the problems

of this approach[7, 8]. Two of the important problems are about high computational costs of pruning and structural instability. As shown in [4], constructing optimal binary decision trees is NP-complete. In this context, this means that it is difficult to determine which leaves should be pruned. CART uses the combination of cross validation method and minimal cost complexity. The difficulty is to calculate the complexity because we should choose the pruned leaves.

PRIMEROSE method also has the similar problems since reduction technique corresponds to pruning. While reduction technique examines the dependencies of attributes, pruning techniques are mainly based on the trade-off between accuracy and structural complexity.

Note that reduction technique only uses topological characteristics of the training samples. And dependencies and independencies of the attributes are important factors, since dependent attributes will not change accuracy of the induced rules. Moreover,as shown in [2], if the attributes are independent and quantized to k levels, there is no peaking phenomenon of accuracy in the Bayesian context, as discussed in the test-sample accuracy of decision trees.

Hence extracting independent variables is very important in probabilistic domain. These facts suggests that when the attributes are the mixture of dependent and independent ones, PRIMEROSE performs much better.On the other hand, when almost all of the attributes are independent, PRIMEROSE is much worse since we cannot use information about dependencies.

CONCLUSION

We introduce a new approach to knowledge acquisition, PRIMEROSE, and develop an program based on this method to extract rules for an expert system from clinical database. It is applied to three medical domains. The results show that the derived rules performs a little better than CART and AQ15 and that the estimation of statistical measures performs well.

Acknowledgements

The authors would like to thank Prof.Ziarko, Prof.Grzymala-Busse and Prof.Nitin Indurkhya for giving me some comments on the manuscript. This research is supported by Grants-in-Aid for Scientific Research No.04229105 from the Ministry of Education, Science and Culture, Japan.

References

[1] Breiman,L.,Freidman,J.,Olshen,R.,and Stone,C. *Classification And Regression Trees.* Belmont,CA:Wadsworth International Group, 1984.

[2] Chandrasekaran,B.and Jain,A.K. Quantization complexity and independent measurements *IEEE Trans.Comput.*,**23**,102-106,1974.

[3] Efron B. *The Introduction to the Bootstrap* Chapman-Hall, 1994. Pennsylvania: CBMS-NSF, 1982.

[4] Hyafil,L and Rivest,R.L. Constructing Optimal Binary Decision Trees is NP-complete. *Information Processing Letters*,1976.

[5] Matsumura,Y, et al. Consultation system for diagnoses of headache and facial pain: RHINOS,*Medical Informatics*,**11**,145-157,1986.

[6] Michalski,R.S.,et al. The Multi-Purpose Incremental Learning System AQ15 and its Testing Application to Three Medical Domains, *Proc. of AAAI-86*, 1041-1045,Morgan Kaufmann,1986.

[7] Mingers,J. An Empirical Comparison of Selection Measures for Decision Tree Induction. *Machine Learning*,**3**,319-342, 1989.

[8] Mingers,J. An Empirical Comparison of Pruning Methods for Decision Tree Induction. *Machine Learning*,**4**,227-243, 1989.

[9] Pawlak,Z *Rough Sets*,Kluwer Academic Publishers, 1991.

[10] Quinlan, J.R. Induction of decision trees, *Machine Learning*, **1**, 81-106, 1986.

[11] Tsumoto,S. and Tanaka,H. PRIMEROSE: Probabilistic Rule Induction based on Rough Sets and Resampling MEthods, *Proc. of RSKD'93*, 1993.

[12] Walker,M.G. and Olshen,R.A. Probability Estimation for Biomedical Classification Problems. *Proc. of SCAMC-92*,McGrawHill,1992.

[13] Ziarko,W. Variable Precision Rough Set Model, *Journal of Computer and System Sciences*,**46**,39-59,1993.

1994 Proceedings Authors

Subject Index